Manual of
Neonatal
Care

Manual of Neonatal Care

Fourth Edition

Editors

John P. Cloherty, M.D.
and
Ann R. Stark, M.D.

Joint Program in Neonatology
Harvard Medical School
Beth Israel Deaconess Medical
  Center
Brigham and Women's Hospital
Children's Hospital
Boston

LIPPINCOTT WILLIAMS & WILKINS
A **Wolters Kluwer** Company

Philadelphia · Baltimore · New York · London
Buenos Aires · Hong Kong · Sydney · Tokyo

Acquisitions Editor: Paula Callaghan
Manufacturing Manager: Dennis Teston
Production Manager: Maxine Langweil
Cover Designer: Jeane Norton
Indexer: Keith Shostak
Compositor: Compset
Printer: RR Donnelley Crawfordsville

Printed in the United States of America

9 8 7 6 5 4

Library of Congress Cataloging-in-Publication Data
Manual of neonatal care / Joint Program in Neonatology, Harvard
   Medical School . . . [et al.]. : edited by John P. Cloherty and Ann R.
   Stark.—4th ed.
      p.   cm.
   Includes bibliographical references and index.
   ISBN 0-781-71578-4 (alk. paper)
      1. Neonatology—Handbooks, manuals, etc.   I. Cloherty, John P.
II. Stark, Ann R.   III. Joint Program in Neonatology.
      [DNLM: 1. Infant, Newborn, Diseases—handbooks.   2. Neonatology-
-handbooks.   WS 39 M2945 1997]
RJ251.M26   1997
618.92'01 — dc21
DNLM/DLC
for Library of Congress   97-22777
                                                          CIP

Care has been taken to confirm the accuracy of the information presented and to describe generally accepted practices. However, the authors, editors, and publisher are not responsible for errors or omissions or for any consequences from application of the information in this book and make no warranty, expressed or implied, with respect to the contents of the publication.

The authors, editors, and publisher have exerted every effort to ensure that drug selection and dosage set forth in this text are in accordance with current recommendations and practice at the time of publication. However, in view of ongoing research, changes in government regulations, and the constant flow of information relating to drug therapy and drug reactions, the reader is urged to check the package insert for each drug for any change in indications and dosage and for added warnings and precautions. This is particularly important when the recommended agent is a new or infrequently employed drug.

Some drugs and medical devices presented in this publication have Food and Drug Administration (FDA) clearance for limited use in restricted research settings. It is the responsibility of the health care provider to ascertain the FDA status of each drug or device planned for use in their clinical practice.

To Laura, Gregory, Maryann, Joan, Danny, Tommy, Anne, David, Monica, Victoria, Chrissy, Ann, and Peter

Contents

Contributing Authors

Charles L. Anderson, Jr., M.D., M.P.H.

Assistant Professor of Pediatrics, Boston University School of Medicine, Boston (former Fellow, Joint Program in Neonatology)

Ester L. Awnetwant, M.S., R.D.

Neonatal Dietician, Department of Nutrition, Brigham and Women's Hospital, Boston

Angela M. Bader, M.D.

Assistant Professor of Anesthesia, Harvard Medical School; Department of Anesthesia, Brigham and Women's Hospital, Boston

Charles Berde, M.D., Ph.D.

Associate Professor of Anesthesia (Pediatrics), Harvard Medical School; Senior Associate in Anesthesia, Director, Pain Treatment Services, Children's Hospital, Boston

Thomas M. Berger, M.D.

Neonatologische und Padiatrische Intensivmedizin Kinderspital Luzern Kantonsspital Luzern Switzerland (former Fellow, Joint Program in Neonatology)

Diana W. Bianchi, M.D.

Associate Professor of Pediatrics and Obstetrics and Gynecology, Tufts University School of Medicine; Chief, Division of Genetics, New England Medical Center, Boston (former Attending Neonatologist and Geneticist, Joint Program in Neonatology)

Sandra K. Burchett, M.D.

Assistant Professor of Pediatrics,
Harvard Medical School;
Assistant in Medicine,
Associate, Department of
Infectious Diseases,
Children's Hospital, Boston

Kimberlee Chatson, M.D.

Instructor in Pediatrics,
Harvard Medical School;
Associate Director, Special Care
Nursery,
Winchester Hospital, Winchester;
Associate Neonatologist, Joint
Program in Neonatology, Boston

Helen A. Christou, M.D.

Instructor in Pediatrics,
Harvard Medical School;
Associate Neonatologist, Joint
Program in Neonatology, Boston

John P. Cloherty, M.D.

Associate Clinical Professor of
Pediatrics,
Harvard Medical School;
Associate Neonatologist, Joint
Program in Neonatology, Boston

William D. Cochran, M.D.

Associate Clinical Professor of
Pediatrics,
Emeritus,
Harvard Medical School;
Associate Neonatologist, Joint
Program in Neonatology, Boston

Sharon B. Collier, R.D.

Clinical Nutrition Manager,
Clinical Nutrition Service,
Children's Hospital, Boston

Kimberly Cox, R.N.

Staff Nurse,
Newborn Intensive Care Unit,
Children's Hospital, Boston

Eric C. Eichenwald, M.D.

Assistant Professor of Clinical
Pediatrics,
Harvard Medical School;
Associate Director, Newborn
Intensive Care Unit,
Brigham and Women's Hospital,
Boston

Francesco Emma, M.D.

Fellow, Division of Nephrology,
Children's Hospital, Boston
(former Fellow, Joint Program in
Neonatology)

James Fackler, M.D.

Assistant Professor,
Anesthesiology and Critical Care
Medicine,
Johns Hopkins University School
of Medicine;
Clinical Director,
Pediatric Intensive Care Unit,
Johns Hopkins Hospital,
Baltimore
(former Director, Multidisciplinary
Intensive Care Unit)

Michael E. Fant, M.D., Ph.D.

Associate Professor of Pediatrics,
Washington University School of
Medicine;
Division of Newborn Medicine,
St. Louis Children's Hospital,
St. Louis
(former Fellow, Joint Program in
Neonatology)

Bruce B. Feinberg, M.D.

Assistant Professor of Obstetrics
and Gynecology,
Harvard Medical School;
Attending Physician,
Department of Obstetrics and
Gynecology,
Brigham and Women's Hospital,
Boston

Emily Feinberg, M.S.N., C.N.P.

S.C.D. Candidate,
Harvard School of Public Health;
Neonatal Intensive Care Unit,
Brigham and Women's Hospital,
Boston

James Filiano, M.D.

Associate Professor of Pediatrics/
Neurology,
Dartmouth Medical School;
Department of Pediatrics,
Children's Hospital at Dartmouth,
Lebanon
(former Assistant Neurologist,
Children's Hospital, Boston)

Linda M. Gallagher, M.Ed., R.D.

Clinical Nutrition Manager,
Clinical Nutrition Service,
Children's Hospital, Boston

Allen M. Goorin, M.D.

Assistant Professor of Pediatrics,
Harvard Medical School;
Associate in Medicine
(Hematology, Oncology),
Children's Hospital,
Dana Farber Cancer Institute,
Boston

Jed B. Gorlin, M.D.	Assistant Professor, Department of Laboratory Medicine and Pediatrics, University of Minnesota; Associate Medical Director, Memorial Blood Center, Minneapolis (former Director, Clinical Cryobiology Laboratory, Children's Hospital, Boston)
James E. Gray, M.D., M.S.	Instructor in Pediatrics, Harvard Medical School; Director, Newborn Services, Beth Israel Deaconess Medical Center; Associate Neonatologist, Joint Program in Neonatology, Boston
Nicholas G . Guerina, M.D., Ph.D.	Assistant Professor of Pediatrics, Tufts University School of Medicine; Division of Newborn Medicine, New England Medical Center, Boston (former Associate Neonatologist, Joint Program in Neonatology)
Louise Wilkins-Haug, M.D., Ph.D.	Assistant Professor of Obstetrics and Gynecology, Harvard Medical School; Director, Antenatal Diagnostic Center, Brigham and Women's Hospital, Boston
Linda J. Heffner, M.D., Ph.D.	Associate Professor of Obstetrics and Gynecology, Harvard Medical School; Director of Maternal-Fetal Medicine, Brigham and Women's Hospital, Boston
Michael T. Hinkes, M.D.	Instructor in Pediatrics, Harvard Medical School; Associate Neonatologist, Joint Program in Neonatology, Boston
Kenneth M. Huttner, M.D., Ph.D.	Assistant Professor of Pediatrics, Harvard Medical School; Associate Neonatologist, Joint Program in Neonatology, Boston
Susan D. Izatt, M.D.	Assistant Professor of Pediatrics, Case Western Reserve School of Medicine; Neonatology Division, Rainbow Babies and Children's Hospital of The University of Cleveland, Cleveland (former Associate Neonatologist, Joint Program in Neonatology)

Lawrence C. Kaplan, M.D.

Associate Clinical Professor of
Pediatrics,
Yale University School of
Medicine;
Director, Yale Center for
Children with Special Health Care
Needs,
Medical Director of Spina Bifida
Program,
Yale New Haven Children's
Hospital, New Haven
(former Chief, Birth Defect Clinic,
Children's Hospital, Boston)

James R. Kasser, M.D.

Associate Professor of Orthopedic
Surgery,
Harvard Medical School;
Chairman of Orthopedic Surgery,
Children's Hospital, Boston

Constance H. Keefer, M.D.

Instructor in Pediatrics,
Harvard Medical School;
Director of Newborn Nurseries,
Brigham and Women's Hospital,
Boston

Sherwin V. Kevy, M.D.

Associate Professor of Pediatrics,
Emeritus,
Harvard Medical School;
Director of Transfusions,
Children's Hospital, Boston

Melanie S. Kim, M.D.

Associate Professor of Pediatrics,
Boston University School of
Medicine;
Boston Medical Center, Boston

Mark S. Korson, M.D.

Instructor in Pediatrics,
Harvard Medical School;
Assistant in Medicine (Genetics),
Children's Hospital, Boston

Stella Kourembanas, M.D.

Associate Professor of Pediatrics,
Harvard Medical School;
Associate Neonatologist,
Joint Program in Neonatology,
Boston

Karl C. K. Kuban, M.D., S.M., Epi.

Assistant Professor of Pediatrics
and Neurology,
Tufts University School of
Medicine;
New England Medical Center,
Floating Hospital, Boston
(former Assistant in Neurology,
Children's Hospital, Boston)

Mark E. Lawson, M.D., M.P.H.

Assistant Professor of Pediatrics, Texas Tech University School of Medicine; Neonatologist, R.E. Thomason General Hospital, El Paso (former Fellow, Joint Program in Neonatology)

Shoo Lee, M.B.B.S., F.R.C.P.C.

Director, Center for Evaluation Science, British Columbia Research Institute for Child and Family Health, Vancouver, British Columbia (former Associate Neonatologist, Joint Program in Neonatology)

Harvey L. Levy, M.D.

Associate Professor of Pediatrics, Harvard School of Medicine; Senior Associate in Medicine, Division of Genetics, Children's Hospital, Boston

Mark Levy, M.D.

Fellow, Multidisciplinary Intensive Care Unit, Children's Hospital, Boston

Helen G. Liley, M.D., Ch.B.

Medical Director, Neonatal Unit, Christchurch Women's Hospital, Christchurch, New Zealand (former Associate Neonatologist, Joint Program in Neonatology)

Denise Maguire, R.N.C., M.S.

Clinical Nurse Specialist, Department of Nursing Education, Research and Program Development, All Children's Hospital, St. Petersburg (former Nurse Manager, Special Care Nursery, Beth Israel Deaconess Medical Center, Boston)

Karen R. McAlmon, M.D.

Instructor in Pediatrics, Harvard Medical School; Director, Special Care Nursery, Winchester Hospital, Winchester; Associate Neonatologist, Joint Program in Neonatology, Boston

Marie C. McCormick, M.D., Sc.D.

Sumner and Esther Feldberg Professor of Maternal and Child Health, Harvard School of Public Health; Professor of Pediatrics, Harvard Medical School; Associate Director, Infant Follow-Up Program, Children's Hospital, Boston

Virginia G. Nichols, M.D.	Assistant Professor of Pediatrics, Bowman Gray School of Medicine of Wake Forest University, Winston-Salem (former Associate Neonatologist, Joint Program in Neonatology)
Irene E. Olsen, M.S., R.D.	Neonatal Dietician, Beth Israel Deaconess Medical Center, Boston
Stephanie J. Packard, A.D.N.	Staff Nurse III, Newborn Intensive Care Unit, Children's Hospital, Boston
Richard B. Parad, M.D., M.P.H.	Instructor in Pediatrics, Harvard Medical School; Associate Neonatologist, Joint Program in Neonatology, Boston
William F. Powers, M.D., M.P.H.	Director, Special Care Nursery, Good Shepherd Hospital, Barrington, Illinois (former Associate Neonatologist, Joint Program in Neonatology)
DeWayne M. Pursley, M.D., M.P.H.	Instructor in Pediatrics, Harvard Medical School; Neonatologist-in-Chief, Beth Israel Deaconess Medical Center; Associate Neonatologist, Joint Program in Neonatology, Boston
John T. Repke, M.D.	Associate Professor of Obstetrics, Gynecology and Reproductive Biology, Harvard Medical School; Director, Center for Labor and Birth, Brigham and Women's Hospital, Boston
Douglas K. Richardson, M.D., M.B.A.	Associate Professor of Pediatrics, Harvard Medical School; Director of Research in Neonatology, Beth Israel Deaconess Medical Center; Associate Neonatologist, Joint Program in Neonatology, Boston
Steven A. Ringer, M.D., Ph.D.	Assistant Professor of Clinical Pediatrics, Harvard Medical School; Director of Newborn Services, Brigham and Women's Hospital, Boston

David H. Rowitch, M.D., Ph.D.

Instructor in Pediatrics,
Harvard Medical School;
Associate Neonatologist, Joint
Program in Neonatology, Boston

Sylvia Schechner, M.D., M.P.H.

Assistant Clinical Professor of
Pediatrics,
Harvard Medical School;
Associate Neonatologist, Joint
Program in Neonatology, Boston

Mary Deming Scott, M.D.

Instructor in Pediatrics,
Harvard Medical School;
Department of Medicine,
Children's Hospital, Boston

Gary A. Silverman, M.D., Ph.D.

Associate Professor of Pediatrics,
Harvard Medical School;
Associate Neonatologist, Joint
Program in Neonatology, Boston

Charles F. Simmons, Jr., M.D.

Assistant Professor of Pediatrics,
Harvard Medical School;
Director, Neonatal-Perinatal
Fellowship Program,
Associate Neonatologist, Joint
Program in Neonatology, Boston

Evan Y. Snyder, M.D., Ph.D.

Assistant Professor of Neurology,
Harvard Medical School;
Associate Neonatologist, Joint
Program in Neonatology, Boston

Ann R. Stark, M.D.

Associate Professor of Pediatrics,
Harvard Medical School;
Clinical Director, Newborn
Medicine,
Children's Hospital;
Clinical Director, Joint Program in
Neonatology, Boston

Jane E. Stewart, M.D.

Instructor in Pediatrics,
Harvard Medical School;
Associate Director, Neonatal
Intensive Care Unit,
Beth Israel Deaconess Medical
Center;
Associate Director, Infant
Follow-Up Program,
Children's Hospital;
Associate Neonatologist, Joint
Program in Neonatology, Boston

Jeffrey W. Stolz, M.D., M.P.H.

Instructor in Pediatrics,
Harvard Medical School;
Associate Director, Neonatal
Intensive Care Unit,
Beth Israel Deaconess Medical
Center;
Associate Neonatologist, Joint
Program in Neonatology, Boston

Yao Sun, M.D.

Instructor in Pediatrics,
Harvard Medical School;
Associate Neonatologist, Joint
Program of Neonatology, Boston

Miles K. Tsuji, M.D.

Neonatologist, Center for Women
and Infants,
St. Joseph's Hospital, Milwaukee
(former Associate Neonatologist,
Joint Program in Neonatology)

Linda J. Van Marter, M.D., M.P.H.

Assistant Professor of Pediatrics,
Harvard Medical School;
Associate Neonatologist, Joint
Program in Neonatology, Boston

Toni B. Vento, R.N.C., M.S.

Developmental Specialist,
Newborn Intensive Care Unit;
Nurse Coordinator,
Community Outreach and
Education Program,
Children's Hospital, Boston

Stephanie Burns Wechsler, M.D.

Lecturer, Division of Pediatric
Cardiology,
Department of Pediatrics and
Communicable Diseases,
University of Michigan Medical
School, Ann Arbor

Gil Wernovsky, M.D.

Associate Professor of Pediatrics,
University of Pennsylvania School
of Medicine;
Director, Cardiac Intensive Care
Unit,
Associate Physician in Cardiology,
The Children's Hospital of
Philadelphia, Philadelphia
(former Assistant Director, Cardiac
Intensive Care Unit, Children's
Hospital, Boston)

Richard E. Wilker, M.D.

Instructor in Pediatrics,
Harvard Medical School;
Chief of Neonatology,
Newton-Wellesley Hospital,
Newton;
Associate Neonatologist, Joint
Program in Neonatology, Boston

Linda Zaccagnini, R.N.

Neonatal Nurse Practitioner, Newborn Intensive Care Unit, Beth Israel Deaconess Medical Center, Boston

Preface

The fourth edition of the *Manual of Neonatal Care* of the Joint Program in Neonatology (JPN) builds on the three previous editions (1980, 1985, 1991) and updates our practice in perinatal and neonatal medicine. The JPN has grown to 28 attending neonatologists and 12 fellows who care for over 14,000 newborns delivered annually at the Beth Israel Deaconess Medical Center (BIDMC), the Brigham and Women's Hospital (BWH, formerly the Boston Lying-In Hospital and Boston Hospital for Women), and more than 450 patients referred annually to the NICU at Children's Hospital (CH).

Our commitment to values including clinical excellence, collaboration with colleagues, and support of families, is evident throughout our book. BIDMC and BWH are referral centers for women with pregnancies complicated by maternal illness, fetal abnormalities, and anticipated neonatal problems. Obstetricians and neonatologists work together to provide prenatal and intrapartum care. This perinatal experience is reflected in the chapters on Fetal Assessment and Prenatal Diagnosis, Maternal Conditions That Affect the Fetus, and Genetic Issues Presenting in the Nursery. The NICU at CH provides telephone consultation to pediatricians at local community hospitals, and transports and cares for critically ill newborns delivered at hospitals throughout New England. Frequent problems seen in this outborn population include perinatal asphyxia, congenital heart disease, severe respiratory disorders, malformations, and metabolic disor-

ders. The practical approaches we have developed to address these problems are described in the *Manual*. Close involvement with the families of our patients is valued in our three NICUs. This is reflected in the chapters on Breast-Feeding, Developmentally Supportive Care, and Management of Neonatal Death and Bereavement Follow-Up.

This version of the *Manual* is completely updated and extensively revised. We have added new chapters on preeclampsia and related conditions, extracorporeal membrane oxygenation (ECMO), arterial and venous thrombosis, care of the very low-birth-weight infant, and neonatal anesthesia and sedation. The chapter on congenital heart disease has been markedly enhanced and includes excellent diagrams of cardiac malformations that will facilitate explanations for caregivers and parents. The chapter on infections has been expanded with new information on many conditions, including human immunodeficiency virus, toxoplasmosis, and Lyme disease. The chapters on hyperbilirubinemia, respiratory disorders, neurology and metabolic disorders have also been extensively expanded and updated.

In the *Manual*, we describe our current and practical approaches to evaluation and management of conditions encountered in the newborn. We recognize that many areas of controversy exist, that there is often more than one approach to a problem, and that our knowledge continues to grow. We acknowledge the efforts of many individuals to advance the care of newborns and the training of physicians in newborn medicine. We are indebted to Clement Smith and Nicholas M. Nelson for their insights into newborn physiology; Stewart Clifford, William D. Cochran, John Hubbell, and Manning Sears for their contributions to the care of infants at Boston Lying-In Hospital; and H. William Taeusch, Jr., Barry T. Smith, Michael Epstein, and Merton Bernfield who served as Directors of the JPN. We are grateful to Mary Ellen Avery for the markedly improved outcomes of premature infants facilitated by her seminal observation that surfactant deficiency results in Respiratory Distress Syndrome, her international leadership as an advocate for newborn infants, her role in establishing the JPN in 1974, and the personal support and advice she has provided to so many, including the editors.

We welcome the opportunity to thank the many others who helped in the preparation of the *Manual.* Individuals who assisted with previous editions, reviewed sections of the present edition, or helped make this work possible include Ann Colangelo, Frederic Frigoletto, Donald Fyler, Luke Gillespie, Donald Goldmann, Kenneth McIntosh, Alexander Nadas, Istvan Seri, Richard Slavin, and Joseph Volpe.

We appreciate our many local and national colleagues for their contribution of chapters or for permission to use data, illustrations, or tables. For their thoughtful questions and field-testing of management algorithms, we note the efforts of JPN fellows in 1995-1997, during the preparation of this edition: Sanjay Aurora, Timothy Baba, Wanda Barfield, Dara Brodsky, Donna Caliguri, Sule Cataltepe, Helen Christou, Anne Cullen, Thomas Diacovo, Marty Ellington, Jay Hagerty, Anne Hansen, Petra Huppi, Bertha Kao, Bilal Khodr, Mark Lawson, Kimberly Lee, Simon Manning, Camilia Martin, Geeta Mathur, Brendan Murphy, Manuel Peregrino, Diana Perry, Mariel Poortenga, Karen Puopolo, David Rowitch, Manisha Sakore, Timothy Watkins, John Zupancic. We thank Laura Mulhall, Stephanie Lightman, and Julie Ristaino for their administrative assistance and secretarial work, without which this would have been an impossible task. Finally, we gratefully acknowledge the nurses, residents, parents, and babies who provide the inspiration for and measure the usefulness of the information contained in this book.

John P. Cloherty, M.D.
Ann R. Stark, M.D.

Manual of
Neonatal
Care

1. FETAL ASSESSMENT AND PRENATAL DIAGNOSIS

Assessment and Prenatal Diagnosis [1]
Louise Wilkins-Haug and Linda J. Heffner

I. **Gestational-age assessment** is important to obstetrician and pediatrician and must be made with a reasonable degree of precision. Elective obstetric interventions such as diagnostic amniocentesis must be timed appropriately. When premature delivery is inevitable, the gestational age of the fetus is important with regard to prognosis and may influence the management of labor and delivery, as well as the initial neonatal treatment plan.

   A. **The clinical estimate** of gestational age is usually made through careful history of the last menstrual period. Recording of basal body temperature is also accurate and helpful, particularly when menstrual periods have been irregular. These historical data, when accompanied by physical examinations, are the baseline criteria for estimating gestational age. An additional, objective estimate is often important when interpreting adequacy of fetal growth or the results of fetal functional tests.

   B. **Ultrasonic estimation** of gestational age. During the second and third trimesters, measurements of the biparietal diameter (BPD) of both the fetal skull and the fetal femur length are useful in estimating gestational age. Strict criteria must be observed in making and measuring the cross-sectional images through the fetal head in order to ensure accuracy. Nonetheless, due to normal biologic variability in fetal growth and head shape, the accuracy with which gestational age can be estimated by BPD decreases with increasing gestational age. For measurements made at 14 to 20 weeks of gestation, the variation is ±10 to 11 days; at 20 to 28 weeks, it is ±14 days; and at 29 to 40 weeks, the variation is ±21 days. The length of the calcified fetal femur is often measured and used in validating BPD measurements or used alone in circumstances where BPD cannot be measured (e.g., deeply engaged fetal head) or is inaccurate (e.g., hydrocephalus).

II. **Prenatal diagnosis** of fetal disease or malformation has markedly improved for two reasons. We understand the genetic or developmental basis for more disorders, and we have improved the procedures necessary to detect them. Two types of tests are available: screening tests and diagnostic procedures. Screening tests, which are run on a sample of the mother's blood, are safe but relatively nonspecific. A positive screening test, a suspicious history, or a questionable ultrasonic examination may lead patient and physician to decide upon a diagnostic procedure. Diagnostic procedures, which necessitate obtaining a sample of fetal material, pose some risk to both mother and fetus but can confirm or rule out the disorder in question.

   A. **Screening** by maternal serum analysis during pregnancy individualizes a woman's risk of carrying a fetus with a neural tube defect (NTD) or trisomy 21 (Down syndrome).

   1. **Maternal serum alpha-fetoprotein (MSAFP) measurement** between 16 and 18 weeks' gestation is used to screen for NTDs. Ultrasonic examination and amniocentesis performed after finding an MSAFP level elevated above 2.5 multiples of the median detect 70 to 85% of fetuses with open spina bifida and 95% of fetuses with anencephaly. In approximately 50% of women with elevated levels, ultrasonic examination reveals another cause, most commonly an error in gestational age. Ultrasound will often detect an NTD if present.

   2. **MSAFP/triple panel.** Low levels of MSAFP may be associated with chromosomal abnormalities. Altered levels of human chorionic gonadotropin

(hCG) and unconjugated estriol (UE3) also may be associated with fetal chromosomal abnormalities. On average, a fetus with trisomy 21 results in hCG levels that are higher than expected and UE3 levels that are decreased. A triple panel screen in combination with maternal age can be used to estimate the risk of fetal trisomy 21 for an individual woman.

B. Diagnostic tests are used in women with a positive family history of genetic disease, a positive screening test, or at-risk features. Amniocentesis is the standard of care for women over 35 years of age. When a significant malformation or a genetic disease is diagnosed prenatally, the information gives obstetrician and pediatrician time to educate parents, discuss options, and establish an initial neonatal treatment plan before the infant is delivered. In some cases, treatment may be given in utero (see Chap. 8).

1. **Amniocentesis.** Amniotic fluid is removed from around the fetus via a needle guided by ultrasonic monitoring. Amniotic fluid removed (about 20 ml) is replaced within 24 hours. Amniocentesis can be performed as early as 10 to 14 weeks' gestation. Loss of the pregnancy following an ultrasound-guided second-trimester amniocentesis (16 to 20 weeks) occurs in 0.5 to 1.0% cases in most centers.

   a. **Amniotic fluid can be analyzed** for a number of compounds, including AFP, acetylcholinesterase (AChE), bilirubin, and pulmonary surfactant. Increased levels of AFP along with the presence of AChE signify NTDs with more than 98% sensitivity when the fluid sample is uncontaminated by fetal blood. AFP levels are also elevated by anencephaly, abdominal wall defects, congenital nephrosis, and intestinal atresia. In cases of isoimmune hemolysis, increased levels of bilirubin reflect erythrocyte destruction. Amniotic fluid bilirubin proportional to the degree of hemolysis is dependent upon gestational age and can be used to predict fetal well-being (Liley curve). Pulmonary surfactant can be measured once or sequentially to assess fetal lung maturity (see Tests for Pulmonary Surfactant).

   b. **Fetal cells** can be extracted from the fluid sample and analyzed for chromosomal and genetic makeup.

      (1) Among second-trimester amniocenteses, 73% of clinically significant **karyotype abnormalities** relate to one of five chromosomes: 13, 18, 21, X, or Y. These can be rapidly detected using fluorescent in situ hybridization, with sensitivities in the 90% range.

      (2) **DNA analysis** is diagnostic for an increasing number of diseases.

         (a) For genetic diseases in which the DNA sequence has not been determined, **indirect DNA studies** use restriction fragment length polymorphism (RFLP) analysis of affected individuals and family members. Both crossing over between the gene in question and the RFLP probe and the need for multiple informative members from a family limit the number of diagnoses that can be made.

         (b) **Direct DNA methodologies** can be used when the gene sequence producing the disease in question is known. Disorders secondary to deletion of DNA (e.g., alpha-thalassemia, Duchenne and Becker muscular dystrophy, cystic fibrosis, and growth hormone deficiency) can be detected by the altered size of DNA fragments produced following a polymerase chain reaction (PCR). Direct detection of a DNA mutation can also be accomplished by allele-specific oligonucleotide (ASO) analysis. If the PCR-amplified DNA is not altered in size by a deletion or insertion, recognition of a mutated DNA sequence can occur by hybridization with the known mutant allele. ASO analysis allows direct DNA diagnosis of Tay-Sachs disease, alpha- and beta-thalassemia, cystic fibrosis, and phenylketonuria.

(3) **DNA sequencing** for many genetic disorders has revealed that several mutations of a specific gene can result in the same clinical disease. For example, cystic fibrosis can result from at least 200 different mutations. Thus, for any specific disease, prenatal diagnosis by DNA testing may require both direct and indirect methods.

2. **Chorionic villus sampling (CVS).** A sample of placental tissue is obtained via a catheter placed under ultrasonic guidance either transcervically or transabdominally. Performed at 10 to 12 weeks' gestation, CVS provides the earliest possible detection of a genetically abnormal fetus through analysis of trophoblast cells. CVS can also be used to obtain a fetal karyotype in the third trimester when amniotic fluid is not available or fetal blood sampling cannot be performed. Two large studies found rates of pregnancy loss were 0.6 and 0.9% higher following CVS than after second-trimester amniocentesis. The possible complications of amniocentesis and CVS are similar; in addition, an association may exist between CVS and fetal limb-reduction defects and oromandibular malformations.

a. Direct preparations of rapidly dividing cytotrophoblasts can be prepared, making a full karyotype analysis available in 2 days. Although the rapidly dividing cytotrophoblasts minimize maternal cell contamination, most centers also analyze cultured trophoblast cells, which are embryologically closer to the fetus. This procedure takes an additional 10 to 14 days.

b. In approximately 2% of CVS samples, both karyotypically normal and abnormal cells are identified. Because CVS-acquired cells reflect placental constitution, in these cases amniocentesis is often performed as a follow-up study to analyze fetal cells. About one-third of CVS mosaicisms are confirmed in the fetus via amniocentesis.

3. **Percutaneous umbilical blood sampling (PUBS)** is performed under ultrasonic guidance from the second trimester until term. PUBS can provide diagnostic samples for cytogenetic, hematologic, immunologic, or DNA studies; it can also provide access for treatment in utero. An anterior placenta facilitates obtaining a sample close to the cord insertion site. Fetal sedation is not needed. PUBS has a 1 to 2% risk of fetal loss along with complications that can lead to a preterm delivery in another 5% (see Chap. 26).

4. **Pre-implantation biopsy.** Early in gestation (eight-cell stage in humans), an individual cell can be removed without known harm to the embryo. In women at risk for X-linked recessive disorders, only XX-containing embryos can be prepared for transfer following in vitro fertilization. Difficulties remain when more cells are needed for molecular diagnoses. An alternative approach is analysis of the second polar body, which contains the same genetic material as the ovum. This alternative technique has been used by couples at risk for cystic fibrosis, alpha-1-antitrypsin deficiency, and hemophilia.

5. **Fetal cells and maternal circulation.** The small number of fetal cells present in the maternal circulation can be separated and analyzed to identify chromosomal abnormalities.

III. **Fetal size and growth-rate abnormalities** may have significant implications for perinatal prognosis and care (see Chap. 3), and appropriate fetal assessment is important in establishing a diagnosis and a perinatal treatment plan.

A. **Intrauterine growth restriction (IUGR)** may be due to conditions in the fetal environment (e.g., chronic deficiencies in oxygen or nutrients or both) or due to problems intrinsic to the fetus itself [2]. So that appropriate care can begin as soon as possible, it is important to identify constitutionally normal fetuses that are affected. Because their risk of mortality is increased several-fold before and during labor, these fetuses may need preterm intervention for best survival rates. Once delivered, these newborns are at increased risk for immediate complications including hypoglycemia and pulmonary hemorrhage, so these fetuses should be delivered at an appropriately equipped facility.

Intrinsic causes of IUGR include chromosomal abnormalities (such as trisomies), congenital malformations, and congenital infections (e.g., cytomegalovirus or rubella). Prenatal diagnosis of malformed or infected fetuses is important so that appropriate interventions can be made. Prior knowledge that a fetus is affected with a malformation (e.g., anencephaly) or chromosomal abnormality (e.g., trisomy 18) that is incompatible with life allows the parents to be counseled before birth and may influence the management of labor and delivery.

1. **Definition of IUGR.** There is no universal agreement on the definition of IUGR. Strictly speaking, any fetus who does not reach his or her intrauterine growth potential is included. Historically, fetuses weighing less than the tenth percentile for gestational age or less than two standard deviations below the mean for gestational age have been classified as IUGR. However, many of these fetuses are merely constitutionally small. We consider all fetuses less than the tenth percentile for gestational age as small for gestational age and restrict the use of the term IUGR for those fetuses in whom corroborative evidence is present.

2. **Diagnosis of IUGR.** Clinical diagnostics detect no more than one-half of growth-restricted fetuses; ultrasound is far more sensitive. IUGR may be diagnosed with a single scan when a fetus less than the tenth percentile demonstrates corroborative signs of a compromised intrauterine environment such as oligohydramnios or an elevated head-abdomen ratio or when the pregnancy is complicated by maternal risk factors such as hypertension. Serial scans documenting absent or poor intrauterine growth regardless of the weight percentile also indicate IUGR. Composite growth profiles derived from a variety of measurements and repeated serially provide the greatest sensitivity and specificity in diagnosing IUGR.

B. **Macrosomia.** Macrosomic fetuses (>4000 gm) are at increased risk of shoulder dystocia and traumatic birth injury. Conditions such as maternal diabetes, post-term pregnancy, and maternal obesity are associated with an increased incidence of macrosomia. Unfortunately, efforts to use a variety of measurements and formulas have met with only modest success in predicting the condition.

IV. **Functional maturity** of the lungs is the most critical variable in determining neonatal survival in the otherwise normal fetus. A number of tests can be performed on amniotic fluid specifically to determine pulmonary maturity (see Tests for Pulmonary Surfactant).

V. **Assessment of fetal well-being.** Acute compromise is detected by studies that assess fetal function. Some are used antepartum, while others are used to monitor the fetus during labor.

A. **Antepartum tests** generally rely on biophysical studies, which require a certain degree of fetal neurophysiologic maturity. The following tests are not used until the third trimester; fetuses may not respond appropriately earlier in gestation.

1. **Fetal movement** monitoring is the simplest method of fetal assessment. The mother lies quietly for an hour and records each perceived fetal movement. Although she does not perceive all fetal movements that might be noted by ultrasonic observation, she will record enough to provide meaningful data.

Fetuses normally have a sleep-wake cycle, and mothers generally perceive a diurnal variation in fetal activity. Active periods average 30 to 40 minutes. Periods of inactivity greater than 1 hour are unusual in a healthy fetus and should alert the physician to the possibility of fetal compromise.

2. **The nonstress test (NST)** is a reliable means of fetal evaluation. It is simple to perform, relatively quick, and noninvasive, with neither discomfort nor risk to mother or fetus.

The NST is based on the principle that fetal activity results in a reflex acceleration in heart rate. The required fetal maturity is typically reached by about 32 weeks of gestation. Absence of these accelerations in a fetus who previously demonstrated them may indicate that hypoxia has sufficiently depressed the central nervous system to inactivate the cardiac reflex.

The test is performed by monitoring fetal heart rate either through a Doppler ultrasound device or through skin-surface electrodes on the maternal abdomen. Uterine activity is simultaneously recorded through a tocodynamometer, palpation by trained test personnel, or the patient's report of activity. The test result may be reactive, nonreactive, or inadequate. The criteria for a **reactive** test are as follows: (1) heart rate between 120 and 160, (2) normal beat-to-beat variability (5 beats per minute), and (3) two accelerations of at least 15 beats per minute lasting for not less than 15 seconds each within a 20-minute period. A **nonreactive** test fails to meet the three criteria. If an adequate fetal heart tracing cannot be obtained for any reason, the test is considered **inadequate**.

Statistics show that a reactive result is reassuring, with the risk of fetal demise within the week following the test at approximately 3 in 1000. A nonreactive test is generally repeated later the same day or is followed by another test of fetal well-being.

3. **The contraction stress test (CST)** may be used as a backup or confirmatory test when the NST is nonreactive or inadequate.

The CST is based on the idea that uterine contractions can compromise an unhealthy fetus. The pressure generated during contractions can briefly reduce or eliminate perfusion of the intervillous space. A healthy fetoplacental unit has sufficient reserve to tolerate this short reduction in oxygen supply. Under pathologic conditions, however, respiratory reserve may be so compromised that the reduction in oxygen results in fetal hypoxia. Under hypoxic conditions, the fetal heart rate slows in a characteristic way relative to the contraction. Fetal heart rate begins to decelerate 15 to 30 seconds after onset of the contraction, reaches its nadir after the peak of the contraction, and does not return to baseline until after the contraction ends. This heart-rate pattern is known as a **late deceleration** because of its relationship to the uterine contraction. Synonyms are **type II deceleration** or **deceleration of uteroplacental insufficiency**.

Like the NST, the CST monitors fetal heart rate and uterine contractions. A CST is considered completed if uterine contractions have spontaneously occurred within 30 minutes, lasted 40 to 60 seconds each, and occurred at a frequency of three within a 10-minute interval. If no spontaneous contractions occur, they can be induced with intravenous oxytocin, in which case the test is called an **oxytocin challenge test**.

A CST is **positive** if late decelerations are consistently seen in association with contractions. A CST is **negative** if at least three contractions of at least 40 seconds each occur within a 10-minute period without associated late decelerations. A CST is **suspicious** if there are occasional or inconsistent late decelerations. If contractions occur more frequently than every 2 minutes or last longer than 90 seconds, the study is considered a **hyperstimulated test** and cannot be interpreted. An **unsatisfactory test** is one in which contractions cannot be stimulated or a satisfactory fetal heart-rate tracing cannot be obtained.

A negative CST is even more reassuring than a reactive NST, with the chance of fetal demise within a week of a negative CST about 0.4 per

1000. If a positive CST follows a nonreactive NST, however, the risk of stillbirth is 88 per 1000, and the risk of neonatal mortality is also 88 per 1000. Statistically, about one-third of patients with a positive CST will require cesarean section for persistent late decelerations in labor.

4. **The biophysical profile** combines an NST with other parameters determined by real-time ultrasonic examination. A score of 0 or 2 is assigned for the absence or presence of each of the following: a reactive NST, adequate amniotic fluid volume, fetal breathing movements, fetal activity, and normal fetal musculoskeletal tone. The total score determines the course of action. Reassuring tests (8 to 10) are repeated at weekly intervals, while less reassuring results (4 to 6) are repeated later the same day. Very low scores (0 to 2) generally prompt delivery. The likelihood that a fetus will die in utero within 1 week of a reassuring test is about the same as that for a negative CST, approximately 0.6 to 0.7 per 1000.

5. **Doppler study** of fetal umbilical artery blood flow velocity is considered an investigational tool but may provide indirect evidence of placental function. Poorly functioning placentas with extensive vasospasm or infarction have an increased resistance to flow that is particularly noticeable in diastole. Thus, a decreased velocity of flow may indicate placental insufficiency, and reversed diastolic flow indicates serious compromise.

B. **Intrapartum assessment** of fetal well-being is important in the management of labor.

1. **Continuous electronic fetal monitoring** is widely used despite the fact that it has not been shown to reduce perinatal mortality or asphyxia relative to auscultation by trained personnel but has increased the incidence of operative delivery. When used, the monitors simultaneously record fetal heart rate and uterine activity for ongoing evaluation.

   a. **The fetal heart rate** can be monitored in one of three ways. The noninvasive methods are **ultrasonic** monitoring and **surface-electrode** monitoring from the maternal abdomen. The most accurate but invasive method is to place a small **electrode** into the skin of the fetal presenting part to record the fetal electrocardiogram directly. Placement requires rupture of the fetal membranes. When the electrode is properly placed, it is associated with a very low risk of fetal injury. Approximately 4% of monitored babies develop a mild infection at the electrode site, and most respond to local cleansing.

   b. **Uterine activity** can also be recorded either indirectly or directly. A **tocodynamometer** can be strapped to the maternal abdomen to record the timing and duration of contractions as well as crude relative intensity. When a more precise evaluation is needed, an **intrauterine pressure catheter** can be inserted following rupture of the fetal membranes to directly and quantitatively record contraction pressure. Invasive monitoring is associated with an increased incidence of chorioamnionitis and postpartum maternal infection.

   c. **Parameters** of the fetal monitoring record that are evaluated include the following:

      (1) **Baseline heart rate** is normally between 120 and 160 beats per minute. Baseline bradycardia may result from congenital heart block associated with congenital heart malformation or maternal systemic lupus erythematosus. Tachycardia may result from fetal dysrhythmia, maternal fever, or chorioamnionitis.

      (2) **Beat-to-beat variability** is recorded from a calculation of each RR interval. The autonomic nervous system of a healthy, awake fetus constantly varies the heart rate from beat to beat by roughly 5 to 10 beats per minute. Reduced beat-to-beat variability may result from depression of the fetal central nervous system due to hypoxia, fetal sleep, fetal immaturity, or maternal narcotic or sedative use.

(3) Accelerations of the fetal heart rate are reassuring, as they are during an NST.

(4) Decelerations of the fetal heart rate may be benign or indicative of fetal distress depending on their characteristic shape and timing in relation to uterine contractions.

    (a) Early, type I, or head-compression decelerations are symmetric in shape and closely mirror uterine contractions in time of onset, duration, and termination. They are benign and usually accompany good beat-to-beat variability. The heart rate may slow to 60 to 80 beats per minute before returning to baseline. These decelerations are more commonly seen late in labor when the fetal head is compressed within the bony pelvis and vagina, resulting in a parasympathetic effect.

    (b) Late, type II, or uteroplacental insufficiency decelerations indicate fetal distress. Fetal heart rate decelerates 10 to 30 seconds after the contraction starts and does not return to baseline until after the contraction ends. A fall in the heart rate of only 10 to 20 beats per minute below baseline (even if still within the range of 120 to 160) is significant. With increasingly severe hypoxia, (1) beat-to-beat variability will be lost, (2) decelerations will last longer, (3) they will begin sooner following the onset of a contraction, (4) they will take longer to return to baseline, and (5) the minimum rate to which the fetal heart slows will be lower. Repetitive late decelerations demand action. If maternal interventions such as oxygen supplementation fail, then a fetal scalp pH (see **V.B.2**) should be done to more precisely assess the level of fetal distress.

    (c) Variable, type III, or cord-pattern decelerations vary in their shape and in their timing relative to contractions. They are a cause for concern if they are severe (down to a rate of 60 beats per minute or lasting for 60 seconds or longer, or both), associated with poor beat-to-beat variability, or mixed with late decelerations. This pattern may result from compression of the umbilical cord, and a shift in maternal or fetal position or both will often cause the pattern to resolve.

2. A fetal scalp blood sample for pH determination is obtained to confirm or dismiss suspicion of fetal distress. An intrapartum scalp pH above 7.25 is normal. A pH between 7.20 and 7.25 is worrisome. If the pH is between 7.10 and 7.20, the clinical circumstances will dictate appropriate action. Fetuses with a scalp pH below 7.10 should be delivered immediately by the most expedient route.

References
1. Creasy, R.K., Resnik, R., eds. *Maternal–fetal medicine: Principles and practice.* Philadelphia: Saunders, 1994, 1237 pp.
2. Hay, W.W., Jr, et al. Fetal growth: Its regulation and disorders. *Pediatrics* 1997; 99:585.

Tests for Pulmonary Surfactant
Douglas K. Richardson

I. Physiologic basis. Fluid formed in the fetal lung flows up the airways and into the amniotic fluid, carrying with it some pulmonary surfactant. Newborns with inadequate amounts of alveolar surfactant commonly develop respiratory distress syndrome (RDS). Fetal tests are based on quantitation of surface-active phospholipids or on functional assessment such as formation of stable foams.

A. Procedure. Fluid obtained by amniocentesis or by removal from the vagina after rupture of membranes can be tested for the presence of pulmonary surfactant.

B. Guidelines for interpretation

1. Fetal pulmonary maturity rises steadily with increasing gestational age, although individual fetuses can vary substantially. Female fetuses tend to be approximately 1 week in advance of males. Black fetuses also tend to mature earlier. Infants of diabetic mothers (IDMs) are more susceptible to RDS than other newborns of the same gestational age.

2. Tests assay only one component of surfactant. The maturity of other, unmeasured surfactant components is probably closely correlated with gestational age. Thus, immature test results in a near-term fetus (advanced gestational age) may not indicate serious risk of RDS, while mature test results in a very preterm pregnancy (early gestational age) may not be reassuring.

3. No simple cutoff value determines zero risk of RDS. Rather, risk decreases in a continuous gradient with increasing levels of surfactant. Clinical complications (e.g., asphyxia, infection, etc.) elevate the risk and may precipitate frank RDS in infants with transitional levels of pulmonary maturity. Thus, estimation of RDS risk involves careful interpretation of the test result within the context of clinical presentation. Obstetricians obtain surfactant tests to guide decisions on whether to delay delivery and whether to use glucocorticoids to accelerate lung maturation. In those circumstances, the likelihood of RDS must be weighed against other medical risks to the fetus and mother.

II. The lecithin-sphingomyelin (L/S) ratio is performed by chromatography. Specific techniques vary among laboratories and may affect the results. Estimation of risk of RDS from the L/S ratio should therefore reflect the experience of the laboratory and the clinical service.

A. Clinical significance of specific results. Generally, pulmonary status is considered mature with an L/S ratio of greater than 2:1. As discussed below, many factors enter into consideration of the value for a given mother and fetus.

B. Interpretation of contaminated samples. The complicating effects of blood and meconium are due to the presence of lecithin and sphingomyelin in these substances. The L/S ratio in these contaminants has never been found to be higher than 2. Therefore, blood and meconium tend to elevate an immature L/S ratio (<2) and depress a mature L/S ratio (>2). Consequently, a contaminated specimen with an L/S ratio over 2 is probably mature, and one under 2 is probably immature. Amniotic fluid obtained vaginally by speculum examination is as reliable as a sample obtained transabdominally.

C. Exceptions to the prediction of pulmonary maturity with an L/S ratio over 2:1

1. **Definite exceptions**
   a. IDMs
   b. Intrapartum asphyxia
   c. Erythroblastosis fetalis

2. **Possible exceptions**
   a. Intrauterine growth restriction
   b. Abruptio placentae
   c. Preeclampsia
   d. Hydrops fetalis

D. Predicting lung maturity in the IDM (see Chap. 2, Diabetes Mellitus). Several cases of RDS have been documented in IDMs with L/S ratios over 2 or even 2.5. This is thought to be due to poor surfactant activity. Our experience with IDMs has been that an L/S ratio between 2 and 3.5 is associated with a 7 to 10% risk of RDS. If the L/S ratio is greater than 3.5, the risk of RDS is extremely low. In addition, the presence of phosphatidylglycerol in amniotic fluid may be particularly reassuring in the IDM.

III. **TDx-Fetal Lung Maturity (FLM II).** The FLM assays the surfactant-albumin ratio using fluorescence polarization technology. This commercial test (Abbott Diagnostics) has come into widespread use because it is simple, automated, and provides results in one-half hour. It seems as effective as the L/S ratio under routine conditions. It has recently been revised and recalibrated as the FLM II.

   A. **Interpreting FLM II results.** Reference intervals for FLM II used at Brigham and Women's Hospital are immature <40 mg/gm; indeterminate 40 to 59 mg/gm; mature ≥60 mg/gm. These are more conservative than the values proposed by Abbott Laboratories.

   B. **Limitations.** Samples with visible bilirubin or contaminated with blood or meconium should not be used. Insufficient published experience exists to interpret the FLM II test in fetuses of diabetic mothers, very immature fetuses, or in the presence of specific disease states such as preeclampsia.

IV. **Other measures of surfactant.** Many variations of the L/S ratio assay as well as tests of other surfactant components have been developed. Perinatal centers usually rely on more sensitive tests such as the L/S ratio, saturated phosphatidylcholine concentration (which is unaffected by contamination with blood or meconium), or combinations such as the lung profile (see **V**).

V. **Combination testing.** The high rate of false prediction of RDS in zones of transitional maturity has led to the use of test combinations such as the lung profile. The presence of phosphatidylglycerol or the concentration of saturated phosphatidylcholine has been used to improve the predictive value of the L/S ratio or FLM II.

2. MATERNAL CONDITIONS THAT AFFECT THE FETUS

Diabetes Mellitus
John P. Cloherty

I. **Background.** Improvements in prolonging pregnancy and assessing fetal pulmonary maturity have significantly reduced the incidence of respiratory distress syndrome (RDS) in the infants of diabetic mothers (IDMs). Infants of mothers with severe renal and vascular disease are often delivered early because of maternal problems (e.g., hypertension, renal failure) or fetal distress and are more likely to have perinatal complications such as asphyxia, RDS, jaundice, or poor feeding.

II. **Classification.** Diabetic mothers are grouped by White's classification (Table 2-1), and perinatal outcome is related to White class. The risk of complications is minimal in gestational diabetes, although macrosomia and neonatal hypoglycemia are sometimes seen. The most difficult maternal, fetal, and neonatal problems occur in women with renal, cardiac, or retinal disease [see **III.D, III.F, IV.B.4.d.(3)**]. Class F disease (renal) is associated with the need for early delivery, class H (cardiac disease) with maternal death, and class R with the risk of progressive retinopathy during pregnancy (see **III.D**).

III. **Maternal-fetal problems during pregnancy and delivery**
   A. In the first half of pregnancy, hypoglycemia and ketonuria are common. Pregnancy-related nausea and vomiting may make control more difficult. However, moderate hypoglycemia unassociated with hypotension may not be harmful to the fetus.
   B. In the second trimester, the **insulin requirement** increases and sometimes is associated with **ketoacidosis,** which may result in high fetal mortality.
   C. In the third trimester, a problem is **sudden fetal demise.** Such deaths are sometimes associated with ketoacidosis, preeclampsia, or maternal vascular disease of the decidua and myometrium, but some are unexplained. The incidence of unexpected demise has declined with the increased use of tests for fetal assessment, but it still occurs occasionally.
   D. In the third trimester, class F mothers may have anemia, hypertension, and decreased renal function. Class H women have a high risk of myocardial failure with infarction. Class R women risk neovascularization, vitreous hemorrhage, or retinal detachment. Infants are often delivered by cesarean section.
   E. Fetal macrosomia and enlargement of umbilical cord and placenta may be seen in gestational diabetes and in class A, B, C, and some D diabetic pregnancies. [See **IV.B.4.e.(2)** and **VI.H** for the ramifications of macrosomia.]
   F. Diabetic women with vascular disease (especially class F) have an increased risk of intrauterine growth restriction (IUGR) (20%). IUGR is associated with a small infarcted placenta, decreased uteroplacental perfusion, and increased incidence of intrauterine fetal death, fetal distress, neonatal complications, and poor outcome.
   G. Many diabetic pregnancies are associated with **polyhydramnios.** Although usually not a sign of significant fetal anomaly as it is in nondiabetic pregnancies, polyhydramnios may be associated with premature rupture of membranes, early cord prolapse, or abruptio placentae. Women with the best metabolic control have the lowest incidence of polyhydramnios.
   H. The **placenta** has extramedullary hematopoiesis in diabetic pregnancies, and this observation may be helpful in the postpartum investigation of late stillbirths.
IV. **Pregnancy management**

Table 2-1. White's classification of maternal diabetes (revised*)

Gestational diabetes (GD):	Diabetes not known to be present before pregnancy Abnormal glucose tolerance test in pregnancy
GD diet	Euglycemia maintained by diet alone
GD insulin	Diet alone insufficient; insulin required
Class A:	Chemical diabetes; glucose intolerance prior to pregnancy; treated by diet alone; rarely seen Prediabetes; history of large babies more than 4 kg or unexplained stillbirths after 28 weeks
Class B:	Insulin-dependent; onset after 20 years of age; duration less than 10 years
Class C:	C_1: Onset at 10 to 19 years of age C_2: Duration 10 to 19 years
Class D:	D_1: Onset before 10 years of age D_2: Duration 20 years D_3: Calcification of vessels of the leg (macrovascular disease) D_4: Benign retinopathy (microvascular disease) D_5: Hypertension (not preeclampsia)
Class F:	Nephropathy with over 500 mg per day of proteinuria
Class R:	Proliferative retinopathy or vitreous hemorrhage
Class RF:	Criteria for both classes R and F coexist
Class G:	Many reproductive failures
Class H:	Clinical evidence of arteriosclerotic heart disease
*Class T:	Prior renal transplantation

Note: All classes below A require insulin. Classes R, F, RF, H, and T have no criteria for age of onset or duration of disease but usually occur in long-term diabetes.
Source: Modified from J. W. Hare. Gestational Diabetes. In *Diabetes Complicating Pregnancy: The Joslin Clinic Method*. New York: Alan R. Liss, 1989.

A. **Patient education.** The importance of good control cannot be overemphasized in counseling diabetic women. The first-trimester spontaneous abortion rate in **well-controlled** diabetic pregnancies is the same as in nondiabetic ones, but the incidence is significantly increased in poorly controlled diabetic pregnancies. Good control also may decrease the incidence of major congenital anomalies (see **VI.F**) and improve perinatal outcome.

B. **Specific management**
   1. **Diabetic control.** Patients found to have gestational diabetes are managed by dietary therapy. If it is insufficient, insulin is used. Oral agents are contraindicated; they cross the placenta and may be associated with severe neonatal hypoglycemia if used near the time of birth. Controlled gestational diabetics should be followed weekly because 15% will eventually require insulin. All diabetic patients should maintain fasting glucose levels of less than 105 mg/dl and postprandial levels of less than 120 mg/dl. Hemoglobin A_1 (HbA_1) is measured to assess control over longer periods.
   2. **First-trimester testing.** Tests include HbA_1, thyroid-function studies, 24-hour urine for total protein and creatinine clearance, and an ophthalmologic evaluation. The estimated date of conception is determined by history of last menstrual period and ultrasonic examination.

3. **Second-trimester testing.** Maternal serum alpha-fetoprotein is assayed at 16 to 18 weeks (see Chap. 1). Ultrasonography is done at 18 weeks to rule out anomalies, assess fetal growth, and confirm gestational age; it can diagnose 95% of the major anomalies of the central nervous system, heart, skeleton, gastrointestinal tract, and urinary tract (see Chap. 1).

4. **Third-trimester testing**
   a. Mothers are monitored for glycemic control, polyhydramnios, preeclampsia, premature labor, and renal function.
   b. Fetuses are monitored for well-being, size, and pulmonary maturity. Ultrasonography is repeated at 26 to 28 weeks and weekly nonstress tests (NSTs) begun. Before 30 weeks, the oxytocin challenge test is probably more reliable than the NST. Biophysical profiles are also used to evaluate fetal well-being (see Chap. 1).
   c. Amniocentesis is performed at 38 weeks to assess pulmonary maturity unless there is reason to deliver earlier. In our laboratory, in nondiabetic pregnancies with a lecithin-sphingomyelin (L/S) ratio greater than 2:1, there is a 5% incidence of RDS; with a saturated phosphatidylcholine (SPC) level greater than 500 μg/dl, there is a 1 percent incidence (see Chap. 1, Tests for Pulmonary Surfactant, **II.E** and **V**). The levels of L/S and SPC considered mature in an IDM depend on the laboratory. In our experience, 10% of IDMs with L/S ratios between 2.0 to 3.5:1.0 have RDS, and 1% of IDMs with L/S ratios greater than 3.5:1.0 have RDS. An SPC level of 500 μg/dl is usually considered mature in non-IDMs; in our hospital, however, 11 percent of IDMs with SPC levels between 501 and 1000 μg/dl had RDS, and 1% of IDMs with SPC levels over 1000 μg/dl had RDS. We consider an IDM to have mature indices when the L/S ratio is over 3.5 and the SPC level is over 1000 μg/dl. Data tables give the risk of RDS so that the risks of a premature delivery can be properly evaluated (Table 2-2).
   d. **Nonemergency delivery**
      (1) Insulin-requiring pregnancies should continue to 38 to 39 weeks as long as (1) there are no maternal contraindications, and (2) there is evidence of fetal growth and well-being. This practice will result in more vaginal deliveries, more mature babies, and a lower perinatal mortality and morbidity because the increased incidence of RDS in IDMs is in premature infants (Fig. 2-1). Timing of delivery is decided individually by weighing the data on maternal health and on relative fetal and neonatal risks (e.g., gestational age, pulmonary maturity).

Table 2-2. Lecithin-sphingomyelin ratio, saturated phosphatidylcholine level, and respiratory distress syndrome in infants of diabetic mothers at the Boston Hospital for Women 1977–1980

SPC level (μg/dl)	L/S ratio			Mild, moderate, or severe RDS/total
	<2.0 : 1.0	2.0–3.4 : 1	≥3.5 : 1.0	
Not done	0/1	0/12	0/13	0/26 (0%)
≤500	6/6	1/9	1/2	8/17 (47%)
501–1000	0/2	3/20	1/15	4/37 (11%)
>1000	0/0	2/22	0/142	2/164 (1.2%)
Total (RDS)	6/9 (67%)	6/63 (10%)	2/172 (1.2%)	14/244 (5.7%)

SPC = saturated phosphatidylcholine; L/S = lecithin/sphingomyelin; RDS = respiratory distress syndrome.

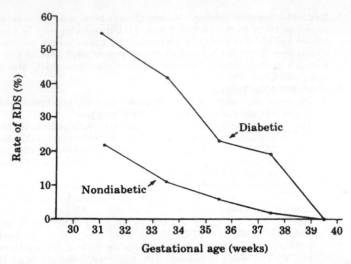

Fig. 2-1. Rate of respiratory distress syndrome (RDS) versus gestational age in nondiabetic and diabetic pregnancies at the Boston Hospital for Women from 1958–1968. (Reprinted with permission from M. Robert, Association between maternal diabetes and the respiratory distress syndrome in the newborn. N. Engl. J. Med. 294:357, 1976.)

(2) Before delivery, physicians should communicate clearly so that problems can be anticipated. The following should be discussed: (1) outcome of previous pregnancies, (2) gestational age and fetal assessment, (3) control of diabetes during pregnancy, (4) present maternal diabetic and medical state, (5) maternal HbA$_1$ levels in pregnancy, (6) results of fetal monitoring for malformations or distress, (7) fetal size, (8) evidence for pulmonary maturity, and (9) monitoring during labor.

(3) Mothers with vascular complications (e.g., White's class F) who have proteinuria of over 400 mg per day in the first half of pregnancy without urinary tract infection and have hypertension and a creatinine clearance under 90 ml/min will often require hospitalization at 26 weeks' gestation for bed rest and antihypertensive medication. They are at greatest risk for uncontrollable hypertension and decreasing renal function and are the most likely to demonstrate IUGR and fetal distress, leading to early delivery. Data (after 24 weeks' gestation) from the Joslin Clinic show no increased mortality but more prematurity and low birth weights.

e. **Emergency delivery** may be necessary even with pulmonary immaturity because of severe maternal problems (e.g., hypertension, decreasing renal function, preeclampsia) or because of IUGR or fetal distress.

(1) Because of the difficulty in controlling maternal diabetes while waiting for an effect, we usually do not use steroids to accelerate fetal pulmonary maturity unless the L/S ratio is less than 2:1, the SPC level is less than 500 μg/dl, and the patient is at very high risk to deliver in the following 7 days.

(2) The route of delivery is selected based on obstetric indications. If the infant appears macrosomic based on clinical and ultrasonographic examination (>4000 gm), cesarean section is usually in-

dicated. Prolongation of gestation beyond 38 weeks does not increase the incidence of dystocia and birth trauma.

(3) Intrapartum maternal blood glucose is kept around 120 mg/dl and fetal well-being assessed by electronic monitoring and measurement of fetal scalp pH. About 25% of diabetic women undergo primary cesarean section because of intrapartum fetal distress. Because of failure in induction, dystocia, or fetal distress in our insulin-requiring diabetics, 47% undergo primary cesarean section. Twenty-five percent have repeat cesarean section, and 28% have vaginal delivery.

V. Evaluation of the infant

A. The **evaluation** of the infant begins **prior to the actual delivery.** If pulmonary maturity is not certain, amniotic fluid can be obtained by aspiration of the amniotic sac before it is opened at cesarean section. Fluid may be evaluated by Gram stain, culture, shake test, L/S ratio, or SPC content.

B. **After the baby is born,** assessment is made on the basis of Apgar scores to determine the need for any resuscitative efforts (see Chap. 4). The infant should be dried and placed under a warmer. The airway is bulb suctioned for mucus, but the stomach is not aspirated, because of the risk of reflex bradycardia and apnea from pharyngeal stimulation in the first 5 minutes of life. A screening physical examination for the presence of major congenital anomalies should be performed and the placenta examined. A glucose level and pH may be determined on cord blood.

C. **In the nursery,** supportive care should be given while a continuous evaluation of the infant is made. This includes providing warmth, suction, and oxygen as needed, while checking vital signs (e.g., heart and respiratory rates, temperature, perfusion, color, and blood pressure). Cyanosis should make one consider cardiac disease, RDS, transient tachypnea of the newborn, or polycythemia. An examination should be repeated for possible anomalies because of the 6 to 9% incidence of major congenital anomalies in IDMs. Special attention should be paid to the brain, heart, kidneys, and skeletal system. Reports indicate that IDMs have a 47% risk of significant hypoglycemia, 22% risk of hypocalcemia, 19% risk of hyperbilirubinemia, and a 34% risk of polycythemia; therefore, the following studies are performed:

1. **Blood glucose** levels are checked at 1, 2, 3, 6, 12, 24, 26, and 48 hours. Glucose is measured with Chemstrip B-G (Bio-Dynamics, BMC, Indianapolis, Indiana). Readings under 40 mg/dl should be checked rapidly by a clinical laboratory or by Ames eyetone instrument (Ames Company, Division of Miles Laboratories, Inc., Elkhart, Indiana) (see Chap. 29).

2. **Hematocrit** levels are checked at 1 and 24 hours (see Chap. 26).

3. **Calcium** levels are checked if the baby appears jittery or is sick for any reason (see **VI.C** and Chap. 29).

4. **Bilirubin** levels are checked if the baby appears jaundiced.

The infant is fed orally or given IV glucose by 1 hour of age (see **VI.B.5** and Chap. 29). Every effort is made to involve the parents in infant care as soon as possible.

VI. Specific problems frequently observed in IDMs

A. **Respiratory distress.** With changes in pregnancy management resulting in longer gestations and more vaginal deliveries, the incidence of RDS in IDMs has fallen from 28% during 1950 to 1960 to 4% in 1990, with the major difference in the incidence of RDS between diabetics and nondiabetics in infants born before 37 weeks' gestation. Most of the deaths from RDS also are in infants under 35 weeks' gestation who were delivered by cesarean section because of fetal distress or maternal indications.

Delayed lung maturity in IDMs may occur because hyperinsulinemia blocks cortisol induction of lung maturation. Causes of respiratory distress besides RDS are cardiac or pulmonary anomalies (4%), hypertrophic cardiomyopathy (1%), transient tachypnea of the newborn, and polycythemia.

Pneumonia, pneumothorax, and diaphragmatic hernia also should be considered. The following studies should be done in infants with respiratory distress:

1. **Chest x-ray** to evaluate aeration, presence of infiltrates, cardiac size and position, and the presence of pneumothorax or anomalies.
2. **Blood gases** to evaluate gas exchange and the presence of right-to-left shunts.
3. **Electrocardiogram, blood pressure measurements,** and an **echocardiogram** if hypertrophic cardiomyopathy or a cardiac anomaly is thought to be present.
4. **Blood cultures,** with spinal-fluid examination and culture if the infant's condition allows and infection is a possibility. (See Chap. 24 for the differential diagnosis and management of respiratory disorders.)

B. **Hypoglycemia.** Hypoglycemia is defined as a blood glucose level under 40 mg/dl in any infant, regardless of gestational age and whether symptomatic or not. Previously, we used a level of under 30 mg/dl as the definition of hypoglycemia (see Chap. 29).

1. With under 30 mg/dl as the definition, the incidence of hypoglycemia in IDMs is from 30 to 40%. The onset is frequently within 1 to 2 hours of age and is most common in macrosomic infants.
2. The **pathogenesis** of neonatal hypoglycemia in IDMs is explained by Pederson's maternal hyperglycemia–fetal hyperinsulinism hypothesis. The correlation between fetal macrosomia, elevated HbA_1 in maternal and cord blood, and neonatal hypoglycemia, as well as between elevated cord blood c-peptide or immunoreactive insulin levels and hypoglycemia, suggests that control of maternal blood sugar in the last trimester may decrease the incidence of neonatal hypoglycemia in IDMs. Mothers should not receive large doses of glucose before or at delivery because this may stimulate an insulin response in the hyperinsulinemic offspring. We attempt to keep maternal glucose level at delivery around 120 mg/dl. Hypoglycemia in small-for-gestational-age (SGA) infants born to mothers with vascular disease may be due to inadequate glycogen stores; it may also present later (e.g., at 12 to 24 hours of age). Other factors that may cause hypoglycemia in IDMs are decreased catecholamine and glucagon secretion as well as inadequate substrate mobilization (diminished hepatic glucose production and decreased oxygenation of fatty acids).
3. **Symptomatic, hypoglycemic** IDMs usually are quiet and lethargic rather than jittery. Symptoms such as apnea, tachypnea, respiratory distress, hypotonia, shock, cyanosis, and seizures may occur. If symptoms are present, the infant is probably at greater risk for sequelae than if asymptomatic. The significance of **asymptomatic hypoglycemia** is unclear, but conservative management to maintain the blood sugar level in the normal range (>40 mg/dl) appears to be indicated.
4. **Diagnosis.** Our neonatal protocol was explained in **V.C.1.** The blood glucose level is measured more often if the infant is symptomatic, if the infant has had a low level, and to see the response to therapy.
5. **Therapy**
   a. **Asymptomatic infants with normal blood glucose levels**
      (1) In our nursery, we begin feeding "well" IDMs by bottle or gavage with dextrose 10% (5 ml/kg body weight) at or before 1 hour of age. Infants weighing less than 2 kg should have parenteral dextrose starting in the first hour of life. Larger infants can be fed hourly for three or four feedings until the blood sugar determinations are stable; infants should be switched to formula feeding (20 cal/oz) if the feedings are 2 hours apart or more. This schedule prevents some of the insulin release associated with oral feeding of pure glucose. The feedings can then be given every 2 hours, and later every 3 hours. As the interval between feedings increases, the volume is increased.

(2) If by 2 hours of age the blood glucose level is under 30 mg/dl despite feeding, or if feedings are not tolerated, as indicated by large volumes retained in the stomach, parenteral treatment is indicated. If the blood glucose level is under 40 mg/dl at 3 hours of age, parenteral treatment is probably indicated.

b. Symptomatic infants, infants with a low blood glucose level after enteral feeding, sick infants, or infants less than 2 kg in weight

(1) The basic treatment element is **IV glucose administration** through reliable access.

(a) Administration of IV glucose is usually by peripheral IV catheter. Peripheral lines may be difficult to place in obese IDMs, and sudden interruption of the infusion may cause a reactive hypoglycemia in these hyperinsulinemic infants. Rarely in emergency situations with symptomatic babies, we have used umbilical venous catheters in the inferior vena cava until a stable peripheral line is placed.

(b) **Specific treatment** is determined by the baby's condition. If the infant is in **severe distress** (e.g., seizure or respiratory compromise), 0.5 to 1.0 gm of glucose per kilogram of body weight is given by an IV push of 2 to 4 ml/kg 25% dextrose in water (D/W) at a rate of 1 ml/min. For example, a 4-kg infant would receive 8 to 16 ml of 25% D/W over 8 to 16 minutes. This is followed by a continuous infusion at a rate of 4 to 8 mg of glucose per kilogram of body weight per minute. The concentration of dextrose in the IV fluid will depend on the total daily fluid requirement. For example, on day 1, the usual fluid intake is 65 ml/kg, or 0.045 ml/kg/minute. Therefore, 10% D/W would provide 4.5 mg of glucose per kilogram per minute, and 15% D/W would provide 6.75 mg of glucose per kilogram per minute. In other words, 10% D/W at a standard IV fluid maintenance rate usually supplies sufficient glucose to raise the blood glucose level above 40 mg/dl. The concentration of dextrose and the infusion rates, however, are increased as necessary to maintain the blood glucose level in the normal range.

The **usual method** is to give 200 mg of glucose per kilogram of body weight (2 ml/kg 10% dextrose) over 2 to 3 minutes. This is followed by a maintenance drip of 6 to 8 mg of glucose per kilogram per minute (10% dextrose at 80 to 120 ml/kg/day) (see Chap. 29).

(c) **If the infant is asymptomatic** but has a blood glucose level in the hypoglycemic range, an initial push of concentrated sugar should **not** be given, in order to avoid a hyperinsulinemic response. Rather, an initial infusion of 5 to 10 ml of 10% D/W at 1 ml/min is followed by continuous infusion at 4 to 8 mg/kg per minute. Blood glucose levels must be carefully monitored at frequent intervals after beginning IV glucose infusions, both to be certain of adequate treatment of the hypoglycemia and to avoid hyperglycemia and the risk of osmotic diuresis and dehydration.

(d) **Parenteral sugar should never be abruptly discontinued,** because of the risk of a reactive hypoglycemia. As oral feeding progresses, the rate of the infusion can be decreased gradually, and the concentration of glucose infused reduced by using 5% D/W. It is vital to measure blood glucose levels during tapering of the IV infusion.

(e) In difficult cases, hydrocortisone (5 mg/kg per day IM in two divided doses) has occasionally been helpful. In our experience, other drugs (epinephrine, diazoxide, or growth hormone) have not been necessary in the treatment of the hypoglycemia of IDMs.

(f) In a **hypoglycemic infant,** if difficulty is experienced in achieving vascular access we administer crystalline glucagon IM or SQ (300 µg/kg to a maximum dose of 1.0 mg), which causes a rapid rise in blood glucose levels in large IDMs who have good glycogen stores; the response is not reliable in smaller infants of maternal classes D, E, F, and others. The rise in blood glucose may last 2 to 3 hours and is useful until parenteral glucose can be started. This method is rarely used.

(g) The hypoglycemia of most IDMs usually responds to the above treatment and resolves by 24 hours. Persistent hypoglycemia is usually due to a continued hyperinsulinemic state and may be manifested by glucose utilization of over 8 mg of glucose per kilogram per minute (see Table 29-1). Efforts should be made to decrease islet cell stimulation (e.g., keeping blood glucose adequate but not high, moving a high umbilical artery line to a low line, etc.).

(h) If the hypoglycemia lasts over 7 days, consider other etiologies (see Chap. 29).

C. Hypocalcemia (see Chap. 29, Hypocalcemia, Hypercalcemia, and Hypermagnesemia) is found in 22 percent of IDMs and is not related to hypoglycemia. Hypocalcemia in IDMs may be caused by a delay in the usual postnatal rise of parathyroid hormone or vitamin D antagonism at the intestinal level from elevated cortisol and hyperphosphatemia due to tissue catabolism. There is no evidence of elevated serum calcitonin concentrations in these infants in the absence of prematurity or asphyxia. Other causes of hypocalcemia such as asphyxia and prematurity may be seen in IDMs. The nadir in calcium levels occurs between 24 and 72 hours, and 20 to 50% of IDMs will become hypocalcemic as defined by a total serum calcium level under 7 mg/dl.

Hypocalcemia in "well" IDMs usually resolves without treatment, and we do not routinely measure serum calcium levels in asymptomatic IDMs. Infants who are sick for any reason—prematurity, asphyxia, infection, respiratory distress—or IDMs with symptoms of lethargy, jitteriness, or seizures that do not respond to glucose should have their serum calcium levels measured. If an infant has symptoms that coexist with a low calcium level, has an illness that will delay onset of calcium regulation, or is unable to feed, treatment with calcium may be necessary (see Chap. 29). Hypomagnesemia should be considered in hypocalcemia in IDMs because the hypocalcemia may not respond until the hypomagnesemia is treated.

D. Polycythemia (see Chap. 26, Polycythemia) is common in IDMs. In infants who are small for gestational age, polycythemia may be related to placental insufficiency, causing fetal hypoxia and increased erythropoietin. In IDMs it may be due to reduced oxygen delivery secondary to elevated HbA_1 in both maternal and fetal serum. If fetal distress occurred, there may be a shift of blood from the placenta to the fetus.

E. Jaundice. Hyperbilirubinemia (bilirubin >15 mg/dl) is seen with increased frequency in IDMs. Bilirubin levels over 16 mg/dl were seen in 19 percent of IDMs at the Brigham and Women's Hospital. Bilirubin production is increased in IDMs as compared with infants of nondiabetic mothers. Insulin causes increased erythropoietin. When measurement of carboxyhemoglobin production is used as an indicator of increased heme turnover, IDMs are found to have increased production as compared with controls. There may be decreased erythrocyte life span because of less deformable cell membranes, possibly related to glycosylation of the erythrocyte cell membrane. This mild hemolysis is compensated for but may cause increased bilirubin production. Other factors that may account for jaundice are prematurity, impairment of the hepatic conjugation of bilirubin, and an increased enterohepatic circulation of bilirubin due to poor feeding. Infants born to well-controlled diabetic mothers have fewer problems with hyperbilirubinemia. The increasing gestational age of IDMs at delivery has contributed to the decreased incidence of hyperbilirubinemia. Hyperbilirubinemia in IDMs is diagnosed and treated as in any other infant (see Chap. 18).

F. Congenital anomalies are found more frequently in IDMs than in infants of nondiabetic mothers.

   1. Incidence. As mortality from other causes such as prematurity, stillbirth, asphyxia, and RDS falls, malformations become the major cause of perinatal mortality in IDMs. Infants of diabetic fathers show the same incidence of anomalies as the normal population; consequently, the maternal environment may be the important factor. Most studies show a 6 to 9% incidence of major anomalies in IDMs, compared with a usual major anomaly rate for the general population of 2% (see Chap. 8). The types of anomalies seen in IDMs involve the central nervous system (anencephaly, meningocele syndrome, holoprosencephaly); cardiac, vertebral, skeletal, and renal systems; situs inversus; and caudal regression syndrome (sacral agenesis). The central nervous system and cardiac anomalies make up two-thirds of the malformations seen in IDMs. Although there is a general increase in the anomaly rate in IDMs, no anomaly is specific for IDMs, although half of all cases of caudal regression syndrome are seen in IDMs.

   2. There have been several studies correlating poor metabolic control of diabetes in early pregnancy with malformations in the IDM. Among more recent studies, one performed by the Joslin Clinic again showed a relationship between elevated HbA_1 in the first trimester and major anomalies in IDMs. The data are consistent with the hypothesis that poor metabolic control of maternal diabetes in the first trimester is associated with an increased risk for major congenital malformations.

G. Poor feeding is a major problem in IDMs, occurring in 37% of a series of 150 IDMs at the Brigham and Women's Hospital. Sometimes poor feeding is related to prematurity, respiratory distress, or other problems; however, it is often present in the absence of other problems. In our most recent experience (unpublished), it was found in 17% of class B to D IDMs and in 31% of class F IDMs. Infants born to class F mothers are often premature. There was no difference in the incidence of poor feeding in large-for-gestational-age infants versus appropriate-for-gestational-age infants, and there was no relation to polyhydramnios. Poor feeding is a major reason for prolonged hospital stays and parent-infant separation.

H. Macrosomia, defined as a birth weight over the ninetieth percentile or over 4000 gm, may be associated with an increased incidence of primary cesarean section or obstetric trauma such as fractured clavicle, Erb's palsy, or phrenic nerve palsy due to shoulder dystocia. The incidence of macrosomia was 28% at the Brigham and Women's Hospital from 1983 to 1984. An association was found between third-trimester elevated maternal blood sugar and macrosomia. There also was an association between hyperinsulinemia in IDMs and macrosomia and between macrosomia and hypoglycemia. Macrosomia is not usually seen in infants born to class F mothers.

I. Myocardial dysfunction. Transient hypertrophic subaortic stenosis resulting from ventricular septal hypertrophy in IDMs has been reported. Infants may present with congestive heart failure, poor cardiac output, and cardiomegaly. The cardiomyopathy may complicate the management of other illnesses such as RDS. The diagnosis is made by echocardiography, which shows hypertrophy of the ventricular septum, the right anterior ventricular wall, and the left posterior ventricular wall, in the absence of chamber dilation. Cardiac output decreases with increasing septal thickness.

Most symptoms resolve by 2 weeks of age, and septal hypertrophy resolves by 4 months. Most infants will respond to supportive care. Inotropic drugs are contraindicated unless myocardial dysfunction is seen on echocardiography; propranolol is the most useful agent. The differential diagnosis of myocardial dysfunction due to diabetic cardiomyopathy of the newborn includes (1) postasphyxial cardiomyopathy, (2) myocarditis, (3) endocardial fibroelastosis, (4) glycogen storage disease of the heart, and (5) aberrant left coronary artery coming off the pulmonary artery (see Chap. 25). There is some evidence that good diabetic control during pregnancy may reduce the incidence and severity of hypertrophic cardiomyopathy.

J. Renal vein thrombosis. Renal vein thrombosis may occur in utero or postpartum. Intrauterine and postnatal diagnosis may be made by ultrasonographic examination. Postnatal presentation may include hematuria, flank mass, hypertension, or embolic phenomena. Most renal vein thrombosis can be managed conservatively, allowing preservation of renal tissue (see Chaps. 31 and 33).

K. Other thrombosis (see Chap. 26, Major Arterial and Venous Thrombosis Management).

L. Small left colon syndrome presents as generalized abdominal distension because of inability to pass meconium. Meconium is obtained by passage of a rectal catheter. An enema performed with meglumine diatrizoate (Gastrograffin) will make the diagnosis and often results in evacuation of the colon. The infant should be well hydrated before Gastrograffin is used. The infant may have some problems with passage of stool in the first week of life, but this usually resolves after treatment with half-normal saline enemas (5 ml/kg) and glycerine suppositories. Other causes of intestinal obstruction should be considered (see Chap. 33).

M. Genetics. The parents of IDMs are often concerned about the eventual development of diabetes in their children. There are conflicting data on the incidence of insulin-dependent diabetes in IDMs. In the general population, a person has a less than 1% chance of becoming a type I diabetic. The offspring of one parent with type I diabetes has a 5–10% risk of developing the disease. If both parents have type I diabetes, the risk is about 20%. In type II diabetes, the average person has a 12–18% chance of developing the disease. If one parent has it, the risk to offspring is 30%; if both parents have it, the risk is 50–60%.

N. Perinatal survival. Despite all problems, a diabetic woman has a 95% chance of having a healthy child if she is willing to participate in a program of pregnancy management and surveillance at an appropriate perinatal center. In a series of 215 IDMs at the Brigham and Women's Hospital from 1983 to 1984, the total perinatal mortality, from 23 weeks of gestation to 28 days postpartum, was 28 per 1000. There was one intrauterine demise of a singleton near term.

References
Cloherty, J. P. Neonatal Management. In F. Brown (Ed.), Diabetes Complicating Pregnancy: The Joslin Clinic Method, 2nd ed. New York: Wiley-Liss, 1995.
Landon, M. B. Diabetes in pregnancy. Clin. Perinatol. 20:507–661, 1993.
Reece, E. A., et al. Infant of the diabetic mother. Semin. Perinatol. 18:459, 1994.

Thyroid Disorders
Mary Deming Scott

I. Thyroid metabolism in pregnancy [7,9]. Many thyroid function tests change in pregnant women, primarily because of an estrogen-induced increase in thyroxine-binding globulin (TBG). Concentrations of free thyroxine (T_4), T_4 production rate, and thyroid-stimulating hormone (TSH) remain constant, but radioactive iodine uptake (RAIU), basal metabolic rate, response to TSH-releasing hormone (TRH), T_4, and total triiodothyronine (T_3) all increase.

The placenta is relatively impermeable to T_4, T_3, reverse T_3, and TSH, although small amounts of maternal T_4 crossing the placenta may be protective in fetuses with thyroid synthetic defects. TRH, thyroid-stimulating immunoglobulins (TSIs), and thyroid-blocking immunoglobulins (TBIIs) all cross the placenta, and maternal TSIs and TBIIs can cause transient hyper- or hypothyroidism in the newborn.

II. **Maternal hypothyroidism.** Women with treated hypothyroidism often deliver normal infants. However, untreated maternal hypothyroidism may result in an increased frequency of first-trimester miscarriages and intrauterine growth restriction (IUGR) in liveborn infants. Pregnant women who have primary hypothyroidism should have thyroid function tests at 6 weeks, 4 months, and 6 months of gestation, with additional TBII and TSI screening in the last trimester. The thyroxine dose may need to be increased up to 100% during pregnancy to keep TSH in the normal range [7]. In women with thyroiditis who make TBIIs, placental transfer of the immunoglobulins may cause fetal hypothyroidism. An increase in the thyroxine dose may help protect the fetus [6].

III. **Maternal hyperthyroidism** [7]. Graves' disease complicates 1 in 1000 pregnancies.
   A. **Obstetric management.** Thioamides should be used at the lowest dose needed to achieve maternal control (for an excellent review, see reference 7). Propylthiouracil (PTU) crosses the placenta, as do iodides and TSIs, and the fetus may be goitrous and hypothyroid or may have thyrotoxicosis. Because maternal hypothyroidism is poorly tolerated by the fetus, mothers should be kept mildly thyrotoxic, with TSIs measured near term in mothers with Graves' disease. If TSIs are elevated, the neonate should be closely watched for the development of thyrotoxicosis in the first 2 weeks of life. Propranolol can cause IUGR.
   D. **Intrapartum management.** Propranolol can cause impaired responses to hypoxia, bradycardia, and hypoglycemia in the fetus. Approximately 10% of infants born to mothers with Graves' disease will be small for gestational age (SGA), particularly if thyrotoxicosis was present for over 30 weeks of pregnancy, or if the mother had a TSI level of 30% or more at delivery, Graves' disease of 10 or more years' duration, or onset of Graves' disease before age 20.
   C. **Thyroid function in neonates.** Thyroid dysfunction is seen in 17% of infants born to mothers with Graves' disease, but only 10% of these neonates are SGA. Fetal thyroid dysfunction is related to the duration of thyrotoxicosis in pregnancy, maternal TSH receptor antibody levels at delivery, and the dosage level of maternal antithyroid drugs.
   D. **Breast-feeding and maternal medications.** Nursing mothers may take PTU because little passes into breast milk, and it does not appear to affect thyroid function in infants [7]. Thyroxine is also acceptable. Methimazole passes readily into breast milk and can cause hypothyroidism in the infant; it should not be used [7].

IV. **Fetal and neonatal goiter**
   A. **PTU-induced fetal goiter.** At PTU doses of less than 200 mg/day, PTU-induced goiter is rarely obstructive. Only 1% of PTU-exposed infants have transient neonatal hypothyroidism, and no intellectual deficits have been reported. After delivery, neonates eliminate PTU in 2 to 4 weeks, with normal thyroid function tests by 4 to 6 weeks (Table 2-3). Newborns with PTU-induced goiter should be treated with thyroxine for about 1 month. Enlarging fetal goiters in PTU-treated mothers may be due to either TSI-induced hyperthyroidism or PTU-induced hypothyroidism. Fetal blood sampling is diagnostic (see Chap. 1, **II.B.3**). Third-trimester goitrous fetal hypothy-

Table 2-3. Normal thyroid function parameters in infants aged 2 to 6 weeks[a]

Serum constituent	Concentration
T_4	84–210 nmol/L (6.5–16.3 μg/dl)
T_3	1.5–4.6 nmol/L (100–300 ng/dl)
Free T_4[b]	12–28 pmol/L (0.9–2.2 ng/dl)
TSH	1.7–9.1 mU/L (1.7–9.1 units/ml)
TBG	160–750 nmol/L (1.0–4.5 mg/dl)
Thyroglobulin[c]	15–375 pmol/L (10–250 ng/ml)

[a]Data from Nichols Institute reference values unless indicated otherwise.
[b]Measured by direct dialysis.
[c]Thyroglobulin from Vulsma et al., N. Engl. J. Med. 321:13, 1989.
Source: From D. A. Fisher. Management of congenital hypothyroidism. J. Clin. Endocrinol. Metab. 72:525, 1991.

roidism has been successfully treated with weekly intraamniotic injections of 250 to 500 μg of L-thyroxine [1,9].

   B. Other forms of goiter. Neonatal goiter may be seen in inherited hypothyroidism or after maternal ingestion of iodine. The differential diagnosis includes hemangiomas or lymphangiomas. Iodine-induced goiter resolves over 2 to 3 months, with resolution accelerated by thyroxine treatment. T_4, T_3, and TSH determinations should be obtained from the infant prior to treatment to exclude permanent defects in T_4 synthesis.

V. Neonatal hyperthyroidism. Neonates born to mothers with Graves' disease may be initially hypothyroid or euthyroid due to transplacental passage of PTU. If maternal TSI activity is near or above 500% 3 to 14 days postpartum, the infant may become thyrotoxic and remain so for 6 to 12 weeks. The half-life of TSIs is 12 days.

   A. Clinical findings. Thyrotoxic newborns may have advanced bone age, microcephaly, low birth weight, irritability, tachycardia and congestive heart failure, goiter, vomiting and diarrhea, hepatosplenomegaly, failure to thrive despite hyperphagia, flushing, hypertension, exophthalmos, and craniosynostosis. Arrhythmias and cardiac failure may be fatal [3]. Hyperviscosity syndromes, including seizures, may be related to intrauterine hypoxia [5]. Measurements of TSIs, T_4, free T_4, and T_3 can be diagnostic.

   B. Supportive treatment, including nutrition with hypercaloric formula, may be sufficient in this self-limited disorder.

   1. In severe cases **PTU** (5 to 10 mg/kg/day in three divided doses) **or methimazole** (0.5 to 1.0 mg/kg/day in three divided doses) may be used. If there is no response in 36 to 48 hours, the drug dose is increased by 50%.

   2. An **iodine** preparation such as Lugol's (or strong iodine) solution containing 4.5 to 5.5 gm of elemental iodine and 9.5 to 10.5 gm of potassium iodide per deciliter is given in a dose of 1 drop tid. If there is no response in 48 hours, the dose is increased by 25% per day until control is obtained. Iopanoic acid (Telepaque) or sodium ipodate (Oragrafin) at 600 mg/m2/day may be preferable to iodine solutions. Sodium ipodate decreases serum T_3 by 50% within 24 hours and appears to be safe and effective in newborns [5].

   3. Approximately 2 mg/kg/day of **propranolol** (range 1 to 3.5 mg/kg/day) in three divided doses is used to control tachycardia and congestive heart failure.

   4. Treatment goal is good weight gain and control of tachycardia and irritability. The T_4 value should be around 10. Treatment may be required for 4 to 12 weeks. Once control is gained, the infant can be discharged with close follow-up. Iodine solutions are given for only 10 to 14 days. Infants are weaned off propranolol as indicated by heart rate and then the dose of PTU is tapered as allowed by T_4 level and clinical situation. Heart rate monitoring may be useful. At the end of treatment, L-thyroxine is sometimes given to keep the T_4 in the 10 range.

VI. Congenital hypothyroidism (CH) [2,3,9,11]

A. Thyroid embryogenesis occurs during the first trimester, with TSH and T_4 becoming measurable by 9 to 11 weeks. The neuroendocrine axis matures until term, particularly with regard to autoregulation of T_4 synthesis. Fetal TSH, TBG, T_3, and T_4 levels increase progressively through gestation. In SGA fetuses, TSH levels are higher and T_4 and free T_4 levels are lower than in normal-sized infants. The elevation of TSH and fall of T_4 may be due to fetal hypoxemia and acidemia.

B. Neonatal physiology. Normally there is a surge in TSH at birth, resulting in the release of T_4. TSH is elevated to the 40 µU/ml range on days 1 and 2 of life and declines to less than 20 µU/ml by age 3 days in both term and premature infants.

C. The incidence of CH is 1 in 4000, with female predominance. CH is relatively common in Hispanic and Native American infants and rare in African-American newborns. CH is also seen more frequently in infants with Down syndrome, trisomy 18, neural tube defects, congenital heart disease, metabolic disorders, familial autoimmune thyroid disorders, and Pierre Robin syndrome.

D. Screening [8]. Newborn screening for CH is routine in developed countries. Most North American programs use a spot T_4 measurement and TSH confirmation of low T_4 values.

1. **Screening and early discharge.** With many neonates discharged on day 1 or 2 of life, obtaining early TSH measurements has increased the false-positive rate for CH screening. Since T_4 is also elevated on days 1 and 2 of life, mild cases of CH may be missed if T_4 is within the low-normal range. If the infant is tested before 24 hours of age, we have the infant retested at 3 to 4 days of life (recommendation of Massachusetts State Newborn Screening Program, Dr. M. Mitchell and Dr. H. Levy).

2. If early signs of hypothyroidism appear (prolonged jaundice, delayed stooling, hypothermia, poor tone, mottled skin, poor feeding), screening should be repeated at the first office visit with the pediatrician (at 1 to 2 weeks of age) even if the original screen was normal. Screening programs miss some cases of CH due to laboratory error, improper or no specimen collection, hospital transfers, sick neonates, and home deliveries, so pediatricians must ensure screening is accomplished correctly on all newborns.

E. Infants with abnormal thyroid-function results (T_4 <6, TSH >20) should have the tests repeated (Fig. 2-2). Bone age evaluation (e.g., knee, foot) may show delay in epiphyseal maturation. RAIU with I-123 may be helpful in differentiating aplasia from synthetic defects. Absent uptake may also be seen in TSH receptor defects and iodide trapping defects. TSH receptor blockade by maternal TSH receptor–blocking antibodies in maternal autoimmune thyroid disease may also cause absent RAIU. Thyroglobulin levels will be low in agenesis or thyroxine synthetic defects and elevated in thyroid dysgenesis, depending on the quantity of thyroid tissue and TSH stimulation. TRH testing (7 µg/kg given IV; TSH release measured at 30 minutes and 1 to 2 hours) will show a subnormal response in pituitary CH (<10 µU/ml) and a delayed response in hypothalamic CH.

Infants with severe hypothyroidism at diagnosis (T_4 <2 µg/dl and knee epiphyses <0.05 cm²) have lower intelligence when tested at age 12 years than less severely affected infants.

F. Etiologies of CH

1. **Permanent conditions**

   a. **Thyroid dysgenesis** (aplasia, hypoplasia, ectopic thyroid) has an incidence of 1 in 4000 births; it is usually sporadic but may be familial

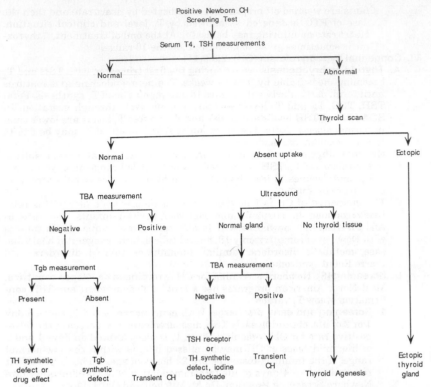

Fig. 2-2. Possible initial approaches to a newborn infant with presumptive positive test results for congenital hypothyroidism (CH) from a screening laboratory. All such infants require measurements of serum thyroxine (T_4) and thyroid-stimulating hormone (TSH) concentrations. Those infants with low T_4 and elevated TSH concentrations can be further screened by a thyroid scan using technetium or radioiodine 123. Finding an ectopic gland provides a definitive diagnosis. Infants with absent uptake or a normally appearing thyroid gland by scan can be evaluated further by ultrasound scanning and measurements of TBA and serum thyroglobulin (Tgb) concentrations. Infants with TBA-induced transient CH may have a normal scan if their CH is partially compensated. This initial evaluation should be accomplished within 2 to 5 days. (From D. A. Fisher. Management of congenital hypothyroidism. *J. Clin. Endocrinol. Metab.* 72:525, 1991.)

if the cause is cytotoxic antibodies crossing the placenta in mothers with autoimmune thyroid disease. The female-male ratio is 2:1. Infants have no goiter, low T_4 and free T_4, low T_3, elevated TSH, normal TBG, no or ectopic RAIU, and an increased response to TRH at 30 minutes.

   b. **Thyroid hormone synthetic defects** (autosomal recessive) have an incidence of 1 in 30,000. Check for family history of goiter or of consanguinity. RAIU scans are typically normal, and a gland is present on ultrasound. Thyroglobulin may be low, T_3, T_4, and free T_4 are low, TSH is high, TBG is normal, and there is an increased response to TRH at 30 minutes. A goiter is usually present.

   c. **Hypothalamic-pituitary hypothyroidism.** The incidence is 1 in 50,000. T_4, free T_4, and T_3 are low, with low-to-normal TSH, normal

TBG, and a low or delayed response to TRH infusion. Infants with suspected hypothalamic or pan-hypopituitarism also may have hypoglycemia and microphallus. Cortisol and growth hormone measurements should be obtained and an MRI scan done to visualize the hypothalamus and pituitary. Goiter is not present.

d. **TBG deficiency** (X-linked). The incidence is 1 in 5000 births, with marked male predominance. Infants have no goiter, low T_4 and mildly low free T_4, and normal T_3 and TSH. Low TBG is diagnostic. The infants are euthyroid. No treatment is indicated.

e. **Hypothyroxinemia, delayed TSH elevation.** The incidence is 1 in 100,000. On initial screening, TSH is normal, with low T_4 and free T_4, low T_3, and normal TBG. TSH is elevated on the confirmatory test, and TRH testing reveals an increased TSH response at 30 minutes.

2. **Transient conditions** are seen frequently in sick or premature neonates.
   a. **Transient hypothyroidism due to thyroid-blocking antibodies** [11] has an incidence of 1 in 50,000. This is seen in maternal autoimmune thyroid disease. Antibodies freely cross the placenta and are secreted in breast milk. Antibodies may inhibit TSH binding to receptors (TBII), inhibit TSH-mediated thyroid cell growth (TGII), or block the effects of TSH on cell function. Antibodies with blocking or stimulating properties may be found in the same mother and may have different or subsequent effects on the fetus, exerting their influence for up to 9 months after birth; hypothyroidism may persist for that length of time. T_4, free T_4, and T_3 are low, TSH is increased, TBG is normal, and antibodies are present in both mother and infant. TRH test shows an increased TSH response. RAIU may be absent, but a gland will be present on ultrasound.
   b. **Transient hypothyroidism due to iodine exposure.** Sick and premature infants are at risk from iodine-containing disinfectant solutions. The incidence is 1 in 200 to 1 in 8000. T_4 is low and TSH high on initial screens, with high urinary iodine levels. Confirmatory tests show normal T_3, T_4, free T_4, TBG, TSH, and TRH. Use of iodine containing solutions should be minimized in susceptible infants; when used, the solution should be rinsed off promptly [11].
   c. **Transient hypothyroxinemia** in sick newborns or those with hypothalamic immaturity has an incidence of 5 in 100, and up to 30% in premature infants. T_4 and free T_4 are low, but T_3 and TSH values are normal. Most values normalize within a few months.

G. **Treatment and monitoring of CH** [11]. Treatment with L-thyroxine should be initiated at 10 to 15 µg/kg, using the highest dose for infants with the lowest T_4 and highest TSH values and most delayed bone ages. A term infant receiving 50 µg/day will have normal T_4 and TSH levels within 2 weeks. Keeping T_4 in the upper half of the normal range (10 to 16 µg/dl) should keep TSH levels below 20 µU/ml in a majority of infants, but up to 20% of infants with CH will continue to have abnormal T_4-to-TSH feedback for the first decade of life.

Thyroxine doses should be adjusted at 6-week intervals for the first 6 months of life and at 2-month intervals during the next 12 months to keep T_4 in the 10 to 16 µg/dl range and TSH below 5 mU/L. Thyroxine must be crushed and fed directly to the infant. It cannot be made into a liquid or put safely into a bottle. A recent review of thyroxine therapy is found in reference 11. Infants with transient hypothyroidism (low T_4, elevated TSH) must be treated as primary hypothyroidism patients until it is certain they have only transient disease. All infants being treated for CH should have a brief trial off medication between 3 and 4 years of age to see if they have transient disease [11]. The question of whether T_4 supplementation of premature infants (<30 weeks' gestation or 1000 gm) with low T_4 and normal TSH levels might improve outcome has not been settled. The present opinion of the New England Hypothyroid Collaborative is that there is no benefit to routine T$_4$ supplementation of these infants. A recent study suggests that treating these infants might improve developmental outcome [10]. Prospective studies are under way.

References

1. Davidson, K. M., et al. Successful in utero treatment of fetal goiter and hypothyroidism. N. Engl. J. Med. 324:543, 1991.
2. Fisher, D. A. Hypothyroidism. Pediatr. Rev. 15:227, 1994.
3. Fisher, D. A. The Thyroid. In S. A. Kaplan (ed.), Clinical Pediatric Endocrinology. Philadelphia: Saunders, 1990.
4. Franklin, J. A. The management of hypothyroidism. N. Engl. J. Med. 330:1731, 1994.
5. Joshi, R., and Kulin, H. E. Treatment of neonatal Graves disease with sodium ipodate. Clin. Pediatr. 32:181, 1993.
6. Larsen, P. R. Monitoring thyroxine treatment in pregnancy. Thyroid 2:153, 1992.
7. Kaplan, M. M. Thyroid Disease in Pregnancy. In N. Gleicher (ed.), Principles and Practice of Medical Therapy in Pregnancy. Norwalk, Conn.: Appleton & Lange, 1992.
8. Newborn screening for congenital hypothyroidism: Recommended guidelines. Pediatrics 91:1203, 1993.
9. Polk, D. H. Diagnosis and management of altered fetal thyroid status. Clin. Perinatol. 21:647, 1994.
10. Reuss, M. L., et al. The relation of transient hypothyroxinemia in preterm infants to neurologic development at two years of age. N. Engl. J. Med. 13:821, 1996. See editorial comment, p. 857.
11. Toft, A. D. Thyroxine therapy [Review]. N. Engl. J. Med. 331:174, 1994.

Preeclampsia and Related Conditions
Bruce B. Feinberg and John T. Repke

I. **Terminology** of preeclampsia and related conditions
  A. Pregnancy-induced hypertension: hypertension without proteinuria
  B. Preeclampsia: hypertension with proteinuria
  C. Eclampsia: preeclampsia with seizure activity
II. **Incidence and epidemiology.** Preeclampsia complicates 6% of pregnancies beyond 20 weeks' gestation; severe preeclampsia, less than 1%. Eclampsia itself is much less frequent, occurring in 0.1% of pregnancies. Six epidemiologic characteristics stand out.
  A. parity (e.g., two-thirds of patients are nulliparous)
  B. partial adaptive protection from recurrence in subsequent pregnancies of the same paternity
  C. extremes of maternal age
  D. gestations with large placental mass (e.g., multiple gestations, molar gestation)
  E. underlying vascular disease (e.g., chronic hypertension, renal disease, autoimmune diseases, and diabetes mellitus)
  F. family history of preeclampsia
III. **Four etiologies have been proposed:** (1) an increased ratio of thromboxane to prostacyclin, which may lead to vasoconstriction, hypertension, and end-organ changes; (2) increased circulating lipid peroxides, which may inhibit endogenous nitric oxide, a vasodilator, leading to vasoconstriction and hypertension; (3) endothelial-cell injury, with causative agent not yet identified; and (4) vasculitis due to circulating immune complexes, although supporting evidence for the last is inconsistent.
IV. **Diagnosis.** The clinical spectrum of preeclampsia ranges from mild to severe. Most patients have mild disease that develops late in the third trimester.

A. Criteria for the **diagnosis of mild preeclampsia**
1. Hypertension defined as a blood pressure of 140/90 mm Hg, or as an increase in systolic pressure of at least 30 mm Hg or an increase of at least 15 mm Hg in diastolic pressure over baseline first-trimester readings, with the diagnostic readings taken twice at least 6 hours apart.
2. Proteinuria defined as at least 300 mg of protein in a 24-hour period or 100 mg/dL in at least two random urine samples taken 6 hours apart.
3. Nondependent edema (e.g., periorbital, hands) is sometimes listed, but it is common and not as useful.
B. Criteria for the **diagnosis of severe preeclampsia**
1. Diastolic blood pressure greater than 110 mm Hg
2. Proteinuria greater than 5 grams per 24-hour collection
3. Visual disturbances, such as scotomata, diplopia, blindness
4. Headache
5. Epigastric pain
6. Pulmonary edema
7. Oliguria: less than 500 ml of urine per 24-hour collection
8. Laboratory abnormalities: elevated values for liver transaminases, serum creatinine, serum uric acid; thrombocytopenia; hyperbilirubinemia
9. Intrauterine growth restriction (IUGR)
C. HELLP syndrome (**h**emolysis, **e**levated **l**iver enzymes, and **l**ow **p**latelets) represents **advanced preeclampsia** associated with disseminated intravascular coagulation (DIC) and reflects systemic end-organ damage.
V. **Complications of preeclampsia** result in a maternal mortality rate of 3 per 100,000 live births in the United States. Maternal morbidity may include central nervous system complications (e.g., strokes, seizures, intracerebral hemorrhage, and blindness), DIC, hepatic failure or rupture, pulmonary edema, and abruptio placentae leading to maternal hemorrhage and/or acute renal failure. Fetal mortality markedly increases with rising maternal diastolic blood pressure and proteinuria. Diastolic blood pressures greater than 95 mm Hg are associated with a threefold rise in the fetal death rate. Fetal morbidity may include IUGR, fetal acidemia, and complications from preterm birth.
VI. **Considerations in management**
A. **The definitive treatment** for preeclampsia is delivery. However, the severity of disease, ripeness of maternal cervix, gestational age at diagnosis, and pulmonary maturity of the fetus influence obstetric management. Delivery is usually indicated if there is evidence of distress in a viable fetus, regardless of gestational age or fetal pulmonary maturity.
B. **Conservative therapy** of severe preeclampsia early in gestation has been suggested, but risks include serious sequelae such as acute renal failure, DIC, HELLP syndrome, abruptio placentae, eclampsia, and intrauterine fetal death. Patients with preterm gestations and mild preeclampsia may be able to continue their pregnancies for weeks with close observation. In these patients, factors that will influence early delivery include the subsequent development of severe preeclampsia, nonreassuring fetal observation, or evidence of adequate fetal pulmonary maturation.
VII. **Clinical management of preeclampsia**
A. **Antepartum conservative management** generally includes hospitalization with bed rest and close maternal and fetal observation.
1. Monitoring of maternal blood pressure, proteinuria, symptoms of severe preeclampsia, daily weight
2. Laboratory monitoring of renal function, serum electrolytes, creatinine, uric acid, liver transaminases, CBC with platelets, plus a coagulation profile if there is thrombocytopenia or transaminase elevation
3. Fetal observation with frequent testing for fetal heart tones, plus semiweekly evaluation such as nonstress testing (see Chap. 1, Assessment and Prenatal Diagnosis), along with fetal ultrasonic evaluation for interval growth and amniotic-fluid volume every 2 to 3 weeks

4. Because preeclampsia does not eliminate the risk of neonatal respiratory distress syndrome, we use glucocorticosteroids to enhance fetal lung maturity if no maternal contraindications exist. Antihypertensive agents are not given to the mother because they have not been shown to improve outcome in cases of mild preeclampsia.
5. When early delivery is indicated, we induce labor. Cesarean delivery is performed in cases of suspected fetal distress, where further fetal evaluation is not possible, or where a rapidly deteriorating maternal condition mandates expeditious delivery.

B. Intrapartum management
1. Magnesium sulfate, used to prevent seizures, is started when the decision to proceed with delivery is made and continued for at least 24 hours postpartum, or until symptoms are resolving in the mother.
2. Careful monitoring of fluid balance is critical because preeclampsia is associated with decreased intravascular volume and oliguria. Many patients also have albuminuria and may develop capillary leak, increasing the risk of pulmonary edema.
3. Severe hypertension may be controlled with agents including hydralazine, labetalol, nifedipine, or nitroglycerin. We avoid sodium nitroprusside before delivery because of potential fetal cyanide toxicity. It is important to avoid large or abrupt reductions in blood pressure since decreased intravascular volume and poor uteroplacental perfusion can lead to acute fetal distress.
4. Because of the risk of acute fetal distress, we use continuous intrapartum fetal heart rate monitoring. Patterns that suggest fetal compromise include persistent tachycardia, decreased short- and long-term variability, and recurrent late decelerations not responsive to standard resuscitative measures. Reduced fetal heart rate variability may also result from maternal administration of magnesium sulfate.

C. Postpartum management. The mother's condition may worsen immediately after delivery. Signs and symptoms usually begin to resolve within 24 to 48 hours postpartum, however, and completely resolve within 1 to 2 weeks. Since postpartum eclamptic seizures occur within the first 48 hours and usually within the first 24 hours after delivery, magnesium sulfate is continued for at least 24 hours. Close monitoring of fluid balance is continued.

VIII. Recurrence rates. Patients who have preeclampsia in their first pregnancy are at increased risk for hypertensive disease in a subsequent pregnancy. Recurrence risk is as high as 65% in women with severe preeclampsia or eclampsia in their first pregnancy. This risk is greater when preeclampsia or eclampsia develop earlier in gestation. Preeclampsia may be linked to the development of chronic hypertension later in the mother's life.

IX. New treatments
A. Because preeclampsia is associated with an increased thromboxane-prostacyclin ratio, selective use of low-dose aspirin has been evaluated. Although no studies support benefits in the management of existing preeclampsia, recent studies suggest the incidence of preeclampsia is reduced when aspirin is given prophylactically to patients at risk for development of the disease.
B. Antenatal calcium supplementation may reduce the incidence of hypertensive disorders of pregnancy without apparent maternal, fetal, or neonatal side effects.

X. Implications for the newborn
A. Infants born to mothers with moderate or severe preeclampsia often show IUGR (see Chaps. 1 and 3) and are frequently delivered prematurely. They may tolerate labor poorly and require resuscitation.
B. Medications used ante- or intrapartum may affect the fetus.
1. Short-term sequelae of hypermagnesemia such as hypotonia and respiratory depression are sometimes seen (see Chap. 29). Long-term mater-

nal administration of magnesium sulfate has rarely been associated with neonatal parathyroid abnormalities and other abnormalities of calcium homeostasis.

2. Antihypertensive medications, including calcium-channel blockers, may have fetal effects. Antihypertensive medications and magnesium sulfate generally are not contraindications to breast-feeding.

3. Low-dose aspirin therapy does not increase the incidence of intracranial hemorrhage, asymptomatic bruising, bleeding from circumcision sites, or persistent pulmonary hypertension.

4. About one-third of infants born to mothers with preeclampsia have decreased platelet counts at birth, but the counts generally increase rapidly to normal levels. About 40 to 50% of newborns have neutropenia that generally resolves before 3 days of age. These infants may be at increased risk of neonatal infection.

Reference

Cunningham, F. G., et al. Hypertensive Disorders in Pregnancy. In P. C. MacDonald et al., William's Obstetrics (19th ed.). East Norwalk, Conn.: Appleton & Lange, 1993. Pp. 763–817.

3. ASSESSMENT OF THE NEWBORN

History and Physical Examination of the Newborn
William D. Cochran

I. **History.** The family, maternal, pregnancy, and perinatal history should be reviewed (Table 3-1) [7].

II. **Routine physical examination of the neonate.** Although no statistics are available, the first routine examination probably reveals more abnormalities than any other routine examination done.

   A. **General examination.** At the initial examination, attention should be directed to determining (1) whether any congenital anomalies are present, (2) whether the infant has made a successful transition from fetal life to air breathing, (3) to what extent gestation, labor, delivery, analgesics, or anesthetics have affected the neonate, and (4) whether he or she has any sign of infection or metabolic disease.

   1. The baby should be naked. Naked newborns are easily chilled, so they should not be kept uncovered for a long time unless they are in or under a warming device. A general appraisal of a naked newborn allows one to assess quickly whether any major anomalies are present, whether jaundice or meconium staining is present, and whether the infant is having trouble making the adjustment to breathing air. At least half of all infants will exhibit jaundice, although usually only at its peak on the third or fourth day of life. Visible jaundice usually means the bilirubin level is at least 5 mg/dl.

   2. It is usually wise to examine infants in the order listed because they will be quieter at the beginning, when you most need their cooperation. If the infant being examined is fretful, offer the baby a pacifier or nipple.

   B. **Cardiorespiratory system**

   1. **Color.** Skin color is probably the single most important index of cardiorespiratory function. Good color in caucasian infants means an overall reddish pink hue, except for possible cyanosis of the hands, feet, and occasionally the lips (acrocyanosis). The mucous membranes of dark-skinned infants are more reliable indicators of cyanosis than skin. Infants of diabetic mothers and premature infants are pinker than average, and postmature infants are paler.

   2. **Respiratory rate** is usually 40 to 60 breaths per minute. All infants are **periodic** rather than regular breathers, and premature infants are more so than term infants. Thus, babies may breathe at a fairly regular rate for a minute or so and then have a short period of no breathing (usually 5 to 10 seconds). **Apnea,** often defined as periods of no breathing during which an infant's color changes from normal to grades of cyanosis, is not normal, whereas periodic breathing is. Apnea is thus an abnormal prolongation of periodic breathing (see Chap. 24, Apnea).

   3. In a warm infant there should be no expiratory grunting and little or no flaring of the nostrils. When crying, infants (especially premature infants) exhibit mild chest retraction; if unaccompanied by grunting, such retraction may be considered normal.

   4. When an infant is pink and breathing without retractions or grunting at a rate of less than 60 breaths per minute, the respiratory system is usually intact. Significant respiratory disease in the absence of tachypnea is rare unless the infant also has severe central nervous system (CNS) depression. Rales, decreased heart or breath sounds, or asymmetry of breath sounds are occasionally found in an asymptomatic infant and may

Table 3-1. Important aspects of maternal and perinatal history

FAMILY HISTORY
Inherited diseases (e.g., metabolic disorders, hemophilia, cystic fibrosis, polycystic
  kidneys, history of perinatal deaths)

MATERNAL HISTORY
Age
Blood type
Transfusions
Blood group sensitizations
Chronic maternal illness
Diabetes
Hypertension
Renal disease
Cardiac disease
Bleeding disorders
Sexually transmitted diseases, including herpes and HIV/AIDS
Infertility
Recent infections or exposures

PREVIOUS PREGNANCIES: PROBLEMS AND OUTCOMES
Abortions
Fetal demise
Neonatal deaths
Prematurity
Postmaturity
Malformations
Respiratory distress syndrome
Jaundice
Apnea

DRUG HISTORY
Medications
Drug abuse
Alcohol
Tobacco

CURRENT PREGNANCY
Probable gestational age
Quickening (normally 16–18 weeks)
Fetal heart heard with fetoscope (normally 18–20 weeks)
Results of any fetal testing (e.g., amniocentesis, ultrasonic examination, estriols,
  fetal monitoring, tests of fetal lung maturity, and prenatal infection screening
  [hepatitis, group B streptococci, syphilis, etc.])
Preeclampsia
Bleeding
Trauma
Infection
Surgery
Polyhydramnios
Oligohydramnios
Glucocorticoids
Labor suppressant
Antibiotics

LABOR AND DELIVERY (PERINATAL)
Presentation
Onset of labor
Rupture of membranes
Duration of labor

Table 3-1. (*continued*)

LABOR AND DELIVERY (PERINATAL) (*continued*)
Fever
Fetal monitoring
Amniotic fluid (blood, meconium, volume)
Analgesic
Anesthesia
Maternal oxygenation and perfusion
Method of delivery
Initial delivery room assessment (shock, asphyxia, trauma, anomalies, temperature, infection)
Apgar scores
Resuscitation
Placental examination

reveal occult disease that is confirmed by chest x-ray (e.g., dextrocardia, pneumothorax, pneumomediastinum).

5. The **heart** should be examined. The examiner should observe precordial activity, rate, rhythm, the quality of the heart sounds, and the presence or absence of murmurs.
   a. It should be determined whether the heart is on the right or left side. This is done by auscultation and by palpation.
   b. The **heart rate** is normally 120 to 160 beats per minute. It varies with changes in the infant's activity, increasing when he or she is crying, active, or breathing rather rapidly, and decreasing when the baby is quiet and breathing slowly. To some, this physiologic slowing provides an important indicator that there is no significant cardiac stress. An occasional term or postmature infant may, at rest, have a heart rate well below 100. In a normal infant, the heart rate will increase if the baby is stimulated.
   c. **Murmurs** mean less in the newborn period than at any other time. Infants can have extremely serious heart anomalies without any murmurs. On the other hand, a closing ductus arteriosus may cause a murmur that is only transient, but at the time is very loud and worrisome. Gallop sounds may be an ominous finding, while the presence of a split S2 may be reassuring.
   d. If there is any question after auscultation and observation that the heart is abnormally placed, abnormally large, or overactive, a **chest x-ray** is the best means of further assessment. Distant heart sounds, especially if accompanied by respiratory symptoms, are often secondary to pneumothorax or pneumomediastinum.
   e. The **femoral pulses** should be felt, although often they are weak in the first day or two. If there is doubt about the femoral pulses by time of discharge, the blood pressure in the upper and lower extremities should be checked. In infants with coarctation, pulses and pressures may be normal in the first few days of life while the ductus is still open (see Chap. 25).

C. **Abdomen.** The abdominal examination of a newborn differs from that of older infants in that observation can again be used to greater advantage.
   1. The anterior abdominal organs (e.g., liver, spleen, bowel) can often be seen through the abdominal wall, especially in thin or premature infants. The edge of the liver is occasionally seen, and intestinal patterning is easily visible. Asymmetry due to congenital anomalies or masses often is first appreciated by observation.
   2. When palpating the abdomen, start with gentle pressure or stroking, moving from lower to upper quadrants to reveal the edges of the liver or spleen. Try to appreciate mushiness when palpating over the intestine compared with the firmer feel over the liver or other organs or masses.

The normal newborn liver extends 2.0 to 2.5 cm below the costal margin. The spleen is usually not palpable. Remember there may be situs inversus.

3. After the abdomen has been gently palpated, **deep palpation** is possible, not only because of the lack of developed musculature but also because there is no food and little air in the intestine. Abnormal, absent, or misplaced kidneys and other deep masses should be felt for. Only during the first day or two of life is it possible for the kidneys to be routinely palpated with relative ease and reliability (see Chap. 31).

D. **Genitalia and rectum**
   1. **Male**
      a. Males almost invariably have marked **phimosis.**
      b. The **scrotum** is often quite large, since it is an embryonic analogue of the female labia and therefore has responded to maternal hormones.
      c. **Hydroceles** are not uncommon, but unless they are communicating types, they will disappear in time without being the forerunner of an inguinal hernia.
      d. The **testes** should be palpated, with the epididymis and vas identified. The testis is best found by running a finger from the internal ring down on either side of the upper shaft of the penis, thus pushing and trapping the testes in the scrotum. Each testis should be the same size, and they should not appear blue (a sign of torsion) through the scrotal skin.
      e. If present, the degree of **hypospadias** should be noted.
      f. The length and width of the penis should be measured. Length under 2.5 cm is abnormal and requires evaluation (see Chap. 30). Torsion of the penis is seen in 1.5% of normal males [2].
   2. **Female**
      a. Female genitalia at term are most noticeable for their enlarged **labia majora.**
      b. Occasionally, a **mucosal tag** from the wall of the vagina is noted.
      c. A **discharge** from the vagina, usually creamy white in color and consistency, is commonly found and, on occasion, replaced after the second day by pseudomenses.
      d. The **labia** should always be spread, and cysts of the vaginal wall, imperforate hymen, or other less common anomalies should be sought.
   3. The **anus** and **rectum** should be checked carefully for patency, position, and size (normal diameter is 10 mm) [4]. Occasionally, large fistulas are mistaken for a normal anus, but if one checks carefully, it will be noted that a fistula will be either anterior or posterior to the usual location of a normal anus.

E. **Skin** (see Chap. 34). The epidermis of a newborn (especially a premature infant) is thin; therefore, the oxygenated capillary blood makes it very pink. Common abnormalities include tiny **milia** (plugged sweat glands) on the nose, unusually brown-pigmented nevi scattered around any body part, and what are referred to as **mongolian spots.** Mongolian spots are bluish, often large areas most commonly seen on the back, buttocks, or thighs that fade slightly over the first year of life.

   Erythema toxicum may be noted occasionally at birth, although it is more common in the next day or two. These papular lesions with an erythematous base are found more on the trunk than the extremities and fade without treatment by 1 week of age. Look for **jaundice.**

F. Palpable **lymph nodes** are found in about one-third of normal neonates. They are usually under 12 mm in diameter and are often found in the inguinal, cervical, and occasionally the axillary area [1].

G. **Extremities, spine, and joints** (see Chap. 28)
   1. **Extremities.** Anomalies of the digits (too few, too many, syndactyly, or abnormal placement), club feet, and hip dislocation are the common problems. Because of fetal positioning, many infants have forefoot ad-

duction, tibial bowing, or even tibial torsion. Forefoot adduction, if correctable with stretching, will often correct itself in weeks and is no cause for concern. Mild degrees of tibial bowing or torsion are also normal.

2. To check for **hip dislocation** (if present, remember that the head of the femur will most often have been displaced superiorly and posteriorly), place the infant's legs in the frogleg position. With the third finger on the greater trochanter and the thumb and index finger holding the knee, attempt to relocate the femoral head in the acetabulum by pushing upward away from the mattress with the third finger and toward the mattress and laterally with the thumb at the knee. If there has been a dislocation, a distinct upward movement of the femoral head will be felt as it relocates in the acetabulum. Hip "clicks," due to movement of the ligamentum teres in the acetabulum, are much more common than dislocated hips (hip "clunks") and are not a cause for concern. It has been shown that not all dislocated hips are present at birth, hence the recent designation "developmental dysplasia of the hip."

3. **Back.** The infant should be turned over and held face down on your hand. The back, especially the lower lumbar and sacral areas, should be examined. Special care should be taken to look for pilonidal sinus tracts and small soft midline swellings that might indicate a small meningocele or other anomaly (see Chap. 27).

H. Head, neck, and mouth

1. **Head**
   a. The average full-term **head circumference** is 33 to 38 cm.
   b. The infant's **scalp** should be inspected for cuts or bruises due to forceps application or fetal monitor leads. Check laterally for erosions from the bony spines of the maternal pelvis, which may be difficult to see under hair. Scalp aplasia may also be present.
   c. **Caput succedaneum** (edema of the scalp from labor pressure) should be checked to see if there are underlying early cephalohematomas; **ocphalohcmotomas** usually do not become full blown until the third or fourth day.
   d. **Mobility of the suture lines** will rule out **craniosynostosis.** Mobility is checked by putting each thumb on opposite sides of the suture and then pushing in alternately while feeling for motion.
   e. The degree of **molding of the skull bones** themselves should be noted, and it may be considerable. Usually, such molding will subside within 5 days.
   f. Occasional infants have **craniotabes,** a soft ping-pong ball effect of the skull bones (usually the parietal bones). It is most common in postmature or dysmature infants. If present, craniotabes is usually only an incidental finding that disappears in a matter of weeks, even if marked at birth.
   g. **Fontanelles.** As long as the head circumference is within normal limits and there is motion of the suture lines, one need pay little attention to the size (large or small) of the fontanelles. Very large fontanelles reflect a delay in bone ossification and may be associated with hypothyroidism (see Chap. 2, Thyroid Disorders), trisomy syndromes, intrauterine malnutrition, hypophosphatasia, rickets, and osteogenesis imperfecta [5]. Normal tension is that in which the tension softens when the infant is raised to the sitting position.
   h. **Ears.** Note size, shape, position, and presence of auditory canals as well as preauricular sinus or pits.

2. The **neck** should be checked for range of motion, goiter, and thyroglossal or branchial-arch sinus tracts. Occasionally, marked asymmetry is noted with a deep concavity on one side. Although the uninitiated might interpret this as possible agenesis of a muscle or muscle group, it is most commonly due to persistent fetal posture with the head tilted to one side

(asynclitism). This is most easily confirmed by noting that the mandibular gum line is not parallel to the maxillary line, further evidence of unequal pressure on the jaw as a result of the head's being held tilted in utero over time (see Chap. 28).

3. The **mouth** should be checked to ensure that there are neither hard nor soft palatal clefts, no gum clefts, and no deciduous teeth present. Rarely, cysts appear on the gum or under the tongue. **Epstein's pearls** (small white inclusion cysts clustered about the midline at the juncture of the hard and soft palate) are normal.

I. **Neurologic examination.** Much has been written about neonatal neurologic examinations, but more will have to be learned before the examination becomes an accurate evaluation—especially one with prognostic significance—when done at birth. A carefully performed, detailed examination will reveal more than a superficial one. Many senior physicians can recall an infant with hydranencephaly or a similar gross internal neurologic lesion that was completely missed by careful neurologic examination only to be found later by ultrasound of the head or even simple transillumination.

1. Probably the most reliable information that can be obtained quickly is gained while handling the infant during the preceding parts of the examination. With experience, the examiner is able to carry out at least two examinations concurrently, that is, the examination of organ and physiologic systems and a simultaneous neurologic evaluation. Symmetry of movement and posturing, body tone, and response to being handled and disturbed (i.e., crying appropriately and quieting appropriately) can all be evaluated while other body parts are being tested.

2. The amount of crying should be carefully noted as well as the pitch. When the infant is crying, seventh nerve weaknesses should be sought (the affected side of the mouth does not pull down). Erb's palsy, if present, will usually be revealed by lack of motion of the shoulder and arm; the arm will lie beside the body in repose rather than being normally flexed with fist near mouth. Jitteriness that is present but disappears in the prone position is usually benign (see Chap. 27, Neonatal Seizures). Persistent crying should make one search for the cause of pain (e.g., fracture).

3. The essentials of a neurologic examination (beyond that acquired while carrying out other components of the physical examination) may be covered by doing the following:

   a. Put your index fingers in the infant's palms to obtain the plantar grasp. Then hold the infant's fingers between your thumb and forefinger and pull him or her to a sitting position. Note the degrees of head lag and head control; remember a crying infant often throws the head back in anger. The infant should be held in a sitting position and the trunk moved forward and back enough to test head control again. Then let the trunk and head slowly fall back.

   b. To test the Moro reflex, pull your fingers quickly from his or her grasp just before the head touches the mattress, allowing the infant to fall onto the back. Usually the Moro reflex will result, although a "complete" Moro is demonstrable in only about 20% of cases.

   c. Touching the upper lip laterally will cause most infants to turn toward the touch and open their mouths; the hungrier and more vigorous the infant, the more intense is the rooting response. Placing a nipple in the mouth will initiate a sucking response.

4. **Stepping (and placing)** can be elicited by holding the infant upright with the feet on the mattress and then leaning the baby forward. This forward motion often sets off a slow alternate stepping action. However, a normal infant frequently will not perform the reflex.

5. The complete **behavioral examination** is more dependent on infant-examiner interaction. Much depends on the infant's relative wakefulness, whether the baby has just been fed or not, and to a degree, on the analge-

sia and anesthesia used during delivery. Eye opening is elicited when the infant is sucking or being held vertically. Some infants will appear alert and listen when they are spoken to in a pleasant voice. Almost all infants enjoy being cuddled. If some of these behavioral responses cannot be elicited, they may indicate either temporary or permanent problems. The more detailed behavioral examination also involves habituation to repeated stimuli of various sorts (noxious and otherwise) that will not be discussed here [3].

J. Head circumference and length. These measurements are usually last in the examination. The head circumference of a term (38- to 40-week) infant of normal weight (2.7 to 3.6 kg, or 6 to 8 lb) is usually 33 to 38 cm (13 to 15 in.). Crown-foot length is 48 to 53 cm (19 to 21 in.).

K. Eye examination [6]. The eyes should be examined for the presence of scleral hemorrhages, icterus, conjunctival exudate, iris coloring, and pupillary size, equality, extraocular muscle movement, and centering. The red reflex should be obtained, and cataracts sought. Glaucoma is manifest by a large cloudy cornea. The normal cornea in a neonate measures less than 10.5 mm in horizontal diameter. In the first 2 days of life, puffy eyelids sometimes make examination of the eyes impossible. If so, it should be noted so that the eyes will be examined upon follow-up.

III. Discharge examination. At discharge, the infant should be reexamined with the following points considered:

A. Heart—development of murmur, cyanosis, failure, femoral pulses

B. CNS—fullness of fontanelles, sutures, activity

C. Abdomen—any masses previously missed, stools, urine output

D. Skin—jaundice, pyoderma

E. Cord—infection

F. Infection—signs of sepsis

G. Feeding—spitting, vomiting, distension, degree of weight loss (or gain), dehydration

H. Parental competence to provide adequate care

I. Follow-up—arrangements made with infant's primary physician

References

1. Bamji, M., et al. Palpable lymph nodes in healthy newborns and infants. *Pediatrics* 78:573, 1986.
2. Ben-Ari, J., et al. Characteristics of the male genitalia in the newborn: Penis. *J. Urol.* 135:521, 1985.
3. Brazelton, T. B. *Neurobehavioral Assessment Scale.* Philadelphia: Lippincott, 1973.
4. El-Haddao, M., et al. The anus in the newborn. *Pediatrics* 76:927, 1985.
5. Faix, R. G. Fontanelle size in black and white term newborn infants. *J. Pediatr.* 100:304, 1982.
6. Nelson, L. B. *Pediatric Ophthalmology.* Philadelphia: Saunders, 1984.
7. Scanlon, J. W. *A System of Newborn Physical Examination.* Baltimore: University Park Press, 1979.

Identifying the High-Risk Newborn and Evaluating Gestational Age, Prematurity, Postmaturity, Large-for-Gestational-Age, and Small-for-Gestational-Age Infants
DeWayne M. Pursley and John P. Cloherty

I. High-risk newborns are associated with certain conditions; when one or more occur, nursery staff should know in order to anticipate possible difficulties.

Cord blood and placentas should be saved for all problem newborns, including infants transferred from other facilities. An elusive diagnosis such as toxoplasmosis may be made based on placental pathology.

The following factors are associated with high-risk newborns:

A. Maternal conditions	Associated risk for fetus or neonate
1. Age at delivery	
a. Over 40 years	Chromosomal abnormalities, small for gestational age (SGA)
b. Under 16 years	Preeclampsia, prematurity, child abuse
2. Personal factors	
a. Poverty	Prematurity, infection, SGA
b. Smoking	SGA (e.g., weight decrease of roughly 150 to 250 gm), increased perinatal mortality
c. Drug, alcohol abuse	SGA, fetal alcohol syndrome, withdrawal syndrome, sudden infant death syndrome, child abuse
d. Poor diet	Slightly SGA, fetal wasting in severe malnutrition
e. Trauma (acute, chronic)	Fetal demise, prematurity
3. Medical history	
a. Diabetes mellitus	Congenital anomalies, stillbirth, respiratory distress syndrome (RDS), hypoglycemia
b. Thyroid disease	Goiter, hypothyroidism, hyperthyroidism
c. Renal disease	SGA, stillbirth, prematurity
d. Urinary tract infection	Prematurity, sepsis
e. Heart, lung disease	SGA, stillbirth, prematurity
f. Hypertension (chronic, preeclampsia)	SGA, stillbirth, asphyxia, prematurity
g. Anemia	SGA, stillbirth, asphyxia, prematurity, hydrops
h. Isoimmunization (red cell antigens)	Stillbirth, anemia, jaundice, hydrops
i. Isoimmunization (platelets)	Stillbirth, bleeding
j. Thrombocytopenia	Stillbirth, bleeding
4. Obstetric history	
a. Infertility	Congenital anomalies, low birth weight, increased perinatal mortality
b. Past history of infant with jaundice, RDS, or anomalies	Same with current pregnancy
c. Maternal medications	See specific medication insert and see Appendix
d. Bleeding in early pregnancy	Stillbirth, prematurity
e. Hyperthermia	Fetal demise, fetal anomalies
f. Low urinary estriols	Stillbirth, SGA
g. Bleeding in third trimester	Stillbirth, anemia
h. Premature rupture of membranes, fever, infection	Infection
i. TORCH infections	See Chap. 23, Viral Infections in the Newborn
B. Fetal conditions	**Associated risk for fetus or neonate**
1. Multiple gestation	Prematurity, twin-transfusion syndrome, asphyxia, birth trauma
2. Intrauterine growth restriction (IUGR)	Fetal demise, stillbirth, congenital anomalies, asphyxia, hypoglycemia, polycythemia
3. Macrosomia	Congenital anomalies, birth trauma, hypoglycemia
4. Abnormal fetal position	Congenital anomalies, birth trauma, hemorrhage
5. Abnormality of fetal heart rate or rhythm	Hydrops, asphyxia, congestive heart failure, heart block
6. Acidosis	Asphyxia, RDS

7. Decreased activity	Fetal demise, stillbirth, asphyxia
8. Polyhydramnios	Anencephaly, other central nervous system (CNS) disorders, neuromuscular disorders, problems with swallowing (e.g., agnathia, esophageal atresia, cord around neck), chylothorax, diaphragmatic hernia, omphalocele, gastroschisis, trisomy, tumors, hydrops, isoimmunization, anemia, cardiac failure, intrauterine infection, inability to concentrate urine, maternal diabetes
9. Oligohydramnios	IUGR, placental insufficiency, postmaturity, fetal demise, intrapartum distress, renal agenesis, pulmonary hypoplasia, deformations

C. Conditions of labor and delivery — **Associated risk for fetus or neonate**

1. Premature labor	Respiratory distress, asphyxia, infection
2. Labor occurring 2 weeks or more after term	Stillbirth, asphyxia, meconium aspiration (see **VI**)
3. Maternal fever	Infection
4. Maternal hypotension	Stillbirth, asphyxia
5. Rapid labor	Birth trauma, intracranial hemorrhage (ICH)
6. Long labor	Stillbirth, asphyxia, birth trauma
7. Abnormal presentation	Birth trauma, asphyxia
8. Uterine tetany	Asphyxia
9. Meconium-stained amniotic fluid	Stillbirth, asphyxia, meconium-aspiration syndrome, persistent pulmonary hypertension
10. Prolapsed cord	Asphyxia, ICH
11. Cesarean section	RDS, transient tachypnea of newborn, blood loss
12. Obstetric analgesia and anesthesia	Respiratory depression, hypotension, hypothermia
13. Placental anomalies	
a. Small placenta	SGA
b. Large placenta	Hydrops, maternal diabetes
c. Torn placenta	Blood loss
d. Vasa praevia	Blood loss

D. Immediate neonatal conditions — **Associated risk for fetus or neonate**

1. Prematurity	RDS, ICH, infection
2. Low 1-minute Apgar score	RDS, asphyxia, ICH
3. Low 5-minute Apgar score	Developmental delay
4. Pallor or shock	Blood loss
5. Foul smell of amniotic fluid or membranes	Infection
6. SGA	See **IV**
7. Postmaturity	See **VI**

II. Gestational age estimation and birth-weight classification

  A. Attempts should be made to classify neonates by gestational age.

    1. Assessment based on **obstetric information** is covered in Chap. 1, Assessment and Prenatal Diagnosis, **I.** Examples include data from early clinical and ultrasonic examinations and dates of first recorded fetal activity and first recorded fetal heart sounds [8].

    2. **Newborn information** can be obtained by use of the modified Dubowitz examination [2] (Figs. 3-1, 3-2), which has been further modified to achieve greater accuracy. Remember there are limitations to the method, especially in sick newborns. Charts and postnatal grids also exist for very low-birth-weight newborns (Figs. 3-3, 3-4).

    3. **Infant classification by gestational age**

      a. Preterm—less than 37 weeks

Neuromuscular Maturity

	-1	0	1	2	3	4	5
Posture							
Square Window (wrist)	>90°	90°	60°	45°	30°	0°	
Arm Recoil			180°	140°-180°	110°-140°	90-110°	<90°
Popliteal Angle	180°	160°	140°	120°	100°	90°	<90°
Scarf Sign							
Heel to Ear							

Physical Maturity

	-1	0	1	2	3	4	5
Skin	sticky friable transparent	gelatinous red, translucent	smooth pink, visible veins	superficial peeling &/or rash, few veins	cracking pale areas rare veins	parchment deep cracking no vessels	leathery cracked wrinkled
Lanugo	none	sparse	abundant	thinning	bald areas	mostly bald	
Plantar Surface	heel-toe 40-50mm: -1 <40mm: -2	>50mm no crease	faint red marks	anterior transverse crease only	creases ant. 2/3	creases over entire sole	
Breast	imperceptible	barely perceptible	flat areola no bud	stippled areola 1-2mm bud	raised areola 3-4mm bud	full areola 5-10mm bud	
Eye/Ear	lids fused loosely:-1 tightly:-2	lids open pinna flat stays folded	sl. curved pinna; soft, slow recoil	well-curved pinna; soft but ready recoil	formed & firm instant recoil	thick cartilage ear stiff	
Genitals male	scrotum flat, smooth	scrotum empty faint rugae	testes in upper canal rare rugae	testes descending few rugae	testes down good rugae	testes pendulous deep rugae	
Genitals female	clitoris prominent labia flat	prominent clitoris small labia minora	prominent clitoris enlarging minora	majora & minora equally prominent	majora large minora small	majora cover clitoris & minora	

Maturity Rating

score	weeks
-10	20
-5	22
0	24
5	26
10	28
15	30
20	32
25	34
30	36
35	38
40	40
45	42
50	44

Expanded NBS includes extremely premature infants and has been refined to improve accuracy in more mature infants.

Fig. 3-1. New Ballard Score. (From J. L. Ballard et al. New Ballard Score, expanded to include extremely premature infants. *J. Pediatr.* 119:417, 1991.)

    b. Term—37 to 41 6/7 weeks

    c. Postterm—42 weeks or more

  B. Although there is no universal agreement on birth-weight classification, the commonly accepted definitions are as follows:

    1. Macrosomia—4000 gm or more

    2. Normal birth weight (NBW)—2500 to 3999 gm

    3. Low birth weight (LBW)—less than 2500 gm. These infants can be further classified by maturity and appropriateness for gestational age:

      a. Premature but appropriate size for gestational age **(preterm AGA)**

      b. Premature but with weight small for gestational age **(preterm SGA)**

      c. Term but small for gestational age **(term SGA)**

    4. Very low birth weight (VLBW)—less than 1500 gm

III. Prematurity [3,7]. A **preterm neonate**'s birth occurs through the end of the last day of the thirty-seventh week (259th day) following onset of the last menstrual period.

  A. Incidence. Approximately 9% of all U.S. births are premature, and almost 2% are less than 32 weeks' gestation [11]. In some population segments, demographics play a major role in the incidence of prematurity.

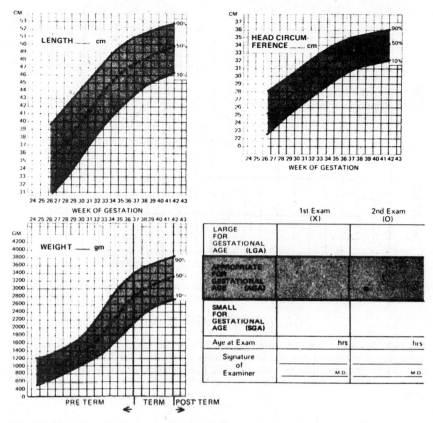

Fig. 3-2. Sample of a form used to classify newborns based on maturity and intrauterine growth. (Reproduced with permission from a form developed by Jacob L. Kay, M.D., Seton Medical Center, Austin, Texas, with Mead Johnson & Co., Evansville, Indiana.)

B. Etiology is unknown in most cases. Premature (and, in many cases, LBW) delivery is associated with the following conditions [6]:

1. **Low socioeconomic status,** whether measured by family income, educational level, residency, social class, or occupation

2. **Black women** experience more than twice the rate of premature delivery than do white women, delivering almost a third of all premature infants [11].

3. **Women under age 16 or over 35** are more likely to deliver LBW infants; age is more significant in whites than in blacks.

4. **Maternal activity** requiring long periods of standing or substantial amounts of physical stress is probably associated with IUGR and prematurity. This is not significant in mothers from higher socioeconomic groups who have good medical care.

5. **Acute or chronic maternal illness** (see **I.A.3**) is associated with early delivery.

6. **Multiple-gestation births** occur prematurely in about half of all cases. Because birth-weight–specific mortality is no higher in these infants

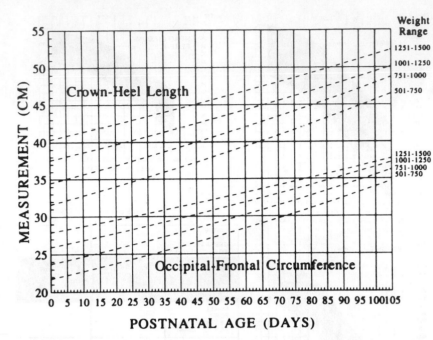

POSTNATAL AGE (DAYS)

Fig. 3-3. Average crown-heel length and occipital-frontal circumference (centimeters) versus postnatal age (days) for infants with birth-weight ranges 501 to 750 gm, 751 to 1000 gm, 1001 to 1250 gm, and 1251 to 1500 gm. (From K. Wright et al. New postnatal growth grids for very low birth weight infants. *Pediatrics* 91:922, 1993.)

compared with singletons, their higher rate of neonatal mortality is primarily due to prematurity.

7. **Prior poor birth outcome** is the single strongest predictor of poor birth outcome. A premature first birth is the best predictor of a preterm second birth [6].

8. **Obstetric factors** such as uterine malformations, uterine trauma, placenta previa, abruptio placentae, incompetent cervix (sometimes occurs in diethylstilbestrol-exposed women), premature rupture of membranes, and amnionitis also contribute to prematurity.

9. **Fetal conditions** such as erythroblastosis, fetal distress, or IUGR may require preterm delivery.

10. **Inadvertent early delivery** because of incorrect estimation of gestational age is another cause of prematurity.

C. **Problems of prematurity**, which are related to difficulty in extrauterine adaptation due to immaturity of organ systems, are noted here but discussed in greater detail in other chapters.

1. **Respiratory.** Premature infants may adapt poorly to air breathing and present with perinatal depression in the delivery room (see Chap. 4). **RDS** may occur because of surfactant deficiency (see Chap. 24), and **apnea** may occur because of immaturity in mechanisms controlling breathing (see Chap. 24). Premature infants are also at risk for bron-

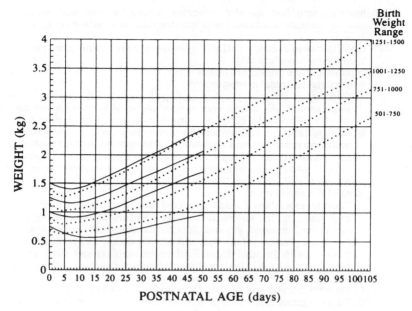

Fig. 3-4. Average daily weight (grams) vs. postnatal age (days) for infants with birth weight ranges 501–701 g, 751–1000 g, 1001–1250 g, and 1250–1500 g (dotted lines), plotted with the curves of Dancis et al. for infants with birth weights 750, 1000, 1250, and 1500 g (solid lines).

chopulmonary dysplasia, Wilson-Mikity disease, and chronic pulmonary insufficiency.

2. **Neurologic.** Premature infants risk acute neurologic problems such as ICH and perinatal depression (see Chap. 27).

3. **Cardiovascular.** Premature infants may be hypotensive due to hypovolemia (such loss is exaggerated by their small size) or cardiac dysfunction and/or vasodilation due to sepsis. Patent ductus arteriosus is common and may result in congestive heart failure (see Chap. 25).

4. **Hematologic** problems, especially anemia resulting from diverse possible causes, are seen frequently (see Chap. 26). Premature infants are more likely to have hyperbilirubinemia (see Chap. 18, **V**).

5. **Nutritional.** Premature infants require specific attention to the type, amount, and route of feeding (see Chap. 10).

6. **Gastrointestinal.** Prematurity is the single greatest risk factor for necrotizing enterocolitis (see Chap. 32).

7. **Metabolic** problems, especially in glucose and calcium metabolism, are more common in premature infants (especially those who are malnourished, sick, or who emerged from an abnormal uterine environment [see Chap. 29]).

8. **Renal.** Immature kidneys are characterized by low glomerular filtration rate and an inability to handle water, solute, and acid loads; fluid and electrolyte management can be difficult (see Chaps. 9, 31).

9. **Temperature regulation.** Premature infants are especially susceptible to hypothermia and hyperthermia (see Chap. 12).

10. **Immunologic.** Because of deficiencies in both humoral and cellular response, premature infants are at greater risk for infection than are term infants.
11. **Ophthalmologic.** Retinopathy of prematurity may develop in the immature retina (see Chap. 35).

D. **Management of the premature infant**
   1. **Immediate postnatal management**
      a. **Delivery** in an appropriately equipped and staffed hospital is most important. Risks to the very premature or sick preterm infant are greatly increased by delays in initiating necessary specialized care.
      b. **Resuscitation and stabilization** require the immediate availability of qualified personnel and equipment. Anticipation and prevention are always preferred over reaction to problems already present. Adequate oxygen delivery and maintenance of proper temperature are immediate postnatal goals (see Chap. 4).
   2. **Neonatal management**
      a. **Thermal regulation** should be directed toward achieving a neutral thermal zone, i.e., the environmental temperature at which oxygen consumption is minimal yet sufficient to maintain body temperature. For the small preterm infant, this will require either an overhead radiant warmer (with the advantages of infant accessibility and rapid temperature response) or a closed incubator (with the advantages of diminished insensible water loss and barrier to infection) (see Chap. 12).
      b. **Oxygen therapy and assisted ventilation** (see Chap. 24)
      c. **Patent ductus arteriosus** usually requires only conservative management: adequate oxygenation, fluid restriction, and possibly intermittent diuresis. In more symptomatic cases, a prostaglandin antagonist such as indomethacin may be necessary. In the most symptomatic infants, surgical ligation may become necessary (see Chap. 25).
      d. **Fluid and electrolyte therapy** must account for potentially high insensible water loss while maintaining proper hydration and normal glucose and plasma electrolyte concentrations (see Chap. 9).
      e. **Nutrition,** which may be limited by the inability of many preterm infants to suck and swallow effectively or to tolerate enteral feedings, may require gavage feeding or parenteral nutrition (see Chap. 10).
      f. **Hyperbilirubinemia,** which is inevitable in the smallest infants, can usually be managed effectively by careful monitoring of bilirubin levels and judicious use of phototherapy. In the most severe cases, exchange transfusion may be necessary (see Chap. 18).
      g. **Infection** is always possible after preterm delivery. Broad-spectrum antibiotics should be begun when suspicion is strong. Consider antistaphylococcal antibiotics for VLBW infants who have undergone multiple procedures or have remained for long periods in the hospital and are at increased risk of nosocomial infection (see Chap. 23).
      h. **Immunization.** Hepatitis B (HBV), DPT (diphtheria, pertussis, and tetanus), polio, and HIB vaccines are given in full doses to premature infants based on their chronologic age (i.e., weeks after birth), not postconceptional age [12].
         (1) If the infant is hospitalized at the appropriate chronologic age, acellular DPT and hemophilis B vaccine are given (usually at 2, 4, and 6 months). Pertussis vaccine is contraindicated in infants with possible or documented evolving neurologic disorders; these infants must receive **pediatric DT,** not **adult dT** vaccine. Infants with stable neurologic conditions may receive acellular DPT.
         (2) Oral polio vaccine should not be given. Administer inactivated polio vaccine (IPV) [12].
         (3) Preterm infants exposed to a mother who tests positive for hepatitis B surface antigen **(HBsAg-positive)** should receive hepa-

titis B immune globulin within 12 hours of birth with the appropriate dose of HBV vaccine given concurrently at a different site, or as soon as possible thereafter, and always within the first month of life (see Chap. 23, Viral Infections in the Newborn).

The optimal time to initiate HBV vaccination in preterm infants with birth weight less than 2 kg and **HBsAg-negative** mothers has not been determined. Seroconversion rates in VLBW infants in whom vaccination was initiated shortly postpartum have been reported to be lower than rates either in preterm infants vaccinated later or in term infants vaccinated shortly postpartum. Hence, initial vaccination in preterm infants with birth weight less than 2 kg and HBsAg-negative mothers should be delayed until just before hospital discharge if the infant weighs 2 kg or more, or until approximately 2 months, when other immunizations are given [see **III.D.2.h.(1)**].

(4) Preterm infants with chronic respiratory disease should receive influenza immunization at 6 months if they are not hospitalized. We have concerns about using live viruses in the neonatal intensive care unit (NICU). Therefore, to protect hospitalized infants with respiratory or other chronic conditions who are younger than 6 months, family and other caretakers should be immunized against influenza. See Chap. 23 for discussion of respiratory syncytial versus immune globulin intravenous (RSV-IGIV).

(5) Immunizations should be given at least 48 hours prior to discharge so that any febrile response will occur in the hospital.

E. Survival of premature infants [1,4]. Tables 3-2 and 3-3 show the survival rates of infants of various birth weights admitted to the NICU facilities of Beth Israel Hospital, Brigham and Women's Hospital, and Children's Hospital (Joint Program in Neonatology). **Admission** is defined as death or admission for more than 24 hours. Admission criteria include prematurity less than 35 weeks, respiratory distress, major congenital anomalies, and perinatal depression. Infants requiring observation or stabilization and admitted for fewer than 24 hours **(triage infants)** are not included in the analysis. The

Table 3-2. Birth weight-specific survival of inborn infants in the Joint Program of Neonatology (JPN), January 1, 1995 to December 31, 1996

Birth weight (gm)	Admissions	Deaths	% Survival
<500	9	3	67
500–599	25	8	68
600–699	44	14	68
700–799	46	9	80
800–899	52	3	94
900–999	79	9	89
1000–1499	370	6	98
1500–1999	548	2	99
2000–2499	569	2	99
>2500	1150	10	99

Note: *Admission* is defined as death or admission for more than 24 hours. All babies <35 weeks are admitted. For babies >35 weeks, admission criteria include respiratory distress, major congenital anomalies, and perinatal depression. Delivery room deaths not included.

Table 3-3. Very low-birth-weight (≤1500 gm) and extremely low-birth-weight (≤1000 gm) infant survival, admissions in selected years to neonatal intensive care units of Joint Program in Neonatology: Total number of admissions (deaths), percent survival

Year	≤1500 gm	≤1000 gm
1975	99 (44) 56%	43 (32) 24%
1982	177 (39) 78%	66 (27) 60%
1983	208 (53) 75%	100 (40) 60%
1987	258 (55) 79%	121 (47) 61%
1988	312 (72) 77%	141 (58) 59%
1993	348 (41) 88%	132 (34) 74%
1994	342 (33) 90%	144 (28) 80%

inborn population, from which the Brigham and Women's Hospital and Beth Israel Hospital infants are drawn, represents approximately 30,000 births. These hospitals serve metropolitan Boston women as well as high-risk maternal referrals from other areas of New England. Infants admitted to Children's Hospital were transferred from other hospitals in New England and the eastern United States. The leveling off of VLBW survival in the 1980s (see Table 3-3) has been witnessed in other perinatal centers [4]. A recent reduction in VLBW mortality nationwide is largely related to a decline in deaths due to RDS and may be associated with artificial surfactant therapy.

F. Long-term problems of prematurity. Premature infants are vulnerable to a wide spectrum of morbidity. Although severe impairment occurs in a small population, the prevalence of lesser morbidities is less clearly defined, although large controlled multicenter trials are now providing a more comprehensive picture both of these sequelae and of the effects of intervention [5,9,10].

   1. **Developmental disability** (see Chap. 14)
      a. **Major handicaps** (cerebral palsy, mental retardation)
      b. **Sensory impairments** (hearing loss, visual impairment) (see Chap. 35)
      c. **Minimal cerebral dysfunction** (language disorders, learning disability, hyperactivity, attention deficits, behavior disorders)
   2. **Retinopathy of prematurity** (see Chap. 35)
   3. **Chronic lung disease** (see Chap. 24)
   4. **Poor growth** (see Chap. 14)
   5. **Increased rates of postneonatal illness and rehospitalization**
   6. **Increased frequency of congenital anomalies**
   7. **Increased risk of child abuse and neglect**
IV. Infants who are SGA (see Chap. 1, Assessment and Prenatal Diagnosis)
   A. Definition. There is no uniform definition of SGA, although most reports define it as two standard deviations below the mean for gestational age or as below the tenth percentile. Numerous "normal birth curves" have been defined using studies of large infant populations (see Fig. 3-2).
   B. Etiology. Approximately one-third of LBW infants are SGA. There is an association of the following factors with SGA infants:
      1. **Maternal factors**
         a. Genetic size
         b. Age
         c. Race
         d. Unwed state
         e. High altitude
         f. Underweight before pregnancy (e.g., malnutrition)

g. Chronic disease
h. Factors interfering with placental flow and oxygenation
  (1) Heart disease
  (2) Renal disease
  (3) Hypertension (chronic or preeclampsia)
  (4) Smoking
  (5) Sickle-cell anemia and other hemoglobinopathies
  (6) Pulmonary disease
  (7) Collagen-vascular disease
  (8) Diabetes (e.g., classes D, E, F, and R) (see Chap. 2, Diabetes Mellitus)
  (9) Preeclampsia (see Chap. 2, Preeclampsia and Related Conditions
  (10) Postmaturity
  (11) Multiple gestation
  (12) Uterine anomalies
  (13) Maternal vascular disease
  (14) Antiphospholipid antibodies
i. Parity
j. Infertility
k. Previous spontaneous abortions
l. Poor weight gain while pregnant
m. Working during pregnancy (see **III.B.4**)
n. Exposure to teratogens such as alcohol, drugs, and radiation
2. Placental lesions
  a. Secondary to maternal vascular disease
  b. Multiple gestation
  c. Malformations
  d. Tumor
3. Fetal factors
  a. Constitutional—normal, genetically small infant
  b. Chromosomal abnormality is the cause in under 5% but is increased in the presence of malformation or symmetric SGA.
  c. Malformations, especially abnormalities of CNS and skeletal system
  d. Congenital infection, especially rubella (60% of infants are SGA) and cytomegalovirus (40% of infants are SGA) (see Chap. 23, Viral Infections in the Newborn)
  e. Multiple gestation
C. Management of the SGA infant
  1. During pregnancy (see Chap. 1, Assessment and Prenatal Diagnosis)
    a. Identification, evaluation, and monitoring. Determination of the cause should be attempted when IUGR is detected. The investigation includes a search for relevant factors (listed in **IV.B**) and usually includes ultrasonic examination. An attempt should be made to assess fetal well-being. Antepartum fetal monitoring, including nonstress testing, oxytocin challenge testing, a biophysical profile, and serial ultrasonic examinations, is often used (see Chap. 1, Assessment and Prenatal Diagnosis). Doppler evaluation of placental flow may be used to evaluate uteroplacental insufficiency. Treatment should be initiated when available. Determination of pulmonary maturity should be considered if early delivery is contemplated (see Chaps. 1, 24).
    b. Early delivery is necessary if the risk to the fetus staying in utero is considered greater than the risk of early delivery. Generally, indications for delivery are arrest of fetal growth, fetal distress, and pulmonary maturity near term, especially in a mother with hypertension. Acceleration of pulmonary maturity with steroids should be considered if amniotic fluid analyses suggest pulmonary immaturity. If there is poor placental blood flow, the fetus may not tolerate labor and may require cesarean delivery.

2. **During delivery.** Very SGA infants are at risk for perinatal problems and often require specialized care in the first few days of life; if possible, delivery should occur at a center with a high-risk nursery. The delivery team should be prepared to manage fetal distress, perinatal depression, meconium aspiration, hypoxia, and heat loss.

3. **In the nursery**

   a. If not yet known, **the cause of IUGR should be investigated;** in many cases the etiology will remain unclear.

      (1) **Newborn examination.** The infant should be evaluated for any of the previously listed causes of poor fetal growth, especially chromosomal abnormalities, malformations, and congenital infection.

         (a) Infants who had growth restriction due to factors influencing the last part of pregnancy (e.g., maternal renal disease, preeclampsia, or other factors interfering with placental circulation) will have a relatively normal head circumference, some reduction in length, but a more profound reduction in weight (see Figs. 3-2, 3-3). Use of the ponderal index (weight in grams × 100/length in centimeters) or the weight-length ratio will quantify weight loss. The infant may have little subcutaneous tissue, peeling loose skin, a wasted appearance, and meconium staining.

         (b) When IUGR begins in early pregnancy, head circumference, length, and weight may all be decreased proportionally, and the ponderal index may be normal. As compared with infants whose IUGR begins in late pregnancy, these infants are more likely to have significant intrinsic fetal problems (e.g., chromosomal defects, malformations, and congenital infection).

      (2) **Pathologic examination of the placenta** for infarction or congenital infection may be helpful.

      (3) Generally, **serologic screening** for congenital infection is **not indicated** unless history or examination suggests infection as a possible cause.

   b. **Evaluation for complications related to IUGR**

      (1) Congenital anomalies
      (2) Perinatal depression
      (3) Meconium aspiration
      (4) Pulmonary hemorrhage
      (5) Persistent pulmonary hypertension
      (6) Hypothermia
      (7) Hypoglycemia
      (8) Hypocalcemia
      (9) Hyponatremia
      (10) Polycythemia

   c. **Infants of hypertensive mothers** may show leukopenia, neutropenia, and thrombocytopenia. The thrombocytopenia is often associated with maternal thrombocytopenia, but the neutropenia and leukopenia are not. The neutropenia is unassociated with a shift to immature forms, as is seen in bacterial infections.

   d. **Specific management considerations**

      (1) **Feeding.** Start feeding milk at 1 hour of age, then continue feedings every 2 to 3 hours. If oral feedings are not tolerated, feed by gavage or intravenously. If there was significant perinatal depression, the infant should be fed only intravenously for 1 to 2 days. SGA infants require more calories per kilogram for growth than AGA infants. The serum sodium concentration should be monitored (see Chap. 9).

      (2) **Blood glucose level** should be monitored every 2 to 4 hours until stable.

(3) **Serum calcium level** may be depressed if the infant was asphyxiated or premature.
D. **Long-term problems of SGA infants.** It is difficult to determine specific effects of IUGR both because studies do not control well for parental height and socioeconomic status and because there are often overlapping effects from prematurity and asphyxia. SGA infants are at risk for poor postnatal growth and neurologic and developmental handicaps. These handicaps occur even in the absence of specific fetal disease (e.g., chromosomal abnormalities). This is especially true in infants who have proportional IUGR, suggesting early onset, and in those who suffered perinatal asphyxia or hypoglycemia (or both) at birth. For any weight group, the total percentage of infants who either die before 1 year of age or are handicapped at 1 year is similar for SGA and AGA infants. However, SGA infants have less risk of neonatal death compared with premature AGA infants of the same birth weight but a greater risk of morbidity at 1 year of age.
E. **Management of subsequent pregnancies** is important because IUGR commonly recurs. Specific recommendations include the following:
    1. The mother should be cared for by personnel experienced with high-risk pregnancies.
    2. The health of mother and fetus should be assessed throughout pregnancy by ultrasonic and nonstress tests (see Chap. 1, Assessment and Prenatal Diagnosis).
    3. Early delivery should be considered if fetal growth is poor.
V. **Infants who are large for gestational age (LGA)** (see Chap. 1)
    A. **Definition.** The newborn's birth weight is two standard deviations above the mean or above the ninetieth percentile (see Fig. 3-2).
    B. **Etiology**
        1. Constitutionally large infants (large parents)
        2. Infants of diabetic mothers (e.g., classes A, B, and C)
        3. Some postterm infants
        4. Transposition of the great vessels
        5. Erythroblastosis fetalis
        6. Beckwith-Wiedemann syndrome
        7. Parabiotic syndrome (twins)
    C. **Management**
        1. The baby should be evaluated for problems listed in **V.B.**
        2. Look for possible evidence of birth trauma, including brachial plexus injury and perinatal depression (see Chaps. 20, 27).
        3. The blood sugar level should be monitored. The infant should be fed early because some LGA infants may have hyperinsulinism and hence be prone to hypoglycemia (infants of diabetic mothers, infants with Beckwith's syndrome, or infants with erythroblastosis [see Chap. 2, Diabetes Mellitus, and Chap. 29, Hypoglycemia and Hyperglycemia]).
        4. Evaluate for polycythemia (see Chap. 26).
VI. **Postmaturity**
    A. **Definition.** The newborn's gestation exceeds 42 weeks.
    B. **Etiology.** The cause of prolonged pregnancy is unknown in the majority of cases. The following are known associations:
        1. **Anencephaly.** An intact fetal pituitary-adrenal axis is involved in the initiation of labor.
        2. **Trisomies 16 and 18**
        3. **Seckel's syndrome** (bird-headed dwarfism)
    C. **Syndrome of postmaturity.** These infants usually have normal length and head circumference. If they have postmaturity syndrome, however, they will have lost weight. Infants with this syndrome are distinct from SGA infants because they were doing well until pregnancy advanced beyond 42 weeks' gestation and they became nutritionally deprived. SGA infants, of course, also may have these signs and symptoms. Postmature infants are classified as follows:

  1. **Stage 1**
     a. Dry, cracked, peeling, loose, and wrinkled skin
     b. Malnourished appearance
     c. Decreased subcutaneous tissue
     d. Skin too big for baby
     e. Open-eyed and alert baby
  2. **Stage 2**
     a. All features of stage 1
     b. Meconium staining
     c. Perinatal depression (in some cases)
  3. **Stage 3**
     a. The findings in stages 1 and 2
     b. Meconium staining of cord and nails
     c. A higher risk of fetal, intrapartum, or neonatal death
 D. **Placenta.** There is some correlation between low placental weight and increased mortality in postmature infants. One study showed that the average placental weight in nonsurvivors was 452 gm, the average placental weight in survivors was 580 gm, and when the placental weight was over 700 gm, there were no deaths.
 E. **Risk.** There is an increase in mortality with postmaturity. Koosterman showed that careful induction of labor or cesarean delivery after 42 weeks resulted in a decreased mortality compared with the results seen following conservative expectant therapy.
 F. **Management**
  1. **Prepartum management**
     a. Careful **estimation of true gestational age,** including data from ultrasonic examination(s)
     b. Careful **monitoring of fetal well-being** (see Chap. 1, Assessment and Prenatal Diagnosis)
  2. **Intrapartum management** involves use of fetal monitoring and preparation for possible perinatal depression and meconium aspiration.
  3. **Postpartum management**
     a. **Evaluation for complications related to postmaturity.** The following conditions occur more frequently in postmature infants:
        (1) Congenital anomalies
        (2) Perinatal depression
        (3) Meconium aspiration
        (4) Persistent pulmonary hypertension
        (5) Hypoglycemia
        (6) Hypocalcemia
        (7) Polycythemia
     b. **Early feeding** for proper nutritional support is important.

References
  1. Allen, M. C., et al. The limit of viability—neonatal outcome of infants born at 22–35 weeks' gestation. *N. Engl. J. Med.* 329:597, 1993.
  2. Ballard, J. L., et al. New Ballard Score, expanded to include extremely premature infants. *J. Pediatr.* 119:417, 1991.
  3. *Guidelines for Perinatal Care.* American Academy of Pediatrics and the American College of Obstetricians and Gynecologists, P.O. Box 1034, Evanston, Ill., 1992.
  4. Hack, M., et al. Outcomes of extremely-low-birth-weight infants between 1982 and 1988. *N. Engl. J. Med.* 321:1642, 1989.
  5. Hack, M., et al. School-age outcome in children with birth weights under 750 g. *N. Engl. J. Med.* 331:753, 1994.
  6. Institute of Medicine. *Preventing Low Birth Weight.* Washington, D.C.: National Academy Press, 1985.
  7. Klaus, M., et al. *Care of the High-Risk Neonate.* Philadelphia: Saunders, 1993.

8. Kramer, M. S., et al. The validity of gestational age estimation by menstrual dating in term, preterm, and post-term gestations. *J.A.M.A.* 260:3306, 1988.
9. McCormick, M., et al. Early educational intervention for very low birth weight infants: Results from the Infant Health and Development Program. *Pediatrics* 123:527, 1993.
10. McCormick, M. Survival of very tiny babies—good news and bad news. *N. Engl. J. Med.* 331:802, 1994.
11. National Center for Health Statistics. Advanced Report of Final Natality Statistics, 1983. Monthly Vital Statistics Report Series 34, No. 6 (Suppl.), U.S. Dept. of Health and Human Services publication (PHS) 85-1120. Hyattsville, Md.: USDHHS, Sept. 20, 1985.
12. *Report of Committee on Infectious Disease: The Red Book.* Evanston, Ill.: Academy of Pediatrics, 1994.

4. RESUSCITATION IN THE DELIVERY ROOM

Steven A. Ringer

I. **General principles.** A person skilled in basic neonatal resuscitation should be present at every delivery. Delivery of all high-risk infants should be attended by skilled personnel whose sole responsibility is the newborn.

The highest standard of care requires the following: (1) knowledge of perinatal physiology and principles of resuscitation; (2) mastery of the technical skills required; and (3) a clear understanding of the roles of other team members, which allows accurate anticipation of each person's reactions in a specific instance. Certification of each caregiver by the Newborn Resuscitation Program of the American Academy of Pediatrics/American Heart Association ensures that each employs a consistent approach to resuscitations.

   A. **Perinatal physiology.** Resuscitation efforts at delivery are designed to help the newborn make the respiratory and circulatory transitions that must be accomplished rapidly and effectively: The lungs expand, clear fetal lung fluid, and establish effective air exchange, and the right-to-left circulatory shunts terminate. The critical period for these physiologic changes is during the first several breaths, which result in lung expansion and elevation of the partial pressure of oxygen (PO_2) in both the alveoli and the arterial circulations. Elevation of the PO_2 from the fetal level of approximately 25 mm Hg to values of 50 to 70 mm Hg is associated with (1) decrease in pulmonary vascular resistance, (2) decrease in right-to-left shunting via the ductus arteriosus, (3) increase in venous return to the left atrium, (4) rise in left atrial pressure, and (5) cessation of right-to-left shunt through the foramen ovale. The end result is conversion from fetal to transitional to neonatal circulation pattern. Adequate systemic arterial oxygenation results from perfusion of well-expanded and well-ventilated lungs and adequate circulation.

   Conditions at delivery may compromise the fetus's ability to make the necessary transitions. Human fetuses respond to hypoxia by becoming apneic. If the insult is brief and occurs just before delivery, recovery from this **primary apnea** is generally accomplished with stimulation and oxygen exposure. If hypoxia continues, the fetus will irregularly gasp and lapse into **secondary apnea.** Infants born during this period require resuscitation with assisted ventilation and oxygen (see **III.B**).

   B. **Goals of resuscitation** are directed toward the following:
   1. **Minimizing immediate heat loss** by drying and providing warmth, thereby decreasing oxygen consumption by the neonate.
   2. **Establishing normal respiration and lung expansion** by clearing the upper airway and using positive-pressure ventilation if necessary.
   3. **Increasing arterial PO$_2$** by providing adequate alveolar ventilation, including added oxygen if necessary.
   4. **Supporting adequate cardiac output.**

II. **Preparation.** Anticipation is key in ensuring that adequate preparations have been made for a neonate likely to require resuscitation at birth.
   A. **Perinatal conditions associated with high-risk deliveries.** Ideally, the obstetrician should notify the pediatrician well in advance of the actual birth. The pediatrician may then review the obstetric history and events leading to the high-risk delivery and prepare for the specific problems that may be anticipated. If time permits, the problems should be discussed with the parent(s). The following antepartum and intrapartum events warrant the presence of a resuscitation team at delivery.

  1. Evidence of fetal distress
   a. Serious heart-rate abnormalities, e.g., sustained bradycardia
   b. Scalp pH of 7.20 or less
   c. Nonreassuring heart-rate pattern (see Chap. 1)
  2. Evidence of fetal disease or potentially serious conditions (see Chap. 3)
   a. Thick or particulate meconium in amniotic fluid (see Chap. 24)
   b. Prematurity (<36 weeks), postmaturity (>42 weeks), anticipated low birth weight (<2.0 kg), or high birth weight (>4.5 kg)
   c. Major congenital anomalies diagnosed prenatally
   d. Hydrops fetalis
   e. Multiple gestation (see Chap. 7)
   f. Cord prolapse
   g. Abruptio placentae
  3. Labor and delivery conditions
   a. Significant vaginal bleeding
   b. Abnormal fetal presentation
   c. Prolonged, unusual, or difficult labor
B. The following conditions do not require a pediatric team to be present, but personnel should be available for assessment and triage.
  1. Neonatal conditions
   a. Unexpected congenital anomalies
   b. Respiratory distress
   c. Unanticipated neonatal depression, e.g., Apgar score of less than 6 at 5 minutes
  2. Maternal conditions
   a. Signs of maternal infection
    (1) Maternal fever
    (2) Membranes ruptured for more than 24 hours
    (3) Foul-smelling amniotic fluid
    (4) History of sexually transmitted disease
   b. Maternal illness or other conditions
    (1) Diabetes mellitus
    (2) Rh or other isoimmunization
    (3) Chronic hypertension or pregnancy-induced hypertension
    (4) Renal, endocrine, pulmonary, or cardiac disease
    (5) Alcohol or other substance abuse
C. Necessary equipment must be present and operating properly. Each delivery room should be equipped with the following:
  1. Radiant warmer with procedure table or bed. The warmer must be turned on and checked before delivery. Additional heat lamps for warming a very low-birth-weight (VLBW) infant should be available.
  2. Oxygen source (100%) with adjustable flowmeter and adequate length of tubing. A humidifier and heater may be desirable.
  3. Flow-through **anesthesia bag** with adjustable pop-off valve or self-inflating bag with reservoir. The bag must be appropriately sized for neonates and capable of delivering 100% oxygen.
  4. Face mask(s) of appropriate size for the anticipated infant
  5. A bulb syringe for suctioning
  6. Stethoscope with infant- or premature-sized head
  7. Equipped emergency box
   a. Laryngoscope with no. 0 and no. 1 blades
   b. Extra batteries
   c. Uniform diameter endotracheal tubes (2.5-, 3.0-, and 3.5-mm internal diameters), two each
   d. Drugs, including epinephrine (1:10,000), sodium bicarbonate (0.50 mEq/ml), naloxone, albumin 5%, and NaCl 0.9%
   e. Umbilical catheterization tray with no. 3.5 and no. 5 French catheters

f. Syringes (1.0, 3.0, 5.0, 10.0, and 20.0 ml), needles (18 to 25 gauge), T-connectors, and stopcocks

8. Transport incubator with battery-operated heat source and portable oxygen supply should be available if delivery room is not close to the nursery.

9. The utility of equipment for continuous monitoring of cardiopulmonary status in the delivery room is hampered by difficulty in effectively applying monitor leads. Pulse oximetry is more easily performed and may become the method of choice.

D. Preparation of equipment. Upon arrival in the delivery room, check that the transport incubator is plugged in, warming up, and has a full oxygen tank. The specialist should introduce himself or herself to the obstetrician and anesthesiologist, the mother (if she is awake), and the father (if he is present). While the history or an update is obtained, the following should be done:

1. Ensure that the radiant warmer is on, and that dry, warm blankets are available.

2. Turn on the oxygen source and adjust the flow to 5 to 8 L/minute.

3. Test the anesthesia bag for pop-off control and adequate flow. Be sure the proper-sized mask is present.

4. Make sure the laryngoscope light is bright and has an appropriate blade (no. 1 for full-term neonates, no. 0 for premature neonates).

5. Set out an appropriate endotracheal tube for the expected birth weight (3.5 mm for full-term infants, 3.0 mm for premature infants >1250 gm, and 2.5 mm for smaller infants). The tube should be 13 cm long. An intubation stylet may be used, if the tip is kept at least 0.5 cm from the distal end of the endotracheal tube.

6. If the clinical situation suggests extensive resuscitation, the following may be required:

    a. Set up an umbilical catheterization tray for venous catheterization.

    b. Draw up sodium bicarbonate (0.5 mEq/ml) solution, 1:10,000 epinephrine, and isotonic saline for catheter flush solution.

    c. Check that other potentially necessary drugs are present and ready for administration.

E. Universal precautions. Exposure to blood or other body fluids is inevitable in the delivery room. Universal precautions must be practiced by wearing caps, goggles or glasses, gloves, and impervious gowns until the cord is cut and the newborn is dried and wrapped.

III. During delivery, the team should be aware of the type and duration of anesthesia, extent of maternal bleeding, and newly recognized problems such as meconium in the amniotic fluid or nuchal cord.

A. Immediately following delivery, begin a process of **evaluation, decision, and action (resuscitation).**

1. Place the newborn on the warming table.

2. Dry the infant completely and discard the wet linens, including those upon which the infant is lying. Make sure the infant is warm. Extremely small infants may require extra warming with rubber gloves filled with warm water (see Chap. 6).

3. Place the infant with head in midline position, with slight neck extension.

4. Suction the mouth, oropharynx, and nares thoroughly with a suction bulb. Deep pharyngeal stimulation with a suction catheter may cause arrhythmias that are probably of vagal origin. Avoid this type of suctioning: use a suction bulb instead.

If thick meconium (not just stained fluid) is present, suction the oropharynx and trachea as quickly as possible (see **IV.A** and Chap. 24, Meconium Aspiration).

B. Sequence of intervention. While Apgar scores (Table 4-1) are assigned at 1 and 5 minutes, resuscitative efforts should begin during the initial neonatal stabilization period.

Table 4-1. Apgar scoring system

Sign	Score		
	0	1	2
Heart rate	Absent	Under 100 beats per minute	Over 100 beats per minute
Respiratory effort	Absent	Slow (irregular)	Good crying
Muscle tone	Limp	Some flexion of extremities	Active motion
Reflex irritability	No response	Grimace	Cough or sneeze
Color	Blue, pale	Pink body, blue extremities	All pink

Source: From V. Apgar. A proposal for a new method of evaluation of the newborn infant. *Anesth. Analg.* 32:260, 1953.

First, assess whether the infant is **breathing spontaneously.** Next, assess whether the **heart rate is greater than 100 beats per minute (bpm).** Finally, evaluate whether the infant's **overall color** is pink (acrocyanosis is normal). If any of these three characteristics is abnormal, take steps to correct the deficiency, and reevaluate every 15 to 30 seconds until all characteristics are present and stable. In this way, adequate support will be given while overly vigorous interventions are avoided when newborns are making adequate progress on their own. This approach will help avoid complications such as laryngospasm and cardiac arrhythmias from excessive suctioning or pneumothorax from injudicious bagging. Some interventions are required in specific circumstances.

1. **Infant breathes spontaneously, heart rate is greater than 100 bpm, and color is becoming pink (Apgar score of 8 to 10).** This situation is found in over 90% of all term newborns. Following (or during) warming, drying, positioning, and oropharyngeal suctioning, the infant should be assessed. If respirations, heart rate, and color are normal, the infant should be wrapped and returned to the parents.

   Some newborns do not immediately establish spontaneous respiration but will rapidly respond to tactile stimulation, including vigorous flicking of the soles of the feet or rubbing the back (e.g., cases of **primary apnea**). More vigorous or other techniques of stimulation have no therapeutic value and are potentially harmful. If breathing does not start after two attempts at tactile stimulation, **secondary apnea** probably exists, and respiratory support should be initiated.

2. **Infant breathes spontaneously, heart rate is greater than 100 bpm, but the overall color remains cyanotic (Apgar score of 5 to 7).** This situation is not uncommon and may follow primary apnea. The newborn should be given blow-by oxygen (100%) at a rate of 5 L/minute by mask or by tubing held about 1 cm from the face. If color improves, oxygen should be gradually withdrawn while color is reassessed. If cyanosis recurs, the oxygen source should be moved closer to the infant. Continuous positive airway pressure by face mask has no role here.

3. **The infant is apneic despite tactile stimulation or has a heart rate of less than 100 bpm despite apparent respiratory effort (Apgar score of 3 to 4).** This represents **secondary apnea** and requires treatment with bag-and-mask ventilation. A bag of approximately 750-ml volume should be connected to oxygen (100%) at a rate of 5 to 8 L/minute and to a mask of appropriate size. The mask should cover the chin and nose but leave eyes uncovered. After positioning the newborn's head in the midline with slight extension, the initial breath should be delivered at a pressure of 30 to 40 cm H_2O. This will establish functional residual capacity, and subsequent inflations will be effective at lower inspiratory pressures.

The inspiratory pressures for subsequent breaths should be 15 to 20 cm H_2O except in infants with known or suspected disease causing decreased pulmonary compliance. In those cases, continued inspiratory pressures of 20 to 40 cm H_2O may be required. A rate of 40 to 60 breaths per minute should be used, and the infant should be reassessed in 15 to 30 seconds. Support should be continued until respirations are spontaneous, and the heart rate is greater than 100 bpm.

Such moderately depressed infants will be acidotic but generally able to correct this respiratory acidosis spontaneously after respiration is established. This process may take up to several hours, but unless the pH remains less than 7.25, acidosis does not need further treatment.

4. **The infant is apneic, and the heart rate is below 100 bpm despite 15 to 30 seconds of assisted ventilation (Apgar score of 0 to 2).** If the heart rate is increasing, bag-and-mask ventilation should be continued, and the heart rate rechecked in 15 to 30 seconds. If the heart rate is 80 to 100 bpm but not increasing, ventilation must be continued and the following steps taken.

   a. **Adequacy of ventilation** should be assessed by observing chest-wall motion at the cephalad portions of the thorax and listening for equal breath sounds laterally over the right and left hemithoraces at the midaxillary lines. The infant should be ventilated at 40 to 60 breaths per minute using the minimum pressure (usually 15 to 20 cm H_2O) that will move the chest and produce audible breath sounds. Infants with respiratory distress syndrome, pulmonary hypoplasia, or ascites may require higher pressures.

      Be certain that 100% oxygen is being delivered and that the mask has a good seal with the face. Recheck head position and clear the airway again. Continue bag-and-mask ventilation and reassess in 15 to 30 seconds. The most important measure of ventilation adequacy is infant response. If, despite good air entry, the heart rate fails to increase and color remains poor, intubation may be considered (see Chap. 36). Air leak (e.g., pneumothorax) should be ruled out.

   b. **Intubation is absolutely indicated** only when a diaphragmatic hernia or similar anomaly is suspected or known to exist. It may be warranted when bag-and-mask ventilation is ineffective, when an endotracheal tube is needed for emergency administration of drugs, or when the infant requires transportation for more than a short distance after stabilization. Even in these situations, effective ventilation with a bag and mask may be done for long periods, and it is preferable to repeated unsuccessful attempts at intubation or attempts by unsupervised personnel unfamiliar with the procedure.

      Intubation should be accomplished rapidly (limiting each attempt to 20 seconds with intervening bag-and-mask ventilation) by a skilled person. The heart rate should increase to over 100 bpm, and color should rapidly improve with adequate ventilation. Intubation can be readily learned and maintained through practice utilizing one of several commercially available models or through humane use of ketamine-anesthetized kittens.

      The key to successful intubation is to correctly position the infant and laryngoscope and to know the anatomic landmarks. If the baby's chin, sternum, and umbilicus are all lined up in a single plane, and if, after insertion into the infant's mouth, the laryngoscope handle and blade are aligned in that plane, the intubator can only see one of four anatomic landmarks: from cephalad to caudad, the posterior tongue, the vallecula and epiglottis, the larynx (trachea and vocal cords), or the esophagus. The successful intubator will view the laryngoscope tip and a landmark, and should then know whether the landmark being observed is cephalad or caudad to the larynx. The intubator can adjust the position of the blade by several millimeters and locate the vocal cords. The endotracheal tube can then be inserted under direct visualization.

c. **Circulation.** If, after intubation and 15 to 30 seconds of ventilation with 100% oxygen, the heart rate remains below 60 bpm, or is 60 to 80 and not increasing, cardiac massage should be instituted. The best technique is to stand at the foot of the infant and place both thumbs at the junction of the middle and lower thirds of the sternum, with the fingers wrapped around and supporting the back. Alternatively, one can stand at the side of the infant and compress the lower third of the infant's sternum with the index and third fingers of one hand. In either method, compress the sternum 1 to 2 cm 90 times per minute in a ratio of three compressions for each breath. Apply ventilation in the period following every third compression. Determine effectiveness by palpating the femoral or brachial pulse or umbilical cord.

After 15 to 30 seconds, suspend both ventilation and compression for 6 seconds as heart rate is assessed. If the rate is greater than 80 bpm, chest compression should be discontinued and ventilation continued until respiration is spontaneous. If no improvement is noted, compression and ventilation should be continued for successive periods of 30 seconds interposed with 6-second periods of assessment.

Infants requiring ventilatory and circulatory support are markedly depressed and require immediate, vigorous resuscitation (Fig. 4-1). Resuscitation may require at least three trained people working together.

d. **Medication.** If, despite adequate ventilation with 100% oxygen and chest compressions, a heart rate of more than 80 bpm has not been achieved by 1 to 2 minutes after delivery, **or if the initial heart rate is zero,** medications such as chronotropic and inotropic agents should be given to support the myocardium, correct acidosis, and ensure adequate fluid status. (See Table 4-2 for drugs, indications, and dosages.) Medications provide substrate and stimulation for the heart so that it can support circulation of oxygen and nutrients to the brain. For rapid calculations, use 1, 2, or 3 kg as the estimate of birth weight.

(1) The most accessible intravenous route for neonatal administration of medications is catheterization of the umbilical vein (see Chap. 36), which can be done rapidly and aseptically. Although the saline-filled catheter can be advanced into the inferior vena cava (i.e., 8 to 10 cm), in 60 to 70% of neonates the catheter may become wedged in an undesirable or dangerous location (e.g., hepatic, portal, or pulmonary vein). Therefore, insertion of the catheter approximately 2 to 3 cm past the abdominal wall (4 to 5 cm total in a term neonate), just to the point of easy blood return, is safest prior to injection of drugs. In this position, the catheter tip will be in or just below the ductus venosus; it is important to flush all medications through the catheter because there is no flow through the vessel after cord separation.

(2) **Drug therapy** as an adjunct to oxygen is to support the myocardium and correct acidosis. Continuing bradycardia is an indication for **epinephrine** administration. A dose of 0.1 to 0.3 ml/kg (up to 1.0 ml) of a 1:10,000 epinephrine solution should be given through the umbilical venous catheter and flushed into the central circulation. This dose may be repeated every 5 minutes if necessary.

When access to central circulation is difficult or delayed, consider delivering epinephrine by means of the endotracheal tube for transpulmonary absorption. Studies in asphyxiated animals have demonstrated the rapid absorption and action of endotra-

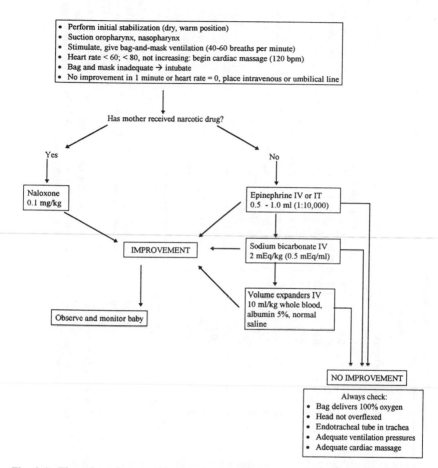

Baby limp and blue; heart rate <100

- Perform initial stabilization (dry, warm position)
- Suction oropharynx, nasopharynx
- Stimulate, give bag-and-mask ventilation (40-60 breaths per minute)
- Heart rate < 60; < 80, not increasing: begin cardiac massage (120 bpm)
- Bag and mask inadequate → intubate
- No improvement in 1 minute or heart rate = 0, place intravenous or umbilical line

Has mother received narcotic drug?

Yes / No

Naloxone 0.1 mg/kg

Epinephrine IV or IT 0.5 - 1.0 ml (1:10,000)

IMPROVEMENT

Sodium bicarbonate IV 2 mEq/kg (0.5 mEq/ml)

Observe and monitor baby

Volume expanders IV 10 ml/kg whole blood, albumin 5%, normal saline

NO IMPROVEMENT

Always check:
- Bag delivers 100% oxygen
- Head not overflexed
- Endotracheal tube in trachea
- Adequate ventilation pressures
- Adequate cardiac massage

Fig. 4-1. Flow sheet for resuscitation of the newborn. (Modified from Perinatal Continuing Education Program, University of Virginia. Courtesy of J. Kattwinkel.)

cheally administered epinephrine, leading to increased heart rate and arterial blood pressure even in the presence of severe acidosis. Case reports support the same effect in newborns, although larger experiences and controlled studies are lacking. Nevertheless, it appears that intratracheal administration of 0.1 to 0.2 ml/kg of 1:10,000 epinephrine is more rapid and safer than intracardiac administration. In emergent situations, use estimated volumes of 0.5 to 1.0 ml of solution in small infants and 1.5 to 2.0 ml in larger infants; higher doses (1 to 2 ml/kg) may be given if no response is seen with standard doses. Epinephrine can be diluted with normal saline to a final volume of 1 to 2 ml.

If two doses of epinephrine do not produce improvement, consider other causes for continuing depression. Documented or sus-

Table 4-2. Neonatal resuscitation

Drug/Therapy	Dose/kg	Weight (kg)	Volume (ml) IV	Volume (ml) IT	Method	Indication
Epinephrine 1:10,000 0.1 mg/ml	0.01 to 0.03 mg/kg IV IT dose is 2 to 3 ×IV	1 2 3 4	0.2 0.4 0.6 0.8	0.5 1.0 1.5 2.0	Give IV push or IT diluted with 1 to 2 ml of normal saline; *do not* give into an artery; *do not mix* with bicarbonate; repeat in 5 min PRN	Asystole or severe bradycardia
Sodium bicarbonate 0.5 mEq/ml	2 mEq/kg IV	1 2 3 4	4 8 12 16		Give IV over 2 minutes; do not mix with epinephrine, calcium, or phosphate; assure adequate ventilation; repeat in 5 to 10 min PRN	Metabolic acidosis
Naloxone (Narcan) 0.4 mg/ml	0.1 to 0.2 mg/kg	1 2 3 4	0.25 to 0.5 0.50 to 1.0 0.75 to 1.5 1.0 to 2.0		Give IV push, IM, SQ, or IT; repeat PRN 3 times if no response; *if maternal narcotic addiction is suspected do not give*; do not mix with bicarbonate (see Chap. 19)	Narcotic depression
Volume expanders Normal saline 5% Albumin Plasma Whole blood	10 ml/kg	1 2 3 4	10 ml 20 ml 30 ml 40 ml		Give IV over 5 to 10 minutes Slower in premature infants	Hypotension due to intravascular volume loss (see Chap. 17)
Dopamine	Begin at 5 µg/kg/min IV (may increase up to 20 µg/kg/min)		$\dfrac{6 \times \text{wt (kg)} \times \text{desired dose (µg/kg/min)}}{\text{desired fluid rate (ml/hr)}} =$		mg of dopamine per 100 ml of solution; give as continuous infusion with pump	Hypotension due to poor cardiac output (see Chap. 17)

Cardioversion/defibrillation (see Chap. 25)	1 to 4 Joules/kg; increase 50% each time		Ventricular fibrillation, ventricular tachycardia
ET tube (see Chap. 36)	Internal diameter (mm)		Distance of tip of ET tube (for nasal intubation add 2 cm.)
	2.5 uncuffed	<1000 gm	7 cm
	3.0 uncuffed	1000 to 2000 gm	8 cm
	3.5 uncuffed	2000 to 4000 gm	9 cm
	3.5 to 4.0 uncuffed	>4000 gm	10 cm
Laryngoscope blades (see Chap. 36)	0 (straight)	<2000 gm	
	1 (straight)	>2000 gm	

IM = intramuscular; IT = intratracheal; IV = intravenous; SQ = subcutaneous.

pected acidosis should be treated with 2 mEq of bicarbonate per kg body weight. The **bicarbonate** may be given as 4 ml/kg of **0.5 mEq/ml of sodium bicarbonate** administered over 2 to 4 minutes through the umbilical vein.

Because there are potential risks as well as benefits for all medications (see Table 4-2), drug administration through the umbilical vein should be reserved for those newborns in whom bradycardia persists despite adequate oxygen delivery and ventilation. If an adequate airway has been established, adequate ventilation achieved, and the heart rate exceeds 100 bpm, the infant should be moved to the neonatal intensive care unit (NICU), where physical examination, determination of vital signs, and test results such as chest radiographic appearance will more clearly identify needs for specific interventions.

(3) **Volume expansion.** If oxygenation and blood pH are satisfactory, but blood pressure is still low and peripheral perfusion poor, volume expansion may be indicated through the use of 5% albumin, packed red blood cells, or whole blood (see **IV.B** and Chap. 17). Additional indications for volume expansion include evidence of acute bleeding or poor response to resuscitative efforts. Volume expansion should be carried out cautiously in newborns in whom hypotension may be caused by asphyxial myocardial damage rather than hypovolemia. It is important to use the appropriate gestational age– and birth weight–related blood-pressure norms to determine volume status (see Chap. 26, Anemia).

(4) **Reversal of narcotic depression.** If the mother has received narcotic analgesia within a few hours of delivery, the newborn may manifest respiratory depression due to transplacental passage. The depression usually presents as apnea, bradycardia, and cyanosis that easily correct with bag-and-mask ventilation but recur upon cessation of support. These infants should be treated with naloxone (0.4 mg/ml), in a dose of 0.25 ml/kg (e.g., 0.1 mg/kg). Naloxone should not be used if the mother is a chronic user of narcotics. Respiratory support should be maintained until spontaneous respirations occur.

IV. Special situations

A. Meconium aspiration (see Chap. 24)

1. In the presence of thick meconium, the obstetrician should suction the mouth and pharynx with a bulb syringe or suction catheter after delivery of the head and before breathing begins.

2. The newborn should immediately be handed to the pediatrician to intubate the trachea and aspirate meconium, preferably before the first breath. In many cases, even if the infant has gasped, some meconium may still be removed with direct tracheal suction. New devices have been manufactured that have an adapter at one end that fits a suction catheter and an adapter at the other end that fits the endotracheal tube. The resuscitator should avoid suction techniques that could allow self-contamination with blood or vaginal contents.

3. For infants at risk of meconium aspiration syndrome who show initial respiratory distress, care should be taken at all times in the delivery room and NICU to provide adequate oxygen and prevent even transient hypoxemia.

4. If the meconium staining is thin or watery, the infant should be evaluated by the pediatric team, but special management is not usually indicated.

B. Shock. Some newborns present with pallor and shock in the delivery room (see Chaps. 17, 26). Shock may result from significant intrapartum blood loss due to placental separation, fetal-maternal hemorrhage, avulsion of the umbilical cord from the placenta, vasa or placenta previa, incision

through an anterior placenta at cesarean section, twin-twin transfusion, or rupture of an abdominal viscus (liver or spleen) during a difficult delivery. These newborns will be pale, tachycardic (over 180 bpm), tachypneic, and hypotensive with poor capillary filling and weak pulses.

After starting respiratory support, immediate transfusion with O-negative packed red blood cells and 5% albumin may be necessary. A volume of 20 ml/kg can be given through an umbilical venous catheter. If clinical improvement is not seen, causes of further blood loss should be sought, and more vigorous blood and colloid replacement should be continued. It is important to remember that the hematocrit may be normal immediately after delivery if the blood loss was acute during the intrapartum period.

If a blood bank is not available in an emergency situation, autologous blood from the placenta may be obtained by preparing the fetal surface of the placenta with Betadine and using a heparin-rinsed sterile needle and syringe. In inexperienced hands, this procedure is fraught with risks of transfusing thrombi or other tissue, so it should be reserved for situations where no other therapeutic option exists. The use of colloid solutions is almost always sufficient for acute stabilization. The risk of transmission of hepatitis B, HIV, or other infectious agents by blood transfusion from mother to infant must be considered when choosing a method of acute volume expansion. Although all these agents can cross the placenta and lead to antenatal infection, direct inoculation of maternal blood certainly increases the risk of neonatal exposure and infection.

C. **Air leak.** If an infant fails to respond to resuscitation despite apparently effective ventilation, chest compressions, and medications, consider the possibility of air-leak syndromes. Pneumothoraces (uni- or bilateral) and pneumopericardium should be ruled out by transillumination or diagnostic thoracentesis (see Chap. 24).

D. **Prematurity.** Premature infants require additional special care in the delivery room, including precautions to prevent heat loss. Apnea due to respiratory insufficiency is more likely at lower gestational ages, and support should be provided. Surfactant-deficient lungs are poorly compliant, and higher ventilatory pressures may be needed.

V. **Apgar scores.** Evaluation and decisions regarding resuscitation measures should be guided by assessment of respiration, heart rate, and color. Apgar scores are conventionally assigned after birth and recorded in the newborn's chart. The Apgar score consists of the total points assigned to five objective signs in the newborn. Each sign is evaluated and given a score of 0, 1, or 2. Total scores at 1 and 5 minutes after birth are usually noted. If the 5-minute score is 6 or less, the score is then noted at successive 5-minute intervals until it is greater than 6 (see Table 4-1). A score of 10 indicates an infant in perfect condition; this is quite unusual because most babies have some degree of acrocyanosis. The scoring, if done properly, yields the following information:

1. **One-minute Apgar score.** This score generally correlates with umbilical cord blood pH and is an index of intrapartum depression. It does not correlate with outcome. Babies with a score of 0 to 4 have been shown to have a significantly lower pH, higher partial pressure of carbon dioxide ($PaCO_2$), and lower buffer base than those with Apgar scores greater than 7. In the VLBW infant a low Apgar **may not** indicate severe depression. As many as 50% of infants with gestational ages of 25 to 26 weeks and Apgar scores of 0 to 3 have a cord pH of greater than 7.25. Therefore, a VLBW infant with a low Apgar score cannot be assumed to be severely depressed. Nonetheless, such infants should be resuscitated actively and will usually respond more promptly and to less invasive measures than newborns whose low Apgar scores reflect acidemia.

2. **Apgar scores beyond 1 minute** are reflective of the infant's changing condition and the adequacy of resuscitative efforts. Persistence of low Apgar scores indicates need for further therapeutic efforts. The most common problem is inadequate pulmonary inflation and ventilation. It

is important to verify a good seal with the mask, correct placement of the endotracheal tube, and adequate peak inspiratory pressure applied to the bag if the Apgar score fails to improve as resuscitation proceeds.

The more prolonged the period of severe depression (i.e., Apgar score ≤3), the more likely is an abnormal long-term neurologic outcome. Nevertheless, many newborns with prolonged depression (>15 minutes) are normal in follow-up. Moreover, most infants with long-term motor abnormalities such as cerebral palsy have not had periods of neonatal depression after birth (see Chap. 27, Perinatal Asphyxia). Apgar scores were designed to monitor neonatal transition and the effectiveness of resuscitation, and their utility remains essentially limited to this important role.

Reference

Bloom, R. S., and Cropley, C. *Textbook of Neonatal Resuscitation.* Dallas: American Heart Association, 1994.

5. NURSERY CARE OF THE WELL NEWBORN*

Constance H. Keefer

I. **Initial period**
   A. **Protective gloves** should be worn when one is handling newborns who have not been bathed and when in contact with an infant's blood, saliva, meconium, or stool.
   B. The **newborn's temperature should be stabilized** with warming lights or an incubator; initial skin care should be deferred until temperature is stable.
   C. On admission to the nursery, repeat part of the initial physical examination (see Chap. 3, History and Physical Examination of the Newborn), looking for the following:
      1. Respiratory distress (see Chap. 24)
      2. Poor color, including pallor, plethora, or cyanosis other than acrocyanosis
      3. Diaphoresis (see Chap. 29)
      4. Jitteriness. If present, check blood glucose level with Dextrostix. When it is below 40 mg/dl, give dextrose (5%) in water and recheck the level (see Chap. 29, Hypoglycemia and Hyperglycemia).
      5. Hypotonia
      6. Hypertonia
      7. Malformations (major and minor)
   D. Classify weight as appropriate, small, or large for gestational age (AGA, SGA, and LGA, respectively; see Chap. 3).
      1. If the infant is SGA, check for possible causes and complications [see Chap. 3, Identifying the High-Risk Newborn, **IV.B** and **IV.C.3.a.(1)**].
      2. If the infant is LGA, check for hypoglycemia.
   E. **Skin care.** Examine skin for signs of trauma and infection (see Chaps. 9, 23).
      1. Use cotton cloth with tap water and nonmedicated soap to remove blood and meconium. Do not remove the vernix caseosa. Afterward, skin can be cleaned as needed with soap and water.
      2. If the nursery is having problems with *Staphylococcus aureus* **infections,** a hexachlorophene soap can be used until the epidemic has passed. Remember, hexachlorophene can be absorbed through intact skin and is potentially toxic to neonates. Leave on skin five minutes and rinse well.
      3. **Skin abrasions** should be carefully cleaned with soap and water. Topical antibiotics may be reasonable to use in infants who will have short hospital stays. Use of topical antibiotics for routine skin care in infants who have prolonged hospitalizations has been associated with the emergence of multiple antibiotic-resistant organisms. Such medications should only be used for specific indications.
   F. **Cord care.** We use a plastic cord clamp (double-grip umbilical cord clamp, Hollister, Inc., Libertyville, Illinois), which is removed 24 hours after birth. There are several methods of cord care, and no single method has proved superior. We use one application per day of topical antibiotic cream (bacitracin), alcohol after diaper changes, and exposure to the air for drying.
   G. **Eye care.** Either silver nitrate drops 1% or erythromycin ointment is applied in the delivery room within 1 hour of life to prevent gonococcal ophthalmia (see Chap. 23).
   H. **Vitamin K** (1.0 mg vitamin K_1 oxide, phytonadione) is administered within 2 hours of life to prevent hemorrhagic disease. The association of vitamin K administration to newborns with increased cancer rates in childhood, found

*This is a revision of a chapter by Dr. E. Manning Sears in the 3rd edition of the *Manual of Neonatal Care.*

in several small studies, was not substantiated in a National Institute of Child Health and Human Development (NICHD) case-control study of the Collaborative Perinatal Project [4,22] (see Chap. 26, Bleeding).

II. Subsequent period

A. Weight should be checked daily.

B. Length and head circumference should be measured at admission.

C. Record time and amount for stools and urine, as well as pulse, respiration rate, and axillary temperature at least every 8 hours. Pulse and respiration should be recorded every 4 hours for infants with any risk factors for infection or pulmonary or cardiac disease. One-third of newborns admitted to newborn intensive care nurseries (NICUs) were considered healthy at birth.

D. Feeding. The first feedings are at the breast or with formula (see Chaps. 10, 11).

   1. Breast-feeding is preferred if there are no contraindications [5] (see Chap. 11).

   a. Facilitation. Have the mother and infant begin as soon as possible and discourage use of formula in the first 2 weeks. Routine postpartum nursing care should include assessment of and instruction in nursing technique. Discharge packs should not include formula [1,28].

   b. Contraindications to breast-feeding are rare and include the following:

   (1) Maternal infection

   (a) Active untreated tuberculosis (see Chap. 23)

   (b) Herpes simplex. Breast-feeding is allowed if infant contact with the lesion is prevented and a good hand-washing technique is practiced after contact with the lesion (see Chap. 23).

   (c) Human immunodeficiency virus (HIV) (see Chap. 23)

   (d) Hepatitis virus (see Chap. 23). Maternal hepatitis B infection is not a contraindication to breast-feeding when the infant is immunized with hepatitis B immune globulin (HBIG) and hepatitis B vaccine [31].

   (e) Breast-feeding by a mother with cytomegalovirus (CMV) infection *does not* cause apparent infection in the infant [31] (see Chap. 23).

   (2) Maternal medications—[6] (see Appendix and Chap. 19)

   (3) Phenylketonuria, galactosemia, or other inborn errors of metabolism (see Chap. 29)

   (4) Breast milk jaundice is not a cause of jaundice in the first 4 days of life. When it occurs, discontinuation of breast-feeding is necessary for only 48 hours (see Chap. 18).

   2. If formula is used for feeding, the brand should be randomly assigned and based on cow's milk unless otherwise specified by the pediatrician or mother (see Chap. 10).

E. Infant sleep position should generally be on the **side** for the first few days of life. After that, the supine position is the one recommended by the American Academy of Pediatrics [2,7,17,25,36]. The infant should sleep on a firm infant mattress with only a thin covering between the infant and the mattress.

   1. Certain infants with craniofacial anomalies or regurgitation problems should not sleep in a supine position.

F. Family-focused care, practiced in our nurseries, includes maternal and infant care provided by the same nurse [29,35] and documented in one pathway chart [16]. The infant is kept in the mother's room as much as possible, consistent with the health of the infant and parental ability to care for him or her.

III. Nursery assessment should include a review of maternal records; reasons for incomplete prenatal care should be explored by a social worker. The initial physician's examination (see Chap. 3 for details) should be completed within the first 24 hours of life.

IV. Interventions

A. Circumcision [14,32]
  1. The following policy for nonritual circumcision exists in our nurseries [8]:
    a. There is no absolute medical indication for routine neonatal circumcision.
    b. Pros and cons of circumcision should be discussed with parents prior to birth [21,30].
    c. Infants who have potential problems that may make lifelong penile hygiene difficult should probably have a circumcision.
    d. In certain infants circumcision should not be performed routinely:
      (1) Infants with chordee or hypospadias because foreskin may be used in later repair
      (2) Infants with ambiguous genitalia
      (3) Infants with bleeding disorders
    e. Circumcision should not be performed during the immediate postpartum stabilization period and should be done by well-trained personnel.
      Note: Because of shortened length of stays, we have changed our policy to allow circumcision to be done (a) prior to the initial pediatric examination, when the obstetrician confirmed normal genitalia, and (b) anytime after the infant has achieved stabilization, not necessarily after the age of 12 hours. Restrictions in oral intake are no longer necessary before the circumcision.
  2. Circumcision and complications
    a. Pain. Local anesthesia may reduce the physiologic response to circumcision but has inherent risks [8]. More data are needed before penile nerve block can be advocated routinely for newborn circumcision (see Chap. 37). Topical anesthetic cream, effective through intact skin, is being tested in newborns and in our nurseries appears to be effective and safe [12] (see Chap. 37).
    b. Risks of surgery. There is a 0.2 to 0.6 percent complication rate. Risks include the following.
      (1) Hemorrhage
      (2) Infection
      (3) Surgical trauma (partial amputation, denudation) [33]
      (4) Late complications—meatal stenosis and ulceration
  3. Care of the uncircumcised penis [26] includes gentle, never forced, retraction of the foreskin for cleaning. Complete retraction is often not possible in neonates.
B. Hepatitis B immunization for prophylaxis is offered to all newborns [31] (see Chap. 23). Parental consent is necessary. Some pediatricians defer the immunization to the 2-week visit.
C. Indications for **social service consultation** include incomplete prenatal care, maternal substance abuse, and maternal medical diagnoses such as depression, other psychiatric diagnosis, and mental retardation. Other indicators for consultation include inadequate housing and maternal support and young maternal age (teenage mothers).
V. Screening
A. Cord blood—save for 2 weeks
  1. Blood type and Coombs' test on infants born to Rh-negative mothers, mothers with a positive finding on antibody screening, and also type O mothers if the infant is to be discharged prior to the age of 24 hours (see Chap. 18)
  2. Blood type and Coombs' test if jaundice is noted within 24 hours after birth
  3. Later screening for intrauterine infection if indicated. Note cord blood should not be used for syphilis testing because of a high false-positive rate [31].

B. Metabolic disease screening [9,10]. In Massachusetts, blood is collected after the age of 24 hours to screen for phenylketonuria, maple syrup urine disease, galactosemia, homocystinuria, hypothyroidism, biotinidase deficiency, hemoglobinopathies, congenital adrenal hyperplasia, and toxoplasmosis (see Chaps. 2, 23, 29). The routine is to obtain a specimen between 24 and 72 hours of life, as close to 48 hours as possible. Screening for cystic fibrosis is being considered in Massachusetts [13,20].

1. Infants who are transferred to other institutions, admitted to NICU, or discharged before 24 hours are the most likely to miss the screening [19].

   a. Infants discharged before the age of 24 hours should have a specimen collected while in the hospital and a follow-up sample obtained between days 3 and 7 [23] (see Chap. 2, Thyroid Disorders).

   b. We obtain a blood sample from sick infants prior to transfer from our institution and remind the receiving institution to get another sample. Sick or premature infants should have a specimen drawn at 48–72 hours of age, a second specimen at 2 weeks of age or at discharge, whichever is earlier. If the birth weight is <1500 gm, obtain specimens at 2, 6, and 10 weeks of age, or until the baby weighs 1500 gm. Specimen should be obtained prior to blood transfusion.

2. Newborn screening for galactosemia, if serum galactose level is used as the marker, will miss infants with galactosemia who are fed lactose-free formulas from birth.

C. Congenital hip dislocation. Ultrasonic screening is recommended for infants at high risk because of an abnormality found at hip examination, a positive family history, or the presence of other musculoskeletal abnormalities (see Chaps. 3, 28).

VI. Administrative policies in effect in our nurseries:

A. Visitors to mother and infant

1. Father or significant other anytime, and healthy siblings of any age, adults, and other children over 12 years old during visiting hours

2. During unusual viral epidemics, visiting may need to be curtailed.

B. Readmission to the regular nursery is restricted to infants younger than 2 weeks who have been diagnosed with hyperbilirubinemia requiring phototherapy.

C. A **healthy infant** may be a **visitor** to a readmitted mother if the mother is able to care for the infant or has a responsible adult to care for the infant on a 24-hour basis.

D. Security

1. Infants are given two identical ankle bands at birth that match the number on a wrist band given to the mother.

2. Fathers or a designated other are given an identification sticker for a photographic identification (e.g., driver's license) or identification band for access to the hospital after visiting hours and for taking the infant from the nursery.

3. All staff are required to wear a picture identification card. Parents are instructed to allow the infant to be taken only by someone with appropriate picture identification.

4. We now take Polaroid pictures of all babies at the time of admission to the nursery, to place in the chart.

VII. Parental education includes instruction by the primary nurse on feeding and infant care, distribution of booklets and pamphlets on care of the healthy newborn [15], and the availability of hospital television with continuous maternal and child-health teaching programs.

VIII. Discharge plan

A. The discharge examination is covered in Chap. 3, History and Physical Examination of the Newborn, III. The physician or primary nurse should answer parents' questions and review the following issues: observation for possible jaundice, skin infection, subtle signs of infant illness (e.g., fever, fussiness, lethargy, change in feeding behavior), adequacy of intake in breast-fed infants (e.g., minimum of 8 nursings, 6 wet diapers, and 2 stools each 24 hours), use of car seat and seat belts and smoke detectors, lowering of hot-water temperature, and forbidding smoking in the home [34].

B. **Pediatric follow-up appointment** should be made prior to discharge.
   1. Two-week visits are routine for healthy infants leaving after 48 hours.
   2. High-risk infants need a follow-up visit for weight check or other examination prior to 2 weeks.
   3. Breast-fed infants, especially if small, preterm, or firstborn, should be monitored closely for signs of dehydration until the milk comes in and weight stabilizes. These infants are usually seen 2 to 3 days after discharge.
C. **Discharge of low-risk infants before 24 hours,** with home visitation at 3 days by a nurse, has been demonstrated to be safe [27,35]. It should be done only when the mother, the pediatrician, and the obstetrician are comfortable with the plan. Decisions should be based on medical rather than financial grounds. We use the following guidelines [18]:
   1. The prenatal course, including prenatal preparation for early discharge, is uncomplicated.
   2. The prenatal screening results are available to the pediatrician in the hospital.
   3. Maternal ability and support to care adequately for the infant are demonstrated.
   4. The infant's 5-minute Apgar score is higher than 6, gestation was longer than 37 weeks, weight is above 2500 gm, physical examination reveals low risk, and the ability to maintain temperature and feed adequately is demonstrated.
   5. Typing and Coombs' test are performed on cord blood when the mother is Rh negative, is type O, or has abnormal antibodies.
   6. State metabolic screening is performed, time noted, and plans are made for repeat screening at 3 to 7 days.
   7. Posthospital pediatric care is identified and arrangements are made for evaluations of the heart, hips, jaundice, feeding, and weight.
   8. Maternal contact telephone number is documented in the chart.
D. Copies of initial and discharge summaries are given to parents or sent to the physician or clinic rendering follow-up care. These should include all test results, social service referrals, and plans for any special follow-up care. Early discharge has been associated with problems such as hyperbilirubinemia, kernicterus, sepsis, feeding problems resulting in severe weight loss, missed metabolic diseases, and late diagnosis of congenital heart disease [3].
E. Infants should be taken home only in an appropriate infant car seat [11].

References

1. Ambulatory Pediatric Association. The World Health Organization code of marketing of breastmilk substitutes. *Pediatrics* 68:432, 1981.
2. American Academy of Pediatrics. *Back to Sleep.* Elk Grove, Ill.: American Academy of Pediatrics, 1995.
3. American Academy of Pediatrics. *Pediatrics* 96:746, 1995.
4. American Academy of Pediatrics. Controversies concerning vitamin K and the newborn. *Pediatrics* 91:1001, 1993.
5. American Academy of Pediatrics. Encouraging breast-feeding. *Pediatrics* 65:657, 1980; reaffirmed, *Pediatrics* 88:867, 1991.
6. American Academy of Pediatrics. Transfer of drugs and other chemicals into human milk. *Pediatrics* 93:137, 1994.
7. American Academy of Pediatrics. Positioning and SIDS. *Pediatrics* 89:1120, 1992.
8. American Academy of Pediatrics. Report of the task force on circumcision. *Pediatrics* 84:388, 1989.

9. American Academy of Pediatrics. Newborn screening fact sheet. *Pediatrics* 98:473, 1996.
10. American Academy of Pediatrics. Newborn screening for sickle disease and other hemoglobinopathies. *Pediatrics* 84:813, 1989.
11. American Academy of Pediatrics. Family shopping guide to car seats. AAP Safe Ride Program. 141 Northwest Point Blvd., P.O. Box 927, Elk Grove Village, Ill.: 60009-0927.
12. Benini, F., et al. Topical anesthesia during circumcision in newborn infants. *JAMA* 270:850, 1993.
13. Bronstein, M. N., et al. Pancreatic insufficiency, growth, and nutrition in infants identified by newborn screening as having cystic fibrosis. *J. Pediatr.* 120:533, 1992.
14. Brown, M. S., and Brown, C. A. Circumcision decision: Prominence of social concerns. *Pediatrics* 80:215, 1987.
15. *Caring for Your Newborn.* Corporate Communications, Brigham and Women's Hospital, 75 Francis Street, Boston, MA 02115.
16. Coffey, R. J., et al. An introduction to critical paths. *Qual. Management Health Care* 1:45, 1992.
17. Elders, J. M. Reducing the risk of sudden infant death syndrome. *JAMA* 272: 1646, 1994.
18. Freeman, R. K., and Poland, R. L. (Eds.). *Guidelines for Perinatal Care* (3d Ed.). Elk Grove Village, Ill.: American Academy of Pediatrics and American Academy of Obstetricians and Gynecologists, 1992.
19. Gray, J. E., et al. Failure to screen newborns for inborn disorders: Lessons from current experience. *Early Human Development* 48:279, 1997.
20. Hammond, K. B., et al. Efficacy of statewide neonatal screening for cystic fibrosis by assay of trypsinogen concentrations. *N. Engl. J. Med.* 325:769, 1991.
21. Herzog L. Urinary tract infections and circumcision: A case-control study. *Am. J. Dis. Child.* 143:348, 1989.
22. Klebanoff MA, et al. The risk of childhood cancer after neonatal exposure to vitamin K. *N. Engl. J. Med.* 329:905, 1993.
23. Massachusetts Department of Public Health. *Newborn Screening Program Specimen Collection Protocol.* Massachusetts Dept. of Public Health, Regional Newborn Screening Program, 305 South St., Boston, MA 02130-3523. March 1994.
24. Massachusetts Task Force on Early Identification of Hearing Loss. *Early Identification of Hearing Loss in Children: Position Statement.* Presented to Massachusetts Department of Public Health, Boston, MA, June 1992.
25. Mitchell, A., and Mandel, F. Critical review: Does the prone sleep position cause SIDS? *Pediatr. Alert* 17:41, 1992.
26. Newborns: Care of the Uncircumcised Penis. *Pediatrics* 80:765, 1987. Department of Publications, American Academy of Pediatrics, 141 Northwest Point Blvd., Elk Grove, Ill. 60007.
27. Norr, K. F., et al. Early discharge with home follow-up: Impacts on low-income mothers and infants. *J. Obstet. Gynecol. Neonatal Nurs.* 17:133, 1988.
28. Perez-Escamilla, R., et al. Infant feeding policies in maternity wards and their effect on breast-feeding success: An analytical overview. *Am. J. Public Health* 84:89, 1994.
29. Phillips, C. R. *Family-Centered Maternity/Newborn Care: A Basic Text.* St. Louis: Mosby-Year Book, 1991.
30. Poland, R. L. The question of routine neonatal circumcision. *N. Engl. J. Med.* 322:1312, 1990.
31. *Report of the Committee on Infectious Diseases.* Elk Grove, Ill.: American Academy of Pediatrics, 1997.
32. Schoen, E. J. The status of circumcision of newborns. *N. Engl. J. Med.* 322:1308, 1990.
33. Sotolongo, J. R., et al. Penile denudation injuries after circumcision. *J. Urol.* 133:102, 1985.

34. Stein, M. T. The Hospital Discharge Examination: Getting to Know the Individual Child. In S. Dixon and M. T. Stein (Eds.), *Encounters with Children: Pediatric Behavior and Development.* St. Louis: Mosby-Year Book, 1992.
35. Williams, L. R., and Cooper, M. K. Nurse-managed postpartum home care. *J. Obstet. Gynecol. Neonatal Nurs.* 21:25, 1993.
36. SIDS and Sleeping Disorders. (Editorial comment.) In J. A. Stockman (Ed.), *Yearbook of Pediatrics.* St. Louis: Mosby Year Book, 1996. P. 255.

6. CARE OF THE EXTREMELY LOW-BIRTH-WEIGHT INFANT

Steven A. Ringer

I. **Introduction.** Extremely low-birth-weight infants (ELBW), birth weight lower than 1000 gm, comprise a unique subclass of the population of very low-birth-weight infants (see Chap. 3). This chapter presents our initial approach to management of these patients.

II. **Prenatal considerations.** If possible, extremely premature infants should be delivered in a facility with a level III neonatal intensive care unit (NICU). The safety of maternal transport must be weighed against the risks of infant transport (see Chap. 13). Prenatal administration of glucocorticoids to the mother reduces the risk of respiratory distress syndrome (RDS) and other sequelae of prematurity.

A. **Neonatology consultation.** If delivery of an extremely premature infant is threatened, a neonatologist should be consulted and discussions undertaken, preferably with both parents present. Although intrapartum consultations are often interrupted for obstetric care, the neonatologist should address the following:

1. **Survival.** To most parents, the impending delivery of a premature infant is frightening, and the greatest initial concern is infant survival. Each consultation must address this concern. Although most data on survival are based on precisely measured birth weight, usually only a gestational age assessment is available prenatally.

   We use survival data from our experience (see Table 3-2) in counseling, with a rough conversion of gestational age (best estimate) to birth weight: 600 gm = 24 weeks; 750 gm = 25 weeks; 850 gm = 26 weeks; 1000 gm = 27 weeks. One recent study [1] reported that the survival rate for infants at less than 23 weeks' gestational age was zero and at 23, 24, and 25 weeks the rates were 15, 55, and 79%, respectively.

   We attempt resuscitation of all newborns who are potentially viable. Parents are counseled that resuscitation will be attempted unless the infant appears extremely immature or clearly weighs less than 500 gm. The moments following delivery are often a poor time to make decisions about viability, so resuscitation is followed by continuous reassessment in the NICU. Many infants are found to be too immature to survive after just a few hours. In our NICU most of these infants die by 18 hours, and often as soon as 2 to 3 hours after birth.

2. **Morbidity.** We try to inform parents as fully as possible about prognosis. Before delivery, particular attention is paid to the problems that might appear at birth or shortly thereafter. We explain the risk of RDS and the potential need for ventilatory support. In our NICU, all infants of 24 weeks' gestation require some ventilatory support; at 25 to 26 weeks, this proportion drops to 80 to 90%; at 27 to 28 weeks, only 50 to 60% of infants require ventilatory support.

   We also inform parents of the likelihood of infection and the risk of intraventricular hemorrhage (IVH), as well as planned early screening tests for these problems.

3. **Potential morbidity.** We avoid immediately giving parents lists of potential sequelae because they may be too overwhelmed to process extensive information during the period surrounding premature birth. However, we discuss problems that occur in many ELBW infants, including apnea of prematurity, IVH, nosocomial sepsis (or evaluations for possible sepsis), and long-term sensory disabilities, including retinopathy of prematurity and subsequent visual deficits and hearing loss [2].

4. Parents' desires. During the consultation, the neonatologist tries to understand parental wishes about resuscitative efforts and subsequent support when chances for infant survival are slim. We encourage parents to voice their understanding of the planned approach. It is important to clarify for parents their role in decision making as well as the limitations of that role. The strength of parental wishes may guide caregivers in determining how long to continue resuscitation attempts.

III. Delivery room care. The pediatric team should include an experienced pediatrician or neonatologist, particularly when the fetus is less than 26 weeks' gestational age. The approach to resuscitation is similar to that in more mature infants (see Chap. 4). Special attention should be paid to the following:

A. Warmth and drying. The ELBW neonate is very susceptible to rapid cooling. The infant should be placed under a preheated warmer and quickly dried. Warming lights should be placed near the radiant warmer. We sometimes provide additional warming by filling latex gloves with warm water and placing them around the infant.

B. Respiratory support. Most ELBW infants require ventilatory support because of pulmonary immaturity and limited respiratory muscle strength. If the neonate cries vigorously, we administer blow-by oxygen as required and observe the infant for signs of tiring. Many are apneic at birth or cry weakly and require bag-and-mask ventilation. The resolution of bradycardia is the best indicator of adequate response to resuscitation. If the infant's lungs are deficient in surfactant, high inflating pressures will be needed even after the first several breaths. Because these infants generally require continued respiratory support and benefit from early application of end-expiratory pressure, we generally perform endotracheal intubation and ventilation shortly after birth. We administer surfactant when the infant is admitted to the NICU, and endotracheal tube position has been radiographically or clinically confirmed; other centers may provide surfactant treatment in the delivery room.

The pediatrician should assess the response to resuscitation and gauge the need for further interventions. If the infant fails to respond, the team should recheck that all support measures are being effectively administered. Support for apnea or poor respiratory effort must include intermittent inflating breaths. Face-mask continuous positive airway pressure (CPAP) alone is not adequate support, and we do not consider an infant who fails to respond to this limited intervention too immature to be resuscitated. If no response occurs after a reasonable length of time, we consider withdrawing support.

C. Care after resuscitation. Immediately after resuscitation the infant should be wrapped in warmed towels and placed in a prewarmed transport incubator for transfer to the NICU. We always show the baby to the parents in the delivery room (while in the transport incubator) because this is important for the beginning of parent-infant interaction. In the NICU, the infant is moved to a radiant warmer where a complete assessment is done and treatment initiated. The infant's temperature should be rechecked at this time and closely monitored.

IV. Care in the intensive care unit. Careful attention to detail and frequent monitoring are the basic components of care of the ELBW infant, because critical changes can occur rapidly. Large fluid losses, balances between fluid intake and blood glucose levels, delicate pulmonary status, and the immaturity and increased sensitivity of several organ systems all require close monitoring. Monitoring itself, however, may pose increased risks because of small blood volumes, tiny-caliber vessels, and limited skin integrity. Issues in routine care that require special attention in ELBW infants include the following:

A. Survival. The first 24 hours are the most critical for survival. Infants who require significant respiratory, cardiovascular, and/or fluid support are assessed continuously, and their chances for survival are estimated. If caregivers and the parents determine that death is imminent, continued treatment is futile, or treatment is likely to result in survival of a neurologically devastated infant, if parents agree we withdraw ventilator support and redirect care to comfort measures only.

B. Respiratory support. Most ELBW infants require initial respiratory support.

1. **Conventional ventilation.** We generally use conventional ventilation and prefer synchronized intermittent mandatory ventilation (SIMV) (see Chap. 24, Mechanical Ventilation).

2. **Surfactant therapy** (see Chap. 24, Respiratory Distress Syndrome/Hyaline Membrane Disease). We administer surfactant to infants with RDS who are ventilated with a mean airway pressure of at least 7 cm H_2O and an inspired oxygen concentration (FiO_2) of 0.30 or higher in the first 2 hours of life. We give the first dose as soon as possible after birth.

3. **High-frequency oscillatory ventilation (HFOV)** is used in infants who fail to improve after surfactant administration and conventional ventilation at high peak inspiratory pressures and in infants with air leak, especially pulmonary interstitial emphysema (see Chap. 24).

C. Fluids and electrolytes (see Chaps. 9, 31). Fluid requirements increase tremendously as gestational age decreases below 28 weeks, due to both an increased surface area–body weight ratio and immaturity of the skin. Renal immaturity may result in large losses of fluid and electrolytes that must be replaced.

1. **Rate of administration.** Table 6-1 presents initial rates of fluid administration for different gestational ages and birth weights. We monitor weight, blood pressure, urine output, and serum electrolyte levels frequently. Fluid rate is adjusted to avoid dehydration or hypernatremia. We generally measure electrolytes before the age of 12 hours (6 hours for infants <800 gm), and repeat as often as every 6 hours until the levels are stable. By the second day, many infants have a marked diuresis and natriuresis and require continued frequent assessment and adjustment of fluids and electrolytes. Insensible water loss diminishes as the skin thickens and dries.

2. **Fluid composition.** Initial intravenous (IV) fluids should consist of dextrose solution in a concentration sufficient to maintain serum glucose levels higher than 40 mg/dl. Immature infants often do not tolerate dextrose concentrations higher than 10% at high fluid rates, so we generally use dextrose 7.5% or 5% solutions. This should provide a glucose administration rate of 4 to 10 mg/kg per minute. If hyperglycemia results, we lower dextrose concentrations, but avoid hypoosmolar solutions (dextrose <5%). If hyperglycemia persists at levels above 180 mg/dl with glycosuria, we begin an insulin infusion at a dose of 0.1 unit/kg per hour and adjust as required (see Chap. 29).

3. **Skin care.** Immaturity of skin with susceptibility to damage requires close attention to maintenance of skin integrity (see Chap. 34).

D. Cardiovascular support

1. **Blood pressure.** We accept mean blood pressures of 24 to 48 mm Hg for infants 24 to 26 weeks' gestational age if the infant appears well perfused

Table 6-1. Fluid administration rates for the first 2 days of life for infants on radiant warmers*

Birth weight (gm)	Gestational age (wk)	Fluid rate (ml\kg\d)	Frequency of electrolyte testing
500–600	23	140–200	q6h
601–800	24	120–130	q8h
801–1000	25–26	90–110	q12h

*Rates may be 25–30% lower if incubator or shield is used. Urine output and serum electrolytes should be closely monitored.

and has a stable heart rate. Hypotension is treated with fluid administration and pressor support. Corticosteroids may be useful in infants with hypotension refractory to this strategy (see Chap. 17).
2. **Patent ductus arteriosus (PDA).** The incidence of symptomatic PDA is as high as 70% in infants with a birth weight lower than 1000 gm, and this often becomes apparent on days 1 to 3. In very small infants, the murmur may be difficult to hear and the signs may be less specific. We rely primarily on clinical criteria when PDA is suspected and provide early treatment with indomethacin (see Chap. 25).

E. **Blood transfusions** are often necessary in infants who are ill because of large phlebotomy losses. We limit donor exposure by setting aside a specific unit of blood for each patient likely to need several transfusions during hospitalization (see Chap. 26).

F. **Nutritional support**
   1. **Initial management.** We begin parenteral nutrition at 2 to 3 days when serum electrolyte levels are stable. Clinically stable infants may begin feedings at this time.
   2. During the second week we attempt to establish adequate nutrition. In infants who are stable, feedings are advanced to volumes that will provide calories adequate for growth. We generally use continuous feedings and monitor for signs of feeding intolerance such as abdominal distention, vomiting (which is rare), and increased gastric residuals. Although intolerance may be a sign of a more serious gastrointestinal disorder such as necrotizing enterocolitis, ELBW infants have poor gastrointestinal motility. At least two-thirds of our ELBW infants have episodes of feeding intolerance that result in interruption of feeds. We try to give trophic feedings (10 ml/kg/day) of breast milk as half to full strength, 20 calories/oz formula in all VLBW infants by day 3–5 (see Chap. 10).

References
1. Allen, M. C., et al. The limit of viability—neonatal outcome of infants born at 22 to 25 weeks' gestation. *N. Engl. J. Med.* 329:1597, 1993.
2. Hack, M., et al. Very low birthweight outcomes of the National Institute of Child Health and Human Development Neonatal Network. *Pediatrics* 87:587, 1991.
3. Phelps, D. L., et al. 28-day survival rates of 6676 neonates with birthweight of 1250 grams or less. *Pediatrics* 87:7, 1991.

7. MULTIPLE BIRTHS

William F. Powers

I. **Epidemiology**
   A. **Twins.** Twins are the most common and best studied form of multiple birth. Recent U.S. data show that for the overall population, the rate of twin pregnancy is 11 per 1000 pregnancies. The rate of twin pregnancy is slightly higher among African Americans (13 per 1000). The rate rises with increasing parity, with older maternal age, and after infertility treatment; the rate of twin pregnancies is increasing, partly due to a rise in the latter two factors.
   B. **Higher-order births.** The U.S. rate of triplet and higher-order multiple births is also increasing. This trend is probably related to the use of fertility services.

II. **Types of multiple gestations**
   A. **Monozygous (MZ) twins** develop from one fertilized egg that splits within the first 15 to 16 days of development. These twins can differ phenotypically even though they are genetically identical. The rate of MZ twins is relatively constant in all demographic groups, at 3.5 to 4.0 per 1000 pregnancies.
   B. **Dizygous (DZ) twins** develop from two fertilized eggs. The rate of DZ twinning is variable and is influenced by heredity (transmitted autosomally but expressed in the mother), race (low among Asians), maternal age and parity (increased with advancing age and parity), nutrition (decreased with maternal malnutrition), and use of reproductive technologies and fertility drugs (e.g., clomiphene, gonadotropins). In the United States, roughly two-thirds of twins are dizygous, a rate of about 8 per 1000 pregnancies.
   C. **Naturally occurring higher-order fetuses** can be monozygous or multizygous (see **IV.C**). & conjoined twins ,

III. **Placentation**
   A. **MZ twinning.** The type of placentation, which is tied to the timing of the ovum's split, affects perinatal mortality rates.
      1. Twenty to 30% of MZ twin pregnancies have **dichorionic-diamnionic placentation,** which results when division occurred in the first several days after fertilization. Such placentation results in the lowest perinatal mortality rate.
      2. Roughly 65% of MZ twins have **monochorionic-diamnionic placentation,** which results when division occurred later than 3 days after fertilization. Placental vascular communications are frequent, and twins with this placentation have a higher perinatal mortality rate.
      3. **Monochorionic-monoamnionic placentation** is far less frequent (1 to 4% of MZ pregnancies), and results from division after the amnion has formed. Because no amnion separates the fetuses, cords can become entangled and knotted; this type of placentation is associated with a 50 to 60% perinatal mortality rate.
   B. **DZ twinning.** Dichorionic placentas occur in all DZ twins and in those MZ twins resulting from a very early division; there are always two amnions. Dichorionic placentas may fuse if implantation was adjacent. The blood vessels of the two fetuses almost never fuse.
   C. The type of placenta can be determined prenatally or at delivery.
      1. **Ultrasonography** can identify the **pattern of placentation,** and the information can be useful in planning the management of complicated multiple pregnancies.

    2. After delivery, the placenta and membranes can be examined. In monochorionic twins the two layers of amnion appear translucent when peeled apart and leave a single, fairly smooth chorionic surface on the placenta. In dichorionic twins the two amnions and two chorions that form the dividing membrane are more opaque and difficult to separate. When peeled off, they disrupt the placental surface.

IV. **The diagnosis of zygosity** can be determined at birth for many twins (and higher-order births) on the basis of gender combination, examination of the placenta, and blood typing.

    A. Twins of unlike gender are DZ. Monochorionic twins are MZ. Like-gender, dichorionic twins with different blood types are DZ. Like-gender, dichorionic twins with the same blood type are probably MZ.

    B. Immunologic studies can prove monozygosity (e.g., for transplantation). Adult twins classify themselves correctly on the basis of similarities with an error of 2 to 5%.

    C. Twins induced by fertility drugs are usually multizygous. Triplets and higher-order births can be a hybrid of cleaved embryos (analogous to MZ twins) and multiple embryos (analogous to DZ twins).

V. **Diagnosis of multifetal pregnancy.** Early diagnosis is important because of the increased incidence of antepartum and peripartum complications.

    A. **Early signs** include increased uterine size for dates, palpation of excess fetal parts or auscultation of multiple heart beats, and maternal serum alpha-fetoprotein level higher than two multiples of the median for gestational age. Diagnosis may be suggested by a maternal family history of twins.

    B. Ultrasonography can confirm the diagnosis.

VI. **Risks of multifetal pregnancies.** Multifetal pregnancies present both maternal and fetal risks.

    A. **Maternal risks** include hyperemesis gravidarum, anemia, preeclampsia, and gestational diabetes.

    B. **Common fetal risks** include congenital anomalies, fetal growth disturbances, vascular communications, fetal demise, premature delivery with low birth weight, increased risk associated with being born second, and high perinatal and neonatal mortality rates. Risks such as locking, knotting of cords, conjoined twins, and vasa praevia are less common.

    C. **Anomalies.** Congenital anomalies occur more frequently in twins compared with singletons, though the magnitude of the increased risk varies among studies.

        1. The same factor(s) that cause MZ twinning might cause the increased frequency of early malformations, including sacrococcygeal teratoma, sirenomelia sequence, VATER association, anencephaly, holoprosencephaly, and exstrophy of the cloaca.

        2. Eighty to 90% of MZ twins are discordant for anomalies, suggesting that uterine environmental factors are important. In concordant cases one twin may be less affected. For example, congenital heart disease is concordant in 25% of MZ twins, but only 5% of DZ twins. Cleft lip and palate are concordant in 40% of MZ twins, but only 8% of DZ twins. When twins discordant for severe malformations are recognized early in pregnancy, selective termination of the affected fetus can be considered.

    D. **Growth disturbances** in multiple gestations

        1. **Normal growth patterns** for twins and triplets

            a. Through 29 weeks' gestation, the mean weight of each twin approximates that of a singleton of comparable gestational age. Subsequently, the rate of twin weight gain is less; after 33 weeks, the mean weight of a twin is less than the fifth percentile for singletons. The average twin weight at term is approximately 2600 gm, compared with 3200 gm in a singleton infant.

            b. Monochorionic twins generally weigh less than dichorionic twins.

    c. After about the twenty-eighth week, the mean fetal weight of triplets fails to keep pace with that of singletons.

  2. Discordant growth. Twins with birth weights different by more than 25% have infant mortality rates 40 to 80% higher than twins whose birth weight disparity is less than 10%.

E. Placental vascular shunts in twin pregnancies occur in almost all monochorionic placentas but rarely in dichorionic ones. They are a major cause of discordant fetal growth and perinatal complications.

  1. As long as blood flow is balanced in the anastomoses (e.g., artery-to-artery and/or vein-to-vein), they pose only a potential threat. However, if perfusion pressure changes (i.e., at delivery or after demise of one fetus), these shunts can cause acute problems, including exsanguination of the second twin into the first.

  2. Artery-to-vein anastomoses are much more important, forming the basis of the twin-transfusion syndrome. These anastomoses are common and usually occur at a placental cotyledon. Variation in size, number, and direction determine their consequences. When monochorionic twins exhibit a hemoglobin difference of more than 5 gm/100 ml, a clinical diagnosis of twin-transfusion syndrome is suggested. This should be suspected clinically when one twin appears plethoric and the other pale.

    a. With chronic intrauterine transfer of blood, the donor fetus will have severe growth restriction, anemia, hypovolemia, renal insufficiency, oligohydramnios, and amnion nodosum. Severe oligohydramnios can lead to development of complications of prolonged compression, including pulmonary hypoplasia, abnormal facies, and extremity deformation.

    b. Recipient fetuses develop polycythemia (which can lead to neonatal jaundice or thrombosis), cardiac hypertrophy, hypervolemia, pulmonary and systemic arterial medial hypertrophy, and polyhydramnios. At times, the volume excess may lead to cardiac decompensation, secondary hepatic dysfunction, hypoalbuminemia, and edema. Hydrops fetalis can occur.

    c. When the difference in neonatal hemoglobin concentration is large but the intrapair birth-weight difference is small, it is probable that the transfer of blood happened acutely.

  3. Emboli or thromboplastic material from a deceased monochorionic MZ fetus can enter the circulation of the surviving twin, placing this fetus at risk of either infarcts or disseminated intravascular coagulation. The surviving twin also could partially exsanguinate into the dead fetus. Either pathophysiology can result in tissue destruction in the survivor, leading to such defects as porencephalic cyst, hydranencephaly, limb amputation, aplasia cutis, gastroschisis, or intestinal atresia.

  4. Pregnancy management in which one fetus dies involves balancing the risks to the mother and cotwin of prolonging the pregnancy against the risks of delivering a preterm infant.

F. Preterm birth. Twelve and 55% of twins are born at under 32 and under 37 weeks' gestation respectively. Over 95% of twins born after 32 weeks survive infancy. Birth before 32 weeks is associated with a risk of infant death that rises with each week of shortened gestation (see Table 3-2).

G. The second twin

  1. The second twin has an increased likelihood of malpresentation, operative delivery, and exposure to longer periods of hypoxia and anesthesia than the first twin does.

  2. The optimal interdelivery period is roughly 15 minutes, and survival of the second twin is progressively lower after 30 minutes. Continuous fetal monitoring can identify a second twin who is tolerating a longer interdelivery interval and does not need urgent delivery.

  3. Some twin pregnancies are discordant for pulmonary maturity at the time of delivery. For planned premature delivery, fetal lung maturation of each twin is measured to assess the associated risks. The second twin is more likely to have respiratory distress syndrome (RDS) when premature. After accounting for the second twin's higher risk for depression and malpresentation (20% of first twins are nonvertex, while more than 40% of second twins are nonvertex), this twin, when vaginally delivered, still remains at increased risk for RDS. Neither malpresentation nor depression are independently associated with RDS. The second twin's increased risk for depression appears more closely associated with its greater likelihood of malpresentation.

   H. Perinatal mortality among twins is 4 to 11 times that of singletons. The major determinants are preterm birth and the resultant low birth weight. Triplets and quadruplets are at even greater risk of death because they are often born more prematurely and with lower birth weights.

VII. Pediatric management of multiple-gestation neonates

   A. A pediatric team should attend all deliveries; if problems are anticipated, a team should be present for each fetus. It is important to remember that the second twin is at greater risk for asphyxia, bleeding, and intracranial hemorrhage.

   B. The infants are examined for signs of prematurity and growth retardation so these problems can be managed appropriately. All twins, and especially those who are growth retarded, are at increased risk for consequences of placental insufficiency. Screening for polycythemia and hypoglycemia should be considered in multiple births.

   C. Infants are also examined for congenital anomalies. The survivor(s) of multiple gestations with intrauterine demise of one fetus must be examined specifically for disruptive structural defects and the consequences of thromboembolic phenomena. Cerebral ultrasonography and screening for coagulopathy should be considered.

   D. Blood pressure and hematocrit are measured to detect twin-transfusion syndrome. If present, consider the risks to both the donor (hypovolemia, anemia, renal insufficiency, and growth retardation) and the recipient (congestive heart failure and hepatic dysfunction) twin; evaluate and treat each appropriately.

   E. Attempt to determine zygosity by gender-pair combination, placental examination, and blood typing.

   F. Assess the adequacy of family support. If necessary, assist the parents in securing home help and financial assistance, particularly with higher-order births.

   G. If one twin dies, encourage the grieving process and do not assume grief will be minimized by the presence of a surviving infant (see Chap. 22).

VIII. Long-term outcomes

   A. Twins who survive the neonatal period remain at risk of postneonatal death (from day 28 to 1 year). The relative risk of postneonatal death for twins is almost three times that of singletons. These postneonatal deaths are strongly related to low (<2500 gm) or very low (<1500 gm) birth weights.

   B. When birth weight differs by more than 35 percent, the twin who was smaller, upon reaching adulthood, generally is shorter, weighs less, has diminished head circumference, and has significantly lower intelligence. Overall, despite an initial postnatal period of rapid growth, the mean weights for twins remain below those for singletons at a given age. In addition, those with intrauterine growth retardation and a low birth weight are at increased risk for developmental morbidity.

   C. Cerebral palsy and mental retardation are more prevalent in twins. Although this increased risk is partially due to low birth weight, even twins of normal birth weight are at greater risk. MZ twins, males, and twins who survive the fetal demise of a cotwin are at particularly high risk.

Reference

1. Keith, L. G., et al. (Eds.), *Multiple Pregnancy: Epidemiology, Gestation and Perinatal Outcome.* New York: Pantheon, 1995.

8. GENETIC ISSUES PRESENTING IN THE NURSERY

Diana W. Bianchi

I. **Introduction.** Although as many as 40% of pediatric hospital admissions have a genetic basis, it is usually the infant with major malformations or an inborn error of metabolism who presents in the nursery setting. **Major malformations** are defined as anomalies that are prenatal in origin and have cosmetic, medical, or surgical significance. The birth of an infant with major malformations, whether diagnosed antenatally or not, evokes an emotional parental response. The medical staff must ensure that the affected infant has an expedient but thorough evaluation so appropriate diagnostic procedures and therapy may proceed.

II. **Incidence.** Major malformations occur in 2 to 3% of live births and have surpassed prematurity as the leading cause of neonatal death.

III. **Etiology.** The etiologies of congenital anomalies are shown in Table 8-1. Note that the cause is unknown in the majority of cases. Only about 10% are associated with a chromosomal abnormality.

IV. **Approach to the infant**
   A. **History**
      1. **Prenatal.** The obstetric chart should be reviewed for the presence or absence of the following:
         a. History of possible teratogenic exposure, including chronic maternal illness, e.g., diabetes, phenylketonuria, myasthenia gravis, myotonic dystrophy, or systemic lupus erythematosus (Table 8-2).
         b. Specific exposure to drugs or alcohol during pregnancy (see Table 8-2 and ref. 8).
         c. Abnormal uterine shape
         d. Infections during pregnancy
         e. Fetal growth pattern (e.g., relationship of uterine size to gestational age)
         f. Results of antenatal ultrasonic examinations (were anomalies, polyhydramnios, or oligohydramnios diagnosed?)
         g. Results of maternal serum screening (see Chap. 1). A **low alpha-fetoprotein** (AFP) level may be seen in the presence of trisomy 18 or 21.

Table 8-1. Etiology of congenital anomalies: Brigham and Women's Hospital malformations surveillance data from 69,227 newborns

	Number	Percent
Single gene (mendelian inheritance)	48	4.1
Chromosome abnormality	157	10.1
Familial	225	14.4
Multifactorial	356	22.8
Teratogens	49	4.1
Uterine factors	39	2.5
Twinning	6	0.4
Unknown	669	43.1
Total	1549	100

Source: Data from K. Nelson and L. B. Holmes. *N. Engl. J. Med.* 320:19, 1989.

Table 8-2. Known human teratogens

DRUGS	MATERNAL CONDITIONS
Aminopterin/amethopterin	Alcoholism
Androgenic hormones	Insulin-dependent diabetes mellitus
Busulfan	Maternal phenylketonuria
Chlorobiphenyls	Myasthenia gravis
Cocaine	Myotonic dystrophy
Cyclophosphamide	Smoking
Diethylstilbestrol	Systemic lupus erythematosus
Iodide	
Isotretinoin (13-*cis*-retinoic acid)	INTRAUTERINE INFECTIONS
Lithium	Cytomegalovirus
Phenytoin	Herpes simplex
Propylthiouracil	Rubella
Tetracycline	Syphilis
Trimethadione	Toxoplasmosis
Valproic acid	Varicella
Warfarin	Venezuelan equine encephalitis virus
HEAVY METALS	OTHER EXPOSURES
Lead	Gasoline fumes
Mercury	Heat
	Hypoxia
RADIATION	
Cancer therapy	

A **high AFP** level may indicate impending fetal demise, open neural tube defect, abdominal wall defect, congenital nephrosis, epidermolysis bullosa, or Turner's syndrome. A high human chorionic gonadotropin (HCG) level is also associated with trisomy 21 [7].

   h. Quality and frequency of fetal movements

2. Family history. The parents and, if possible, the grandparents should be asked the following:

   a. Have there been any prior affected infants in the family?

   b. Is there a history of infertility, multiple miscarriages, neonatal death, or newborns with other malformations?

   c. What is the ethnic background of both mother and father?

   d. Is there a history of consanguinity?

3. Perinatal events

   a. Fetal position in utero

   b. Significant events during labor and type of delivery

   c. Length of umbilical cord (e.g., positive association between fetal motor activity and cord length)

   d. Placental appearance

4. Neonatal course

B. Physical examination. A complete physical examination is **essential** to making an accurate diagnosis. Often, however, the critically ill neonate is partially hidden by monitoring equipment. Beware of making a diagnosis when (1) the midface is obscured by adhesive tape securing endotracheal and nasogastric tubes, (2) the extremities cannot be visualized because there are peripheral intravenous (IV) lines in place, and (3) the infant has received pancuronium bromide. Edema resulting from muscular paralysis can cause considerable distortion of facial features.

   1. Anthropometrics. Specific physical parameters that should be measured include length, head circumference, outer and inner canthal distance, palpebral fissure length, interpupillary distance, ear length, philtrum length, internipple distance, chest circumference, upper-lower segment ratio, and hand and foot length. Normal standards exist for all these measurements in infants of 27 to 41 weeks' gestation [6].

2. Aspects of the physical examination to be emphasized include a thorough inspection of the skin, the position of the hair whorls, head shape and facial characteristics, and dermatoglyphics, and a description of the extremities. The dermatoglyphic pattern of low-arch dermal ridges is particularly useful in the bedside diagnosis of trisomy 18 (Table 8-3).

C. Laboratory and other studies
   1. **Placental pathology,** if possible
   2. **Chromosome studies.** Skin and peripheral blood are the most available sources of cells for chromosome analysis. Generally, 1 ml of peripheral blood is collected in a green-top tube (sodium heparin being the anticoagulant). The sample should be kept at room temperature. It does not matter if the infant has received transfusions. Results are usually available within 48 hours. Although 0.6% of newborns have abnormal chromosomes, only a third of these will have serious malformations. See Table 8-3 for a summary of physical findings in the three major live-born autosomal trisomies. For all newborns with **conotruncal heart malformations** (e.g., interrupted aortic arch, truncus arteriosis, tetralogy of Fallot), ex-

Table 8-3. Physical findings in the three major live-born autosomal trisomies

	Trisomy 13	Trisomy 18	Trisomy 21
Birth weight:	Normal range	Growth retarded	Normal range
Skin:	Scalp defects		
CNS:	Major malformations: Holoprosencephaly Neural tube defects	Microcephaly	
Facies:	Abnormal midface	Micrognathia	Upslanting eyes
	Microphthalmia		Flattened facies
	Cleft lip/palate		Epicanthal folds
			Prominent tongue
			Small ears
Heart:	VSD, PDA, ASD Dextrocardia	VSD, ASD, PDA	AV canal VSD, PDA
Abdomen:	Polycystic kidneys	Omphalocele	
Extremities:	Polydactyly	Camptodactyly Overlapping fingers	Brachydactyly Simian crease in 45 percent
		Abnormal dermato-glyphics	Fifth finger clinodactyly
		Nail hypoplasia	Wide space between first and second toe
Neurologic:		Hypertonic	Muscular hypotonia Weak Moro reflex

VSD = ventricular septal defect; ASD = atrial septal defect; PDA = patent ductus arteriosus; AV = atrioventricular.

Table 8-4. DNA mutations presenting as serious neonatal illness

Hemophilia
Ornithine transcarbamylase deficiency
Autosomal dominant polycystic kidney disease
Alpha-1-antitrypsin deficiency
Chronic granulomatous disease
21-OH deficiency (congenital adrenal hyperplasia)
Cystic fibrosis
Phenylketonuria
Myotonic dystrophy
Osteogenesis imperfecta
Spinal muscular atrophy

amine the karyotype with specific emphasis on long-arm deletions of chromosome 22 [3]. For newborns with severe unexplained **hypotonia,** consider a diagnosis of Prader-Willi syndrome; look for long-arm deletions of chromosome 15 [2].

3. **DNA-based diagnosis and/or banking.** An increasing number of diseases presenting in the nursery result from single-gene mutations [5]. Many are potentially lethal. Obtaining blood or skin fibroblasts for DNA studies may facilitate genetic counseling and prenatal diagnosis in future pregnancies. The relevant disorders are listed in Table 8-4. DNA mutation analysis for infants suspected to have cystic fibrosis is preferable to the sweat test, especially for premature infants [10]. DNA studies are also useful in the determination of twin zygosity and paternity.

4. **Radiographic studies** are important in the overall assessment.

   a. **Ultrasonic examinations** can detect cranial malformations, congenital heart disease, and liver and renal anomalies.

   b. **Radiographs** can define bony malformations or skeletal dysplasias (see ref. 9).

5. **Ophthalmologic examination** is indicated if there is suspicion of congenital infection, or there are CNS or craniofacial anomalies.

6. **Determination of TORCH titers** is only indicated if the physical findings are suggestive of congenital infection (see Chap. 23, Viral Infections in the Newborn).

7. **Measurement of urinary organic acids** is useful to diagnose metabolic disease in the dysmorphic newborn with metabolic acidosis (see Chap. 29, Inborn Errors of Metabolism).

V. **Diagnosis.** After all results are known, a diagnosis may be possible [1,4,5]. In many cases it is not possible to make a diagnosis in the nursery. Because of major changes in facial features over the first year of life, certain diagnoses may become apparent later. Careful **follow-up** is vital.

VI. **Counseling.** If a diagnosis is made, genetic counseling should be offered to discuss prognosis and potential therapy. A future counseling session should be scheduled to provide a **recurrence risk** and give information about the **possibility of prenatal diagnosis.**

VII. **Perinatal death of an infant with malformations**

   A. Have a complete **autopsy** performed, including radiographs and photographs.

   B. Obtain a sterile **skin biopsy specimen** for tissue culture. Cultured fibroblasts may serve as a source of chromosomes, enzymes, or DNA (see Chap. 29).

   C. Arrange a follow-up meeting with the family to summarize the results of studies.

References

1. Baraitser, M., et al. *A Colour Atlas of Clinical Genetics.* London: Wolfe Medical Publications, 1983.
2. Butler, M. G. Prader-Willi syndrome. *Am. J. Med. Genet.* 35:319, 1990.
3. Goldmuntz, E., et al. Microdeletions of chromosomal region 22q11 in patients with congenital conotruncal cardiac defects. *J. Med. Genet.* 30:807, 1993.
4. Jones, K. L. *Smith's Recognizable Patterns of Human Malformation* (5th Ed.). Philadelphia: Saunders, 1994.
5. McKusick, V. A. *Mendelian Inheritance in Man* (8th Ed.). Baltimore: Johns Hopkins University Press, 1988.
6. Merlob, P., et al. Arthropometric measurements of the newborn infant (27 to 41 gestational weeks). *Birth Defects* 20:1, 1984.
7. Norton, M. E. Biochemical and ultrasound screening for chromosomal abnormalities. *Semin. Perinatol.* 18:256, 1994.
8. Shephard, T. H. *Catalog of Teratogenic Agents* (5th Ed.). Baltimore: Johns Hopkins University Press, 1986.
9. Taybi, H., et al. *Radiology of Syndromes and Metabolic Disorders* (2d Ed.). Chicago: Year Book Medical, 1985.
10. Tizzano, E. F., et al. Cystic fibrosis: Beyond the gene to therapy. *J. Pediatr.* 120:337, 1992.

9. FLUID AND ELECTROLYTE MANAGEMENT

Charles F. Simmons, Jr.

Dramatic changes in body composition and skin, renal, and neuroendocrine function accompany the transition to extrauterine life. The skin regulates fluid and electrolyte balance in newborns. Developmental immaturity in extremely premature neonates contributes substantially to possible mortality and morbidity.

I. **Principles of water and electrolyte metabolism.** Fluid and electrolyte therapy must be individualized, and an infant's requirements can be determined only by careful assessment of clinical and laboratory status.

    A. **Compartmentation of total-body water (TBW).** TBW is divided into **intracellular fluid (ICF)** and **extracellular fluid (ECF)** (Fig. 9-1). ECF is composed of intravascular and interstitial fluid, and is readily assessed when evaluating fluid and electrolyte therapy. The goals of therapy are (1) to maintain an appropriate ECF volume, which is determined primarily by total-body sodium, and (2) to maintain appropriate ICF and ECF osmolality, determined by the amount of TBW relative to solutes.

    B. **Perinatal changes in TBW.** In term infants, a physiologic diuresis of TBW and ECF occurs within 3 to 5 days after birth. This results in a weight loss of 5 to 10% [7,9,10]. The diuresis may be desirable in preterm infants because excessive parenteral fluid and sodium administration may be detrimental in these neonates [2,5,18]. At lower gestational ages, ECF accounts for a greater proportion of birth weight (see Fig. 9-1). Therefore, very low-

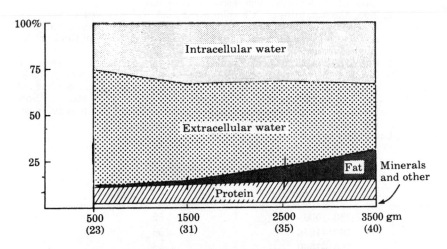

Fig. 9-1. Body composition in relation to fetal weight and gestational age. (From H. S. Dweck. *Clin. Perinatol.* 2:183, 1975; data from E. M. Widdowson. Growth and Composition of the Fetus and Newborn. In N. S. Assali [Ed.], *Biology of Gestation*, Vol. 2. New York: Academic Press, 1968.)

birth-weight (VLBW) infants must lose a greater percentage of birth weight (5 to 15%) during the first week of life to maintain ECF proportions equivalent to those of term infants.

C. Renal and hormonal maturation. Renal function matures with increasing gestational age. Consequently, urinary water and electrolyte losses can exhibit great variability. Premature infants often manifest immature sodium and water homeostasis. Contributing factors include (1) decreased glomerular filtration, (2) reduced maximal proximal and distal tubule sodium reabsorption, (3) diminished renal capacity for concentration and dilution of urine, and (4) decreased bicarbonate reabsorption and potassium and hydrogen ion secretion [11,12]. Profoundly immature renal function often leads to water and electrolyte imbalance in extremely premature newborns (see Chaps. 6, 31).

D. Extrarenal sources of water and electrolyte loss. Insensible water loss in VLBW infants can exceed 150 ml/kg per day because of radiant warmers, phototherapy, loss of skin integrity, or extreme prematurity [3,4,8,13,15,19,20] (Table 9-1). Losses of other fluids such as cerebrospinal fluid (ventriculostomy drainage or repeated lumbar punctures), stool (diarrhea or ostomy drainage), and nasogastric tube or thoracostomy tube drainage should be quantitated, characterized, and replaced if significant.

II. Assessment of fluid and electrolyte status

A. History. Newborn fluid and electrolyte status partially reflects maternal hydration and drug administration. Excessive use of oxytocin, diuretics, and hypotonic intravenous (IV) fluid can lead to maternal and fetal hyponatremia.

B. Physical examination

1. Body weight. Acute changes in TBW result in weight changes. Therefore, body weight should be measured at least daily. The distribution of water in body compartments reflects the distribution of total-body solutes and vascular permeability characteristics. Thus, acute changes in body weight may not reflect changes in intravascular volume. For example, neuromuscular paralysis or peritonitis can lead to increased body weight and interstitial edema but decreased intravascular volume.

2. Skin. Abnormalities of ECF volume can lead to altered skin turgor, alterations of anterior fontanelle tension, variations in mucous membranes, and edema. These findings are not sensitive indicators of fluid or electrolyte balance.

3. Cardiovascular. Tachycardia can result from ECF excess (e.g., congestive heart failure) or hypovolemia. **Delayed capillary refill time** (reperfusion after pressure-induced skin blanching) can signify reduced cardiac output, and **hepatomegaly** can suggest an increased ECF volume. **Blood pressure changes** occur late in the sequence of responses to reduced cardiac output.

C. Laboratory evaluation

Table 9-1. Insensible water loss (IWL)*

Birth weight (gm)	IWL (ml/kg/d)
750–1000	82
1001–1250	56
1251–1500	46
>1501	26

*Values represent mean IWL for infants in incubators during the first week of life. IWL is *increased* by phototherapy (up to 40 percent), radiant warmers (up to 50 percent), and fever. IWL is *decreased* by the use of humidified gas with respirators and heat shields in incubators [3,4,8,15].

1. **Serum electrolytes and plasma osmolarity** reflect the composition and tonicity of ECF.
2. **Urine electrolytes and specific gravity** can reflect renal capacity to concentrate or dilute urine and reabsorb or excrete sodium. If the patient's hydration and ECF tonicity are normal, urine electrolytes do not correlate well with replacement needs. **Diuretic therapy** results in wide diurnal variation in urine electrolyte composition and increased sodium, potassium, calcium, and chloride excretion.
3. **Urine output** falls with ECF depletion (dehydration), often to less than 1 ml/kg per hour. In neonates with immature renal function, urine output may not decrease despite ECF volume depletion.
4. **Fractional excretion of sodium (FE-Na)** reflects the balance between glomerular filtration and tubular reabsorption of sodium. FE-Na is determined after measuring sodium (Na) and creatinine (Cr) concentrations in both urine and plasma:

$$\% \text{ filtered Na excreted} = \frac{\text{excreted Na}}{\text{filtered Na}} \times 100$$

$$= \frac{\text{urine Na} \times \text{plasma Cr}}{\text{urine Cr} \times \text{plasma Na}} \times 100$$

Newborns with FE-Na values less than 1 percent manifest their oliguria due to prerenal factors reducing renal blood flow, such as hypovolemia or poor cardiac output. Values higher than 2.5% occur with acute renal failure and in infants receiving diuretics. FE-Na is frequently higher than 2.5% in infants less than 32 weeks' gestation, irrespective of fluid and electrolyte status: FE-Na is less helpful in the evaluation of oliguria in these infants. Diuretic use in any infant will make the measurement meaningless.

5. **Blood urea nitrogen (BUN) and serum creatinine** values provide indirect information about ECF volume and glomerular filtration. Values in the early postnatal period reflect placental clearance.
6. **Arterial pH, carbon dioxide tension (PCO$_2$), and sodium bicarbonate** determinations can provide indirect evidence of intravascular volume depletion because poor tissue perfusion leads to high-anion-gap metabolic acidosis (lactic acidosis).

III. **Management of fluids and electrolytes.** The goal of early management is to allow initial loss of ECF over the first 5 to 6 days as reflected by weight loss, while maintaining normal tonicity and intravascular volume as reflected by blood pressure, heart rate, urine output, serum electrolyte levels, and pH. Subsequent fluid management should maintain water and electrolyte balance, including requirements for body growth.

A. **The term infant.** Body weight decreases by 3 to 5% over the first 5 to 6 days. Subsequently, fluids should be adjusted so that changes in body weight are consistent with caloric intake. Clinical status should be monitored for maldistribution of water (e.g., edema). Sodium supplementation is not usually required in the first 24 hours unless ECF expansion is necessary. Small-for-gestational-age term infants may require early sodium supplementation to maintain adequate ECF volume.

B. **The premature infant.** Body weight may be allowed to decrease 5 to 15% over the first 5 to 6 days. Table 9-2 summarizes initial fluid therapy. Fluids should then be adjusted to maintain stable weight until an anabolic state is achieved and growth occurs. Response to fluid and electrolyte therapy should be assessed frequently during the first 2 days of life. **Physical examination, urine output and specific gravity, and serum electrolyte determinations may initially be required as frequently as every 6 to 8 hours in in-**

Table 9-2. Initial fluid therapy[a]

Birth weight (kg)	Dextrose (gm/100 ml)	Fluid rate (ml/kg/d)		
		<24 hr	24–48 hr	>48 hr
<1.0	5–10	100–150[b]	120–150	140–190
1.0–1.5	10	80–100	100–120	120–160
>1.5	10	60–80	80–120	120–160

[a]Infants in humidified incubators. Infants under radiant warmers usually require higher initial fluid rates.
[b]Very low-birth-weight infants frequently require even higher initial rates of fluid administration, and frequent reassessment of serum electrolytes, urine output, and body weight.

fants who weigh less than 1000 gm. Losses of water through skin and urine may exceed 200 ml/kg per day, which can represent up to **one-third of TBW per day** [15]. IV sodium supplementation is not required for the first 24 hours unless ECF volume loss exceeds 5% of body weight per day [13] (see Chap. 6).

IV. **Approach to disorders of sodium and water balance.** Abnormalities can be grouped into disorders of **tonicity** or **ECF volume.** The conceptual approach to disorders of tonicity (e.g., hyponatremia) depends on whether the newborn exhibits a state of normal ECF (euvolemia), ECF depletion (dehydration), or ECF excess (edema).
   A. **Isonatremic disorders**
      1. **Dehydration**
         a. **Predisposing factors** frequently involve equivalent losses of sodium and water (via thoracostomy, nasogastric, or ventriculostomy drainage) or third-space losses that accompany peritonitis, gastroschisis, or omphalocele. Renal sodium and water losses in the VLBW infant can lead to hypovolemia despite normal body tonicity.
         b. **Diagnosis.** Dehydration is usually manifested by weight loss, decreased urine output, and increased urine specific gravity. However, infants fewer than 32 weeks' gestation may not demonstrate oliguria in response to hypovolemia. Poor skin turgor, tachycardia, hypotension, metabolic acidosis, and increasing BUN may coexist. A low FE-Na (<1 percent) is consistent with dehydration, although this is usually only seen in infants beyond 32 weeks' gestational age (see **II.C.4**).
         c. **Therapy.** Sodium and water administration should first correct deficits and then be adjusted to equal maintenance needs plus ongoing losses. Therapy of acute isonatremic dehydration may require IV infusion of 10 ml of 5% albumin or normal saline solution per kilogram if acute weight loss exceeds 10% of body weight with signs of poor cardiac output.
      2. **Edema**
         a. **Predisposing factors** include administration of isotonic crystalloid or colloid, congestive heart failure, sepsis, and neuromuscular paralysis.
         b. **Diagnosis.** Edema may accumulate periorbitally and in the extremities. Increased weight and hepatomegaly often accompany edema.
         c. **Therapy.** Sodium restriction is necessary (to decrease total-body sodium), as well as water restriction, depending on subsequent electrolyte response.
   B. **Hyponatremic disorders** (Table 9-3). Consider **factitious hyponatremia** due to hyperlipidemia or **hyperosmolar hyponatremia** due to osmotic agents. True hypoosmolar hyponatremia can then be evaluated.
      1. **Hyponatremia due to ECF volume depletion**

Table 9-3. Hyponatremic disorders

Clinical diagnosis	Etiology	Therapy
Factitious hyponatremia	Hyperlipidemia	
Hypertonic hyponatremia	Mannitol	
	Hyperglycemia	
ECF volume normal	SIADH	Restrict water intake
	Pain	
	Opiates	
	Excess intravenous fluids	
ECF volume deficit	Diuretics	Increase sodium intake
	Congenital adrenal	
	hyperplasia	
	Severe glomerulotubular	
	imbalance (immaturity)	
	Renal tubular acidosis	
	Gastrointestinal losses	
	Necrotizing enterocolitis	
	(third-space loss)	
ECF volume excess	Congestive heart failure	Restrict water intake
	Neuromuscular blockade	
	(e.g., pancuronium)	
	Sepsis	

a. **Predisposing factors** include diuretics, osmotic diuresis (glycosuria), VLBW with renal water and sodium wasting, adrenal or renal tubular salt-losing disorders, gastrointestinal losses (vomiting, diarrhea), and third-space losses of ECF (skin sloughing, early necrotizing enterocolitis).
b. **Diagnosis.** Decreased weight, poor skin turgor, tachycardia, rising BUN, and metabolic acidosis are frequently observed. If renal function is mature, the newborn may develop decreased urine output, increased specific gravity, and a low FE-Na.
c. **Therapy.** If possible, reduce ongoing sodium loss. Administer sodium and water to replace deficits and then adjust to balance maintenance needs plus ongoing losses.
2. **Hyponatremia with normal ECF volume**
   a. **Predisposing factors** include excess IV administration of fluids and the syndrome of inappropriate antidiuretic hormone secretion (SIADH). Factors that cause SIADH include pain, opiate administration, intraventricular hemorrhage (IVH), asphyxia, pneumothorax, and positive-pressure ventilation.
   b. **Diagnosis of SIADH.** Weight gain usually develops without edema. The infant who has received excess IV fluids without SIADH should demonstrate appropriately low urine specific gravity and high urine output. SIADH leads to **decreased urine output** and **increased urine osmolarity.** Urinary sodium excretion in infants with SIADH varies widely and reflects sodium intake. The diagnosis of SIADH presumes no volume-related stimulus to antidiuretic hormone (ADH) release, such as reduced cardiac output or abnormal renal, adrenal, or thyroid function.
   c. **Therapy.** Water restriction is therapeutic unless (1) serum sodium concentration is less than approximately 120 mEq/L or (2) neurologic signs such as obtundation or seizure activity develop. In these instances, furosemide 1 mg/kg IV q6h can be initiated while replacing

urinary sodium excretion with hypertonic NaCl (3%). This strategy leads to loss of free water with no net change in total-body sodium. Fluid restriction alone can be utilized once serum sodium concentration exceeds 120 mEq/L and neurologic signs abate.

3. **Hyponatremia due to ECF volume excess**
   a. **Predisposing factors** include sepsis with decreased cardiac output, late necrotizing enterocolitis, congestive heart failure, abnormal lymphatic drainage, and neuromuscular paralysis.
   b. **Diagnosis.** Weight increase with edema is observed. Decreasing urine output, increasing urine specific gravity and BUN concentration, and a low FE-Na are often present in infants with mature renal function.
   c. **Therapy** should be directed toward the underlying disorders. Water restriction can help alleviate hypotonicity. Sodium restriction may be required, and efforts to improve cardiac output may be beneficial.

C. **Hypernatremic disorders**
   1. **Hypernatremia with normal or deficient ECF volume**
      a. **Predisposing factors** include increased renal and insensible water loss in VLBW infants. Skin sloughing can accelerate water loss. ADH deficiency secondary to IVH can occasionally exacerbate renal water loss.
      b. **Diagnosis.** Weight loss, tachycardia and hypotension, and metabolic acidosis can develop. Decreasing urine output and increasing urine specific gravity may occur. Urine may be dilute if the newborn exhibits central or nephrogenic diabetes insipidus. **Hypernatremia in the VLBW infant in the first 24 hours of life is almost always due to free-water deficits.**
      c. **Therapy.** The rate of free-water administration should be increased. If signs of ECF depletion or excess develop, sodium intake should be adjusted. **The development of hypernatremia does not necessarily imply excess total-body sodium.**
   2. **Hypernatremia with ECF volume excess**
      a. **Predisposing factors** include excessive administration of isotonic or hypertonic fluids. Hypernatremia and edema can be exaggerated in infants with sodium retention, because of reduced cardiac output.
      b. **Diagnosis.** Weight increase associated with edema is observed. The infant may exhibit normal heart rate, blood pressure, and urine output and specific gravity, but an elevated FE-Na.
      c. **Therapy.** Restrict sodium administration by reducing fluid sodium concentration, restricting the rate of fluid administration, or both.

V. **Oliguria** exists if urine flow is less than 1 ml/kg per hour. Although delayed micturition in a healthy infant is not of concern until 24 hours after birth, urine output in a critically ill infant should be assessed by 8 to 12 hours of life, using urethral catheterization if indicated. Diminished urine output may reflect abnormal prerenal, renal parenchymal, or postrenal factors (Table 9-4). The most common causes of neonatal acute renal failure are asphyxia, sepsis, and severe respiratory illness. It is important to exclude other potentially treatable etiologies in oliguric infants. (See Chap. 31.)

A. **History and physical examination.** The maternal and infant history should be assessed for maternal diabetes (renal vein thrombosis), birth asphyxia (acute tubular necrosis), and oligohydramnios (Potter's syndrome). Force of the infant's urinary stream (posterior urethral valves), rate and nature of fluid administration and urine output, and the use of nephrotoxic drugs (aminoglycosides, indomethacin, furosemide) should be evaluated. **Physical examination** should determine blood pressure and ECF volume status; evidence of cardiac disease, abdominal masses, or ascites; and the presence of any congenital anomalies associated with renal abnormalities (e.g., Potter's syndrome, epispadias).

B. **Diagnosis**

Table 9-4. Etiologies of Oliguria

Prerenal	Renal parenchymal	Postrenal
Decreased inotropy	Acute tubular necrosis Ischemia (hypoxia, hypovolemia)	Posterior urethral valves
Decreased preload	Disseminated intravascular coagulation Renal artery or vein thrombosis	Neuropathic bladder
Increased peripheral resistance	Nephrotoxin Congenital malformation Polycystic disease Agenesis Dysplasia	Prune-belly syndrome Uric acid nephropathy

1. **Initial laboratory examination** should include urinalysis and BUN, creatinine, and FE-Na determinations. These values often aid in diagnosis and provide baseline values for further management.

2. **Fluid challenge,** consisting of a total of 20 ml of normal saline or 5% albumin per kilogram, is administered as two infusions at 10 ml/kg per hour if no suspicion of structural heart disease or heart failure exists. Decreased cardiac output not responsive to ECF expansion may require the institution of inotropic/chronotropic pressor agents. Dopamine at a dose of 1 to 5 μg/kg per minute may increase renal blood flow and a dose of 2 to 15 μg/kg per minute may increase total cardiac output. These effects may augment glomerular filtration and urine output. (See Chap. 17.)

3. **If no response to fluid challenge occurs,** diuresis may be induced with **furosemide** 2 mg/kg IV. Although rarely required, **mannitol** 0.5g/kg IV given **slowly** over 1 to 2 hours may induce osmotic diuresis without a significant increase in serum osmolality.

4. Patients who are unresponsive to increased cardiac output and diuresis should be evaluated with **abdominal ultrasound** to define renal, urethral, and bladder anatomy. IV pyelography, renal scanning, angiography, or cystourethrography may be required (see Chap. 31).

C. **Management.** Oliguria due to prerenal factors should respond to increased cardiac output. Postrenal obstruction requires urologic consultation, with possible urinary diversion and surgical correction. If parenchymal acute renal failure is suspected, management minimizes excessive ECF expansion and electrolyte abnormalities [1,16]. Any reversible causes of declining glomerular filtration rate (GFR), such as use of nephrotoxic drugs, should be eliminated if possible.

1. **Monitoring** should include daily weight measurements, input and output assessments, and BUN, creatinine, and serum electrolyte determinations.

2. **Fluid restriction.** Insensible fluid loss plus urine output should be replaced. Potassium supplementation should be withheld unless hypokalemia develops. Sodium should be administered to replace urinary losses unless edema develops.

3. **Drug dosage** and frequency should be adjusted for drugs eliminated by renal excretion. Interpretation of serum drug concentrations can guide the clinician to adjust dosing intervals.

4. **Peritoneal or hemodialysis** may be indicated in patients whose GFR progressively declines with complications related to ECF volume or electrolyte abnormalities (see Chap. 31).

VI. **Metabolic acid–base disorders**

A. Normal acid–base physiology. Metabolic acidosis results from excessive loss of buffer or from an increase of volatile or nonvolatile acid in the extracellular space. Normal sources of acid production include the metabolism of amino acids containing sulfur and phosphate, as well as hydrogen ion released from bone mineralization. Intravascular buffers include bicarbonate, phosphate, and intracellular hemoglobin. Maintenance of normal pH depends on excretion of volatile acid (e.g., carbonic acid) from the lungs, skeletal exchange of cations for hydrogen, and renal regeneration and reclamation of bicarbonate. The contribution of the kidneys to maintenance of acid–base balance includes resorption of the filtered load of bicarbonate, secretion of hydrogen ions as titratable acidity (e.g., $H_2PO_4^-$), and excretion of ammonium ions.

B. Metabolic acidosis (see Chap. 29, Inborn Errors of Metabolism)

1. **Anion gap.** Metabolic acidosis can result from accumulation of acid or loss of buffering equivalents. Determination of the anion gap will assist in distinguishing which process is causative. Sodium, chloride, and bicarbonate are the primary ions of the extracellular space and exist in approximately electroneutral balance. The difference between the sodium concentration and the sum of the chloride and bicarbonate concentrations, commonly known as the **anion gap,** reflects the unaccounted-for anion composition of the ECF. Acidosis caused by accumulation of organic acids results in an increased anion gap, whereas acidosis due to loss of buffer does not increase the anion gap. Normal values for the neonatal anion gap are 5 to 15 mEq/L and vary directly with serum albumin concentration.

2. **Metabolic acidosis associated with an increased anion gap (>15 mEq/L).** Disorders (Table 9-5) include renal failure, inborn errors of metabolism, lactic acidosis, late metabolic acidosis, and toxin exposure. Lactic acidosis results from diminished tissue perfusion and resultant anaerobic metabolism in infants with asphyxia or severe cardiorespiratory disease. Late metabolic acidosis typically occurs during the second or third week of life in premature infants who ingest formula containing high concentrations of casein. An increased acid load is produced by the metabolism of sulfur-containing amino acids in casein and by increased hydrogen ion release due to the rapid mineralization of bone. Subsequently, inadequate hydrogen ion excretion by the premature kidney results in acidosis.

3. **Metabolic acidosis associated with a normal anion gap (<15 mEq/L)** results from loss of buffer through the renal or gastrointestinal systems (see Table 9-5). Premature infants of less than 32 weeks' gestation frequently manifest a proximal or distal renal tubular acidosis (RTA). Distal RTA is suggested if urine pH is persistently higher than 7.0 in an in-

Table 9-5. Metabolic acidosis

Increased anion gap (>15 mEq/L)	Normal anion gap (<15 mEq/L)
Acute renal failure	Renal bicarbonate loss
Inborn errors of metabolism	Renal tubular acidosis
Lactic acidosis	Acetazolamide
Late metabolic acidosis	Renal dysplasia
Toxins (e.g., benzyl alcohol)	Gastrointestinal bicarbonate loss
	Diarrhea
	Cholestyramine
	Small-bowel drainage
	Dilutional acidosis
	Hyperalimentation acidosis

fant with metabolic acidosis. A urinary pH less than 5.0 documents normal distal-tubule hydrogen ion secretion but does not establish the capacity of the proximal tubule to reabsorb a filtered load of bicarbonate. IV infusion of sodium bicarbonate in infants with proximal RTA will result in a urinary pH higher than 7.0 prior to attaining a normal serum bicarbonate concentration (22 to 24 mEq/L).

4. **Therapy.** Whenever possible, therapy should be directed at the underlying cause. **Lactic acidosis** due to low cardiac output or to decreased peripheral oxygen delivery should be treated with specific measures. The use of a low-casein formula may alleviate late metabolic acidosis. The treatment of normal-anion-gap metabolic acidosis should focus on decreasing the rate of bicarbonate loss (e.g., decreased small-bowel drainage) or the provision of buffer equivalents. IV sodium bicarbonate or sodium acetate (which is compatible with calcium salts) is most commonly used for this purpose if the arterial pH is less than 7.25. The bicarbonate deficit may be estimated from the following formula:

$$\text{Deficit} = 0.4 \times \text{body weight} \times (\text{desired bicarbonate} - \text{actual bicarbonate})$$

The premature infant's acid–base status can change rapidly, and frequent monitoring is warranted. The infant's ability to tolerate an increased sodium load and to metabolize acetate is an important variable that influences acid–base status during treatment.

C. **Metabolic alkalosis.** The etiology of metabolic alkalosis can often be clarified by determining urinary chloride concentration. Alkalosis accompanied by ECF depletion is associated with decreased urinary chloride, whereas states of mineralocorticoid excess are usually associated with increased urinary chloride (Table 9-6). Therapy is for the underlying disorder.

VII. **Disorders of potassium balance.** Potassium is the fundamental intracellular cation. Serum potassium concentrations (3.5 to 5.5 mEq/L) do not necessarily reflect total-body potassium because the distribution of extracellular and intracellular potassium also depends on the pH of body compartments. **An increase of 0.1 pH unit in serum results in approximately a 0.6 mEq/L fall in serum potassium concentration due to an intracellular shift of potassium ions.** Total-body potassium is regulated by balancing potassium intake (normally 1 to 2 mEq/kg per day) and potassium excretion through urine and the gastrointestinal tract.

A. **Hypokalemia** can lead to arrhythmias, ileus, renal concentrating defects, and obtundation in the newborn.

1. **Predisposing factors** include nasogastric or ileostomy drainage, chronic diuretic use, and renal tubular defects.

2. **Diagnosis** is made from analysis of serum and urine electrolytes, pH, and an ECG to detect possible conduction defects (prolonged QT interval and U waves).

Table 9-6. Metabolic alkalosis

Low urinary chloride (<10 mEq/L)	High urinary chloride (>20 mEq/L)
Diuretic therapy (late)	Bartter's syndrome with mineralocorticoid excess
Correction of chronic respiratory acidosis	Alkali administration
Nasogastric suction	Massive blood product transfusion
Vomiting	Diuretic therapy (early)
Secretory diarrhea	Hypokalemia

3. **Therapy** should reduce renal or gastrointestinal losses of potassium. Intake of potassium salts should be gradually increased as needed.
B. **Hyperkalemia.** The normal serum potassium level in a nonhemolyzed blood specimen at normal pH is 3.5 to 5.5 mEq/L; hyperkalemia is a serum potassium level higher than 6 mEq/L.
   1. **Predisposing factors.** Hyperkalemia can occur unexpectedly in any patient but should be **anticipated** and **screened** for in the following scenarios:
      a. Increased potassium release secondary to tissue destruction, trauma, cephalhematoma, hypothermia, bleeding, intravascular or extravascular hemolysis, asphyxia/ischemia, and IVH
      b. Decreased potassium clearance as seen with renal failure, oliguria, hyponatremia, and congenital adrenal hyperplasia syndrome
      c. Miscellaneous associations including dehydration, birth weight lower than 1500 gm, blood transfusion, *inadvertent administration of excess potassium chloride,* bronchopulmonary dysplasia (BPD) with potassium chloride supplementation, and exchange transfusion
      d. Up to 50% of VLBW infants born before 25 weeks' gestation manifest serum potassium levels higher than 6 mEq/L in the first 48 hours of life [11,17]. **The most common cause of sudden unexpected hyperkalemia in the neonatal intensive care unit (NICU) is medication error.**
   2. **Diagnosis** is based on determination of nonhemolyzed serum and urine electrolytes, as well as serum pH and calcium concentrations. The hyperkalemic infant may be asymptomatic or may present with a spectrum of signs including bradyarrhythmias or tachyarrhythmias, cardiovascular instability, or collapse. The ECG findings appear to be related to the level of serum potassium and may include peaking of T waves (increased rate of repolarization), flattening of P waves and increasing PR interval (suppression of arterial conductivity), QRS widening and slurring (conduction delay in ventricular conduction tissue as well as in the myocardium itself), and finally supraventricular/ventricular tachycardia, bradycardia, or ventricular fibrillation. The ECG findings may be the first indication of hyperkalemia or may be observed after diagnosis (see Chap. 25). **Once the diagnosis of hyperkalemia has been made, remove all sources of exogenous potassium (change all IV solutions and analyze for potassium content, check all feedings for potassium content), rehydrate the patient if necessary, and treat arrhythmia-promoting factors.** The pharmacologic therapy of hyperkalemia in term and preterm neonates consists of three components:
      a. Goal 1: Stabilization of conducting tissues. This can be accomplished by sodium or calcium ion administration. **Calcium gluconate given carefully at 1 to 2 ml/kg IV** may be the most useful in the NICU. Treatment with hypertonic NaCl solution is not done routinely. However, if the patient is both hyperkalemic and hyponatremic, infusion of normal saline solution may be beneficial. Use of antiarrhythmic agents such as **lidocaine** and **bretylium** should be considered for refractory ventricular tachycardia. (See Chap. 25.)
      b. Goal 2: Dilution and intracellular shifting of potassium. Increased serum potassium in the setting of dehydration should respond to the usual fluid resuscitation measures. Alkalemia will promote intracellular potassium-for-hydrogen-ion exchange. **Sodium bicarbonate 1 to 2 mEq/kg IV** may be used for induction of metabolic alkalosis, although the resultant pH changes may not be sufficient to markedly shift potassium ions. Sodium treatment as described in **I** may be effective. **Rapid administration of sodium bicarbonate in infants, especially those born before 34 weeks' gestation and younger than 3 days, should be avoided.** Respiratory alkalosis may be produced in an intubated infant by hyperventilation, although the risk of hypocarbia di-

minishing cerebral perfusion may make this option more suited to emergency situations. Theoretically, every 0.1 pH unit increase leads to a decrease of 0.6 mEq/L in serum potassium.

Insulin enhances intracellular uptake of potassium by direct stimulation of the membrane-bound sodium-potassium ATPase. Insulin infusion with concomitant glucose administration to maintain normal blood glucose concentration is relatively safe as long as frequent monitoring of serum or blood glucose levels is maintained. **This therapy may begin with a bolus of insulin and glucose (0.05 unit of human regular insulin per kilogram with 2 ml of dextrose 10% in water [10% D/W]) per kilogram followed by continuous infusion of 10% D/W at 2 to 4 ml/kg per hour and human regular insulin (10 units/100 ml) at 1 ml/kg per hour.** The insulin may be made up in a 5% albumin solution to minimize nonspecific protein binding to IV tubing. Alternatively, the tubing may be flushed with the insulin diluted in 10% D/W. Adjustments in infusion rate of either glucose or insulin in response to hyperglycemia or hypoglycemia may be simplified if the two solutions are prepared individually (see Chap. 29).

Beta-2-adrenergic stimulation enhances potassium uptake, probably via stimulation of the sodium-potassium ATPase. The immaturity of the beta-receptor response in preterm infants may contribute to non-oliguric hyperkalemia in these patients. To date, beta stimulation is not primary therapy for hyperkalemia in the pediatric population. However, the presence of cardiac dysfunction and hypotension may indicate the use of dopamine or other adrenergic agents which could, through beta-2 stimulation, lower serum potassium.

c. Goal 3: Enhanced potassium excretion. Diuretic therapy (e.g., **furosemide 1 mg/kg IV**) may increase potassium excretion by increasing flow and sodium delivery to the distal tubules. In the absence of adequate urine output, and in the clinical setting of reversible renal disease (e.g., indomethacin-induced oliguria), **peritoneal dialysis** and **double volume exchange transfusion** are potentially lifesaving options. The former has been successfully performed in infants weighing less than 1000 gm and should not be excluded if the patient's clinical status and etiology of hyperkalemia suggest a reasonable chance for good long-term outcome. **With double volume exchange transfusion, fresh whole blood (<24 hours old) or deglycerolized red blood cells reconstituted with fresh-frozen plasma should be used.** Aged banked blood may have potassium levels as high as 10 to 12 mEq/L; aged, washed packed red blood cells will have low potassium levels (see Chap. 26).

Enhancement of potassium excretion using cation exchange resins such as sodium or calcium polystyrene sulfonate has been studied primarily in adults. The resins can be administered orally per gavage (PG) or rectally. A study involving uremic as well as control rats demonstrated that sodium polystyrene sulfonate (Kayexelate) administered by rectum with sorbitol was toxic to the colon, but rectal administration after suspension in distilled water produced only mild mucosal erythema in 10 percent of animals. Another possible complication of resins is bowel obstruction secondary to bezoar or plug formation.

The reported experience with resin use in neonates covers those born at 25 to 40 weeks' gestation. PG administration of sodium polystyrene sulfonate is **not recommended in preterm infants because they are prone to hypomotility and are at risk for necrotizing enterocolitis. The rectal administration of sodium polystyrene sulfonate (1 gm/kg at 0.5 gm/ml of normal saline solution) with a minimum retention time of 30 minutes should be effective in lowering serum potassium levels by approximately 1 mEq/L. The enema should be inserted 1 to 3 cm** using a thin Silastic feeding tube. There is published evidence on the effectiveness of this treatment in infants. With the elimination of sorbitol as a solubilizing reagent, sodium polystyrene sulfonate prepared in water or normal saline solution and delivered rectally should be a therapeutic agent with acceptable risk-benefit ratio.

The clinical condition, ECG, and actual serum potassium level all affect the choice of therapy for hyperkalemia. Figure 9-2 contains guidelines for treatment of hyperkalemia.

VIII. Common clinical situations

    A. VLBW infant. Increased free-water loss through skin and urine often leads to **hypernatremia** and the need for frequent serum electrolyte determina-

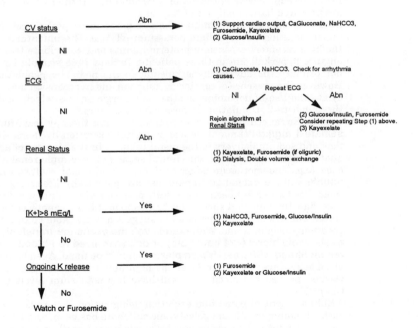

Remove all sources of exogenous potassium.

CV status — Abn → (1) Support cardiac output, CaGluconate, NaHCO3, Furosemide, Kayexelate
(2) Glucose/Insulin

Nl

ECG — Abn → (1) CaGluconate, NaHCO3. Check for arrhythmia causes.
    Repeat ECG
    Nl   Abn
Rejoin algorithm at Renal Status
(2) Glucose/Insulin, Furosemide Consider repeating Step (1) above.
(3) Kayexelate

Nl

Renal Status — Abn → (1) Kayexelate, Furosemide (if oliguric)
(2) Dialysis, Double volume exchange

Nl

[K+]>8 mEq/L — Yes → (1) NaHCO3, Furosemide, Glucose/Insulin
(2) Kayexelate

No

Ongoing K release — Yes → (1) Furosemide
(2) Kayexelate or Glucose/Insulin

No

Watch or Furosemide

In general, if [K+] acceptable for 6 hours cease therapy but continue monitoring.

Drug doses:
CaGluconate	1-2ml/kg IV
NaHCO3	1-2 mEq/kg IV
Furosemide	1 mg/kg IV
Glucose/Insulin	Bolus: D10W 2ml/kg

Bolus: D10W 2ml/kg
Humulin 0.05 U/kg
Infusion: D10W 2-4 ml/kg/hr
Humulin, 10 U/100 ml D10W or 5% Albumin, 1 ml/kg/hr
Kayexelate   1 gm/kg PR, used cautiously in the setting of an immature ischemic GI tract

Fig. 9-2. Treatment of hyperkalemia. (CV = cardiovascular; Nl = normal; Abn = abnormal). For a given algorithm outcome proceed by administering the entire set of treatments labeled (1). If unsuccessful in lowering [K+] or improving clinical condition, proceed to the next set of treatments, e.g., (2) then (3).

tions (q6–8h) and increased rates of parenteral fluid administration. In addition, **impaired glucose tolerance** can lead to hyperglycemia, requiring reduced rates of parenteral glucose infusion (see Chap. 29, Hypoglycemia and Hyperglycemia). This combination frequently leads to administration of reduced dextrose concentrations (below 5%) in parenteral solutions. Avoid the infusion of parenteral solutions containing less than 200 mOsmol/L (i.e., <3% D/W), to minimize local osmotic hemolysis and thus reduce renal potassium load.

Hyperkalemia in these infants often is due to a shift from intracellular to extracellular potassium, reduced peripheral glucose and potassium uptake in insulin-sensitive tissues, and reduced renal excretion of potassium [17]. The use of insulin infusions to treat hyperkalemia may be necessary but elevates the risk of iatrogenic hypoglycemia. The therapeutic use of cation exchange resin sodium polystyrene sulfonate can occasionally be beneficial in infants born before 32 weeks' gestation despite the obligate sodium load and frequent irritation of bowel mucosa by rectal administration. Sodium restriction can reduce the risk of bronchopulmonary dysplasia [6].

B. **Bronchopulmonary dysplasia** (see Chap. 24, Chronic Lung Disease). Chronic lung disease requiring **diuretic** therapy often leads to hypokalemic, hypochloremic metabolic alkalosis. Affected infants frequently have a chronic respiratory acidosis with partial metabolic compensation. Subsequently, vigorous diuresis can lead to total-body potassium depletion and contraction of ECF volume, establishing a superimposed metabolic alkalosis. If the alkalosis is severe, alkalemia (pH >7.45) can supervene and result in central hypoventilation. If possible, gradually reduce urinary sodium and potassium loss by reducing the diuretic dose, and/or increase potassium intake by administration of potassium chloride (up to 1 mEq/kg per day). Rarely, administration of ammonium chloride (0.5 mEq/kg) is required to treat the metabolic alkalosis. Long-term use of loop diuretics such as furosemide promotes excessive urinary calcium losses and nephrocalcinosis. Urinary calcium losses may be reduced through concomitant thiazide diuretic therapy (see Chap. 24).

References

1. Anand, S. K. Acute renal failure in the neonate. *Pediatr. Clin. North Am.* 29:791, 1982.
2. Bell, E. F., et al. Effect of fluid administration on the development of symptomatic patent ductus arteriosus and congestive heart failure in premature infants. *N. Engl. J. Med.* 302:598, 1980.
3. Bell, E. F., et al. The effects of thermal environment on heat balance and insensible water loss in low-birth-weight infants. *J. Pediatr.* 96:452, 1980.
4. Bell, E. F., et al. Heat balance in premature infants: Comparative effects of convectively heated incubator and radiant warmer, with or without plastic heat shield. *J. Pediatr.* 96:460, 1980.
5. Brown, E. R., et al. Bronchopulmonary dysplasia: Possible relationship to pulmonary edema. *J. Pediatr.* 92:982, 1978.
6. Costarino, A. T., Jr., et al. Sodium restriction versus daily maintenance replacement in very low birth weight premature neonates: A randomized, blind therapeutic trial. *J. Pediatr.* 120:99, 1992.
7. Cheek, D. B., et al. Further observations on the corrected bromide space of the neonate and investigation of water and electrolyte status in infants born of diabetic mothers. *Pediatrics* 28:861, 1961.
8. Fanaroff, A. A., et al. Insensible water loss in low birth weight infants. *Pediatrics* 50:236, 1972.
9. Fink, C. W., et al. The corrected bromide space (extracellar volume) in the newborn. *Pediatrics* 26:397, 1960.
10. Fisher, D. A., et al. Control of water balance in the newborn. *Am. J. Dis. Child.* 106:137, 1963.

11. Gruskay, J., et al. Nonoliguric hyperkalemia in the premature infant weighing less than 1000 grams. *J. Pediatr.* 113:381, 1988.
12. Leake, R. D. Perinatal nephrobiology: A developmental perspective. *Clin. Perinatol.* 4:321, 1977.
13. Lorenz, J. M., et al. Water balance in very low-birth-weight infants: Relationship to water and sodium intake and effect on outcome. *J. Pediatr.* 101:423, 1982.
14. Norman, M. E., et al. A prospective study of acute renal failure in the newborn infant. *Pediatrics* 63:475, 1979.
15. Okken, A., et al. Insensible water loss and metabolic rate in low birth weight newborn infants. *Pediatr. Res.* 13:1072, 1979.
16. Rahman, N., et al. Renal failure in the perinatal period. *Clin. Perinatol.* 8:241, 1981.
17. Shaffer, S. G., et al. Hyperkalemia in very low birth weight infants. *J. Pediatr.* 121:275, 1992.
18. Skorecki, K. L., et al. Body fluid homeostasis in man. A contemporary overview. *Am. J. Med.* 70:77, 1981.
19. Stevenson, J. G. Fluid administration in the association of patent ductus arteriosus complicating respiratory distress syndrome. *J. Pediatr.* 90:257, 1977.
20. Wu, P. Y. K., et al. Insensible water loss in pre-term infants: Changes with postnatal development and non-ionizing radiant energy. *Pediatrics* 54:704, 1974.

10. NUTRITION

Yao Sun, Ester L. Awnetwant, Sharon B. Collier, Linda M. Gallagher, Irene E. Olsen, and Jane E. Stewart

Newborns rapidly adapt from a relatively constant intrauterine supply of nutrients to intermittent feedings of milk. Normal infants double their birth weight by about 5 months. However, preterm infants or those with medical or surgical conditions commonly exhibit impaired sucking or absorption or may have increased nutritional needs.

I. Principles of nutritional support
A. Growth
1. **Growth patterns.** From about 24 to 37 to 39 weeks' gestation, fetal growth increases at a rate of approximately 15 gm/kg per day (or 1.5% fetal weight per day), with slower growth near term. Term neonates initially lose about 5 to 8% of their birth weight, largely in body water; if breastfed, these infants regain their birth weight by about 10 days and then grow rapidly.

   Preterm infants lose 10 to 20% of their birth weight with increased extracellular water losses due to immature skin and kidneys. Preterm infants take longer to regain their birth weight and may not establish consistent growth for several weeks.
2. **Fetal body composition** changes, with deposition of fat and glycogen dependent on gestational age and body weight. Term infants normally have sufficient glycogen and fat to meet energy demands during the relative starvation of the first days of life. In contrast, preterm infants rapidly deplete their limited endogenous nutrient stores, becoming hypoglycemic and catabolic unless appropriate nutrition is provided (see Fig. 9-1).
B. Nutritional goals for preterm infants are normal growth and development. For these infants, a widely accepted approach uses intrauterine growth and nutrient accretion-rate data as reference standards for assessing growth and nutrient requirements.
C. Nutritional assessment
1. **Growth parameters.** Under most circumstances, we recommend daily measurement of weight and weekly measurement of body length and head circumference for all hospitalized infants. **The growth chart is the single most useful tool for the assessment of nutritional status,** and data should be recorded on a grid for intrauterine growth or for growth of preterm infants (Fig. 10-1).
2. **Metabolic parameters.** All infants receiving parenteral nutrition (PN) and enterally fed babies considered at high nutritional risk are monitored according to the schedule indicated in Table 10-1.
3. **Indications of inappropriate or inadequate nutrition**
   a. Poor growth—inadequate energy intake
   b. Elevated BUN, metabolic acidosis—excessive protein intake
   c. Poor growth, low BUN and albumin—inadequate protein intake
   d. Elevated alkaline phosphatase level (with normal direct bilirubin) and low or normal levels of serum calcium and phosphorus—inadequate calcium and/or phosphorus intake or vitamin D deficiency
   e. Elevated triglyceride level—fat intolerance
   f. Elevated direct bilirubin, alkaline phosphatase, transaminase—cholestasis (often associated with PN and/or fasting)

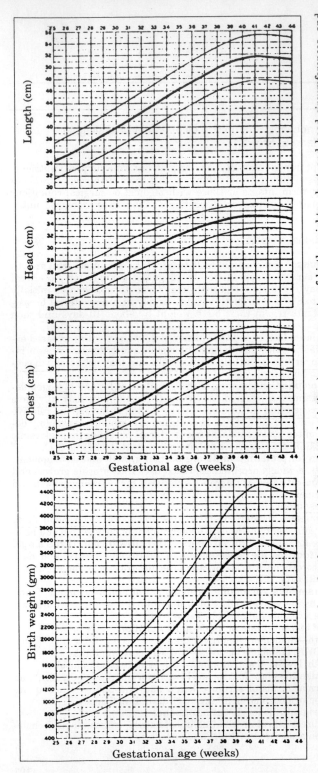

Fig. 10-1. Smoothed curve values for the mean (±2 standard deviations) measurements of birth weights, chest and head circumferences, and crown–heel length made on 300 infants of known gestational age. From R. H. Usher and F. H. McLean. Intrauterine growth of live-born Caucasian infants at sea level. Standards obtained from measurements in seven dimensions of infants born between 25 and 44 weeks of gestation. From R. Usher et al. *J. Pediatr.* 74:901, 1969.

Table 10-1. Schedule for metabolic monitoring of infants receiving
parenteral nutrition

Measurement	Frequency of measurement
BLOOD	
Glucose, electrolytes, including total carbon dioxide or pH	Daily for 2 to 3 days, then twice weekly
Blood urea nitrogen, creatinine, calcium, phosphorus, magnesium, total protein, albumin, transaminases, (ALT, AST), bilirubin, alkaline phosphatase, cholesterol, triglycerides, hematocrit	Weekly or every other week
URINE	
Specific gravity, reducing substances, total volume	Daily

g. Poor growth, decreased feeding, skin lesions, poor wound healing, hair
loss, decreased protein synthesis, immunosuppression—inadequate
zinc intake or absorption

II. Nutrient requirements. Estimated needs for **normal newborns** are summarized
as the *Recommended Dietary Allowances* (Table 10-2). Sources for nutrition recommendations for **preterm infants** include the ESPGAN-CON 1987 [2], AAP-
CON 1993 [1], and Tsang and colleagues [4] (Table 10-3). Because of limited
data, **the needs for preterm infants are recommendations only.** The recommendations that we use [4] were based on a consensus consideration of the recommended daily allowances for infants 0 to 6 months old, vitamin content of human milk, decreased vitamin stores in premature infants, assumed higher
nutritional needs, and available data on serum blood values reflecting vitamin
intake.

A. Energy. Average energy content of human milk is 67 kcal/dl, and healthy
term babies grow well with intakes of at least 80 to 90 kcal/kg per day. **Low-
birth-weight (LBW) infants have greater needs in order to sustain greater
growth velocity.** Energy intake (E_{intake}) may be estimated as follows (Table
10-4):

$$E_{intake} = E_{stored} + E_{expended} + E_{excreted}$$

1. **Energy stored** can be estimated from fetal fat- and protein-accretion data.
2. **Energy expenditure** may be increased by cold temperature, infection, surgery, or the increased respiratory and metabolic activity accompanying
chronic lung disease (CLD) or congestive heart failure (CHF). Small-for-
gestational-age (SGA) neonates also frequently expend more energy because of increased metabolic needs and higher energy costs for synthesis
of new tissue.
3. **Energy excreted** is increased in premature infants because of poor fat and
carbohydrate digestion and absorption and in infants with short-bowel
syndrome or malabsorption.
4. These estimates suggest that preterm infants in a thermoneutral environment need approximately **50 kcal/kg per day for maintenance of body
weight,** assuming adequate protein is provided. Growth requires an additional 5 to 6 kcal/gm of weight gain. **A growth rate of 15 gm/kg per day
theoretically requires 50 kcal/kg per day (maintenance) plus 75 to 90**

Table 10-2. Recommended daily dietary allowances for normal infants

Infant age (yr)	Weight (kg)	Keals	Protein (gm)	Vitamin A (µg RE)[a]	Vitamin D (µg)[b]	Vitamin E (mg α-TE)[c]	Vitamin K (µg)	Vitamin C (mg)	Thiamine (mg)	Riboflavin (mg)	Niacin (mg NE)[d]	Vitamin B6 (mg)	Folacin (µg)	Vitamin B12 (µg)	Calcium (mg)	Phosphorus (mg)	Magnesium (mg)	Iron (mg)	Zinc (mg)	Iodine (µg)	Selenium (µg)
				Fat-soluble vitamins				Water-soluble vitamins							Minerals and trace elements						
0.0–0.5	6	kg × 108	kg × 2.2	375	7.5	3	5	30	0.3	0.4	5	0.3	25	0.3	400	300	40	6	5	40	10

ESTIMATED SAFE AND ADEQUATE DAILY DIETARY INTAKES OF SELECTED VITAMINS AND MINERALS[e]

Infant age (yr)	Biotin (µg)	Pantothenic acid (mg)	Copper (mg)	Manganese (mg)	Fluoride (mg)	Chromium (µg)	Molybdenum (µg)
	Vitamins		Trace elements[f]				
0.0–0.5	10	2	0.4–0.6	0.3–0.6	0.1–0.5	10–40	15–30

[a]Retinol equivalents: 1 retinol equivalent = 1 µg retinol or 6 µg β-carotene.
[b]As cholecalciferol: 10 µg cholecalciferol = 400 IU of vitamin D.
[c]Alpha-tocopherol equivalents: 1 mg of D-alpha-tocopherol = 1 alpha-TE.
[d]Niacin equivalent: 1 NE is equal to 1 mg of niacin or 60 mg of dietary tryptophan.
[e]Because there is less information on which to base allowances, these figures are not given in the main table of RDA and are provided here in the form of ranges of recommended intakes.
[f]Since the toxic levels for many trace elements may be only several times usual intakes, the upper levels for the trace elements given in this table should not be habitually exceeded.
Source: Food and Nutrition Board, National Academy of Sciences–National Research Council, 1989.

kcal/kg per day (growth), for 125 to 140 kcal/kg per day. In practice, lesser energy intake (90 to 120 kcal/kg per day) may sustain intrauterine growth rates if energy expenditure is minimal and fat is well absorbed, or if PN is used. Sick or stressed infants may require higher intakes. A recommended upper limit of energy intake is 165 to 180 kcal/kg per day because energy above this value may not be adequately utilized for growth.

B. Water (see Chap. 9). The first step in nutritional support is to determine an infant's water requirements, which depend on gestational age, postnatal age, and environmental conditions. Term infants fed on demand typically ingest at least 150 ml/kg per day. During the first week of life, very low-birth-weight (VLBW) newborns may require fluid intakes of more than 200 ml/kg per day because of increased water loss (see **I.A.1**). Environmental factors (phototherapy, radiant warmers, low humidity) also increase insensible losses, raising water requirements. Conversely, restriction of water intake along with increased caloric density of feedings may be necessary for infants with respiratory distress syndrome, CLD, CHF, patent ductus arteriosus, or renal insufficiency.

C. Protein

1. **Digestion and absorption.** Up to the age of 3 months, peptic activity is low, with minimal protein digestion in the stomach. However, intestinal intraluminal digestion by proteases and peptidases is relatively efficient, even in preterm infants.

2. **Amount of protein.** The recommended allowance for protein in term infants is 2.2 gm/kg per day. We aim for 3.0 to 3.6 gm/kg per day for VLBW infants (3.6 to 3.8 gm/kg per day for extremely low-birth-weight [ELBW] infants). Ziegler advised protein intakes of 3.8 gm/kg per day for VLBW infants (4.0 gm/kg per day for ELBW infants) based on intrauterine accretion rates for protein [5].

   Because recommendations may not be met in full by commercial preterm formulas or supplemented human milk, a **protein supplement** (e.g., Promod) may be required to support adequate growth. On the other hand, higher intakes have been associated with potentially deleterious metabolic consequences such as azotemia. Careful monitoring is warranted if protein supplements are used.

   If energy intake is low, dietary protein cannot be utilized fully for tissue synthesis, causing decreased nitrogen retention and azotemia. When dietary energy available for growth is adequate, the same protein intake produces greater weight gain and nitrogen retention. We recommend that 7 to 12% of daily calories be derived from protein.

3. **Type of protein.** Precipitation of whole milk at pH 4.0 to 5.0 produces casein curds and a suspension of more easily digestible whey proteins.

   a. **Human milk,** considered the highest-quality protein source for human infants, is whey-predominant (whey-casein ratio of 80:20) and contains relatively little methionine, phenylalanine, and tyrosine. The relatively high cysteine content and very low methionine-cysteine ratio of human milk are adapted to newborns' limited capability to convert methionine to cysteine. Human milk is also an unusually rich source of taurine, an amino acid important in brain development and the conjugation of bile acids.

   b. Cow's milk is casein-predominant (whey-casein ratio of 18:82). Commercial cow's milk–based formulas are made more easily digestible by heat treatment. They may be supplemented with whey protein, cysteine, and taurine to simulate human milk more closely.

   c. Standard commercial formulas sustain satisfactory growth in healthy term infants. Because several amino acid pathways are incompletely developed in preterm infants, elevated plasma levels of methionine, phenylalanine, and tyrosine, hyperammonemia, and acidosis can develop when infants are fed casein-predominant milk. Cysteine, taurine, and glycine may be essential for preterm infants.

Table 10-3. Comparison of enteral intake recommendations of the **premature infant** per kilogram per day[a]

(Handwritten annotations: "Preterm formula" over the two formula columns; "Calculated for ≅ 150 ml/kg/day"; ✗ and ★ marks over the Mature Human milk and Preterm Human milk columns)

Nutrient	Unit	Tsang et al. [4]	AAP-CON [1][b]	ESPGAN-CON [2][b]	24 kcal/oz Similac Special Care w/Iron	24 kcal/oz Enfamil Premature w/Iron	Preterm Human milk[c]	Preterm Human milk plus (4 Packets Enfamil HMF/dl)	Mature Human milk	Mature Human milk plus (4 packets Enfamil HMF/dl)
Protein	gm/kg/day		3.5–4.0	2.7–3.7	3.3	3.6	2.4	3.4	1.54	2.6
Infants <1000 gm	gm/kg/day	3.6–3.8								
Infants >1000 gm	gm/kg/day	3.0–3.6								
Carbohydrate	gm/kg/day	—	10.8–15.6	8.4–16.8	12.7	13.3	11	14.9	10.6	14.5
Fat	gm/kg/day	—	5.4–7.2	4.3–8.4	6.5	6.1	5.3	5.3	5.7	5.8
Vitamin A	IU/kg/day	700–1500	e	360–600	828	1500	72	1488	328	1742
Vitamin D	IU/day	150–400[e,f]	500/day	800–1600/day[f]	183	324	12	324	3	315
Vitamin E	IU/kg/day	6–12	0.84	6	4.8	7.6	0.6	7.5	0.34	7.2
Vitamin K	µg/kg/day	8–10	e	4.8–18.0	15	9.6	3	9.5	0.3	6.8
Ascorbate (vitamin C)	mg/kg/day	18–24	23–45	8.4–48.0	45	24	6.7	23.9	6	23.2
Thiamine	µg/kg/day	180–240	e	24–300	305	240	13	238	31	256
Riboflavin	µg/kg/day	250–360	e	72–720	755	360	41	353	51	363
Pyridoxine	µg/kg/day	150–210	e	42–300	305	180	9	178	30	200
Niacin	mg/kg/day	3.6–4.8	e	1–6	6.1	4.8	0.3	4.8	0.2	4.7
Pantothenate	mg/kg/day	1.2–1.7	e	>0.36	2.3	1.44	0.3	13.7	0.27	1.33
Biotin	µg/kg/day	3.6–6.0	e	>1.8	45	4.8	0.8	4.8	0.6	4.6
Folate	µg/kg/day	25–50	50/day[f]	>72	45	42	5	42.5	7.4	45
Vitamin B$_{12}$	µg/kg/day	0.3	e	>0.18	0.68	0.3	0.03	0.3	0.07	0.34
Sodium	mEq/kg/day	2–3	2.5–3.5	1.2–2.8	2.3	2.0	1.9	2.3	1.1	1.6

Potassium	mEq/kg/day	2–3	2–3	2.2–4.6	4.0	3.2	1.9	2.5	2	2.6
Chloride	mEq/kg/day	2–3	—	1.6–3.0	2.8	2.9	2.5	3.2	1.8	2.3
Calcium	mg/kg/day	120–230	210	84–168	219	198	38	171	41	174
Phosphorus	mg/kg/day	60–140	140	60–108	110	100	22	88.5	21	87.5
Magnesium	mg/kg/day	7.9–15.0	7–10	7.2–14.4	15	8.2	5	6.4	5.1	6.5
Iron	mg/kg/day	2	2–3	1.8	2.3	2.2	0.14	0.14	0.04	0.04
Zinc	µg/kg/day	1000	600	660–1320	1830	1800	560	1618	180	1062
Copper	µg/kg/day	120–150	108	108–144	305	150	57	148	37	128
Selenium	µg/kg/day	1.3–3.0	—	—	2.2	2.2	—	—	2.2	2.2
Chromium	µg/kg/day	0.1–0.5	—	—	—	0.5	—	—	—	—
Manganese	µg/kg/day	7.5	6	2.5–6.6	15	7.6	0.5	7.6	0.9	8
Molybdenum	µg/kg/day	0.3	—	—	—	0.3	—	—	—	—
Iodine	µg/kg/day	30–60	6	12–54	7.5	30	27	27	16	16
Taurine	mg/kg/day	4.5–9.0	—	—	8.1	7.2	—	—	5.9	5.9
Carnitine	mg/kg/day	2.9	—	—	7.1	2.4	—	—	—	—
Inositol	mg/kg/day	32–81	—	—	6.8	20	—	—	22	22
Choline	mg/kg/day	14.4–28.0	—	—	12.2	14.4	—	—	13.2	13.2

HMF = human milk fortifier.

a Recommendations and calculated intakes of formulas and human milk are based on 150 ml/kg/d.

b Recommendations per 100 calories were converted to 120 cal/kg/d values for comparison.

c Adapted from [3].

d Aim for 400 IU/d.

e Specific recommendations for these nutrients are not available from the American Academy of Pediatrics; references are made to the needs of "full-term infants."

f Total recommended vitamin D is IU/day.

Table 10-4.   Estimated energy intake in growing preterm infants

	kcal/kg/d enteral feeds
Resting energy expenditure	47
Minimal activity[a]	4
Occasional cold stress[a]	10
Fecal loss of energy (10% to 16% of total intake)	15
Growth[b] (includes dietary-induced thermogenesis)	45
Total	121

[a]As an infant matures, energy expended in activities such as crying and nursing increases; energy expended due to cold stress decreases.
[b]Calculated assuming 3.0 to 4.5 kcal/gm weight gain at a rate of gain at 10 to 15 gm/kg/d.
Source: From M. Klaus and A. Fanaroff (Eds.). *Care of the High-Risk Neonate.* Philadelphia: Saunders, 1993.

D. Fat. Approximately one-half of the calories in human milk and most commercial formulas is derived from fat. However, fat intake of more than 60% of total calories may lead to ketosis.

1. **Linoleic acid and related unsaturated C18, C20, and C22 compounds** are essential fatty acids (EFAs); they must be provided in the diet. It is recommended that infant formulas supply at least 3% of total energy as linoleic acid (300 mg/100 kcal). Preterm infants are more vulnerable to EFA deficiency because of inefficient fat absorption, increased fat requirements for rapid brain growth and myelinization, and limited adipose reserves. VLBW infants should be provided with an EFA source by the first week of life.

2. **Fat digestion** is largely determined by intraluminal concentrations of lipases and bile acids. In newborns, digestion is initiated in the stomach by lingual lipase and continues in the duodenum by pancreatic lipases and a bile salt–activated lipase from human milk. Fat absorption is limited by the following:

   a. **Type of fatty acids.** Triglycerides containing palmitic acid esterified at the 2 position (the predominant form in human milk) are better absorbed than are other forms. In general, unsaturated fatty acids are better absorbed than saturated fatty acids. Medium-chain triglycerides (MCTs) are more easily digested and absorbed than long-chain triglycerides. MCTs are absorbed directly into the portal circulation and are not dependent on concentrations of lipases or bile salts. However, MCTs do not contain EFAs.

   b. **Bile salt deficiency** occurs with prematurity and cholestasis. Duodenal bile acid concentrations are decreased in preterm infants because of ineffective ileal resorption of bile acids and reduced synthesis. Feeding human milk can increase total bile acid concentration and bile acid pool size.

E. Carbohydrate. Nearly all the carbohydrate in human milk and standard infant formulas is lactose, whereas the carbohydrate in preterm formula is approximately half lactose and half glucose polymers. Generally, intestinal mucosal disaccharidase activity increases rapidly after 20 weeks' gestation and is very active by the twenty-eighth week. Lactase activity rises more slowly but increases in response to preterm birth. Glycosidases, which act on glucose polymers, are active in very preterm infants; hence, they tolerate these polymers well.

F. Minerals
  1. Sodium, potassium, and chloride
    a. Dietary recommendations for these electrolytes are 2 to 3 mEq/kg per day, but requirements may be considerably higher in ELBW infants because of significant renal losses.
    b. Human milk contains about 1.1 to 1.9 mEq/100 cal (mature and preterm milk, respectively) of sodium, which is often insufficient for the VLBW infant.
  2. Calcium. About 99% of body calcium is located in bone. Prolonged deficiency of dietary calcium or abnormal intestinal or renal losses eventually demineralize bone, causing osteopenia and rickets (see Chap. 29).

  The calcium present in human milk (40 mg/100 cal) is well absorbed by the healthy preterm infant, but these infants are very susceptible to calcium deficiency. Third-trimester calcium accretion (120 to 150 mg/kg per day) is greater than the amount of calcium a preterm infant can ingest from human milk, even with maximal absorption. Human milk fortifier (HMF) must be added to support bone mineralization. Both Premature Enfamil and Similac Special Care approximate the recommendation (see Table 10-3).
  3. Phosphorus (see Chap. 29). Inorganic phosphate is distributed mostly in bone (80%) and muscle (9%). Human milk contains approximately 21 mg/100 cal. The intrauterine accretion rate is about 75 to 85 mg/kg per day. The recommended phosphate intake is higher for preterm infants, and the addition of HMF to human milk is necessary; premature formulas are sufficient (see Tables 10-3, 10-5).
  4. The intrauterine accretion rate for **magnesium** is approximately 3 to 4 mg/kg per day. Human milk (roughly 5 mg/100 cal) and premature infant formulas (6.8 to 12.0 mg/100 cal) can provide sufficient magnesium for preterm infants.
  5. Iron stores, primarily accrued during the third trimester, are generally adequate for term infants until the age of 4 months. Breast-fed term infants need iron supplementation then. Term infants fed formula should receive iron-fortified formula. Because **preterm neonates have diminished stores, we provide them with iron once tolerance of full feeds is achieved** (e.g., 24 kcal/oz at 150 ml/kg per day) (Table 10-6). The purpose of early iron supplementation is to increase storage and reduce the risk of later deficiency with its sequelae. Infants who receive multiple transfusions can receive the same iron supplementation because transfusions should not decrease the need for dietary iron or impair its absorption. Iron supplementation will not prevent the physiologic anemia of prematurity (see Chap. 26).
G. Vitamins. Vitamins are essential metabolic cofactors that must be provided. The vitamin content of preterm human milk changes considerably over the course of lactation. For example, vitamins A, E, and B_{12} decrease during lactation, while thiamine and vitamin B_6 increase. This should be considered when estimating micronutrient intakes for preterm infants.
  1. Fat-soluble vitamins (e.g., A, D, E, and K) can be stored in tissue, and the potential for toxicity is well recognized.
    a. Vitamin A (retinol). The benefits of supplementing vitamin A to decrease the incidence of CLD in VLBW infants remain controversial, although low serum vitamin A levels have been observed in infants with CLD. Because VLBW infants have virtually no hepatic reserves of vitamin A, they are particularly susceptible to a deficiency. An intake of 1500 IU of vitamin A per kilogram per day is recommended for preterm infants.
    b. Vitamin D (calciferol) is synthesized in skin exposed to sunlight (ultraviolet light), but adequate levels generally also require a dietary source. Vitamin D at 400 IU per day can maintain adequate vitamin D status and prevent rickets.

Table 10-5. Oral dietary supplements

	Supplements		Preterm human milk (100 ml)[a] (approximate value)	
Nutrient	Enfamil Human Milk Fortifier (Mead Johnson) per 4 packets	Similac Natural Care (Ross)/dl	Plus 4 packets Enfamil HMF (Mead Johnson)/dl	Diluted 1:1 with Natural Care (Ross)/dl
Energy (kcal)	14	81	81	77
Protein (gm)	0.7	2.2	2.3	1.9
Fat (gm)	<0.1	4.4	3.5	4.0
Carbohydrate (gm)	2.7	8.6	10	7.9
MINERALS				
Calcium (mg)	90	171	115	100
Phosphorus (mg)	45	85	59	50
Magnesium (mg)	10	10	4.3	6.5
Sodium (mEq)	0.3	1.5	1.5	1.37
Potassium (mEq)	0.4	2.7	1.7	2.0
Chloride (mEq)	0.5	1.8	2.14	1.8
Zinc (mg)	0.71	1.2	1.08	0.7
Copper (μg)	62	203	100	120
Manganese (μg)	4.7	10	5.07	5.0
VITAMINS				
A (IU)	950	548	1000	298
D (IU)	210	122	213	65
E (IU)	4.6	3.2	4.9	1.8
K (IU)	4.4	10	6.4	5.9
Thiamine (μg)	151	203	160	105
Riboflavin (μg)	210	500	240	264
Niacin (μg)	3000	4032	3200	2118
Pantothenate (μg)	730	1532	960	868
Pyridoxine (μg)	114	203	120	104
Biotin (μg)	2.7	30	3.3	15.2
Vitamin B_{12} (μg)	0.18	0.45	0.20	0.25
Vitamin C (mg)	11.6	30	16	17
Folate (μg)	25	30	28	17

[a]Source: From R. C. Tsang et al. (Eds.). *Nutritional Needs of the Premature Infant: Scientific Basis and Practical Guidelines.* Baltimore: Williams & Wilkins, 1993.

Table 10-6. Iron Supplementation Guidelines in the Premature Infant*

| | Birth weight | | | | |
	<1000 gm	1000–1500 gm	1500–1800 gm	>1800 gm	Notes
Total dose	4 mg/kg/day	3–4 mg/kg/day	2–3 mg/kg/day	2 mg/kg/day	—
Formula Low iron	Supplement with elemental iron 4 mg/kg/day	Supplement with elemental iron 3–4 mg/kg/day	Supplement with elemental iron 2–3 mg/kg/day	Supplement with elemental iron 2 mg/kg/day	—
Iron fortified	Supplement with elemental iron 2 mg/kg/day	Additional elemental iron 1–2 mg/kg/day	Additional 1 mg/kg/day as needed	No additional supplementation	—
Human milk (HM) only	Elemental iron 4 mg/kg/day (see Notes)	Elemental iron 3–4 mg/kg/day (see Notes)	Elemental iron 2 mg/kg/day (see Notes)	Elemental iron 2 mg/kg/day	Infants under 1800 gm should be on 24 cal/oz HM (with human milk fortifier) before iron supplementation is begun
Combination (formula plus HM) Low iron	Supplement with elemental iron 4 mg/kg/day	Supplement with elemental iron 3–4 gm/kg/day	Supplement with elemental iron 2–3 mg/kg/day	Supplement with elemental iron 2 mg/kg/day	—
Iron fortified	Calculate for total iron dose of 4 mg/kg/day	Calculate for total dose of 3–4 mg/kg/day	Additional 1 mg/kg/day as needed	No additional supplementation	—

*Early initiation of iron supplementation in the premature infant reduces the risk of later iron deficiency and its sequelae. These guidelines are based on an intake of 150 ml/kg/day of 24 cal/oz. The clinician must consider iron content in formula when determining additional iron supplementation. Low iron and iron-fortified formulas provide 0.3 and 2.2 mg/kg/day, respectively.

c. Vitamin E (D-alpha-Tocopherol)

   (1) Iron catalyzes lipid oxidation through generation of free radicals. Adequate vitamin E is necessary to prevent peroxidation of erythrocyte membranes and resultant hemolytic anemia when preterm infants are given iron supplements. We advocate early iron supplementation (see **II.F.5**) because all current formulas provide a vitamin E–polyunsaturated fatty acid (mg/gm) ratio of less than 0.4, sufficient to prevent lipid peroxidation.

   (2) The recommendation for **preterm infants is 6 to 12 IU of vitamin E per kilogram per day.** Current formulas provide amounts of vitamin E at the lower range of the recommendations. Some premature infants may require additional supplementation if they are receiving elemental iron at levels of 4 mg/kg per day or higher.

   (3) At present, there is no proven benefit of vitamin E for the prevention and/or treatment of retinopathy of prematurity, CLD, intraventricular hemorrhage, or thrombocytosis.

d. Vitamin K is required for the hepatic synthesis of coagulation factors II, VII, IX, and X; **administration at birth of vitamin K (0.5 to 1.0 mg intramuscularly [IM]) can prevent hemorrhagic disease of the newborn.** Continuing requirements of vitamin K for preterm infants have not been determined (see Chaps. 5, 26).

2. Toxicity of **water-soluble vitamins** is unusual because of high renal clearance and low storage capacity.

   a. Vitamin B complex includes B_1 (thiamine), B_2 (riboflavin), B_3 (niacin), pantothenic acid, B_6 (pyridoxine), biotin, B_{12} cobalamin), and folic acid. Few data exist to assess whether vitamin B complex is adequately provided to LBW infants by available preterm formulations or supplemented human milk. We do not supplement folic acid above the level in current premature formulas (see Tables 10-3, 10-5). When human milk is exposed to ultraviolet light or heat, losses of riboflavin, pyridoxine, and folate may occur, although there is no evidence of subsequent vitamin deficiencies.

   b. No studies have evaluated the adequacy of vitamin C (ascorbic acid) in current formulations for preterm infants.

H. Trace elements are accumulated primarily during the third trimester, predisposing preterm infants to deficiency. Most current preterm formulas contain adequate amounts of trace elements (see Table 10-3), including zinc, copper, selenium, chromium, manganese, molybdenum, and iodine.

I. Nutrient and multivitamin supplementation. Many ill and preterm infants require additional amounts of specific dietary components.

1. Major nutrients. Several oral dietary supplements are listed in Table 10-7.

   a. MCT oil is a convenient and usually well-tolerated source of additional energy used to provide up to approximately 55% of calories from fat. The addition of about 0.25 ml of MCT oil per 30 ml of formula increases the energy content by about 2 kcal/30 ml.

   b. Polycose (glucose polymer) is hydrolyzed by maltase and theoretically is more efficiently absorbed than are lactose and sucrose. If supplemented at more than 4 kcal per 30 ml of formula, Polycose may increase intestinal motility or cause diarrhea.

   c. The use of fat or carbohydrate to increase energy content above 4 kcal/30 ml significantly decreases the protein-energy ratio, with possible harmful effects (see **II.C.2**). In general, we first increase caloric density by concentrating formula to 24 kcal/30 ml; if needed, MCT oil and/or Polycose is added in increments of 2 kcal/30 ml.

   d. We often add Promod (1 gm protein/tsp) to supplemented human milk to increase protein content closer to 4.0 gm/kg per day, especially in ELBW infants.

   e. Human milk fortifiers (HMFs). Preterm infants weighing up to 1800 gm fed human milk need HMFs to promote optimal growth and bone mineralization. Because of possible toxicity, HMFs should be used very

Table 10-7. Oral dietary supplements available for use in infants

Nutrient	Product	Source	Energy content
Fat	MCT oil (Mead Johnson)	Medium-chain triglycerides	8.3 kcal/gm 7.7 kcal/ml
	Microlipid (Sherwood)	Long-chain triglycerides	4.4 kcal/ml
	Corn oil	Long-chain triglycerides	9 kcal/gm 8.4 kcal/ml
Carbohydrate	Polycose (Ross)	Glucose polymers	4 kcal/gm 8 kcal/tsp (powder) 2 kcal/ml (liquid)
Protein	Promod (Ross)	Whey concentrate	4.2 kcal/gm 5.7 kcal/tsp

cautiously in infants weighing more than 1800 gm or infants consuming more than 160 ml/kg per day. Hypercalcemia has occurred in VLBW infants receiving human milk with HMF, possibly due to excessive intake of vitamin D and/or calcium.

HMF is also useful when feeding preterm infants specialized formulas not originally designed for preterm infants (e.g., Pregestimil, Nutramigen, and Portagen).

2. **Vitamins.** Not all preterm infant formulas provide nutrients in recommended ranges. Vitamin supplementation may be initiated when the infant reaches full volume feeds.

   a. **Human milk.** For infants up to 1800 gm, 4 packages of HMF per 100 ml should be added to human milk. If the milk is supplemented with HMF, no additional vitamin supplementation is required. If unsupplemented human milk is used in premature infants over 1800 gm, 1 ml per day of Pediatric MVI should be given.

   b. **Premature infant formulas.** If the infant is receiving at least 150 ml/kg per day in enteral feeds, no vitamin supplementation is required for Enfamil Premature 24. Similac Special Care 24 provides 180 IU vitamin D/kg per day: vitamin D may need to be supplemented to provide a total of 400 IU per day.

   c. **Specialized formulas.** These formulas are suboptimal for growth and nutrition of LBW infants and should not be used as long-term primary nutrition.

      (1) **Pregestimil:** increase 4 kcal per oz by concentration and 2 kcal per oz with HMF to total of 26 kcal per oz. Provides suboptimal vitamin D and high vitamin K intake.

      (2) **Nutramigen:** increase 4 kcal per oz by concentration and 2 kcal per oz with HMF to total of 26 kcal per oz. Provides suboptimal vitamin D and high vitamin K intake.

      (3) **Portagen:** increase 2 kcal per oz by concentration and 2 kcal per oz with HMF to total of 24 kcal per oz. Has high vitamin K, protein, magnesium, and manganese compared to preterm formulas. Provides suboptimal vitamin D intake.

      (4) Supplementing specialty formulas with HMF is contraindicated in infants with cow's milk protein allergy.

3. **Iron** (see Table 10-6 for supplementation guidelines). Iron-deficiency anemia is treated with 6 mg elemental iron/kg per day.

4. After 6 months of age, we recommend **fluoride** supplementation (0.25 mg per day) for breast-fed infants when the mother drinks water containing less than 0.3 ppm of fluoride (spring, well, or some community water) and for term infants fed formula diluted with nonfluoridated water.

III. Infant diets

A. Human milk is preferred for term infants; **when fortified, human milk is also the nutritionally optimal diet for preterm infants** (see Chap. 11).

1. Alternatives to breast-feeding or when appropriate, supplementation of human milk should be considered in the following instances:
   a. Parental choice
   b. Lack of milk available due to maternal illness or geographic separation from infant
   c. Presence of certain maternal diseases (e.g., active tuberculosis or human immunodeficiency virus [HIV] infection)
   d. Maternal medications for which breast-feeding is contraindicated
   e. Infants with special nutrient needs (Table 10-8)

2. Neonatal physiology and the **composition of human milk** are mutually adapted (see Table 10-3).
   a. Mature human milk contains an average energy density of 67 kcal/dl (20 kcal/30 ml); protein content of 0.9 to 1.3 gm/dl (7 to 10% of total calories), fat content of 3.8 to 4.5 gm/dl (about 50% calories), and carbohydrate content of 6.8 gm/dl (about 40% of calories).
   b. Several factors may alter the composition of human milk:
      (1) The mother's health and nutritional status
      (2) Protein, sodium, mineral, and immunoglobulin contents are highest in colostrum, intermediate in transitional milk, and lowest in mature milk.
      (3) "Hindmilk" (milk expressed at the end of a feeding) has a higher fat content and lower protein content than does "foremilk."
      (4) Milk of women delivering prematurely differs from milk of women delivering at term (see Table 10-3). Milk produced by mothers of premature infants contains increased amounts of protein, sodium, and zinc, but a decreased amount of vitamin A. The composition of preterm milk changes to approach that of term milk after a few weeks.
   c. **Human milk has many properties not reproduced by commercial formulas:**
      (1) Factors protective for infection—leukocytes, immunoglobulins (especially secretory IgA), lactoferrin, lysozymes, and complement; serious infections may be less frequent in breast-fed infants.
      (2) Growth and differentiation factors, e.g., epidermal growth factor, which may promote intestinal maturation
      (3) Enzymes, e.g., bile salt–stimulated lipase (see **II.D.2**).

3. Our protocol for collection and storage of human milk is outlined in Chap. 11. Freezing human milk destroys cells, and heat sterilization destroys most bioactive proteins.

4. **We routinely supplement human milk for preterm infants.**
   a. Fresh or frozen/thawed human milk has potentially important physiologic properties (see **III.A.2.c**).
   b. Preterm human milk (e.g., milk expressed by mothers of preterm infants) may contain more protein, sodium, chloride, and magnesium than term milk. However, composition varies.
   c. Protein deficiency, rather than insufficient energy retention per se, can cause poor growth in human milk–fed preterm infants. Mineral deficiency causes metabolic bone disease (see Chap. 29). Addition of a fortifier to human milk (see Tables 10-3, 10-5) raises energy, protein, mineral, and vitamin contents to levels more appropriate to the needs of preterm infants. Because addition of HMF may result in hypercalcemia, we monitor calcium and phosphorus weekly or biweekly. Use of a liquid supplement (Similac Natural Care) may not be ideal because it dilutes human milk properties.

5. When human milk is fed via continuous infusion, incomplete delivery of nutrients may occur because nonhomogenized fat clings to the tubing. In

Table 10-8. Indications for use of infant formulas

Clinical condition	Suggested formula	Rationale
Allergy to cow's milk protein or soy protein	Pregestimil, Nutramigen, Alimentum, Neocate	Protein hydrolysate due to protein sensitivity
Bronchopulmonary dysplasia	High-energy, nutrient-dense	Increased energy requirement, fluid restriction
Biliary atresia	Pregestimil	Impaired intraluminal digestion and absorption of long-chain fats
Chylothorax (persistent)	Portagen	Decrease lymphatic absorption of fats
Congestive heart failure	High-energy formula	Lower sodium content; increased energy requirement
Constipation	Standard formula, increase sugar (Polycose)	Mild laxative effect
Cystic fibrosis	Pregestimil or standard formula with pancreatic enzyme supplementation	Impaired intraluminal digestion and absorption of long-chain fats
Diarrhea Chronic nonspecific	Standard formula	Appropriate distribution of calories
	Lactofree	If malabsorbing lactose
Intractable	Pregestimil	Impaired digestion of intact protein, long-chain fats, and disaccharides
Galactosemia	Lactofree	Lactose free
Gastroesophageal reflux	Standard formula	Thicken with 1–3 tsp of cereal per ounce; small, frequent feedings
GI bleeding (due to cow's milk protein intolerance)	Soy formula or other cow's milk–free formula	Milk protein intolerance
Hepatic insufficiency	Portagen, Pregestimil	Impaired intraluminal digestion and absorption of long-chain fats
Hypoparathyroidism, late-onset hypocalcemia	PM 60/40	Low phosphate content
Lactose intolerance	Lactofree	Impaired digestion or utilization of lactose
Lymphatic anomalies	Portagen	Impaired absorption of long-chain fats
Necrotizing enterocolitis	Pregestimil (when feeding is resumed), breast milk	Impaired digestion

(*continued*)

Table 10-8. *Continued*

Clinical condition	Suggested formula	Rationale
Renal insufficiency	PM 60/40	Low phosphate content, low renal solute load

Source: Modified from J. Gryboski and W. A. Walker. *Gastrointestinal Problems in the Infant* (2d Ed.). Philadelphia: Saunders, 1983.

addition, nutrients in the fortifier may also settle in the tubing. Small frequent bolus feedings may be better than continuous feedings, when clinically appropriate.

B. Infant formulas. In the United States, the American Academy of Pediatrics (AAP) provides specific guidelines for the composition of infant formulas so **commercial formulas approximate human milk** in general composition. Table 10-9 describes the composition of commonly available formulas, many of which are derived from modified cow's milk (see **II.C.3** for comparison with human milk). Formula selection should be based on an infant's gestational age, energy needs, digestive and absorptive capacities, and disease entities.

1. **Standard (modified cow's milk–based) formulas** have an energy density of 67 kcal/dl (20 kcal/30 ml), equivalent to human milk; 81 kcal/dl (24 kcal/30 ml) formulations are also available for infants with increased energy or nutrient needs (e.g., increased energy expenditure or need for catch-up growth) or infants taking in limited fluid volumes. **The nutrient composition of standard formulas is suboptimal for premature infants.**

2. **Soy protein–based, lactose-free formulas** were developed for term infants with cow's milk protein allergy. Soy protein is supplemented to improve its biologic quality. Carbohydrate is provided as glucose polymers (corn syrup solids) and/or sucrose. The fat composition is similar to that of standard milk-based formulas.

   a. **We recommend soy formulas in the following instances** (see Table 10-8):

      (1) Secondary lactose intolerance following gastroenteritis, primary lactase deficiency, and galactosemia

      (2) Allergy or intolerance to cow's milk protein or prophylaxis for potentially allergic infants (e.g., those with a family history of atopy)

   b. **We do not recommend soy formulas for routine use in preterm infants.**

      (1) Botanical phytate-protein-mineral complexes may impair mineral absorption, leading to hypophosphatemia and metabolic bone disease.

      (2) Growth and nitrogen retention may be inadequate.

      (3) Vitamin content is low relative to current recommendations.

3. **Lactose-free cow's milk–based formulas** were developed for term infants with lactose intolerance. Carbohydrate is provided as glucose polymers.

4. **Preterm formulas** are designed to meet the nutritional and physiologic needs of preterm infants and have some common features:

   a. Whey-predominant, taurine-supplemented protein, which is better tolerated and produces a more normal plasma amino acid profile than casein-dominant protein

   b. Carbohydrate mixtures of 40 to 50% lactose and 50 to 60% glucose polymers to compensate for infants' relative lactase deficiency

   c. Fat mixtures containing approximately 50% MCTs to compensate for limited pancreatic lipase secretion and small bile acid pools

   d. Higher concentrations of electrolytes, minerals, vitamins, and protein to meet the increased needs associated with rapid growth, poor intestinal absorption, and limited fluid tolerance

   e. Availability as 67 and 81 kcal/dl (20 and 24 kcal/oz)

5. **Specialized formulas** have been designed for a variety of congenital and

neonatal disorders, including allergy, malabsorption syndromes, and several inborn errors of amino acid, organic acid, urea, or carbohydrate metabolism (see Table 10-9). These formulas were not designed to meet the special nutritional needs of preterm infants. Preterm infants fed these formulas require vigilant nutritional monitoring and assessment for protein, mineral, and multivitamin supplementation.

a. **Pregestimil** is a readily digestible formula designed for infants with disorders of digestion and absorption. The protein is casein, which is enzymatically hydrolyzed to free amino acids and small peptides and treated to reduce allergenicity. Fat is provided as 50% MCT. The primary carbohydrate source is glucose polymers. It is high in fat-soluble vitamins and EFAs. We use Pregestimil for term infants (and for short intervals for preterm infants) with malabsorption problems (e.g., cystic fibrosis) or short-bowel syndrome, or those recovering from conditions associated with impaired intestinal function. Pregestimil is provided in a powder and can be concentrated for increased calories and nutrition.

b. **Alimentum** is indicated for similar absorptive problems. The main difference between Alimentum and Pregestimil is the carbohydrate: Alimentum contains sucrose. Also, Alimentum is a ready-to-feed liquid formula that cannot be concentrated.

c. **Nutramigen** was developed as a hypoallergenic formula with the same protein hydrolysates as Pregestimil. The fat source is corn and soy oils, and it is lactose- and sucrose-free. Nutramigen can be useful in managing patients with protein allergies or lactose intolerance.

d. **Neocate** is designed for infants with severe cow's milk protein allergy. In contrast to Pregestimil, Alimentum, and Nutramigen, Neocate contains 100% free amino acids as a protein source rather than hydrolyzed casein.

e. **Portagen** was designed for patients who cannot efficiently digest or absorb conventional dietary fat or have certain lymphatic anomalies or disruptions. Portagen contains carbohydrate as 75% glucose polymers and 25% sucrose. The protein is casein. It contains slightly less fat than standard formulas, but 85% of its total fat content is MCTs. The EFA content of Portagen is 3.4% of total calories, just over the 3% minimum recommendation. EFA deficiency has been documented in hyperbilirubinemic patients receiving Portagen because of its unsatisfactory blend of MCTs and long-chain triglycerides. The linoleic acid content of Pregestimil is 7% of total calories; this is our preferred formula for infants with chronic liver disease or pancreatic insufficiency. Portagen is useful in infants with persistent chylothorax in order to minimize thoracic duct flow and for infants with fatty acid metabolism defects.

f. **Similac PM 60/40** was one of the earliest cow's milk–based, whey-predominant formulas. It has a low sodium and phosphate content and a high calcium-phosphorus ratio (2:1), which is useful in situations causing hypocalcemia and hyperphosphatemia:

(1) Renal insufficiency requiring sodium and potassium restriction and low renal solute load

(2) Hypoparathyroidism

g. **Similac 27** is a high-energy (90 kcal/dl, 27 kcal/30 ml) product with carbohydrate (lactose), protein (whey-predominant), and fat composition similar to a full-term formula. However, Similac 27 is significantly higher in many nutrients, including protein, calcium, phosphorus, and electrolytes. This formula may be useful for fluid-restricted infants with CHF or bronchopulmonary dysplasia (BPD).

IV. **Enteral feeding methods.** The method chosen for each infant should be individualized on the basis of gestational age, clinical condition, and extrauterine adaptation. Very sick or VLBW infants may not tolerate enteral feedings for pro-

Table 10-9. Human milk and formula composition

Formula (distributor)	kcal/30 ml	Protein (gm/dl)	Fat (gm/dl)	Carbohydrate[a] (gm/dl)	Minerals (mg/dl)			Electrolytes (mEq/dl)			Vitamins (IU/dl)			Folate (mg/dl)	Osmolality (mOsmol/kg)	Renal solute load (mOsmol/L)[c]
					Ca	P	Fe[b]	Na+	K+	Cl	A	D	E			
BREAST MILK (Composition varies)	20	1.1	4.5	7.1	33	15	0.03	0.8	1.4	1.1	250	2.2	0.18	5.0	290–300	75
STANDARD COW'S MILK–BASED FORMULAS																
Similac 20 (Ross)	20	1.5	3.6	7.2	51	39	0.15 (1.2)	0.8	1.9	1.3	203	41	2.0	10	300	100
Enfamil (Mead Johnson)	20	1.5	3.8	6.9	46	32	0.11 (1.3)	0.8	1.8	1.2	210	41.5	2.1	10.5	300	134
Similac 24 (Ross)	24	2.2	4.3	8.5	73	56	0.18 (1.5)	1.2	2.7	1.9	244	49	2.4	12	380	146
Enfamil 24 (Mead Johnson)	24	1.8	4.5	8.3	56	38	0.13 (1.5)	1.0	2.2	1.4	251	50	2.5	13	360	161
MILK PROTEIN, LACTOSE-FREE																
Lactofree (Mead Johnson)	20	1.5	3.7	6.7	55	37	1.2	0.9	1.9	1.3	201	40	1.3	10.7	200	130
SOY FORMULAS																
Isomil (Ross)	20	1.8	3.7	6.8	71	51	1.2	1.4	1.9	1.2	203	41	2.0	10.0	240	116
Prosobee (Mead Johnson)	20	2.0	3.6	6.8	63	50	1.3	1.0	2.1	1.6	208	41.5	2.1	10.5	200	178
PRETERM FORMULAS[d]																
Similac Special Care (Ross)	20	1.8	3.6	7.1	120	60	0.2	1.2	2.2	1.5	453	100	2.7	24.7	235	124

Similac Special Care (Ross)	24	2.2	4.4	8.6	146	73	0.3 (1.5)	1.5	2.7	1.9	552	122	3.2	30	300	149
Enfamil Premature (Mead Johnson)	20	2.0	3.4	7.4	112	56	0.17 (1.27)	1.13	1.8	1.6	833	180	4.2	23	260	176
Enfamil Premature (Mead Johnson)	24	2.4	4.1	8.9	134	68	0.2	1.4	2.3	2.0	970	220	3.7	29	310	210
SPECIALIZED FORMULAS																
Pregestimil (Mead Johnson)	20	1.9	3.8	6.9	63	42	1.3	1.4	1.9	1.6	250	51	2.5	10.5	320	169
Alimentum (Ross)	20	1.8	3.7	6.8	70	50	1.2	1.3	2.0	1.5	200	36	2.0	10	370	120
Neocate	20	2.1	2.7	7.1	84	63	1.2	1.0	2.5	1.3	250	53	0.7	6.2	342	—
Nutramigen (Mead Johnson)	20	1.9	2.6	9.1	63	42	1.3	1.4	1.9	1.6	208	42	2.1	10.5	320	172
Portagen (Mead Johnson)	20	2.4	3.2	7.8	63	48	1.3	1.6	2.2	1.6	530	53	2.1	10.5	230	200
Similac PM 60/40 (Ross)	20	1.6	3.8	6.9	38	19	0.15	0.7	1.5	1.1	203	41	2.0	10.0	280	96
Similac 27 (Ross)	27	2.5	4.8	9.6	82	64	0.2	1.4	3.1	2.1	274	55	2.7	14.0	430	164

Ca = calcium; P = phosphorus; Fe = iron; Na$^+$ = sodium; K$^+$ = potassium; Cl = chloride.

[a]See text for types of carbohydrates used in formula.

[b]In instances where high and low Fe formulations are available, the low Fe value appears.

[c]Estimated renal solute load = [Protein (gm) $\times$ 4] + [Na(mEq) + K (mEq) + Cl (mEq)].

[d]20 kcal/30 ml formulations are also available.

longed periods. **Whenever possible, however, the enteral route is preferred.**
Enteral feeding is generally safer, less expensive, more nutritionally complete,
and more physiologic. Moreover, lack of enteral feeding, despite PN, can lead to
intestinal mucosal atrophy. We encourage starting low volume "trophic" feedings
as soon as possible. Trophic feedings may be tolerated before the infant is able to
obtain significant nutrition from enteral feedings (see **IV.E.3**).

A. Breast and bottle feedings. In preterm infants, breast-feeding or feeding by
   a soft nipple specifically designed for preterm babies often is possible by 32
   to 34 weeks' gestational age, when coordination of suck and swallow may be
   present. Considerations for bottle feeding include the following:

   1. **Temperature.** The milk or formula can be offered at body or room temper-
      ature.

   2. **Position.** The hungry infant should be held in a comfortable, secure posi-
      tion, either reclining or sitting in the feeder's lap. The bottle should be
      held so that the air rises to the upturned bottom and the infant sucks in
      milk and not air. The bottle should never be propped for a young infant;
      the benefit derived from cuddling and body contact is as important as
      caloric intake.

   3. **Schedule**
      a. Bottle feedings can be offered either on a schedule of every 3 to 4 hours
         (the usual practice in a nursery) or on infant demand.
      b. The fluid for the initial bottle feeding is sterile water. If water is toler-
         ated without aspiration or regurgitation, the infant can be rapidly ad-
         vanced to full-strength formula or human milk.

B. Gavage (orogastric or nasogastric [NG] tube) feeding

   1. **Candidates**
      a. Infants less than 32 weeks' gestational age
      b. Preterm infants expending significant energy in the process of sucking
         may require a combination of nipple and gavage feedings
      c. Infants with impaired suck and swallow mechanisms due to conditions
         including encephalopathy, hypotonia, or maxillofacial abnormalities

   2. **Method**
      a. With the infant's head placed to the side, pass a 5F or 8F polyethyl-
         ene feeding tube through the nose or mouth; the distance from the
         nose to the ear and to the xiphoid should first be marked on the tube.
         Check catheter position by injecting air and auscultating over the
         stomach.
      b. After the catheter is placed, residual gastric aspirate is checked, the
         volume recorded, and the aspirate returned to prevent metabolic com-
         plications from continued acid and electrolyte removal.
      c. A measured amount of fluid is poured into a syringe attached to the
         tube and allowed to drip in by gravity. Never inject the fluid under
         pressure.
      d. When the tube is removed, it is pinched closed to avoid dripping fluid
         into the pharynx.

   3. **Feeding schedule** (see **IV.E** regarding VLBW infants). The fluid volume
      ordered depends on the estimated stomach volume. Undistended stomach
      volume varies from 3 ml in 800-gm neonates to 40 ml in 4000-gm neo-
      nates.
      a. Orders for gavage feeding should include the type of formula, the fre-
         quency and fluid volume for the initial feedings, and the increments of
         feedings to be given over the following 12 to 24 hours.
      b. When the gastric residual measured before a feeding is higher than ex-
         pected, the residual should be returned to the stomach and the amount
         of fluid reduced by that volume. Should residuals persist, one should
         look for signs of GI or systemic illness. Positioning the infant in the
         prone position after feedings may facilitate stomach emptying, reduc-
         ing gastric residual.
      c. Sterile water is recommended for the initial oral feeding; if aspirated, it

causes less pulmonary irritation than either dextrose 5% in water (5% D/W) or formula. Once human milk or formula is introduced, increase strength and volume by recommended increments (see **IV.E.4**) until fluid and caloric requirements are met.

C. **Continuous NG feeding**

1. **Candidates.** We reserve continuous feeding through an indwelling NG tube for infants who do not tolerate intermittent gavage feeding (e.g., those with gastric distention or regurgitation).

2. **Method**

   a. A 5F Silastic tube designed as an indwelling feeding tube is passed through the nose into the stomach in the same manner as for intermittent gavage. With an indwelling NG tube, extreme care must be taken to tape the tube securely to the infant's nose and head (or to the endotracheal tube if the infant is intubated); otherwise, manipulation of the infant or tube could dislodge the tube into the esophagus or pharynx, where infusion of formula could result in aspiration.

   b. Formula is administered at a constant slow rate by pump.

3. **Feeding schedule.** The formula is pumped at a constant rate, starting at rates seen in Table 10-10. See **IV.E.5** regarding advancement.

   a. Extension tubing from the pump to the gastric tube is changed every 8 to 12 hours, and the indwelling tube itself is changed every few days to 1 week.

   b. A fresh supply of formula or milk is flushed through the pump and tubing every 3 to 4 hours.

   c. Check gastric residuals every 2 to 4 hours, with adjustments in subsequent feedings the same as those made with gavage feedings. If the infant is receiving total nutrition by the enteral route (full feeds), residuals should not exceed the volume of feeding fluid given in 1 to 2 hours.

D. **Continuous transpyloric feedings**

1. **Candidates.** There are only a few indications for transpyloric feeding by indwelling nasoduodenal or nasojejunal tubes, and infants requiring long-term transpyloric feeding should be considered for a surgically placed feeding tube.

   a. Infants who cannot tolerate intragastric nutrition owing to severe gastric retention or regurgitation

   b. Anatomic abnormalities of the GI tract such as microgastria

2. **Method**

   a. A weighted feeding tube of a length approximately equal to the distance from the tip of the infant's nose to the knee is passed in the same manner as for gavage feeding (see **IV.B.2**). The infant may be placed on the right side and the tube allowed to migrate through the pylorus into the duodenum, which usually occurs within a few hours.

   b. We routinely utilize **fluoroscopy** or **ultrasound** to guide placement.

   c. Tube position is verified by a pH reading higher than 5.0 and by the yellow color of the aspirate; verification by radiography may be necessary.

3. **Feeding schedule.** The same formulas and feeding schedules as for NG feedings are used; the formula is administered at a constant, slow rate by a pump, starting at rates seen in Table 10-10.

   a. Orders include volumes, rates of administration, and infusion pump settings. Take care not to deliver excessively rapid or large volumes to the intestine, and regularly observe for abdominal distention and diarrhea.

   b. Gastric residuals should be checked for occasionally; formula in the stomach may indicate a malpositioned tube, intestinal obstruction, or ileus.

   c. The indwelling nasojejunal tube is not changed routinely. Connecting tubing and formula supplies are changed as for continuous NG feeding.

Table 10-10.   Tube feeding guidelines[a-d]

Birth weight (gm)	Initial Rate (ml/kg/day)	Volume Increase (ml/kg/day)
<800	10	10–20
800–1000	10–20	10–20
1001–1250	20	20–30
1251–1500	30	30
1501–1800	30–40	30–40
1801–2500	40	40–50
>2500	50	50

[a]This table does not apply to infants capable of po feeding.
[b]The above guidelines must always be individualized based on the infant's clinical status/severity of illness.
[c]Consider advancing feeding volume more rapidly than the above guidelines once tolerance of ≥100 cc/kg/day is established, but would not exceed increments of 30 cc/kg/day in most infants weighing less than 1500 gm.
[d]The recommended volume goal for feedings is 140 to 160 cc/kg/day.

E. Special considerations for feeding preterm infants
1. Preferences for feeding methods and schedules vary considerably among neonatal intensive care units (NICUs). We frequently use intermittent gavage for VLBW infants. We generally start continuous NG feedings in extremely small, premature infants (<1000 gm) and in premature infants who were unstable perinatally.
   a. **Intermittent bolus feedings** may be physiologically better because they stimulate feeding-associated release of GI hormones, which may play a role in further development and maturation of the GI tract.
   b. Conversely, **continuous feedings** are usually better tolerated in VLBW infants, with fewer GI side effects such as reflux and gastric distention. In addition, bolus feedings can decrease pulmonary compliance in the postprandial period compared with continuous feedings. The significance of these effects must be considered in the overall context of providing optimal nutritional support with minimal clinical compromise.
2. **Initiation of feeding.** The decision to start enteral feeding in premature infants is based on an **assessment of clinical and metabolic stability.** We delay initiation of feedings in infants who are hemodynamically unstable and in those with conditions, including perinatal asphyxia or sepsis, that may compromise bowel function or integrity. We do not withhold enteral feeding for any predetermined period if the infant is medically stable.
   a. We routinely begin enteral feedings on day 1 for nondistressed, larger preterm infants (>1500 gm, >32 weeks' gestation).
   b. For nondistressed infants weighing less than 1500 gm at birth, enteral feedings are started when there is no cardiovascular instability, respiratory distress, significant apnea, or evidence of asphyxia.
   c. Some extremely small infants with intrauterine growth restriction (IUGR) can be fed safely earlier than more premature infants of the same weight, although they should also have feedings advanced cautiously.
   d. Although umbilical arterial catheters (UACs) have been associated with necrotizing enterocolitis (NEC), controlled trials of feeding with UACs in place have not shown an increased incidence of NEC. We have recently started trophic feeding in infants with UACs in place (see **E.3**).
   e. If an infant with patent ductus arteriosus shows clinical compromise, we generally withhold feedings.
3. **Trophic feedings** (also referred to as "gut priming" or "early minimal enteral feedings"). The structural and functional integrity of the GI tract is

dependent on enteral nutrition. When the tract is deprived, intestinal mucosal atrophy and villous flattening occur. Trophic feedings (less than or equal to 10 ml/kg per day) can be given soon after birth to premature infants whose illness severity otherwise prevents advancement of enteral feeding volume. These feedings stimulate the GI tract in preparation for more substantial enteral nutrition later.

  a. Findings related to trophic feedings
   (1) Stimulation of GI hormonal response
   (2) Promotion of maturation of GI motor patterns
   (3) Improve feeding tolerance
   (4) Facilitation of earlier progression to full enteral feedings
   (5) Improved weight gain
   (6) Fewer days on parenteral nutrition
  b. Guidelines for trophic feedings
   (1) Start as soon as possible after birth when the infant is medically stable, ideally by day of life 2 to 3.
   (2) Use full-strength human milk or full-strength 20 kcal per oz preterm formula in a volume less than or equal to 10 cc/kg per day. We administer trophic feedings every 4, 6, or 8 hours.
   (3) Volume of feedings may be advanced when the infant is considered ready for enteral nutrition. If the infant's clinical condition deteriorates and enteral feedings may not be appropriate, we consider reducing feeding volume to trophic feeding levels (10 cc/kg per day or less).
   (4) We do not use trophic feedings in infants with suspected or confirmed necrotizing enterocolitis, severe hemodynamic instability, undergoing treatment with indomethacin, evidence of ileus, or clinical signs of intestinal pathology.
 4. Choice of feeding interval
  a. An every-3-hour schedule is suggested for infants with birth weights less than 1500 gm, hyperbilirubinemia, hypoglycemia, asphyxia, or a history of feeding intolerance.
  b. A 3- to 4-hour feeding schedule is suitable for most other infants.
 5. Feeding advancement. Advancing a premature infant to total enteral nutrition (full feeds) can be done in many ways, and there are very few data to support any one method as optimal. The following recommendations reflect our current practice.
  a. Few controlled studies address the issue of whether to first advance feeding concentration versus feeding volume. We generally use full-strength human milk and full-strength formula before increasing feeding volume. Other methods of advancement, however, may be well tolerated (e.g., advancement of volume at half-strength concentration, or alternating advancement of volume and concentration (Table 10-10).
  b. Intravenous fluid and nutrient intakes must be adjusted downward as enteral feeding increases (i.e., if previously on total PN). As enteral feedings are increased, we reduce the IV fluid rate milliliter per milliliter so that daily fluid volume remains the same.
F. Feeding intolerance, gastroesophageal reflux (GER), and GI dysmotility
 1. Signs of feeding intolerance in newborns include poor suckling, swallowing difficulties, choking, vomiting, abdominal distention, gastric stasis or gastroparesis, and reducing substances or blood in the stool (see Chaps. 32, 33).
 2. Associations
  a. Persistent or severe feeding intolerance may indicate anatomic abnormalities, NEC, sepsis, or metabolic abnormalities (see Chaps. 23, 29, 32, 33).
  b. Functional feeding intolerance and gastric stasis frequently are associated with prematurity, CNS or neuromuscular disease, GI repairs, and CLD.

3. **Symptomatic GER** often complicates oral feedings for these infants and may lead to apnea, airway obstruction, and failure to grow.

   a. GER, a physiologic event in infancy, decreases in frequency as the pressure of the lower esophageal sphincter rises over the first several months. Pathologic GER is frequently associated with delayed gastric emptying and esophageal motility disorders.

   b. Other signs of pathologic GER, especially in preterm infants, include signs of possible aspiration (e.g., increased pulmonary secretions, episodes of pulmonary deterioration, apnea, airway obstruction, bradycardic episodes) and signs of esophagitis (e.g., refusal to eat, irritability, arching of the back during feedings, failure to grow).

4. **Treatment** for symptomatic GER and gastric stasis

   a. Positioning the infant is a simple and frequently effective maneuver. LBW infants reflux less frequently when prone than when placed on either side. Prone position with the head elevated about 30 degrees is preferred for infants with symptomatic GER. Upright positioning in "achalasia chairs" may actually exacerbate GER.

   b. Frequent feedings with small volumes can decrease gastric distention.

   c. Thickening the feeding fluid with cereal may be effective.

   d. Esophagitis can potentiate GER. Antacids or H_2 antagonists (cimetidine or ranitidine) diminish gastric acid and may relieve esophagitis.

   e. Drugs that promote gastric emptying and GI motility, such as metoclopramide and cisapride, are used occasionally for severe GER.

      (1) Persistent functional feeding intolerance, even in preterm babies and term infants with neuromuscular disease, may respond to metoclopramide 0.03 to 0.10 mg/kg per dose orally or cisapride 0.1 to 0.3 mg/kg per dose orally.

      (2) Metoclopramide toxicity can produce extrapyramidal reactions (especially dystonia-dyskinesia) and methemoglobinemia. Cisapride may cause diarrhea.

   f. Transpyloric feeding (see **IV.D**)

   g. Persistent clinically compromising GER may require fundoplication.

G. **Nutritional management of NEC**

1. **Withholding feedings.** In infants with NEC, nutrient delivery must be by the parenteral route. The duration of withholding of enteral feedings ranges from 2 to 3 days for suspected NEC to 10 to 14 days for confirmed NEC.

2. When it is appropriate to resume enteral feedings, start with small volumes (5 to 10 ml/kg per day) of full-strength or half-strength formula or breast milk.

   a. Human milk or premature formula may be well tolerated following mild NEC; however, in infants with more severe NEC an elemental formula such as Pregestimil may be used. In order to receive adequate nutrition, premature infants should be switched back to fortified human milk or premature formula when they are near or at full feeds.

   b. Increases in strength and volume are based on both feeding tolerance and severity of the NEC insult. Once feeding tolerance has been established, follow the general guidelines for advancement (see Table 10-10); some infants may require slower feeding advancement.

   c. If feeding intolerance recurs, consider evaluation for post-NEC complications such as intestinal strictures.

H. **Short-bowel syndrome** (SBS). When an extensive length of small bowel is removed, malabsorption can occur, with subsequent malnutrition. Infants with SBS are prone to deficiencies of sodium, zinc, copper, manganese, magnesium, iron, selenium, and chromium.

1. **Early initiation of enteral feedings.** After the postoperative recovery period for gut resection, early feedings with small amounts of formula can enhance the rate of intestinal adaptation. Formula selection depends on the length and type of residual bowel. In general, because carbohydrate

and fat malabsorption is common following resection, an elemental formula (e.g., Pregestimil) is initially preferred.

2. **Diluted feedings by continuous infusion** are often best tolerated. While continuing with PN, enteral feedings can be advanced by volume to establish tolerance. When one-fourth to one-half total fluids are provided enterally, increases of concentration can occur. Fat- and water-soluble vitamin supplementation may be warranted.

3. Once enteral feedings are established, advancement may proceed (see **IV.E.5**). The rate of PN administration is reduced as feeding volume is increased so that total daily fluid intake remains the same.

I. **SGA infants (see Chap. 3).** Nutritional efforts should be aggressive because SGA infants do not demonstrate as much catch-up growth in the first year as do appropriate-for-gestational-age (AGA) infants of similar gestational age. SGA infants with head-sparing asymmetric growth restriction display more catch-up growth than do infants with symmetric growth restriction. The continued use of premature formula after 35 weeks' corrected gestational age may be beneficial to improve bone mineralization and to enhance nutritional intake for optimal growth. Nutrition affects neurologic outcome more significantly in SGA than in AGA infants; head circumference growth may be the best indicator.

V. **PN** is the IV delivery of energy and nutrients.

A. **Indications**

1. Because of the nutritional complexity, risks of complications, and expense, **PN should be reserved for infants in whom an adequate enteral diet is not possible.** Very-short-term (e.g., <3 days) PN has no clear benefits, particularly for larger neonates with greater energy and nutrient reserves. PN should be considered for infants who are metabolically stable and who may be in the following classifications:

   a. Weighing less than 1800 gm and not expected to receive significant enteral nutrition for more than 3 days

   b. Weighing more than or equal to 1800 gm and not expected to receive significant enteral nutrition for more than 5 to 7 days

2. **Choice between peripheral and central PN**

   a. PN solutions can be infused into peripheral veins or a central vein, usually the vena cava. Central PN allows the use of more hypertonic solutions but incurs greater risks. It is possible to support growth, even fetal growth rates, by the use of peripheral PN with a fat emulsion, thereby avoiding the complications associated with prolonged use of central venous catheters. Peripheral PN may not, however, support adequate growth in extremely premature infants with high metabolic demands.

   b. Placement of a central venous catheter is warranted under the following circumstances:

      (1) An extended period (e.g., >1 week) of bowel rest in some postoperative infants and in infants with NEC

      (2) Nutritional requirements exceeding the capabilities of peripheral PN. Significantly increased energy demands, especially combined with decreased fluid-volume tolerance, may necessitate dextrose concentrations higher than 10.0 to 12.5%.

      (3) Imminent lack of peripheral venous access

B. **Nutritional goals**

1. Preterm infants who receive 60 kcal/kg per day of IV glucose and 2.5 gm/kg per day of amino acid solution show a positive nitrogen balance. Higher energy intakes improve nitrogen retention and spare fat reserves.

2. In general, PN can support growth at slightly lower energy intakes than can enteral feedings because energy is not lost in absorption and digestion.

3. Intrauterine weight gain rates provide practical guidelines for estimating

appropriate PN intake, but needs must be individualized for each patient. For example, infants subjected to metabolic stress, such as surgery, may require more energy and protein.

C. Nutrient sources
  1. Carbohydrate. Glucose (dextrose) is the carbohydrate source for IV solutions, with the glycerol in lipid emulsions making a small caloric contribution.
  a. IV dextrose has an energy density of **3.4 kcal/gm.**
  b. The osmolality of glucose limits the concentrations that can be infused safely by means of peripheral vein to 10.0 to 12.5% D/W. We use concentrations up to 12.5% D/W for umbilical arterial infusions and up to 25% D/W for central venous infusions. In unusual cases, higher concentrations of glucose have been delivered through central venous lines (e.g., during renal failure when fluid volume must be severely restricted).
  c. The signs of glucose intolerance are hyperglycemia, hyperosmolality, and secondary glycosuria and osmotic diuresis. The quantity of dextrose that an infant can tolerate varies, especially with gestational age.
  d. It is helpful to refer to dextrose infusions in terms of **milligrams of glucose per kilogram per minute** (mg/kg/min), which expresses the total glucose load and accounts for infusion rate, dextrose concentration, and patient weight (Fig. 10-2).
    (1) Term infants usually tolerate initial infusions of 7 to 8 mg/kg per minute and these rates can be rapidly increased to 11 to 14 mg/kg per minute without displaying glucose intolerance.
    (2) Glucose tolerance is related to gestational age. Premature infants have decreased peripheral glucose utilization, and because of hepatic insensitivity to insulin, may have persistent hepatic glucose production in the setting of hyperglycemia. LBW infants usually tolerate an initial infusion rate of 6 to 8 mg/kg per minute and a gradual increase up to 11 to 14 mg/kg per minute. At this level, hyperglycemia becomes prevalent. VLBW infants may develop significant and persistent hyperglycemia if infusion rates exceed 6 to 7 mg/kg per minute, which is equivalent to 10% D/W infused at about 100 ml/kg per day.
    (3) As the rate of glucose infusion increases, both metabolic rate (oxygen consumption) and carbon dioxide production rise as carbohydrate is converted to fat. Thus, very high glucose infusion rates may compromise infants with lung disease by increasing oxygen consumption and carbon dioxide production; these effects can be limited by replacing some carbohydrate with fat.
  2. Protein. Crystalline amino acid solutions provide the nitrogen source in PN.
  a. The energy density of amino acids is **4 kcal/gm.**
  b. Two pediatric amino acid formulations are commercially available in the United States (Aminosyn-PF, Abbott Laboratories; Trophamine, McGaw). In theory, these products are better adapted to the needs of newborns than are standard adult amino acid solutions, which are based on the composition of egg albumin. The optimal amino acid composition for neonatal PN is yet to be defined, and no products designed for preterm infants are currently available.
  c. Benefits of pediatric amino acid solutions
    (1) Produces a plasma amino acid pattern that approximates postprandial plasma of healthy, breast-fed neonates
    (2) Promotes weight gain and positive nitrogen balance
    (3) Minimizes the abnormalities in liver function observed with long-term PN support
    (4) Increases calcium and phosphorus solubility due to lower pH

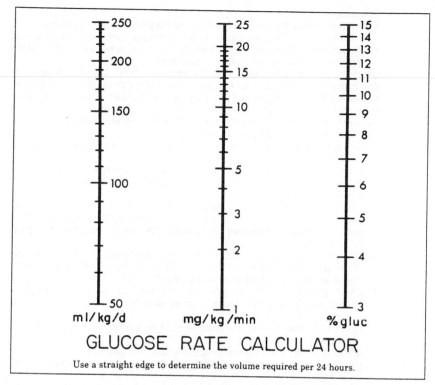

250
200
150
100
50
ml/kg/d

25
20
15
10
5
3
2
1
mg/kg/min

15
14
13
12
11
10
9
8
7
6
5
4
3
%gluc

GLUCOSE RATE CALCULATOR

Use a straight edge to determine the volume required per 24 hours.

Fig. 10-2. Interconversion of glucose infusion units. (From M. H. Klaus and A. A. Faranoff, eds. *Care of the High-Risk Neonate,* 2nd ed. Philadelphia: Saunders, 1979, 430.)

d. **Major differences between pediatric and adult amino acid formulations**

(1) **Addition of taurine** (see **II.C.3**), which is a conditionally essential amino acid normally synthesized from methionine via cysteine. Taurine forms a less hepatotoxic conjugated bile acid, and therefore may be advantageous in decreasing the risk of cholestasis.

(2) **Contains histidine and tyrosine,** which are essential in infants

(3) **Addition of glutamic and aspartic acids,** found in very high concentrations in human milk.

(4) **Lower amounts of methionine and phenylalanine** because serum levels were very high with adult amino acid preparations, and a **lower amount of glycine,** because its conjugated form of bile acid is more hepatotoxic

e. Standard PN solutions contain 0.5 to 3.0 gm of amino acids per deciliter, but the delivered concentration is tailored to the needs of the individual patient.

3. **Fat.** Soybean oil–based Intralipid (Cutter Medical) and Soyacal (Alpha Therapeutic) and safflower oil–based Liposyn (Abbott Laboratories) are the currently available lipid emulsions. **Ten percent lipid emulsions have an energy density of 1.1 kcal/ml** (0.9 kcal from lipid and 0.2 kcal from glycerol and phospholipid stabilizer); **20% lipid emulsions yield 2.0 kcal/ml** because the glycerol and stabilizer are not doubled in the 20% emulsion.

4. **Electrolytes**
   a. **Sodium and potassium concentrations may be adjusted daily** to meet individual needs. Electrolytes are added at the time solutions are prepared.
   b. **Metabolic acidosis** in VLBW infants may be treated by increasing the proportion of anions provided as **acetates**.
5. **Calcium, phosphorus, and magnesium** (see Chap. 29). **The amount of calcium and phosphate that can be administered IV is limited by the precipitation of calcium phosphate.** Unfortunately, the variables that determine calcium and phosphate compatibility in parenteral solutions are complex, and what constitutes maximal safe concentrations is controversial. We use the following guidelines:
   a. **Calcium.** Our standard solution contains 30 mg/dl (1.5 mEq/dl) of elemental calcium.
   b. **Phosphate.** Approximately 21 mg/dl of phosphate is routinely added to solutions as 1.0 mEq potassium phosphate (0.68 mM phosphate; 1 mM phosphate = 31 mg).
   c. These standard mineral concentrations provide about one-third of the daily intrauterine accretion rates for calcium and phosphorus. Thus, **preterm infants receiving prolonged PN are at risk for metabolic bone disease** (see Chap. 29).
   d. Metabolic bone complications can be diminished by **increasing the mineral content of PN solutions to 50 to 60 mg of calcium per deciliter and 40 to 45 mg of phosphate per deciliter.**
   e. **Calcium-phosphorus precipitation.** The solubility of calcium and phosphorus in PN solutions depends on several factors, primarily the concentration of each mineral.
      (1) The calcium-phosphate ratio should be about 1.3:1 by weight (1:1 molar).
      (2) More acidic solutions increase calcium and phosphorus solubility.
      (3) The amount of magnesium can affect calcium and phosphorus solubility.
      (4) Higher temperature can also be a contributing factor to precipitation. Therefore, both very slow infusion rates and solutions at room temperature can pose another risk for precipitation.
   f. **The suggested higher intakes of calcium and phosphate for preterm infants should be given through a central venous line,** not a peripheral vein, because of increased risk of tissue injury with IV extravasation.
   g. **We do not use 3:1 solutions (PN mixed in one bag with lipids),** for the following reasons:
      (1) The pH of lipids is more basic and increases the pH of the total solution, which decreases the solubility of calcium and phosphorus, limiting the amount of these minerals in the solution. This is of primary concern with long-term use of PN (e.g., >5 days).
      (2) If the calcium and phosphorus in a 3:1 solution precipitated, it would be undetectable, since the solution is already cloudy.
      (3) 3:1 solutions require a larger-micron filter or no filter, which may pose a greater sepsis risk.
   h. **Magnesium** 0.3 to 0.6 mEq/dl is added to solutions. Higher concentrations (1.0 mEq/dl) in our nurseries have been associated with hypermagnesemia and intestinal dysmotility in VLBW infants.
6. **Vitamins and trace elements**
   a. Recommendations for IV vitamin intakes for infants, including preterm infants, were recently revised. The current vitamin formulation (MVI Pediatric, Astra) does not maintain blood levels of all vitamins within an acceptable range for preterm infants. Table 10-11 provides guidelines on how to best use the available formulations for term and preterm infants. Vitamin A is the most difficult vitamin to provide in adequate amounts to the VLBW infant without providing excess

amounts of all other vitamins. Vitamin A is also subject to loss via photodegradation and adsorption to plastic tubing and solution-containing bags. This is of particular concern with long-term PN use.

b. Trace-mineral parenteral requirements have been estimated for preterm infants. Trace-element preparations are added to provide the following concentrations per 100-ml solution: zinc, 300 μg; copper, 20 μg; chromium, 0.2 μg; manganese, 5 μg; selenium, 1.5 μg. These standard additions are designed to meet the needs of infants receiving PN at about 150 ml/kg per day. Significantly different fluid requirements or altered rates of excretion necessitate modifications.

c. Copper and manganese are eliminated in bile.

  (1) Caution is required in administering IV copper to infants with impaired biliary excretion, including infants with PN cholestasis.

  (2) Manganese should be withheld when cholestatic liver disease is present.

d. At present, **several potentially important micronutrients, including carnitine, iodide, and molybdenum, are not contained in neonatal PN solutions.** The lack of these nutrients is most concerning for those patients requiring PN for longer than 1 to 2 weeks and not receiving enteral feedings.

  (1) Carnitine deficiency may occur owing to impaired biosynthetic capacity and limited uptake and tissue stores. A deficiency state may impair fatty acid oxidation. Supplementation of PN may be beneficial to increase utilization of endogenous fat stores, to eliminate fatty liver deposition in those receiving concentrated dextrose solutions, and to enhance utilization of IV lipids.

  (2) Significant iodine absorption likely occurs through the skin with the use of iodine-containing disinfectants or detergents. The recommendation is to add 1.0 μg/kg per day for those on long-term PN, which takes into account the transdermal absorption and avoids the risk of excess iodine intake.

  (3) Molybdenum deficiency has not been described in the pediatric population, and therefore becomes necessary only after long-term PN support. The recommended dose is 0.25 μg/kg per day.

D. A suggested schedule for PN follows, and should be modified according to the requirements and tolerance of each infant and tapered as enteral feeding begins. Convenient daily nutrient calculations appear in Table 10-12.

1. Dextrose

  a. Six to 8 mg/kg per minute of dextrose (10% D/W) at a rate of approximately 80 to 120 ml/kg per day is generally well tolerated initially.

  b. Advance by about 2 mg/kg per minute every 24 hours either by increasing dextrose concentration (e.g., 7.5% D/W to 10% D/W) or by increasing infusion rate. ELBW infants may require slower advancement to maintain euglycemia. The upper limit of tolerance is usually 11 to 14 mg/kg per minute.

  c. Newborns with birth weights lower than 1000 gm may have fluid requirements in excess of 200 ml/kg per day. These infants are relatively intolerant to the standard neonatal dextrose infusions.

  (1) When **hyperglycemia is severe or persistent, an insulin infusion may be useful.** We also occasionally use insulin to allow higher caloric intake while maintaining euglycemia. We initiate an infusion of short-acting insulin at a rate of 0.01 to 0.05 unit/kg per hour, with insulin dose titrated to maintain blood glucose concentrations of 100 to 200 mg/dl. A convenient initial solution is 10 units of insulin per kilogram in 100 ml of fluid (0.1 unit/ml). The IV tubing should first be thoroughly flushed with the solution (see Chap. 29).

  (2) For the smallest preterm infants, we rarely use 2.5% D/W with sodium, potassium, calcium salts, or amino acids to adjust osmolality. The risk of hemolysis and hyperkalemia sometimes associated

Table 10-11. Suggested intakes of parenteral vitamins in infants

| Vitamin | Estimated needs | | Forty percent of a single-dose vial MVI Pediatric (Astra) per kilogram of body weight | 1.5 ml MVI Pediatric per 100 ml PN administered at a rate of 150 ml/kg/d[a] |
	Term infants (dose/d)	Preterm infants (dose/ kg/d)		
LIPID SOLUBLE				
A (μg)[b]	700	500	280	315
D (IU)[b]	400	160	160	180
E (IU)[b]	7	2.8	2.8	3.2
K (μg)	200	80	80	90
WATER SOLUBLE				
Thiamine (mg)	1.2	0.35	0.48	0.54
Riboflavin (mg)	1.4	0.15	0.56	0.63
Niacin (mg)	17	6.8	6.8	7.65
Pantothenate (mg)	5	2.0	2.0	2.25
Pyridoxine (mg)	1.0	0.18	0.4	0.45
Biotin (μg)	20	6.0	8.0	9.0
Vitamin B_{12} (μg)	1.0	0.3	0.4	0.45
Vitamin C (mg)	80	25	32	36
Folate (μg)	140	56	56	63

[a]Assumes 150 ml/kg is the average PN administration rate.
[b]700 μg retinol equivalent = 2300 IU; 7 mg alpha-tocopherol = 7 IU; 10 μg vitamin D = 400 IU.
Source: From H. L. Greene et al. Guidelines for the use of vitamins, trace elements, calcium, magnesium, and phosphorus in infants and children receiving total parenteral nutrition. *Am. J. Clin. Nutr.* 48:1324, 1988.

with this approach must be weighed against the risk of swings in glucose level that sometimes accompany insulin infusion.

2. **Protein.** Crystalline amino acid solutions provide nitrogen in PN. We generally initiate protein within the first 48 hours.
   a. Infants weighing less than or equal to 1000 gm
      (1) Begin with 0.5–1.0 gm/kg per day.
      (2) Advance by 0.25 to 0.50 gm/kg per day up to 2.5 to 3.5 gm/kg per day. Positive nitrogen balance can be achieved with a minimum of 60 kcal/kg per day and 2.0 to 2.5 gm/kg per day of amino acids. Intrauterine accretion rates for nitrogen can be attained with 70 kcal/kg per day and 2.7 to 3.0 gm/kg per day of amino acids.
   b. Infants weighing more than 1000 gm
      (1) Begin with 1.0 gm/kg per day.
      (2) Advance by 1.0 gm/kg per day up to 2.5 to 3.0 gm/kg per day.
3. **Fat**
   a. The use of 20% lipid solution is preferable to conserve fluid volume. For the VLBW infant, however, it may be necessary to use 10% solution infused over 24 hours. Twenty percent lipid may decrease the incidence of hyperlipidemia because the ratio of phospholipid to triglyceride is

Table 10-12. Nutritional calculations

Intravenous Intake

Carbohydrate

$$\frac{\text{Carbohydrate}}{\%\ \text{dextrose}} \times \underline{\hspace{3cm}} \times .34\ \text{kcal/gm} \div 100 = \underline{\hspace{3cm}}$$
$$\text{ml/kg/d of solution} \qquad\qquad\qquad \text{total CHO kcal/kg/d}$$

Example: Dextrose 10% at 150 ml/kg/d = 51 kcal/kg/d

$$\frac{\text{Protein}}{\%\ \text{amino acid}} \times \underline{\hspace{3cm}} \times 4.0\ \text{kcal/gm} \div 100 = \underline{\hspace{3cm}}$$
$$\text{ml/kg/d of solution} \qquad\qquad\qquad \text{total protein kcal/kg/d}$$

Example: 2.5% amino acid solution at 150 ml/kg/d = 15 kcal/kg/d

$$\text{Fat 10\% Intralipid} \underline{\hspace{3cm}} \times 1.1\ \text{kcal/ml} = \underline{\hspace{3cm}}$$
$$\text{ml/kg/d of solution} \qquad\qquad \text{total kcal fat/kg/d}$$

Example: 10% intralipid at 24 ml/d = 26.4 kcal/kg/d

$$\text{20\% Intralipid} \underline{\hspace{3cm}} \times 2.0\ \text{kcal/ml} = \underline{\hspace{3cm}}$$
$$\text{ml/kg/d of solution} \qquad\qquad \text{total kcal fat/day}$$

Example: 20% Intralipid at 24 ml/kg/d = 48 kcal/kg/d

Total intravenous kcals/kg/d =

$$\underline{\hspace{2.5cm}} + \underline{\hspace{2.5cm}} + \underline{\hspace{2.5cm}}$$
$$\text{total CHO kcal/kg/d} \quad \text{total protein kcal/kg/d} \quad \text{total fat kcal/kg/d}$$

Enteral Intake

$$(\underline{\hspace{2.5cm}} + \underline{\hspace{2.5cm}})$$
$$\text{Basic formula kcal/oz} \quad \text{Additive kcal/oz}$$
$$\times \underline{\hspace{2.5cm}} \times 1\ \text{oz/30 ml} = \underline{\hspace{2.5cm}}$$
$$\text{ml/day of solution} \qquad\qquad \text{total kcal day}$$

Example: Similac 24 kcal/oz with 2 kcal/oz polycose and 2 kcal/oz MCT oil
at 150 ml/kg/day = [24 kcal/oz + 2 kcal/oz + 2 kcal/oz] × 150 ml/kg/d × 1oz/30 ml
= 140 kcal/kg/d

Caloric Content of Ingredients

Dextrose = 3.4 kcal/gm	Polycose = 2 kcal/ml (liquid)
Protein = 4.0 kcal/gm	Polycose = 8 kcal/1 tsp (powder)
10% Intralipid = 1.1 kcal/ml	MCT oil = 7.7 kcal/ml
20% Intralipid = 2.0 kcal/ml	HMF = 3.5 kcal/package

lower than in the 10% emulsion, which results in less inhibition of lipoprotein lipase activity due to infused phospholipid.

  b. Infants weighing less than 1000 gm

    (1) Begin with 0.5 gm/kg per day.

    (2) Advance by 0.25 to 0.50 gm/kg per day up to 2.0 to 3.0 gm/kg per day.

  c. Infants weighing more than 1000 gm

    (1) Begin with 1.0 gm/kg per day.

    (2) Advance by 1.0 gm/kg per day up to 3.0 gm/kg per day.

  d. Infuse lipids over 24 hours for optimal tolerance.

4. Weaning PN. When advancing enteral feedings, reduce the rate of PN administration to achieve the desired total fluid volume. Nutrient intake from both enteral and PN sources are assessed in relation to overall nutrition goals: PN components may be adjusted (e.g., increase protein concentration) as the PN intake volume decreases to strive for optimum nutrition. Peripheral PN may limit the ability to concentrate components as infusion rates decrease.

E. Peripheral PN procedures

  1. Dextrose and amino acids are mixed in the same bottle, which is then connected to the distal end of an infusion line with a 0.22-micron, in-line air-eliminating filter.

2. The lipid emulsion is connected to the infusion line beyond the filter through the upper portion of a T- or Y-connector. The amino acid, dextrose, and fat solutions can then be infused together through a peripheral IV catheter.

3. Either 10% or 20% fat emulsions can be used in peripheral venous lines.

4. **Limit concentration to 10% or 12.5% dextrose** to maintain an osmolality close to 1000 mOsm.

5. **Limit concentration to 2% amino acids** unless adequate energy can be provided from carbohydrates and fats to prevent protein catabolism (probably in the range of 35 to 50 kcal/kg per day). Solution osmolality will be increased with higher concentrations, but not as greatly as with dextrose.

6. **Limit concentration to 40 mEq potassium and 30 mEq calcium per liter.** If infiltration occurs (a known risk with peripheral access), a higher electrolyte concentration can cause greater damage to surrounding tissue.

7. Infusion pumps are required to maintain a constant rate of fluid administration.

8. We recommend that the entire infusion set, including tubing up to the IV needle, be changed every 72 hours, except for the lipid emulsion tubing, which is changed every 24 hours. Parenteral solutions and lipid emulsions are changed daily.

9. We do not add heparin to peripheral PN solutions, although some centers routinely heparinize peripheral lines.

F. Central PN procedures

1. The catheter can be placed percutaneously or surgically (see Chap. 36). We prefer to use very thin number 2.0F Silastic catheters for percutaneous central venous access in VLBW infants. For larger infants, 2.7F catheters (e.g., Cook, Broviac) can be used. Larger catheters should be used cautiously because of the association with superior vena cava syndrome and vessel wall erosion.

2. The catheter is inserted through the antecubital, saphenous, internal or external jugular, subclavian, or less frequently, the umbilical or femoral vein. The catheter should be placed so that the tip lies at the junction of the right atrium and the superior or inferior vena cava.

3. We recognize the risks of using UACs to infuse PN solutions in VLBW neonates, including arterial thrombosis and infection. Difficulty in maintaining peripheral or other central access may necessitate their use.

4. Solutions are infused by pumps through a Y- or T-connector, as with peripheral PN (see **V.E**).

5. **If possible, the continuity of the central line should not be broken for blood drawing, medication infusion, or blood transfusion** because of the increased risk of infection.

6. **Heparin is added** at a concentration of 0.5 to 1.0 unit per milliliter of solution.

G. General PN procedures

1. Most medications are not given in PN solutions. If necessary, the PN catheter is flushed with saline solution, then the medication is infused in a compatible IV solution.

2. All solutions are prepared in the pharmacy under laminar-flow hoods and protected from ambient light to avoid photodegradation.

3. Minerals, vitamins, and trace elements are added in the pharmacy.

4. Because lipid peroxidation may increase with light, consider protecting emulsions from ambient light, including phototherapy.

H. Complications. Infants receiving PN are closely monitored (see Table 10-1).

1. **PN-associated cholestatic hepatitis** (see Chap. 18) is common and more often transient than progressive. Experimentally, even short-term PN can reduce bile flow and bile salt formation.

   a. **Risk factors** include prematurity, duration of PN administration, duration of fasting (since lack of enteral feeding also produces bile inspissation and cholestasis), underlying disease, infections, and narcotic administration.

   b. **Recommended management**

(1) Evaluate other possible causes of hepatic dysfunction.

(2) Attempt enteral feeding slowly and decrease PN. Even minimal enteral feedings may stimulate bile secretion.

(3) Reduce the amino acid infusion to the lower end of the recommended range, particularly if infusion rate has exceeded 3 gm/kg per day.

(4) Decrease dextrose infusion rates; high rates may produce steatosis.

(5) Continue lipid infusion, maintaining serum triglyceride concentrations of 200 mg/dl or lower.

2. **Cholelithiasis.** Risk factors include prolonged fasting, ileal disease or resection, and exposure to opiates or anticholinergic drugs.

3. **PN-associated hepatic steatosis.** PN enhances hepatic fatty acid synthesis and decreases triglyceride secretion. Experimentally, steatosis is associated with glucose overfeeding. Substituting IV lipid for some dextrose-derived calories can decrease hepatic fat accumulation. Lipids should not exceed 3.0 gm of fat per kilogram per day.

4. **Metabolic bone disease** (see Chap. 29)

5. **Metabolic abnormalities**

   a. Azotemia, hyperammonemia, and hyperchloremic metabolic acidosis have become uncommon since introduction of the current crystalline amino acid solutions. Term infants usually tolerate amino acid infusions of up to 3.0 gm/kg per day without overt metabolic derangement.

   b. VLBW newborns may develop metabolic acidosis even at low amino acid infusion rates (1.0 to 1.5 gm/kg per day). Treatment is either a temporary decrease of the infusion rate or a temporary substitution of acetate for chloride anions in the solution.

6. **Metabolic disturbances related to lipid emulsions,** which may require limiting lipid content

   a. **Hyperlipidemia and hypercholesterolemia.** The incidence is inversely related to gestational age. Treatment is a decrease in infusion rate sufficient to normalize serum lipid levels. It may help to shorten the lipid infusion time to 18 to 20 hours, and then check triglyceride levels 4 hours after lipid is stopped.

   b. **Hyperbilirubinemia.** Since free fatty acids can potentially displace bilirubin from albumin-binding sites, the safety of IV fat emulsions during neonatal hyperbilirubinemia has been questioned. At low infusion rates, displacement is not significant.

   c. **Severe thrombocytopenia or abnormal bleeding may be contraindications** to using lipids because decreased platelet adhesion has been reported with high triglyceride levels.

   d. Severe pulmonary insufficiency and hypoxemia (FiO_2 requirements >0.60) may warrant limited lipid use because of possible deleterious pulmonary effects, including fat accumulation in alveolar macrophages or lung arteries or capillaries, although this is seen in infants who have not received IV lipids.

   e. **Lipid tolerance may be impaired in sepsis,** which is associated with decreased lipoprotein activity, impaired triglyceride clearance, and fatty acid oxidation. It may be necessary to **limit the lipid infusion to 2.0 gm/kg per day if the triglyceride level is elevated.**

   f. Acute reactions (respiratory distress, cyanosis, fever, rash, vomiting) are associated with older formulations that are not currently available.

   g. Measuring triglyceride concentration assesses lipid clearance from plasma. However, the lipids may not be utilized for energy requirements because storage may occur instead of oxidation. Observing plasma samples for turbidity to monitor lipid tolerance is subjective and may give false-negative readings. It is possible to have elevated triglyceride concentrations without plasma turbidity.

VI. The need to optimize preterm infants' nutritional care and status continues after discharge.

A. Growth patterns. Growth patterns represent minimum goals, and failure to achieve the minimums should prompt nutritional assessment. Further evaluation for failure to thrive will depend on clinical judgment.

   1. Infants should gain at least 20 to 30 gm/day from term to 3 months corrected age, 15 gm/day from 3 to 6 months corrected age, and 10 gm/day from 6 to 9 months corrected age.
   2. Growth should be maintained or cross upward on standardized growth curves.
   3. Weight-length ratio should stay equal to or greater than twenty-fifth percentile.
   4. Head circumference should be proportional to weight gain and linear growth. Head circumference growth that has not achieved normal percentiles by 8 months corrected age has been associated with poor cognitive function and academic achievement, and behavioral problems. The rate of head circumference growth should be more than 0.5 cm/wk from term to 3 months corrected age and more than 0.25 cm/wk from 3 to 6 months corrected age.

B. Nutritional considerations in discharge planning. In addition to monitoring growth data, consider the type and volume of formula, appropriate vitamin and mineral supplements, length of feedings, oral feeding skill development, and medical factors that affect nutritional status.

C. Calorically enhanced feedings may be warranted to optimize growth after nursery discharge through the continued use of enhanced-caloric-density formula or human milk. This is most appropriate in infants in need of catch-up growth, SGA infants, infants with poor weight gain prior to discharge, and infants with inadequate volume intake to support appropriate growth. These infants may receive formulas concentrated to 24 kcal/oz or human milk calorically enhanced by the addition of dry formula powder, corn oil, or Polycose.

D. Use of preterm formulas. We do not normally recommend the use of HMF or preterm formulas after discharge because excessive nutrient intake is possible (e.g., vitamin D). Similac Neocare is designed to provide the former premature infant with more nutrients than the full-term infant formulas (e.g., protein, calcium, phosphorus, and zinc).

E. Multivitamin supplementation should be given to exclusively breast-fed infants, and to formula-fed infants until intake is more than 750 ml/day or a weight of 3.5 kg is reached.

F. Iron. All premature infants should be discharged with an iron supplement. The AAP recommends that iron supplementation be continued throughout the first year of life.

   1. All premature infants being fed human milk should receive iron supplements after discharge.
   2. All premature infants being fed formula should receive iron-fortified formula, and additional iron supplementation when indicated, after discharge.
   3. The total dose of iron for discharge should be individualized based on the infant's serum hematocrit and reticulocyte count.

G. In some states, **outpatient nutrition services** may be requested through the local Early Intervention Program (EIP) or associated community health center.

References

1. American Academy of Pediatrics, Committee on Nutrition (AAP-CON). *Pediatric Nutrition Handbook.* Evanston, Ill.: 1993.
2. European Society of Paediatric Gastroenterology and Nutrition, Committee on Nutrition of the Preterm Infant (ESP-AN-CON). *Nutrition and Feeding of Preterm Infants.* Oxford: Blackwell Scientific, 1987.
3. Greer, F. R. Formulas for the healthy term infant. *Pediatr. Rev.* 16:107, 1995.
4. Tsang, R. C., et al. (Eds.). *Nutritional Needs of the Premature Infant: Scientific Basis and Practical Guidelines.* Baltimore: Williams & Wilkins, 1993.
5. Zeigler, E. E. Malnutrition in the premature infant. *Acta Pediatr. Scand. Suppl.* 374:58–66, 1991.

11. BREAST-FEEDING

Susan D. Izatt

I. **Introduction.** Breast-feeding helps to foster mother–child interaction. In addition, data support the reduction of ear and respiratory infections, diarrheal illness, and atopic skin disorders among breast-fed infants.
II. **Prenatal preparation.** The obstetrician should ask about any history of breast surgery or disease and examine the nipples and breasts. Flat or inverted nipples can be treated prenatally. Information on support groups and prenatal classes should be made available.
III. **Postpartum education and management**
   A. **Physiology of lactation.** Circulating hormones cause preparatory changes in the breast. **Colostrum** is secreted as early as the second trimester because of placental lactogen. After delivery, **prolactin** stimulates milk production. Nursing is the most effective stimulant of continued prolactin production. Tactile stimulation of the nerve endings in the areola and nipple induce **oxytocin** release from the pituitary gland, which causes myoepithelial cells to contract and eject milk. Milk ejection, or the **letdown reflex,** is a neuroendocrine reflex that is affected negatively by maternal stress or pain.
   B. **Guidelines for initial breast-feeding of the healthy term infant**
      1. Infants should nurse as soon as possible after delivery, preferably within the initial alert state, and subsequently should nurse on demand. No supplemental feedings should be given unless medically indicated.
      2. We recommend nursing from each breast for 10 to 15 minutes. The new mother should be aware that the letdown reflex may take 3 to 5 minutes to be elicited.
      3. The infant's gums must be 0.5 to 1.0 cm behind the nipple-areola junction for efficient and comfortable nursing. Alternating positions will avoid stress on the areola from a single latch-on site.
   C. **Common maternal problems in the immediate postpartum period**
      1. **Nipple sensitivity** is a discomfort at latch-on that resolves with letdown. Sensitivity usually subsides over 1 to 2 weeks as the protective keratin layer builds up. Care includes nursing first on the more comfortable side, allowing nipples to air dry after nursing, and minimizing drying agents such as soap. **Sore nipples** are experienced throughout a feeding. The nipple may crack. The cause is often incorrect positioning of the infant. Nipple care is similar to that for nipple sensitivity.
      2. **Engorgement** presents 2 to 3 days post partum as bilateral generalized breast swelling. The mother may have a low-grade fever. Areolar engorgement makes latching on very difficult. Manual expression of milk or compression of the areola may make latching on easier for the infant. Engorgement due to increased breast blood flow will respond to warm packs and showers. Frequent breast-feeding is the best treatment.
      3. **Plugged ducts** present as isolated, tender lumps in an otherwise well mother. Nursing should continue. Manual massage of the area before and during nursing may promote duct drainage.
      4. **Mastitis** presents several weeks post partum as a tender, inflamed lump in a woman who may be febrile and have flu-like symptoms. She should continue breast-feeding and see her physician, who will prescribe an appropriate antibiotic.
IV. **Early infant concerns and management**
   A. **On-demand breast-feeding** by the nursing mother generally averages 8 to 12 feedings per day. Frequent nursing is the best way to increase the milk supply.

B. **Duration of feedings** should be sufficiently long for the fat-rich hindmilk to be released.

C. **Proper suck.** A fully open mouth, splayed lips, and pausing as the infant opens the mouth signifies effective nursing.

D. **An adequate output** for a well-fed infant is 6 to 8 wet diapers per day and a minimum of two stools per day.

E. **Activity and vigor** suggest a well-fed baby. If an infant is slow to gain weight but demonstrates good activity and adequate output, breast-feeding technique may require adjustment but not supplementation. Infants who do not demonstrate the above signs of a well-fed baby and lose weight require immediate evaluation.

F. **The first growth spurts** typically occur at 8 to 12 days and 3 to 4 weeks, but they may occur at any time. On-demand nursing will increase milk supply to meet the infant's needs.

V. **Special situations for breast-feeding**

A. **Cesarean delivery.** Nursing should begin as soon as possible after delivery, preferably while regional anesthesia is still in effect. If general anesthesia was used, the mother will first need to wake fully. Analgesics are not contraindicated in the nursing mother and may be helpful with incisional pain. Careful positioning of the infant will make the initial nursing experience more comfortable.

B. **Maternal medications.** Although many drugs are transferred to milk, breast-feeding is rarely contraindicated.

C. **Physiologic jaundice** is not a contraindication to breast-feeding. Frequent breast-feeding should be encouraged to enhance gut motility and bilirubin excretion (see Chap. 18).

D. **Multiple births.** These infants can be breast-fed because the supply of milk increases to meet the demand.

E. **Maternal viral infections** can be transmitted through breast milk, and breast-feeding may be contraindicated (see Chap. 23).

1. Mothers with active **herpetic** lesions on the breast should pump the milk and discard it until the lesions have dried. Active lesions elsewhere should be covered.

2. **HIV infection** can be transmitted via breast milk, although the risk has not been quantified. In the United States, HIV-infected mothers should not nurse. The World Health Organization recommends breast-feeding regardless of HIV status in areas where malnutrition and infectious diseases are important causes of infant mortality. Breast-feeding mothers in the United States who are at high risk for exposure to HIV should be counseled.

3. **Maternal hepatitis B** infection should not prevent breast-feeding in most circumstances. However, infants should receive hepatitis B immune globulin and hepatitis vaccine prior to receiving breast milk.

4. **Cytomegalovirus** transmission through human milk does not cause disease in term infants. Premature infants are at greater potential risk because of low concentrations of transplacentally acquired maternal antibodies.

F. **Immunizations** may be given to lactating women who have not received recommended immunizations before or during pregnancy.

VI. **Separation of mother and infant** poses specific challenges to the mother who desires to breast-feed. Separation commonly occurs with the delivery of a premature infant or an infant requiring special care.

A. **Initiation and maintenance of lactation during separation**

1. **Expression of breast milk** is best performed by an electric pump, although manual pumps and expression by hand can be used.

2. **Pumping routine**

a. Pumping should begin within 24 hours after delivery.

b. Pumping should be done a minimum of six times per day if possible, every 2 to 3 hours during the day and once at night. Frequent pumping maintains milk volume over long-term separation.

   c. Letdown may be inhibited. A quiet private site, sensory stimuli such as a picture of the infant, heat, and gentle massage of the nipple-areolar area may ease the letdown reflex.

   d. Failure of letdown may be assisted with **oxytocin nasal solution** (Syntocinon nasal spray, Sandoz Pharmaceuticals, East Hanover, New Jersey). Continued usage is not recommended.

  3. Decrease in milk production commonly occurs because of stress and long-term pumping. Mothers using a pump may notice a decrease in breast milk production at 3 to 4 weeks.

   a. Generally, milk production will increase as the infant begins to nurse at breast.

   b. Significant reduction in milk production has been treated with **metoclopramide** (Reglan, A. H. Robins Company, Richmond, Virginia). The American Academy of Pediatrics does not recommend the use of metoclopramide during lactation because of the theoretical risks of central nervous system effects. None have been described.

B. Storage of breast milk

  1. Containers include plastic bottles, disposable plastic nurser bags, and glass bottles. Glass containers may initially bind leukocytes found in breast milk, but they are released after 24 hours. No container is superior, but plastic bottles are unbreakable and leakproof. The containers used for storage of milk for a sick or premature infant should be sterile. Dishwashers that reach water temperatures of 180°F are adequate.

  2. The general practice is to store fresh breast milk at 39°F for 1 to 2 days.

  3. Breast milk may be frozen in a self-defrosting freezer for 6 months if kept in the back and off the bottom, away from the warming section of the defrost unit.

  4. Breast milk should be refrigerated or kept cool immediately after expression until it is used or frozen. Frozen milk should not be allowed to defrost during transport.

  5. Containers should be labeled with the date and should hold small volumes of breast milk suitable for single feedings.

  6. Frozen breast milk may be defrosted by thawing in the refrigerator or by holding under lukewarm water for 5 to 10 minutes. Thawed milk can be stored in a refrigerator for up to 48 hours. Microwave heating or boiling of breast milk is not recommended. As breast milk separates during freezing, it should be shaken before use. Once warmed to room temperature, it should be used immediately or discarded.

C. Breast-feeding the premature infant requires patience and support. Attention to ways that mother–infant interactions can be promoted should be considered at all points in the hospitalization.

  1. Kangaroo care or similar skin-to-skin techniques should begin as soon as the infant is stable.

  2. Gavage feedings should be given while the infant is being held by the mother near her naked breast. This should both promote rooting reflexes in the infant and encourage the letdown response in the mother.

  3. When a suck is demonstrated, the infant should be allowed to go to breast. Consistent oxygen saturation is maintained by premature infants during breast-feeding with no detrimental effects upon weight gain.

   a. The infant will likely suck only several times during the first nursing sessions. The mother should be assured that this is normal, as anxiety could inhibit letdown and compromise further sessions. The standard gavage feeding should be given after the nursing session.

   b. The mother should be encouraged to nurse at all feedings deemed appropriate for oral feeding. Minimizing rubber-nipple feedings will ease the transition to breast-feeding.

   c. The suck-swallow reflex will improve as the infant matures, and more feedings will be taken orally. Discharge planning includes increased breast-feeding sessions without supplementation to assess both weight gain and maternal confidence in breast-feeding skills. Rooming-in of mother–infant nursing pairs before discharge should be encouraged if feasible.

D. Discharge planning and follow-up is essential. The nursing mother should receive clear information on maternal care and signs of infant well-being. With support from the health-care team, many premature infants are discharged to home fully breast-feeding. Relactation support may be needed after discharge.

1. **Relactation with a nursing supplementer.** The supplementer consists of a plastic bottle and a thin tube that are worn by the mother at each nursing session. The tubing leads from the bottle to the mother's nipple-areolar area. When the baby nurses, the tubing is located above the nipple against the hard palate and allows supplementary feeding to reach the infant. Weaning of supplemental volumes can be done as the milk supply increases.

2. **Relactation may be supported with supplementation.** The infant should nurse at the breast for each feeding. Following a feeding, the infant is given a prescribed amount of breast milk or formula in a bottle. The mother should pump her breasts for 5 minutes after each nursing session to increase her milk supply. As the mother feels her milk supply is increasing and the infant requires less supplemental volume, the supplemental feedings can be weaned. This is best performed with supervision by a health-care professional such as a lactation consultant.

References

Powers, N. G., Slusser, W. Breastfeeding update 2: Immunology, nutrition, and advocacy. *Pediatr. Rev.* 18:147–161, 1997.

Slusser, W., Powers, N. G. Breastfeeding update 1: Immunology, nutrition, and advocacy. *Pediatr. Rev.* 18:111–119, 1997.

12. TEMPERATURE CONTROL

Kimberlee Chatson, Michael E. Fant, and John P. Cloherty

I. **Thermoregulation** in adults is achieved by both metabolic and muscular activity (e.g., shivering). During pregnancy, maternal mechanisms maintain intrauterine temperature. After birth, neonates must adapt to their relatively cold environment by the metabolic production of heat because they are not able to generate an adequate shivering response.

Term newborns have a source for thermogenesis in brown fat, which is highly vascularized and innervated by sympathetic neurons. When these infants face cold stress, norepinephrine levels increase and act in the brown-fat tissue to stimulate lipolysis. Most of the **free fatty acids (FFA)** are reesterified or oxidized; both reactions produce heat. Hypoxia or beta-adrenergic blockade decreases this response.

II. **Temperature maintenance in premature vs. term neonates**
   A. Most infants provided with reasonable warmth are able to maintain a normal temperature without sacrificing the calories needed for growth. Premature infants have special problems that put them at a disadvantage in temperature maintenance.
   1. They have a higher ratio of skin surface area to weight.
   2. They have decreased subcutaneous fat, with less insulative capacity.
   3. Their stores of brown fat are less well developed and therefore less able to mobilize norepinephrine and FFAs.
   4. They are unable to take in enough calories to provide nutrients for thermogenesis and growth.
   5. Oxygen consumption is limited in some premature infants because of pulmonary problems.
   B. **Temperature.** Infants who are asphyxiated will often be hypothermic. A measure of resuscitation adequacy is the infant's temperature after stabilization. Attention paid in the delivery room to the issues of sick neonates is important (see **V.B** and Chaps. 4, 13).
   C. **Cold stress.** Premature infants subjected to acute hypothermia respond with peripheral vasoconstriction, causing anaerobic metabolism and metabolic acidosis, which can cause pulmonary vessel constriction, leading to further hypoxia, anaerobic metabolism, and acidosis. Hypoxia further compromises the infant's response to cold. Premature infants are therefore at great risk for hypothermia and its sequelae (i.e., hypoglycemia, metabolic acidosis, increased oxygen consumption).
   The most common problem facing premature infants is **caloric loss from unrecognized chronic cold stress,** resulting in excess oxygen consumption and inability to gain weight.
   D. **Neonatal cold injury** occurs in low-birth-weight infants (LBW) and in term infants with central nervous system (CNS) disorders. It occurs more often in home deliveries, emergency deliveries, and settings where inadequate attention is paid to the thermal environment and heat loss. These infants have a bright red color because of the failure of oxyhemoglobin to dissociate at low temperature. There may be central pallor or cyanosis. The skin may show edema and sclerema. Core temperature is often below 32.2°C (90°F). Symptoms may include the following: (1) hypotension, (2) bradycardia, (3) slow, shallow, irregular respiration, (4) decreased activity, (5) poor suck, (6) decreased response to stimulus, (7) decreased reflexes, and (8) abdominal distention or vomiting. Metabolic acidosis, hypoglycemia, hyperkalemia, azotemia, and oliguria are present. Sometimes there is generalized bleeding, including pulmonary hemorrhage.

These infants should be warmed slowly in incubators set 1.5°C higher than the abdominal temperature. If the infant is hypotensive, saline or 5% albumin (10 to 20 ml/kg) should be given with sodium bicarbonate to correct metabolic acidosis. Evaluate and treat infection, bleeding, or injury. Some professionals believe that rewarming should be rapid [1].

E. **Hyperthermia,** elevated core body temperature, may be caused by a relatively hot environment, infection, dehydration, CNS dysfunction, or medications. Placing newborns in sunlight to control bilirubin is hazardous and may be associated with significant hyperthermia.

If environmental temperature is the cause of hyperthermia, the trunk and extremities are the same temperature and the baby is vasodilated. In sepsis, the baby may be vasoconstricted and the extremities 2 to 3°C colder than the trunk.

III. There are three major **mechanisms of heat loss** in neonates:
A. **Radiation.** Heat dissipates from the infant to a colder object in the environment.
B. **Convection.** Heat is lost from the skin to moving air. The amount lost depends on air speed and temperature.
C. **Evaporation.** The amount of loss depends primarily on air velocity and relative humidity. Wet infants in the delivery room are especially susceptible to evaporative heat loss.

IV. **Neutral thermal environments minimize heat loss.** Thermoneutral conditions exist when heat production (measured by oxygen consumption) is minimum and core temperature is within normal range (see Table 12-1).

V. **Treatment to prevent heat loss**
A. **Healthy infant**
1. Newborns should be dried and wrapped in a warmed blanket after delivery.
2. Examination in the delivery room should be done with the infant under radiant heaters. A skin probe with servocontrol to keep skin temperature at 36.5°C (97.7°F) should be used for prolonged examinations.
3. A cap is very useful in preventing significant heat loss through the scalp.
4. If the temperature is stable, the infant can be placed in a crib with blankets.

B. **Sick infant**
1. The infant should be dried.
2. Heated incubators should be used for transport.
3. Radiant warmers should be used during procedures.
4. Sick or premature infants require a thermoneutral environment; the incubator should be kept at an appropriate temperature (see Table 12-1) if a skin probe cannot be used because of the potential damage to skin in small premature infants.
5. Servocontrolled open warmer beds may be used for very sick infants when access is important. The use of plastic tenting (Saran Wrap) has been shown to be effective in preventing both convection heat loss and insensible water loss (see Chap. 9).
6. A small, clear plastic heat shield around small infants prevents convection heat loss by limiting air movement. It also prevents body heat from radiating to cold walls because the shield will be heated by the incubator air. This may help prevent apnea related to sudden changes in temperature. Clothing the infant helps but sometimes makes observation difficult.
7. Premature infants who are in relatively stable condition can be dressed in clothes and double-layered caps. We try to do this as soon as possible even if the infant is on a ventilator or an open bed. If infants are in an incubator, we dress them and cover them with blankets. We monitor heart rate and respiration because observation is difficult in a clothed infant (see Chap. 14).

VI. **Hazards of temperature control methods**

Table 12-1. Neutral thermal environmental temperatures

Age and weight	Temperature*	
	At start (°C)	Range (°C)
0–6 hours		
Under 1200 gm	35.0	34.0–35.4
1200–1500 gm	34.1	33.9–34.4
1501–2500 gm	33.4	32.8–33.8
Over 2500 gm (and >36 weeks' gestation)	32.9	32.0–33.8
6–12 hours		
Under 1200 gm	35.0	34.0–35.4
1200–1500 gm	34.0	33.5–34.4
1501–2500 gm	33.1	32.2–33.8
Over 2500 gm (and >36 weeks' gestation)	32.8	31.4–33.8
12–24 hours		
Under 1200 gm	34.0	34.0–35.4
1200–1500 gm	33.8	33.3–34.3
1501–2500 gm	32.8	31.8–33.8
Over 2500 gm (and >36 weeks' gestation)	32.4	31.0–33.7
24–36 hours		
Under 1200 gm	34.0	34.0–35.0
1200–1500 gm	33.6	33.1–34.2
1501–2500 gm	32.6	31.6–33.6
Over 2500 gm (and >36 weeks' gestation)	32.1	30.7–33.5
36–48 hours		
Under 1200 gm	34.0	34.0–35.0
1200–1500 gm	33.5	33.0–34.1
1501–2500 gm	32.5	31.4–33.5
Over 2500 gm (and >36 weeks' gestation)	31.9	30.5–33.3
48–72 hours		
Under 1200 gm	34.0	34.0–35.0
1200–1500 gm	33.5	33.0–34.0
1501–2500 gm	32.3	31.2–33.4
Over 2500 gm (and >36 weeks' gestation)	31.7	30.1–33.2
72–96 hours		
Under 1200 gm	34.0	34.0–35.0
1200–1500 gm	33.5	33.0–34.0
1501–2500 gm	32.2	31.1–33.2
Over 2500 gm (and >36 weeks' gestation)	31.3	29.8–32.8
4–12 days		
Under 1500 gm	33.5	33.0–34.0
1501–2500 gm	32.1	31.0–33.2
Over 2500 gm (and >36 weeks' gestation)		
4–5 days	31.0	29.5–32.6
5–6 days	30.9	29.4–32.3
6–8 days	30.6	29.0–32.2
8–10 days	30.3	29.0–31.8
10–12 days	30.1	29.0–31.4

continued

Table 12-1. *Continued*

| Age and weight | Temperature* | |
	At start (°C)	Range (°C)
12–14 days		
Under 1500 gm	33.5	32.6–34.0
1501–2500 gm	32.1	31.0–33.2
Over 2500 gm (and >36 weeks' gestation)	29.8	29.0–30.8
2–3 weeks		
Under 1500 gm	33.1	32.2–34.0
1501–2500 gm	31.7	30.5–33.0
3–4 weeks		
Under 1500 gm	32.6	31.6–33.6
1501–2500 gm	31.4	30.0–32.7
4–5 weeks		
Under 1500 gm	32.0	31.2–33.0
1501–2500 gm	30.9	29.5–35.2
5–6 weeks		
Under 1500 gm	31.4	30.6–32.3
1501–2500 gm	30.4	29.0–31.8

*In their version of this table, Scopes and Ahmed had the walls of the incubator 1 to 2°C warmer than ambient air temperatures. Generally speaking, the smaller infants in each weight group will require a temperature in the higher portion of the temperature range. Within each time range, the younger infants require the higher temperatures. Source: From M. Klaus and A. Fanaroff, The Physical Environment. In *Care of the High Risk Neonate.* 4th ed. Philadelphia: Saunders, 1993.

A. **Hyperthermia.** A servocontrolled warmer can generate excess heat, causing severe hyperthermia if the probe becomes detached from the infant's skin. Temperature alarms are subject to mechanical failure.

B. **Undetected infections.** A servocontrol may mask the hypothermia or hyperthermia associated with infection. A record of both environmental and core temperatures, along with observation for other signs of sepsis, will help detect this problem.

C. **Dehydration.** Radiant heaters can cause increased insensible water loss (IWL). By measuring **radiant power density (RPD)** and monitoring the weight and surface area of the infant, it is possible in a predictable manner to estimate IWL due to radiant warming.

References
Klaus, M. A., Martin, R. J., Fanaroff, A. A. (Eds.). The physical environment. In *Care of the High Risk Neonate* (4th Ed.). Philadelphia, Saunders, 1993.

LeBlanc, M. H. Thermoregulation: incubators, radiant warmers, artificial skins, and body hoods. *Clin. Perinatol.* 18:403, 1991.

Scopes, J. W., Ahmed, I. Range of critical temperatures in sick and premature newborn babies. *Arch. Dis. Child.* 47:417–419, 1966.

13. NEONATAL TRANSPORT

Virginia G. Nichols

I. Transport for ill neonates. Transport systems were developed as part of regional programs designed to reduce neonatal mortality and morbidity. Newborns are transported to Level III centers when maternal transport cannot be safely accomplished before delivery or when the management of a sick infant exceeds the ability of a Level I or II hospital.

II. Communication. Effective transport requires reliable communication at several levels.

    A. Hospital to hospital. Referral and educational networks among Level I, II, and III nurseries differ among the states. In some states, these structures are formalized and sometimes regulated. In others, networks are shaped by individually forged relationships. It is always important that Level I and II nurseries know how to contact regional Level III NICUs quickly; the NICUs must be responsive, recognizing the diagnostic and therapeutic capabilities of the referring nurseries.

    B. Within the Level III hospital. Communication must be efficient among subspecialty services at the receiving hospital. The medical control officer assumes responsibility for streamlining the flow of information to and from the referring physician and for identifying the appropriate admitting unit.

III. Transport team organization. The transport director is responsible for the quality of care; the director should be a clinician with both firsthand knowledge of the tertiary hospital and regular contact with referring hospitals.

    A. Personnel. Transport teams generally consist of at least two members skilled in neonatal clinical care. Members can include nurses, respiratory therapists, nurse practitioners, neonatologists, subspecialty fellows, and pediatric residents. Residents should be at least at the PL-3 level. Skills of team members must be assessed, and arrangements made for advice and supervision.

    B. Logistics

        1. Call triage. Efficient mechanisms for rapid triage of incoming calls are vital. The medical control officer initiates transport and locates the neonatologist or appropriate consultant for the referring physician, providing a single entry point.

        2. On-site versus off-site. The decision to keep a transport team on site should be based on activity level and local traffic patterns. In general, a team should depart within 30 minutes from the time of the call.

        3. Equipment. The team should be self-sufficient in terms of equipment, medications, and other supplies. Packs especially designed for neonatal transport are commercially available. These packs or other containers should be stocked by members of the transport team. The weight of the stocked packs should be documented for air transport. Commercial air transport services often request the use of equipment provided on board; unless the plane or helicopter has been specifically stocked for neonates, the team should bring its own supplies (see Tables 13-1, 13-2, 13-3).

        4. Carriers

            a. Ground transport. Many hospitals own, maintain, and insure ambulances or vans and train their drivers. Other hospitals contract with commercial ambulance services that agree to install the apparatus necessary to secure a transport incubator and to train their drivers appropriately. Vehicles must accommodate two or three team members in addition to the incubator and supply packs. The vehicle must supply

Table 13-1. Medications used by transport personnel

Albumin 5%	Gentamicin
Ampicillin	Heparin
Atropine	Isoproterenol
Calcium	Lidocaine
Calcium gluconate	Midazolan
Dexamethasone	Morphine
Dextrose 50% in water	Naloxone
Dextrose 10% in water	Normal saline
Diphenylhydantoin	Pancuronium
Digoxin	Phenobarbital
Dobutamine	Potassium chloride
Dopamine	Prostaglandin E_1 (on ice)
Epinephrine	Sodium bicarbonate
Erythromycin eye ointment	Sterile water
Fentanyl	Vitamin K_1

Table 13-2. Supplies used by transport personnel

Airways	Kelly clamp
Alcohol swabs	Lubricating ointment
Armboards	Monitor leads and transducers
Batteries	Needles: 18, 20, 26 gauge
Benzoin	Oxygen tubing
Betadine swabs	Replogle nasogastric tube
Blood culture bottles	Scalpel blades, no. 11
Blood pressure cuff	Sterile gown
Butterfly needles: 23 and 25 gauge	Stopcocks
Chest tubes: 10 and 12F, and connectors	Stylus
Chemstrip	Suction catheters: 6, 8, and 10F and traps
Clipboard with transport data forms, permission forms, progress notes, and booklet for parents	Suture material (silk 3-0, 4-0, on curved needle)
Culture tubes	Syringes: 1, 3, 10, 50 ml
Endotracheal tubes: 2.5, 3.0, 3.5, 4.0 mm	Tape
Face mask, term and premature	T-connectors
Feeding tubes: 5 and 8F	Thermometer
Gauze pads	Tubes for blood specimens
Gloves, sterile and exam	Umbilical catheters: 3.5 and 5F
Heimlich valves	Urine collection bags
Intravenous catheters: 22 and 24 gauge	Xeroform gauze
Intravenous tubing	

Table 13-3. Equipment for transport

Transport incubator equipped with
  monitors for heart rate, vascular pressures, oxygen saturation, temperature
  suction device
  infusion pumps
  gel-filled mattress
  adaptors to plug into both hospital and vehicle power
Airway equipment
  anesthesia bag with manometer
  laryngoscopes with no. 0 and no. 1 blades
  Magill forceps
Instrument tray for chest tubes and vascular catheters
Stethoscope
Tanks of oxygen and compressed air

---

oxygen, compressed air, heat, light, and a source of electrical power. The carrier must be ready to depart within 30 minutes.

  b. Air transport is more complicated. In regions where long distances frequently require flights, transport systems may maintain planes or helicopters. Alternatively, arrangements can be made with a commercial air transport service. In general, we avoid flights when transport can be accomplished safely by ground. Team members should be knowledgeable about the effects of alterations in the partial pressure of oxygen and gas expansion (see Table 13-4).

C. Legal and regulatory issues. The transport process may raise several legal issues, which vary from state to state. We periodically review all routine procedures and documentation forms with hospital legal counsel and provide the team with access to legal advice by phone when problems occur.

  1. Malpractice coverage is required for all team members. Each tertiary hospital should decide whether transport is considered an off-site or extended on-site activity because this can affect the necessary coverage.

  2. Carrier regulations vary from state to state and may conflict with transport goals. For example, some states require that an ambulance stop at the scene of an unattended accident until a second ambulance arrives. If this is an issue, it should be reviewed with the medical director of the commercial carrier.

  3. Consent should be obtained for procedures and transport prior to initiation of therapy, although this may be impossible in an emergency. Consent to remove the infant from the referring hospital must also be obtained. In extreme emergencies, any therapy, including the transport itself, can be initiated without consent if the patient will be substantially harmed by lack of therapy or transport. In that case, the documentation should be meticulous and the consent obtained as soon as possible. The hospital's risk management office should be apprised.

D. Documentation should be complete for every transport. We document all interactions between the two hospitals, including content and timing of the referral call, clinical guidance given, and transport team activity in the referral hospital and en route to the receiving hospital.

IV. Transport protocol

  A. Before departure

The process begins when an ill neonate is identified, and the referring physician's call is received by the medical control officer. If a transport team is required, the team and carrier are mobilized while the control officer gathers more information about the infant and advises the referring physician on

Table 13-4. FiO_2 required to maintain a constant PaO_2 at increasing altitude

Sea level	2000	4000	6000	8000	10,000	12,000	14,000	16,000	18,000	20,000
0.21	0.23	0.24	0.27	0.29	0.31	0.34	0.37	0.41	0.45	0.49
0.30	0.32	0.35	0.38	0.41	0.45	0.49	0.53	0.59	0.64	0.71
0.40	0.43	0.47	0.51	0.55	0.60	0.65	0.71	0.78	0.85	0.94
0.50	0.54	0.58	0.63	0.69	0.75	0.81	0.89	0.98		
0.60	0.65	0.70	0.76	0.83	0.99	0.98				
0.70	0.76	0.82	0.89	0.96						
0.80	0.86	0.94								
0.90	0.97									
1.00										

Column header: F_1O_2 at altitude (ft) of

Key: FiO_2 = fractional concentration of inspired oxygen; PaO_2 = arterial oxygen tension.

continuing management. Both the history and the advice are documented, and the time of the call is recorded.

1. **Recommendations** focus on basic cardiovascular, respiratory, and metabolic stabilization; recommendations for airway management and vascular access should be specific. All recommendations are documented.

2. The **neonatologist** discusses the patient's condition and potential therapies with team members prior to their departure. The time of departure is documented. We ask the referring physician for copies of the baby's chart and a copy of the mother's obstetrical chart, including results of prenatal screening tests, and a signed consent for transfer. If the parents do not speak English, we request an interpreter other than a family member who can convey complex medical information.

B. **En route**

While the team is en route, we generally contact the referring hospital for an update of the patient's condition, to offer further advice on management, and to obtain more details of the obstetrical and neonatal history. During this period, we prepare for the patient's arrival in the NICU.

C. **At the referring hospital**

Team members identify themselves to the referring physician, the nurse, and the parents if they are present in the nursery. The team should rapidly assess the infant's condition and plan needed diagnostic studies (e.g., blood gases, radiographs), airway management, and vascular access. Before procedures are performed, consent for treatment should be obtained from the parents. If the infant is acutely ill, therapy should be initiated, and the referring physician should communicate with the parents as soon as possible.

1. **Vascular access.** A peripheral venous catheter is frequently adequate to provide fluids and medications during the return transport. Umbilical venous catheters may be placed for immediate delivery of fluids and medications, and venous blood-gas samples can be used with an oxygen saturation monitor to assess respiratory status. Unless use of a central catheter is deemed urgent, we defer placement until the infant is in the NICU.

2. **Respiratory stabilization.** We select appropriate respiratory support on the basis of clinical condition and results of blood gas analysis obtained immediately upon arrival. If the infant is likely to require intubation and mechanical ventilation, we prefer to initiate these procedures at the referring hospital rather than risk respiratory failure en route.

3. **Cardiovascular stabilization.** We assess blood pressure and perfusion immediately upon arrival. A venous or arterial blood-gas sample for pH and serum bicarbonate can provide additional guidance. Infusions of normal saline or colloid, bicarbonate, or pressor support are provided as needed. If PGE_1 therapy is begun for suspected congenital heart disease, we intubate and mechanically ventilate the infant in anticipation of apnea and prepare infusions of volume and pressor support if they are required for hypotension.

4. **Metabolic stabilization.** We perform rapid estimation of serum glucose by Chemstrip from a heelstick sample. Profound hypoglycemia is treated with a slow bolus of 10% dextrose infusion (see Chap. 29), and the response is monitored. A serum glucose test can generally be deferred. If metabolic acidosis is suspected, a venous blood-gas sample can be used to assess need for treatment.

5. Because accurate determination of **sepsis risk** is difficult for a given infant, nearly all sick infants are treated with antibiotics during stabilization and transport. Samples for blood culture should be obtained before antibiotics are begun. In rare cases when meningitis is strongly suspected, we perform a lumbar puncture to obtain CSF samples before beginning antibiotics. The benefit derived from this procedure, however, must be weighed against the time requirement and potential clinical compromise of the infant before transport.

D. **Preparing to leave the referring hospital**

The decision to leave requires a realistic assessment of the acuteness of illness and the benefit to be gained by further interventions in the referring hospital. It is important to remember that a complete diagnosis is generally not necessary to provide appropriate initial respiratory and cardiovascular stabilization. On the other hand, it is rarely necessary to depart so hurriedly that stabilization is incomplete.

1. The extent of **monitoring** required during transport depends on the patient's condition and the duration of the trip. We always use cardiac monitors that can be powered from either a battery pack or the ambulance's power source. If an umbilical artery catheter is in place, we use a transducer to monitor blood pressure and detect disconnection. We often use an oxygen-saturation monitor, although the monitors may malfunction during ambulance rides. We monitor temperature with the incubator's servo-control device. The team should be able to clearly observe the infant to assess skin color and perfusion and to detect changes in clinical condition.

2. **Report to NICU.** Prior to departure, the team should telephone the tertiary hospital. Plans for interventions that may be necessary en route can be reviewed with the NICU staff, who can then prepare for all contingencies for admission.

3. **Parental consent.** A team member should speak briefly with the parents as soon as possible after arrival and again before departure. We obtain consent for transfer of the infant even if this has already been done by the referring physician. We also obtain consent for possible blood transfusions. If immediate surgery is anticipated, we try to facilitate the telephone consent process by contacting the surgeon and anesthesiologist so they can speak to the parents.

4. **Parents and transport.** We discourage parents from accompanying the infant, although parents are legally entitled to do so in some states. We provide a brochure that contains instructions for calling the NICU and specific directions for getting there.

E. **Returning to the Level III hospital**

If stabilization is complete, the return trip is generally uneventful. The benefit of obtaining vital signs en route should be weighed against the thermal loss incurred by opening the incubator. Continuous direct observation of the infant is the most important form of monitoring. We prepare medications or fluids that may be required during transport and place syringes inside the incubator. Transport teams may use cellular telephones in the ambulance to maintain contact with the NICU and seek advice for unexpected events.

F. **Arrival at the NICU**

1. **The primary caretakers** should receive clinical information about the infant from team members, as well as accurate and complete documentation of the team's activities.

2. The **parents** should be telephoned by a team member to tell them that their child has arrived safely. This can allay parental anxiety and help to establish a working relationship.

3. **Quality assurance** tools may be used to monitor transport activities. These and any other documentation of the admission should be completed shortly after the team returns.

4. The transport process provides opportunities for **outreach education.** A mechanism should be in place to encourage feedback to and from physicians and nurses in the referring hospital.

5. The transport team can facilitate **good communication** by identifying both the referring physician and the pediatrician who will be the primary physician.

V. **Specialized therapy**

A. **Anemia** (see Chap. 26). A variety of conditions may result in neonatal anemia, including twin-to-twin transfusion, perinatal hemorrhage, and hydrops fetalis. Acute hemorrhage may not be reflected in the hematocrit for several hours but may be suggested by the history and clinical presentation. In such cases, cross-matching of blood for transfusion should begin at the referral hospital while the transport team is en route. Emergently ill infants should be transfused with non-cross-matched Type O-negative packed cells until matched blood is available.

B. In infants in whom **congenital diaphragmatic hernia** is suspected (Chap. 33), we perform immediate endotracheal intubation and mechanical ventilation and place a nasogastric tube to prevent gaseous distention of herniated viscera during respiratory support.

C. **Abdominal wall defects** (see Chap. 33). Both omphalocele and gastroschisis are treated by placing a nasogastric tube and immediately wrapping exposed viscera with warm, sterile, saline-soaked gauze. An outer wrapping with a plastic bag or wrap will decrease heat and insensible water losses.

D. **Tracheoesophageal fistula and esophageal atresia** (see Chap. 33). Positive-pressure ventilation should be avoided if possible in order to avoid overdistention of the GI tract. It is sometimes possible to safely ventilate the infant by advancing the tip of the endotracheal tube past the opening of the fistula, but this approach risks selectively intubating a single mainstem bronchus. In all cases, a Replogle-type (sump) tube should be placed gently in the esophageal pouch to minimize aspiration risk.

E. Infants with **neural tube defects** (see Chap. 27) should be carefully wrapped in warm saline-soaked gauze and plastic wrap for protection and to minimize heat and fluid loss, as well as to prevent contamination with stool.

F. When **cyanotic congenital heart disease** is a possible diagnosis (see Chap. 25), prostaglandin E_1 (PGE_1) must be available during transport, and administration should begin at the referring hospital. Apnea, hyperthermia, and hypotension are common side effects of PGE_1. Endotracheal intubation is usually warranted for transport of an infant requiring PGE_1 infusion.

G. **Air transport**

1. **Partial pressure of oxygen.** Barometric pressure drops as altitude increases, leading to a decrease in oxygen tension. This is important even in aircraft with pressurized cabins because pressure is usually maintained at a level equal to 8000 to 10,000 feet above sea level. To correct for this, FiO_2 must be increased to result in an adequate PaO_2. The easiest and most expeditious way to monitor and adjust FiO_2 is to use transcutaneous monitoring techniques. If oxygen saturation monitoring is unavailable, PaO_2 is estimated using the alveolar gas equation. Values of FiO_2 needed to maintain a constant PaO_2 at any altitude are shown in Table 13-4.

2. **Gas expansion.** As barometric pressure decreases, gases trapped in closed spaces will expand. Even a small pneumothorax or normal gaseous distention of the intestinal tract may become clinically significant and should be drained or vented before transport. All infants undergoing air transport should have a nasogastric tube placed prior to departure.

References

Jaimovich, D. G., Vidyasagar, G. (Eds.). Transport medicine. *Pediatr. Clin. North Am.* 40(2):1993.

Task Force on Interhospital Transport, American Academy of Pediatrics. *Guidelines for Air and Ground Transport of Neonatal and Pediatric Patients.* Chicago: American Academy of Pediatrics, 1993.

14. DEVELOPMENTALLY SUPPORTIVE CARE*

Toni B. Vento and Emily Feinberg

I. **Introduction.** As neonates of ever younger gestational age survive, there is increasing interest in their long-term outcomes. Developmentally supportive care (DSC) modifies both the NICU environment and the manner in which care is delivered in order to offer a preventive approach to the physical and mental health of infants and their families. This approach, especially as developed by Als [1–5], has shown promise in improving the outcomes of very-low-birth-weight infants.

II. **Direct care supportive of infant development.** The general role of the caregiver in DSC is to estimate when stress is so great that it inhibits growth and to support the infant without compromising necessary medical treatment. Individualized care has been shown to be particularly important for infants with chronic lung disease, in whom decreasing unnecessary energy expenditures can decrease oxygen consumption and improve weight gain.

   A. **Structuring the 24-hour day.** The primary team coordinates interventions into clusters of care that are timed in accordance with the infant's sleep-wake cycles, state of alertness, medical needs, and feeding competence. The goal is to structure an individualized schedule that provides restfulness and integrates the infant into his or her family unit through their involvement with care.

   B. **Delivery of care.** Caregivers support development by viewing their interactions with the infant as a dialogue; taking the time to appreciate the infant's initiations as well as responses to care and modifying delivery accordingly are part of the process. For instance, a caregiver can use a soft voice or gentle touch or provide periods of recovery between manipulations. Other supports include nonnutritive sucking and hand-holding.

   C. **Transition periods.** Careful attention is directed to transition periods, for example, when an infant wakes or moves toward alertness. Increased support during these periods may be especially important for very premature infants and those with impaired central nervous systems, as these infants demonstrate greater disorganization.

   D. **Alert periods.** As an infant becomes alert, it is important to watch for behavioral cues so that caregivers can balance sensory input with the infant's current level of competence. Periods of alertness may support greater therapeutic and social interaction.

III. **A physical environment supportive of infants.** Most premature infants demonstrate sensitivity to the NICU environment; adverse responses to light, noise, and routine handling have been well documented. Modifying the environment and supporting parental nurturance of infants are essential to optimal infant development over time.

   A. **The physical environment.** Individualized bedside lighting is preferred to bright overhead lighting. Noise level can be reduced by creating a space for admissions and special procedures, educating staff and visitors about infants' responses to high noise levels, and dampening sounds from equipment such as telephones and monitor alarms. For example, covering an incubator with a heavy blanket provides protection from both light and noise. Safety is ensured by cardiac and respiratory monitoring; the Brigham and Women's Hospital nursery has covered incubators in this way since 1984 without incident.

*This is a revision of Chapter 35, Developmentally Supportive Care by Gretchen Lawhon and Alexandra Melzar, that appeared in the third edition of this book.

B. The social environment. Infants should be cared for in the context of their families. Each bedspace can be individualized by the presence of sheepskin bedding, pacifiers, or other items brought by parents. Along with family-specific areas for sleeping and showering, the simple presence of a recliner chair at each bedspace supports the comfort of the postpartum mother and other family members who are with the infant for extended periods. Siblings who have been screened for communicable illnesses present no increased risk to the infant.

IV. Caregiving considerations

A. Positioning. Aids such as blanket rolls, swaddling, and hands-on containment give support to comfortably aligned positions during sleep, routine care, and special procedures. Lying on the side or prone is more effective than supine positioning in optimizing oxygenation status in the premature infant.

B. Feeding. The feeding method and frequency of feedings are individualized to move toward demand feeding controlled by the infant. Feeding competence is helped by decreasing environmental stimulation and by securely containing the infant in a semiupright, flexed position. (See Chap. **10.VI.C** for detail on feeding methods.)

C. Suctioning has been demonstrated to lead to abrupt changes in blood flow in the brain. Support by a second caregiver helps to contain and stabilize the infant throughout the procedure. It is also recommended that suctioning be done when needed rather than on schedule.

D. Skin-to-skin holding. Such holding (kangaroo care) takes advantage of the soothing effects of touch and provides body warmth to the infant. Rhythmic respiratory movements appear to support increased respiratory stability with decreased incidence of apnea and bradycardia. Physical contact also appears to result in more restful infant sleep and a sense of calm in the parent. Successful breast-feeding is increased in mothers who hold their infants skin-to-skin. Opportunities for such holding should be discussed with families, including those of intubated VLBW infants.

E. Bathing. Full immersion of the infant's body to the shoulder and neck level in a suitable tub is recommended for all infants with intact skin. Placing the loosely swaddled infant in warm water and providing hands-on containment supports infant relaxation and temperature stability. Parents often view bathing as an integral part of infant care and should be given the opportunity to bathe their infant as soon as possible.

V. Implementation of developmentally supportive care. Implementation requires availability of resources and a collaborative approach. The primary team, including the family, should work toward establishing an individualized care plan, which can be reviewed daily at rounds. Regular meetings should include the family; this is especially important as the time for discharge approaches. In addition, a professional trained in infant development who is not a direct caregiver should be available as a resource. A multidisciplinary developmental-care committee may also be useful. Formal training in behavioral observation and assessment should be available to all staff.

VI. Discharge planning (see Chap. 16). Ongoing collaboration with families supports them in appreciating their infants' strengths and in developing strategies for dealing with changing infant abilities and environments; this element of developmental care moves families naturally toward discharge.

If formal behavioral assessments are necessary for referrals or as baselines for other follow-up care, several options exist that can be performed before discharge.*†

---

*Formal training in the Brazelton Newborn Assessment Scale is available by contacting Child Development Unit, The Children's Hospital, 300 Longwood Avenue, Boston, MA 02115, tel: (617) 735-6948.

†Formal training in the Assessment of Preterm Infant Behavior (APIB) and the Newborn Individualized Developmental Care and Assessment Program (NIDCAP) is available by contacting National APIB and NIDCAP Training Centers, Enders Pediatric Research Laboratories, Room EN-029, The Children's Hospital, 300 Longwood Avenue, Boston, MA 02115, tel: (617) 735-8249.

Acknowledgment
The authors were supported in part by Grant HO 24590003 EEPCD, OSERS, U.S. Department of Education. The authors would like to express their sincere thanks to Heidelise Als, Ph.D., and Deborah Buehler, Ph.D., for their guidance and assistance with this manuscript. Thank you, Gretchen Lawhon and Alexandra Melzar Briggs, for paving the way for this chapter.

References

1. Als, H. Individualized, family-focused developmental care for the very low birthweight preterm infant in the NICU. In S. L. Friedman and M. D. Sigman (Eds.). *Advances in Applied Developmental Psychology.* Norwood, N.J.: Ablex Publishing Company, 1992, 341.

2. Als, H., et al. *Newborn Individualized Developmental Care and Assessment Program (NIDCAP).* Unpublished training guide. 1986.

3. Als, H., et al. Individualized behavioral and environmental care for the very low birth weight preterm infant at high risk for bronchopulmonary dysplasia: Neonatal Intensive Care Unit and developmental outcome. *Pediatrics* 78:1123, 1986.

4. Als, H., et al. Individualized developmental care for the very low birthweight preterm infant: Medical and neurofunctional effects. *JAMA* 272:853, 1994.

5. Als, H., et al. Manual for the assessment of preterm infants' behavior (APIB). In H. E. Fitzgerald, B. M. Lester and M. W. Yogman (Eds.). *Theory and Research in Behavioral Pediatrics.* New York: Plenum Press, 1982, 65.

6. Harrison, H. The principles for family-centered neonatal care. *Pediatrics* 92:643, 1993.

7. Lawson, K., et al. Environmental characteristics of a neonatal intensive care unit. *Child Dev.* 48:1633, 1977.

8. Long, J. G., et al. Noise and hypoxemia in the intensive care nursery. *Pediatrics* 65:143, 1980.

15. FOLLOW-UP CARE OF VERY-LOW-BIRTH-WEIGHT INFANTS

Marie C. McCormick and Jane E. Stewart

I. Introduction. Appropriate follow-up for very-low-birth-weight (VLBW) infants requires a broad-based concept of outcome, including developmental progression, age-appropriate assessment, and management techniques. We consider health status to include (1) specific conditions or types of morbidity, (2) the effects of health problems on the usual activities of daily living, and (3) mental or social health or both. We are also concerned about how problems in these areas affect the child, as well as the family and other social units.

II. Follow-up programs support optimization of health status for NICU graduates and provide feedback information for improvement of medical care. Activities can include the following:

   A. Management of sequelae associated with prematurity. As ever smaller infants survive, the risk of chronic sequelae increases. At discharge, many infants experience symptoms related to such conditions as chronic lung disease (CLD), necrotizing enterocolitis (NEC), and intraventricular hemorrhage (IVH). Although symptoms related to most of these problems will diminish over the first 2 years of life, specialized medical management may be required.

   B. Consultative assessment and referral. Regardless of specific morbidity at the time of discharge, NICU graduates require surveillance for the emergence of a variety of problems that may require referral to and coordination of multiple preventive and rehabilitative services.

   C. Monitoring outcomes. Information on health problems and use of services by NICU graduates is integral to both the assessment of the effect of services and the counseling of parents regarding an individual child's future.

III. Program structure

   A. The **population** requiring follow-up care differs with each NICU and the availability and quality of community resources. Most programs use some combination of birth weight and specific complications as criteria. The criteria must be explicit and well understood by all members of the NICU team, with mechanisms developed for identifying and referring appropriate children. We currently target all graduates with a birth weight of under 1500 gm.

   B. Visits depend on the infant's needs and community resources. Most programs recommend a first visit within a few weeks of discharge to assess the transition to home. If not dictated by problems, future visits are scheduled to assess progress in key activities. In the absence of acute care needs, we assess patients routinely at 6-month intervals.

   C. Because the focus of follow-up care is enhancement of individual and family function, **personnel** must have breadth of expertise, including (1) clinical skill in the management of sequelae of prematurity, (2) the ability to perform neurologic and cognitive diagnostic assessment, (3) familiarity with general pediatric problems presenting in premature infants, (4) the ability to manage children with complex medical, motor, and cognitive problems, and (5) knowledge of the availability of and access to community programs.

   D. Methods for assessing an individual's progress depend on the need for direct assessment by health professionals and the quality of primary care and early intervention services. A variety of indirect approaches now exist for children with few problems and access to adequate community resources that provide information needed by NICU programs; such approaches operate at minimal inconvenience to parents.

155

IV. Specific conditions or types of morbidity. The increase in survival of VLBW infants has not resulted in an increased proportion of children with severe disabilities; the number of children surviving with such conditions has not been quantified, however. The majority of NICU graduates will be free of severe disabilities. The following conditions are the most common:

A. Neurologic problems

1. **Definition and prevalence.** Intracranial events are a major cause of both neonatal mortality and long-term morbidity. The risk of neurologic problems is increased by extreme prematurity, intracranial hemorrhage, periventricular leukomalacia or evidence of cerebral white-matter injury, severe asphyxia, severe IUGR, and prolonged sequelae such as CLD.

    a. **Severe neurologic problems** include significant cerebral palsy, major seizure disorders, hydrocephalus, sensorineural loss (blindness and deafness), and severe mental retardation (IQ less than 70). The prevalence of handicaps increases with decreasing birth weight: 17% of those weighing less than 800 gm, 9% of those weighing 801 to 1000 gm, and 3 to 5% of those weighing 1000 to 1500 gm. About 10% of surviving children with birth weight less than 1500 gm will be severely handicapped, a percentage that has not changed appreciably for about 20 years.

    b. **Less severe, relatively common neurologic abnormalities** are also seen in infants. These include transient changes in muscle tone (increased and decreased) of various muscle groups and muscle weaknesses leading to strabismus. In older children, high rates (30 to 50%) of minor neurologic abnormalities, fine motor coordination difficulties, and perceptual problems have been reported, although their functional significance is unclear.

2. **Assessment.** (For NICU assessment of intracranial hemorrhage and retinopathy of prematurity, see Chaps. 27 and 35.) All infants should have ophthalmologic examinations and hearing assessments with evoked potentials prior to discharge. Repeat vision and hearing screening is done in the first year of life for infants with normal discharge findings to detect the possible emergence of such problems as strabismus, recurrent otitis media, or language delay. The detection of neuromuscular problems in infancy requires careful neurologic examination. For children beyond the first year, specific subscales of routine tests of development are used for assessment.

3. **Management.** Both transient and long-term motor problems in infants require assessment and treatment by physical therapists. These services are usually provided at home through local programs. Infants with sensorineural handicaps require coordination of appropriate clinical services and developmental programs. For older children, consultation with the schools and participation in an educational plan are important.

B. Respiratory problems (see Chap. 24)

1. **Definition and prevalence.** Residual respiratory problems in NICU graduates include CLD, recurrent apnea, and airway obstruction. Later in childhood, graduates may experience higher rates of reactive airway disease. The proportion of infants discharged with CLD varies from 5 to 35% among hospitals, although most infants will have shown resolution of symptoms by 2 years of age. The prevalence of reactive airway disease is estimated to be 20% of VLBW children, twice that of normal-birth-weight (NBW) children.

2. **Assessment**

    a. **Respiratory effort:** resting respiratory rate, use of accessory muscles, prolonged expiratory phase or expiratory wheezing, presence of rales.

    b. **Oxygenation:** periodic measurement of hemoglobin or hematocrit, pulse oximetry, arterial blood gases, or combination.

    c. **Pharmacotherapy:** serum levels of drugs when appropriate; monitoring for side effects.

d. Physical growth (see **V.A**)

3. **Management** includes the use of bronchodilators, fluid restriction, diuretics, adequate caloric intake for weight gain, chest physiotherapy, and oxygen as needed. Parents are instructed in monitoring respiratory rate, use of apnea monitors, use of CPR, and avoidance of respiratory irritants (e.g., smoking). For older children, asthma management protocols may be needed.

C. Other health problems

1. **Definition and prevalence.** VLBW survivors have higher rates of general morbidity than do children of normal birth weight, but specific conditions and relationship to prematurity are not yet established. These infants are four times more likely to be rehospitalized during the first year than NBW infants; up to 60% are rehospitalized at least once by the time they reach school age. About half of this medical care is due to sequelae of prematurity. The increased risk of hospitalization persists into early school age; 7% of VLBW children are hospitalized in a given year, compared with 2% of NBW children.

   The risk of illness not requiring hospitalization has not been established, but a predisposition to infections such as otitis media may occur. VLBW children do not appear to be at increased risk for nonintentional injury. Intentional injury or child abuse may be more frequent in NICU graduates, but the data are subject to criticism. The risk of morbidity among older children is currently being elucidated; they appear to be at twice the risk of NBW children for reactive airway disease.

2. **Detection and management.** The increased risk of morbidity for VLBW infants requires access to high-quality pediatric care. This is both most important and most problematic for infants from disadvantaged families, where the risk conferred by low birth weight is compounded by the risks associated with poverty. Primary care provided to these infants should include the completion of recommended immunizations on a schedule consistent with chronological age and annual influenza shots for children with pulmonary problems.

V. Limitations in daily activities. The concept of limitations in daily living has been developed to capture the personal impact of health problems. For infants, important daily activities include physical growth, psychosocial development, and the degree to which greater difficulty is encountered or increased help is needed than is normal for age in routine issues like feeding, elimination, and achieving regular sleep patterns. As children grow older, the scope of activities broadens to include play, sports, and participation in school and work.

A. Physical growth

1. **Definition and prevalence.** The normal growth patterns of premature infants are being established. One or more periods of rapid, catch-up growth generally occur during the first 3 years; only about 20% of VLBW infants are below the third percentile by the age of 3 years. The pattern favors head growth followed by gains in weight and height. By the time they reach school age, the average head size is normal for age, whereas height and weight may fall into less than the 50th percentile (but in a normal-for-age range). Those at risk for poor growth include infants with chronic disease, malformations, and environmental deprivation (nonorganic failure to thrive).

2. **Detection.** Routine growth measurements should be plotted on standard curves; percentiles for both chronological age and age corrected for duration of gestation should be recorded. Monitoring for iron deficiency anemia is also recommended.

3. **Management** entails a careful history of feeding practices, including amount and types of food. For children with chronic illnesses, aggressive management with high-calorie formulas may be needed. In addition, careful attention should be given to appropriate supplements such as iron, vitamins, and fluoride.

B. Psychosocial development

1. **Definition and prevalence.** The psychosocial development of VLBW infants has attracted a great deal of attention. Most commonly, progress is assessed by use of some form of intelligence or development quotient (IQ or DQ) on an established scale. VLBW infants tend to average somewhat lower on such scales than NBW infants, but they still fall within the normal range. The percentage of infants with scores lower than 68 to 70 (below two standard deviations) is between 5 and 20% in different studies; the lower the birth weight, the higher the proportion of infants seen in this range (but they are still in the minority). Most studies reflect the status of children under the age of 2 years. Among older children, the percentage severely affected (i.e., in the same range) appears to be the same, but the percentage with school failure or school problems is as high as 50%, with rates of 20% even among children with average IQ scores.

   Children at greater risk for developmental problems include ELBW infants; those with evidence of intracranial problems such as hemorrhage, cerebral white-matter injury, and shunting for hydrocephalus; those with severe chronic sequelae such as CLD; and those with severe IUGR. Developmental problems related to these risk factors may emerge relatively early. Toward the end of the second year, problems related to environmental factors such as poverty (with its increased risk of low birth weight) also may contribute to delayed development. The risk factors for school problems in the presence of normal IQs are still being established.

2. **Detection** combines routine inquiry about the achievement of developmental milestones with periodic assessment. For screening purposes in primary care, the Denver Developmental Screening Instruments provide a useful start, although they must be used with caution in premature infants. However, their use does not substitute for periodic assessment by well-standardized, more diagnostic observational instruments such as the Bayley Scales of Infant Development II, or the Wechsler scales for children with developmental achievement. School functioning may be assessed with standard scales such as the Woodcock-Johnson. For specific areas of performance, or for children with sensorineural handicaps, special testing by experienced assessors is needed.

3. **Management** requires coordination of therapeutic modalities and health professionals over time. Physical therapists may provide early regimens to enhance the normal motor activities necessary for other aspects of development. Specialists in the development of infants and preschool children may provide programs for parents to enhance the child's acquisition of developmental skills, especially when the parents have had limited experience. More intensive interventions used with combined home visits and educational day care have proven successful in enhancing development, but they remain expensive for many communities. When the child reaches school age, careful coordination in planning individualized educational plans is needed.

C. Other activities

1. **Definition and prevalence.** Parents report a variety of problems for VLBW infants. These infants may be difficult to feed, requiring prolonged periods to finish a meal and more frequent feedings than usual. Problems in regulation of state may cause difficulty in establishing sleeping patterns, over- or underreaction to stimuli, and perceptions of temperamental difficulties. Abnormal patterns of parent–infant interaction may be established that exacerbate problems. The prevalence and risk factors for these problems are still being established. Anecdotal experience suggests that they are fairly frequent but may not be revealed without specific questions during interviews. In addition, the health problems noted previously may reduce VLBW children's abilities to engage in many usual activities.

2. **Detection.** Few established scales of documented clinical utility are available. Detection generally relies on sensitive inquiry.
3. **Management.** For many parents, reassurance that such problems are relatively frequent among premature infants and therefore may represent their norm is sufficient. For others, specific management techniques, psychotherapy, or parent support groups may be indicated.

VI. Emotional and behavioral health

A. **Overview.** Routine consideration of pediatric emotional and behavioral issues is relatively recent. Most current information relates to behavior problems.

B. **Behavior problems**

1. **Definition and prevalence.** Because children often lack the ability to communicate emotions, early specialists in pediatric mental health relied on aberrant behaviors to signal mental health problems. Such behaviors included those thought to be associated with increased aggression or withdrawal. On standardized measures of behavior, about 15% of general populations of preschool children have abnormal scores (7 to 10% severely affected), with recent evidence suggesting that such abnormalities are associated with a high risk of future problems such as delinquency.

VLBW children are at increased risk for behavior problems related to hyperactivity and/or attention deficit. The risk factors for behavior problems also include stress within the family, maternal depression, and smoking. Behavior problems can contribute to school difficulties. In relation to both school problems and other health issues, VLBW children are seen as less socially competent than NBW children.

2. **Detection.** In the United States, the most commonly used scales are those developed by Achenbach to elicit parental and teacher concerns. The youngest children for which such standardized scales are available are 2 years old.

3. **Management** depends on the nature of the problem and the degree of functional disruption. Some problems may be managed with special educational programs; others may involve referral to appropriate psychotherapy services, medication, or both.

VII. Overall perceived health. Self-rating of health or, in the case of children, parental rating of health has proved a powerful predictor of health care use in general populations. VLBW infants may be perceived as less healthy than their peers, largely as a result of experiences and parental anxiety in the neonatal period rather than because of their current health status. For older children, parental ratings tend to be consistent with the current level of health problems experienced by the child. Risk factors for such parental ratings of the health of VLBW children include poor maternal health, which suggests familial aggregation of poor health.

VIII. Family and social impact

A. **Overview.** The assessment of the social effects of low-birth-weight survivors has been extended to include the financial and other burdens associated with caring for these infants that may fall to the family or to the medical or educational systems. To date, data are rudimentary.

B. **Definition and prevalence.** Most attention has focused on the costs of initial hospitalization, with much less information available on subsequent medical care. However, the monthly costs for medical services for VLBW infants until age 3 may average 3 to 200 times that of a healthy term child (i.e., $60 to $1200 versus $22 to $26). This may well be an underestimate, because the study involved did not assess the full range of direct and indirect costs that may be associated with caring for such infants.

C. **Detection and management.** Unless specific questions are asked, the stresses of caring for such children may be minimized by parents. Careful nursing and social work evaluations are needed to elicit difficulties and plan support where appropriate and available (see Chap. 16).

References
Achenbach, T. M., Edelbrock, C., Howell, C. T. Empirically based assessment of the behavioral/emotional problems of 2- and 3-year-old children. *J. Abnorm. Child Psychol.* 15:629–650, 1987.
Escobar, G. J., Littenberg, B., Pettiti, D. B. Outcome among very low birthweight infants; A meta-analysis. *Arch. Dis. Child.* 66:204–211, 1991.
McCormick, M. C., Stewart, M. C., Cohen, R., et al. Follow-up of NICU graduates: Why, what, and by whom. *J. Intensive Care Med.* 10:213–225, 1995.

16. DISCHARGE PLANNING

Kimberly Cox and Linda Zaccagnini

The survival rate for low-birth-weight (less than 2500 gm), moderately low-birth-weight (1500–2500 gm), very-low-birth-weight (less than 1500 gm), and extremely low-birth-weight (less than 1000 gm) infants has increased in the past three decades. The infant who weighs less than 750 gm has a greater than 30% chance of survival, while survival rates for the infant weighing more than 1000 gm are 90% (see Table 3-2 in Chap. 3). Greater survival rates for preterm infants have created a population with unique long-term health care needs. Changes in the health care system in the United States are encouraging earlier discharge and more out-of-hospital care.

Effective discharge planning ensures continuity of care from hospital to home. The plan must provide for individualized family and infant needs and prepare family members and health care providers for infant care requirements.

I. **Features of a good discharge plan**
   A. Individualized to meet infant and family needs and resources
   B. Begins early
   C. Includes clearly identified goals
   D. Decreases fragmentation and duplication of services
   E. Decreases delays in accessing care and progressing through the provider system
   F. Anticipates potential delays in development and directs care toward prevention and early intervention
   G. Is community based
   H. Increases quality of care
II. **System assessment.** Assign a primary team upon admission to assist the family in developing trusting relationships with staff. This enhances communication and minimizes the number of staff with whom the family will need to interact. It is important to know how your facility functions, who assumes responsibility for various components of discharge planning, and how communication is carried out. Early planning will expedite discharge. Delays in discharge can be costly, and readmissions can be traumatic to the infant and the family.
   A. A **primary physician** or **nurse practitioner** is assigned to the infant at admission. That person is responsible for daily management of issues. In teaching institutions where staff rotate monthly, families may need to adjust to many different primary providers. It is helpful for an assigned primary attending physician or practitioner to follow up infants with complex cases throughout their stay and provide continuity.
   B. **Primary and associate nurses** follow up the family through the NICU stay, coordinating and implementing the care plan developed by the team.
   C. **Social workers** support the family in crisis and assist in locating available resources.
   D. **Discharge planners** vary from institution to institution. They may be specialized advance practice nurses, clinical specialists, primary nurses, social workers, or a combination of players.
   E. **Respiratory, physical, and occupational therapists** can teach families skills and can transfer care to community resources.
   F. **Payer resources.** HMOs and third-party payers may have case managers or resource personnel to assist and approve coordination of services. Preferred providers may be contractually required to be used. Case managers can clarify coverage issues or advise of availability.

III. **Family assessment** may begin prior to admission. Ongoing communication between professionals and the family will allow providers to develop a multidisciplinary, individualized care plan that includes discharge planning. Involving the family in developing the plan optimizes its success by individualizing the plan and adding to the parents' feeling of control. The transition to home can go smoothly, even in the most complex cases, with early planning, ongoing teaching, and attention to the family's needs and resources.

A. **Family dynamics.** Include the following issues when assessing the family's readiness for discharge:

1. Willingness to assume responsibility for care
2. Previous or present experiences with infant care and medical procedures
3. The actual as well as perceived complexity of the skills required to care for the infant
4. Family structure
5. Financial concerns
6. Home setting
7. Coping skills
8. Supports
9. Medical and psychological history (ongoing illness may impact caretaking needs)
10. Cultural beliefs (bonding, roles, and available supports)
11. Language barriers (may require an interpreter)

B. **Home environment.** Structural components of the home may need alteration. Confirm electrical, water, heating, and cooling resources.

C. **Stress and coping.** In the NICU, discuss what it will be like to have the infant at home. Consider who will be involved for the extended duration and for available support. Referral to a parent group or specialized support group may be helpful. Explore the availability of community services for counseling and social needs. The following are common issues:

1. **Grief.** Parents need to cope with the loss of their "perfect" infant. The four psychological effects of a high-risk pregnancy are denial, blame and guilt, feelings of failure, and ambivalence.
2. **Abandonment and isolation.** Much attention and support are available while the infant is hospitalized. After discharge, parents may feel alone and abandoned.
3. **Siblings** may delay reacting until the new baby comes home and then respond with regressive or acting-out behaviors.
4. **Parenting disorders.** When the child is well, parents may be so overburdened with the memories of severe illness that they never treat the infant as a healthy child.
5. **Privacy.** Infants requiring complex care at home may require "blocks" of nursing or ancillary care at home; these disrupt space and privacy. An array of "strangers" in the home adds stress to the family.

D. **Financial resources.** Complete a financial assessment early. Early delivery or complex care can alter the family's plans for work and child care. Loss of work, income changes, cost of copayments, and inability to make career moves because of insurance coverage all impact the family's financial stability.

IV. **Infant's readiness for discharge**

A. **Healthy, growing, preterm infants** are considered ready for discharge when they meet the following criteria:

1. Ability to maintain temperature in an open crib
2. Ability to take all feedings by bottle or breast without respiratory compromise
3. No apnea or bradycardia for 5 days (see Chap. 24, Apnea)
4. Steady weight gain

B. **Infants with specialized needs** require a complex, flexible, ongoing discharge and teaching plan. Discharge specifics may not be identified until just prior to discharge. It is important to consider the relative fragility and stability of various systems and the complexity of interventions. Include assessment of behavioral and developmental issues, and evaluate parental recognition and response.

C. Discharge screening. Complete routine screening tests and immunizations according to individual institutional guidelines.

1. **Hearing screening** (see Chap. 35)
2. **Eye exams** (see Chap. 35)
3. Perform **cranial ultrasound** (see Chap. 27) screening for intraventricular hemorrhage or periventricular leukomalacia for all infants who
   a. weigh less than 1500 gm
   b. are under 34 weeks gestational if mechanically ventilated
   Perform **head ultrasound** at
   a. day of life 1–3
   b. day of life 7–10
   c. day of life 21–28
4. **Immunizations.** Administer according to American Academy of Pediatrics guidelines based on chronological, not postconceptional, age (see Chap. 3).

V. Follow-up care for the infant with special needs may involve many different services and providers to meet all of the child's needs.

A. Primary care is usually provided through a pediatrician, family practitioner, or nurse practitioner. Ongoing communication between NICU staff and the primary care provider begins long before discharge. This maintains continuity and improves the infant's chances of receiving appropriate medical care after discharge.

B. Specialty services may be required.

C. Infant follow-up programs affiliated with many Level III nurseries offer multidisciplinary services including developmental assessments, hearing and visual screening, physical therapy assessments, and referrals to community-based providers and support groups (see Chap. 15).

D. Early intervention programs are community based and offer multidisciplinary services for children from birth to age 3. Children deemed at biological, environmental, or emotional risk are eligible. Programs are partially federally funded and are offered free or on a sliding scale. They provide multidisciplinary services including physical therapy, early childhood education, social services, and parental support groups. Services may be home-based or center-based. Make referrals early in the child's hospital stay, as some centers have long waiting lists.

VI. Preparing the home for the infant's discharge

A. Home care services are becoming more widely available; however, their ability to provide specialized pediatric or neonatal services is variable. Assess individual programs separately before making a referral.

B. Skilled nursing care

1. **Public health nurses** may do home visits before discharge to assess the family's readiness and the home situation. They may also do well-baby and basic health care teaching.
2. **Visiting nurse associations** provide home visits for reinforcement of teaching, health and psychosocial assessments, and short-term treatments or nursing care. They usually charge service fees.
3. **Home health care agencies** provide skilled nursing care, home health aids, physical and/or occupational therapy, and medical equipment and supplies. Fees for service and insurance coverage are highly variable.

C. Respite care. Many parents do not realize how emotionally and physically draining it can be to care for a child with complex medical needs. The usual support people, such as relatives, friends, and babysitters, may be uncomfortable or be unable to deal with the added responsibility. Explore resources for respite care before discharge.

D. **Notify emergency care providers** including community hospital emergency wards and local EMT or fire responders of the child's presence, medical needs, and likely problems. This will assure appropriate emergency response.

E. **Local utility companies** (telephone, electricity, fuel) should be notified in writing of the child's presence in the home so they will assign priority resumption of services if there is an interruption.

F. **Supplies and equipment**

  1. Order **supplies and equipment** well before discharge to assure availability. Have caregivers care for their child using the home monitors and oxygen equipment in the NICU. This increases their skill and confidence.

  2. **Medications and special formulas** or dietary supplements should also be ordered early and delivered to the home. Many preparations are not readily available in the community.

  3. It is helpful to locate a **home health agency** that can be contracted to coordinate equipment delivery and repair, reorder and deliver medical supplies and medications, and arrange for home care providers. It enables the family to deal with only one person for all of their home care needs.

VII. **Preparing the family for discharge**

A. **Simplify care** by thoroughly reviewing the infant's care regimen. Alter medication schedules to fit the family's schedule. Eliminate unnecessary medications. Formulas and additives can be changed to less expensive or more easily obtained products, such as substituting corn oil for medium chain triglyceride (MCT) oil. Get the infant used to the daily schedule that will be followed at home.

B. Begin **teaching** early to allow the caregivers adequate time to process information, practice skills, and formulate questions. Make teaching protocols detailed and thorough. Include written information for the family to take home to use as reference (see Figs. 16-1, 16-2, and 16-3). Standardize information to ensure that every family member receives the same essential information. Address well-baby care, developmental issues, and necessary medical information. Include several family members in the learning process so that the parents can get needed support.

C. **Provide transitional programs** for parents. Schedule blocks of hands-on care or have the parents room in with the infant in the NICU. This maximizes parental confidence and competence and helps strengthen the parent–infant bond.

D. **Retrotransfer** to a Level II nursery in the community. This may allow the family to spend more time with the infant, and facilitate learning in a less acute environment.

E. It is vital to **include the family** in formulating all plans and, whenever possible, choosing care providers.

VIII. **Alternatives to home discharge** may be temporary or permanent. Integrating the child into the home may be difficult because of medical needs or family dynamics. Decisions regarding alternative placement may be painful for the family. Alternatives vary widely from community to community.

A. **Specialized foster care** places the special-needs infant in a home setting with specially trained caregivers. The ultimate goal is to place the infant back with the family.

B. **Pediatric rehabilitation hospitals** can be used for the high-risk infant who requires ongoing but less acute hospital care.

C. **Pediatric nursing homes** provide extended care at a skilled level.

D. **Hospice care** may be institutional or home based. It focuses on maximizing the quality of life when cure is no longer possible.

IX. **Financial concerns**

A. Neonatal intensive care, especially for very-low-birth-weight infants, ranks among the most costly of all hospital admissions. Health insurance may not cover 100% of costs.

CHILDREN'S HOSPITAL
DEPARTMENT OF NURSING
CONTINUING CARE PROGRAM

DISCHARGE PLAN

ADMISSION DATE_____

DISCHARGE DATE_____

ATTENDING PHYSICIAN_____

RESIDENT PHYSICIAN _____

PRIMARY NURSE _____ DISCHARGE DIAGNOSES

OTHER SERVICES _____   (primary) _____

_____   (secondary) _____

_____   (tertiary) _____

DISCHARGE TO HOME_____ OTHER_____   __ _____

DIET _____

(see page ____2 or ____page 3 for additional information)

TREATMENT   TIME OR FREQUENCY

_____   _____

_____   _____

_____   _____

(see page ____2 or ____page 3 for additional information)

MEDICATIONS (List all current)

　　　　　name of drug　　　　　　dose　　　　time　　　　　　special instructions

_____ _____ _____ _____

_____ _____ _____ _____

_____ _____ _____ _____

_____ _____ _____ _____

(see page ____2 or ____page 3 for additional information)

____ (prescriptions given to patient/parents)

COMMUNITY PROVIDERS

agency name & address_____   contact person _____

_____   telephone _____ start date _____

_____   service/frequency requested _____

agency name & address_____   contact person _____

_____   telephone _____ start date _____

_____   service/frequency requested _____

FOLLOW UP MEDICAL/CLINIC APPOINTMENTS

1. Clinic _____   2. Clinic _____

　　Date_____   　　Date_____

　　Contact person _____RN/MD   　　Contact person _____RN/MD

　　tel # _____   　　tel # _____

_____ Check if page 2 is attached.

I ACKNOWLEDGE MY PARTICIPATION IN, REVIEW OF AND AGREEMENT WITH THE ABOVE PLAN. I HAVE RECEIVED A
WRITTEN COPY, MY QUESTIONS HAVE BEEN ANSWERED, AND I UNDERSTAND THE CONTENTS. I UNDERSTAND
THAT, IN ORDER TO ARRANGE NECESSARY SERVICES, RELEVANT MEDICAL AND OTHER INFORMATION IS BEING
RELEASED TO THE ABOVE-LISTED PROVIDERS.

_____   _____

(signature of patient/parent/legal guardian)　　　　(date)   (signature of discharging nurse)　　　　(tel. #)　　　(date)

If patient/parent/legal guardian does not sign above,   _____

state reasons for not signing, including any objections to   (signature of preparing nurse)

the plan: _____

_____

IMPORTANT!! BE SURE TO BRING THIS FORM WITH YOU ON YOUR NEXT VISIT TO THE CLINIC OR YOUR DOCTOR.

Fig. 16-1. Discharge plan.

BRIGHAM AND WOMEN'S HOSPITAL
A Teaching Affiliate of Harvard Medical School
75 Francis Street, Boston, Massachusetts 02115

NEWBORN DISCHARGE INSTRUCTION SHEET

BABY'S CAREGIVERS
Private Pediatrician or Health Center _____
Attending Neonatologist _____
Social Worker _____
Primary Nurse(s) _____
Other _____

PREPARATION FOR DISCHARGE
I am comfortable with these aspects of my baby's care: (Comments)

- ☐ Bathing/skin care _____
- ☐ Breastfeeding _____
- ☐ Bottlefeeding/type of formula _____
- ☐ Assessing baby's breathing pattern _____
- ☐ Taking baby's temperature _____
- ☐ Bowel patterns _____
- ☐ Urination _____
- ☐ Baby's behavior _____
- ☐ Car seat use _____
- ☐ CPR _____
- ☐ When to contact baby's doctor _____
- ☐ Other _____

MEDICATIONS THAT BABY IS TAKING

MEDICATION AND CONCENTRATION	BABY IS GETTING MEDICATION BECAUSE	AMOUNT TO GIVE	HOW LONG TO GIVE WHEN TO GIVE HOW TO GIVE	SPECIAL THINGS TO WATCH FOR
1.				
2.				
3.				

☐ Prescriptions given   ☐ Medications Given   ☐ Special instructions attached

BABY'S FOLLOW-UP CARE

	Appointment Date	Phone Number
Private Pedi/Health Center		
Early Intervention		
Visiting Nurse or Public Health Nurse		
Follow-up programs		
Other		

BABY'S PROBLEMS IN THE HOSPITAL HAVE BEEN:

- ☐ Prematurity/Gestational Age at birth _____ weeks
- ☐ Respiratory distress syndrome (RDS)
- ☐ Patent Ductus Arteriosus (PDA)
- ☐ Bronchopulmonary Dysplasia (BPD)
- ☐ Cardiac _____
- ☐ Retinopathy of prematurity (ROP)
- ☐ Intraventricular hemorrhage (IVH)
- ☐ Apnea of prematurity
- ☐ Necrotizing enterocolitis (NEC)
- ☐ Other _____

Birth weight ___ lbs ___ oz
Discharge weight ___ lbs ___ oz
Birthdate _____
Discharge date from NICU _____

Hepatitis B vaccine given _____
                                Date

This information has been reviewed with me and my questions have been answered.

_____ _____ _____ RN
Date   Parent signature   RN signature

Fig. 16-2. Newborn discharge instruction sheet.

THE CHILDREN'S HOSPITAL
DEPARTMENT OF NURSING
CONTINUING CARE PROGRAM

PT. NAME

PARENT

**ADDITIONAL DISCHARGE
INSTRUCTIONS**

ADDRESS

TEL. #

COMMUNITY PROVIDERS

agency name & address _____   contact person _____

_____   telephone _____ start date _____

_____   service/frequency requested _____

agency name & address _____   contact person _____

_____   telephone _____ start date _____

_____   service/frequency requested _____

agency name & address _____   contact person _____

_____   telephone _____ start date _____

_____   service/frequency requested _____

EQUIPMENT/SUPPLIES (list all items ordered)

home care company name _____ tel. # ___-___-___ contact person _____

delivery date _____ delivery to home ___ hospital ___ other _____

items ordered & quantity _____

_____

_____

_____

_____

_____

OTHER (Include insurance and financial information, as needed)

_____

_____

_____

_____

Received and discussed as part of
the discharge plan:

_____

(patient/parent initials)   (date)

_____

(nurse initials)   (date)

Fig. 16-3. Additional discharge instruction sheet.

At Brigham and Women's Hospital

◆	Newborn ICU	(617) 732-5420
◆	To contact the doctor that cared for your baby in NICU,	
◆	call NICU Medical Director's Office	(617) 732-5209
◆	OB Social Service Office	(617) 732-6462
◆	To schedule outpatient hearing screen, call	(617) 732-5601
◆	Birth Certificate Office	(617) 732-6071

Outside of Brigham and Women's Hospital

The following is a list of some resources of which we are aware in the Greater Boston area. Please be aware that we do not imply any approval, but are merely trying to assist you in finding community resources. When you call, tell them what services you want and ask about qualifications of providers and fees (some are free while many will bill your insurer or offer a sliding scale); if they cannot help you, ask them if they can refer you to other sources.

◆	Battered Women's Hotline (24-hour)	(617) 661-7203
◆	Children's Hospital (Boston) Emergency Room	(617) 735-6611
◆	Poison Control Center	(617) 232-2120
	(if calling from outside Boston area, call:)	1-800-682-9211
◆	If you are fearful of losing control with your child, call the Parental Stress Line	1-800-632-8188
◆	If you would like to talk to a parent who has gone through a NICU experience, call NICU: Parent Support, Inc.	(617) 698-1172
◆	If you need information about where to get help for substance abuse problems, call the Statewide Alcohol and Drug Hotline	1-800-327-5050

Breastfeeding Support/Electric Breastpump Rentals

◆	RMS Medical Sales	(508) 660-1607
	Walpole, MA	(508) 668-1806
	White River Portable Electric Pumps delivered to over 70 Greater Boston area cities and towns.	
◆	Harvard Community Health Plan	(617) 431-5245
	The Wellesley Center	
	Breastfeeding classes and consultation for members and non members. Ask for Marsha Walker.	(617) 698-1172
◆	Medela Breastpump Rental Stations	1-800-435-8316
◆	Egnel Breastpump Rental Stations	1-800-323-8750
◆	Newborn Support Services	(617) 232-5344
	Brookline, MA	
◆	La Leche League of Mass/Vermont	(617) 334-3035

WHEN TO CALL YOUR BABY'S DOCTOR

-If you notice any sudden changes in baby's usual patterns of behavior:
  - ◆ increased sleepiness
  - ◆ increased irritability
  - ◆ feeding poorly

-If you notice any of the following:
  - ◆ breathing difficulties
  - ◆ blueness around lips, mouth, or eyes
  - ◆ fever (by rectal temperature) over 100° or under 97°
  - ◆ vomiting or diarrhea
  - ◆ dry diapers for longer than 12 hours
  - ◆ no bowel movement for longer than 4 days
  - ◆ black or bright red color seen in stool

Fig. 16-4. Parent resources with important telephone numbers and additional instructions from Brigham and Women's Hospital NICU.

BODY TEMPERATURE CONTROL

THE FOLLOWING GUIDELINES MAY HELP YOU TO KEEP YOUR BABY COMFORTABLE BOTH IN AND OUT OF DOORS:

Air Temperature	Clothing Needs
80°	a T-shirt and diaper
between 75° and 80°	one more layer of clothing than you wear
between 70° and 75°	two more layers of clothing than you wear
below 70°	two more layers of clothing than you wear, plus a blanket and a hat

PROTECTING YOUR BABY FROM INFECTION

Your baby's immune system is still quite immature; this makes him especially vulnerable to colds and other communicable diseases. To protect your baby from infections we advise that you:

♦ avoid taking baby to crowded indoor places
♦ avoid contact with anyone who has a cold, flu or other active infection
♦ do not allow anyone to smoke around baby
♦ encourage anyone who comes into close contact with baby to wash their hands

SAFETY

♦ It is a Massachusetts state law that all children 12 year old and under must be fastened in in a properly adjusted carseat or safety belt. It is strongly recommended that children under 40 pounds always ride in carseats.

Fig. 16-4. *Continued*

B. **Home care benefits** are often limited. Prior authorization is almost universally required. Services may be restricted to a particular provider or to a finite period.
C. **Alternative funding**
1. **Social Security.** Several states have programs that waive parental income criteria and provide Medicaid benefits to infants and children or to those whose hospitalization may be extended if home care services are not provided.
2. **State government financial assistance.** The maternal and child health agencies in most state governments will provide some financial assistance for follow-up of certain infants whose families meet state-established financial criteria. Services vary from state to state but may include physical therapy services, equipment, and diagnostic and treatment services.
3. **Private charities** such as the Easter Seal Society and the March of Dimes Birth Defects Foundation have local chapters that provide specialized services on an ability-to-pay or free basis.
4. **Public health departments** may offer immunizations and well-child clinics at no cost or very low cost.
5. **Women, Infants and Children Program (WIC)** is federally funded and provides nutrition education and supplemental formula to financially eligible pregnant women and to children up to 5 years of age who are assessed as being at risk.
D. **Social services or continuing care departments** are invaluable in determining existing coverage and in accessing alternative sources of financial support.

References

Damato, E. Discharge planning from the neonatal intensive care unit. *J. Perinatal. Neonatal. Nurs.* 5(1):43, 1991.

Hulseman, M. L., Lee, N. The neonatal ICU graduate: Part I. Common problems. *Am. Fam. Physician* 45(3):1301, 1992.

Hulseman, M. L., Lee, N. The neonatal ICU graduate: Part II. Fundamentals of outpatient care. *Am. Fam. Physician* 45(4):1696, 1992.

Hutt, H. L. Home care. In C. Kenner, A. Brueggemeyer, L. P. Gunderson (Eds.). *Comprehensive Neonatal Nursing.* Philadelphia: Saunders, 1991.

Kenner, C., Bagwell, G. Assessment and management of the transition to home. In C. Kenner, A. Brueggemeyer, L. P. Gunderson (Eds.). *Comprehensive Neonatal Nursing.* Philadelphia: Saunders, 1991.

Leonard, C. High risk infant follow-up programs. In R. Ballard (Ed.). *Pediatric Care of the ICN Graduate.* Philadelphia: Saunders, 1988.

17. SHOCK

Stella Kourembanas

I. **Background.** Shock is an acute, complex state of circulatory dysfunction resulting in insufficient oxygen and nutrient delivery to satisfy tissue requirements.
II. **Causes of shock**
  A. **Hypovolemia** is the most common cause of shock in the neonate (see Chap. 26). The decrease in blood volume can result from loss of whole blood, plasma, or extravascular fluid.
    1. Placental hemorrhage, as in abruptio placentae or placenta previa
    2. Fetal-to-maternal hemorrhage (diagnosed by the Kleihauer-Betke test of the mother's blood for fetal erythrocytes)
    3. Twin-to-twin transfusion (see Chap. 7)
    4. Intracranial hemorrhage (see Chap. 27)
    5. Intraabdominal bleeding from liver laceration caused by gastrointestinal surgery or traumatic breech delivery. Necrotizing enterocolitis or other causes of peritonitis can cause plasma loss
    6. Massive pulmonary hemorrhage (see Chap. 24)
    7. Disseminated intravascular coagulation (DIC) or other severe coagulopathies
    8. Plasma loss into the extravascular compartment, as seen with low oncotic pressure states or capillary leak syndrome (e.g., sepsis)
    9. Excessive extravascular fluid losses, as seen with dehydration from insensible water loss or inappropriate diuresis, commonly seen in very premature infants.
  B. **Distributive causes.** Abnormalities of circulatory distribution can cause inadequate tissue perfusion. This may result from increased venous capacitance, vasomotor paralysis from pharmacologic agents, or shunting past capillary beds. Etiologies of maldistribution include the following:
    1. **Sepsis.** The precise mechanisms underlying circulatory dysfunction in septic shock are not clear. Multiple factors can interact to alter blood flow: (1) direct depressive effect of microbial products, including endotoxin on the cardiovascular system and/or (2) release of other vasoactive agents, including nitric oxide, serotonin, prostaglandins, histamine, and endorphins resulting in peripheral vasodilatation and relative hypovolemia.
    2. **Drugs** that decrease vascular tone include muscle relaxants and anesthetics. Vancomycin has been reported to cause acute circulatory failure in newborn infants.
  C. **Cardiogenic shock.** Although an infant's myocardium normally exhibits good contractility, various perinatal insults, congenital abnormalities, or arrhythmias can result in heart failure.
    1. Intrapartum asphyxia can cause poor contractility and papillary muscle dysfunction with tricuspid regurgitation, resulting in low cardiac output.
    2. Myocardial dysfunction can occur secondary to infectious agents (bacterial or viral) or metabolic abnormalities such as hypoglycemia. Cardiomyopathy can be seen in infants of diabetic mothers (IDMS) with or without hypoglycemia (see Chap. 2).
    3. Obstruction to blood flow resulting in decreased cardiac output can be seen with many congenital heart defects (see Chap. 25).
      a. **Inflow obstructions**
        (1) Total anomalous pulmonary venous return
        (2) Cor triatriatum
        (3) Tricuspid atresia

(4) Mitral atresia

(5) Acquired inflow obstructions can occur from intravascular air or thrombotic embolus, or from increased intrathoracic pressure caused by high airway pressures, pneumothorax, pneumomediastinum, or pneumopericardium.

b. Outflow obstructions

(1) Pulmonary stenosis or atresia

(2) Aortic stenosis or atresia

(3) Hypertrophic subaortic stenosis seen in IDMs with compromised left ventricular outflow, particularly when cardiotonic agents are used

(4) Coarctation of the aorta or interrupted aortic arch

(5) Arrhythmias, if prolonged. Supraventricular arrhythmias such as paroxysmal atrial tachycardia are most common.

III. Pathophysiology of circulatory failure

A. Hypovolemic shock. In the compensated phase, central venous pressure (CVP) and urine output are decreased, and tachycardia and increased systemic vascular resistance are present. In very premature infants, acute hypotension with bradycardia can occur without preceding tachycardia.

B. Distributive shock presents initially with a hyperdynamic state of tachycardia, normal blood pressure and urine output, and bounding pulses. The arteriovenous oxygen saturation difference, when measured, is narrow. Eventually, cardiogenic shock ensues.

C. In cardiogenic shock, compensatory mechanisms can have deleterious effects. Increased vascular resistance maintains adequate blood supply to vital organs but increases left ventricular afterload and cardiac work. Decreased renal perfusion from low cardiac output results in sodium and water retention, causing increased central blood volume, increased left ventricular pressure and volume, and therefore pulmonary edema, with hypoxia and acidosis further compromising cardiac function. Tachycardia, hypotension, oliguria, and acidosis dominate the presentation of cardiogenic shock.

IV. Clinical presentation. In addition to hypotension and tachycardia (except in very premature infants; see **III.A**), shock is manifested principally by (1) pallor and poor skin perfusion, (2) cool extremities, (3) central nervous system signs (see **III.A**), and (4) decreased urine output. Organ dysfunction occurs because of inadequate blood flow and oxygenation, and cellular metabolism becomes predominantly anaerobic, producing lactic and pyruvic acid. Hence, metabolic acidosis often indicates inadequate circulation.

A. Brain: irritability, lethargy, seizures, and coma

B. Heart: decreased cardiac output and increased pulmonary blood volume

C. Lungs: release of vasoactive substances, pulmonary edema, and decreased compliance

D. Gastrointestinal tract: mucosal dysfunction, diarrhea, sepsis, hemorrhage, and perforation

E. Kidneys: reduced glomerular filtration rate (GFR) and urinary output, loss of renal tubular epithelium, uremia, electrolyte abnormalities, and hypotension

V. Treatment always begins by ensuring a patent airway, assessing ventilation, and providing supplemental oxygen. Heart rate, blood pressure, and oxygenation should be monitored continuously. An infusion of 10 ml/kg normal saline or 5% albumin-saline solution will help establish etiology. If hypovolemia exists, the infusion will be therapeutic, at least temporarily, until the underlying cause is corrected.

A. Measurement of central venous pressure (CVP) helps management. CVP is measured by a catheter with its tip in the right atrium or in the intrathoracic superior or inferior vena cava. The catheter can be placed through the umbilical vein or percutaneously through the external or internal jugular or subclavian vein. In many infants, maintaining CVP at 5 to 8 mm Hg with volume infusions is associated with improved cardiac output. If CVP exceeds 5 to 8 mm Hg, additional volume will usually not be helpful. CVP is influenced by noncardiac factors such as ventilator pressures and by cardiac factors such as tricuspid valve function. Both types of factors may affect the interpretation and usefulness of CVP measurements.

B. Correction of negative inotropic factors such as hypoxia, acidosis, hypoglycemia, and other metabolic derangements will improve cardiac output. **Sodium bicarbonate** infusion at a dose of 1 to 2 mEq/kg is indicated for metabolic acidosis with pH below 7.20 if there is adequate ventilation (PCO_2 under 40 mm Hg). More sodium bicarbonate can be infused if the pH remains low. In addition, hypocalcemia frequently occurs in infants with circulatory failure, especially after the administration of large amounts of solutions containing albumin; this must be corrected. In this setting, calcium frequently produces a positive inotropic response. **Calcium gluconate** 10% (1 ml/kg) can be infused slowly on an empirical basis or after measurement of the ionized calcium level (see Chap. 29).

C. **Positive inotropic agents** should be used to increase cardiac output.
   1. **Sympathomimetic amines** are commonly used in infants. The advantages include rapidity of onset, ability to control dosage, and ultrashort half-lives.
      a. **Dopamine** is a naturally occurring catecholamine. Exogenous dopamine activates receptors in dose-dependent fashion. At low doses (0.5 to 2 μg/kg/minute), dopamine stimulates peripheral dopamine receptors (DA_1 and DA_2) and increases renal, mesenteric, and coronary blood flow with little effect on cardiac output. In intermediate doses (2 to 6 μg/kg/minute), dopamine has positive inotropic and chronotropic effects (beta-1 and beta-2). At high doses (over 6 to 10 μg/kg/minute), dopamine stimulates alpha-1 and alpha-2 adrenergic receptors and serotonin receptors, resulting in vasoconstriction and increased peripheral vascular resistance. High-dose dopamine also increases venous return. In preterm infants, dopamine may stimulate the alpha receptors at lower doses. The increase in myocardial contractility depends in part on myocardial norepinephrine stores.
      b. **Dobutamine** is a synthetic catecholamine. Its inotropic effects, unlike those of dopamine, are independent of norepinephrine stores. In doses of 5 to 15 μg/kg/minute, dobutamine increases cardiac output (alpha-1 receptors) with little effect on heart rate. Dobutamine can decrease systemic vascular resistance (beta-receptors). Dobutamine is often used with dopamine to improve cardiac output and to avoid the extreme vasoconstriction associated with high doses of dopamine.
      c. **Epinephrine** increases myocardial contractility and peripheral vascular resistance (beta- and alpha-receptors). It is not a first-line drug in newborns; however, it may be effective in patients who do not respond to dopamine and dobutamine. Epinephrine may be helpful in conditions such as sepsis when low perfusion is due to peripheral vasodilatation. The starting dose is 0.05 to 0.1 μg/kg/minute and can be increased rapidly as needed.
   2. **Other agents**
      a. **Corticosteroids** may be useful in extremely premature infants with hypotension refractory to volume expansion and vasopressors, but this usage has not been tested in clinical trials. We have used doses of 1 mg/kg of hydrocortisone. If it works, we repeat it every 12 hours for 2–3 days. Steroids have been used in sepsis, but their efficacy remains controversial, perhaps because administration is initiated late in the clinical course after the cascade of inflammatory mediators has begun.

References
Helbock, H.J., et al. Glucocorticoid-responsive hypotension in ELBW newborns. *Pediatrics* 92:715, 1993.
Seri, I. Cardiovascular, renal, and endocrine actions of dopamine in neonates and children. *J. Pediatr.* 126:333–344, 1995.

18. NEONATAL HYPERBILIRUBINEMIA

Michael T. Hinkes and John P. Cloherty

I. **Background.** General discussions of this topic are found in references [1,2,8,9,12]. The normal adult serum bilirubin level is less than 1 mg/dl. Adults appear jaundiced when the serum bilirubin level is greater than 2 mg/dl, and newborns appear jaundiced when it is greater than 7 mg/dl. Between 25 and 50% of all term newborns and a higher percentage of premature infants develop clinical jaundice. Also, 6.1% of well term newborns have a maximal serum bilirubin level over 12.9 mg/dl. A serum bilirubin level over 15 mg/dl is found in 3% of normal term babies.

   A. **Source of bilirubin.** Bilirubin is derived from the breakdown of heme-containing proteins in the reticuloendothelial system. The normal newborn produces 6 to 10 mg of bilirubin per kilogram per day, as opposed to the production of 3 to 4 mg/kg per day in the adult.

   1. The major heme-containing protein is **red blood cell (RBC) hemoglobin.** Hemoglobin released from senescent RBCs in the reticuloendothelial system is the source of 75% of all bilirubin production. One gram of hemoglobin produces 34 mg of bilirubin. Accelerated release of hemoglobin from RBCs is the cause of hyperbilirubinemia in isoimmunization (e.g., Rh and ABO incompatibility), erythrocyte biochemical abnormalities (e.g., G6PD and pyruvate kinase deficiencies), abnormal erythrocyte morphology (e.g., hereditary spherocytosis), sequestered blood (e.g., bruising and cephalohematoma), and polycythemia.

   2. The other 25% of bilirubin is called **early labeled bilirubin.** It is derived from hemoglobin released by ineffective erythropoiesis in the bone marrow, from other heme-containing proteins in tissues (e.g., myoglobin, cytochromes, catalase, and peroxidase), and from free heme.

   B. **Bilirubin metabolism.** The heme ring from heme-containing proteins is oxidized in reticuloendothelial cells to **biliverdin** by the microsomal enzyme heme oxygenase. This reaction releases **carbon monoxide (CO)** (excreted from the lung) and **iron** (reutilized). Biliverdin is then reduced to bilirubin by the enzyme **biliverdin reductase.** Catabolism of 1 mole of hemoglobin produces 1 mole each of CO and bilirubin. Increased bilirubin production, as measured by CO excretion rates, accounts for the higher bilirubin levels seen in Asian, Native American, and Greek infants.

   1. **Transport.** Bilirubin is nonpolar and insoluble in water and is transported to liver cells bound to serum **albumin.** Bilirubin bound to albumin does not usually enter the central nervous system and is thought to be nontoxic. Displacement of bilirubin from albumin by drugs, such as the sulfonamides, or by free fatty acids (FFA) at high molar ratios of FFA : albumin, may increase bilirubin toxicity (Table 18-1).

   2. **Uptake.** Nonpolar, fat-soluble bilirubin (dissociated from albumin) crosses the hepatocyte plasma membrane and is bound mainly to cytoplasmic **ligandin** (Y protein) for transport to the smooth endoplasmic reticulum. Phenobarbital increases the concentration of ligandin.

   3. **Conjugation.** Unconjugated (indirect) bilirubin (UCB) is converted to water-soluble conjugated (direct) bilirubin (CB) in the smooth endoplasmic reticulum by **uridine diphosphate glucuronyl transferase (UDPG-T).** This enzyme is inducible by phenobarbital and catalyzes the formation of bilirubin monoglucuronide. The monoglucuronide may be further conjugated to bilirubin diglucuronide. Both mono- and diglucuronide forms of CB are able to be excreted into the bile canaliculi

Table 18-1. Drugs that cause significant displacement of bilirubin from albumin in vitro

Sulfonamides
Moxalactam
Fusidic acid
Radiographic contrast media for cholangiography (sodium iodipamide, sodium ipodate, iopanoic acid, meglumine ioglycamate)
Aspirin
Apazone
Tolbutamide
Rapid infusions of albumin preservatives (sodium caprylate and N-acetyltryptophan)
Rapid infusions of ampicillin
Long-chain free fatty acids (FFA) at high molar ratios of FFA: albumin

Source: From P. Roth and R. A. Polin, Controversial topics in kernicterus. *Clin. Perinatol.* 15:970, 1988.

against a concentration gradient. Inherited deficiencies of the conjugating enzyme UDPG-T (Crigler-Najjar syndrome) can cause severe hyperbilirubinemia in neonates.

4. **Excretion.** CB in the biliary tree enters the gastrointestinal (GI) tract and is then eliminated from the body in the stool, which contains large amounts of bilirubin. CB is not normally resorbed from the bowel unless it is converted back to UCB by the intestinal enzyme **beta-glucuronidase.** Resorption of bilirubin from the GI tract and delivery back to the liver for reconjugation is called **enterohepatic circulation.** Intestinal bacteria can prevent enterohepatic circulation of bilirubin by converting CB to **urobilinoids,** which are not substrates for beta-glucuronidase. Pathologic conditions leading to increased enterohepatic circulation include decreased enteral intake, intestinal atresias, meconium ileus, and Hirschsprung's disease.

5. **Fetal bilirubin metabolism.** Most UCB formed by the fetus is cleared by the placenta into the maternal circulation. Formation of CB is limited in the fetus because of decreased fetal hepatic blood flow, decreased hepatic ligandin, and decreased UDPG-T activity. The small amount of CB excreted into the fetal gut is usually hydrolyzed by beta-glucuronidase and resorbed. Bilirubin is normally found in amniotic fluid by 12 weeks' gestation and is usually gone by 37 weeks' gestation. Increased amniotic fluid bilirubin is found in hemolytic disease of the newborn and in fetal intestinal obstruction below the bile ducts.

II. **Physiologic hyperbilirubinemia.** The serum UCB level of most newborn infants rises to over 2 mg/dl in the first week of life. This level usually rises in full-term infants to a peak of 6 to 8 mg/dl by 3 days of age and then falls. A rise to 12 mg/dl is in the physiologic range. In premature infants, the peak may be 10 to 12 mg/dl on the fifth day of life, possibly rising over 15 mg/dl without any specific abnormality of bilirubin metabolism. Levels under 2 mg/dl may not be seen until 1 month of age in both full-term and premature infants. This "normal jaundice" is attributed to the following mechanisms:

A. **Increased bilirubin production** due to
1. Increased RBC volume/kilogram and decreased RBC survival (90-day vs. 120-day) in infants compared with adults.
2. Increased ineffective erythropoiesis and increased turnover of non-hemoglobin heme proteins.

B. Increased enterohepatic circulation caused by high levels of intestinal beta-glucuronidase, preponderance of bilirubin monoglucuronide rather than diglucuronide, decreased intestinal bacteria, and decreased gut motility with poor evacuation of bilirubin-laden meconium.

C. **Defective uptake** of bilirubin from plasma caused by decreased ligandin and binding of ligandin by other anions.

D. **Defective conjugation** due to decreased UDPG-T activity.

E. **Decreased hepatic excretion** of bilirubin.

III. **Nonphysiologic hyperbilirubinemia** (Fig. 18-1 and Table 18-2). Nonphysiologic jaundice may not be easy to distinguish from physiologic jaundice. The following situations suggest nonphysiologic hyperbilirubinemia and require investigation:

A. **General conditions**

1. Onset of jaundice before 24 hours of age.

2. Any elevation of serum bilirubin that requires phototherapy (see Fig. 18-3 and **VI.D**).

3. A rise in serum bilirubin levels of over 0.5 mg/dl/hour.

4. Signs of underlying illness in any infant (vomiting, lethargy, poor feeding, excessive weight loss, apnea, tachypnea, or temperature instability).

5. Jaundice persisting after 8 days in a term infant or after 14 days in a premature infant.

B. **History**

1. A family history of jaundice, anemia, splenectomy, or early gallbladder disease suggests hereditary hemolytic anemia (e.g., spherocytosis).

2. A family history of liver disease may suggest galactosemia, alpha-1-antitrypsin deficiency, tyrosinosis, hypermethioninemia, Gilbert's disease, Crigler-Najjar syndrome types I and II, or cystic fibrosis.

3. Ethnic or geographic origin associated with hyperbilirubinemia (East Asian, Greek, and American Indian).

4. A sibling with jaundice or anemia may suggest blood group incompatibility, breast-milk jaundice, or Lucey-Driscoll syndrome.

5. Maternal illness during pregnancy may suggest congenital viral or toxoplasmosis infection. Infants of diabetic mothers tend to develop hyperbilirubinemia (see Chap. 2, Maternal Diabetes).

6. Maternal drugs may interfere with bilirubin binding to albumin, making bilirubin toxic at relatively low levels (sulfonamides) or may cause hemolysis in a G-6-PD-deficient infant (sulfonamides, nitrofurantoin, antimalarials).

7. The labor and delivery history may show trauma associated with extravascular bleeding and hemolysis. Oxytocin use may be associated with neonatal hyperbilirubinemia, although this is controversial. Asphyxiated infants may have elevated bilirubin levels caused either by inability of the liver to process bilirubin or by intracranial hemorrhage. Delayed cord clamping may be associated with neonatal polycythemia and increased bilirubin load.

8. The infant's history may show delayed or infrequent stooling, which can be caused by poor caloric intake or intestinal obstruction and lead to increased enterohepatic circulation of bilirubin. Poor caloric intake may also decrease bilirubin uptake by the liver. Vomiting can be due to sepsis, pyloric stenosis, or galactosemia.

9. **Breast-feeding.** A distinction has been made between breast-milk jaundice, in which jaundice is thought to be due to the breast milk itself, and breast-feeding jaundice, in which low caloric intake may be responsible.

a. **Breast-milk jaundice** is of late onset. By day 4, instead of the usual fall in the serum bilirubin level, the bilirubin level continues to rise and may reach 20 to 30 mg/dl by 14 days of age. If breast-feeding is continued, the levels will stay elevated and then fall slowly at 2 weeks of age, returning to normal by 4 to 12 weeks of age. If breast-

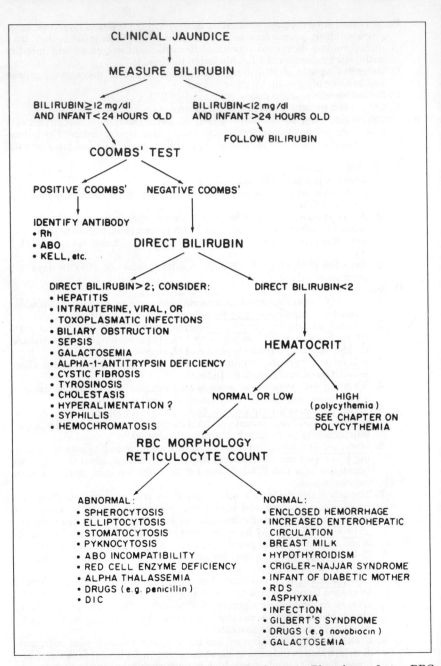

Fig. 18-1. Diagnosis of the etiology of hyperbilirubinemia. Rh = rhesus factor; RBC = red blood cell; DIC = disseminated intravascular coagulation; RDS = respiratory distress syndrome.

feeding is stopped, the bilirubin level will fall rapidly in 48 hours. If nursing is then resumed, the bilirubin may rise 2 to 4 mg/dl but usually will not reach the previous high level. These infants show good weight gain, have normal liver function test results, and show no evidence of hemolysis. Mothers with infants who have breast-milk jaundice syndrome have a recurrence rate of 70% in future pregnancies. The mechanism of true breast-milk jaundice is unknown but is thought to be due to an unidentified factor (or factors) in breast milk interfering with bilirubin metabolism. Additionally, compared with formula-fed infants, breast-fed infants are more likely to have increased enterohepatic circulation because they ingest the beta-glucuronidase present in breast milk, are slower to be colonized with intestinal bacteria that convert CB to urobilinoids, and excrete less stool. There are reports of kernicterus in otherwise healthy, breast-fed, term newborns [14].

   b. **Breast-feeding jaundice.** Infants who are breast-fed have bilirubin levels slightly higher in the first 3 to 4 days of life than bottle-fed infants. The differences in the levels of bilirubin are not clinically significant. The main factor thought to be responsible for breast-feeding jaundice is a decreased intake of milk that leads to increased enterohepatic circulation.

C. **The physical examination.** Jaundice is detected by blanching the skin with finger pressure to observe the color of the skin and subcutaneous tissues. Jaundice progresses in a cephalocaudal direction. The highest bilirubin levels are associated with jaundice below the knees and in the hands. Although transcutaneous bilirubinometry and the card ictometer have been used successfully to screen for jaundice in term infants, they have not been used extensively by clinicians in our nurseries.

   Jaundiced infants should be examined for the following physical findings:
   1. **Prematurity.**
   2. **Small size for gestational age (SGA),** which may be associated with polycythemia and in utero infections.
   3. **Microcephaly,** which may be associated with in utero infections.
   4. **Extravascular blood:** bruising, cephalohematoma, or other enclosed hemorrhage.
   5. **Pallor** associated with hemolytic anemia or extravascular blood loss.
   6. **Petechiae** associated with congenital infection, sepsis, or erythroblastosis.
   7. **Hepatosplenomegaly** associated with hemolytic anemia, congenital infection, or liver disease.
   8. **Omphalitis.**
   9. **Chorioretinitis** associated with congenital infection.
   10. Evidence of **hypothyroidism** (see Chap. 2).

D. **Clinical tests** (Figs. 18-1, 18-3, and 18-4). The following tests are indicated in the presence of nonphysiologic jaundice:
   1. **Total serum bilirubin.**
   2. **Blood type, Rh, and direct Coombs' test of the infant** to test for isoimmune hemolytic disease. Infants of women who are Rh-negative should have a blood type, Rh, and Coombs' test performed at birth. Routine blood typing and Coombs' testing of all infants born to O-positive mothers to determine whether there is risk for ABO incompatibility is probably unnecessary. Such testing is reserved for infants with clinically significant jaundice, those in whom follow-up is difficult, or those whose skin pigmentation is such that jaundice may not be easily recognized. Blood typing and Coombs' testing should be considered for infants who are to be discharged early, especially if the mother is Type O (see Chap. 5).
   3. **Blood type, Rh, and antibody screen of the mother** should have been done during pregnancy and the antibody screen repeated at delivery.

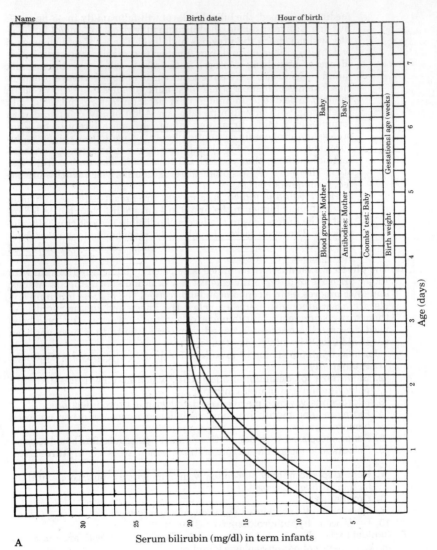

A   Serum bilirubin (mg/dl) in term infants

Fig. 18-2. Serum bilirubin levels plotted against age in term infants **(A)** and premature infants **(B)** with erythroblastosis. Levels above the top line are predictive of an ultimate bilirubin level that will be over 20 unless the natural course is altered by treatment. Levels below the bottom line predict that the level will not eventually reach 20. Between the lines is an intermediate zone, in which the ultimate level could be below or above 20. These charts were developed before phototherapy was used in this country and before the discovery of many factors that might lead to kernicterus at low bilirubin levels; however, the charts still offer good guidelines to the natural progression of bilirubin levels in infants with Rh incompatibility. (From F. H. Allen, Jr., and L. K. Diamond, *Erythroblastosis Fetalis: Including Exchange Transfusion Technique.* Boston: Little, Brown, 1957, 57.)

Name   Birth date   Hour of birth

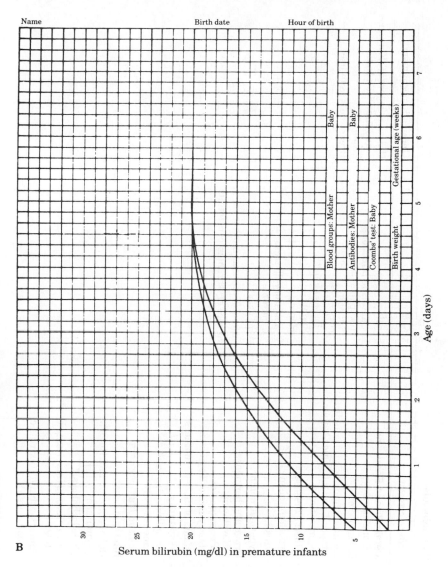

B

Serum bilirubin (mg/dl) in premature infants

Fig. 18-2. *Continued.*

4. **Peripheral smear for RBC morphology and reticulocyte count** to detect causes of Coombs'-negative hemolytic disease (e.g., spherocytosis).
5. **Hematocrit** will detect polycythemia or suggest blood loss from occult hemorrhage.
6. Identification of **antibody on infant's RBCs** (if result of direct Coombs' test is positive).

Table 18-2. Causes of neonatal hyperbilirubinemia

Overproduction	Undersecretion	Mixed	Uncertain mechanism
Fetomaternal blood group incompatibility (e.g., Rh, ABO)	**Metabolic and Endocrine Conditions**	Sepsis	Chinese, Japanese, Korean, and American Indian infants
Hereditary spherocytosis eliptocytosis, somatocytosis	Galactosemia	Intrauterine infections Toxoplasmosis	Breast-milk jaundice
Nonspherocytic hemolytic anemias	Familial nonhemolytic jaundice types 1 and 2 (Crigler-Najjar syndrome)	Rubella CID Herpes simplex	
G-6-PD deficiency and drugs	Gilbert's disease	Syphilis Hepatitis	
Pyruvate-kinase deficiency	Hypothyroidism	Respiratory distress syndrome	
Other red-cell enzyme deficiencies	Tyrosinosis	Asphyxia	
Alpha thalassemia	Hypermethioninemia	Infant of diabetic mother	
Delta-beta thalassemia	Drugs and hormones	Severe erythroblastosis fetalis	
Acquired hemolysis due to vitamin K_3, nitrofurantoin, sulfonamides, antimalarials, penicillin oxytocin?, bupivacaine, or infection	Novobiocin Pregnanediol Lucey-Driscoll syndrome Infants of diabetic mothers Prematurity Hypopituitarism and anencephaly		
Extravascular Blood	**Obstructive Disorders**		
Petechiae	Biliary atresia*		
Hematomas	Dubin-Johnson and Rotor's syndrome*		
Pulmonary, cerebral, or occult hemorrhage	Choledochal cyst*		
	Cystic fibrosis (inspissated bile)*		
	Tumor* or band* (extrinsic obstruction)		

Polycythemia
Fetomaternal or fetofetal transfusion
Delayed clamping of the umbilical cord

Increased Enterohepatic Circulation
Pyloric stenosis*
Intestinal atresia or stenosis including annular pancreas
Hirschsprung's disease
Meconium ileus and/or meconium plug syndrome
Fasting or hypoperistalsis from other causes
Drug-induced paralytic ileus (hexamethonium)
Swallowed blood

Alpha-1-antitrypsin deficiency*
Parenteral nutrition

Key: G-6-PD = glucose-6-phosphate dehydrogenase; CID = cytomegalovirus inclusion disease, as in TORCH.
*Jaundice may not be seen in the neonatal period.
Source: Modified from G. B. Odell, R. L. Poland, and E. Nostrea, Jr., Neonatal Hyperbilirubinemia. In M. H. Klaus and A. Fanaroff (Eds.), *Care of the High Risk Neonate*. Philadelphia: Saunders, 1973. Chap. 11.

7. **Direct bilirubin** determination is necessary when jaundice persists beyond the first 2 weeks of life or whenever there are signs of cholestasis (light-colored stools and bilirubin in urine).

8. In prolonged jaundice, tests for liver disease, congenital infection, sepsis, metabolic defects, or hypothyroidism are indicated. Total parenteral nutrition is a well-recognized cause of prolonged direct hyperbilirubinemia.

9. **A G-6-PD screen** may be helpful, especially in male infants of Asian, Mediterranean, or Middle Eastern ethnicity. Term black infants with G-6-PD deficiency usually do not have a significant increase in jaundice. Screening of the parents for G-6-PD deficiency is helpful. Infants who had G-6-PD deficiency and were discharged early have been reported with severe hyperbilirubinemia and significant sequelae [13].

IV. **Diagnosis of neonatal hyperbilirubinemia** (see Table 18-2 and Fig. 18-1).

V. **Bilirubin toxicity.** This area remains highly controversial. The problem is that bilirubin levels that are toxic to one infant may not be toxic to another, or even to the same infant in different clinical circumstances. Currently, major debate surrounds the toxicity of bilirubin in otherwise healthy full-term infants and in premature, low-birth-weight infants. For recent detailed reviews and analyses of these debates, see references [14,17,18,25] and the accompanying commentaries, editorials, and rebuttals.

Bilirubin levels refer to total bilirubin. Direct bilirubin is not subtracted from the total unless it constitutes more than 50% of total bilirubin.

A. Bilirubin entry into the brain occurs as free (unbound) bilirubin or as bilirubin bound to albumin in the presence of a disrupted blood–brain barrier. It is estimated that 8.5 mg of bilirubin will bind tightly to 1 gm of albumin (molar ratio of one), although this binding capacity is less in small and sick prematures. Free fatty acids and certain drugs (see Table 18-1) interfere with bilirubin binding to albumin, while acidosis affects bilirubin solubility and its deposition into brain tissue. Factors that disrupt the blood–brain barrier include hyperosmolarity, anoxia, and hypercarbia, and the barrier itself may be more permeable in premature infants.

B. **Kernicterus** is a pathologic diagnosis and refers to **yellow staining** of the brain by bilirubin together with evidence of **neuronal injury.** Grossly, bilirubin staining is most commonly seen in the basal ganglia, various cranial nerve nuclei, other brain stem nuclei, cerebellar nuclei, hippocampus, and anterior horn cells of the spinal cord. Microscopically, there is necrosis, neuronal loss, and gliosis.

C. **Acute bilirubin encephalopathy** is classically seen in term infants dying of Rh hemolytic disease with high (>20 mg/dl) bilirubin levels who have kernicterus on autopsy. The clinical presentation of acute bilirubin encephalopathy can be divided into three phases:

1. Hypotonia, lethargy, high-pitched cry, and poor suck.

2. Hypertonia of extensor muscles (with opisthotonus, rigidity, oculogyric crisis, and retrocollis), fever, and seizures. Many infants die in this phase. All infants who survive this phase develop chronic bilirubin encephalopathy.

3. Hypotonia replaces hypertonia after about 1 week of age.

D. **Chronic bilirubin encephalopathy** is marked by athetosis, partial or complete sensorineural deafness, limitation of upward gaze, dental dysplasia, and mild intellectual deficits.

E. **Bilirubin toxicity and hemolytic disease.** There is general agreement that in Rh hemolytic disease there is a direct association between marked elevations of bilirubin and signs of bilirubin encephalopathy with kernicterus at autopsy. Studies and clinical experience have shown that in full-term infants with hemolytic disease, if the total bilirubin level is kept under 20 mg/dl, bilirubin encephalopathy is unlikely to occur. Theoretically, this should apply to other causes of isoimmune hemolytic disease, such as ABO incompatibility, and to hereditary hemolytic processes such as hereditary

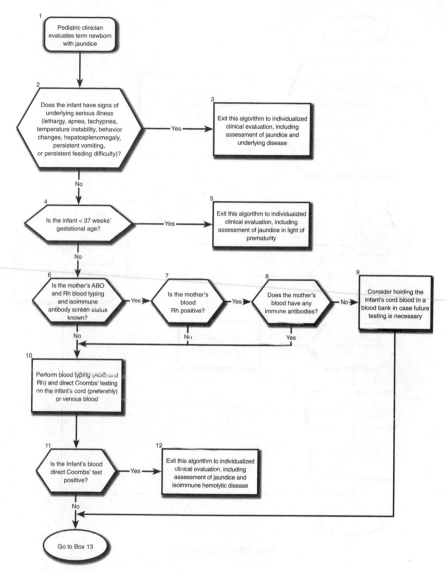

Fig. 18-3. Algorithm: Management of hyperbilirubinemia in the healthy term infant. From American Academy of Pediatrics [2].

spherocytosis, pyruvate kinase deficiency, or glucose-6-phosphate dehydrogenase (G-6-PD) deficiency.

F. Bilirubin toxicity and the healthy full-term infant [2,9,17,18]. In contrast to infants with hemolytic disease, there is little evidence showing adverse neurologic outcome in healthy term neonates with bilirubin levels below 25 to 30 mg/dl [16]. A large prospective cohort study failed to demonstrate a clinically significant association between bilirubin levels above 20 mg/dl and definite

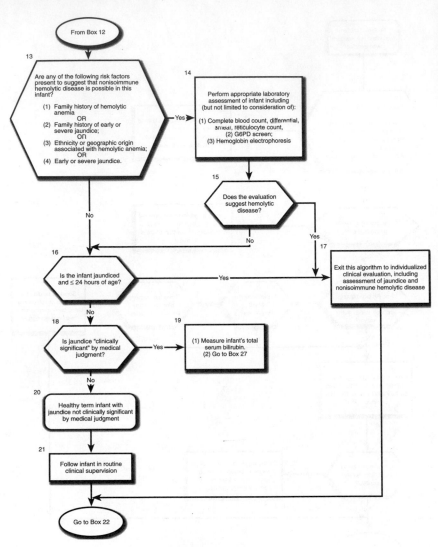

Fig. 18-3. *Continued.*

neurologic abnormality, long-term hearing loss, or IQ deficits. However, an increase in minor motor abnormalities of unclear significance was detected in those with serum bilirubin levels over 20 mg/dl [15]. Hyperbilirubinemia in term infants has been associated with abnormalities in brain-stem audiometric evoked responses (BAER), cry characteristics, and neurobehavioral measures. However, these changes disappear when bilirubin levels fall and there are no measurable long-term sequelae [23]. Kernicterus has been reported in jaundiced healthy, full-term, breast-fed infants [14].

G. **Bilirubin toxicity and the low-birth-weight infant** [25]. Initial early studies of babies of 1250 to 2500 gm and 28 to 36 weeks' gestational age showed no

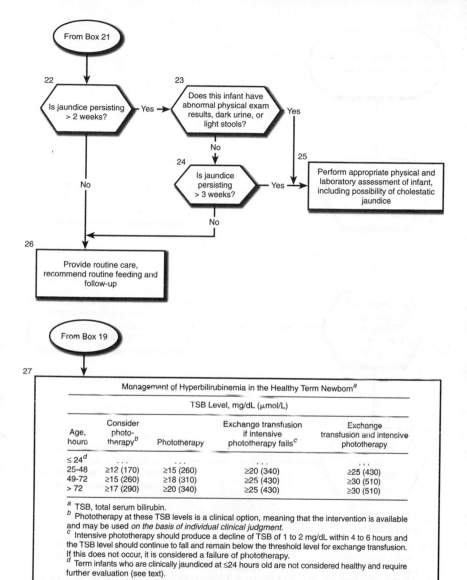

Fig. 18-3. *Continued.*

relationship between neurologic damage and bilirubin levels over 18 to 20 mg/dl. Later studies, however, began to report "kernicterus" at autopsy or neurodevelopmental abnormalities at follow-up in premature infants under 1250 gm who had bilirubin levels previously thought to be safe (e.g., under 10 to 20 mg/dl). Because kernicterus in preterm infants is now considered uncommon, hindsight suggests that this so-called "low bilirubin ker-

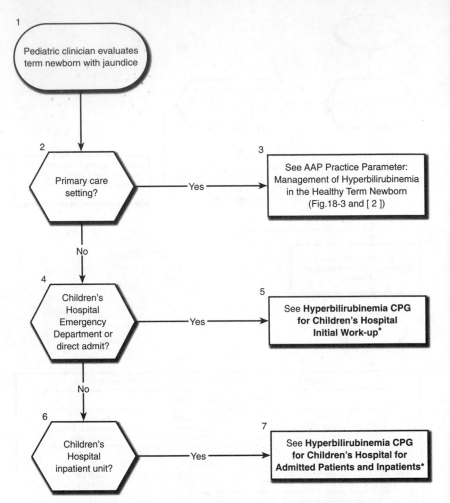

Fig. 18-4A. Children's Hospital hyperbilirubinemia clinical practice guide for evaluation of infants with jaundice who have been discharged from the birth hospital.

*These algorithms have been locally tailored for Children's Hospital, Boston, using the *American Academy of Pediatrics' Practice Parameter: Management of Hyperbilirubinemia in the Healthy Term Newborn* [2].

CLINICAL PRACTICE GUIDELINES DISCLAIMER STATEMENT: "This Clinical Practice Guideline is designed to provide clinicians an analytical framework for evaluation and treatment of a particular diagnosis or condition. This Clinical Practice Guideline is not intended to establish a protocol for all patients with a particular condition, nor is it intended to replace a clinician's clinical judgment. A clinician's adherence to this Clinical Practice Guideline is voluntary. It is understood that some patients will not fit the clinical conditions contemplated by this Clinical Practice Guideline and that the recommendations contained in this Clinical Practice Guideline should not be considered inclusive of all proper methods or exclusive of other methods of care reasonably directed to obtaining the same results. Decisions to adopt any specific recommendation of this Clinical Practice Guideline must be made by the clinician in light of available resources and the individual circumstances presented by the patient."

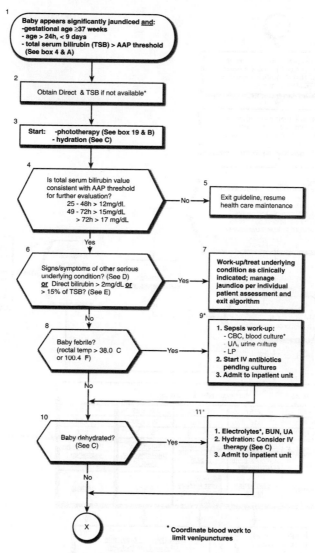

1
Baby appears significantly jaundiced **and:**
-gestational age ≥37 weeks
- age > 24h, < 9 days
- total serum bilirubin (TSB) > AAP threshold
  (See box 4 & A)

2
Obtain Direct & TSB if not available*

3
Start: -phototherapy (See box 19 & B)
           - hydration (See C)

4
Is total serum bilirubin value
consistent with AAP threshold
for further evaluation?
     25 - 48h > 12mg/dL
     49 - 72h > 15mg/dL
     > 72h > 17 mg/dL

5
Exit guideline, resume
health care maintenance

—No→

↓ Yes

6
Signs/symptoms of other serious
underlying condition? (See D)
or Direct bilirubin > 2mg/dL **or**
> 15% of TSB? (See E)

7
Work-up/treat underlying
condition as clinically
indicated; manage
jaundice per individual
patient assessment and
exit algorithm

—Yes→

↓ No

8
Baby febrile?
(rectal temp > 38.0 C
or 100.4 F)

9*
1. Sepsis work-up:
   - CBC, blood culture*
   - UA, urine culture
   - LP
2. Start IV antibiotics
   pending cultures
3. Admit to inpatient unit

—Yes→

↓ No

10
Baby dehydrated?
(See C)

11*
1. Electrolytes*, BUN, UA
2. Hydration: Consider IV
   therapy (See C)
3. Admit to inpatient unit

—Yes→

↓ No

(X)

* Coordinate blood work to
  limit venipunctures

Fig. 18-4B. Hyperbilirubinemia CPG Children's Hospital initial work-up.

nicterus" was largely due to factors other than bilirubin alone. For example, unrecognized intracranial hemorrhage, inadvertent exposure to drugs that displace bilirubin from albumin, or the use of solutions (e.g, benzyl alcohol) that can alter the blood–brain barrier may have accounted for developmental handicaps or kernicterus in infants with low levels of serum bilirubin. In addition, premature infants are more likely to suffer from anoxia, hypercarbia, and sepsis, which also open the blood–brain barrier and lead to enhanced bilirubin deposition in neural tissue. Finally, the pathologic changes seen in postmortem preterm infant brains has been more consistent with

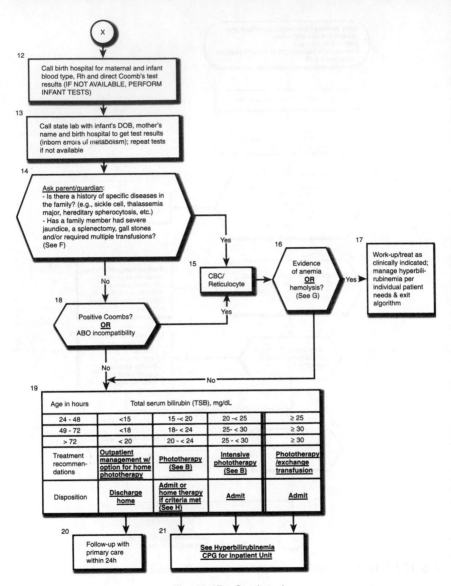

Fig. 18-4B. *Continued.*

nonspecific damage than with true kernicterus. Thus, bilirubin toxicity in low-birth-weight infants may not be a function of bilirubin levels per se but of their overall clinical status.

VI. Management of unconjugated hyperbilirubinemia. Given the uncertainty of determining what levels of bilirubin are toxic, these are general clinical guidelines only and should be modified in any sick infant with acidosis, hypercap-

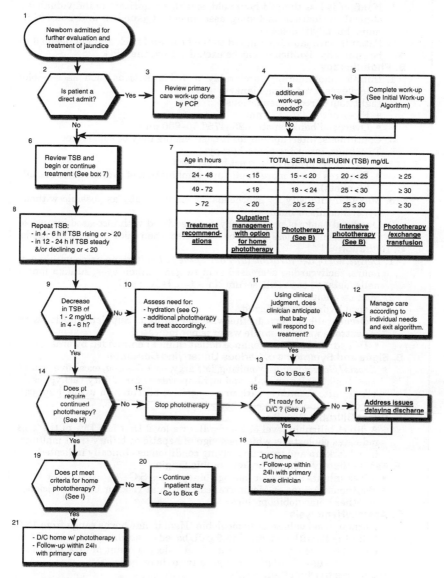

Fig. 18-4C. Hyperbilirubinemia CPG Children's Hospital for admitted patients or inpatients.

nia, hypoxemia, asphyxia, sepsis, hypoalbuminemia (<2.5 mg/dl), or signs of bilirubin encephalopathy.

A. General principles. Management of unconjugated hyperbilirubinemia is clearly tied to the etiology. Early identification of known causes of nonphysiologic hyperbilirubinemia (see III) should prompt close observation for de-

Annotations for Hyperbilirubinemia CPG (Fig. 18-4A and B)

A. Exclusion Statement

1. If infant is less than 24 hours old, exit this algorithm to individualized clinical evaluation, including assessment of jaundice and non-isoimmune hemolytic disease.
2. Patients with jaundice limited to the head and neck and not deemed to be clinically significant may be excluded from the CPG.

B. Phototherapy

1. Initiate phototherapy (preferably with blanket) as soon as feasible; shield eyes if not using blanket.
2. Light source recommendations:
   - Fiber optic (425–475 nm)
   - Overhead banks/spots (425–475/550–600 nm).
3. Continuous; interruptions for breast-feeding may be considered.
4. To achieve intensive phototherapy:
   - Maximal surface area must be exposed
   - Requires two or more lights (any combination of overheads, spots, bili blankets).
5. Maximal intensity for overheads: as close to baby as possible without hyperthermia or burn.
6. Overhead banks of phototherapy are associated with increased insensible fluid loss, and this loss should be considered when calculating intake needs.

C. Hydration

1. *Definition of dehydration (any one of the following):* no urine within 4–6 hours, tachycardia, decreased skin turgor, sunken eyes, sunken fontanelle, delayed cap refill, serum Na > 145, HCO_3 < 17.
2. Management:
   - Oral hydration preferred.
   - Breast milk preferred; otherwise, use formula. Supplementation with dextrose water or sterile water is not indicated.
   - IV hydration if maintenance deficit cannot be provided by oral route.

D. Signs and Symptoms of Serious Underlying Condition

- *Sepsis / Galactosemia:* vomiting, lethargy, poor feeding, excessive weight loss, hepatosplenomegaly, apnea, temperature instability, tachypnea.
- *Cholestatic Jaundice:* dark urine, positive bilirubin in urine, light-colored stools, persistent jaundice > 3 weeks.

E. Direct Bilirubin Results

A direct bilirubin level of 2.0 mg/dL or a level that is ≥ 15% of the TSB indicates cholestasis which is a sign of hepatic or biliary tract malfunction. Work-up and treat underlying condition as clinically indicated.

F. Family History—Ethnic or Geographic Origin

- Black infants at risk for hemoglobinopathies S,C
- Southeast Asians or Mediterranean origin at risk for G6PD deficiency or other hemoglobinopathies.

G. Anemia/Hemolysis

Normal blood values for hemoglobin (Hgb) in newborns range from 13.7 to 20.1 g/dL with a mean of 16.8 g/dL based on studies of cord blood levels in term newborns. An elevated reticulocyte count of >6% accompanied by a Hgb of <13 g/dL is suggestive of hemolysis.

H. Response to Phototherapy [2]

Bili	Age	Action
<18	—	Wean to single phototherapy
≤12	—	Discharge home
≤14	49–72h	Discontinue phototherapy, discharge home*
≤15	>72h	Discontinue phototherapy, discharge home*

*Check rebound TSB 12–24 hours after discharge.

Fig. 18-4C. *Continued.*

I. Home Phototherapy
- Parents must agree.
- Community pediatrician must agree.
- Insurance approval.
- Treatment and monitoring must be readily accessible.

J. Discharge Criteria
- Infant feeds normally and family has access to lactation consultation if breast-feeding.
- Parents have received education as to normal infant well-being, including feeding, voiding, stooling, sleep patterns and position, signs of acute illness, and infant safety.
- Follow-up appointments have been scheduled with primary pediatrician and appropriate home health services, and parents agree to such care.
- Hearing screening test should be scheduled as part of follow-up after discharge for infants who reached TSB levels exceeding indication for exchange transfusion.

Fig. 18-4C. *Continued.*

velopment of jaundice, appropriate laboratory investigation, and timely intervention. Any medication (see Table 18-1) or clinical factor that may interfere with bilirubin metabolism, bilirubin binding to albumin, or the integrity of the blood–brain barrier should be discontinued or corrected. Infants who are receiving inadequate feedings, or who have decreased urine and stool output, need increased feedings both in volume and in calories to reduce the enterohepatic circulation of bilirubin. Infants with hypothyroidism need adequate replacement of thyroid hormone. If levels of bilirubin are so high that the infant is at risk for kernicterus, bilirubin may be removed mechanically by exchange transfusion, its excretion increased by alternative pathways using phototherapy, or its normal metabolism increased by drugs such as phenobarbital.

B. Infants with hemolytic disease
1. In **Rh disease** we start intensive phototherapy immediately. An exchange transfusion is performed if the bilirubin level is predicted to reach 20 mg/dl (see Fig. 18-2, A and B).
2. In **ABO hemolytic disease** we start phototherapy if the bilirubin level exceeds 10 mg/dl at 12 hours, 12 mg/dl at 18 hours, 14 mg/dl at 24 hours, or 15 mg/dl at any time. If the bilirubin reaches 20 mg/dl, an exchange transfusion is done.
3. In hemolytic disease of other causes we treat as if it were Rh disease (Tables 18-3, 18-4, 18-5).

C. Healthy term infants (Fig. 18-3). The American Academy of Pediatrics (AAP) has published a set of practice parameters for the treatment of unconjugated hyperbilirubinemia in healthy, full-term neonates [2,3].
1. Bilirubin levels are not routinely measured on our healthy term infants unless jaundice occurs in the first 2 days of life. Most of our term infants are sent home by 24 to 48 hours of age; therefore, parents should be informed about neonatal jaundice prior to discharge from the hospital.
2. In healthy term infants who are jaundiced, we follow the guidelines published by the AAP (Fig. 18-3) [2] and have a local clinical practice guideline based on these recommendations (Fig. 18-4). For example, if the bilirubin level of a 2½-day-old is 25 to 30 mg/dl, intensive phototherapy will be started as preparations are made to perform an exchange transfusion. If a repeat bilirubin determination 4 to 6 hours later shows the bilirubin remaining above 25 mg/dl, an exchange transfusion will be performed. However, if total serum bilirubin declines to under 25 mg/dl, exchange transfusion will be held as intensive phototherapy continues.
3. In healthy term **breast-fed infants** with hyperbilirubinemia, preventive measures are the best approach and include encouragement of frequent

nursing (at least every 3 hours) and, if necessary, supplementation with formula (not dextrose water) (see **III.B.9**) [14].

4. Guidelines for phototherapy and exchange transfusion are identical for breast-fed and formula-fed infants. However, in **breast-fed infants,** a decision is often made whether or not to discontinue breast-feeding and supplement with formula if phototherapy is needed. In a recent randomized controlled trial of breast-fed infants with bilirubin levels of at least 17 mg/dl, 3% of those who switched to formula and received phototherapy reached bilirubin levels above 20 mg/dl compared with 14% of those who continued nursing while they were receiving phototherapy. In infants not receiving phototherapy, 19% of those who switched to formula reached bilirubin levels over 20 mg/dl compared with 24% of those who simply continued nursing. No infant in any group had a bilirubin over 23 mg/dl, and none required exchange transfusion [14,15].

In general, **our current practice** is that if the bilirubin reaches a level that would require phototherapy and is predicted to exceed 20 mg/dl, we will start phototherapy, discontinue breast-feeding for 48 hours, and supplement with formula. The mother requires much support through this process and is encouraged to pump her breasts until breast-feeding can be resumed.

5. Failure of bilirubin levels to fall after the interruption of breast-feeding may indicate other causes of prolonged indirect hyperbilirubinemia, such as hemolytic disease, hypothyroidism, and familial nonhemolytic jaundice (Crigler-Najjar syndrome).

D. Premature infants. There are no consensus guidelines for phototherapy and exchange transfusion in low-birth-weight infants. The following statement from the *Guidelines for Perinatal Care* from the American Academy of Pediatrics and the American Academy of Obstetricians and Gynecologists [1] emphasize our current lack of knowledge in this area:

"Some pediatricians use guidelines that recommend aggressive treatment of jaundice in low-birth-weight neonates, initiating phototherapy early and performing exchange transfusions in certain neonates with very low bilirubin levels (<10 mg/dl). However, this approach will not prevent kernicterus consistently. Some pediatricians prefer to adopt a less aggressive therapeutic stance and allow serum bilirubin concentrations in low-birth-weight neonates to approach 15 to 20 mg/dl (257 to 342 µmol/liter), before considering exchange transfusions. At present, both of these approaches to treatment should be considered reasonable. In either case, the finding of low bilirubin kernicterus at autopsy in certain low-birth-weight neonates cannot necessarily be interpreted as a therapeutic failure or equivalent to bilirubin encephalopathy. Like retinopathy of prematurity, kernicterus is a condition that cannot be prevented in certain neonates, given the current state of knowledge. Although there is some evidence of an association between hyperbilirubinemia and neurodevelopmental handicap less severe than classic bilirubin encephalopathy, a cause-and-effect relationship has not been established. Furthermore, there is no information presently available to suggest that treating mild jaundice will prevent such handicaps" [1].

Our current practice for treating jaundiced premature infants is as follows:

1. **Infants <1000 gm.** Phototherapy is started within 24 hours, and exchange transfusion is performed at levels of 10 to 12 mg/dl.
2. **Infants 1000 to 1500 gm.** Phototherapy at bilirubin levels of 7 to 9 mg/dl and exchange transfusion at levels of 12 to 15 mg/dl.
3. **Infants 1500 to 2000 gm.** Phototherapy at bilirubin levels of 10 to 12 mg/dl and exchange transfusion at levels of 15 to 18 mg/dl.
4. **Infants 2000 to 2500 gm.** Phototherapy at bilirubin levels of 13 to 15 mg/dl and exchange transfusion at levels of 18 to 20 mg/dl.

VII. Phototherapy. Although bilirubin absorbs visible light with wavelengths of about 400 to 500 nm, the most effective lights for phototherapy are those with high-energy output near the maximum adsorption peak of bilirubin (450 to 460 nm). Special blue lamps with a peak output at 425 to 475 nm are the most efficient for phototherapy. Cool white lamps with a principal peak at 550 to 600 nm and a range of 380 to 700 nm are usually adequate for treatment.

A. Photochemical reactions. When bilirubin absorbs light, three types of photochemical reactions occur.

1. **Photoisomerization** occurs in the extravascular space of the skin. The natural isomer of unconjugated bilirubin (4Z,15Z) is instantaneously converted to a less toxic polar isomer (4Z,15E) that diffuses into the blood and is excreted into the bile without conjugation. However, excretion is slow, and the photoisomer is readily converted back to unconjugated bilirubin, which is resorbed from the gut if the baby is not having stools. After about 12 hours of phototherapy, the photoisomers make up about 20% of total bilirubin. Standard tests do not distinguish between naturally occurring bilirubin and the photoisomer, so bilirubin levels may not change much even though the phototherapy has made the bilirubin present less toxic. Photoisomerization occurs at low-dose phototherapy (6 u W/cm2/nm) with no significant benefit from doubling the irradiance.

2. **Structural isomerization** is the intramolecular cyclization of bilirubin to **lumirubin.** Lumirubin makes up 2 to 6% of serum concentration of bilirubin during phototherapy and is rapidly excreted in the bile and urine without conjugation. Unlike photoisomerization, the conversion of bilirubin to lumirubin is irreversible, and it cannot be reabsorbed. It is the most important pathway for the lowering of serum bilirubin levels and is strongly related to the dose of phototherapy used in the range of 6 to 12 u W/cm2/nm.

3. The slow process of **photo-oxidation** converts bilirubin to small polar products that are excreted in the urine. It is the least important reaction for lowering bilirubin levels.

B. Indications for phototherapy

1. Phototherapy should be used when the level of bilirubin may be hazardous to the infant if it were to increase, even though it has not reached levels requiring exchange transfusion (see **VI**).

2. Prophylactic phototherapy may be indicated in special circumstances, such as extremely-low-birth-weight infants or severely bruised infants. In hemolytic disease of the newborn, phototherapy is started immediately while the rise in the serum bilirubin level is plotted (see Fig. 18-2) and during the wait for exchange transfusion.

3. Phototherapy is usually contraindicated in infants with direct hyperbilirubinemia caused by liver disease or obstructive jaundice because indirect bilirubin levels are not usually high in these conditions and because phototherapy may lead to the **"bronze baby" syndrome.** If both direct and indirect bilirubin are high, exchange transfusion is probably safer than phototherapy because it is not known whether the bronze pigment is toxic.

C. Technique of phototherapy [1,2,8,9,12]

1. We have found that **light banks** with alternating special blue (narrow-spectrum) and daylight fluorescent lights are effective and do not make the baby appear cyanotic. The irradiance can be measured at the skin by a radiometer and should exceed 5 u W/cm2 at 425 to 475 nm. There is not much benefit in exceeding 9 u W/cm2/nm. Bulbs should be changed at intervals specified by the manufacturer. Our practice is to change all the bulbs every 3 months because this approximates the correct number of hours of use in our unit.

2. For infants under radiant warmers, we lay infants on fiberoptic blankets and/or use **spot phototherapy** overhead with quartz halide white light having output in the blue spectrum.

3. **Fiberoptic blankets** with light output in the blue-green spectrum have proved very useful in our unit, not only for single phototherapy but also

for delivering **"double phototherapy"** in which the infant lies on a fiberoptic blanket with conventional phototherapy overhead.

4. Infants under phototherapy lights are kept naked except for eye patches and a face mask used as a diaper to insure light exposure to the greatest skin surface area. The infants are turned every 2 hours. Care should be taken to ensure that the eye patches do not occlude the nares, as asphyxia and apnea can result.

5. If an incubator is used, there should be a 5- to 8-cm space between it and the lamp cover to prevent overheating.

6. The infants' temperature should be carefully monitored and servocontrolled.

7. Infants should be weighed daily (small infants are weighed twice each day). Between 10 and 20% extra fluid over the usual requirements is given to compensate for the increased insensible water loss in infants in open cribs or warmers who are receiving phototherapy. Infants also have increased fluid losses caused by increased stooling (see Chap. 9).

8. Skin color is not a guide to hyperbilirubinemia in infants undergoing phototherapy; consequently, bilirubin level should be monitored at least every 12 to 24 hours.

9. Once a satisfactory decline in bilirubin levels has occurred (e.g., exchange transfusion has been averted), we allow infants to be removed from phototherapy for feedings and brief parental visits.

10. **Phototherapy is stopped** when it is believed that the level is low enough to eliminate concern about the toxic effects of bilirubin, when the risk factors for toxic levels of bilirubin are gone, and when the baby is old enough to handle the bilirubin load. A bilirubin level is usually checked 12 to 24 hours after phototherapy is stopped. In a recent study of infants with nonhemolytic hyperbilirubinemia, phototherapy was discontinued at mean bilirubin levels of 13.0 ± 0.7 mg/dl in term and 10.7 ± 1.2 mg/dl in preterm infants. Rebound bilirubin levels 12 to 15 hours later averaged less than 1 mg/dl, and no infant required reinstitution of phototherapy [10].

11. **Home phototherapy** is effective and is cheaper than hospital phototherapy, and is easy to implement with the use of fiberoptic blankets. Most candidates for home phototherapy are breast-fed infants whose bilirubin problems can be resolved with a brief interruption of breast-feeding and increased fluid intake. Constant supervision is required, and all the other details of phototherapy, such as temperature control and fluid intake, are also required. The Academy of Pediatrics has issued guidelines for home phototherapy but has not endorsed its use.

12. It is contraindicated to put jaundiced infants under direct sunlight, as severe hyperthermia may result.

D. Side effects of phototherapy [12]

1. Insensible water loss is increased in infants undergoing phototherapy, especially those under radiant warmers. The increase may be as much as 40% for term and 80 to 190% in premature infants. Incubators with servocontrolled warmers will decrease this water loss. Extra fluid must be given to make up for these losses (see Chap. 9, Fluid and Electrolyte Management of the Newborn).

2. Watery diarrhea and increased fecal water loss may occur. The diarrhea may be caused by increased bile salts and unconjugated bilirubin in the bowel.

3. Low calcium levels have been described in preterm infants under phototherapy.

4. Retinal damage has been described in animals whose eyes have been exposed to phototherapy lamps. The eyes should be shielded with eye patches. Follow-up studies of infants whose eyes have been adequately shielded show normal vision and electroretinography.

5. Tanning of the skin of black infants. Erythemia and increased skin blood flow may also be seen.
6. "Bronze baby" syndrome (see **VII.B.3**).
7. Mutations, sister chromatid exchange, and DNA strand breaks have been described in cell culture. It may be wise to shield the scrotum during phototherapy.
8. Tryptophan is reduced in amino acid solutions exposed to phototherapy. Methionine and histidine are also reduced in these solutions if multivitamins are added. These solutions should probably be shielded from phototherapy by using aluminum foil on the lines and bottles.
9. No significant long-term developmental differences have been found in infants treated with phototherapy compared with controls.
10. Phototherapy upsets maternal-infant interactions and therefore should be used only with adequate thought and explanation.

VIII. Exchange transfusion
  A. Mechanisms. Exchange transfusion removes partially hemolyzed and antibody-coated RBCs as well as unattached antibodies and replaces them with donor RBCs lacking the sensitizing antigen. As bilirubin is removed from the plasma, extravascular bilirubin will rapidly equilibrate and bind to the albumin in the exchanged blood. Within half an hour after the exchange, bilirubin levels return to 60% of preexchange levels, representing the rapid influx of bilirubin into the vascular space. Further increases in postexchange bilirubin levels are due to hemolysis of antibody-coated RBCs sequestered in bone marrow or spleen, from senescent donor RBCs, and from early labeled bilirubin.

  B. Indications for exchange transfusion
    1. When phototherapy fails to prevent a rise in bilirubin to toxic levels (see **VI** and Figs. 18-2, 18-3, 18-4).
    2. Correct anemia and improve congestive heart failure in hydropic infants with hemolytic disease.
    3. Stop hemolysis and bilirubin production by removing antibody and sensitized RBCs.
    4. Figure 18-2 shows the natural history of bilirubin rise in infants with Rh sensitization without phototherapy. In hemolytic disease, immediate exchange transfusion is usually indicated if
      a. The cord bilirubin level is over 4.5 mg/dl and the cord hemoglobin level is under 11 gm/dl.
      b. The bilirubin level is rising over 1 mg/dl per hour despite phototherapy.
      c. The hemoglobin level is between 11 and 13 gm/dl and the bilirubin level is rising over 0.5 mg/dl per hour despite phototherapy.
      d. The bilirubin level is 20 mg/dl, or it appears that it will reach 20 mg/dl at the rate it is rising (see Fig. 18-2).
      e. There is progression of anemia in the face of adequate control of bilirubin by other methods (e.g., phototherapy).
    5. Repeat exchanges are done for the same indications as the initial exchange. All infants should be under intense phototherapy while decisions regarding exchange transfusion are being made.

  C. Blood for exchange transfusion
    1. We use fresh (<7 days old) irradiated reconstituted whole blood (hematocrit 45 to 50) made from PRBCs and fresh frozen plasma collected in citrate-phosphate-dextrose (CPD). Cooperation with the obstetrician and the blood bank is essential in preparing for the birth of an infant requiring exchange transfusion (see Chap. 26).
    2. **In Rh hemolytic disease,** if blood is prepared before delivery, it should be type O Rh-negative cross-matched against the mother. If the blood is obtained after delivery, it also may be cross-matched against the infant.
    3. **In ABO incompatibility,** the blood should be type O Rh-negative or Rh-compatible with the mother and infant, be cross-matched against the

mother and infant, and have a low titer of naturally occurring anti-A or anti-B antibodies. Usually, type O cells are used with AB plasma to ensure that no anti-A or anti-B antibodies are present.

4. In other isoimmune hemolytic disease, the blood should not contain the sensitizing antigen and should be cross-matched against the mother.

5. In nonimmune hyperbilirubinemia, blood is typed and cross-matched against the plasma and red cells of the infant.

6. Exchange transfusion usually involves double the volume of the infant's blood and is known as a two-volume exchange. If the infant's blood volume is 80 ml/kg, then a two-volume exchange transfusion uses 160 ml/kg of blood. This replaces 87% of the infant's blood volume with new blood.

D. Technique of exchange transfusion

1. Exchange is done with the infant under a servocontrolled radiant warmer and cardiac and blood pressure monitoring in place. Equipment and personnel for resuscitation must be readily available, and an intravenous line should be in place for the administration of glucose and medication. The infant's arms and legs should be properly restrained.

2. An assistant should be assigned to the infant to record volumes of blood, observe the infant, and check vital signs.

3. The glucose concentration of CPD blood is about 300 mg/dl. After exchange, we measure the infant's glucose to detect rebound hypoglycemia.

4. Measurement of potassium and pH of the blood for exchange may be indicated if the blood is over 7 days old or if metabolic abnormalities are noted following exchange transfusion.

5. The blood should be warmed to 37°C.

6. Sterile techniques should be used. Old, dried umbilical cords can be softened with saline-soaked gauze to facilitate locating the vein and inserting the catheter. If a dirty cord was entered or there was a break in sterile technique, we treat with oxacillin and gentamicin for 2 to 3 days.

7. We do most exchanges by the **push-pull technique** through the umbilical vein inserted only as far as required to permit free blood exchange. A catheter in the heart may cause arrhythmias. (See Chap. 36 for insertion of an umbilical venous catheter.)

8. **Isovolumetric** exchange transfusion (simultaneously pulling blood out of the umbilical artery and pushing new blood in the umbilical vein) may be tolerated better in small, sick, or hydropic infants.

9. If it is not possible to insert the catheter in the umbilical vein, exchange transfusion can be accomplished through a central venous pressure line placed through the antecubital fossa or into the femoral vein via the saphenous vein.

10. In the push-pull method, blood is removed in aliquots that are tolerated by the infant. This usually is **5 ml** for infants under 1500 gm, **10 ml** for infants 1500 to 2500 gm, **15 ml** for infants 2500 to 3500 gm, and **20 ml** for infants over 3500 gm. The rate of exchange and aliquot size have little effect on the efficiency of bilirubin removal, but smaller aliquots and a slower rate place less stress on the cardiovascular system. The recommended time for the exchange transfusion is 1 hour.

11. The blood should be gently mixed after every deciliter of exchange to prevent the settling of RBCs and the transfusion of anemic blood at the end of the exchange.

12. After exchange transfusion, phototherapy is continued and bilirubin levels are measured every 4 hours.

13. When the exchange transfusion is finished, a silk purse-string suture should be placed around the vein; the tails of the suture material should be left. This localization of the vein will facilitate the next exchange transfusion.

14. When the catheter is removed, the tie around the cord should be tightened snugly for about 1 hour. It is important to remember to loosen the tie after 1 hour to avoid necrosis of the skin.

E. **Complications of exchange transfusions**
   1. **Hypocalcemia and hypomagnesemia.** The citrate in CPD blood binds ionic calcium and magnesium. Hypocalcemia associated with exchange transfusion may produce cardiac and other effects (see Chap. 29). We usually do not give extra calcium unless the electrocardiogram (ECG) and clinical assessment suggest hypocalcemia. The fall in magnesium associated with exchange transfusion has not been associated with clinical problems.
   2. **Hypoglycemia.** The high glucose content of CPD blood may stimulate insulin secretion and cause hypoglycemia 1 to 2 hours after an exchange. Blood glucose is monitored for several hours after exchange and the infant should have an intravenous line containing glucose (see Chap. 29).
   3. **Acid-base balance.** Citrate in CPD blood is metabolized to alkali by the healthy liver and may result in a late metabolic alkalosis. If the baby is very ill and unable to metabolize citrate, the citrate may produce significant acidosis.
   4. **Hyperkalemia.** Potassium levels may be greatly elevated in stored PRBCs, but washing the cells before reconstitution with fresh frozen plasma removes this excess potassium. Washing by some methods (IBM cell washer) may cause hypokalemia. If blood is over 24 hours old, it is best to check the potassium level before using it (see Chap. 9).
   5. **Cardiovascular.** Perforation of vessels, embolization (with air or clots), vasospasm, thrombosis, infarction, arrhythmias, volume overload, and arrest.
   6. **Bleeding.** Thrombocytopenia, deficient clotting factors (see Chap. 26).
   7. **Infections.** Bacteremia, hepatitis, CMV, HIV (AIDS), and malaria (see Chap. 23).
   8. **Hemolysis.** Hemoglobinemia, hemoglobinuria, and hyperkalemia caused by overheating of the blood have been reported. Massive hemolysis, intravascular sickling, and death have occurred from the use of hemoglobin SC donor blood.
   9. **Graft-versus-host disease.** This is prevented by using **irradiated blood.** Before blood was irradiated, a syndrome of transient maculopapular rash, eosinophilia, lymphopenia, and thrombocytopenia without other signs of immunodeficiency was described in infants receiving multiple exchange transfusions. This did not usually progress to graft-versus-host disease.
   10. **Miscellaneous.** Hypothermia, hyperthermia, and possibly necrotizing enterocolitis.

IX. **Other treatment modalities**
A. **Increasing bilirubin conjugation. Phenobarbital,** in a dose of 5 to 8 mg/kg every 24 hours, induces microsomal enzymes, increases bilirubin conjugation and excretion, and increases bile flow. It is useful in treating the indirect hyperbilirubinemia of Crigler-Najjar syndrome type II (but not type I) and in the treatment of the direct hyperbilirubinemia associated with hyperalimentation. Phenobarbital given antenatally to the mother is effective in lowering bilirubin levels in erythroblastotic infants, but concerns about toxicity prevent its routine use in pregnant women in the United States. Phenobarbital does not augment the effects of phototherapy.
B. **Decreasing enterohepatic circulation.** In breast-fed and formula-fed infants with bilirubins above 15 mg/dl, oral agar significantly increases the efficiency and shortens the duration of phototherapy. In fact, oral agar alone was as effective as phototherapy in lowering bilirubin levels [6]. Although oral agar may prove to be an economical therapy for hyperbilirubinemia, we have limited experience with its use in our nurseries.

C. **Inhibiting bilirubin production.** Metalloprotoporphyrins (e.g., tin and zinc protoporphyrins) are competitive inhibitors of heme oxygenase, the first enzyme in converting heme to bilirubin. They have been used to treat hyperbilirubinemia in Coombs'-positive ABO incompatibility and in Crigler-Najjar type I patients. In addition, a single dose of tin mesoporphyrin given shortly after birth substantially prevented the development of hyperbilirubinemia and the duration of phototherapy in Greek preterm (30 to 36 weeks) infants [22]. However, these agents are still experimental and are not yet in routine use.

D. **Inhibiting hemolysis.** High-dose intravenous immune globulin has been used to reduce bilirubin levels in infants with isoimmune hemolytic disease [20]. The mechanism is unknown, but the immune globulin could act by occupying the Fc receptors of reticuloendothelial cells, thereby preventing them from taking up and lysing antibody-coated RBCs. This therapy has not been used in our nurseries to control hyperbilirubinemia.

X. **Direct or conjugated hyperbilirubinemia** (CB) [7] is due to failure to excrete CB from the hepatocyte into the duodenum. It is manifested by a CB level over 2.0 ml/dl or a CB level greater than 15% of the total bilirubin level. It may be associated with hepatomegaly, splenomegaly, pale stools, and dark urine. CB is found in the urine; UCB is not. The preferred term to describe it is **cholestasis,** which includes retention of conjugated bilirubin (CB), bile acids, and other components of bile.

A. **Differential diagnosis**

   1. **Liver cell injury (normal bile ducts)**

      a. **Toxic.** Intravenous hyperalimentation in low-birth-weight infants is a major cause of elevated CB in the newborn intensive care unit. It appears to be unrelated to the parenteral use of lipid. Sepsis and ischemic necrosis may cause cholestasis.

      b. **Infection.** Viral: hepatitis (B, non-A, non-B, A?), giant-cell neonatal hepatitis, rubella, cytomegalovirus, herpes, Epstein-Barr virus, coxsackievirus, adenovirus, echoviruses 14 and 19. Bacterial: syphilis, *Escherichia coli,* group B β-hemolytic *Streptococcus, Listeria,* tuberculosis, *Staphylococcus.* Parasitic: *Toxoplasma.*

      c. **Metabolic.** Alpha-1-antitrypsin deficiency, cystic fibrosis, galactosemia, tyrosinemia, hypermethionemia, fructosemia, storage diseases (Gaucher's, Niemann-Pick, glycogenosis type IV, Wolman's), Roter syndrome, Dubin-Johnson syndrome, Byler disease, Zellweger syndrome, idiopathic cirrhosis, porphyria, hemochromatosis, trisomy 18.

   2. **Excessive bilirubin load (inspissated bile syndrome).** Seen in any severe hemolytic disease but especially in infants with erythroblastosis fetalis who have been treated with intrauterine transfusion. In addition, a self-limited cholestatic jaundice is frequently seen in infants supported on extracorporeal membrane oxygenation (ECMO) (see Chap. 24). The cholestasis may last as long as 9 weeks and is thought to be secondary to hemolysis during ECMO [23].

   3. **Bile flow obstruction (biliary atresia, extrahepatic or intrahepatic).** The extrahepatic type may be isolated or associated with a choledochal cyst, trisomy 13 or 18, or polysplenia. The intrahepatic type may be associated with the Alagille syndrome, intrahepatic atresia with lymphedema (Aagenaes syndrome, nonsyndromic paucity of intrahepatic bile ducts, coprostanic acidemia, choledochal cyst, bile duct stenosis, rupture of bile duct, lymph node enlargement, hemangiomas, tumors, pancreatic cyst, inspissated bile syndrome, and cystic fibrosis.

   4. In the newborn intensive care unit, the most common causes of elevated CB, in decreasing order of frequency, are hyperalimentation, idiopathic hepatitis, biliary atresia, alpha-1-antitrypsin deficiency, intrauterine infection, choledochal cyst, galactosemia, and increased bilirubin load from hemolytic disease.

B. Diagnostic tests and management
  1. Evaluate for hepatomegaly, splenomegaly, petechiae, chorioretinitis, and microcephaly.
  2. Evaluate liver damage and function by measurement of serum glutamic oxaloacetic transaminase (SGOT) level, serum glutamic pyruvic transaminase (SGPT) level, alkaline phosphatase level, prothrombin time (PT), partial thromboplastin time (PTT), and serum albumin level.
  3. Stop parenteral hyperalimentation with amino acids. If this is the cause, the liver dysfunction will usually resolve.
  4. Test for bacterial, viral, and intrauterine infections (see Chap. 23).
  5. Serum analysis for alpha-1-anitrypsin deficiency.
  6. Serum and urine amino acids determinations (see Chap. 29).
  7. Urinalysis for glucose and reducing substances (see Chap. 29).
  8. If known causes are ruled out, the problem is to differentiate idiopathic neonatal hepatitis from bile duct abnormalities such as intrahepatic biliary atresia or hypoplasia, choledochal cyst, bile plug syndrome, extrahepatic biliary atresia, hypoplasia, or total biliary atresia.
      a. Abdominal ultrasound should be done to rule out a choledochal cyst or mass.
      b. We use a hepatobiliary scan with technetium [^{99m}Tc]diisopropyliminodiacetic (DISIDA) as the next step to visualize the biliary tree.
      c. Iodine-131–rose bengal fecal excretion test may be useful if the [^{99m}Tc]DISIDA scan is not available.
      d. A nasoduodenal tube can be passed and fluid collected in 2-hour aliquots for 24 hours. If there is no bile, treat with phenobarbital, 5 mg/kg per day for 7 days, and repeat the duodenal fluid collection.
      e. If the duodenal fluid collections, scans, and ultrasound suggest no extrahepatic obstruction, a **percutaneous needle liver biopsy** is done. If the biopsy shows no features of extrahepatic obstruction, the child may be observed with careful follow-up. Sometimes features of both bile duct disease and hepatocellular disease are present, and the pathologist will be unable to give a definite diagnosis.
      f. If the ultrasound, scans, or fluid collections suggest extrahepatic obstruction disease, the baby will need an exploratory laparotomy, cholangiogram, and open liver biopsy to enable a definite diagnosis.
      g. If the diagnosis of extrahepatic obstruction disease cannot be ruled out, the baby must have the studies outlined, because surgical therapy for choledochal cyst is curative if done early and hepatoportoenterostomy has better results if done early.
XI. Hydrops [5,11,26] is a term used to describe generalized subcutaneous edema in the fetus or neonate. It is usually accompanied by ascites and often by pleural and/or pericardial effusions. Hydrops fetalis is discussed here, because in the past, hemolytic disease of the newborn was the major cause of both fetal and neonatal hydrops. However, because of the decline in Rh sensitization, nonimmune conditions are now the major causes of hydrops in the United States.
  A. Etiology. The pathogenesis of hydrops includes anemia, cardiac failure, decreased colloid oncotic pressure (hypoalbuminemia), increased capillary permeability, asphyxia, and placental perfusion abnormalities. There is a general, but not a constant, relationship between the degree of anemia, the serum albumin level, and the presence of hydrops. There is no correlation between the severity of hydrops and the blood volume of the infant. Most hydropic infants have normal blood volume (80 mg/kg).
      1. **Hematologic** due to chronic in utero anemia (10% of cases). Isoimmune hemolytic disease (e.g., Rh incompatibility), homozygous alpha thalassemia, homozygous G-6-PD deficiency, chronic fetomaternal hemorrhage, twin-to-twin transfusion, hemorrhage, thrombosis, bone marrow failure (chloramphenicol, maternal parvovirus infection), bone marrow replacement (Gaucher's disease), leukemia.

2. **Cardiovascular** due to heart failure (20% of cases) (see Chap. 25).
   a. **Rhythm disturbances.** Heart block, supraventricular tachycardia, atrial flutter.
   b. **Major cardiac disease.** Hypoplastic left heart, Epstein's anomaly, truncus arteriosus, myocarditis (coxsackievirus), endocardial fibroelastosis, cardiac neoplasm (rhabdomyoma), cardiac thrombosis, arteriovenous malformations, premature closure of foramen ovale, generalized arterial calcification, premature restructure of the foramen ovale.
3. **Renal** (5% of cases). Nephrosis, renal vein thrombosis, renal hypoplasia, urinary obstruction.
4. **Infection** (8% of cases). Syphilis, rubella, cytomegalovirus, congenital hepatitis, herpesvirus, adenovirus, toxoplasmosis, leptospirosis, Chagas' disease, parvovirus (see Chap. 23).
5. **Pulmonary** (5% of cases). Congenital chylothorax, diaphragmatic hernia, pulmonary lymphangiectasia, cystic adenomatoid malformations, intrathoracic mass.
6. **Placenta or cord** (rare cause). Chorangioma, umbilical vein thrombosis, arteriovenous malformation, chorionic vein thrombosis, true knot in umbilical cord, cord compression, choriocarcinoma.
7. **Maternal conditions** (5% of cases). Toxemia, diabetes, thyrotoxicosis.
8. **Gastrointestinal** (5% of cases). Meconium peritonitis, in utero volvulus, atresia.
9. **Chromosomal** (10% of cases). Turner syndrome; trisomy 13, 18, 21; triploidy; aneuploidy.
10. **Miscellaneous** (10% of cases). Cystic hygroma. Wilms' tumor, angioma, teratoma, neuroblastoma, CNS malformations, amniotic band syndrome, lysosomal storage disorders, congenital myotonic dystrophy, skeletal abnormalities (osteogenesis imperfecta, achondrogenesis, hypophosphatasia, thanatophoric dwarf, arthrogryposis), Noonan syndrome, acardia, absent ductus venosus, renal venous thrombosis, cystic hygroma.
11. **Unknown** (20% of cases).

B. **Diagnosis.** A pregnant woman with polyhydramnios, severe anemia, toxemia, or isoimmune disease should undergo ultrasonic examination of the fetus. If the fetus is hydropic, a careful search by ultrasound and real-time fetal echocardiography may reveal the cause and may guide fetal treatment. The accumulation of pericardial or ascitic fluid may be the first sign of impending hydrops in a Rh-sensitized fetus. Investigations should be carried out for the causes of fetal hydrops mentioned in **A.** The usual investigation includes the following:
   1. **Maternal** blood type and Coombs' test as well as red cell antibody titers, complete blood count and red blood cell indices, hemoglobin electrophoresis, Kleihauser-Betke stain of maternal blood for fetal red cells, VDRL, studies for viral infection and toxoplasmosis (see Chap. 23), sedimentation rate, lupus tests.
   2. **Fetal** echocardiography for cardiac abnormalities and ultrasound for other structural lesions.
   3. **Amniocentesis** for karyotype, metabolic studies, fetoprotein, cultures and polymerase chain reaction (PCR) for viral infections and restriction endonucleases as indicated.
   4. **Fetal blood sampling (PUBS)** (see Chap. 1, [26]). Karyotype, CBC, hemoglobin electrophoresis, cultures, and PCR, DNA studies, albumin.
   5. **Neonatal.** Following delivery, many of the same studies may be carried out on the infant. A complete blood count, blood typing, and Coombs' test; ultrasound studies of the head, heart, and abdomen; and a search for the causes listed in **A** should be done. Examination of pleural and/or ascitic fluid, liver function tests, urinalysis, viral titers, chromosomes, placental examination, and x-rays may be indicated. If the infant is stillborn or dies, a detailed autopsy should be done.

Table 18-3. Common antigens other than Rh implicated in hemolytic disease of the newborn

Antigen	Alternative symbol or name	Blood group system
Do^a		Dombrock
Fy^a		Duffy
Jk^a		Kidd
Jk^b		Kidd
K	K:1	Kell
Lu^a	Lu:1	Lutheran
M		MNSs
N		MNSs
S		MNSs
s		MNSs

C. Management

1. A hydropic fetus is at great risk for intrauterine death. A decision must be made about intrauterine treatment if possible, e.g., fetal transfusion in isoimmune hemolytic anemia (see Chap. 1) or maternal digitalis therapy for supraventricular tachycardia (see Chap. 25). If fetal treatment is not possible, the fetus must be evaluated for the relative possibility of intrauterine death versus the risks of premature delivery. If premature delivery is planned, pulmonary maturity should be induced with steroids if it is not present (see Chap. 24). Intrauterine paracentesis or thoracentesis just prior to delivery may facilitate subsequent newborn resuscitation.

2. Resuscitation of the hydropic infant is complex and requires advance preparation whenever feasible. Intubation can be extremely difficult with massive edema of the head, neck, and oropharynx and should be done by a skilled operator immediately after birth. (A fiberoptic scope may facilitate placement of the endotracheal tube.) A second individual should provide rapid relief of hydrostatic pressure on the diaphragm and lungs by paracentesis and/or thoracentesis with an 18- to 20-gauge angiocatheter attached to a three-way stopcock and syringe. After entry into the chest or abdominal cavity, the needle is withdrawn so that the plastic catheter can remain without fear of laceration. Cardiocentesis may also be required if there is electromechanical dissociation due to cardiac tamponade.

3. Ventilator management can be complicated by pulmonary hypoplasia, barotrauma, pulmonary edema, or reaccumulation of ascites and/or pleural fluid. If repeated thoracenteses cannot control hydrothorax, chest tube drainage may be indicated. Judicious use of diuretics (e.g., furosemide) is often helpful in reducing pulmonary edema. Arterial access is needed to monitor blood gases and acid-base balance.

4. Because hydropic infants have enormous quantities of extravascular salt and water, fluid intake is based on an estimate of the infant's "dry weight" (e.g., 50th percentile for gestational age). Free water and salt are kept at a minimum (e.g., 40 to 60 ml/kg/day as dextrose water) until edema is resolved. Monitoring the electrolyte composition of serum, urine, ascites fluid, and/or pleural fluid, and careful measurement of intake, output, and weight are essential for guiding therapy. Normoglycemia is achieved by providing glucose at a rate of 4 to 8 mg/kg per minute. Unless cardiovascular and/or renal function are compromised,

Table 18-4. Other antigens involved in hemolytic diseases of the newborn

Antigen	Alternative symbol or name	Blood group system
Co^a		Colton
Di^b		Diego
Ge		Gerbich
Hy	Holley	
Jr		
Js^b	Matthews, K:7	Kell
k	Cellano, K:2	Kell
Kp^b	Rautenberg, K:4	Kell
Lan	Langereis	
Lu^b		Lutheran
LW	Landsteinder-Weiner	
P, P1, P^k	Tj^a	P
U		MNSs
Yt^a		Cartwright

edema will eventually resolve and salt and water intake can then be normalized.

5. If the hematocrit is under 30%, a partial exchange transfusion with 50 to 80 ml/kg packed red cells (hematocrit 70%) should be performed to raise the hematocrit and increase oxygen carrying capacity. If the problem is Rh isoimmunization, the blood should be type O Rh-negative. We often use O-negative cells and AB serum prepared before delivery and cross-matched against the mother. An isovolumetric exchange (simultaneous removal of blood from the umbilical artery while blood is transfused in the umbilical vein at 2 to 4 ml/kg per minute) may be better tolerated in infants with compromised cardiovascular systems.

6. Inotropic support (e.g., dopamine) may be required to improve cardiac output. Central venous and arterial lines are needed for monitoring pressures. Most hydropic infants are normovolemic, but manipulation of the blood volume may be indicated after measurement of arterial and venous pressures and after correction of acidosis and asphyxia. If a low serum albumin level is contributing to hydrops, fresh-frozen plasma may help. Care must be taken not to volume-overload an already failing heart, and infusions of colloid may need to be followed by a diuretic.

7. Hyperbilirubinemia should be treated as in **VI.**

8. Many infants with hydrops will survive if aggressive neonatal care is provided.

XII. **Isoimmune hemolytic disease of the newborn** [4]

A. **Etiology.** Maternal exposure (via blood transfusion, feto-maternal hemorrhage, amniocentesis, or abortion) to foreign antigens on fetal RBCs causes the production and transplacental passage of specific maternal IgG antibodies directed against the fetal antigens, resulting in the immune destruction of fetal RBCs. The usual antigen involved prenatally is the Rh(D) antigen, and postnatally, the A and B antigens. A positive Coombs' test result in an infant should prompt identification of the antibody. If the antibody is not anti-A or anti-B, then it should be identified by testing the mother's serum against a panel of red cell antigens or the father's red cells. This may have implications for subsequent pregnancies. Since the dramatic decline in Rh hemolytic disease with the use of Rhogam, maternal antibody against A or

Table 18-5. Infrequent antigens implicated in hemolytic diseases of the newborn

Antigen	Alternative symbol or name	Blood group system
Be^a	Berrens	Rh
Bi	Biles	
By	Batty	
C^w	Rh:8	Rh
C^x	Rh:9	Rh
Di*^{a}		Diego
Evans		Rh
E^w	Rh:11	Rh
Far	See Kam	
Ga	Gambino	
Go^a	Gonzales	Rh
Good		
Heibel		
Hil	Hill	MNSs Mi sub +
Ht^a	Hunt	
Hut	Hutchinson	MNSs Mi sub
Js^a	Sutter	Kell
Kam (Far)	Kamhuber	
Kp^a	Penney	Kell
Mit	Mitchell	
Mt^a	Martin	MNSs#
Mull	Lu:9	Lutheran
Mur	Murrell	MNSs Mi sub
Rd	Radin	
Re^a	Reid	
R^N	Rh:32	Rh
Vw(Gr)	Verweyst (Graydon)	MNSs Mi sub
Wi^a	Wright	
Zd		

This may not be a complete list. Any antigen that the father has and the mother does not have and that induces an IOG response in the mother may cause sensitization.

B antigens (ABO incompatibility) is now the most common cause of isoimmune hemolytic disease. In addition, other relatively uncommon antigens (Kell, Duffy, E, C, and c) now account for a greater proportion of cases of isoimmune hemolytic anemia (Tables 18-3, 18-4, 18-5).

B. Fetal management. All pregnant women should have blood typing, Rh determination, and an antibody screening performed on their first prenatal visit. This will identify the Rh-negative mothers and identify any antibody due to Rh or any rare antigen sensitization. In a Caucasian population in the United States, 15% of people lack the D antigen (dd). Of the remainder, 48% are heterozygous (dD) and 35% are homozygous (DD). Approximately 15% of matings in this population will result in a fetus with the D antigen and a mother without it.

1. If the mother is **Rh-positive** and her **antibody screening is negative,** it may be advisable to repeat the antibody screening later in pregnancy, but this will have a low yield.

2. If the mother is **Rh-negative/antibody screen negative** and the father of the fetus is Rh-negative, she should be retested at 28 and 35 weeks' gestation (see **D** for prenatal Rhogam). If the father is Rh-positive, she should be retested at 18 to 20 weeks and monthly thereafter.

3. If the mother is **Rh-negative/antibody screen positive**, the antibody titer is repeated at 16 to 18 weeks, at 22 weeks, and every 2 weeks thereafter. Amniocentesis is usually done for antibody titers over 1:16 or at a level at which the local center has had a fetal demise (each center should have its own standards for action on various titers). Irrespective of antibody titers, if there is a prior history of a severely isoimmunized fetus, serial amniocentesis may be indicated beginning at 16 to 18 weeks to measure the optical density at a wavelength of 450 nm (bilirubin) to assess the risk for fetal death from hydrops. If the fetus is less than 24 weeks (optical density is less accurate) or if placental trauma is likely with amniocentesis, direct percutaneous fetal blood sampling for blood type, direct Coombs' test, hematocrit, CBC, and blood gases may be preferable.

4. Fetuses at high risk for death may be treated by early delivery if the risk of fetal demise or intrauterine transfusion exceeds the risk of early delivery. In our institution, this is usually 30 weeks, but this requires careful fetal monitoring, induction of pulmonary maturity, and close cooperation between obstetrician and neonatologist. If the hydropic fetus is too immature for early delivery to be considered, **intrauterine transfusion** is indicated. Transfusion can be carried out by intraperitoneal or intravascular routes, although intravascular transfusion may be the only option in a moribund hydropic infant who has ascites, is not breathing, and is unable to absorb intraperitoneal blood. Intrauterine transfusions are repeated whenever fetal hemoglobin levels fall below about 10 gm/dl. Following transfusion, serial ultrasound examinations are done to assess changes in the degree of hydrops and fetal well-being. Some infants who have undergone multiple intrauterine transfusions will be born with all adult O-negative RBCs because all the fetal cells are destroyed. Although one should be prepared, not all infants will need postnatal exchange transfusion. These infants are at risk to develop conjugated hyperbilirubinemia.

C. **Neonatal management.** About half the infants with a positive Coombs' test result from Rh hemolytic disease will have minimum hemolysis and hyperbilirubinemia (cord bilirubin level <4 mg/dl and hemoglobin level >14 gm/dl). These infants may require no treatment or only phototherapy. One-fourth of infants with Rh hemolytic disease present with anemia, hemoglobin level less than 14 gm/dl, and hyperbilirubinemia (cord bilirubin >4 mg/dl). They have increased nucleated red cells and reticulocytes on blood smear. These infants may have thrombocytopenia and a very elevated white blood cell count. They have an enlarged liver and spleen, and they require early exchange transfusion and phototherapy (see **VI.B, VII,** and **VIII**). Figure 18-2 and Table 18-3 can be used in deciding what treatment to use. Infants with isoimmune hemolytic anemia may develop an exaggerated physiologic anemia at 12 weeks of age, requiring blood transfusion. Erythropoietin is currently being evaluated for use in preventing this late anemia [21]. High dose intravenous immune gamma-globulin therapy is an experimental therapy for Rh hemolytic disease.

D. **Prevention.** Eliminating exposure of women to foreign red cell antigens will prevent immune hemolytic disease of the newborn. Avoiding unnecessary transfusions and medical procedures that carry the risk of transplacental passage of blood will help decrease sensitization. Rh hemolytic disease is now being prevented by the administration of **Rho(D) immune globulin (Rhogam)** to unsensitized Rh-negative mothers. This is usually done at 28 weeks' gestation and again within 72 hours after delivery.

Other indications for Rho(D) immune globulin (or for using larger doses) are prophylaxis following abortion, amniocentesis, chorionic villus sampling, and transplacental hemorrhage. Interestingly, **ABO incompatibility** between mother and fetus protects against sensitization of an Rh-negative mother, probably because maternal antibodies eliminate fetal RBCs from the maternal circulation before they can encounter antibody-forming lymphocytes.

XIII. **ABO hemolytic disease of the newborn** [10,12]. Since the introduction of Rh immune globulin, ABO incompatibility has been the most common cause of hemolytic disease of the newborn in the United States.

    A. Etiology. The cause is the reaction of maternal anti-A or anti-B antibodies to the A or B antigen on the red cells of the fetus or newborn. It is usually seen only in type A or B infants born to type O mothers because these mothers make anti-A or anti-B antibodies of the IgG class, which cross the placenta, while mothers of type A or B usually make anti-A or anti-B antibodies of the IgM class, which do not cross the placenta. The combination of a type O mother and a type A or type B infant occurs in 15% of pregnancies in the United States. Only one-fifth of infants with this blood group setup (or 3% of all infants) will develop significant jaundice. Some bacterial vaccines, such as tetanus toxoid and pneumococcal vaccine, had A and B substance in the culture media and were associated with significant hemolysis in type A or type B neonates born to type O mothers who were given these vaccines. New preparations of the vaccine are said to be free of these A and B substances.

    B. Clinical presentation. The situation is a type O mother with a type A or type B infant who becomes jaundiced in the first 24 hours of life. Approximately 50% of the cases occur in firstborn infants. There is no predictable pattern of recurrence in subsequent infants. **The majority of ABO-incompatible infants have anti-A or anti-B antibody on their red cells, yet only a small number have significant ABO hemolytic disease of the newborn.** Infants may have a low concentration of antibody on their red cells; consequently, their antibody will not be demonstrated by elution techniques or by a positive direct antiglobulin test (Coombs' test). As the antibody concentration increases, the antibody can be demonstrated first by elution techniques and then by the Coombs' test. Although all ABO-incompatible infants have some degree of hemolysis, significant hemolysis is *usually* associated only with a positive direct Coombs' test result on the infant's red cells. If there are other causes of neonatal jaundice, ABO incompatibility will add to the bilirubin production. In infants with significant ABO incompatibility, there will be many spherocytes on the blood smear and an elevated reticulocyte count. RBCs from infants with ABO incompatibility may have increased osmotic fragility and autohemolysis, as in hereditary spherocytosis (HS). The autohemolysis is not corrected by glucose, as in HS. The family history and long-term course will usually help with the diagnosis of HS.

    C. Management. If blood typing and Coombs' test are done on the cord blood of infants born to type O mothers, these infants can have bilirubin levels monitored and therapy instituted early enough to prevent severe hyperbilirubinemia. However, this approach may not be cost-effective, because most infants do not develop significant jaundice and only 10% of infants with a positive direct Coombs' test result for ABO incompatibility will need phototherapy. In the absence of a routine test on all infants born to type O mothers, one must rely on clinical observation to notice the jaundiced infants. This will depend on the observation of the caregivers and may not be reliable in infants whose skin pigmentation makes the diagnosis of jaundice difficult. A bilirubin level at 12 hours of age, or cord blood typing and a Coombs' test on all black or Asian infants born to type O mothers, may be a reasonable compromise. Infants born to type O mothers who are to have an early discharge (within 24 hours) should be evaluated for ABO incompatibility, and the parents should be made aware of the possibility of jaundice. Many infants have an initial rise in bilirubin that quickly falls to normal levels. If the criteria for Rh disease are used, many will undergo unnecessary treatment. An approach to phototherapy and exchange transfusion management has been outlined in **VI.B.** Kernicterus has been reported in ABO incompatibility. If exchange transfusion is necessary, it should be with type O blood that is of the same Rh type as the infant with a low titer of anti-A or anti-B antibody. We often use type O cells resuspended in type AB plasma. There is no need for prenatal diagnosis or treatment and no need for early delivery.

References

1. AAP and ACOG. *Guidelines for Perinatal Care* (3d Ed.). Elk Grove Village, Ill.: American Academy of Pediatrics, 1992.
2. AAP. Practice parameter: Management of hyperbilirubinemia in the healthy term newborn. *Pediatrics* 94:558, 1994.
3. AAP. *Practice parameter: Management of hyperbilirubinemia in the healthy term newborn. Technical Report.* Elk Grove Village, Ill.: AAP, 1994.
4. Bowman, J. M., Hemolytic disease (erythroblastosis fetalis). In Creasy, R. K., and Resnik, R. (Eds.). *Maternal-Fetal Medicine: Principles and Practice* (3rd Ed.). Philadelphia: Saunders, 1994.
5. Carlton, D. P., et al. Nonimmune hydrops fetalis: A multidisciplinary approach. *Clin. Perinatol.* 16:839, 1989.
6. Coglayan, S., et al. Superiority of oral agar and phototherapy combination in the treatment of neonatal hyperbilirubinemia. *Pediatrics* 92:86, 1993.
7. Fitzgerald, J. F. Cholestatic disorders of infancy. *Pediatr. Clin. North Am.* 35:357, 1988.
8. Gartner, L. M. Neonatal jaundice. *Pediatr. Rev.* 15:422, 1994.
9. Gartner, L. M., et al. Neonatal bilirubin workshop. *Pediatrics* 94:537, 1994.
10. Lazar, L., et al. Phototherapy for neonatal nonhemolytic hyperbilirubinemia. *Clin. Pediatr.* 32:264, 1993.
11. Machin, G. A. Hydrops revisited: Literature review of 1,414 cases published in the 1980's. *Am. J. Med. Gen.* 34:366, 1989.
12. Maisels, M. J. Jaundice. In Avery, G. B., Fletcher, M. A., and MacDonald, M. A. (Eds.). *Neonatology: Pathophysiology and Management of the Newborn* (4th Ed.). Philadelphia: Lippincott, 1994, 630.
13. MacDonald, M. Early discharge and bilirubin toxicity due to G-6-PD deficiency. *Pediatrics* 96:134, 1995.
14. Maisels, M. J., et al. Kernicterus in otherwise healthy, breast-fed term newborns. *Pediatrics* 96:730, 1995.
15. Martinez, J. C., et al. Hyperbilirubinemia in the breast fed newborn: A controlled trial of four interventions. *Pediatrics* 91:470, 1993.
16. Newman, T. B., et al. Neonatal hyperbilirubinemia and long-term outcome: Another look at the collaborative perinatal project. *Pediatrics* 92:651, 1993.
17. Newman, T.B., et al. Does hyperbilirubinemia damage the brain of healthy full-term newborns? *Clin. Perinatol.* 17:331, 1990.
18. Newman, T. B., et al. Evaluation and treatment of jaundice in the term newborn: A kinder, gentler approach. *Pediatrics* 89:809, 1992.
19. Peterec, S. M. Management of neonatal Rh disease. *Clin. Perinatol.* 22:561, 1995.
20. Rubo, J., et al. High dose intravenous immune globulin therapy for hyperbilirubinemia caused by Rh hemolytic disease. *J. Pediatr.* 121:93, 1992.
21. Scaradavon, A., et al. Suppression of erythropoiesis by intrauterine transfusions in hemolytic disease of the newborn: Use of erythropoietin to treat the late anemia. *J. Pediatr.* 123:279, 1993.
22. Valaes, T., et al. Control of jaundice in preterm infants by an inhibitor of bilirubin production: Studies with tin-mesoporphyrin. *Pediatrics* 93:1, 1994.

23. Vohr, B. R. New approaches to assessing the risks of hyperbilirubinemia. *Clin. Perinatol.* 17:293, 1990.
24. Walsh-Sukys, M. C., et al. The natural history of direct hyperbilirubinemia associated with extracorporeal membrane oxygenation. *Am. J. Dis. Child.* 146:1176, 1992.
25. Watchko, J. F. Kernicterus in preterm newborns: Past, present, and future. *Pediatrics* 90:707, 1992.
26. Wilkins, I. Nonimmune hydrops. In Creasy, R. K., and Resnik, R. (Eds.). *Maternal-Fetal Medicine: Principles and Practice* (3rd Ed.). Philadelphia: Saunders, 1994.

19. DRUG ABUSE AND WITHDRAWAL

Sylvia Schechner

I. **Maternal substance abuse.** In the epidemic of substance abuse in the United States, the drugs most often abused are cannabinoids, heroin, and, most recently, cocaine, probably because of its inexpensive alkaloidal free-base form, "crack." There is a 15% overall prevalence of at least one of the above substances in urine samples. Iatrogenic neonatal abstinence syndrome may been seen in infants who required narcotics for surgery, ECMO, or other procedures.

  A. **Take a comprehensive medical and psychosocial history** including a specific inquiry about maternal drug use as part of every prenatal and newborn evaluation.

   1. **Maternal associations with drug abuse**
      a. Poor or no prenatal care
      b. Preterm labor
      c. Placental rupture
      d. Precipitous delivery
      e. Frequent demands or requests for large doses of pain medication
   2. **Signs of maternal drug abuse in the infant**
      a. SGA
      b. Microcephaly
      c. Neonatal stroke or any arterial infarction
      d. Any of the symptoms in Table 19-1

  B. **Diagnostic tests.** Screen urine if drug withdrawal is a possibility. Consider the implications of a positive test result. The following is our statement for testing:

Physician Guidelines for Testing, Reporting, and Care of Neonates Who May Have Been Exposed Prenatally to Controlled Substances

Brigham and Women's Hospital, Boston, MA

   1. **Testing**
      a. **Purpose**

      A positive urine test for controlled substances can serve several purposes: (1) it may help to complete a diagnostic work-up for an infant with symptoms of drug dependency or withdrawal (e.g., seizures or jitteriness); (2) it may serve as a marker for an infant at risk for developmental delay; and (3) it may indicate an at-risk family in need of social services. (A negative test result, however, cannot rule out any of these items.)

      b. **Symptomatic infants**

         i. *Performance of a toxic screen is recommended for infants with any of the following symptoms: (a) severe Intrauterine Growth Retardation (IUGR) which is defined as a birth weight below the third percentile; (b) symptoms consistent with neonatal drug dependency and withdrawal; (c) central nervous system (CNS) irritability; and (d) symptoms consistent with intra-cranial hemorrhage (ICH) such as focal seizures or paresis. These criteria are intended to serve as guidelines only. The attending physician must decide on a case by case basis whether a toxic screen is indicated.*

         ii. *It is hospital policy not to require a separate specific consent from the parents for a toxic screen on a symptomatic infant. As testing of symptomatic infants is done to assist in the medical diagnosis or treatment of the infant, the general parental consent obtained in the initial admission consent form is usually sufficient. Parents, how-*

211

Table 19-1. Reported withdrawal syndromes in newborns after maternal drug ingestion

	Lethargy	Poor state control	Fever	Diaphoresis	Tachycardia	Tachypnea	Cyanosis	High-pitched cry	Altered sleeping	Tremors	Hypotonicity	Hypertonicity	Hyperreflexia	Increased suck
Narcotics														
Heroin			X	X	X	X		X	X	X		X	X	X
Methadone			X	X	X	X		X	X	X		X	X	X
Propoxyphene			X	X	X			X		X		X	X	X
Pentazocine plus tripelennamine ("T's and Blues")				X	X			X		X	X	X		X
("T's and Blues")								X	X				X	
Codeine	X									X		X	X	
Sedatives														
Barbiturates				X					±	X	X	X	X	X
Butalbital (Fiorinal, Esgic)														
Chlordiazepoxide										X				
Diazepam						X	X			X			X	X
Diphenhydramine										X				
Ethanol						X				X	X			
Ethchlorvynol (Placidyl) (plus propoxyphene plus diazepam)						X						X		
Glutethimide (plus heroin)				X				X	X	X			X	X
Hydroxyzine (Vistaril) (600 mg/day plus Pb)								X	X	X				X
Stimulants														
Methamphetamine	X	X							X			X		
Phencyclidine												X	X	X
Cocaine	X	X						X	X	X		X	X	X
Antidepressants														
Tricyclics				X	X	X	X			X	X	X	X	
Antipsychotics														
Phenothiazines								X		X		X	X	X

Key: X = symptom usually present; ± = symptom may be present, but not always; Pb = phenobarbital.

ever, should be informed by the responsible pediatrician (prior to the test if possible) of the purpose of the toxic screen, and that a positive test will be included in any report to the State Department of Social Services. This discussion should be documented in the medical record. In the event that the parents, when informed, object to the performance of the toxic screen, the legal office should be contacted for consultation. The results of the test and any follow-up or

Ineffective suck	Irritability	Jitteriness	Seizures	Nasal congestion	Sneezing/yawning	Ravenous appetite	Vomiting	Excessive regurgitation	Diarrhea	Weight loss	Abdominal distention	Onset	Duration
	X	X	X	X	X	X	X	X	X	X		1–144 hours	7–20 days
	X	X	X	X	X	X	X	X	X	X		1–14 days	20–45 days
	X	X	X	X	X	X			X	±		3–20 hours	56 h–6 days
	X	X	X	X		X		X			X		
X	X	X											
X	X	X					X		X			0.5–30 hours	4–17 days
X	X	X	X			X	X	X	X	X	X	0.5 h–14 days	11 days–6 months
X	X	X	?	X								2 days	24 days
		X										21 days	37 days
X		X					X				X	2–6 hours	10 days–6 weeks
								X				5 days	10 days–5 weeks
	X	X	X	±						±	X	6–12 hours	
X	X	X						X	X			24 hours	9–10 days
X										X		8 hours	45 days
X	X	X	X									15 minutes	156 hours
X					X							5–24 hours	
	X								X	X		18–20 hours	18 days–2 months
X				X	X	X						1–3 days	
X	X	X	X									5–12 hours	96 hours–30 days
X	X	X								X		21 days	>11 days–4 months

treatment should also be discussed with the parents. The obstetrician should also be notified of all positive test results.

c. Asymptomatic infants

    i. *Specific parental consent must be obtained in order to perform a toxic screen on an asymptomatic infant. (The general admission consent form is not sufficient.) As part of the process of seeking consent, the parent or parents should be advised by the attending physician or the physician designee of the purpose of the test and that a positive test will likely result in a referral to the Department* *of Social Services. Documentation of this discussion and the oral, parental response should be made in the infant's medical record. (A separate written consent form signed by the parent is not required.) The obstetrician should also be notified of all positive test results.*

ii. *Testing of an asymptomatic infant may be indicated by the following circumstances: (a) lack of adequate prenatal care; (b) past or present parental history or signs of substance abuse; or (c) abruptio placenta. These criteria are simply guidelines. It is the responsibility of the attending physician to determine on a case by case basis whether testing of an asymptomatic infant may be beneficial.*

2. **Referral**

Physicians, nurses, social workers, and other patient care employees are required by the State of Massachusetts' Protection and Care of Children Act (commonly known as 51A) to report to the Massachusetts Department of Social Services cases of suspected child abuse and neglect, including all infants "determined to be physically dependent upon an addictive drug at birth." Reports generated by this hospital are usually filed by the hospital Social Services Department. The hospital Social Services Department should therefore be notified of all infants with symptoms of physical dependency to an addictive drug so that a 51A report can be filed as legally required.

The hospital Social Services Department should also be notified of all asymptomatic infants with a positive toxic screen and all infants believed to be at risk due to possible parental or family substance abuse. Such cases are not automatically required by law to be reported, and the hospital Social Services Department will conduct a further evaluation to determine whether a potential abuse or neglect situation exists. If such situation is believed to exist, a report will be made. Prior experience indicated that most situations involving an infant with a positive screen (regardless of whether the infant is asymptomatic) will warrant the filing of a report.

Drugs administered during labor may cause difficulty in interpreting urine results. The length of time during which results may be positive varies with the drug.

1. Cocaine: up to 4 days
2. Heroin: 2 to 4 days
3. PCP: 2 to 4 days
4. Marijuana: 2 to 5 days

If the drugs were taken before these times, negative results may be falsely reassuring. Meconium may be useful for screening for cocaine, cannabinoids, heroin, and morphine.

C. A drug-addicted mother is at **increased risk for other diseases** such as sexually transmitted diseases, tuberculosis, hepatitis, and AIDS, especially if she involves herself in intravenous drug use or prostitution. About 30% of pregnant intravenous drug users are seropositive for HIV.

II. **Withdrawal in the infant.** The onset of symptoms for acute narcotic withdrawal varies from shortly after birth to 2 weeks of age, but symptoms usually begin in 24 to 48 hours, depending on the type of drug and when the mother took the last dose. Table 19-1 shows the withdrawal symptoms in newborns. Methadone, heroin, and cocaine are the most common reasons for withdrawal seen in our nurseries.

A. **The severity of withdrawal** depends on the drugs used. Withdrawal from polydrug use is more severe than from methadone, which is more severe than from opiates alone or cocaine alone.

B. **Methadone,** because of its ability to block the euphoric effects of heroin, is used in pregnancy to treat heroin addiction.

1. It can cause withdrawal in 75 to 90% of infants exposed in utero.
2. The severity of the symptoms correlates with the maternal dose.

3. Maintaining a woman on less than 20 mg per day will minimize symptoms in the infant. Higher methadone doses may increase severity and prolong withdrawal.
4. Some infants have late withdrawal, which may be of two types:
  a. Symptoms appear shortly after birth, improve, and recur at 2 to 4 weeks.
  b. Symptoms are not seen at birth but develop 2 to 3 weeks later.
5. Effects in the infant exposed to methadone during pregnancy:
  a. Lower birth weight, length, and head circumference.
  b. Sleep disturbances.
  c. Depressed interactive behavior.
  d. Poor self-calming.
  e. Tremors.
  f. Increased tone.
  g. Abstinence-associated seizures.
  h. Abnormal pneumograms.
  i. Increased incidence of sudden infant death syndrome (SIDS).
  j. Follow-up studies reveal a higher incidence of hyperactivity, learning and behavior disorders and poor social adjustment. This may be due more to environmental factors than as a consequence of in-utero methadone exposure.
C. Differential diagnosis. Consider hypoglycemia, hypocalcemia, hypomagnesemia, sepsis, and meningitis even if the diagnosis of drug-addicted mother is certain.
III. Treatment of infant narcotic withdrawal. The goal is an infant who is not irritable, has no vomiting or diarrhea, can feed well and sleep between feedings, and yet is not heavy sedated (see Fig. 19-2).
  Never give **Narcan** (naloxone) to these infants nor to one whose mother was on methadone; it may precipitate immediate withdrawal or seizures.
A. Symptomatic treatment. Forty percent need no medication. Symptomatic care includes tight swaddling, holding, rocking, placing in a slightly darkened quiet area, and hypercaloric formula (24 cal per 30 ml) as needed.
B. Medication. Infants who are unresponsive to symptomatic treatment will need medication. Base the decision to start medication on objective measurement of symptoms recorded on a withdrawal scoring sheet, such as the one shown in Fig. 19-1. A total abstinence score of 8 or higher for three consecutive scorings indicates a need for pharmacologic intervention. Once the infant scores 8 or higher, decrease the scoring interval from 4-hour to 2-hour intervals. Once the desired effect has been obtained for 72 hours, slowly taper the dose until it is discontinued. Observe the infant for 2 to 3 days prior to discharge.
  For treatment of infants with narcotic withdrawal, we use the following pharmacologic agents in our nurseries:
  1. Neonatal morphine solution (NMS). This solution of morphine sulfate made up in a concentration of 0.4 mg/ml is our treatment of choice for narcotic withdrawal.
    a. It is a pharmacologic replacement.
    b. Controls all symptoms.
    c. Least impairs sucking.
    d. Contains few additives.
  However, high doses are often necessary, and withdrawal is slow.
  This is the equivalent dose of morphine contained in neonatal opium solution (NOS) (see **III.B.2**). Since the only diluent is water, it avoids alcohol, preservatives, or camphor. Ours is made up in the hospital pharmacy. It has greater stability than DTO, and if it is prepared properly there are no problems with overgrowth of mold or microorganisms. The dose is 0.05 ml/kg or 2 drops per kilogram every 4 to 6 hours, increased by 2 drops (or 0.05 ml/kg) at the end of each 4-hour period until the desired response is achieved.

DATE: _____

SYSTEM	SIGNS AND SYMPTOMS	SCORE	AM	PM	COMMENTS
					Daily Weight:
CENTRAL NERVOUS SYSTEM DISTURBANCES	Excessive High-pitched (OR Other) Cry	2			
	Continuous High-pitched (OR Other) Cry	3			
	Sleeps < 1 Hour After Feeding	3			
	Sleeps < 2 Hours After Feeding	2			
	Sleeps < 3 Hours After Feeding	1			
	Hyperactive Moro Reflex	2			
	Markedly Hyperactive Moro Reflex	3			
	Mild Tremors Disturbed	1			
	Moderate-Severe Tremors Disturbed	2			
	Mild Tremors Undisturbed	3			
	Moderate-Severe Tremors Undisturbed	4			
	Increased Muscle Tone	2			
	Excoriation (Specify Area): _____	1			
	Myoclonic Jerks	3			
	Generalized Convulsions	5			
METABOLIC/VASOMOTOR/RESPIRATORY DISTURBANCES	Sweating	1			
	Fever < 101 (99-100.8° F./37.2-38.2° C)	1			
	Fever > 101 (38.4° C. and Higher)	2			
	Frequent Yawning (> 3-4 times/interval)	1			
	Mottling	1			
	Nasal Stuffiness	1			
	Sneezing (> 3-4 times/interval)	1			
	Nasal Flaring	2			
	Respiratory Rate > 60/Min.	1			
	Respiratory Rate > 50/Min. with Retractions	2			

Guidelines for the use of neonatal abstinence scoring system

1. Record time of scoring (end of observation interval).
2. Give points for all behaviors or symptoms observed during the scoring interval, even though they may not be present at the time of recording. (For example, if the baby was diaphoretic at 11 A.M. and is "scored" at noon, when he or she is not, the baby still gets the "sweating" point.)
3. Awaken the baby to test reflexes. Calm before assessing muscle tone, respirations, or Moro reflex. Many of the signs of hunger can appear the same as withdrawal. Appearance after feeding gives a good idea of muscle activity.
4. Count respirations for a full minute. Always take temperature at the same site. The temperatures on the sheet are rectal levels; an axillary temperature that is 2 degrees cooler may also indicate withdrawal.
5. Do not give points for perspiration if it occurs due to swaddling.
6. A startle reflex should not be substituted for the Moro reflex.

7. Record doses administered (dose/time/initials) on sheet. One hour leeway is acceptable in dosing a fairly stable baby.
8. Record daily weight on graphic sheet.
9. Do not hesitate to get your experienced colleagues' opinions.

GASTROINTESTINAL DISTURBANCES

Excessive Sucking	1
Poor Feeding	2
Regurgitation / Projectile Vomiting	2 / 3
Loose Stools / Watery Stools	2 / 3

TOTAL SCORE

INITIALS OF SCORER

NO.	PHARMACOTHERAPY REGIMEN	STATUS OF PHARMACOTHERAPY	RX	STATUS	DOSE	TIME	STATUS	DOSE	TIME	STATUS	DOSE	TIME	STATUS	DOSE	TIME	STATUS
1	TITRATION REGIMENS	Indicate exact dose, time of administration & coded dosing status in the following blocks	#1												AM PM	
		Dosing Code	#2												AM PM	
		Initiation (+)	#3												AM PM	
2		Maintenance (m) Increase (↑) Decrease (↓) Discontinuation (−)	#4												AM PM	

Drug Administered:

SEROLOGIC QUANTITATION OF PHARMACOLOGIC AGENTS

* BEFORE BIRTH   METHADONE _____

− AFTER BIRTH   BENZODIAZEPINES (Specify): _____

BARBITURATES (Specify): _____

OTHERS (Specify): _____

Fig. 19-1. Neonatal abstinence syndrome assessment and treatment. Guidelines for use of the neonatal abstinence scoring system are also included. (Adapted from L. P. Finnigan et al. A scoring system for evaluation and treatment of neonatal abstinence syndrome: A new clinical and research tool. In: Morselli, P. L., Garattini, S., Serini, F. (Eds.) *Basic and therapeutic aspects of perinatal pharmacology*, New York: Raven Press, 1975.)

An alternative dosing scheme for NMS or NOS according to abstinence score is as follows:

Score	NMS or NOS
8–10	0.8 ml/kg/day divided q 4 h
11–13	1.2 ml/kg/day divided q 4 h
14–16	1.6 ml/kg/day divided q 4 h
17 or greater	2.0 ml/kg/day divided q 4 h; increase by 0.4-ml increments until controlled

Add phenobarbital to control irritability when the NMS or NOS dose is greater than 2.0 ml/kg/day (see **III.B.2**). Some babies will need medication more often than every 4 hours.

Once an adequate dose has been found, and infant scores have been less than 8 for 1 to 2 days, wean by 10% (of total dose) daily. If weaning results in scores greater than 8, restart the last effective dose. Discontinue NMS or NOS when the daily dose is less than 0.3 ml/kg/day. The infant should be able to tolerate mild symptomatology during reduction.

If the scores are too low, make sure that the infant is not overdosed. Side effects include sleepiness, constipation, poor suck, and ultimately profound narcosis with obtundation, hypothermia, respiratory depression, apnea, and bradycardia. If this occurs, stop the medication until the abstinence scores are over 8. Use Colace to treat constipation.

2. **Neonatal opium solution (NOS)** (diluted deodorized tincture of opium [DTO]). If NMS is not available, use NOS for treatment of narcotic withdrawal. DTO is a hydroalcoholic solution containing 10% USP laudanum and is equal to morphine 1.0%. This is diluted 25-fold with sterile water to a concentration and potency equal to that of paregoric (0.4 mg/ml of morphine). The diluted mixture should be called NOS, as suggested in the Neonatal Drug Withdrawal Statement of the American Academy of Pediatrics' Committee on Drugs. The NOS dose is the same as that of NMS. This dilution is stable for 2 weeks. Keep the stock solution of tincture of opium in the pharmacy and dilute it there because of the possibility of giving the stronger mixture to the patient in error.

3. **Paregoric** contains opium 0.4%, equivalent to morphine 0.04% (0.4 mg/ml). It also contains anise oil, benzoic acid, camphor, and glycerin in an alcohol base. Dose as for NMS or NOS. Paregoric is readily available and has a long shelf life. Because of the unknown effects of many of the ingredients, we do not use it.

4. **Phenobarbital** (5 to 8 mg/kg/day). Give IM or PO in three divided doses and taper by 10% each day after improvement of symptoms. Phenobarbital is the drug of choice if the infant is thought to be withdrawing from a nonnarcotic drug or from multiple drug use. In narcotic withdrawal, some prefer phenobarbital to NOS to discontinue exposing the developing neonatal brain to narcotics. The possible side effects of phenobarbital include sedation and poor sucking. It does not control the diarrhea that occurs with withdrawal. Using phenobarbital with NOS allows a lower dose of NOS and lessens the side effects. Phenobarbital elixir may contain 20% alcohol, and the parenteral form may contain propylene glycol, ethyl alcohol, and benzyl alcohol.

5. **Chlorpromazine** is no longer routinely used by us because of its unacceptable side effects, including tardive dyskinesia. It is useful to control the vomiting and diarrhea that sometimes occur in withdrawal. The dosage is 1.5 to 3.0 mg/kg/day, administered in four divided doses, initially IM, then PO. Maintain this dose for 2 to 4 days and then taper as tolerated every 2 to 4 days.

6. **Methadone** is not routinely used by us for withdrawal from narcotics. Since methadone is excreted in breast milk, methadone-treated mothers

should not breast-feed. It has a prolonged plasma half-life (24 hours). Doses used by others are 0.5 to 1.0 mg every 4 to 8 hours.

7. **Morphine** in doses of 0.1 to 0.2 mg/kg can be effective in the emergency treatment of seizures or shock due to acute narcotic withdrawal.

8. We do not recommend **diazepam** (Valium), but it has been used for control of symptoms. Some hospitals use it in doses of 0.1 to 0.3 mg/kg IM until symptoms are controlled, halve the dose, then change to every 12 hours, and lower again. The major side effect is respiratory depression. Breakthrough symptoms, including seizures, respiratory depression, and bradycardia have been seen during diazepam use. Also, withdrawal has recurred after termination of therapy. The sodium benzoate included in parenteral diazepam may interfere with the binding of bilirubin to albumin. The manufacturer warns that the safety and efficacy of injectable diazepam have not been established in the newborn (see Appendix).

9. **Lorazepam** is often used for sedation by itself or with NMS or NOS. The parenteral preparation of lorazepam contains benzyl alcohol and polyethylene glycol. It is given as 0.05 to 0.1 mg/kg IV per dose. When used in conjunction with NOS, it may decrease the amount of NOS needed. Limited data are available about its use in newborns.

C. Closely monitor fluid and electrolyte intake and losses. Replace as needed.

D. The narcotic abstinence scoring sheet (see Fig. 19-1) will help establish objective criteria for weaning the infant from the medications. Irritability, tremors, and disturbance of sleeping patterns may last for up to 6 months and should not be a reason for continuing medication. For a general approach to management, see Fig. 19-2.

IV. **Maternal addiction to drugs other than narcotics.** Infants born to mothers using drugs other than narcotics may be symptomatic.

A. **Cocaine** has a potent anorexic effect and may cause prenatal malnutrition, an increased rate of premature labor, spontaneous abortion, placental abruption, fetal distress, meconium staining, and low Apgar scores. Cocaine increases catecholamines, which can increase uterine contractility and cause maternal hypertension and placental vasoconstriction with diminished uterine blood flow and fetal hypoxia.

1. The following are congenital anomalies associated with cocaine use during pregnancy: cardiac anomalies; skull defects; genitourinary malformations; "prune belly" syndrome; intestinal atresias; perinatal cerebral infarctions, usually in the distribution of the middle cerebral artery with resultant cystic lesions; early-onset necrotizing enterocolitis; and retinal digenesis and retinal coloboma.

2. **Effects in the newborns.** Although cocaine-addicted infants do not show the classic signs of narcotic withdrawal, they demonstrate abnormal sleep patterns, tremors, poor organizational response, inability to be consoled, and transiently abnormal EEGs and visual evoked potentials.

3. **Treatment.** The newborn's withdrawal rarely requires pharmacologic treatment. When the pregnant cocaine abuser also uses other drugs, the neonate may have more severe withdrawal; we then use phenobarbital.

   If symptomatic treatment is not adequate (see **III.A**), use phenobarbital or lorazepam for sedation.

4. **SIDS.** Cocaine-exposed infants appear to be at a 3 to 7 times higher risk for SIDS. This may be due to impaired regulation of respiration and arousal.

5. **Long-term disabilities** such as attention deficits, concentration difficulties, abnormal play patterns, and flat, apathetic moods have been reported. Some believe that the neurologic and cognitive outcomes of cocaine exposure are unclear, because standard methods of measuring infant neurologic and behavioral functions are difficult to quantitate. It is also difficult to extricate the effects of cocaine use from the effects of lack of prenatal care, polydrug use, and the increased risks associated

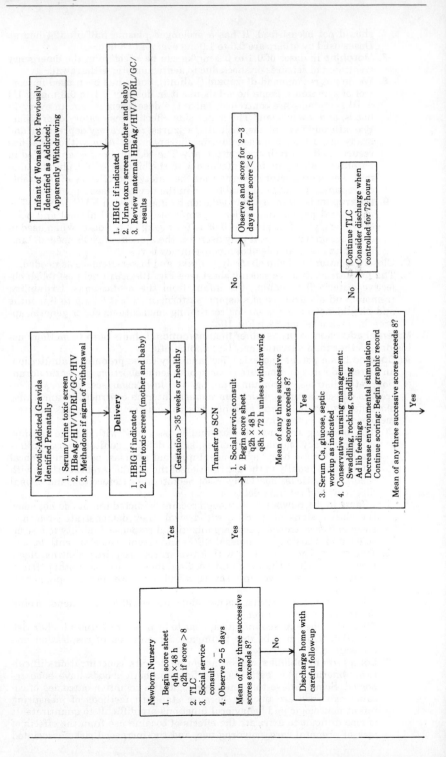

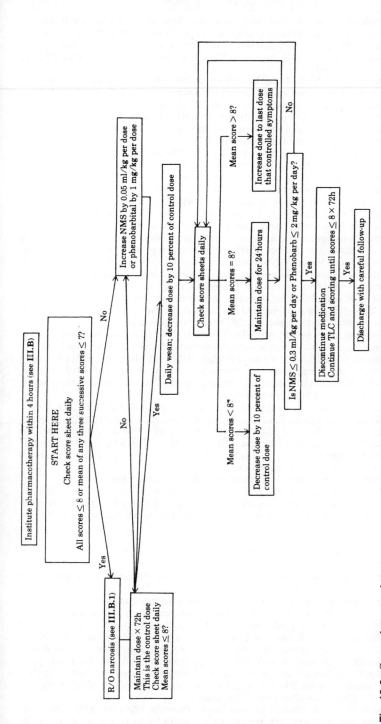

Fig. 19-2. General approach to management of a narcotic-addicted gravida identified antenatally and of a withdrawing infant of a woman not previously identified as addicted. HBsAG = hepatitis B surface antigen, VDRL = Venereal Disease Research Laboratory, TLC = tender loving care, NMS = neonatal morphine solution, RR = respiratory rate, HR = heart rate, GC = gonorrhea, HBIG = hepatitis B immune globulin, HIV = human immunodeficiency virus, SCN = special care nursery.

with a drug-using lifestyle. Convulsions have been seen both in infants of breast-feeding mothers using cocaine and in infants exposed to passive crack smoke inhalation. Because cocaine and its metabolites can be found in breast milk for up to 60 hours after use, breast-feeding is not recommended.

B. Phencyclidine (PCP). A methanolysis of 206 infants exposed to phencyclidine prenatally did not show any congenital anomalies. Infants of PCP-abusing mothers are of normal size. Most of the neonatal manifestations of in utero exposure center on neurobehavioral effects (irritability, jitteriness, hypertonicity). Since phencyclidine is excreted in breast milk, discourage breast-feeding if the mother uses this drug.

C. Marijuana. Prenatal use may result in shorter gestation with prolonged or arrested labor. There may be decreased fetal growth but no increase in major or minor morphologic anomalies. No reported adverse effects have been documented with breast-feeding. However, the drug may persist in milk for days after exposure and become concentrated with long-term use. Encourage abstinence if the infant is to be breast-fed. Some have found low Brazelton scores in these neonates and poor McCarthy scores on follow-up [4].

D. Ethanol. Teratogenic studies are confounded by other risk factors, but there is no established safe level of ethanol use in pregnancy. Symmetric growth retardation can occur in utero, the extent of which depends on the dose and duration of maternal use and on other factors such as concomitant tobacco or other drug use and overall nutrition. Although alcohol passes freely into breast milk, acetaldehyde, the toxic metabolite of ethanol, does not pass into milk. Therefore, the American Academy of Pediatrics considers moderate maternal ethanol use to be compatible with breast-feeding.

  1. Fetal alcohol syndrome (FAS) includes the following features: microcephaly, growth retardation, dysmorphic facial features (such as hypoplastic midface, low nasal bridge, flattened philtrum, thinned upper vermilion, epicanthal fold, shortened palpebral fissure), cardiac problems, hydronephrosis, increased incidence of mental retardation, motor problems, and behavioral issues.

E. Tobacco. Smoking by pregnant women is associated with a higher rate of spontaneous abortions. Placental vascular resistance is increased as a consequence of the effects of nicotine, with resultant chronic ischemia and hypoxia. Nicotine can enter breast milk in relatively low levels and is not well absorbed by the infant's intestinal tract. This does not negate the risks to the infant from passive exposure to smoke.

  1. Effects on newborn infants of regular smokers (1 pack per day)
    a. Typically weigh 150 to 250 grams less than the newborns of nonsmokers. The most pronounced effects of smoking on fetal growth occur after the second trimester. Fetuses may also be at risk by passive exposure.
    b. Increased tremors.
    c. Poor auditory responsiveness.
    d. Increased tone.
    e. No association has been found between maternal smoking during pregnancy and congenital anomalies.
    f. SIDS has been associated, in a dose–response manner, with maternal smoking, possibly secondary to passive exposure to smoke after birth.

V. Disposition. The major problems with infants of a drug-addicted mother are proper disposition and follow-up. Studies show a high incidence of abuse and violence in the childhood and lives of drug-abusing women. This, combined with their own drug use and chaotic lifestyles, places them at risk for inadequate parenting. These factors may be more important to the outcome of the child than the drug abuse. The health of the mother, especially if she has AIDS, is significant for the ultimate well-being of the infant.

A. These infants are difficult to care for, as they are often irritable, have poor sleeping patterns, and will try the patience of any caregiver. They are at increased risk for child abuse. Infants of HIV-positive mothers should be followed up closely because of their increased risk of AIDS (see Chap. 23).

B. Coordination of plans with social service agencies, drug treatment centers, and the courts, when necessary, is essential for proper follow-up and disposition.

C. Many states require that infants who show signs of withdrawal be reported as battered children.

References

1. Chemical dependency and pregnancy. *Clin. Perinatol.* 18(1), 1991.
2. Drug abuse in pregnancy. *Clin. Obstet. Gynecol.* 36(2), 1993.
3. The 100th Ross Conference on Research. Ross Substances, Columbus, Ohio, 1991.
4. Rosen, T. S. Infants of addicted mothers. In: Fanaroff, A. A., Martin, R. J. (Eds.). *Neonatal-Perinatal Medicine,* 6th ed. St. Louis: Mosby, 1997, Chap. 25.
5. Vilandi, F. L. Assessment and management of opoid withdrawal in ill neonates. *Neonatal Network* 14:39, 1995.

20. BIRTH TRAUMA*

Miles K. Tsuji

I. **Background.** **Birth trauma** is defined as injury to the infant resulting from mechanical forces (such as compression or traction) during parturition. Such injuries are not always avoidable and may occur antenatally, during resuscitation, or intrapartum.

A. **Incidence.** Advances in obstetric practice and technology have significantly decreased birth trauma mortality, which now occurs in only 3.7 per 100,000 live births [3,6]. The incidence of nonfatal birth trauma varies depending on the injury type. Caput succedaneum and cephalhematoma are common. More significant injuries occur in 2 to 7 per 1000 live births [3].

B. **Risk factors.** The process of birth is a blend of compressions, contractions, torques, and tractions. When fetal size, presentation, or neurologic immaturity complicates this, such intrapartum forces can lead to tissue damage, edema, hemorrhage, or fracture in the neonate. The use of obstetric instruments may amplify the effect of such forces or may induce injury by itself. Proper use of obstetric instruments may decrease the incidence of asphyxia. Although breech presentation carries the greatest risk of injury, delivery by cesarean section does not guarantee an injury-free infant.

The following circumstances increase the risk of birth injury and may act synergistically:

1. **Primiparity**
2. **Small maternal stature**
3. **Maternal pelvic anomalies**
4. **Prolonged or extremely rapid labor**
5. **Deep transverse arrest** of descent of presenting part of fetus
6. **Oligohydramnios**
7. **Abnormal presentation** (i.e., breech)
8. **Use of midforceps or vacuum extraction**
9. **Versions and extraction**
10. **Very-low-birth-weight infant or extreme prematurity**
11. **Fetal macrosomia**
12. **Large fetal head**
13. **Fetal anomalies**

C. **Evaluation.** Recognition of trauma at birth necessitates a careful physical and neurologic examination of the infant to establish whether there are other injuries. This is also essential in any infant who requires resuscitation in the delivery room when trauma may be occultly responsible. Assess symmetry of structure and function, range of motion of individual joints, and scalp and skull integrity, and perform cranial nerve examinations.

II. **Types of birth trauma**

A. **Head and neck injuries**

1. **Associated with fetal monitoring.** Fetal scalp blood sampling and electrode placement rarely produce hemorrhage, or infection with abscess formation at the monitoring site. Malpositioned electrodes can cause facial or ocular injuries.

2. **Extracranial hemorrhage** (see Chap. 27)

   a. **Classification**

      (1) **Cephalhematoma** is a subperiosteal collection of blood secondary to rupture of the blood vessels between the skull and periosteum;

---

*This is a revision of a chapter by Brian S. Bradley that appeared in the third edition of *Manual of Neonatal Care.*

over days, suture lines delineate its extent. Occipital cephalhematoma can mimic an encephalocele and cranial ultrasound is required for diagnosis. Linear fractures may underlie a cephalhematoma 5 to 20% of the time. Resolution occurs over 1 to 2 months, occasionally with residual calcification.

(2) **Subgaleal hematoma** is blood that invaded the potential space between the skull periosteum and the galea aponeurotica, an area that extends posteriorly from the orbital ridges to the occiput and laterally to the ears. This hematoma is capable of spreading across the entire calvarium. Its growth may be insidious and not recognizable for hours or days, or it may present as hemorrhagic shock and even death. The scalp may pit similarly to edema; ecchymoses may present periorbitally and/or auricularly. Resorption occurs very slowly.

(3) **Caput succedaneum** is a serosanguineous, subcutaneous, extraperiosteal fluid collection with poorly defined margins; it can extend across the midline and over suture lines and is usually associated with head molding. The soft-tissue edema usually resolves over the first few days postpartum. There have been rare instances of scalp necrosis with permanent scarring [1].

(4) **Vacuum caput** is a serosanguineous fluid accumulation well defined by the position of the vacuum extractor on the scalp. Significant hemorrhage is unusual; the fluid collection typically redistributes within hours after birth. Scalp abrasions and lacerations sometimes leading to local infection are rare.

b. **Management.** Most extracranial hemorrhages resolve spontaneously and warrant only observation. Caput succedaneum is least likely to result in complications. Vacuum caput complications are also uncommon. Cephalhematomas may be more significant, and subgaleal hemorrhage may be severe. Significant hemorrhage can produce anemia with secondary hypotension and hyperbilirubinemia. The infant may need transfusion and phototherapy for jaundice. Large blood accumulations raise the possibility of a bleeding disorder. Infection of extracranial hematomas is unusual but can occur if skin integrity has been broken. Avoid aspiration unless there are signs of infection. Infection requires antibiotic therapy and possible drainage. Osteomyelitis and meningitis can occur with infected hematomas in the presence of skull fractures. Cephalhematomas may be associated with skull fractures and skull x-rays and/or computed tomography (CT) are indicated if CNS symptoms are present or fracture is suspected by history or examination.

3. **Intracranial hemorrhage** (see Chap. 27, Intracranial Hemorrhage)
4. **Skull fracture.** Most fractures are linear, parietal, and asymptomatic. Depressed fractures are usually associated with forceps delivery. Occipital bone fractures are usually associated with difficult breech delivery and carry a poor prognosis. The forces responsible for fracture of the skull can also cause brain contusions or disruption of blood vessels, leading to subcutaneous or intracranial bleeding. Fractures may lie occultly beneath a cephalhematoma or present with seizures, hypotension, or death. Linear fractures are most often asymptomatic. An indentation in the skull can range from inward depression of the outer bony layer without true fracture to a complete disruption of bone. Fractures associated with dural laceration can lead to herniation of meninges and brain, progressing to leptomeningeal cysts.

a. **Management.** X-ray studies are used to diagnose skull fracture. Cranial CT will show the presence of intracranial hemorrhage or edema. Linear skull fractures without neurologic sequelae heal quickly and require only observation. A neurosurgeon should evaluate depressions of the skull; occasionally, elevation requires only closed technique without surgery.

Basal skull fractures can produce shock requiring transfusion. Cerebrospinal fluid leakage is an indication for antibiotic treatment and neurosurgical consultation. X-ray studies of fractures should be repeated at 8 to 12 weeks to look for "growing fractures" or leptomeningeal cysts.

5. **Facial or mandibular fractures** may present as facial asymmetry with ecchymoses, edema, crepitance, respiratory distress, or poor feeding. Unrecognized or untreated facial fractures can lead to craniofacial deformities, including mandibular hypoplasia and malocclusion, with ocular, respiratory, and mastication problems.

   a. **Management.** Protect the airway. Immediately consult a plastic surgeon or otorhinolaryngologist and provide radiographic confirmation of fractures. Cranial CT or MRI may help in searching for retroorbital or cribriform plate disruption. Initiate treatment before fractures heal, usually by 7 to 14 days. Use antibiotics to treat all fractures that involve the sinuses or middle ear.

6. **Nasal injuries.** Compression of the nose during the birth process can result in mucosal edema and/or dislocation of the cartilaginous nasal septum from its vomerine groove. Either condition can cause significant respiratory distress and stridor.

   a. **Management.** Diagnose nasal septum dislocation by septal deviation on manual nasal tip compression. Partial obstruction of patent nasal passages is most likely due to nasal edema. Assess patency by holding a mirror or cotton wisp under the nostrils. Repeated nasal suctioning or passage of large catheters to assess patency may exacerbate nasal edema and respiratory distress. Dislocation of the septum requires otorhinolaryngology consultation and realignment of the septum to prevent deformity. Nasal edema resolves over a few days. Investigate persistent nasal obstruction to rule out choanal stenosis. Consider antibiotic coverage.

7. **Ocular injuries.** Retinal and subconjunctival hemorrhages are a common occurrence with vaginal delivery and usually resolve within 24 to 48 hours postpartum without sequelae. Forceps can be responsible for both ocular and periorbital injury. Disruption of Descemet's membrane of the cornea will lead to scarring and eventually to astigmatism and amblyopia. Hyphema, vitreous hemorrhage, local lacerations, palpebral edema, orbital fracture with abnormal extraocular muscle function, and lacrimal gland or duct damage also can occur.

   a. **Management.** Promptly consult an ophthalmologist for significant ocular injuries. Follow-up attempts at funduscopic examination may detect the haziness of evolving corneal injury.

8. **Ear injuries.** Damage to the external pinna may present as hematoma with evolution to a "cauliflower" ear. Lacerations involving the cartilage can develop into refractory perichondritis. Temporal bone injury can lead to middle- and inner-ear complications such as hemorrhage (seen as hemotympanum) and ossicular disarticulation.

   a. **Management.** Aspirate pinna hematomas with a 23-gauge needle before they can organize. For external cartilaginous or inner-ear involvement, consult an otologist. Treat with antibiotics.

9. **Sternocleidomastoid muscle (SCM) injury.** Congenital muscular torticollis is thought to be a muscular compartment syndrome, most likely due to intrauterine positioning. SCM injury during delivery can also be a cause. Head tilt and palpable mass in the SCM may be present at birth or (more commonly) may develop over the first 2 to 3 weeks of life.

   a. **Management.** Promptly begin passive stretching of the muscle several times each day; visual and auditory stimulation should encourage infant head movement that stretches the muscle. Recovery over 3 to 4 months is typical. Up to 20% of affected infants may require surgery to prevent facial asymmetry. Rule out cervical vertebral anomalies and soft-tissue lesions because they can also produce torticollis. (See also Chap. 28.)

10. **Pharyngeal injury** can occur with postpartum suctioning, endotracheal intubation, or nasogastric tube placement. Minor injuries produce only submucosal lesions, but perforation into the mediastinum or pleural cavity can occur. The infant may develop excessive secretions and regurgitation of food.

   a. **Management.** Establish diagnosis by water-soluble contrast x-ray study. Antibiotic treatment and withholding feedings for 2 weeks is successful in most infants. Treat pleural effusions by tube thoracostomy. Large perforations and persistent leakage may require surgical exploration or drainage.

B. **Cranial nerve, spinal cord, and peripheral nerve injuries.** These may be associated with breech delivery. These injuries result from hyperextension, traction, and overstretching with simultaneous rotation; they can range from localized neurapraxia to complete nerve or cord transection. Compression injury from forceps is rarely involved.

   1. **Cranial nerve injuries.** Unilateral branches of the facial (VII) and vagus (X) nerves, in the form of the recurrent laryngeal nerve, are most commonly involved and result in temporary or permanent paralysis.

      a. **Facial nerve injury.** Compression by forceps blades has been implicated in facial nerve injuries, but facial nerve palsy may be unrelated to trauma.

         (1) **Physical findings**
            (a) **Central nerve injury**—asymmetric crying facies. The mouth is drawn to the normal side, wrinkles are deeper on the normal side, and movement of the forehead and eyelid is unaffected. The paralyzed side is smooth with a swollen appearance, the nasolabial fold is absent, and the corner of the mouth droops. There is no evidence of trauma on the face.
            (b) **Peripheral nerve injury**—asymmetric crying facies. Sometimes there is evidence of trauma.
            (c) **Peripheral nerve branch injury**—asymmetric crying facies. The paralysis is limited to the forehead, eye, or mouth.

         (2) **Differential diagnosis**—nuclear agenesis (Möbius' syndrome), congenital absence of facial nerve branches, congenital absence of facial muscles, unilateral absence of orbicularis oris muscle, and intracranial hemorrhage

         (3) **Management.** Protect the open eye with patches and "synthetic tears" (methylcellulose drops) every 4 hours. If the condition has not improved in 7 to 10 days, seek neurologic and surgical consultation. Electrodiagnostic tests may be useful to predict recovery or potential residual effects. Most infants begin to recover in the first week, but full resolution may take several months. Palsy due to trauma will usually resolve or improve. Facial nerve palsy that persists is often due to absence of the nerve. Absence of the orbicularis oris muscle is often confused with facial palsy.

      b. **Recurrent laryngeal nerve injury.** Unilateral abductor paralysis, usually the result of injury to the recurrent laryngeal nerve, presents with a hoarse cry or respiratory stridor. Bilateral paralysis of vocal cords can be caused by trauma to both recurrent laryngeal nerves or more commonly, by a CNS injury such as hypoxia or hemorrhage involving the brain stem. Bilateral paralysis may present with more severe respiratory distress or asphyxia. It occasionally occurs without any trauma or known etiology.

         (1) **Diagnosis.** Direct laryngoscopy can be used to make the diagnosis and to distinguish vocal cord paralysis from other causes of respiratory distress and stridor in the newborn. Appropriate birth history (e.g., excess traction on the head during vertex delivery) sug-

gests the diagnosis. Without appropriate history, consider further evaluation to rule out more unusual causes such as cardiovascular or CNS malformations or a mediastinal tumor.

(2) Management. To minimize the risk of aspiration to infants with unilateral paralysis, give small, frequent feedings. The paralysis usually resolves within 4 to 6 weeks. Bilateral paralysis may necessitate intubation to maintain the airway. The prognosis for bilateral paralysis is variable; if recovery has not occurred by 6 weeks, tracheostomy is often required.

2. Spinal cord injuries. A fetus who is delivered vaginally with a hyperextended head has a high incidence of severe spinal cord injury. Infants born by vaginal breech delivery are also at some risk. Low Apgar scores in the delivery room may reflect injury to the brain stem and/or spinal cord. The infant may be alert, yet flaccid. Cord dural rupture can present as a loud, sharp "snap" heard at the time of delivery. This can occur without vertebral dislocation or damage. Epidural hemorrhage is the most common complication of cord trauma, with edema and temporary denervation subsequent. Motor function will be absent distal to the level of injury, with loss of deep tendon reflexes; interruption of peripheral circulatory control may lead to temperature instability. There will be a sensory level if the cord is transected. Constipation and urinary retention may appear.

  a. Management. If cord injury is suspected, in the delivery room immediately focus efforts on resuscitation and prevention of further insult. Immobilize the head relative to the spine and secure on a flat, firm surface with padding of pressure points. Perform a careful neurologic examination and evaluate the cervical spine with x ray studies to help rule out other causes of hypotonia or spinal dysraphism. CT, myelography, or magnetic resonance imaging (MRI) may be necessary. Daily neurologic assessment with attention to bowel and bladder function will help to predict long-term outcome.

3. Cervical nerve root injuries

  a. Phrenic nerve palsy (C3, 4, or 5) may result from lateral hyperextension of the neck. It is virtually always unilateral and frequently associated with brachial plexus injury (75% of patients). Respiratory distress with ipsilaterally diminished breath sounds may be the presenting sign of diaphragmatic paralysis. This nerve is occasionally damaged by the insertion of chest tubes or by surgery. Congenital absence of the nerve is rare but occurs.

    (1) Management. Chest x-ray films usually show elevation of the affected diaphragm and mediastinal shift to the opposite side. Ultrasonography or fluoroscopic examination confirms the diagnosis by showing paradoxical (upward) diaphragmatic movement during inspiration. Institute pulmonary toilet to avoid pneumonia during the anticipated 1- to 3-month recovery phase. Diaphragmatic plication or phrenic nerve pacing is possible for refractory cases.

  b. Injuries to the brachial plexus may follow traction of the head and neck, arm, or trunk. Large, hypotonic infants are especially vulnerable to excessive separation of bony segments and overstretching.

    (1) Physical findings

      (a) Injury to the fifth and sixth cervical spinal nerves (Duchenne-Erb paralysis). The affected arm is adducted and internally rotated with the elbow extended; the forearm is in pronation; and the wrist is flexed. When passively adducted, the arm falls limply to the side of the body. The Moro, biceps, and radial reflexes are absent on the affected side. The grasp reflex is intact.

      (b) Injury to the seventh and eighth cervical and first thoracic spinal nerves (Klumpke's paralysis). This affects the intrinsic muscles of the hand, and grasp is absent. Biceps and radial reflexes are present. If the cervical sympathetic fibers of the first thoracic spinal nerves are involved, Horner's syndrome is present.

(c) Injury to the entire brachial plexus. The entire arm is flaccid; all reflexes are absent.

(2) Differential diagnosis—cerebral injury, bone or soft-tissue injury of shoulder or upper arm

(3) Diagnosis and management. Perform x-ray studies of the shoulder and upper arm to rule out bony injury. Examine the chest to rule out associated phrenic nerve paralysis (present in 5% of Erb's palsy infants). Delay passive movement to maintain range of motion of the affected joints until the nerve edema resolves (7 to 10 days). Do not use the "Statue of Liberty" splint because of subsequent contractures about the shoulder. Splints may be useful to prevent wrist and digit contractures.

(4) Prognosis. Spontaneous resolution occurs in the majority of patients. However, the degree of recovery varies with the severity of the injury and is difficult to predict in the immediate neonatal period. Definite improvements during the first 1 to 2 weeks predict normal or near-normal function. Lack of improvement by 6 months suggests a permanent deficit. The ultimate length of a permanently denervated limb is markedly shortened. Delayed iris pigmentation or heterochromia iridis may follow Horner's syndrome in the newborn. Recovery is generally better for Erb's palsy. Acute surgical exploration is not indicated. Consider nerve grafting if there is no improvement by 3 months, but some infants will not be treatable because of nerve root avulsion.

C. Bone injuries (see also Chap. 28). Fractures are most often seen following breech delivery or with shoulder dystocia in macrosomic infants, but are occasionally seen with cesarean delivery. Limb traction and rotation are usually responsible.

1. Clavicular fracture. This is the most common neonatal orthopedic injury. The infant may display a pseudoparalysis on the affected side. Crepitus, palpable bony irregularity, and SCM spasm are other physical findings. Greenstick (incomplete) fractures may be asymptomatic.

   a. Management. A chest x-ray film confirms clavicular fracture. If there is diminished arm function, assess the cervical spine, brachial plexus, and humerus. Healing with palpable callus formation occurs in 7 to 10 days, even for displaced fractures, and may make the unaware parent quite anxious when discovered. Arm motion can be limited by pinning the infant's sleeve to the shirt until callus forms. Treat pain.

2. Long-bone injuries. Loss of spontaneous arm or leg movement is usually the first sign of humeral or femoral injury, followed by swelling and pain on passive motion. The obstetrician may hear and feel the "snap" of fracture. Orthopedic consultation is important.

   a. Fractures: management. Fractured humeral and femoral shafts are usually treatable by splinting; they require closed reduction and casting only when the bones are displaced. X-ray studies will help differentiate fracture from septic arthritis. Radial nerve injury may be seen with humeral fracture. Healing with callus formation occurs over 2 to 4 weeks, with complete recovery expected. Treat pain.

   b. Epiphyseal displacement: management. Separation of the humeral or femoral epiphysis occurs at the hypertrophied cartilaginous layer of the growth plate. It is secondary to rotation with strong traction, may be proximal or distal, and may result in limb growth compromise if severe. Initial examination reveals swelling, crepitus, and pain. It may be confused with a dislocation or septic joint. True joint dislocation is rare. Ultrasonography is more useful than radiographic plain films initially because the epiphysis is not ossified at birth. Metaphyseal displacement may be seen with both separation and septic arthritis. Limb immobilization for 10 to 14 days will allow callus formation. For displacement with fractures, be sure to treat pain.

D. Intraabdominal injuries (see Chap. 33). These uncommon injuries involve rupture or subcapsular hemorrhage into the liver, spleen, or adrenal gland. Infants with hepatosplenomegaly are at increased risk of these injuries.

1. **Physical findings.** Presentation may be sudden, with shock and abdominal distention, sometimes accompanied by a bluish discoloration. Hemorrhage confined by the capsule of the liver may present more insidiously, with gradual onset of jaundice, pallor, poor feeding, tachypnea, and tachycardia. Rupture of the hematoma into the abdomen causes discoloration of the abdominal wall and shock. Severe adrenal hemorrhage may present as a flank mass.

2. **Management.** Suspect intraabdominal injuries in any newborn with shock, with or without abdominal distention. For infants who have had a difficult delivery, follow daily with careful, gentle abdominal palpation and serial determinations of hematocrit level. Abdominal ultrasonography may be useful. Paracentesis is diagnostic in infants with intraperitoneal bleeding. Surgical consultation is mandatory as laparotomy is usually required for hepatic or splenic injury and sometimes required for adrenal hemorrhage. Adrenal hemorrhage may also produce adrenal insufficiency requiring hormonal replacement therapy.

E. Soft-tissue injuries
1. **Petechiae and ecchymosis** (see Chap. 26, Bleeding, and Thrombocytopenia) are common manifestations of birth trauma in the newborn. The birth history, the location of the lesions, their early appearance without evolution of new lesions, and the absence of bleeding from other sites help in differentiating petechiae and ecchymoses secondary to birth trauma from those caused by coagulopathy or vasculitis. If the etiology is uncertain, perform studies to rule out coagulation disorders and infectious etiology. These lesions resolve spontaneously within 1 week. Observe for signs of anemia or hyperbilirubinemia if the ecchymoses are extensive. Muscle trauma and soft-tissue injury of the back and lower extremities rarely produce a crush syndrome and disseminated intravascular coagulation. Treatment is supportive.

2. **Lacerations and abrasions** [see Chaps. 3 (History and Physical Exam) and 5] may be secondary to fetal monitoring (scalp electrodes) as well as actual injury during the birth process. Deep wounds (e.g., scalpel cuts during cesarean section) may require suturing. Infection is an ever-present risk, particularly with scalp lesions and underlying caput succedaneum or hematoma. Carefully clean and observe.

3. **Subcutaneous fat necrosis** [see Chaps. 3 (History and Physical Exam), 5, and 34]. Although not detectable at birth, these irregularly shaped, hard, nonpitting, subcutaneous plaques with overlying dusky, red-purple discoloration may be caused by pressure during delivery. They appear during the first 2 weeks of life, usually in large babies, on the cheeks (at the angle of the jaw), arms, back, buttocks, and thighs. These lesions are common; they are usually felt by the mother and cause her concern. They may become calcified and thus can be seen on x-ray studies. They usually resolve completely over several weeks to months.

References
1. Donn, S. M., and Faix, R. G. Long-term prognosis for the infant with severe birth trauma. *Clin. Perinatol.* 10:507, 1983.
2. Faix, R. G., and Donn, S. M. Immediate management of the traumatized infant. *Clin. Perinatol.* 8:487, 1983.
3. Mangurten, H. H. Birth injuries. In: Fanaroff, A. A., and Martin, R. J. (Eds.). *Neonatal Perinatal Medicine* (6th Ed.). St. Louis: Mosby Year Book, 1997.
4. Schullinger, J. N. Birth trauma. *Pediatr. Clin. North Am.* 40:1351, 1993.

5. Volpe, J. J. (Eds.). *Neurology of the Newborn* (3rd Ed.). Philadelphia: Saunders, 1995.
6. Wegman, M. E. Annual summary of vital statistics—1993. *Pediatrics* 92:743, 1994.

21. DECISION MAKING AND ETHICAL DILEMMAS*

Linda J. Van Marter

I. **Background.** Neonatal intensive care units (NICUs) necessitate decision making. Everyday, decisions are made about fluids, nutrition, antibiotics, tests, and other specifics of patient care. Systems are in place; expectations are defined and shared by both professionals and families. However, this apparatus is stressed when decisions with ethical implications are required; these include decisions about instituting, withholding, or withdrawing life-supporting therapy.

Issues such as extreme prematurity, multiple congenital anomalies, severe depression at birth, and chronic ventilator dependency regularly occur and present caregivers with difficult choices. Staff and parents sometimes struggle to identify the choices and then to make decisions. It is important to define the decision-making process; discussions among NICU personnel that incorporates knowledge and values at a time and place distant from a specific patient eases the process when an actual decision needs to be made.

II. **Developing a process for ethical decision making**

A. Develop a written set of guidelines for addressing difficult decisions regarding patient care. Focus on process (who, when, where) as well as on substance (how). Identify areas of consensus and disagreement, as well as the underlying guiding principles: the best interests of the child, the equal role of parents and staff in decision making, the relevance of quality of life, and so on. The guidelines should be available in the NICU and discussed during the orientation of new personnel.

B. Identify common situations (e.g., extreme prematurity, multiple congenital anomalies, severe asphyxia) and have a series of multidisciplinary discussions about these models. Develop a consensus on group values and tolerance for individual differences. In addition, develop models for discussion of cases and establish trust among professionals so that caregivers are prepared when actual situations arise.

C. Identify available resources. Determine the roles of social service, chaplains, hospital attorneys, and the hospital ethics committee. Be knowledgeable about hospital policies already existing regarding orders for DNR ("Do not resuscitate") and withdrawal of life support. Examine the ethics code of national organizations such as the American Medical Association or relevant policies of the American Academy of Pediatrics and applicable federal and state laws.

D. The role of parents needs to be defined. Determine whether parents are the formal decision makers, partners with the caregivers, or the passive recipients of predetermined decisions. Establish who communicates with families and under what circumstances.

E. Decisions should be based on the most accurate, up-to-date medical information. Good ethics starts with good facts. Consult widely, and take the time to accumulate the relevant data. Do not set **certainty** as a goal. It is almost never achievable in the NICU. A reasonable degree of medical certainty is achievable. As the weight of a decision's consequences increases, so should the rigor of the requirement for a reasonable degree of certainty.

F. Decision making should be broad-based and as free from temporal urgency as possible. **Broad-based** means relevant caregivers, family members, and others responsible for the patient's well-being.

*This is a revision of a chapter by Michael F. Epstein in the third edition of *Manual of Neonatal Care.*

G. Decision making identifies options and then uses the guidelines and principles of the unit to choose an option. Most NICUs identify the best interests of the child and the application of a benefit-burden calculus as an operating procedure.

H. Individual caregivers must feel free to remove themselves from patient care if their ethical sense conflicts with the decision of the primary team and parents.

I. People of good conscience can disagree. Therefore, parents and caregivers must be able to appeal decisions to an individual such as the NICU director or hospital attorney or to a group such as an ethics committee. No system will provide absolute certainty that the "right" decision will always be made. However, a system that is inclusive, systematic, and built on an approach that establishes a procedure for approaching issues is most likely to produce acceptable decisions.

III. The decision to redirect life-sustaining care to comfort measures. One of the most difficult issues is deciding when to withhold or withdraw life-sustaining therapies. Philosophies and approaches vary among caregivers and NICUs. The model we use emphasizes an objective interdisciplinary approach to determine the best interests of the child.

A. The goal of the process is to identify the action that is in the baby's best interest. The interests of others, including caregivers and family, are of lesser priority than are the baby's.

B. Decision making is guided by data. Caregivers explore every reasonable avenue to maximize collection of data relevant to the ethical question at hand (e.g., the most accurate possible assessments of the infant's current condition, clinical course, therapeutic options, prognosis).

C. Communication among caregivers and parents is completely open. The process by which decisions are reached is shared with the parents. The primary-care team meets daily with the parents to discuss the baby's progress, current status, plan of care, and to summarize the team's medical and ethical discussions.

D. Parents have an important role as surrogate decision makers for their child. In instances where substantial uncertainty exists as to which option is in the baby's best interest, the parents' wishes are supported.

E. Establishment of brain death is not necessary for withholding or withdrawing life-sustaining treatments. As established by amendments to the Child Abuse and Neglect Prevention and Treatment Act of 1984, medically indicated treatment can be withheld under the following conditions: (1) ongoing treatment is prolonging the baby's death, (2) the baby is in an irreversible coma, or (3) the underlying condition is so significant as to render ongoing treatment futile and inhumane. Under this legislation, subjective judgments regarding anticipated quality of life are not justifiable reasons for withholding or withdrawing life-sustaining treatment.

IV. Our **procedures** for decision making when withdrawing life-sustaining therapy is being considered are as follows:

A. The principal decision makers are the members of the primary-care team (e.g., resident, nurse practitioner, fellow, attending physician, primary nurses, and social worker). The team discusses the data, their implications, and their degree of certainty with the goal of building a consensus regarding the best plan of care for the baby and/or recommendations for the parents. Sometimes there will be strong scientific support for a particular option; in other instances, the best course of action must be estimated. A recommendation to withhold or withdraw life-sustaining treatment is made only if the team reaches consensus. When the team recommends withdrawing life-sustaining treatment, consultations are requested from a senior attending neonatologist and a senior NICU nurse who have not been directly involved in the team's decision making. If these individuals also agree, the recommendation is made to the parents.

B. Objective data including consultations are evaluated in the context of the primary team's meetings. Thorough evaluation of the baby's condition, progress, and current clinical status is emphasized. Information about alternative therapies and prognosis is based on the best available information. When relevant, subspecialty consultations are obtained, and if involved, consultants provide their input to the primary care team and, when appropriate, to the parents.

C. The parents' role as surrogate decision makers is respected. Parental views are always considered; they are most likely to influence decisions when it remains unclear which option (e.g., continuing versus discontinuing life-sustaining support) is in the child's best interest. Parents are not expected to evaluate clinical data in isolation. Even in such instances of medical uncertainty, the primary team objectively assesses what is known as well as what remains uncertain about the baby's condition and/or prognosis, and members provide the parents with this information as well as their best assessment and recommendation.

D. The hospital ethics committee is helpful when the primary team is unable to reach consensus or disagrees with the parents' wishes. In our experience, in most cases there is objective evidence that contributes to developing a plan that is in the baby's best interest and is supported by both caregivers and parents. Therefore, committee consultation is not routinely requested.

Reference
1. Goldworth, A., et al. (Eds.). *Ethics and Perinatology.* New York: Oxford University Press, 1995.

22. MANAGEMENT OF NEONATAL DEATH AND BEREAVEMENT FOLLOW-UP

Stephanie J. Packard and Denise Maguire

I. **Introduction.** Neonatal death is traumatic for both families and caregivers. The goal of management is to establish and reinforce a memory of the infant to facilitate successful grieving. Whether the infant lived many months or just a few minutes, parents cherish their memories and those shared by caregivers. Bereavement follow-up provides an important link that guides families toward recovery.

Many models of follow-up are described. In the traditional model, a physician discusses with the family the medical events surrounding death. Another familiar model features social workers who meet with the family to help with the grieving process. Bereavement follow-up can also be offered through support groups. We use a multidisciplinary approach (e.g., physician, nurse, social worker) that offers continuity consistent with our professional practice model.

II. **The multidisciplinary model.** The primary care team supports the family when the infant dies, discusses the events leading to death, explains autopsy results, presents any implications for future pregnancies, evaluates the need for community referrals, and explores the effects of grieving on family members.

III. **Management of the family with a critically ill infant.** The primary care team collaborates with the parents throughout the period of the infant's hospitalization, establishing a relationship of openness and trust. In the period preceding an infant's death, team members can acknowledge and validate both the family's and the caregivers' loss of control and the inability of the infant to achieve parental expectations.

IV. **Management of the family at the time of death.** The primary team openly anticipates the baby's death with the family, preserves the child's dignity, and reinforces the family's importance in the child's life. Team members perform the following interventions:

A. Assess the family's ability to cope with the infant's impending death.

B. Support the family's need to be with the infant during the period near death, provide an adequate time and place for family members to hold the infant, and acknowledge the needs of each family member at the time of death.

C. Reinforce the family's positive role during the infant's life.

D. Discuss the technical aspects of the infant's death in a manner understandable during a time of great stress.

E. Make every attempt to honor the family's requests around and after the death, including cultural and religious rituals.

F. Arrange to take photographs of the infant with or without the family.

G. Gather mementos for the family: infant identification bands, footprints, hat, blanket.

H. Offer the option of autopsy, underscoring its importance and limitations in the particular case.

I. Discuss the bereavement follow-up meeting as standard care for the family; establish an expectation of continuing contact with the family, starting with telephone contact by primary team members within a week.

J. Encourage the family to utilize bereavement support groups in the community.

V. **Management of the family after the infant's death.** Primary team members continue to support the family, primarily through a meeting several weeks after the death. Assessing the family's stage of grief and helping them understand their thoughts and feelings underlie the following interventions surrounding the meeting:

A. A coordinator assumes responsibility for documentation and arranging the meeting.

B. Resource materials (booklets, list of community bereavement support groups, annotated bibliography) are mailed to the family based on individual circumstances and needs.

C. The coordinator contacts the family within 1 week of the infant's death to reestablish the relationship.

D. Subsequent phone calls are made to set a date for the meeting. In general, the meeting is scheduled 4 to 6 weeks after the infant's death, but it can be earlier or later depending on the individual family. Involvement of extended family and referring caregivers (e.g., obstetricians, antepartum nurses) is encouraged. Some families may choose not to meet; for these families, follow-up continues by telephone, by letter, and through other primary providers such as pediatricians and obstetricians. Referrals to appropriate community agencies are made in collaboration with the family. Meetings often include the following:

1. Review of events that led to the infant's death
2. Review of autopsy results (if applicable)
3. Discussion of the need for genetic counseling
4. Discussion of implications for future pregnancies
5. Assessment of the effects of grief on individual and family dynamics

E. Team members document interventions and assessments made with each family.

F. Notification of the death is made to referring professionals by telephone and by letter.

VI. Staff education and support

A. All new neonatal intensive care unit staff (nurses, physicians, social workers) are oriented to their roles in bereavement follow-up.

B. Caregivers who have never been involved in bereavement follow-up are mentored by experienced staff.

C. The staff reviews expected grief reactions to the death of an infant in order to support newly bereaved parents best.

D. Educational conferences are useful to share information and build knowledge.

References

Maguire, D. P. et al. Developing a bereavement follow-up program. *J. Perinatal Neonatal Nurs.* 2(2):67, 1988.

Williams, W. V. et al. Follow-up research in primary prevention: a model of adjustment in acute grief. *J. Clin. Psychol.* 35(1):35, 1979.

Videka-Sherman, L. et al. The effects of self-help and psychotherapy on child loss: the limits of recovery. *Am. J. Orthopsychiatr.* 55(1):70, 1985.

Forrest, G. C. et al. Support after perinatal death. *Br. Med. J.* 285(6353):1475, 1982.

Harrigan, R. et al. Perinatal grief: response to the loss of an infant. *Neonatal Network* 12(5):25, 1993.

23. INFECTIONS

Viral Infections*
Sandra K. Burchett

Vertically transmitted viral infections of the fetus and newborn can generally be divided into two major categories. The first is congenital infections and consists of viral infections that are transmitted to the fetus in utero. The second is perinatal infections and consists of viral infections that are acquired intrapartum or in the immediate postpartum period. Many, if not all, of these agents can cause both congenital and perinatal infections or may be acquired outside the newborn period. However, classifying these viruses into congenital and perinatal categories emphasizes unique aspects of their pathogenesis in the fetus and newborn infant.

Although classically the congenital infections have been thought of by the acronym **TORCH** (**T** = toxoplasma, **O** = other, **R** = rubella, **C** = cytomegalovirus, **H** = herpes simplex virus), the recognition of other important agents causing vertically transmitted infections makes this term archaic. Also, herpes simplex virus infection does not share many of the features common to the other agents. In what follows, the concept of TORCH is avoided. When congenital or perinatal infections are suspected, the diagnosis of each of the possible infectious agents should be considered separately. Useless information is often obtained when the diagnosis is attempted by drawing a single serum sample to be sent for measurement of TORCH titers.

I. Congenital infections
A. Cytomegalovirus (CMV). CMVs are members of the herpesvirus family and derive their name from the cytopathology of infected cells, which is characterized by cellular enlargement with intranuclear and cytoplasmic inclusions. Human CMV is species-specific with no known vector for transmission in nature. Infection occurs as a result of intimate personal contact or exposure to infected breast milk, blood, or blood products. It is believed that nearly as many as 50% of all individuals acquire CMV infection at some time in their life. Fortunately, most infections are asymptomatic, but significant or life-threatening infection occurs in the immunocompromised or immunosuppressed patient. The fetus is particularly susceptible to severe disseminated CMV disease. Infection can occur at any time in gestation or in the perinatal period.

1. **Intrauterine infection.** Congenital CMV occurs in 1% of all live births in the United States, and 7% of those infected manifest symptomatic disease. Twelve percent of those with symptomatic disease die and 90% of the survivors have significant sequelae. The asymptomatically infected infants (93%) generally do well, but 15% develop sequelae. Therefore, at least 8,000 infants are severely affected by or die from CMV infection in the United States each year. Clinically apparent newborn disease is almost always associated with primary maternal infection in pregnancy. It is estimated that the rate of intrauterine transmission from primary maternal infection is 30 to 40%, and approximately 18% of these newborns develop significant disease. Recurrent maternal infection or viral reactivation can occur during pregnancy, and transmission to the fetus may result. However, in mothers with recurrent infection, the fetus and newborn rarely show clinical symptoms. The risk of transmission to the fetus as a function of gesta-

*This is a revision of Chapter 12 by Dr. Nicholas G. Guerina in the 3rd edition of the *Manual of Neonatal Care.*

tional age is uncertain. Infection during early gestation likely carries a higher risk of severe fetal disease.

  a. Symptomatic CMV infection of the fetus has two presentations.

   (1) Acute fulminant infection involves multiple organ systems. The most common findings in the first 2 weeks following delivery in 34 infected newborns were petechiae or purpura (79%), hepatosplenomegaly (74%), and jaundice (63%); 34% were premature as well. Approximately 33% have intrauterine growth retardation and 25% are premature. These infants are at higher risk of mortality. Noted abnormalities in infants with symptomatic CMV infections include elevated hepatic transaminase and bilirubin levels, anemia, and thrombocytopenia. Bilirubin levels may be elevated at birth or rise over the first postnatal weeks. There is usually an elevated conjugated component that may increase to 50% of the total bilirubin. Hyperbilirubinemia usually persists beyond the period of physiologic jaundice.

   (2) A second presentation includes those infants who are **symptomatic but without life-threatening complications.** These babies may have microcephaly or intrauterine growth retardation. In one series, 12% of infants have chorioretinitis. Intracranial calcifications may also occur anywhere in the brain, although classically calcifications have been found in the periventricular area. Infants surviving symptomatic CMV infection are at high risk for developing significant developmental abnormalities and neurologic dysfunction. These include mental retardation, hearing deficits, language and learning disabilities, motor abnormalities, and visual disturbances. Hearing loss is very common with symptomatic congenital CMV infection, occurring in at least 15% of infants. Since hearing loss is the most common sequela of CMV infection, hearing should be rigorously assessed in the newborn period as well as in early infancy.

  b. In contrast to symptomatic newborn infants, those with **asymptomatic** infection have no mortality, but 5 to 15% may have developmental abnormalities. These include hearing loss, mental retardation, motor spasticity, and microcephaly. Other problems that can be detected later in life include dental defects characterized by abnormal enamel production.

 2. Perinatal infection. Perinatally acquired CMV may occur (1) from intrapartum exposure to the virus within the maternal genital tract, (2) from postnatal exposure to infected breast milk, (3) from exposure to infected blood or blood products, or (4) nosocomially through urine or saliva. The incubation period varies from 4 to 12 weeks. Almost all term infants who acquire infection perinatally from infected mothers remain asymptomatic. Many of these infections arise from mothers with reactivated viral excretion. In these cases, long-term developmental and neurologic abnormalities are infrequently seen. However, symptomatic perinatally acquired infections may occur at a higher frequency in preterm infants. Hearing abnormalities may also be detected in infants with perinatal CMV infection; therefore, hearing should be assessed in infants documented to have acquired CMV.

  a. CMV pneumonitis. CMV has been associated with pneumonitis occurring in infants less than 4 months old. Symptoms and radiographic findings in CMV pneumonitis are similar to those seen in afebrile pneumonia of other causes in neonates and young infants, including *Chlamydia trachomatis,* respiratory viruses, and *Ureaplasma urealyticum.* In general, there is tachypnea, cough, coryza, and nasal congestion. Intercostal retractions and hypoxemia may be present, and apnea may occur. Radiographically, there is hyperinflation, diffuse increased pulmonary markings, thickened bronchial walls, and focal atelectasis. A small number of infants may have symptoms that are severe enough to require mechanical ventilation, and approximately 3% of infants die. Laboratory findings in CMV pneumonitis are nonspecific. Long-term sequelae include recurrent pulmonary problems, including wheezing, and in some cases, repeated hospitalizations for respiratory distress. Whether this reflects congenital or perinatal CMV infection is unclear, but it does pose a risk, especially to the premature infants.

   b. Transfusion-acquired CMV infection. Significant morbidity and mortality can occur in newborn infants receiving CMV-infected blood or blood products. Those most severely affected are preterm, low-birth-weight infants born to CMV-seronegative women. Symptoms typically develop 4 to 12 weeks after transfusion, last for 2 to 3 weeks, and consist of respiratory distress, pallor, and hepatosplenomegaly. Hematologic abnormalities are also seen and include hemolysis, thrombocytopenia, and atypical lymphocytosis. Mortality is estimated to be 20% in very-low-birth-weight infants. Disease can be prevented by the use of blood from donors who are seronegative for CMV. Thus, it is recommended that all blood and blood products for infants in the special care nursery be obtained from seronegative donors or that blood be prepared so as to virtually eliminate the risk of CMV transmission (see Chap. 26, Blood Products Used in the Newborn).

3. Diagnosis. Congenital CMV infection should be suspected in any infant having typical symptoms of infection or if there is a maternal history of seroconversion or a mononucleosis-like illness in pregnancy. The diagnosis of congenital CMV infection is made by the identification of virus in clinical specimens taken from infected newborns within the first 2 weeks of delivery. Virus may be isolated from urine or saliva, but urine has the greatest sensitivity because CMV is concentrated in high titers. Specimens should be maintained at 4°C (ice or refrigerator) for transport and storage, to optimize viral recovery. The identification of CMV in standard tissue culture may take from 2 to 6 weeks. For this reason, the "shell vial" technique has been developed to rapidly identify CMV in clinical specimens. CMV infects tissue culture cells on a coverslip, but replication and the resultant cytopathic effect are not required. Rather, the cells are lysed and reacted with antibody to CMV antigens present early in viral cultures. Virus can be detected with high sensitivity and specificity within 24 to 72 hours of inoculation. To differentiate perinatal from congenital CMV infection, the absence of viral excretion during the first 2 postnatal weeks should be documented.

   The determination of serum antibody titers to CMV has limited usefulness for the neonate, although negative IgG titers in both maternal and infant sera are sufficient to exclude congenital CMV infection. The interpretation of a positive IgG titer in the newborn is almost always complicated by the presence of transplacentally derived maternal IgG. Uninfected infants usually show a decline in IgG within 1 month and have no detectable titer by 4 to 9 months. Infected infants continue to produce IgG throughout the same time period. Tests for CMV-specific IgM have limitations but can help to elucidate infant infection. If the diagnosis of congenital CMV infection is made, the infant should have a thorough physical and neurological exam, a CT of the brain, and ophthalmologic exam, hearing test, a CBC, liver function tests, and CSF exam. Measurement of CMV DNA is helpful for diagnosis and prognosis.

4. Treatment. There is no highly effective antiviral therapy currently available for the treatment of congenital or perinatal CMV infection in newborns. Clinical trials are in progress; however, toxicity (particularly marrow suppression) is a major factor. The most promising antiviral drug is ganciclovir (9-[(13-dihydroxy-2-propoxy)methyl]guanine). This agent is effective in the treatment of chorioretinitis and pneumonitis in immunosuppressed transplant patients. The drug is under investigation for use in newborns with CNS involvement associated with congenital CMV infection. Early results warrant broader study of this agent. A different approach using monoclonal antibody to a segment of CMV is in early trial and may provide a less toxic and equally efficacious modality. Hyperimmune CMV immunoglobulin may also be an alternative.

5. **Prevention**
   a. **Screening.** Currently, screening to identify fetuses at risk for symptomatic CMV infection is not routinely recommended. Approximately 2% of women acquire acute primary CMV infection during pregnancy. In general, these women are asymptomatic, and the overall risk for significant fetal disease is low. Isolation of virus from the cervix or urine of pregnant women cannot be used to predict fetal infection. There simply is not enough information about fetal transmission to provide guidelines for obstetric management. At this time, no recommendations for therapeutic abortion can be made, even if primary maternal CMV infection is documented.
   b. **Immunization.** Passive immunization with hyperimmune anti-CMV immunoglobulin and active immunization with a live attenuated CMV vaccine represent attractive therapies for prophylaxis against congenital CMV infections. However, data from clinical trials are lacking. Immune globulin might be considered as prophylaxis of susceptible women against primary CMV infection in pregnancy. Two live attenuated CMV vaccines have been developed, but their efficacy has not been clearly established. The possibility of reactivation of vaccine-strain CMV in pregnancy with subsequent infection of the fetus must be considered carefully before adequate field trials can be completed in women of childbearing age.
   c. **Breast milk restriction.** Although breast milk is a common source for perinatal CMV infection in the newborn, symptomatic infection is rare, especially in term infants. In this setting, protection against disseminated disease may be provided by transplacentally derived maternal IgG or antibody in breast milk. However, there may be insufficient transplacental IgG to provide adequate protection in preterm infants. In this setting, the use of breast milk from CMV-negative mothers should be encouraged. At present there is no recommended method of minimizing the risk of exposure to CMV in infected breast milk; freezing milk at $-20°C$ will reduce the titer of CMV but will not eliminate active virus.
   d. **Environmental restrictions.** Day-care centers and hospitals are potential high-risk environments for acquiring CMV infection. Not surprisingly, a number of studies confirmed an increased risk for infection in day-care workers. However, there does not appear to be an increased risk for infection in hospital personnel. These studies demonstrated that good hand-washing and infection-control measures practiced in hospital settings may be sufficient to control the spread of CMV to workers. Unfortunately, such control may be difficult to achieve in day-care centers. Good hand-washing technique should be suggested to pregnant women with children in day care, especially if they are known to be seronegative. The determination of the CMV susceptibility of these women by serology may be useful for counseling.
   e. **Transfusion product restrictions.** The risk of transfusion-acquired CMV infection in the neonate should be minimized by the use of

blood and blood products obtained from CMV-negative donors. For packed red blood cell transfusions, deglycerolized frozen cells provide a safe alternative. It is particularly important to use blood from one of these sources in preterm, low-birth-weight infants (see Chap. 26, Blood Products Used in the Newborn).

B. Rubella. This human-specific RNA virus is a member of the Togavirus family. It causes a mild self-limiting infection in susceptible children and adults, but its effects on the fetus can be devastating. Prior to widespread immunization beginning in 1969, rubella was a common childhood illness: 85% of the population was immune by late adolescence and nearly 100% by ages 35 to 40 years. Epidemics occurred every 6 to 9 years, with pandemics arising with a greater and more variable cycle. During pandemics, susceptible women were at significant risk of exposure to rubella, resulting in a high number of fetal infections. A worldwide epidemic from 1963 to 1965 accounted for an estimated 11,000 fetal deaths and 20,000 cases of congenital rubella syndrome. Childhood immunization has dramatically reduced the number of cases of rubella in the United States. However, 12 to 24% of postpubertal individuals are susceptible, and outbreaks of rubella have occurred in several large urban areas over the past 10 years.

1. Congenital rubella syndrome (CRS). Fetal infection can occur at any time during pregnancy, but early-gestation infection may result in multiple organ anomalies. Classically, CRS is characterized by the constellation of cataracts, sensorineural hearing loss, and congenital heart disease. The most common cardiac defects are patent ductus arteriosus and pulmonary artery stenosis. Common early features of CRS are intrauterine growth retardation, retinopathy, microphthalmia, meningoencephalitis, electroencephalographic abnormalities, hypotonia, dermatoglyphic abnormalities, hepatosplenomegaly, thrombocytopenic purpura, radiographic bone lucencies, and diabetes mellitus. The onset of some of the abnormalities of CRS may be delayed months to years. Many additional rare complications have been described, including myocarditis, glaucoma, microcephaly, chronic progressive panencephalitis, hepatitis, anemia, hypogammaglobulinemia, thymic hypoplasia, thyroid abnormalities, cryptorchidism, and polycystic kidney disease. A 20-year follow-up study of 125 patients with congenital rubella from the 1960s epidemic found ocular disease to be the most common disorder (78%), followed by sensorineural hearing deficits (66%), psychomotor retardation (62%), cardiac abnormalities (58%), and mental retardation (42%).

The relative risk of fetal transmission and the development of CRS as a function of gestational age have been studied. With maternal infection in the first 12 weeks of gestation, the rate of fetal infection was 81%. The rate dropped to 54% for weeks 13 to 16, 36% for weeks 17 to 22, and 30% for weeks 23 to 30. During the last 10 weeks of gestation, the rate of fetal infection again rose: 60% for weeks 31 to 36 and 100% for weeks 36 and beyond. When maternofetal transmission occurred during the first 10 weeks of gestation, 100% of the infected fetuses had cardiac defects and deafness. Deafness was found in one-third of fetuses infected at 13 to 16 weeks, but no abnormalities were found when fetal infection occurred beyond the twentieth week of gestation. There are also case reports of vertical transmission with maternal reinfection.

2. Diagnosis of maternal infection. The diagnosis of acute rubella in pregnancy requires serologic testing. This is necessary because the clinical symptoms of rubella are nonspecific and can be seen with infection by other viral agents (e.g., enteroviruses, measles, human parvovirus). Furthermore, a large number of individuals may have subclinical infection. Several sensitive and specific assays exist for the detection of

rubella-specific antibody. Viral isolation from the nose, throat, and/or urine is possible, but this is costly and not practical in most instances.
  a. Symptomatic maternal infection. Symptoms typically begin 2 to 3 weeks after exposure and include malaise, low-grade fever, headache, mild coryza, and conjunctivitis occurring 1 to 5 days prior to the onset of rash. The rash is a salmon-pink macular or maculopapular exanthem that begins on the face and behind the ears and spreads downward over 1 to 2 days. The rash disappears within 5 to 7 days from onset, and posterior cervical lymphadenopathy is common. Approximately one-third of women may have arthralgias without arthritis.
  In women suspected of having acute rubella infection, confirmation can be made by demonstrating a fourfold or higher rise in serum IgG titers when measured at the time of symptoms and approximately 2 weeks later. The results of some assays may not directly correlate with a fourfold rise in titer, so other criteria for a significant increase in antibody may be required. When there is uncertainty about the interpretation of assay results, advice should be obtained from the laboratory running the test and an infectious diseases consultation. It is very important to have the acute serum titer determined again, in tandem with the convalescent titer. In some infants, the relative increase in titer within the first 2 weeks of symptoms may be less obvious because serum IgG has already begun to rise at the time of clinical symptoms. In this situation, repeated measurement of serum titers may be required. Obviously, a prior knowledge of a woman's immune status can be very useful. Also, a single, high-positive, rubella-specific IgM titer may be diagnostic, but problems with the specificity of these assays and the persistence of IgM for many weeks make the interpretation of low-positive values difficult. Additionally, IgM may be present in the setting of reinfection.
  b. Recognized or suspected maternal exposure. Any individual known to have been immunized with rubella vaccine after their first birthday is generally considered immune. However, it is best to determine immunity by measuring rubella-specific IgG, which has become a standard of practice in obstetric care. If a woman exposed to rubella is known to be seropositive, she is immune and the fetus is considered not to be at risk for infection. Reinfections in previously immune women have been rarely documented, but the risk of fetal damage appears to be very small. If the exposed woman is known to be seronegative, a serum sample should be obtained 3 to 4 weeks after exposure, for determination of titer. A negative titer indicates that no infection has occurred, whereas a positive titer indicates infection. Women with an uncertain immune status and a known exposure to rubella should have serum samples obtained as soon as possible after exposure. If this is done within 7 to 10 days of exposure, and the titer is positive, the patient is rubella immune and no further testing is required. If the first titer is negative or was determined on serum taken more than 7 to 10 days after exposure, repeat testing (approximately 3 weeks later) and careful clinical follow-up are necessary. When both the immune status and the time of exposure are uncertain, serum samples for titer determination should be obtained 3 weeks apart. If both titers are negative, no infection has occurred. Alternatively, infection is confirmed if seroconversion or a fourfold increase in titer is observed. Further testing and close clinical follow-up are required if titer results are inconclusive. In this situation, specific IgM determination may be helpful. Again, it should be emphasized that all serum samples should be tested simultaneously by the same laboratory when one is determining changes in

titers with time. This can be accomplished by saving a portion of each serum sample prior to sending it for titer determination. The saved portion can be frozen until convalescent serum samples have been obtained.

3. **Diagnosis of congenital rubella infection**
   a. **Antenatal diagnosis.** The risk of severe fetal anomalies is highest with acute maternal rubella infection during the first 16 weeks of gestation. However, not all early-gestation infections result in adverse pregnancy outcomes. Approximately 20% of fetuses may not be infected when maternal rubella occurs in the first 12 weeks of gestation, and as many as 45% of fetuses may not be infected when maternal rubella occurs closer to 16 weeks of gestation. Unfortunately, there is no foolproof method of determining infected from uninfected fetuses early in pregnancy, but in utero diagnosis is being investigated. One method that has been used with some success is the determination of specific IgM in fetal blood obtained by percutaneous umbilical blood sampling (PUBS). Direct detection of rubella antigen and RNA in a chorionic villous biopsy specimen also has been used successfully. Although these techniques offer promise, their use may be limited by sensitivity and specificity or the lack of widespread availability.
   b. **Postnatal diagnosis.** Guidelines for the establishment of congenital rubella infection or CRS in neonates have been summarized by the Centers for Disease Control. The diagnosis of congenital infection is made by one of the following:
      (1) Isolation of rubella virus (oropharynx, urine)
      (2) Detection of rubella-specific IgM in cord or neonatal blood
      (3) Persistent rubella-specific titers over time (i.e., no decline in titer as expected for transplacentally derived maternal IgG). If, in addition, there are congenital defects, the diagnosis of CRS is made.

4. **Treatment.** There is no specific therapy for either maternal or congenital rubella infection. Maternal disease is almost always mild and self-limiting. If primary maternal infection occurs during the first 5 months of pregnancy, termination options should be discussed with the mother. Over one-half of newborns with congenital rubella may be asymptomatic at birth. If infection is known to have occurred beyond the twentieth week of gestation, it is unlikely that any abnormalities will develop, and parents should be reassured. Nevertheless, hearing evaluations should be repeated during childhood. Closer follow-up is required if early-gestation infection is suspected or the timing of infection is unknown. This is true for asymptomatic infants as well as those with obvious CRS. The principal reason for close follow-up is to identify delayed-onset abnormalities or progressive disorders. In some cases, early interventions such as therapy for glaucoma may be critical. Unfortunately, there is no specific therapy to halt the progression of most of the complications of CRS.

5. **Prevention.** The primary means of prevention of CRS is by immunization of all susceptible persons. Immunization is recommended for all nonimmune individuals 12 months or older. Documentation of maternal immunity is an important aspect of good obstetric management. When a susceptible woman is identified, she should be reassured of the low risk of contracting rubella, but she should also be counseled to avoid contact with anyone known to have acute or recent rubella infection. Individuals with postnatal infection typically shed virus for 1 week before and 1 week after the onset of rash. On the other hand, infants with congenital infection may shed virus for many months, and contact should be avoided during the first year. Unfortunately, once exposure has occurred, little can be done to alter the chances of maternal and subsequently fetal disease. While hyperimmune globulin does not diminish the risk of maternal rubella following exposure or the rate of

fetal transmission, it should be given in large doses to any woman who is exposed to rubella and who does not wish to interrupt her pregnancy. The lack of proven efficacy must be emphasized in these cases. Susceptible women who do not become infected should be immunized soon after pregnancy. There have been reports of acute arthritis occurring in women immunized in the immediate postpartum period, and a small percentage of these women developed chronic joint or neurologic abnormalities or viremia. Vaccine-strain virus also may be shed in breast milk and transmitted to breast-fed infants, some of whom may develop chronic viremia. Thus it may be best to avoid breast-feeding in women receiving rubella vaccine. Conception also should be avoided for 3 months following immunization. Immunization during pregnancy is not recommended because of the theoretical risk to the fetus. Inadvertent immunizations during pregnancy have occurred, and fetal infection has been documented in a small percentage of these pregnancies. However, no cases of CRS have been identified. In fact, the rubella registry at the Centers for Disease Control has been closed, with the following conclusions: The number of inadvertent immunizations during pregnancy is too small to be able to state with certainty that no adverse pregnancy outcomes will occur, but these would appear to be very uncommon. Thus it is still recommended that immunization not be carried out during pregnancy, but when this has occurred, reassurance of little risk to the fetus can be given.

C. **Human immunodeficiency virus (HIV)** [11,13]. As of December 31, 1993, 361,164 cases of the acquired immunodeficiency syndrome (AIDS) in the United States, caused by HIV, have been reported to the Centers for Disease Control. Approximately 1.5% of cases are in children younger than 13 years and 12% are in females. In women of childbearing age, the leading risk behavior is injection drug use, accounting for approximately 52% of cases, followed by heterosexual activity as the only risk behavior in 37% of cases. An estimated 1.5 to 4.0 million individuals are currently infected with HIV. This represents an approximately threefold increase since 1990. The number of cases occurring in infants and children younger than 13 years is rapidly rising, and as of the end of December 1993, there were 5228 children with AIDS in the United States; 50% have died. Nearly 90% of children with AIDS acquired HIV by vertical transmission. In Massachusetts, anonymous newborn screening revealed an overall seropositivity of 2.0 to 2.5 per 1000. This has been consistent over the past 4 years and means that approximately 0.2% of women giving birth are HIV-infected. In inner-city areas, the rate increased to 8.0 per 1000. Seropositivity as high as 6 to 8% has been reported in some major metropolitan areas of the United States. In other parts of the world such as central and eastern Africa, 5 to 40% of women of childbearing age are seropositive for HIV. Thus HIV poses a serious and challenging problem for obstetricians and pediatricians.

1. **The virus.** HIV is a cytopathic RNA retrovirus. HIV-1 is the principal cause of HIV infection in the United States and throughout the world. The virus enters the host CD4+ cell, uses reverse transcriptase to synthesize DNA from RNA, and integrates into the host genome. HIV contains genomic RNA within a core that is surrounded by an inner protein shell and an outer lipid envelope. The genome consists of the three genes found in all retroviruses *(gag, pol, env)* along with at least six additional genes, including gp120, which is necessary for the binding of virus to target cells, and p24, which is the major core protein. The lipid envelope is derived from the host-cell membrane as the virus buds from the infected cell surface.

2. **Pathogenesis.** During host-cell transcription, viral replication occurs until the host cell is destroyed. With components of the immune response destroyed, the host is susceptible to opportunistic infections and

malignancies. In initial HIV infection, a mononucleosis-like syndrome results, the viral inoculum is high, and viremia is present, which allows for seeding of the lymphoid tissue. The host immune response is triggered, viremia is cleared, and 80% of patients become asymptomatic; for 20% a rapidly progressive course ensues. Even in asymptomatic patients, disease progression is maintained, with the median duration of the asymptomatic phase being approximately 10 years in adults, after which the patient becomes symptomatic, generally with opportunistic infections, and death occurs within 5 years. Some suggest that the local cytokine milieu [mainly interleukin (IL-2, IL-12), interferon (IFN-gamma)] produced by cells in the lymphoid tissue holds viral replication to a minimum during the quiescent period. Then, unknown factors may shift the cytokine pool to one in which IL-4 and IL-6 are increased and disease progression continues. Even from early infection, in addition to a decrease in cell number, altered T-cell function occurs. Characteristics of the virus itself may also be relevant. For example, initial infection almost always occurs with a monocytotropic isolate of HIV but with time a lymphocytotropic isolate may develop. With this mutation, the isolate is then also likely to be able to induce syncytia or giant-cell formation. With this change, viral replication is enhanced as is cell death. The other CD4+ cells that may play a prominent role in HIV infection are monocytes and macrophages. These cells are relatively resistant to the cytopathic effects of HIV and thus may act as major viral reservoirs. They also may be important in the transport of HIV to other parts of the body, including the CNS. A small subset of patients may not show CD4+ T-cell decline. Early studies suggest that at least some of these patients may have a mutated viral isolate that may be less likely to induce cytolysis of CD4+ cells, such that the cellular immune system is functional in preventing opportunistic infections. Clearly, better identification and characterization of long-term survivors may lead to development of effective vaccines and other preventive therapies.

Infants with HIV infection may not fit the described pattern. Some infants have a very high viral load when the infant is first diagnosed as infected. Whether this declines with time as the infant's immune system becomes responsive to the infection is unclear, because many investigators would offer antiretroviral therapy to these children as the majority seem to be symptomatic. Issues of when to initiate antiretroviral therapy should be individualized.

3. **Transmission.** There are three principal routes for HIV transmission: sexual contact, parenteral inoculation, and maternal-fetal or maternal-newborn transfer.

   a. **Sexual contact.** This remains the principal mode of transmission of HIV worldwide. In the United States, sexual contact is the major risk behavior for men who have sex with men, but the rate of heterosexual transmission has increased considerably. Both semen and vaginal secretions have been found to contain HIV. The principal risk behavior for mothers of children reported with AIDS is heterosexual contact.

   b. **Parenteral transmission.** Parenteral transmission of HIV results from the direct inoculation of infected blood or blood products. The groups affected have been intravenous (IV) drug users and patients receiving transfusions or factor concentrates. Careful screening of blood donors for risk factors for infection, universal HIV antibody testing of donated blood, and the special preparation of clotting factor to eliminate the risk of viral contamination have greatly reduced the incidence of transfusion-acquired HIV. The most likely reason for false-negative HIV serology is the seronegative window that occurs between the time of initial infection and the production of antiviral antibody. The odds of transfusion-acquired HIV infection from the transfusion of a single unit of tested blood have been estimated to be from 1:250,000 to 1:150,000 (see Chap. 26, Blood Products Used in the Newborn).

c. Congenital and perinatal transmission. In utero and intrapartum transmissions from infected mothers constitute the principal modes of HIV infection in the pediatric population. Breast milk is occasionally a medium of transport. Approximately 90% of pediatric AIDS cases have resulted from maternal transmission. The rate of transmission of HIV from infected mothers to their fetuses and newborn infants has been estimated to be between 15 and 40%. Prospective studies prior to February 1994 suggested that the overall risk for transmission may be closer to 25%. Transmission can occur throughout gestation or at birth. HIV has been isolated from cord blood specimens, and products of conception have demonstrated HIV infection as early as 14 to 20 weeks' gestation. The mechanism of transplacental transfer of HIV is not known, but HIV can infect trophoblast and placental macrophage (hofbauer) cell lines. Neither infection of nor quantity of virus present in the placenta correlate with congenital infection. This may suggest that the placenta in general acts as a protective barrier to transmission or conversely as a focus of potential transmission.

In a study of 100 sets of twins delivered to HIV-infected mothers, twin A was infected in 50% delivered vaginally and 38% delivered by cesarean. Twin B was infected in 19% of both vaginal and cesarean deliveries [13]. This suggested that intrapartum infection occurs and that time of exposure to infected secretions may be a factor because the first twin spends longer in the birth canal and is likely to have more invasive procedures than the second twin. Many infants who ultimately prove to have acquired HIV infection do not show evidence of HIV within the first 2 weeks of life, even by the most sensitive of assays, also suggesting that infants may become infected by intrapartum exposure to maternal secretions. Based on this kind of information, investigators are targeting the intrapartum interval to offer preventive treatments such as antiretroviral therapy or birth canal washes. Mode of delivery (i.e., vaginal versus cesarean) has not been firmly established as a correlate of transmission. It may be that duration of rupture of membranes will be a stronger factor in transmission than mode of delivery. At present, infants with evidence of HIV infection by viral detection methods in the first 3 days of life are defined as having been infected in utero and those with negative results on early tests and positive ones after 1 week of life are defined as infected intrapartum. Intrapartum transmission is likely to account for at least 50% of HIV infections in infants.

Any instrumentation, including fetal scalp electrodes and pH sampling, during the intrapartum period which would expose the fetus to maternal blood and secretions should be avoided at the present time; it is still unclear if cesarean section decreases the risk of HIV transmission. Prolonged rupture of membranes may be associated with increased transmission of HIV. Postpartum, the mother should be advised to avoid allowing her infant to contact her blood or secretions.

Studies have also suggested that in countries where breast-feeding is almost exclusively practiced, the transmission rate may be as much as 14% over the presumed rate seen due to in utero or intrapartum transmission. In one prospective study of women in an endemic area who were not HIV-infected at the time of delivery but who seroconverted postpartum, some infants seroconverted almost simultaneously with their mothers. Several investigators reported on infants born to women who were not HIV-infected, but who were breast-fed by an HIV-infected wet nurse and subsequently acquired HIV infection. It may be that infants who do not have maternally derived, passively transferred antibody to HIV or those infants whose mothers acquire primary HIV infection during lactation are at a higher risk of acquisition of HIV exposure through breast milk than are those who are probably exposed to virions and antibody together. Therefore breast-feeding is contraindicated in countries in which formula preparations are safe and nutritionally replete.

4. **HIV in pregnancy**

a. The HIV-infected pregnant woman should be counseled that completion of pregnancy probably does not worsen her prognosis. HIV-infected women should be carefully screened for other sexually transmitted diseases (gonorrhea, herpes, chlamydia, hepatitis B and C, and syphilis) as well as being tested for antibody to CMV and toxoplasmosis. The mother should also have a tuberculin skin test and, when appropriate, be offered hepatitis B, pneumococcal, and influenza vaccines. If the CD4+ count is below 500 per microliter, she should be offered zidovudine for her own health care. *Pneumocystis carinii* and possibly *Mycobacterium avium intracellulare* prophylaxis should be considered. Since pregnancy itself can lead to altered immunity, the need for pregnant seronegative control subjects in prospective studies may be important. Currently, prospective studies on HIV in pregnancy, such as the Women and Infants Transmission Study (WITS), which is a multicenter National Institutes of Health (NIH)–sponsored investigation, are under way.

b. **Pediatric HIV infection.** The majority of pediatric AIDS cases occur in infants and young children, reflecting the preponderance of congenital and perinatally acquired infections. Fifty percent of pediatric AIDS cases occur in the first year of life, and approximately 80% occur by the age of 3 years. Of these patients, HIV-related symptoms occur in more than 80% in the first year of life (median age at onset of symptoms is 9 months). It is estimated that 20% of infants with congenital/perinatal HIV infection will die within the first year of life, and 60% will have severe symptomatic disease by the age of 18 months. These patients are defined as "rapid progressors." These statistics reflect only pediatric AIDS cases reported to the Centers for Disease Control, and may reflect only the part of the spectrum of disease that is identified. It is possible that many infected children are undiagnosed and remain asymptomatic for years. Some perinatally infected children who are known to be HIV-infected may remain asymptomatic for 7 to 15 years.

The clinical presentation also differs in children compared with adults. The HIV-infected newborn is asymptomatic, but may present with lymphadenopathy and/or hepatosplenomegaly. Generally the infant infected peripartum does not develop symptoms until after the first 2 weeks of life. These include lymphadenopathy and hepatosplenomegaly (as in adults), poor weight gain as might be found in chronic viral infection, and occasionally neuromotor abnormalities or encephalopathy. Before antiretroviral therapy was available to children, 50 to 90% of HIV-infected children had CNS involvement characterized by an encephalopathy that was often clinically devastating. Although the clinical presentation may vary, developmental delay or loss of developmental milestones and diminished cognitive function are common features. All too often an infant is diagnosed with AIDS between the ages of 2 to 6 months when he or she presents with *P. carinii* pneumonia (PCP). This is an interstitial pneumonia often without ascultatory findings. Patients present with low-grade fever, tachypnea, and often, tachycardia. Progressive hypoxia ensues and may result in mortality as high as 90%. PCP is the AIDS-defining illness at presentation in 37% of pediatric patients, with a peak incidence at the age of 4 months. Treatment is intravenous trimethoprim-sulfamethoxazole and steroids. Prophylaxis to prevent such life-threatening possibilities is of course preferable to acquisition of disease. Based on adult studies, early on the Centers for Disease Control recommended offering PCP prophylaxis to HIV-infected infants based on CD4+ lymphocyte number and percent by age. The majority of infants with PCP in the first year of life had CD4+ cell counts lower than 1500 per microliter. It was recognized that fully 50% of infants presenting with PCP had either no CD4+ cell assessment available or the count was above the 1500-per-microliter guideline. It is now recommended by the Public Health Service that all infants born to HIV-infected mothers be started on PCP prophylaxis at the age of 1 month until the infection and immune status of that infant is known.

A second condition possibly unique to pediatric AIDS is the development of chronic interstitial lung disease, referred to as **lymphoid interstitial pneumonitis (LIP)**. LIP is characterized by a diffuse lymphocytic and plasma cell infiltrate. The clinical course of LIP is quite variable but may be progressive, resulting in marked respiratory distress (tachypnea, retractions, wheezing, hypoxemia). There is an association with Epstein-Barr virus infection, but the significance of this is uncertain. After the initial presentation, the prognosis appears to be more favorable for children with symptomatic HIV infection when the AIDS-defining illness is LIP. In addition to LIP, recurrent bacterial infections are a frequent feature of pediatric AIDS, owing in part to the early occurrence of B-cell dysfunction with dysfunctional hypergammaglobulinemia. Both focal and disseminated infections are encountered, with sepsis being most common. The organisms usually isolated from the bloodstream are *Streptococcus pneumoniae, Haemophilus influenzae,* and *Salmonella* species, but a variety of other bacteria have been recovered, especially from hospitalized patients. Other manifestations of HIV infection that may be more common in children are parotitis and cardiac dysfunction.

5. **Diagnosis.** The diagnosis of HIV infection in adults is made by the detection of specific antibody by an enzyme-linked immunosorbent assay (ELISA) with confirmation by Western blot analysis. Testing should be offered to anyone engaging in risk behaviors for HIV transmission. Testing requires counseling and informed consent. Serology is of limited value in diagnosing vertically transmitted HIV infection in infants less than 15 months old, since maternal IgG crosses the placenta and can persist in infants throughout the first year or more of life. In the presence of symptomatology and/or specific laboratory findings strongly indicative of HIV, the diagnosis of HIV can still be made. However, the picture is less clear in infants with minimal or no symptomatology. Thus viral detection tests must be used to identify infected infants born to HIV-seropositive mothers. These include the following:

   a. In vitro cell culture
   b. p24 antigen detection in peripheral blood
   c. Polymerase chain reaction (PCR) to detect viral nucleic acid in peripheral blood
   d. ELISA for the detection of specific IgM and IgA
   e. In vitro stimulation of peripheral blood leukocytes to produce specific antibody
   f. In situ hybridization to detect HIV-specific DNA in infected cells
      Culture is sensitive and specific but is expensive, is technically difficult, and may require weeks before results are obtained. The

p24 antigen assay suffers from a lack of sensitivity, particularly in infants, and can be replaced by acid-dissociated p24 antigen detection, which has a much greater sensitivity. PCR generally correlates with cell culture and may be more quickly obtained. Detection of HIV-specific IgA and IgM has been fraught with problems of both sensitivity and specificity. The sensitivity of in vitro antibody production has been equally problematic. The mainstays of early viral diagnostic testing of the infant born to an HIV-infected mother remain HIV culture, acid-dissociated p24 antigen detection, and PCR to detect both viral RNA and DNA. The importance of obtaining an early diagnosis is clear: to provide even very young infants the benefit of antiretroviral therapy, which is hoped to reduce viral load and possibly prevent or reduce the viral burden at sites such as the CNS.

6. **Treatment.** A major part of the management of HIV infection is symptomatic treatment. At present, there is no cure for HIV infection. Optimization of nutrition, prophylaxis against opportunistic infections (most notably PCP), and the prompt recognition and treatment of HIV-related complications (e.g., opportunistic infections, cardiac dysfunction) are paramount to the improvement in the longevity and the quality of life for HIV-infected patients. In the newborn, special attention should be given to the possibility of congenitally and perinatally transmitted pathogens, such as *Mycobacterium tuberculosis, Toxoplasma,* and sexually transmitted diseases (STDs), that may have a relatively high prevalence in HIV-infected adults.

There are intense efforts to develop methods to treat and prevent HIV infections. Possibilities being investigated include vaccines to actively immunize against HIV and use of the following specific antiretroviral therapies:

a. Drugs that inhibit the action of viral proteins, such as reverse transcriptase or protease

b. Immunotherapy with interferon (IFN-gamma) or neutralizing monoclonal antibodies

c. Gene therapy that targets genetic information to the cell and prevents viral replication

The greatest clinical experience has been with dideoxynucleoside analogues that interfere with viral reverse transcriptase. Of these, zidovudine (ZDV; 3'-azido-2',3'-dideoxythymidine, formerly known as AZT) is of benefit in at least transiently improving or slowing the development of some of the symptoms related to HIV infection in adults. ZDV is taken up by cells, where it is phosphorylated into a 5'-triphosphate form. In this form, ZDV binds to the nucleotide recognition site on reverse transcriptase (competitive inhibition). ZDV is also incorporated into the growing DNA chain, but since it lacks a 3'-OH group, chain elongation is terminated.

ZDV is beneficial in children with symptomatic HIV disease, particularly CNS abnormalities. Intravenous gamma globulin therapy has been used in children with HIV infections. The most apparent use for this therapy is to provide functional IgG, as antibody responses to new antigens are frequently reduced in HIV-infected children. This may lead to a reduction in the frequency and severity of bacterial infections.

7. **Prevention.** In February 1994, a large clinical trial conducted by the AIDS Clinical Trials Group (ACTG) was closed early owing to astonishing results [11]. HIV-infected pregnant women with more than 200 CD4+ T cells were randomized to receive ZDV (at 100 mg 5 times/day) or placebo, beginning at 14 weeks' gestation. The mothers randomized to receive ZDV also received intrapartum ZDV intravenously at 2 mg/kg for the first hour of labor followed by 1 mg/kg/hour until delivery, and their infants orally received ZDV syrup orally at 2 mg/kg every 6 hours

for the first 6 weeks of life. This trial (ACTG 076) closed when approximately 183 babies had been born to each cohort and had been assessed for HIV infection. Only 13 babies (8.3%) in the ZDV-receiving group were infected, whereas 40 babies (25.5%) in the placebo group were infected. As of February 1994, it has been the standard of care to offer ZDV to pregnant HIV-infected women with more than 200 CD4+ T cells following the 076 algorithm. It is likely that the infection rate of babies born to mothers with fewer than 200 CD4+ T cells would also be decreased with ZDV use, but those mothers were not part of the study population.

Clearly this study challenges all health care providers to participate in offering testing and counseling to all pregnant women, especially those who have engaged in high-risk behaviors. Frequently mothers may learn for the first time that they are HIV-infected during their pregnancy. The appropriate social, nonjudgmental support network must be effectively in place to achieve the best pregnancy outcome possible. The mother's health, both medical and emotional, should not be subjugated to that of the fetus; rather optimization of the mother-baby pair is key in effecting the best possible outcome.

Several studies suggested that maternal viral load, along with lower CD4+ T cell counts, is a strong correlate of vertical transmission [6]. Assessment of viral load might also allow for targeting the pregnancies at highest risk of transmission to selected therapeutic strategies. Since HIV may be transmitted at the time of delivery, there has been speculation as to whether the risk of fetal infection may be reduced by cesarean section. Trials have been initiated to test this notion. No recommendations concerning mode of delivery can be made at this time.

Further strategies targeted to reduce the rate of vertical transmission even in the setting of ZDV use are being planned. It is estimated that persons newly infected with HIV will acquire a ZDV-resistant strain approximately 15% of the time; therefore, studies of other antiretroviral agents such as didanosine are being conducted in pregnancy. Resistance develops quickly to other agents such as nonnucleoside reverse transcriptase inhibitors (e.g., nevirapine), but these agents may be quite efficacious in decreasing the viral load at critical time periods -such as the intrapartum interval. Hyperimmune gamma globulin, prepared from healthy HIV-infected volunteers, is also under study to reduce the rate of transmission. Active immunity has also been an avenue of pursuit with vaccines to the surface glycoprotein of HIV (gp120). Infants will also be offered both active and passive immunity with vaccine and gamma globulin, much along the hepatitis B model. Birth canal washes with a virostatic agent have also been proposed as HIV administered by gavage has been found to infect infant monkeys. Hopefully, combinations of these approaches or newer ones will be able to reduce the anticipated 15% rate of transmission of HIV to infants of infected mothers of any CD4+ count, even if receiving ZDV.

Education plays an important role in the prevention of the spread of HIV infection. Informing the public about high-risk behaviors such as IV drug use and unprotected sexual contact is critical in curtailing this epidemic. The health care provider should take advantage of every patient contact to provide preventive education. Eliminating unwarranted fears about casual contact with HIV-infected individuals is also within the purview of the provider.

8. **HIV and the health care worker.** The transmission of HIV from patients to health care providers is very uncommon as is transmission from care providers to patients. The greatest risk for transmission is from parenteral inoculation of infected blood by inadvertent needle sticks or cuts with contaminated sharp instruments. To minimize the risk of transmission of HIV, universal precautions have been recom-

mended for all hospital environments [11]. Particular emphasis in perinatal/neonatal medicine should be placed on the avoidance of blood and bloody secretions in the delivery room by the wearing of gowns, gloves, and eye protection (preferably goggles with side shields). Meconium and gastric aspirates should never be suctioned by mouth; special meconium suction adapters and catheters that can be attached to wall suction are generally available. Of special concern in the nursery is the recapping of needles after drawing blood from umbilical lines. If recapping is required, it is best to use cap-holding devices, to avoid needle sticks. Also, syringes should not be tapped or "flicked" to remove air when obtaining arterial blood gas samples. Specific guidelines have been suggested for the recognition and management of occupational exposures to HIV. Types of exposures include percutaneous injury (needle sticks, cuts with sharp instruments), mucous membrane contact, and skin contact (particularly from skin with cuts, abrasions, or dermatitis, or for prolonged exposure or over a large area) with potentially infectious tissues or body fluids. The guidelines recommend procedures for serologic testing in the worker and the patient contact. The use of ZDV for postexposure prophylaxis is also discussed. Review of these guidelines is recommended for all individuals at risk for occupational exposure to HIV. The average risk of contracting HIV per episode of percutaneous exposure to HIV-infected blood is estimated to be approximately 0.3%. It is unknown if postexposure ZDV will further reduce this risk.

D. Parvovirus [6]. Parvoviruses are small, unenveloped viruses that range in size from 18 to 26 mm and contain single-stranded DNA. Human infections are primarily due to strain B19, which is responsible for several clinical syndromes. Although parvovirus B19 has genotypic variation, no antigenic variation between isolates has been demonstrated. Parvoviruses tend to infect rapidly dividing cells and can be transmitted across the placenta, posing a potential threat to the fetus [11].

1. **Epidemiology.** The seroprevalence of parvovirus B19 IgG reflects the age-related incidence of clinical disease. Approximately 2 to 9 percent of children less than 5 years old have detectable B19 IgG, compared with 15 to 35 percent of those 5 to 18 years old. Rates in adults have varied, with seropositivity for B19 IgG ranging from 30 to 60 percent. Based on studies of household contacts, the incubation period for parvovirus B19 infection appears to be 4 to 14 days, with an attack rate of 50 to 60 percent for all ages. Of infected contacts (IgM-positive), approximately 20 percent may be asymptomatic and 50 percent may not have a rash. Peak occurrence is from around midwinter through spring, with a cyclic peak activity every 5 to 7 years. The virus is probably spread by means of respiratory secretions, which clear in patients with typical erythema infectiosum at or shortly after the onset of rash. Interestingly, recently it was suggested that subjects who lack the P antigen, the cellular receptor for parvovirus B19, are naturally resistant to infection. This antigen is found on erythrocytes, erythroblasts, megakaryocytes, endothelial cells, placenta, and fetal liver and heart cells. This tissue specificity correlates with sites of clinical abnormalities. Lack of the P antigen is extremely rare, but these findings might suggest a basis for future therapy.

2. **Common clinical presentations of parvovirus B19 infection**
   a. **Disease in children.** Parvovirus B19 has been associated with a variety of rashes, including the typical "slapped cheek" rash of erythema infectiosum (fifth disease). In approximately 60% of school-age children with erythema infectiosum, fever occurs 1 to 4 days before the facial rash appears. Associated symptoms include myalgias, upper respiratory or gastrointestinal symptoms, and malaise, but these symptoms generally resolve with the appearance of the

rash. The rash is usually macular, progresses to the extremities and trunk, and may involve the palms and soles. The rash may be pruritic and may recur. These children are likely most infectious before the onset of fever or rash and are *unlikely to be infectious after the onset of the rash.* The incubation period is usually 4 to 14 days, but can extend to 20 days.

b. **Disease in adults.** The typical school-age presentation of erythema infectiosum can occur in adults, but arthralgias and arthritis are more common. As many as 60% of adults with parvovirus B19 infection may have acute joint swelling, most commonly involving peripheral joints (symmetrically). Rash and joint symptoms occur 2 to 3 weeks after infection. Arthritis may persist for years and may be associated with the development of rheumatoid arthritis.

3. **Less common manifestations of parvovirus B19 infection**
    a. **Infection in patients with hemolytic anemia or immunosuppression.** Parvovirus B19 has been clearly identified as a cause of red blood cell aplasia. In particular, parvovirus B19 is the principal cause of aplastic crisis in individuals with chronic hemolytic anemia, including acquired diseases. Severe anemia has been observed in individuals with hemoglobin abnormalities (sickle-cell disease, hemoglobin SC disease, thalassemia), hereditary spherocytosis, and cellular enzyme deficits, such as pyruvate kinase deficiency. A viral prodrome usually occurs within 1 week of anemia. A rash also may occur but is less common. Parvovirus B19 also has been associated with acute and chronic red blood cell aplasia in immunosuppressed patients.

    b. **Fetal infection.** Based primarily on the demonstration of viral DNA in fetal tissue samples, parvovirus B19 has been firmly linked to fetal nonimmune hydrops. The presumed pathogenic sequence is as follows:

    Transplacental transfer of B19 virus → Infection of RBC precursors → Arrested RBC production → Severe anemia → Congestive heart failure → Edema

    The overall rate of vertical transmission of parvovirus from the mother with primary infection to the fetus is approximately one-third. The overall risk of fetal loss after maternal infection is approximately 10%. The risk of fetal hydrops following maternal infection with parvovirus B19 showed that up to 15% of fetuses may be affected with maternal infection during the first 18 weeks of gestation. However, in this study, B19 DNA was demonstrated in approximately one-third of the fetuses, suggesting that the attack rate for severe fetal disease was approximately 5% for maternal infection during the first 18 weeks of gestation. No adverse outcomes were noted for maternal infection occurring beyond 18 weeks, but more recent reports indicated that anemia may result from third-trimester infections [11].

    B19 may infect cells other than those of the hematopoietic system. The finding of an ocular anomaly in one fetus infected with B19 suggests this possibility. Furthermore, B19 DNA has been detected in cardiac tissues from aborted fetuses. It has been suggested that B19 may cause fetal myocarditis and that this may contribute to the development of hydrops. There is one report of B19-associated fetal hydrops dramatically responding to in utero digitalization. Despite this improvement, the fetus died and on postmortem examination was found to have intranuclear viral particles consistent with B19 present in cardiac tissue. Finally, fetal hepatitis with severe liver disease has been documented.

    The possibility of parvovirus B19–induced fetal anomalies has been questioned given the propensity for the virus to infect rapidly growing cells. Although there is one case report implicating B19 as a cause of an ocular anomaly, a study of 130 newborn infants to mothers with documented infection during pregnancy did not show any fetal anomalies [11].

4. **Diagnosis.** Parvovirus B19 is difficult to grow in vitro and will not grow in standard tissue cultures. Determination of serum IgG and IgM levels is the most practical test. Serum B19 IgG is absent in susceptible hosts, and IgM appears by day 3 of an acute infection. Serum IgM may be detected in up to 90% of patients with acute B19 infection, and serum levels begin to fall by the second to third month after infection. Serum IgG appears a few days after IgM and may persist for years. Viral antigens may be directly detected in tissues by radioimmunoassay, ELISA, immunofluorescence, in situ nucleic acid hybridization, or PCR. These techniques may be valuable for certain clinical settings, such as the examination of tissues from fetuses with nonimmune hydrops or determination of infection (PCR).

5. **Treatment.** Treatment is generally supportive. Intravenous gamma globulin (IVIG) has been used with reported success in a limited number of patients with severe hematologic disorders related to persistent parvovirus infection. The rationale for this therapy stems from the observations that (1) the primary immune response to B19 infection is the production of specific IgM and IgG, (2) the appearance of systemic antibody coincides with the resolution of clinical symptoms, and (3) specific antibody prevents infection. However, no controlled studies have been undertaken to establish the efficacy of IVIG prophylaxis or therapy for B19 infections.

Given the potential for severe disease in immunocompromised patients exposed to parvovirus B19, IVIG prophylaxis is a reasonable consideration. Even more compelling is the use of IVIG to treat patients with symptomatic anemia and parvoviremia. IVIG is not currently recommended for prophylaxis in pregnancy.

Intrauterine blood transfusions have been used with success in a few cases of fetal hydrops, but the institution of such therapy must take into account the severity of fetal disease and the risk of the procedure to the fetus and mother. Attempts to identify other causes of fetal hydrops are obviously important. The possible contribution of cardiac dysfunction that may not respond to blood transfusions also should be considered (see Chap. 25).

6. **Management of pregnant women at risk for parvovirus exposure.** Three groups of pregnant women of interest when considering the potential risk of fetal parvovirus disease are pregnant women exposed to an infected household contact, pregnant schoolteachers, and pregnant health care providers. In each, the measurement of serum IgG and IgM levels may be useful to determine the women at risk or acutely infected after B19 exposure. The tests can be arranged through state departments of public health or the Centers for Disease Control, Atlanta, Georgia. In general, requests for these tests should be limited to pregnant women clearly at increased risk for acute parvovirus B19 exposure during the first 18 weeks of gestation. Consultation with an infectious disease service or state department of public health is recommended.

   a. **The pregnant woman exposed to an infected household contact.** The risk of fetal B19 disease is apparently very small for asymptomatic pregnant women in communities where outbreaks of erythema infectiosum occur. In this setting, no special diagnostic tests or precautions may be indicated. However, household contacts with erythema infectiosum place the pregnant women at increased risk for acute B19 infection. The estimated risk of B19 infection in a susceptible adult with a household contact is approximately 50%. Considering an estimated risk of 5% for severe fetal disease with acute maternal B19 infection, the risk of hydrops fetalis is approximately 2.5% for susceptible pregnant women exposed to an infected household contact during the first 18 weeks of gestation. Management of these women may include the following:

(1) Determination of susceptibility or acute infection by serum IgG and IgM

(2) For susceptible or acutely infected women, serial fetal ultrasound to monitor fetal growth and the possible evolution of hydrops

(3) Serial determinations of maternal serum alpha-fetoprotein (AFP) (AFP may rise up to 4 weeks before ultrasound evidence of fetal hydrops), although this use is questioned

(4) Determination of fetal IgM by PUBS. The utility of this is questionable given the relatively high risk-benefit ratio at present, especially since it is unclear that obstetric management will be altered by results. It may be useful to confirm B19 etiology when hydrops fetalis is present.

(5) Intrauterine fetal transfusions of packed red blood cells when B19-associated hydrops fetalis is present

b. The pregnant schoolteacher and health care provider. The epidemiology of community outbreaks of erythema infectiosum suggests that the risk of infection to susceptible schoolteachers is approximately 19% (compared with 50% for household contacts). This would lower the risk of B19 fetal disease in pregnant schoolteachers to less than 1%. It is not obvious that special precautions are necessary in this setting. In fact, there is likely to be widespread inapparent infection in both adults and children, providing a constant background exposure rate that cannot be altered. Considering the high prevalence of B19, the low risk of severe fetal disease, and the fact that attempts to avoid potential high-risk settings only reduce but do not eliminate exposure, exclusion of pregnant schoolteachers from the workplace is not recommended.

A similar approach may be taken for pregnant health care providers where the principal exposure will be from infected children presenting to the emergency room or physician's office. However, in many cases, the typical rash of erythema infectiosum may already be present, at which time infectivity is low. Furthermore, precautions directed at minimizing exposure to respiratory secretions may be taken to decrease the risk of transmission. Particular care should be exercised on pediatric wards where there are immunocompromised patients or patients with hemolytic anemias in whom B19 disease is suspected. These patients may shed virus well beyond the period of initial clinical symptoms, particularly when presenting with aplastic crisis. In this setting, there may be a significant risk for the spread of B19 to susceptible health care workers or other patients at risk for B19-induced aplastic crisis. To minimize this risk, patients with aplastic crises from B19 infections should be maintained on contact precautions, masks should be worn for close contact, and pregnant health care providers should not care for these patients.

II. Perinatal infections

A. Herpes simplex virus (HSV) [2,5,8,11]

1. Pathogenesis and epidemiology. There are two virologically distinct types of HSV—types 1 and 2. HSV-2 is the predominant cause of neonatal disease (80%), but both types produce clinically indistinguishable syndromes. Infection in the newborn occurs as a result of direct exposure, most commonly in the perinatal period from maternal genital disease. The virus can cause localized disease of the skin, eye, or mouth or may disseminate by cell-to-cell contiguous spread or viremia. After adsorption and penetration into host cells, viral replication proceeds, resulting in cellular swelling, hemorrhagic necrosis, formation of intranuclear inclusions, cytolysis, and cell death.

Since HSV-2 is more likely to recur in the genital tract and therefore accounts for the majority of neonatal HSV infections, it is important to understand the potential for neonatal exposure to virus. The seroprevalence of HSV-2 varies according to locale in the United States but is likely to be at least 30%. In a study of 779 women attending a sexually transmitted disease clinic, while 47% had serologic evidence of HSV-2 infection, only 22% had symptoms. The characteristic ulcerations of the genitalia were only present in two-thirds of the genital tracts from which HSV could be isolated, and the others had asymptomatic shedding or atypical lesions. It is estimated that 0.01 to 0.39% of all women shed virus at delivery, and approximately 1% of all women with a history of recurrent HSV infection asymptomatically shed HSV at delivery. However, when the birth canal is carefully visualized and those with asymptomatic lesions excluded, this rate of shedding may be nearer 0.5%. It is critical to recognize that the majority of mothers of infants with neonatal HSV do not have a history of HSV. Infants at greatest risk of acquisition of infection are those born to mothers with newly acquired HSV during pregnancy (primary infection), in whom the rate of transmission of HSV is estimated to be 50%. Additionally, one-third of infants born to mothers with newly acquired HSV-2, although already infected with HSV-1 (nonprimary, first episode), may acquire HSV infection. Infants born to HSV 2–seropositive mothers (recurrent) have an approximate 3% risk of acquiring infection. This may well be due to protective maternal type-specific antibodies in the infant's serum or the birth canal. The overall incidence of newborn infection with HSV is estimated to be 1:2000 to 1:5000 per year.

    a. Intrapartum transmission. This is the most common cause of neonatal HSV and is primarily associated with active shedding of virus from the cervix or vulva at the time of delivery. Up to 95% of newborn infections occur as a result of intrapartum transmission. At least four factors have been identified that relate to intrapartum transmission. First, the amount and duration of maternal virus shedding is likely to be a major determinate of fetal transmission. These are greatest with primary maternal infections. Maternal antibody to HSV is also important and is associated with a decreased risk of fetal transmission. In fact, when maternal antibody is present, the risk of acquisition of HSV, even for the newborn exposed to HSV in the birth canal, is very low. The exact mechanism of action of maternal antibody in preventing perinatal infection is not known, but transplacentally acquired antibody has been shown to reduce the risk of severe newborn disease following postnatal HSV exposure. The risk of intrapartum infection increases with ruptured membranes, especially when ruptured longer than 6 hours. Finally, direct methods for fetal monitoring, such as with scalp electrodes, increase the risk of fetal transmission in the setting of active shedding. Thus it is best to avoid these techniques in women with a history of recurrent infection or suspected primary HSV disease.

    b. Antenatal transmission. In utero infection has been documented but is uncommon. Spontaneous abortion has occurred with primary maternal infection prior to 20 weeks' gestation, but the true risk to the fetus of early-trimester primary infection is not known. Fetal infections may occur by either transplacental or ascending routes and have been documented in the setting of both primary and recurrent maternal disease. There may be a wide range of clinical manifestations from localized skin or eye involvement to multiorgan disease and congenital malformations. Chorioretinitis, microcephaly, and hydranencephaly may be found in a small number of patients.

c. **Postnatal transmission.** There is evidence that a percentage of neonatal HSV infections result from postnatal exposure. Potential sources include symptomatic and asymptomatic oropharyngeal shedding by either parent, hospital personnel, or other contacts; maternal breast lesions; and nosocomial spread. Measures to minimize exposure from these sources are discussed below.

2. **Clinical manifestations.** Data from the National Institute of Allergy and Infectious Diseases (NIAID) Collaborative Antiviral Study Group indicate that morbidity and mortality of neonatal HSV best correlates with three categories of disease. These are infection localized to the skin, eye, and/or mouth; encephalitis with or without localized mucocutaneous disease; and disseminated infection with multiple organ involvement. The NIAID Collaborative Antiviral Study Group reported on the outcome of 210 infants with HSV infection who were randomized to receive either acyclovir or vidarabine antiviral therapy. Eight babies had congenital infection with signs (chorioretinitis, skin lesions, hydrocephalus) at birth. The highest mortality (>50%) was seen in infants having disseminated disease; hemorrhagic shock and pneumonitis were the principal causes of death. Of the survivors for whom follow-up was available, significant neurologic sequelae were seen in a high percentage of the infants with encephalitis and disseminated disease.

a. **Skin, eye, and mouth infection.** Approximately 40% of infants with HSV have disease localized to the skin, eye, or mucocutaneous membranes, and vesicles typically appear on the sixth to ninth day of neonatal life. Often a cluster of vesicles develops on the presenting part of the body, where extended direct contact with virus may occur. Vesicles occur in 90% of infants with localized mucocutaneous infection, and recurrent disease is common. Furthermore, significant morbidity can occur in these infants despite the absence of signs of disseminated disease at the time of diagnosis; up to 10% of infants later show neurologic impairment, and infants with keratoconjunctivitis can develop chorioretinitis, cataracts, and retinopathy. Ophthalmologic and neurologic follow-up is important in all infants with mucocutaneous HSV. Infants with three or more recurrences of vesicles had an increased risk of neurologic complications.

b. **CNS infection.** Approximately one-third of neonates with HSV present with encephalitis in the absence of disseminated disease, and from 40 to 60% of these infants do not have mucocutaneous vesicles. These infants usually become symptomatic at 10 to 14 days of life with lethargy, seizures, temperature instability, and hypotonia. In the setting of disseminated disease, HSV is thought to invade the CNS from hematogenous spread. However, CNS infection in the absence of disseminated disease probably results from retrograde axonal spread. The latter condition most often occurs in infants having transplacentally derived viral neutralizing antibodies, which may protect against widespread dissemination but not influence intraneuronal viral replication. Mortality is high without treatment and is approximately 15% with treatment, and approximately two-thirds of surviving infants have impaired neurodevelopment. Long-term sequelae from acute HSV encephalitis include microcephaly, hydranencephaly, poren-cephalic cysts, spasticity, blindness, chorioretinitis, and learning disabilities.

c. **Disseminated infection.** This is the most severe form of neonatal HSV infection. It accounts for approximately 22% of all infants with neonatal HSV infection, and ends in mortality for 57% of the infants with this presentation. Pneumonitis was associated with greatest mortality. Symptoms usually begin within the first week of neonatal life. The liver, adrenals, and multiple other visceral organs are usually involved. Approximately two-thirds of infants also have encephalitis. Clinical findings include seizures, shock, respiratory distress, disseminated intravascular coagulation (DIC), and pneumonitis. A typical vesicular rash may be absent in up to 20% of infants. Forty percent of the infants who live have morbidity.

3. **Diagnosis.** HSV infection should be considered in the differential diagnosis of ill neonates with a variety of clinical presentations. These include CNS abnormalities, fever, shock, DIC, and/or hepatitis. HSV also should be considered in infants with respiratory distress without an obvious bacterial cause or clinical course and findings consistent with immature lung disease. The possibility of concomitant HSV infection with other commonly encountered problems of the preterm infant should be considered. Viral isolation in the appropriate clinical setting remains critical to the diagnosis. Serology is of little value, because specific IgM may not be detected for up to 3 weeks. However, the number of different viral antigen-specific antibodies produced seems to correlate with the extent of disseminated disease, and the presence of certain antigen-specific antibodies may have long-term prognostic value. For the infant with mucocutaneous lesions, tissue should be scraped from vesicles, placed in the appropriate viral transport medium, and promptly processed for culture by a diagnostic virology laboratory. Alternatively, virus can be detected directly when tissue samples are swabbed onto a glass slide and evaluated by direct fluorescent antibody technique. Virus also can be isolated from the oropharynx and nasopharynx, conjunctivae, stool, and urine. In the absence of a vesicular rash, viral isolation from these sites may aid in the diagnosis of disseminated HSV or HSV encephalitis. With encephalitis, an elevated CSF protein level and pleocytosis are often seen, but initial values may be within normal limits. Thus serial CSF examinations may be very important. Electroencephalography and CT/MRI are also useful in the diagnosis of HSV encephalitis. Viral isolation from CSF is reported to be successful in up to 40% of cases, and rates of detection in CSF by PCR may reach close to 100%. Laboratory abnormalities seen with disseminated disease include elevated hepatic transaminase levels, direct hyperbilirubinemia, neutropenia, thrombocytopenia, and coagulopathy. A diffuse interstitial pattern is usually observed on x-ray films of infants with HSV pneumonitis.

4. **Treatment.** Effective antiviral therapy exists for HSV, but the timing of therapy is critical. Treatment is indicated for all forms of HSV disease. Previously, extensive studies were carried out with vidarabine, which reduced the morbidity and mortality for all forms of neonatal HSV. Unfortunately, with disseminated disease, very high mortality occurs despite therapy. In a collaborative study examining the efficacy of vidarabine in the treatment of neonatal HSV, therapy reduced the mortality from disseminated disease from 90 to 70%. The mortality with encephalitis was reduced from 50 to 15%. Recently the NIAID Collaborative Antiviral Study Group found that acyclovir may be as efficacious as vidarabine for the treatment of neonatal HSV. Furthermore, acyclovir is a selective inhibitor of viral replication with minimal side effects on the host. It can be administered in relatively small volumes over short infusion times. Thus acyclovir has become favored in the treatment of neonatal HSV. Doses of 45 or 60 mg/kg per day are being compared to the standard dose of 30 mg/kg per day. Early studies suggested tolerance and greater efficacy. At present, infants with skin, eye, and mouth (SEM) disease should receive 10 to 15 mg acyclovir per kilogram every

8 hours for 10 to 14 days. Infants with CNS or disseminated disease should receive 10 to 15 mg acyclovir per kilogram every 8 hours for 21 days.
5. **Management of the newborn at risk for HSV** (Table 23-1). The principal problem in developing strategies for the prevention of HSV transmission is the inability to identify maternal shedding of virus at the time of delivery. Viral identification requires isolation in tissue culture, so any attempt to identify women who may be shedding HSV at delivery would require antenatal cervical cultures. Unfortunately, such screening cultures taken prior to labor fail to predict active excretion at delivery.

Until more rapid techniques are made available for the identification of HSV, the only clear recommendation that can be made is to deliver infants by cesarean section if genital lesions are present at the start of labor. The efficacy of this approach may diminish when membranes are ruptured beyond 4 hours. Nevertheless, it is generally recommended that cesarean section be considered even with membrane rupture of longer durations, although data showing efficacy beyond 4 hours are lacking. The upper time limit for membrane rupture has been suggested to be 12 hours to 24 hours. For women with a history of prior genital herpes, careful examination should be performed to determine whether lesions are present when labor commences. If lesions are observed, cesarean section should be carried out. If no lesions are identified, vaginal delivery is appropriate, but cervical tissue should be obtained for culture. At this time there are no data to support the prophylactic use of antiviral agents or immunoglobulin to prevent transmission to the newborn infant.

Infants inadvertently delivered vaginally in the setting of cervical lesions should be isolated from other infants in the nursery, and cultures should be obtained from the oropharynx/nasopharynx and conjunctivae. If the mother can be identified as having recurrent infection, the resultant neonatal infection rate is low, and parents should be instructed to consult their pediatrician when a rash or other clinical changes (lethargy, tachypnea, poor feeding) develop. Weekly pediatric follow-up during the first month is recommended. Infants with a positive culture from any site or the evolution of clinical symptomatology should immediately have cultures repeated and antiviral therapy

Table 23-1. Management of the child born to a woman with active genital HSV infection [11]

Maternal primary or first-episode infection
  Cesarean section within 24 (preferably 4) hours of ruptured membranes
    Culture eyes, nose, mouth, urine, stool at 48 hours
    Treat with acyclovir if culture positive or signs of neonatal HSV[a]
  Unavoidable vaginal delivery
    Culture eyes, nose, mouth, urine, stool, CSF
    Treat with acyclovir
Recurrent infection, active at delivery
  Cesarean section within 24 (preferably 4) hours of ruptured membranes
    Culture eyes, nose, mouth, urine, stool at 48 hours
    Treat with acyclovir if culture positive or signs of HSV infection[a]
  Unavoidable vaginal delivery
    See III.A.5
    Treat with acyclovir only if cultures are positive or signs of neonatal HSV
    infection

---

[a]If infant is to be treated with acyclovir, a CSF analysis, culture and PCR for HSV DNA are indicated.

initiated. These infants should be evaluated for possible disseminated and CNS infection as well.

Currently, there is no indication for isolation of newborns from mothers with genital and/or recurrent mucocutaneous HSV infection. Careful hand-washing and preventing the infant from having direct contact with lesions should be emphasized. Breast-feeding should be avoided if there are breast lesions.

Hospital personnel with orolabial HSV infection represent a low risk to the newborn, although the use of face masks can be recommended if active lesions are present. Of course, hand-washing or use of gloves should again be emphasized. The exception to these guidelines is nursery personnel with herpetic whitlows. Because they have a high risk of viral shedding, and because transmission can occur despite the use of gloves, these individuals should not care for newborns.

B. Varicella-zoster virus [2]. The causative agent of varicella (chickenpox) is a member of the herpesvirus family. The same agent is responsible for herpes zoster (shingles); hence this virus is referred to as **varicella-zoster virus (V-Z virus).** Chickenpox results from primary V-Z virus infection, following which the virus may remain latent in sensory nerve ganglia. Zoster results from reactivation of latent virus later in life.

There are approximately 3 million cases of varicella yearly in the United States, primarily occurring in school-age children. The majority of adults have antibodies to V-Z virus, indicating prior infection, even when there is thought to be no history of chickenpox. It follows that varicella is an uncommon occurrence in pregnancy. The precise incidence of gestational varicella is uncertain but has been estimated to be 0.8 to 5.0 per 10,000. Alternatively, zoster is primarily a disease of adults. The incidence of zoster in pregnancy is also unknown, but the disease is likely to be uncommon as well.

1. **Transmission.** It appears that the primary mode of transmission of V-Z virus is through respiratory droplets from patients with chickenpox. Spread through contact with vesicular lesions also can occur. Typically, individuals with chickenpox are contagious from 1 to 2 days before and 5 days after the onset of rash. Conventionally, a patient is no longer considered contagious when all vesicular lesions have dried and crusted over. The incubation period for primary disease extends from 10 to 21 days, with most infections occurring between 13 and 17 days. Transplacental transfer of V-Z virus may take place, presumably secondary to maternal viremia, but the frequency of this event is unknown. Interestingly, maternal zoster during pregnancy also may result in fetal infection, although this is likely to be an uncommon event.

2. **Perinatal varicella.** Varicella occurs in approximately 25% of newborns whose mothers developed varicella within the peripartum period. The onset of disease usually occurs 13 to 15 days after the onset of maternal rash. Rarely, neonatal disease occurs within 3 days of maternal rash, and the maximum incubation period has been 16 days (mean incubation of 11 days). When rash develops in the newborn within 10 days, it is presumed to result from in utero transmission. The greatest risk for severe disease is seen when maternal varicella occurs within 4 days of delivery. In these cases there is insufficient time for the fetus to acquire transplacentally derived V-Z virus–specific antibodies. Symptoms generally begin 5 to 10 days after delivery, and the expected mortality is approximately 30%.

3. **Congenital varicella.** When in utero transmission of V-Z virus occurs prior to the peripartum period, there is no obvious clinical impact in the majority of fetuses.

    a. **Varicella-associated chromosomal abnormalities.** It appears that chromosomal abnormalities may be common in the patient with congenital varicella. Although these are thought to be transient without adverse effects on the host, the possibility of more permanent abnormalities following in utero fetal infection has been suggested. Possible consequences include a higher incidence of childhood leukemia, but it must be emphasized that there are insufficient data to indicate the incidence of persistent chromosomal abnormalities or to confirm an increase in related disorders later in life.

b. **Congenital malformations.** There is a strong association between gestational varicella and a spectrum of congenital defects comprising a unique syndrome. Characteristic findings include cicatricial skin lesions, ocular defects, CNS abnormalities, intrauterine growth retardation, and early death. The syndrome most commonly occurs with maternal V-Z virus infection in weeks 7 to 20 of gestation. The overall risk of the congenital varicella syndrome following maternal infection in the first trimester is 2 percent. It is primarily seen with gestational varicella but may occur with maternal zoster.

4. **Zoster.** Zoster is uncommon in young infants but may occur as a consequence of in utero fetal infection with V-Z virus. Similarly, children who develop zoster but have no history of varicella most likely acquired V-Z virus in utero. Zoster in childhood is usually self-limiting, with only symptomatic therapy indicated in otherwise healthy children.

5. **Postnatal varicella.** Varicella acquired in the newborn period as a result of postnatal exposure is generally a mild disease. Rarely, severe disseminated disease occurs in newborns exposed shortly after birth. In these instances, treatment with acyclovir may be beneficial (see below). Varicella has been detected in breast milk by PCR; therefore, it may be prudent to defer breast-feeding at least during the period of time in which the mother is likely to be viremic and/or infectious.

6. **Diagnosis.** Infants with congenital varicella resulting from in utero infection occurring before the peripartum period do not shed virus, and the determination of V-Z virus–specific antibodies is often confusing. Thus the diagnosis is made on the basis of clinical findings and maternal history. With neonatal disease, the presence of a typical vesicular rash and a maternal history of peripartum varicella or postpartum exposure are all that is required to make the diagnosis. Laboratory confirmation can be made by (1) culture of vesicular fluid, although the sensitivity of this method is not optimal because the virus is quite labile, and (2) demonstration of a fourfold rise in V-Z virus antibody titer by the fluorescent antibody to membrane antigen (FAMA) assay or by ELISA. Antigen also can be detected in vesicular fluid by countercurrent immunoelectrophoresis, which is very sensitive and specific. Alternatively, indirect immunofluorescence can be used for rapid detection of virus from vesicular material.

7. **Treatment.** Infants with congenital infection, resulting from in utero transmission before the peripartum period, are unlikely to have active viral disease, so antiviral therapy is not indicated. However, infants with perinatal varicella acquired from maternal infection near the time of delivery are at risk for severe disease. In this setting, therapy with acyclovir is generally recommended. Data are not available on the most efficacious and safe dose of acyclovir for the treatment of neonatal varicella, but minimal toxicity has been shown with the administration of 30 mg/kg per day (divided q8h) for the treatment of neonatal HSV infection. This dose given over 7 days may be efficacious for uncomplicated varicella, but a higher dose of 1500 mg/m^2 over a longer duration may be more appropriate for severe (disseminated) disease.

At the present time, there is no established immunotherapy for the treatment of V-Z virus infections, but varicella-zoster immune globulin

(VZIG) may be of prophylactic value. When administered within 72 hours of exposure, VZIG is effective in preventing or attenuating V-Z virus infection. The dose for newborns is 125 units intramuscularly. Vaccination of females who are not immune to varicella should decrease the incidence of congenital and perinatal varicella. Women should not receive the vaccine if they are pregnant or within 3 months before pregnancy. If this inadvertently occurs the women should be enrolled in the National Registry by calling (800) 897-8999.

8. Management of varicella in the nursery. The risk of horizontal spread of varicella following exposure in the nursery appears to be low, possibly due to a combination of factors, including (1) passive protection due to transplacentally derived antibody in infants born to varicella-immune mothers and (2) brief exposure with a lack of intimate contact. Nevertheless, nursery outbreaks do occur, so steps should be taken to minimize the risk of nosocomial spread. The infected infant should be isolated in a separate room, and visitors and caregivers should be limited to individuals with a history of varicella. A new gown should be worn upon entering the room, and good handwashing technique should be used. Bedding and other materials should be bagged and sterilized. VZIG can be given to all other exposed neonates, but this can be withheld from full-term infants whose mothers have a history of varicella. Exposed personnel without a history of varicella should be tested for V-Z virus antibodies, and patient care by these individuals should be restricted as outlined below.

In the regular nursery, all exposed infants will ordinarily be discharged home before they could become infectious. Occasionally, an exposed infant needs to remain in the nursery for more than 8 days, and in this circumstance, isolation may be required. In the special care nursery, exposed neonates are generally cohorted and isolated from new admissions within 8 days after exposure.

Several situations of varicella exposure arise from time to time in the nursery for which the following guidelines may be useful:

a. Antepartum exposure in mothers without a history of varicella. The concern here is for women exposed within 21 days prior to admission to the hospital.

(1) Mother and infant should be discharged as soon as possible from the hospital. If the exposure was from a household contact with current disease, VZIG should be administered to both mother and infant prior to discharge. Alternatively, arrangements to isolate the infectious household contact from the mother and infant may be done prior to discharge.

(2) If exposure occurred 6 days or less prior to admission and the mother is discharged within 48 hours, no further action is required. Otherwise, mothers hospitalized between 8 to 21 days after exposure should be kept isolated from the nursery and other patients.

(3) Personnel without a history of varicella should be kept from contact with a potentially infectious mother. If such an individual is inadvertently exposed, serologic testing (FAMA or ELISA) should be performed to determine susceptibility, and further contact should be avoided until immunity is proved. If the mother at risk for infection has not developed varicella 48 hours after the staff member was exposed, no further action is required. Alternatively, if a susceptible staff member is exposed to any individual with active varicella lesions or in whom a varicella rash erupts within 48 hours of the exposure, contact with any patients should be restricted for that staff member from day 8 through day 21 after exposure. Personnel without a

history of varicella should have serologic testing, and if not immune should be vaccinated.
  - **b. Maternal varicella.** Of concern are mothers with active disease while in the hospital or in whom varicella has occurred within 21 days prior to delivery.
    - **(1) Resolution of the infectious stage prior to hospitalization**
      - **(a)** Maternal isolation is not required.
      - **(b)** Isolate the newborn from other infants (room in with mother).
    - **(2) Active varicella lesions on admission to the hospital**
      - **(a)** Isolate mother.
      - **(b)** Administer VZIG (125 units intramuscularly) to the newborn if maternal disease began less than 5 days before delivery or within 2 days postpartum (not 100% effective).
      - **(c)** Isolate the infant from the mother until she is no longer infectious.
      - **(d)** If other neonates were exposed, VZIG may be administered and these infants may require isolation if they are still hospitalized by day 8 after exposure.
- **C. Hepatitis [11].** Acute viral hepatitis is defined by the following clinical criteria: (1) symptoms consistent with viral hepatitis, (2) elevation of serum aminotransferase levels to more than 2.5 times the upper limit of normal, and (3) the absence of other causes of liver disease. At least five agents have been identified as causes of viral hepatitis: hepatitis A virus (HAV), hepatitis B virus (HBV), hepatitis D virus (HDV), hepatitis C virus (HCV) (posttransfusion non-A, non-B hepatitis virus [NANB]), and hepatitis E virus (HEV) (enteric, epidemic NANB hepatitis virus). HDV, also referred to as the **delta agent,** is a defective virus that may require coinfection or superinfection with HBV. HDV is coated with hepatitis B surface antigen (HBsAg). Specific antibodies to HDV can be detected in infected individuals, but there is no known therapy to prevent infection in exposed HBsAg-positive patients. For the newborn, therapy directed at the prevention of HBV infection also should prevent HDV infection, since coinfection is required.
  - **1. HAV.** This virus is spread by the fecal-oral route and can be detected by the presence of hepatitis A antigen (HAAg) in stool or by the presence of anti-HAV antibody. Anti-HAV IgG is present very early in infection and levels may already be significantly elevated at the time of clinical diagnosis. Thus a fourfold rise in IgG, ordinarily diagnostic of acute infection, may be difficult to demonstrate. However, specific IgM can be determined. The usual incubation period for HAV is approximately 4 weeks (range, 15 to 50 days). Symptoms include fever, malaise, anorexia, nausea, abdominal discomfort, dark urine, and jaundice. Infectivity typically diminishes rapidly. Immunization or prophylaxis against HAV is recommended primarily for travelers to developing countries or individuals at risk from personal contact with infected patients.

    Studies of acute hepatitis during pregnancy failed to demonstrate fetal transmission of HAV, although an increase in preterm deliveries may occur. Nevertheless, acute maternal HAV infection near the peripartum period poses a threat to the neonate. **It is recommended that infants born to a mother who developed acute HAV infection within 2 weeks of delivery receive an intramuscular injection of 0.5 ml of immune serum globulin.** Measures also should be taken to minimize fecal-oral spread of virus from the infected mother to her newborn and within the nursery. Of particular importance here are the appropriate disposal of contaminated materials and good hand-washing practices. Blood transfusion is a rare cause of HAV infection.
  - **2. HBV.** This virus is one of the most common causes of acute and chronic hepatitis worldwide. In endemic populations, the carrier state is high and perinatal transmission is a common event. The risk of chronic in-

fection is inversely proportional to age, with a 90% carriage rate following infection in neonates. The overall incidence of HBV infections in the United States is relatively low but still substantial. There is estimated to be approximately 300,000 infections yearly, with 250 deaths from fulminate disease. As many as 1 million individuals are chronic carriers, approximately 25% of whom develop chronic active hepatitis. Patients with chronic active hepatitis are at increased risk for developing cirrhosis and hepatocellular carcinoma, and approximately 5000 of these patients die each year from HBV-related hepatic complications (primarily cirrhosis). The incubation period for HBV infection is approximately 120 days (range, 45 to 160 days). Transmission occurs by percutaneous or permucosal routes from infected blood or body fluids. Symptoms include anorexia, malaise, nausea, vomiting, abdominal pain, and jaundice.

  a. High-risk groups for HBV infection in the United States include the following:
  - **(1)** Persons born in endemic areas: Alaskan natives and Pacific Islanders and natives of China, Southeast Asia, most of Africa, parts of the Middle East, and the Amazon basin
  - **(2)** Descendants of individuals from endemic areas
  - **(3)** Persons with high-risk behavior: homosexual activity, intravenous drug abuse, and multiple sex partners
  - **(4)** Close contacts with HBV-infected persons (sex partners, family members)
  - **(5)** Selected patient populations, particularly those receiving multiple blood or blood product transfusions
  - **(6)** Selected occupational groups, including health care providers
  b. Diagnosis. The diagnosis is made by specific serology and by the detection of viral antigens. The specific tests are as follows:
  - **(1)** HBsAg determination: usually found 1 to 2 months after exposure and lasts a variable period of time
  - **(2)** Anti-HB surface antigen (anti-HBs): appears after resolution of infection and provides long-term immunity
  - **(3)** Anti-HB core antigen (anti-HBc): present with all HBV infections and lasts for an indefinite period of time
  - **(4)** Anti-HBc IgM: appears early in infection, is detectable for 4 to 6 months after infection, and is a good marker for acute or recent infection
  - **(5)** HB e antigen (HBeAg): present in both acute and chronic infections and correlates with viral replication and high infectivity
  - **(6)** Anti-HB e antigen (anti-HBe): develops with resolution of viral replication and correlates with reduction in infectivity
    Infectivity correlates best with HBeAg positivity, but any patient positive for HBsAg is potentially infectious. Acute infection can be diagnosed by the presence of clinical symptoms and a positive HBsAg or anti-HBc IgM. The **chronic carrier state** is defined as the presence of HBsAg on two occasions, 6 months apart, or the presence of HBsAg without anti-HBc IgM.
  c. Prevention of HBV infection in the neonate. The transmission of HBV from infected mothers to their newborns is thought to result primarily from exposure to maternal blood at the time of delivery. Transplacental transfer appears to occur in Taiwan, but this has not been found in other parts of the world, including the United States. In Taiwan there is a high chronic carrier rate that may be related to the transplacental transfer observed in that country. When acute maternal HBV infection occurs during the first and second trimesters of pregnancy, there generally is little risk to the newborns, because antigenemia is usually cleared by term and anti-HBs is present. Acute maternal HBV infection during late pregnancy or

near the time of delivery, however, may result in a 50 to 75% transmission rate. The principal strategy for the prevention of neonatal HBV disease has been to use immunoprophylaxis for newborns at high risk for infection. Vaccination of these infants is also an important part of perinatal prevention and safeguards against postnatal exposure as well. Immunization of infants effectively reduced the risk of chronic HBV infection in Taiwan. Universal immunization of infants promises to be one of the best options for disease control in the United States, and is now recommended for all infants born to HBsAg-negative mothers. Three doses before the age of 18 months should be given. High-risk populations such as Alaskan natives, Pacific Islanders, and infants of immigrant mothers from areas where HBV is endemic should receive the three-dose series by the age of 6 to 9 months. The recommended schedule is begun during the newborn period or by the age of 2 months; the second dose is given 1 to 2 months later; and the third dose is given at the age of 6 to 18 months. The premature infant should be started on the immunization series at discharge or at approximately 2 months of age, unless born to an HBsAg-positive mother, in which case immunization and treatment with hepatitis B immune globulin (HBIG) should begin immediately (see Table 23-2). Other methods of disease control have been considered and include delivery by cesarean section. In one study in Taiwan, cesarean section in conjunction with maternal immunization dramatically reduced the incidence of perinatally acquired HBV from highly infective mothers. These results are promising and may offer a potential adjunctive therapy for very high-risk situations (e.g., HBsAg/HBe-positive women). Currently, no specific recommendations can be made regarding mode of delivery. **It is recommended that all pregnant women be screened for HBsAg.** Screening should be done early in gestation. If the test result is negative, no further evaluation is recommended unless there is a potential exposure history. When there is any concern about a possible infectious contact, development of acute hepatitis, or high-risk behavior in a nonimmunized woman, testing should be repeated. **All infants born to mothers confirmed to be positive for HBsAg should receive HBIG in addition to recombinant hepatitis B vaccine.** The first immunization and HBIG are given within the first 12 hours of life and the vaccine is repeated at the ages of 1 and

Table 23-2. Doses of hepatitis B vaccines in neonates

	Recombivax HB (Merck)		Energix-B (SmithKline Beecham)	
	μg	ml	μg	ml
Infants of HBsAg-negative mothers	2.5	0.5 of pediatric formulation	10	0.5
Infants of HBsAg-positive mothers (HBIG [0.5 ml] should also be given)	5	1.0 of pediatric formulation 0.5 of adult formulation	10	0.5

Both vaccine regimens use a 3-dose schedule (see text) [2].

6 months. If the mother has immigrated from an endemic area, HBIG also should be given unless the mother is found to be HBsAg-negative (Table 23-2).

Postnatal transmission of HBV by the fecal-oral route probably occurs, but the risk appears to be small. Nevertheless, this possibility adds further support to the need for the immunization of infants born to HBsAg-positive women. Another potential route of infection is by means of breast milk. This mode of transmission appears to be very uncommon in developed countries; there has been no documented increase in the risk of HBV transmission by breast-feeding mothers who are HBsAg-positive. This is true even though HBsAg can be detected in breast milk. Recommendations regarding breast-feeding in developed countries should be individualized depending on how strongly breast-feeding is desired by the mother. The risk is certain to be negligible in infants who have received HBIG and hepatitis vaccine.

d. **Prevention of nosocomial spread.** HBsAg-positive infants pose a definite risk for nosocomial spread in the nursery. To minimize this risk, nursery personnel are advised to wear gloves and gowns when caring for infected infants. Of course, current universal precautions should be in effect in all nurseries, so the risk of exposure to blood and body secretions already should be minimized. Immunization of health care workers is also strongly recommended, but if exposure should occur in a nonimmunized person, blood samples should be sent for hepatitis serology and HBIG administered as soon as possible unless the individual is known to be anti-HBs–positive. This should apply to personnel having close contact without appropriate precautions as well as those exposed parenterally (e.g., from a contaminated needle).

3. **HCV.** Recently, the agent responsible for the majority of NANB hepatitis in transfusion or organ transplant recipients was identified as a single-strand RNA virus related to the *Flavivirus* family.

a. **Epidemiology.** At least five HCV subtypes have been characterized based on sequence heterogeneity of the viral genome. HCV is found worldwide, and different subtypes have been identified from the same area.

(1) **Horizontal transmission.** Injection drug use is now the most common risk behavior for infection. In addition to injection drug users and transfusion recipients, dialysis patients and sexual partners of HCV-infected persons may also be infected, but 50% of identified persons are unable to define a risk factor.

(2) **Vertical transmission.** Studies on the vertical transmission rate of HCV prior to the availability of second-generation ELISAs are problematic. In general, studies that used this test or PCR found an approximately 6% or lower rate of transmission [8]. The transmission rate may well be much higher, and may approach 70% when the pregnant mother has a high viral load as assessed by semiquantitative PCR. Some early investigations suggested that HCV is transmitted at a higher frequency if the mother is also HIV-infected. This has since been found not to be the case.

The mode of transmission is also unknown. Detection of HCV by RNA PCR in cord blood would suggest that at least in some cases, in utero transmission occurs. There is also a case report of one infant having been infected with an HCV strain different from all maternal strains at the time of delivery, suggesting in utero transmission. Conversely, PCR negative infants at birth may develop PCR positivity later in infancy, suggesting perinatal infection. One study found 50% of vaginal samples collected at 30 weeks' gestation from HCV-positive mothers to contain HCV, suggesting the possibility of infection by passage through the birth canal [11].

The potential risk of breast-feeding is not well defined. Two studies were unable to detect HCV in breast milk at any interval postpartum. However, there is one report of PCR detection of HCV in breast milk [11]. It may be wise to discourage breast-feeding until this issue is clarified.

b. **Clinical manifestations.** HCV accounts for 20 to 40% of viral hepatitis in the United States. The incubation period is 40 to 90 days after exposure and manifestations often present insidiously. Serum transaminase levels may fluctuate or remain chronically elevated for up to 1 year. Chronic disease may result in as many as 60% of community-acquired HCV infections. Cirrhosis may result in as many as 20% of chronic disease cases, but may be less likely in pediatric patients. Children can acquire HCV by transfusion or dialysis, in addition to vertical acquisition. At present it is impossible to estimate a rate of chronic carriage or progression to cirrhosis in infants with vertical infection.

c. **Diagnosis.** A second-generation ELISA detects antibodies to three proteins (c100-3, c22-3, and c33c) that are components of HCV. This test may be able to detect infection as early as 2 weeks after exposure. Another serologic assay with even greater sensitivity is the radioimmunoblot assay (RIBA), which detects antibodies to the three antigens detected by the ELISA and a fourth antigen, 5-5-1. Infants born to HCV-infected mothers will show evidence of passively acquired maternal antibody; therefore to determine infection in the infant, RNA PCR, which detects the viral genome itself, must be performed. This assay can detect viremia within 1 week of infection in adults. In adults, approximately 70% of samples with detectable antibody will also be positive by PCR. This is a curious finding in that a serologic response does not provide adequate protection. Persons who have had an acute infection that resolves will become antibody-negative.

d. **Treatment and prevention.** Because blood products were instrumental in transmitting HCV infection, they are now screened for antibody to HCV. Presence of the antibody likely also indicates presence of virus, and the unit is discarded. Before blood products were screened and before the recognition that viremia often accompanied antibody positivity, some had recommended the use of immune globulin for prophylaxis for individuals exposed to HCV. This concept had transcended to the infant of the HCV-infected mother. There is no benefit to immune globulin given to the exposed infant or to the needle stick recipient, as products containing antibody are excluded from the lot. For some persons with chronic HCV infection, alpha interferon, given for as long as a year, may clear the infection. Side effects of this therapy include fever and myalgias, and the risk-benefit ratio must be carefully weighed (see Chap. 26, Blood Products Used in the Newborn).

4. **HEV [6].** Enterically transmitted NANB viral hepatitis (HEV) is a single-stranded RNA virus that is similar to a calcivirus. It is primarily spread by fecal-contaminated water supplies. Epidemics have been documented in parts of Asia, Africa, and Mexico, and shellfish have been implicated as sources of infection. Incubation is 15 to 60 days. The clinical picture in infected individuals is similar to that of HAV infection, with fever, malaise, jaundice, abdominal pain, and arthralgia. HEV infection has an unusually high incidence of mortality in pregnant women. Treatment is supportive. The efficacy of immunoglobulin pro-

phylaxis against this form of hepatitis is unknown, but because the infection is not endemic in the United States, commercial preparations in the U.S. would not be expected to be helpful.

D. Enteroviruses [11]

1. The enteroviruses are RNA viruses belonging to the *Picornaviridae* family. They are classified into four major groups: coxsackieviruses group A, coxsackieviruses group B, echoviruses, and polioviruses. All four groups cause disease in the neonate. Infections occur throughout the year, with a peak incidence between July and November. The viruses are shed from the upper respiratory and gastrointestinal tracts. In most children and adults, infections are asymptomatic or produce a nonspecific febrile illness.

2. **Perinatal infection.** Most infections in newborns are caused by coxsackieviruses B and echoviruses. The mode of transmission appears to be primarily transplacental, although this is less well understood for echoviruses. Clinical manifestations are most commonly seen with transmission in the perinatal period.

   Symptoms in the newborn often appear within the first week postpartum. Clinical presentations vary from a mild nonspecific febrile illness to severe life-threatening disease. There are three major clinical presentations in neonates with enterovirus infections. Approximately 50% have meningoencephalitis, 25% have myocarditis, and 25% have a sepsis-like illness. The mortality (approximately 10%) is lowest for the group with meningoencephalitis. With myocarditis, there is a mortality of approximately 50%. The mortality from the sepsis-like illness is essentially 100%. The majority (70%) of severe enteroviral infections in neonates are caused by echovirus 11.

3. **Diagnosis.** The primary task in symptomatic enterovirus infections is differentiating between viral and bacterial sepsis and meningitis. In almost all cases, presumptive therapy for possible bacterial disease must be initiated. Obtaining a careful history of a recent maternal viral illness, as well as that of other family members, particularly young siblings, and especially during the summer and fall months, may be helpful. The principal diagnostic laboratory aid generally available at this time is viral culture. Material for cultures should be obtained from the nose, throat, stool, blood, urine, and CSF. Usually, evidence of viral growth can be detected within 1 week, although a longer time is required in some cases. PCR is also available.

4. **Treatment.** In general, treatment of symptomatic enteroviral disease in the newborn is supportive only. There are no specific antiviral agents known to be effective against enteroviruses. However, protection against severe neonatal disease appears to correlate with the presence of specific transplacentally derived antibody. Furthermore, the administration of immune serum globulin appears to be beneficial in patients with agammaglobulinemia who have chronic enteroviral infection. Given these observations, **it has been recommended that high-dose immune serum globulin be given to infants with severe, life-threatening enterovirus infections. It may also be beneficial to delay the time of delivery if acute maternal enteroviral infection is suspected, provided there are no maternal or fetal contraindications.** The clinical presentation in infants with a sepsis-like syndrome frequently evolves into shock, fulminant hepatitis with hepatocellular necrosis, and DIC. This expectation dictates close monitoring with early interventions for any signs of cardiovascular instability and coagulopathy. In the initial stages of treatment, broad-spectrum antibiotic therapy is indicated for possible bacterial sepsis. Later, with the recognition of progressive viral disease, some form of antibiotic prophylaxis to suppress intestinal flora may be helpful. Neomycin (25 mg/kg every 6 hours) has been recommended.

E. **Respiratory Syncytial Virus (RSV) [12]**
   Respiratory syncytial virus immunoglobulin for intravenous administration (RSV-IGIV) has been approved by the FDA for use in infants for the prevention of RSV-induced lower respiratory tract disease (e.g., bronchiolitis). RSV-IGIV has been shown to be ineffective in treating established RSV infection.
   RSV-IGIV is administered at a dose of 750 mg/kg intravenously over 4 hours each month during the RSV season (typically mid-November to March/April). RSV-IGIV is supplied in 2.5 g/50 ml vials and 1 g/20 cc vials.
   RSV-IGIV is licensed for administration to any infant or child under 2 years of age who has bronchopulmonary dysplasia or was born ≤35 weeks' gestational age. Because the drug supply is limited, its protection incomplete, and administration difficult, the American Academy of Pediatrics has made recommendations regarding which high-risk infants should receive RSV-IGIV [2].

Recommendations
Due to the difficulty of administration, the use of RSV-IGIV in prophylaxis should be limited to infants at *high risk for severe* RSV disease. Because infants are at low risk of encountering the virus within the NICU, use within the NICU will be restricted to infants whose discharge is imminent.

1. RSV-IGIV **is recommended** during the RSV season (November through April) in infants who:
   • Continue to require supplemental oxygen or diuretic therapy for chronic lung disease.
   • Have demonstrated severe chronic lung disease during their NICU stays (even though they may not still require medical therapy at the time of discharge). Risk factors to be considered include prolonged mechanical ventilation, protracted supplemental oxygen requirement, and tendency toward fluid overload.
2. RSV-IGIV **should be considered** in infants who:
   • Are premature (under 35 weeks) and potentially exposed during a NICU RSV outbreak. RSV is known to be transmitted in the hospital setting and to cause serious disease in high-risk infants. In high-risk hospitalized infants, the major means to prevent RSV disease is strict observance of infection control practices, including the use of rapid means to identify and cohort RSV-infected infants. If an RSV outbreak is documented in a high-risk unit (e.g., pediatric intensive care unit), primary emphasis should be placed on proper infection control practices. The need for and efficacy of RSV-IGIV prophylaxis in these situations has not been documented. Each unit should evaluate the risk to its exposed infants and decide on the need for treatment. If the patient stays hospitalized, this may only require one dose.
3. RSV-IGIV **may also be considered** for use in premature infants <32 weeks' gestation after consideration of additional factors, including:
   • Underlying conditions that predispose to respiratory complications
   • Number of young siblings in the home
   • Day care attendance
   • Exposure to tobacco smoke in the home or other care settings
   • Ease of intravenous access
   • Anticipated cardiac surgery
   • Practicality and tolerability of monthly infusions
   • Distance to and availability of hospital care for severe respiratory illness
4. RSV-IGIV **is not recommended** for:
   • Healthy prematures >32 weeks' gestation
   • Children with cystic fibrosis
   • Term infants following treatment for persistent pulmonary hypertension of the newborn

5. RSV-IGIV **is** **not** **FDA approved** for patients with congenital heart disease (CHD). Available data indicated that RSV-IGIV should not be used in those with cyanotic CHD. However, patients with BPD and/or prematurity who meet the criteria in recommendations 1 and 2 and who also have asymptomatic acyanotic CHD (e.g., patent ductus arteriosus or ventricular septal defect) may benefit from prophylaxis.

Procedure for RSV-IGIV Administration:
1. Check that the patient meets the criteria above.
2. Discuss the option of Respigam therapy with the patient's parents. If parents are opposed to taking the patient for subsequent monthly outpatient infusions, there may be little benefit to initiating therapy in the NICU. Document the discussion about the use of this product in the medical record.
3. Once IV is placed, order 15 cc/kg (<750 mg/kg) Respigam to be administered as follows:

Time (min)	Rate (cc/kg/hr)
0–15*	1.5
15–30*	3
30 to end	6

*Check HR, RR, BP, temperature at 0, 15, 30, 60, 120, and 180 minutes.
Please note: Respigam requires no filtration.
If fluid overload is a concern, this infusion may be slowed to occur over 4–6 hours. Consider administration of furosemide.

(Please see pages 299–300 for list of references.)

Bacterial and Fungal Infections
Nicholas G. Guerina

I. Bacterial Sepsis and Meningitis
A. Introduction. Bacterial sepsis and meningitis continue to be major causes of morbidity and mortality in the newborn. This is despite improvements in antimicrobial therapy, advances in neonatal life support measures, and the prompt recognition of perinatal risk factors for infection. Sepsis neonatorum can be devastating and surviving infants can have significant neurologic sequelae as a consequence of CNS involvement, septic shock, or hypoxemia secondary to severe parenchymal lung disease or persistent pulmonary hypertension.
B. Epidemiology. The overall incidence of neonatal sepsis varies between 1 and 8 cases per 1000 live births. Approximately one-third of septic newborns develop meningitis. Multiple risk factors for perinatal infection have been identified. Generally these factors can be divided between maternal (obstetric) and neonatal factors.
    1. Maternal risk factors. Obstetric factors include premature onset of labor, premature rupture of membranes (PROM), and maternal peripartum infection. The extent to which these factors increase the likelihood of newborn disease is best illustrated by studies in pregnant women with vaginal colonization with group B beta-hemolytic streptococci (GBS). The attack rate for perinatally acquired sepsis in newborns of GBS-colonized women is 1 to 2%, but this rate increases to 15.2% with premature onset of labor (<37 weeks), 10.7% for chorioamnionitis or PROM of more than 24 hours, and 9.7% for maternal postpartum bacteremia [3]. Overt chorioamnionitis or maternal sepsis are relatively uncommon, so the only maternal indicator of intrauterine infection,

aside from preterm labor, may be intrapartum fever. Boyer et al. (see Table 23-3) studied attack rates as a function of peak intrapartum temperature, and length of rupture of membranes, for GBS disease in 32,384 newborns. Their findings are summarized in Table 23-3, along with the attack rates by infant birth weight. The attack rate for neonatal infection increased by more than 10-fold when membranes were ruptured for 24 hours or longer, although the rate started to increase by 18 hours. There was a fourfold increase in attack rate when the peak maternal intrapartum temperature reached 37.5°C and a 10-fold increase for temperatures 38°C or higher.

a. Preterm labor. Although there are many noninfectious causes of preterm labor, the possibility of evolving bacterial disease must always be considered. In the absence of fetal distress, signs or symptoms of chorioamnionitis, or any other developing maternal condition that is hazardous to the fetus or mother, it is often preferred to arrest labor with tocolysis. This is particularly true in early-third-trimester pregnancies, where the high morbidity and mortality of very-low-birth-weight infants obviate against delivery. Alternatively, delivery may be the best option for older fetuses, especially if there are maternal complications (e.g., pregnancy-induced hypertension, toxemia), or the fetal status is uncertain (e.g., decelerations, decreased fetal movement).

(1) Antenatal steroids. One of the common issues in the management of preterm labor is the use of steroids to induce fetal lung maturation. In the presence of intact membranes, steroids can decrease the incidence of respiratory distress syndrome (RDS) in preterm newborns (see Chap. 24, Respiratory Distress Syndrome/Hyaline Membrane Disease). One argument against the use of steroids is the possibility of masking intrauterine infections, but there are few data to support this concept in the setting of intact membranes.

Table 23-3. Attack rates for perinatally acquired group B streptococcal infections in newborn infants

Risk factor	Attack rate (cases/1000 live births)	Death rate of infected infants (%)
Birth weight (gm)		
<1000	26	90
1001–1500	8	25
1501–2000	9	29
2001–2500	4	33
>2500	1	3
Rupture of membranes (hr)		
<6	0.8	33
7–12	1.9	10
13–18	1.5	40
19–24	5.7	27
25–48	8.6	18
>48	10.8	33
Peak intrapartum temperature (°C)		
<37.5	1.5	29
>37.5	6.5	17

Source: From Boyer et al. (*J. Infect. Dis.* 148:795, 1983 and *J. Infect. Dis.* 148:802, 1983); data for 32,384 newborn infants.

b. PROM. This frequently complicates preterm labor by increasing the risk for sepsis. All of the issues discussed for preterm labor apply, only now the increased risk for infection may tip the scales toward early delivery. In the setting of PROM, the use of steroids to facilitate fetal lung maturation is controversial; the incidence of RDS may be decreased with PROM of more than 24 hours, and steroids may complicate the assessment of intrauterine infection. Nonetheless, the potential benefit of antenatal steroid therapy is often thought to outweigh any concerns for their use in the setting of PROM (see Chap. 24).

2. Neonatal risk factors. The single most important neonatal risk factor is low birth weight. The overall rate of sepsis reportedly is eight times higher in 1000- to 1500-gm than 2000- to 2500-gm infants, and meningitis occurs 3 to 17 times more often in infants weighing less than 2500 gm than those weighing 2500 gm or more. In the study of Boyer et al. (see Table 23-3), the attack rate for GBS sepsis was 26 times higher in infants weighing less than 1000 gm than in those weighing more than 2500 gm. Considering low birth weight and maternal risk factors, an attack rate of 7.6 per 1000 and a mortality rate of 33% for GBS-infected infants were observed for the combined risk factors of birth weight lower than 2500 gm, ruptured membranes for more than 18 hours, and intrapartum maternal temperature higher than 37.5°C [7,11]. By comparison, infants without these risk factors had an attack rate of 0.6 per 1000, and a mortality rate in infected infants of 6%. Other perinatal risk factors have been recognized, particularly for neonatal GBS infections (Table 23-4).

C. Microbiology and pathogenesis. Although a variety of bacteria have been isolated from newborns with sepsis, the principal etiologic agent in the United States is GBS. Other bacteria less commonly associated with neonatal sepsis are gram-negative enteric rods, especially *Escherichia coli*; other gram-positive bacteria including *Listeria monocytogenes* and enterococcus; and nontypeable *Haemophilus influenzae*.

1. GBS [1,3,9,11]. GBS is the most common cause of neonatal sepsis and meningitis in the United States. Infection most commonly occurs during the first few days of life (early-onset disease), with a mean age at onset of 20 hours. This form of the disease has an incidence of 2 to 4 per 1000 births. An epidemiologically distinct form of the disease occurs after the first week of life (mean onset, 24 days). This form, referred to as late-onset disease, has an incidence of 1 to 2 per 1000 births.

Table 23-4. Risk factors for early-onset neonatal group B streptococcal (GBS) infection[a]

Intrapartum maternal fever of ≥38°C (100.4°F)

Rupture of membranes ≥18 hours[b]

Mother with a previous infant with GBS infection

Preterm labor (<37 weeks)

Premature rupture (<37 weeks) of membranes for any duration

Multiple gestation[c]

Maternal GBS bacteriuria

---

[a]Intrapartum antibiotics should be started for women presenting with one or more of these risk factors who are colonized with GBS or for whom the GBS status is unknown.
[b]It may be beneficial to start antibiotics if membranes are ruptured for 12 hours and labor is likely to progress to ≥18 hours.
[c]This "risk factor" is controversial; it is considered in the American Academy of Pediatrics guidelines (*Pediatrics* 90:775, 1992) but rejected by the American College of Obstetrics and Gynecology (ACOG Technical Bulletin No. 170, Washington, D.C., 1992).

a. **Microbiology.** At least five capsular serotypes of GBS have been identified (types I through V). These serotypes can be further divided into subclasses based on serologically distinct polysaccharide and protein antigens isolated from capsular and cell wall extracts. All serotypes can cause vaginal colonization and neonatal disease, but the distribution of serotypes isolated from infected neonates depends on the site of infection and the age at onset of disease. Nearly equal distribution of serotypes occurs among newborns with early-onset sepsis, but 85 to 90% of strains isolated from infants with early-onset meningitis, or late-onset disease, have type III capsules.

b. **Pathogenesis and host susceptibility.** Approximately 15 to 20% of women in the United States have vaginal colonization with GBS. Early-onset disease requires exposure to GBS colonizing the vagina, either from infected amniotic fluid or from swallowed inoculum during transit through the vaginal canal. Alternatively, late-onset disease can occur from maternally or nosocomially acquired organisms. Many studies have been designed to elucidate both host and bacterial factors critical for infection. One of the most significant findings is the correlation between the level of maternally derived capsular antibody, and susceptibility of the neonate to infection. Although this finding is best demonstrated for disease caused by serotype III, it may also be important for other serotypes, particularly serotype II. Other factors that may contribute to host susceptibility include deficiencies in the alternative and classic complement pathways, and neutrophil dysfunction.

2. **Escherichia coli K1 (ECK1).** *E. coli* had been recognized as the second most prevalent cause of neonatal sepsis and meningitis in previous decades, but the current incidence may be less than the previous estimates of 1 to 2 per 1000 births. The majority of *E. coli* infections are caused by strains possessing the K1 polysaccharide capsule.

a. **Pathogenicity and host susceptibility.** As for GBS disease, attempts have been made to identify host and bacterial factors associated with ECK1 infections. ECK1 poorly activates the classic complement pathway, so protection depends on antibody-mediated activation of the alternative pathway. Unfortunately, the K1 capsule is a poor immunogen, so virtually no maternally derived antibody is available for the neonate. Other bacterial components may contribute to the virulence of ECK1, including the O antigen serotype, hemolysin production, presence of the ColV plasmid, and expression of different classes of filamentous protein structures known as pili.

3. **Listeria monocytogenes.** It is difficult to know the true incidence of neonatal listeriosis, but recent active surveillance in the United States indicates a rate of 13 per 100,000 live births [11]. In addition, *Listeria* organisms may also be a significant cause of stillbirths and spontaneous abortions. Major epidemics occur, usually associated with contaminated food products. Three major populations are affected in these epidemics: (1) immunosuppressed patients (e.g., renal transplant recipients), (2) pregnant women, and (3) neonates (plus fetuses). As in GBS infections, there is both an early-onset (mean age between 1 and 2 days) and a late-onset (mean age approximately 14 days) form of the disease.

a. **Pathogenesis and host susceptibility.** Several cellular components of *Listeria* have been isolated and characterized, and some of the effects of these structures on the host immune system have been elucidated in vitro and in experimental animal models. Alternatively, immunocompromised or *Listeria*-sensitive hosts may have defects in their immune system allowing *Listeria* organisms to grow unchecked in the host tissues. The specific immune defects or deficiencies critical to *Listeria* infections in pregnant women and neonates are not completely defined. Both cell-mediated and humoral immunity appear to play roles in resistance to listeriosis [5,11]. In vitro and in vivo (animal models) studies suggest that cell-mediated immunity may be altered in pregnancy, and the newborn may have a defect in macrophage–T-cell interaction. Another important aspect of infection in pregnancy relates to the remarkable tropism of *Listeria* organisms for the placenta. Studies in an animal model demonstrated that *Listeria* species can grow to high density in the decidua basalis of the placenta, and in the fetal chorioallantoic plate. This uncontrolled growth can result in spontaneous abortion, stillbirths, or newborn infections by direct spread of *Listeria* to the fetus.

4. **Other bacterial pathogens.** A variety of other bacteria have been isolated from neonates with sepsis. Of these, nontypeable *H. influenzae* and **enterococci** have received increasing attention recently. Infection with nontypeable *H. influenzae* usually occurs in utero or in the immediate postpartum period. Mortality is high; the overall mortality rate is 55%, and can be as high as 90% for newborns of less than 30 weeks' gestation. Enterococcal sepsis and meningitis may have either an early-onset or a late-onset presentation. *Citrobacter diversus* is an uncommon neonatal pathogen that deserves mention. It may be isolated as part of the adult intestinal flora and can be vertically transmitted intrapartum from colonized mothers or by nosocomial spread. Although invasive neonatal disease is uncommon, it is often accompanied by meningitis, and up to three-fourths of infants with meningitis develop brain abscess.

5. **Nosocomial infections.** Nosocomial bacterial infections are significant problems for the neonate requiring extended care in the special care nursery. This is particularly true for very-low-birth-weight infants. The overall incidence of nosocomial infections in neonates is less than 5%, but infection rates for individual nurseries have been much higher [6]. Beyond the first 1 to 2 weeks of life, the neonate who has remained in the special care nursery is likely to be colonized with perinatally (endogenous) and nosocomially acquired flora. This places the neonate at risk of infection due to coagulase-negative staphylococci; enterococci; *Staphylococcus aureus,* including methicillin-resistant strains; and gram-negative bacteria, including multiply resistant enteric strains. In addition, late-onset disease caused by GBS and *Listeria* organisms must be considered. The most frequently identified factors contributing to nosocomial infections are postnatal age (length of stay in nursery), low birth weight, foreign bodies (e.g., intravascular catheters, chest tubes, endotracheal tubes), nursery crowding, surgery, and prolonged treatment with broad-spectrum antibiotics. Strict isolation procedures should be enforced for all infants colonized or infected with multiply resistant bacteria.

a. **Coagulase-negative staphylococcus.** This organism has been recognized as an important cause of nosocomial bacteremia in the neonate in recent years. It is unclear whether there has actually been an increase in the incidence of coagulase-negative staphylococcal bacteremia, or the realization that positive blood cultures represent true infection, not culture contamination. This may be influenced, in part, by the changing population of the neonatal intensive care unit (NICU) with an increase in the proportion of very-low-birth-weight infants. Coagulase-negative staphylococci account for more than 50% of bacteremia in the NICU. Generally, many strains (40 to 80%) are methicillin-resistant. Central venous lines and intralipid infusions are significant risk factors for coagulase-negative staphylococcal infections.

D. **Clinical signs of infection** [5,7,11]. Infection in the newborn may present with nonspecific, often subtle clinical findings. **Respiratory distress** is the most common symptom, occurring in up to 90% of infants with sepsis. The clinical presentation may vary from apnea, mild tachypnea, or a slight increase in oxygen requirement, to severe RDS requiring mechanical ventilation.

Gastrointestinal symptoms in septic infants include vomiting, diarrhea, abdominal distention, ileus, and poor feeding. Sepsis should also be considered in infants with **temperature instability.** The normal neonatal isothermic temperature range is 97°F (36°C) to 99.6°F (37°C). Single temperature values outside the isothermic range are unlikely to be associated with infection, but sepsis should always be considered when abnormal temperatures are sustained over 1 hour. When temperature instability accompanies sepsis, hypothermia is more common in infected preterm infants while fever is more common in term infants. Other clinical findings that should raise the suspicion of sepsis include **hypotension, metabolis acidosic, hyperglycemia, poor feeding, diminished activity or lethargy, seizures, and petechiae or purpura.**

Other causes of the symptoms found in sepsis are transient tachypnea, meconium aspiration, intracranial hemorrhage, drug withdrawal, coarctation of the aorta, cardiac disease, inborn errors of metabolism, bowel perforation, necrotizing enterocolitis, and nonbacterial (viral) sepsis.

E. **Laboratory studies.** No single laboratory test has been found to have acceptable specificity and sensitivity for predicting infection. Therefore, the results of laboratory studies must be assessed in conjunction with the presence of risk factors and clinical signs of sepsis.

1. **Total neutrophil count and immature to total neutrophil ratio.** A total WBC count of less than 5000 per microliter, a total neutrophil count of less than 1000 per microliter, or an immature (band) to total neutrophil ratio of higher than 0.2 have been correlated with an increased risk of bacterial infection. Unfortunately, the positive predictive value of an abnormal WBC count is poor. This is not surprising since many noninfectious conditions can be associated with an abnormal neonatal WBC count. These include maternal fever, difficult or prolonged labor, extended administration of intrapartum oxytocin, neonatal asphyxia, meconium aspiration, pneumothorax, seizures, intraventricular hemorrhage, and hemolytic disease (all associated with neutrophilia and elevated immature to total neutrophil ratio), and maternal toxemia (associated with neutropenia). Thus, the initial WBC with differential cell count may not be helpful in the decision to initiate antibiotic therapy for an asymptomatic newborn infant with identified risk factors for sepsis. Nevertheless, it is common practice to perform these tests as part of the immediate postnatal assessment of the "at-risk" infant. In infants suspected of being infected, a repeat WBC and differential cell count at 8 to 12 hours may have considerably greater predictive value, but the usefulness of repeated tests in term infants who remain asymptomatic is not known.

2. **Cultures.** Cultures are critical in the diagnosis and treatment of bacterial infections. Blood for culture should be obtained from a peripheral site thoroughly cleansed with an antiseptic agent. No less than 0.5 ml of blood per bottle should be cultured. Two blood cultures will increase the yield of positive results. CSF samples should be plated promptly to avoid loss of viability of organisms due to changes in fluid pH. Urine culture has little value in the immediate perinatal period, but may be very important for late-onset neonatal sepsis (over 7 days of age).

3. **Chest x-ray studies.** Infants with respiratory distress should have a chest x-ray to assess lung parenchyma as well as the cardiothymic silhouette. Focal parenchymal lung findings in the first hours of life may simply reflect retained fetal lung fluid or atelectasis which usually resolves within 48 hours. Although uncommon, persistent focal changes consistent with an infiltrative process may require extended antibiotic therapy for possible pneumonia (typically 7 to 10 days).

With GBS sepsis chest x-ray findings and respiratory symptoms may be identical to those of surfactant deficiency (hyaline membrane disease).

4. **Erythrocyte sedimentation rate (ESR), C-reactive protein (CRP) concentration, and haptoglobin.** The sensitivity and specificity of each of these parameters do not justify their measurement in the newborn; however, they may be useful when used in conjunction with each other and the WBC and differential cell count. Philip et al. used a five-part screen to evaluate infants. The abnormal test results indicative of infection were (1) total WBC count of less than 5000 per microliter, (2) bandneutrophil ratio of 0.2 or higher, (3) positive CRP, (4) elevated haptoglobin level, and (5) ESR of 15 mm or more for the first hour. If results of all five tests were normal, the probability that infection was absent was 99%. If three of the five tests were abnormal, the probability of infection was 90% [7].

5. **Gram stain of gastric aspirate.** This assay has a low positive predictive value. Generally, if there are more than 5 neutrophils per high-power field or a large number of bacteria, particularly gram-positive cocci in clumps and chains, the result is positive. The low specificity of the test is not surprising since a positive aspirate reflects an infected intrauterine environment, not a fetal inflammatory response. Thus, stain of the gastric aspirate may add little to what is already known from clinical information. In addition, the inhomogeneity of gastric aspirates may lead to sampling errors.

6. **Antigen detection methods.** Latex particle agglutination (LPA) assays are available for both GBS and ECK1. These tests may complement other laboratory tests, particularly in the setting of antenatal maternal treatment with antibiotics, or parenchymal lung disease with negative blood cultures. The most widely used test is the urine GBS LPA assay. Although this is a sensitive test, specificity problems limit its usefulness; false-positive findings may result from mucocutaneous colonization in the absence of systemic infection. Thus the significance of a positive urine test in a culture-negative asymptomatic infant is uncertain and may simply represent a false-positive result. Countercurrent immunoelectrophoresis (CIE) is generally more specific but less sensitive than LPA.

7. **Lumbar puncture.** Examination of the CSF is necessary when meningitis is suspected, but CNS infection is uncommon in infants who have no clinical signs of sepsis. Thus it is unclear whether **asymptomatic** infants who have risk factors for sepsis need to have a lumbar puncture. This is particularly true for term asymptomatic infants who have a negative blood culture. Since intrapartum antibiotics are likely to diminish the risk for fetal/newborn infection, it may be possible to defer the lumbar puncture for well "pretreated" infants with no abnormal clinical or laboratory findings.

The presence of meningitis must be considered in **symptomatic** infants at risk for sepsis, but these infants most commonly have respiratory distress which may be severe enough to require that the lumbar puncture be deferred. Obtaining CSF studies prior to antibiotic treatment is preferable, when possible, because cultures are unreliable while antibiotics are being administered, and interpretation of the cell count may be limited if the lumbar puncture is "traumatic" or there is a coexisting subarachnoid or intraventricular hemorrhage. In addition, a small percentage of infants may have meningitis with normal CSF cell counts and chemistries. (See **I.G.3.**)

F. **Evaluation and treatment—antenatal.** Evaluation and treatment of neonatal sepsis commonly begins in utero, especially in the presence of established obstetric risk factors for infection. It is clear that the fetus at very high risk for infection should be delivered. However, the true risk of in utero bacterial infection is often difficult to assess, and the risk of other intrapartum or postnatal complications to the preterm infant must be considered. Antenatal/intrapartum administration of antibiotics to the pregnant woman should always be considered when there is increased risk for fetal infection.

1. **Obstetric management strategies to decrease the risk of early-onset neonatal GBS infection** [1,3,4]. Early-onset GBS infection is the most common and best studied neonatal infection: Clinical and laboratory research over the past two decades has contributed greatly to the understanding of pathogenesis and possible mechanisms of prevention. Current preventive strategies focus on (1) the development of polysaccharide vaccines for maternal immunization, and (2) the use of selective intrapartum chemoprophylaxis. Vaccine development is in the early experimental stages for most serotypes but clinical trials have begun for a monovalent vaccine composed of purified type III polysaccharide. Ultimately it is hoped that an effective polyvalent vaccine will be produced and significantly reduce the incidence of neonatal GBS infections.

Selective intrapartum chemoprophylaxis, using an antibiotic active against GBS, was tested in a number of studies, most of which demonstrated a reduction in the incidence of neonatal infection. Only a few of these studies, however, had an appropriate study design and statistical power to demonstrate efficacy. Furthermore, no study has tested all of the risk factors thought to be significant for early-onset GBS disease. Boyer et al. studied the prevention of GBS disease in neonates by selective intrapartum and postpartum chemoprophylaxis. Their experimental design and results are shown in Table 23-5. All infants received postnatal antibiotics, including those born to treated mothers (each received 4 doses of ampicillin). **Intrapartum ampicillin, followed by limited postpartum treatment of the newborn, effectively prevented early-onset GBS disease in colonized mothers presenting with either preterm labor (<37 weeks) or PROM of longer than 12 hours.**

Table 23-5. Experimental design and results of selective intrapartum and postpartum antibiotic therapy for the prevention of neonatal GBS disease

EXPERIMENTAL DESIGN
1. Maternal vaginal and rectal materials for cultures were obtained at 26 to 28 weeks' gestation.
2. Women with positive cultures for GBS who presented with preterm labor (<37 weeks) or premature rupture of membranes of >12 hours were started on ampicillin 2 gm IV followed by 1 gm q4h until delivery.
3. Newborns in the control groups only received antibiotic therapy postpartum.
4. Both randomized and nonrandomized groups were followed.
5. All septic infants received ampicillin and aminoglycoside therapy.
6. Asymptomatic infants born to ampicillin-treated mothers received 4 doses of ampicillin 50 mg/kg IV q12h.

RESULTS

| Randomization | Rate of early-onset GBS disease | |
	Ampicillin	Control
Yes	0/85	5/79
No	0/235	15/1426
Total	0/320	20/1505*

*Attack rate = 13.4/1000 live births.
Source: From K. M. Boyer et al., *N. Engl. J. Med.* 314:1665, 1986.

a. The American College of Obstetrics and Gynecologists (ACOG) and the Centers for Disease Control (CDC) published recommendations for the prevention of early-onset GBS infections in the neonate [1,3]. "Enhanced communication among personnel in multiple disciplines is needed to ensure that programs for prevention of GBS disease succeed. Open communication between clinicians and patients is a critical component of GBS disease prevention. An informational brochure for pregnant women on GBS is available through the CDC (Childhood and Respiratory Diseases Branch, Division of Bacterial and Mycotic Diseases, National Center for Infectious Diseases, Mailstop CO9, Atlanta, GA 30333; Internet address: http://www.cdc.gov/ncidid/diseases/bacter/ strep_b.htm.) The following recommendations for the prevention of GBS disease will need periodic reappraisal to incorporate advances in technology or other refinements in prevention strategies.

(1) Obstetric care practitioners, in conjunction with supporting laboratories and labor and delivery facilities, should adopt a strategy for the prevention of early-onset GBS disease. Patients should be informed regarding the GBS prevention strategy.

(2) Regardless of which prevention strategy is used, women with symptomatic or asymptomatic GBS bacteriuria detected during pregnancy should be treated at the time of diagnosis. Because such women are usually heavily colonized with GBS, they should also receive intrapartum chemoprophylaxis. Women who previously gave birth to an infant with GBS disease should receive intrapartum chemoprophylaxis; prenatal screening is not necessary for these women.

(3) Until further data become available to define the most effective strategy, the following two approaches are appropriate:

(a) Screening-based approach. All pregnant women should be screened at 35 to 37 weeks' gestation for anogenital GBS colonization (Fig. 23-1). Patients should be informed of screening results and of potential benefits and risks of intrapartum antimicrobial prophylaxis for GBS carriers. Information systems should be developed and monitored to ensure that prenatal culture results are available at the time and place of delivery. Intrapartum chemoprophylaxis should be offered to all pregnant women identified as GBS carriers by culture at 35 to 37 weeks' gestation.

(i) If the result of GBS culture is not known at the time of labor, intrapartum antimicrobial prophylaxis should be administered if one of the following risk factors is present: gestation less than 37 weeks, duration of membrane rupture 18 hours or longer, or temperature of 100.4°F (38.0°C) or higher.

(ii) Culture techniques that maximize the likelihood of GBS recovery should be used. These are described in reference 3.

(iii) Oral antimicrobial agents should not be used to treat women who are found to be colonized with GBS during prenatal screening. Such treatment is not effective in eliminating carriage or preventing neonatal disease.

(b) Risk-factor approach. A prophylaxis strategy based on the presence of intrapartum risk factors alone (e.g., gestation shorter than 37 weeks, duration of membrane rupture 18 hours or longer, or temperature ≥100.4°F [≥38.0°C]) is an acceptable alternative (Fig. 23-2).

For intrapartum chemoprophylaxis, intravenous penicillin G (5 mU initially and then 2.5 mU every 4 hours) should be administered

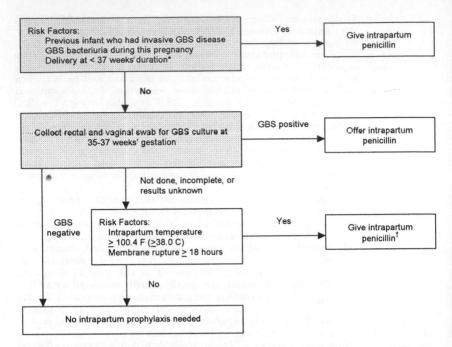

Fig. 23-1. Algorithm for prevention of early-onset group B streptococcal (GBS) disease in neonates using prenatal screening at 35–37 weeks' gestation. *If membranes ruptured at <37 weeks' gestation and the mother has not begun labor, collect group B streptococcal culture and either (a) administer antibiotics until cultures are completed and the results are negative or (b) begin antibiotics only when positive cultures are obtained. No prophylaxis is needed if the culture obtained at 35–37 weeks' gestation was negative.†Broader spectrum antibiotics may be considered at the physician's discretion, based on clinical indications [3].

until delivery (Table 23-6). Intravenous ampicillin (2 gm initially and then 1 gm every 4 hours until delivery) is an acceptable alternative to penicillin G, but penicillin G is preferred because it has a narrow spectrum and thus is less likely to select for antibiotic-resistant organisms. Clindamycin or erythromycin may be used for women allergic to penicillin, although the efficacy of these drugs for GBS disease prevention has not been measured in controlled trials. (Note: Penicillin G does not need to be administered to women who have the clinical diagnosis of amnionitis and who are receiving other treatment regimens that include agents active against streptococci [e.g., ampicillin or clindamycin].)

(c) **Infants without clinical symptoms born to mothers treated at least 4 hours prior to delivery need not necessarily be treated.** By following these guidelines it is hoped that 50 to 75 percent of early-onset GBS infections may be prevented. Failures of this approach are likely to occur for the following reasons:

(i) Early-onset GBS infection can occur in the absence of risk factors.

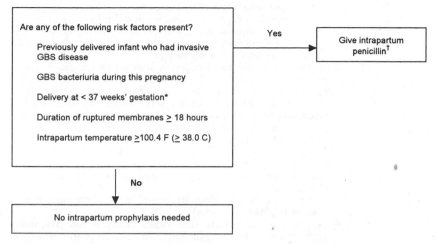

Fig. 23-2. Algorithm for prevention of early-onset group B streptococcal (GBS) disease in neonates using risk factors. *If membranes ruptured at <37 weeks' gestation and the mother has not begun labor, collect GBS culture and either (a) administer antibiotics until cultures are completed and results are negative or (b) begin antibiotics only when positive cultures are obtained. No prophylaxis is needed if culture obtained at 35–37 weeks' gestation was negative. †Broader spectrum antibiotics may be considered at the physician's discretion, based on clinical indications, e.g., if chorioamnionitis is suspected, ampicillin and gentamicin are used [3].

      (ii) The screening culture may give false-negative results for some colonized women.
      (iii) Some women who were not colonized at 26 to 28 weeks may become colonized by delivery.
      (iv) Intrapartum chemoprophylaxis is unlikely to be 100 percent effective.
      Investigations designed to evaluate and compare the two strategies described and others are needed. Such studies will require the participation of multiple institutions and should evaluate multiple outcomes (e.g.,

Table 23-6. Recommended regimens for intrapartum antimicrobial prophylaxis for perinatal group B streptococcal disease

Recommended	Penicillin G, 5 mU IV load, then 2.5 mU every 4 hours until delivery
Alternative	Ampicillin, 2 gm IV load, then 1 gm IV every 4 hours until delivery
If penicillin-allergic Recommended	Clindamycin, 900 mg IV every 8 hours until delivery
Alternative	Erythromycin, 500 mg IV every 6 hours until delivery

Note: If the patient is receiving treatment for amnionitis with an antimicrobial agent active against group B streptococci (e.g., ampicillin, penicillin, clindamycin, or erythromycin), additional prophylactic antibiotics are not needed [3].

perinatal GBS infections, adverse reactions to antimicrobial prophylaxis, and perinatal infections caused by penicillin-resistant organisms). Characterization of protocol failures may contribute to improvement of future prevention strategies.

b. Even if maternal GBS colonization is known to be negative, intrapartum antibiotics may be indicated because infection can be caused by other bacterial pathogens. Broad-spectrum antibiotics should be given to women with intrapartum fever (especially if ≥38°C) or other signs of chorioamnionitis (e.g., elevated maternal WBC count, uterine tenderness). Antibiotics should also be considered if there is unexplained fetal distress (e.g., sustained fetal tachycardia), especially in the presence of other intrapartum risk factors. The choice of antibiotics is based on the likely non-GBS pathogens that may be present, and should include ampicillin and either an aminoglycoside or cephalosporin.

c. Duration of maternal antibiotic treatment for preterm labor before 37 weeks or PROM (>18 hours)

(1) For women known to be GBS vaginal culture–negative, intrapartum antibiotics (broad-spectrum, e.g., ampicillin and gentamicin) should be given if there are clinical findings suggesting maternal or fetal infection (e.g., maternal fever, other indicators for evolving maternal chorioamnionitis, sustained fetal tachycardia).

(2) For women who are GBS-positive or the status is unknown, if delivery is imminent, intrapartum antibiotics for GBS prophylaxis should be given until the infant is delivered. If delivery is delayed (e.g., successful tocolysis), there are no other clinical indicators for maternal or fetal infection, and membranes are intact, antibiotics can be discontinued. If labor does not progress but membranes are ruptured, the duration of antibiotic prophylaxis is less clear. One possible approach is to perform a lower vaginal/rectal culture for GBS and if this is negative and there are no signs of maternal or fetal infection, antibiotics can be discontinued. If the GBS screening result is positive but there are no other signs for infection, antibiotics can be discontinued after 1 week.

G. Evaluation and treatment—postnatal. The evaluation and treatment of the newborn at risk for bacterial disease vary with clinical presentation. Asymptomatic infants, or infants with minimal distress (e.g., mild, transient tachypnea without an oxygen requirement), may only require routine newborn care. At the opposite end of the spectrum are critically ill infants with symptoms that are indistinguishable from sepsis (e.g., severe respiratory distress, persistent pulmonary hypertension, shock). These infants require immediate antibiotic therapy and can challenge the limits of neonatal life support.

1. Assessment of the SYMPTOMATIC newborn. (See I.D.) The clinical signs and symptoms of sepsis in the newborn can be very nonspecific, and infection must be considered in virtually all infants with neonatal distress. This is particularly true with respiratory distress. Meconium aspiration pneumonitis, RDS, birth asphyxia, persistent pulmonary hypertension (primary or secondary to meconium aspiration or asphyxia), and apnea may be indistinguishable from sepsis. A **low Apgar score (<5 at 1 minute)** may also be due to sepsis, especially when there are other risk factors for infection and there is no alternative explanation for the initial depressed activity (e.g., documented umbilical cord compression, shoulder dystocia, maternal intrapartum narcotic administration). Accordingly, a CBC count should be performed, blood drawn for culture, and antibiotic therapy initiated for the symptomatic newborn. Meningitis must also be considered, but the clinical status of the ill neonate often requires that a lumbar puncture be deferred. This should be done as soon as the infant is stable and before antibiotics are stopped. Latex agglutination tests may aid in the diagnosis of GBS and ECK1 infections, especially if intrapartum antibiotics have been administered.

2. **Assessment of the ASYMPTOMATIC newborn who has risk factors for sepsis.** The incidence of infection in **asymptomatic** newborns is low, even if intrapartum risk factors are present. Nevertheless, these infants remain at risk for developing sepsis either from bacteremia present at birth or from bloodstream invasion by bacteria colonizing mucosal surfaces after delivery. Unfortunately, there is no reliable test to predict which infant might develop bacterial sepsis. Even more important, there is no test that can be done in the first hours of life that can predict that an infant is not septic and will not get septic. The pressure of early discharge of infants from the hospital makes it more difficult to screen out infants who will be septic. Over the years we have struggled with this, trying not to be unnecessarily invasive yet not wanting to miss any septic infants. Treating all at-risk but asymptomatic infants with antibiotics for 48 hours (see Table 23-5) may have some impact on early-onset bacterial infections, but the efficacy of this aggressive approach is unknown. In addition, the use of selective intrapartum antibiotic prophylaxis is likely to decrease the incidence of early-onset bacterial infection, making the need for postnatal therapy even more questionable.

For infants with risk factors with no abnormal clinical findings, Tables 23-3 to 23-8 provide information regarding risk factors and the approach to evaluation and treatment. For infants with one major and two minor risk factors, a CBC count and a blood culture should be performed.

The CBC count lacks sensitivity and specificity for infection, but particularly concerning values are WBC counts of 5000 or lower, or immature-total neutrophil ratios (the percent bands divided by the sum of the percent bands plus segmented neutrophils) higher than 0.2. A clustering of several major and minor risk factors should lead to a CBC count, culture of blood and CSF, and immediate antibiotic therapy.

Table 23-7. Risk factors for neonatal sepsis*

Major risk factors	Minor risk factors
Rupture of membranes >24 hours	Rupture of membranes >12 hours
Maternal intrapartum fever >100.4°F/38°C	Maternal intrapartum fever >99.5°F/37.5°C
Chorioamnionitis	Maternal WBC count >15,000/μl
Sustained fetal heart rate >160	Low Apgar score (<5 at 1 min, <7 at 5 min)
	Low birth weight (<1500 gm)
	Preterm labor (<37 weeks)
	Multiple gestation (see comment Table 23-4)
	Foul lochia
	Maternal GBS colonization (see Table 23-4)

*Infants with one major or two minor risk factors should have a CBC count and a blood culture. (See **I.G**)

The asymptomatic infant who has one major factor or two minor risk factors and who has a WBC count below 5000 and an immature-total neutrophil ratio higher than 0.2 should be treated with antibiotics. If the CBC count is a cause to initiate treatment, a second blood sample should be drawn for culture when treatment is started. For infants who are not treated but about whom the clinician is concerned, monitoring vital signs every 4 hours and repeating a CBC count at 12 hours of life may be helpful.

Our general approach is outlined in Table 23-8. Evaluation of the mother 12 to 24 hours postpartum may be helpful (is she sick? is she on antibiotics?).

Antibiotics for rule out (R/O) of sepsis are ampicillin 150 mg/kg IV q12h and gentamicin 2.5 mg/kg IV q12–24h (interval adjusted for gestational age).

3. **Lumbar puncture.** We have struggled about the need to perform lumbar punctures on asymptomatic infants who have risk factors for sepsis. We are aware of the reports of positive CSF cultures in infants who have negative blood cultures, but this has not been our experience in a large neonatal service (14,000 deliveries per year). It is not clear from these reports that the infants were asymptomatic. We have used the following policy for the past 5 years without problems. Once the decision has been made to initiate antibiotic therapy, it has been general practice to perform a lumbar puncture for CSF studies. This procedure is controversial for the **asymptomatic term** newborn. For asymptomatic term newborns, the incidence of bacterial meningitis with a negative blood culture is certain to be small. Support for this comes from a review of our infants evaluated for R/O sepsis, anecdotal experience, and consideration of the pathogenesis of bacterial meningitis in the newborn.

A preliminary retrospective review of available data on infants evaluated for sepsis at Brigham and Women's Hospital was recently conducted. Over a 6-month period an estimated 570 asymptomatic infants were evaluated for possible sepsis based on the criteria set forth by the Joint Program in Neonatology Clinical Working Group (see Tables 23-7, 24-8). Two hundred fifty-eight of these infants were treated with antibiotics for R/O sepsis, and 225 had a lumbar puncture for CSF studies. There were 4 positive CSF cultures in asymptomatic infants, all of whom had negative blood cultures. These CSF cultures were presumed to be contaminants, although one culture grew enterococci, which has been described as a perinatal newborn pathogen. None of these infants were treated for meningitis by the clinicians caring for them (those on the scene did not believe that the infant had meningitis).

A survey was conducted to determine the anecdotal experience of faculty from the Joint Program in Neonatology in treating newborns with sepsis and meningitis. The years of practice and number of infants treated for bacterial infections varied considerably, but no cases of culture-positive meningitis with negative blood cultures could be remembered. Since bacterial meningitis in the absence of documented sepsis is a rare occurrence, it is reasonable to assume that such few cases would not be forgotten.

Neonatal bacterial meningitis is believed to arise from hematogenous spread following the penetration of bacteria through mucous membranes. Uncommonly, bacteremias may be transient, and it has been hypothesized that some cases of late-onset GBS disease result from transient bacteremias in **previously asymptomatic newborns.** However, any infant with sustained or progressive acute meningitis in the perinatal period is likely to be symptomatic and to have sustained bloodstream infection as well. The possibility that the positive blood culture was missed must always be considered.

It is the consensus view of the Joint Program in Neonatology Clinical Working Group that the incidence of blood culture–negative bacterial meningitis in **asymptomatic** term newborns is rare. Thus, the lumbar puncture *may* not be necessary for all infants who receive antibiotics for R/O sepsis. The inclusion of the lumbar puncture as part of the R/O sepsis work-up of **asymptomatic** term infants is optional at the discretion of the primary care physician. It must be emphasized that this applies only to **term** newborn infants who meet the following criteria:

a. There are no clinical symptoms (no respiratory, cardiovascular, neurologic [lethargy, poor feeding], or metabolic abnormalities). (Tachypnea is usually present with sepsis.)

b. There is a low suspicion for sepsis (asymptomatic infant with some risk factors and laboratory values meeting criteria for antibiotic treatment).

c. Adequate blood (at least 0.5 ml) was taken for blood culture.

d. More than one negative blood culture is reassuring.

e. It must be recognized that treatment prior to delivery can cause a newborn to have a negative blood culture even though the culture was positive prior to treatment.

All infants who do not undergo a lumbar puncture but who are subsequently found to have a positive blood culture should have CSF studies performed as soon as the results of the blood culture are known. CSF should be sent for culture, Gram stain, cell count, and protein and glucose measurements. A GBS latex agglutination test on CSF should also be performed unless the organism has been identified as a gram-negative bacteria. It is recognized that some lumbar punctures may be unsuccessful or CSF results may be difficult to interpret. For "dry" taps, repeated attempts at obtaining CSF should be made prior to stopping antibiotics. There may be difficulties in interpreting CSF results. A benign lymphocytosis/histocytosis with total cell counts ranging from 25 to 100 can be seen in the absence of bacterial meningitis. Furthermore, a WBC pleocytosis is common with "traumatic taps" or when there is an accompanying subarachnoid hemorrhage. **In these circumstances there may be no recourse but to extend treatment for possible meningitis.** In nearly all cases, if meningitis is present, GBS will be the offending organism, and therapy will need to be extended for a total of 10 to 14 days.

4. Evaluation and antibiotic therapy for the PRETREATED newborn. Asymptomatic newborns who have risk factors and whose mothers were treated with antibiotics prior to delivery because of a risk for maternal perinatal bacterial infection (e.g., maternal fever, uterine tenderness) should automatically have a CBC count and blood culture performed, and antibiotic therapy initiated (see Tables 23-7, 23-8). However, antibiotics can be discontinued after 48 hours provided cultures remain negative and the infants remain asymptomatic. There is good precedent for this approach. The decision to examine CSF in this setting is an individualized clinical decision. (See **I.G.3.**)

In the study by Boyer and Gotoff (see Table 23-3) [5], newborns at high risk for sepsis were given ampicillin for 48 hours after delivery following intrapartum administration of ampicillin to mothers. Colonization was dramatically reduced and no bacteremia occurred in the group treated with intrapartum ampicillin compared to the control group of infants who received only postpartum antibiotic therapy (0/85 versus 5/79, respectively). All who remained asymptomatic with negative cultures at 48 hours had no further evidence of sepsis or meningitis after the discontinuation of antibiotic therapy. The same outcome was observed for additional nonrandomized infants also followed over the 5-year study period. Although the authors' data concern potential GBS disease, the same outcome would be expected with other perinatal

Table 23-8. Guidelines for management of "well-appearing" infants at risk for sepsis: Joint Program in Neonatology Clinical Working Group Guideline

Maternal GBS colonization (includes GBS bacteriuria)	Sepsis risk factors (1 major or 2 minor risk factors)[a]	Intrapartum antibiotic treatment (begun >4 hours prior to delivery)	Management[b]
+	−	+	Routine care
+	−	−	CBC; blood culture Treat if CBC is abnormal[c]
+	+	+	CBC; blood culture Treat if 1) CBC is abnormal[c] or 2) gestational age <35 weeks or 3) other significant clinical concern[d]
+	+	−	CBC, blood culture Treat
+	− (Intact Membranes C/S)	−	Routine care
−	−	+	Routine care
−	−	−	Routine care
−	+	+	CBC; blood culture Treat if 1) CBC is abnormal[c] or 2) other significant clinical concern[d]
−	+	−	CBC; blood culture Treat if 1) CBC is abnormal[c] or 2) other significant clinical concern[d]

			Evaluation / Treatment
?		+	Routine care
?		–	Routine care
?	Only Risk: ROM >24 hours	+	Routine care
?		–	CBC; blood culture Treat if CBC is abnormal[c]
?	Only Risk: ROM >24 hours	+	CBC; blood culture Treat if 1) CBC is abnormal[c] or 2) gestational age <35 weeks or 3) other significant clinical concern[d]
?		–	CBC, blood culture Treat

[a] These are **GUIDELINES** only, and should not substitute for clinical judgment. A clustering of several major or minor risk factors should lead to immediate culture of blood and CSF and the institution of antibiotics therapy before CBC results are available. **Major:** Delivery <35 weeks, maternal fever ≥100.4°F (38°C), ROM >24 hours, chorioamnionitis, sustained FHR >160, previous child with GBS disease **Minor:** Delivery 35–37 weeks, maternal fever ≥99.5°F (37.5°C), multiple births, ROM >12 hours. *Note:* For infants whose only risk factor is prematurity, the circumstances of delivery should be taken into account when determining the appropriate evaluation and treatment.

[b] For infants to be treated, consider lumbar puncture and treat with ampicillin and gentamicin for 48 hours.

[c] Abnormal CBC is WBC <5000 or I:T [immature polys = (bands + other immature polys) ÷ (immature polys + mature polys)] ratio is >0.2.

[d] Other significant clinical concerns include the following: maternal fever ≥101°F, chorioamnionitis, ROM >24 hours, more than one major sepsis risk factor.

pathogens sensitive to the same antibiotic(s) given antenatally. There are case reports of infants treated for 48 hours who presented 2 to 3 weeks later with GBS meningitis. Perinatal treatment may not decrease the incidence of late meningitis.

This work-up and treatment are not necessary if the mother had routine antibiotic treatment because of cesarean section or cardiac disease (e.g., mitral valve prolapse). Because of the new ACOG guidelines, many uncultured mothers delivering term infants whose only risk factor is ruptured membranes for longer than 18 hours will be treated during labor. If the infant is asymptomatic, membranes are ruptured between 18 and 24 hours, and the infant has no other risk factors, we elect not to treat or perform a culture for these babies. Vital signs are assessed every 4 hours. If the membranes are ruptured longer than 24 hours, a CBC count and blood culture are performed and vital signs are assessed every 4 hours. If the CBC count is abnormal, a second blood culture is done and the baby is started on antibiotics for at least 48 hours. See Table 23-8.

5. **Changing length of treatment for R/O sepsis from 72 hours to 48 hours in asymptomatic newborns.** The recognition of identifiable perinatal risk factors for sepsis and meningitis frequently results in the initiation of antibiotic therapy in the asymptomatic newborn. In most cases, antibiotics are continued for 72 hours pending culture results. The possibility of shortening the length of antibiotic therapy for R/O sepsis to 48 hours was approved by the Joint Program in Neonatology Clinical Working Group under the following conditions:

   a. Cultures remain negative after a full 48 hours' incubation.
   b. The infant is asymptomatic from birth or has had mild transient (<2 hours) symptoms.
   c. The culture is observed for 5 days.

   There is the possibility that an asymptomatic infant could have infection in the lung with a negative blood culture. Clinical judgment (risk factors, abnormal CBC count) may cause one to treat this baby longer. The change in the length of treatment for R/O sepsis is based on a large experience in older infants at several centers including The Children's Hospital in Boston and a review of cultures from newborns at Beth Israel Hospital in Boston. At Beth Israel Hospital, 38 positive blood cultures were recorded for newborns evaluated for R/O sepsis over a 21-month period. With a single exception all cultures turned positive within 48 hours. One culture grew *Staphylococcus* organisms (not *aureus*) on day 3.

6. **Treatment with antibiotics** may not be required, especially if the mother received intravenous antibiotics 4 hours or more prior to delivery.

   a. This approach may be particularly appropriate for term infants when there is prolonged rupture of membranes but no other identified risk factors or abnormal laboratory/clinical findings (see Table 23-7). If, however, the infant is preterm or there are multiple risk factors for sepsis, it may be best to treat with antibiotics for R/O sepsis (antibiotics for 48 hours).

   Obstetricians have different approaches to this matter. Some obtain cultures for all the mothers and some obtain cultures for those with risk factors. Some treat all mothers whose cultures are positive or the results are unknown. To standardize our management of these infants, the Joint Program in Neonatology Clinical Working Group proposed the recommendations in Table 23-8. These recommendations do not substitute for clinical judgment. These apply only to **asymptomatic** infants.

H. **Therapy**
   1. **Antibiotic therapy for neonatal septicemia** (Table 23-9). Presumptive antibiotic therapy in the neonate is directed toward the most commonly

encountered pathogens for a given clinical setting. In the perinatal period the pathogens of greatest concern are GBS, ECK1, and *Listeria* species. These organisms remain the principal pathogens throughout the first month of life for otherwise healthy infants living at home. **Ampicillin** and an aminoglycoside, usually **gentamicin,** are usually effective against these bacteria. This combination also provides broad coverage for many other gram-positive and gram-negative bacteria less commonly isolated from the septic newborn. Another important consideration is the in vivo and in vitro synergy demonstrated for penicillins with aminoglycosides, especially against GBS and *Listeria.* Third-generation cephalosporins also are effective against gram-negative infections, but they have limited activity against *Listeria* organisms, and no study has clearly demonstrated improved morbidity or mortality with their use. Cephalosporins also displace bilirubin from albumin-binding sites, which may place the neonate at increased risk for kernicterus in the setting of hyperbilirubinemia. Nevertheless, with documented gram-negative meningitis, third-generation cephalosporins are recommended on the theoretical basis of greater CSF killing power. **Cefotaxime** is generally recommended as this agent has been used most frequently with proven efficacy for the newborn. The CSF killing power of an antibiotic is defined as

$$KP = \frac{\text{Concentration of antibiotic in CSF}}{\text{MBC of antibiotic for infecting organism}}$$

It is the low minimal bactericidal concentration (MBC), not a high CSF penetration, that gives third-generation cephalosporins a high CSF killing power. Recommended antibiotic regimens for specific perinatal infections are provided in Table 23-9.

2. **Antibiotic therapy for neonates at risk for nosocomial infections.** Although ampicillin and gentamicin provide excellent broad coverage for perinatal pathogens, this combination may not be preferred for neonates at risk for nosocomial infections (usually >1 week in the special care nursery). Considering the predominance of coagulase-negative staphylococci as the principal cause of nosocomial sepsis, **vancomycin** has become the principal agent for presumptive gram-positive bacterial coverage. Presumptive gram-negative coverage is provided with an aminoglycoside. The aminoglycoside of choice is usually **gentamicin,** but resistant organisms may be prevalent in many nurseries. An alternative aminoglycoside is **amikacin**; resistance to this antibiotic has been reported to be low, despite long-term use in the nursery. In addition to blood, cultures of CSF and urine (bladder tap or catheterization) should be obtained.

   Vancomycin is dosed at 15 mg/kg intravenously every 12 hours (preterm) or every 8 hours (term), with the dose adjusted based on serum levels. Vancomycin resistance is being reported.

3. **Immunotherapy for neonatal septicemia** [4,11]. The human neonate may be considered an immunocompromised host with incomplete development of multiple components of the immune system. This is not to say that the newborn cannot limit the spread of disease, but defense mechanisms may frequently be overcome, especially in the low-birth-weight infant. Problems with the immune system of the newborn may relate to decreased quantities and/or functions of multiple cellular and humoral constituents. Based on theoretical considerations, and some experimental evidence, the administration of blood and tissue factors to bolster the neonatal immune system has been proposed. In addition to the specific interventions discussed below, current studies are under way to assess the efficacy of prophylactic administration of recombi-

Table 23-9. Recommended antibiotic regimens for neonatal sepsis and meningitis

Site of organism infection	Antibiotic therapy[a]	Duration of therapy
GBS		
Blood	Penicillin, 200,000 units/kg/d	10–14 d
CNS	Penicillin, 400,000 units/kg/d	14–21 d
ECK1		
Blood	Cefotaxime, 50–100 mg/kg/d, or other third-generation antibiotic	14 d
CNS	Cefotaxime, 100 mg/kg/d (? gentamicin 5 mg/kg/d)	21 d (5–10 d for synergy)
Listeria		
Blood	Ampicillin, 100–200 mg/kg/d (? gentamicin 5 mg/kg/d)	14 d (up to 1 wk for synergy)
CNS	Ampicillin, 200–300 mg/kg/d (? gentamicin 5 mg/kg/d)	14–21 d (up to 1 wk for synergy)

[a]In all cases, therapy with ampicillin and gentamicin is initiated until an organism has been identified and antibiotic sensitivities are determined. Ampicillin dosing is 200–300 mg/kg/d in 2 or 3 divided doses (the higher dosing may be preferable until meningitis has been excluded, but individual doses need not exceed 500 mg). Gentamicin dosing is 2.5 mg/kg every 12 hours, with the interval adjusted based on gestational age and serum levels. In general, the intervals are every 24 hours for infants <1000 gm, every 18 hours for infants <35 weeks' gestation, and every 12 hours for infants ≥35 weeks. Cefotaxime dosing is 100 mg/kg/d in 2 divided doses.

nant human interferon-gamma or granulocyte-macrophage colony-stimulating factor (rhu-GM-CSF) to enhance neutrophil function or produce sustained neutrophilia.

a. Immunoglobulin therapy. This has received much attention in recent years. Shigeoka et al. [9] observed increased survival has been noted when neonates infected with GBS received an exchange transfusion with blood containing elevated levels of GBS capsular antibodies [11]. Thus, some septic newborns may benefit from the administration of *GBS-specific* immunoglobulin preparations, or by an exchange transfusion using blood from donors with high levels of GBS capsular antibodies. Protection against experimental GBS infections also occurred in animals receiving high-titer capsular antibody preparations, provided the therapy was given within the first few hours of infection.

Specific intravenous immunoglobulin (IVIG) preparations are not currently available, and although commercially produced IVIG preparations may be safe, efficacy has not been demonstrated.

The use of IVIG for prophylaxis against infection in preterm infants has been investigated over the past decade. The results of initial studies were conflicting, but two recent multicenter trials failed to demonstrate a reduction in significant morbidity and mortality. At present, the routine use of IVIG for prophylaxis or treatment of sepsis neonatorum is not recommended. In some clinical situations (overwhelming infection, recurrent infection in the small premature infant with low immunoglobulin levels) therapy with IVIG may be indicated. Doses used have been 500 to 1000 mg/kg/dose every 2 weeks [11].

(1) Local immunity. Oral administration of exogenous IgA and IgG can prevent or reduce the symptoms of gastrointestinal disease in preterm infants. IgA-IgG feedings significantly decreased the incidence of necrotizing enterocolitis (NEC). Breast milk may serve as a source of both immunoglobulins and nonimmunoglobulin factors that can bathe the neonatal gastrointestinal mucosa and may decrease the colonization by nosocomial pathogens. In a prospective multicenter study, preterm infants fed breast milk had a significantly lower incidence of NEC compared to those receiving formula alone; the incidence of NEC in infants fed only formula was 6 to 10 times more common for all infants, and 20 times more common for infants of more than 30 weeks' gestation [5].

b. Granulocyte infusions [4,11]. There is some evidence that granulocyte transfusions may significantly improve the survival of the septic newborn who is also neutropenic, and who has insufficient bone marrow reserve to replenish the granulocyte deficit. Christensen et al. demonstrated survival in 7 (100%) of 7 septic newborns who received granulocyte transfusions compared to 1 (11%) of 9 infected infants receiving supportive care alone. The infants in this study had severe depletion of bone marrow neutrophil storage pools (NSP = total metamyelocytes, band, and segmented forms ≤7% of marrow cells). Although a one-to-one correspondence between NSP and the percentage of neutrophils in peripheral smears has not been found, Christensen et al. suggested that neutropenia with an immature-total neutrophil ratio higher than 0.8 reflects severe NSP depletion. Results from several other studies incorporating granulocyte infusions for neonatal sepsis support the findings of Christensen et al. with a single exception. Stork et al. were unable to demonstrate improved survival in a randomized prospective clinical trial of granulocyte infusions in 25 septic newborns with NSP depletion. It is also important to note that only a small number of medical centers are currently established in the preparation and administration of granulocytes, and that infusions may have significant side effects in the neonate.

c. Double volume exchange transfusions [11]. Double volume exchange transfusions using fresh whole blood have been used in neonatal septicemia to attempt to (1) remove bacterial toxins and/or decrease the bacterial burden, (2) improve peripheral and pulmonary perfusion, and (3) bolster the immune system of infected newborns. Unfortunately, there has been no prospective randomized controlled study on the use of exchange transfusions for neonatal sepsis. Reports have suggested that improvements in hemodynamic and possibly pulmonary parameters may result from fresh whole blood exchange transfusions. Furthermore, fresh whole blood transfusions provide an alternative method of providing neutrophils to septic newborns with severe NSP depletion. Clearly further studies are needed to confirm the efficacy of fresh whole blood double volume exchange transfusions in the septic newborn. Based on current knowledge, combined with the potential complications of the procedure, exchange transfusions should only be considered in the critically ill neonate with profound neutropenia and severe NSP depletion, and in whom optimal supportive conventional management is failing.

II. Focal bacterial infections
A. Skin infections (see Chap. 34). The newborn may develop a variety of rashes associated with bacterial disease. Some of these are related to systemic infec-

tion, while others are the direct result of primary cutaneous disease. Skin damage from delivery or from monitors may be the source of infection. The most frequently encountered clinical manifestations of localized skin infections are pustules, vesicles, cellulitis, and abscesses. The common bacteria colonizing the skin of the newborn include coagulase-negative staphylococci, *S. aureus*, streptococci (including GBS), gram-negative enterics (including *E. coli*), and diphtheroids. The colonizing organisms will vary with the vaginal flora present at the time of delivery, and the organisms present in the environment of the nursery. Careful washing of all abrasions and treatment with a topical antibiotic ointment may prevent skin infections from traumatized skin.

1. **Pustules.** Infectious pustules in the newborn are most commonly caused by *S. aureus*, but must be distinguished from the similarly appearing lesions of erythema toxicum. Infectious pustules are often found in the axillae, groin, and periumbilical area.
   a. **Diagnosis.** A lesion can be carefully cleansed with povidone-iodine (Betadine), unroofed, and a Gram stain performed on the contents. With true pustules, numerous polymorphonuclear lymphocytes and gram-positive cocci can be seen. Culture of the material confirms the suspected pathogen. Cells consistent with eosinophils without organisms are seen with erythema toxicum. The eosinophils may best be demonstrated with a Wright stain.
   b. **Treatment.** Topical treatment, with bacitracin or mupirocin, and close observation may be all that is required for a small number of pustules occurring on an otherwise well infant. Oral therapy with a penicillinase-resistant penicillin or first-generation cephalosporin may also be appropriate. More extensive lesions or lesions occurring in an ill infant should be treated with parenteral antibiotic after material for systemic cultures has been obtained.
   c. **Nosocomial outbreaks.** Because of the incubation period, most cases of staphylococcal pustulosis occur in term infants after discharge from the newborn nursery. Pediatricians should report any cases they identify to the hospital of birth. This will allow for the recognition of nosocomial outbreaks in nurseries. When nosocomial outbreaks occur, material for culture should be obtained from the skin and umbilicus of infants in the nursery, and colonized infants should be grouped together. Adjunctive interventions include bathing full-term infants (with intact skin) with a 1:4 or 1:5 dilute solution of hexachlorophene. The application of topical antimicrobial agents (especially mupirocin in a paraffin base) to the umbilicus may be beneficial but studies are limited. Outbreaks usually result from nosocomial spread of *S. aureus* from colonized infants by nursery personnel. They rarely occur as a result of a colonized staff member who is identified as the common source by epidemiologic association. When this occurs, the person should be cultured for nasal carriage, and if *S. aureus* is recovered, colonization can be eradicated by the topical application of mupirocin to the nose 2 to 3 times each day for 5 days.
2. **Bullous lesions.** Some strains of *S. aureus* produce toxins that can cause bullous lesions or scalded skin syndrome. The cutaneous changes are due to the local and systemic spread of toxin, and blood cultures may be negative. Nevertheless, systemic antibiotics (e.g., oxacillin 50 mg/kg every 12 hours or every 6 to 8 hours after the first week of life) should be given until the progression of disease stops and skin lesions are healing.
3. **Cellulitis.** The causative agents are usually streptococci and parenteral antibiotic therapy is required. *S. aureus* and gram-negative enteric bacteria may also be present with cellulitis associated with disruption of the skin.

a. **Omphalitis.** This is characterized by erythema and/or induration with purulent discharge from the umbilical stump. Both gram-negative and gram-positive organisms may be involved, and in the setting of poor maternal immunity and poor aseptic technique, clostridia may be common. Routine cord care is discussed in Chap. 5. Treatment of omphalitis requires a full septic work-up and parenteral antibiotics (usually oxacillin and an aminoglycoside). The seriousness of the condition is emphasized by the complications seen with progressive disease. These are related to contiguous spread to adjacent soft tissues or umbilical blood vessels. Abdominal wall cellulitis, necrotizing fasciitis, peritonitis, and umbilical arteritis or phlebitis with hepatic vein thrombosis or hepatic abscess have all been described.

B. **Ophthalmia neonatorum.** This condition refers to inflammation of the conjunctiva within the first month of life. Causative agents include topical antimicrobial drugs (chemical conjunctivitis), bacteria, and herpesvirus. Bacterial conjunctivitis is caused by *Neisseria gonorrhoeae, Chlamydia trachomatis,* staphylococci, pneumococci, streptococci, *E. coli,* and other gramnegative bacteria. In the United States, where universal prophylaxis with topical antimicrobial solutions or ointments is practiced, the incidence is lower than 2%. The worldwide incidence is estimated to be approximately 20%.

1. **Prophylaxis against infectious ophthalmia.** The efficacy of single-dose topical antimicrobial prophylaxis to prevent ophthalmia neonatorum has been established. Effective agents include silver nitrate 1%, erythromycin 0.5%, tetracycline 1%, and povidone-iodine ophthalmic solution. All of these agents have comparable efficacy in preventing conjunctivitis caused by most bacterial pathogens, including penicillin-sensitive *N. gonorrhoeae.*

a. **Penicillinase-producing N. gonorrhoeae.** Silver nitrate may be the preferred agent for prophylaxis in areas where there is a high incidence of penicillinase-producing strains of *N. gonorrhoeae.* Povidone-iodine is equally effective as silver nitrate or erythromycin in preventing gonococcal conjunctivitis. Since this agent is inexpensive, appears to cause chemical conjunctivitis less commonly than silver nitrate and erythromycin, and is active against all bacteria, a 2.5% povidone-iodine solution may be a reasonable alternative for prophylaxis, especially in developing nations. Iodine may be absorbed across neonatal mucous membranes and concerns have been raised about the possibility of adverse effects on thyroid function. It is not known if this potential problem could result from the small quantity of 2.5% povidine-iodine used for ophthalmic prophylaxis.

Effective prevention of gonococcal ophthalmia neonatorum begins with maternal screening during pregnancy. **All pregnant women should have endocervical cultures for N. gonorrhoeae** as part of prenatal care. Cultures should be repeated at delivery for high-risk women. Treatment of infected pregnant women is the best means of preventing disease in the newborn. Ocular prophylaxis should be provided for all newborns within 1 hour of birth as described above. In addition, infants born to culture-positive mothers should receive a single dose of ceftriaxone 125 mg intramuscularly (or 25 to 50 mg/kg intramuscularly for low-birth-weight infants).

b. **C. trachomatis.** In the United States neonatal conjunctivitis is more commonly caused by chlamydia than *N. gonorrhoeae.* Although *C. trachomatis* is sensitive to erythromycin, tetracycline, and silver nitrate, the effectiveness of topical prophylaxis with these agents has not been established. Prenatal treatment of pregnant women with chlamydial cervicitis can prevent neonatal chlamydial conjunctitis. For infants born to mothers with untreated chlamydial infection, treatment of the infant with a 14-day course of oral erythromycin or sulfonamides is recommended.

c. **General procedure for administering topical ophthalmic prophylaxis.** This should be done using single-dose ampules or ointment containers within the first hour of life. The usual method of application is as follows:

   (1) Cleanse the eyelid and surrounding skin with sterile cotton moistened with sterile water.

   (2) Gently open the infant's eyelids and instill 2 drops of silver nitrate or a ribbon of antibiotic ointment on each conjunctival sac. Allow the silver nitrate to run across the whole conjunctival sac, or apply a 1- to 2-cm ribbon of antibiotic ointment across the lower sac. Carefully manipulate the lids to ensure spread of the applied agent.

   (3) After 1 minute, wipe the excess solution or ointment from the surrounding skin and eyelids with sterile cotton. **Do not irrigate the eyes after this procedure.** Irrigation may reduce the efficiency of prophylaxis without altering the incidence of chemical conjunctivitis.

2. **Treatment of ophthalmia neonatorum**

   a. **Chemical conjunctivitis.** This is predominantly seen with silver nitrate 1%; approximately 90% of infants develop conjunctival hyperemia, edema, and eye drainage within hours of exposure to silver nitrate 1% ophthalmic drops. In some cases periorbital edema also occurs. The reaction is usually self-limiting and resolves within 36 to 48 hours. Gentle wiping of the eyes with sterile cotton moistened with sterile saline solution or water is all that is required.

   Infectious conjunctivitis may also occur within hours of delivery, especially in the setting of PROMs. A Gram stain can help differentiate between chemical and infectious conjunctivitis. With the former, only polymorphonuclear lymphocytes without organisms is seen. If doubt still exists, the exudate should be cultured and presumptive antimicrobial therapy initiated. A broad-spectrum agent such as cefotaxime provides coverage for *S. aureus*, *N. gonorrhoeae*, and most gram-negative organisms. Chlamydia rarely causes conjunctivitis within the first day of life. Herpesvirus should be considered.

   b. **N. gonorrhoeae.** Gonococcal ophthalmia neonatorum usually presents as conjunctivitis with chemosis, purulent exudate, and lid edema starting at 1 to 4 days after birth. Clouding or perforation of the cornea, or pan ophthalmitis may also be present. Rhinitis, scalp infections, anorectal infection, funistitis, sepsis, arthritis, and meningitis have all been described with gonococcal infections in the newborn. The highest incidence of gonococcal infection is in adolescents and young adults (1 to 2%). This rate can be as high as 10% in selected populations of pregnant women, and the recurrence rate in pregnancy can be high. Risk factors for high incidence of perinatal gonococcal infection are low socioeconomic group, prior history of venereal disease, unmarried state, and urban populations. There is an increased risk of gonococcal ophthalmia neonatorum with PROMs in infected women.

      (1) Diagnosis. A Gram stain should be performed on conjunctival scrapings from any infant suspected of having infectious conjunctivitis. Routine bacteriologic cultures as well as prompt plating of exudate on appropriate growth medium (e.g., Thayer-Martin) for the isolation of *Neisseria* are required. Intracellular gram-negative diplococci are characteristically seen on a Gram stain, and if present, the infant should have a blood culture performed and be treated with systemic antibiotics. Presumptive therapy should be initiated if the clinical presentation is most consistent with gonococcal ophthalmia neonatorum, but the Gram stain is equivocal. Maternal cervical cultures should also be obtained. Conjunctivitis can be caused by nongonococcal *Neisseria*, indicating the need for careful confirmation of gonorrhea by appropriate microbiologic techniques.

(2) Treatment. Conventional management consists of cefotaxime 100 mg/kg per day intravenously or intramuscularly in two divided doses. Once-daily dosing of ceftriaxone 125 mg intramuscularly or intravenously (25 to 50 mg/kg per day for low-birth-weight infants) is an alternative acceptable regimen for infants without hyperbilirubinemia. If the gonococcal isolate is penicillin sensitive, aqueous penicillin G 100,000 units/kg/day in 2 divided doses can begin. The duration of treatment is 7 days for localized conjunctival disease and 10 to 14 days for disseminated disease. Frequent saline conjunctival irrigations should be performed in infants with gonococcal ophthalmia neonatorum. Topical antibiotic ointments or drops are probably not necessary for the treatment of *N. gonorrhoeae* infection but tetracycline 1% ointment or erythromycin ointment may be applied hourly at first for 6 hours and then four times a day for 14 days. Mothers should be treated for their own sake and to prevent postnatal infection of the neonate. All sex partners of infected mothers should be evaluated and treated. For any infant suspected of being exposed to gonococcal infection, precautions regarding secretions should be in place for 24 hours after the initiation of ocular and parenteral antimicrobial prophylaxis or treatment.

c. C. trachomatis. In the United States, this is the most common cause of infectious conjunctivitis in the newborn. The highest prevalence of cervical infection occurs in adolescents and ranges from 8 to 37%, and chlamydia is identified in approximately 50% of women with mucopurulent cervicitis. The principal mode of transmission is to the newborn upon vaginal delivery, with the organism being transmitted at a rate of 50 to 75%. Between 20 and 50% of infants born to infected mothers develop conjunctivitis.

Chlamydial conjunctivitis usually appears 5 to 14 days after birth. There may be minimum inflammation or severe conjunctival inflammation with a purulent yellow discharge and swelling of the eyelids. Conjunctival scarring is possible. The cornea is usually not involved, although corneal pannus formation has been described.

(1) Diagnosis. The diagnosis of chlamydial conjunctivitis can be made by the demonstration of basophilic intracytoplasmic inclusion bodies on Giemsa stain of scrapings taken from the palpebral conjunctival surface. The bodies are not found in the cells of the purulent exudate. Both polymorphonuclear and mononuclear lymphocytes are found in the exudate. Three rapid antigen detection methods as well as tissue culture are also available for the diagnosis of chlamydial infection. A direct fluorescent antibody test (DFA), an enzyme-linked immunosorbent assay (ELISA), and a DNA probe are available for chlamydia testing and are very sensitive and specific for the detection of chlamydia from conjunctival material. Tissue culture may not be readily available at all centers, and requires special handling and at least 3 to 5 days for growth and detection.

(2) Treatment. Chlamydial conjunctivitis can best be treated by systemic therapy with erythromycin ethylsuccinate, 50 mg/kg per day in four divided doses for 14 days. This therapy may also eradicate the organism from the upper respiratory tract. A second treatment course may be required for some infants. Mothers and their sex partner(s) should be evaluated and treated for genital infection. The eyes should be cleaned as in the treatment for gonococcal ophthalmia and tetracycline or erythromycin ophthalmic ointment applied four times a day for 3 weeks.

C. Urinary tract infection (UTI)

1. Incidence. This varies somewhat with birth weight but the overall incidence is probably lower than 3% for all neonates. Bacteriuria may signal generalized sepsis with hematogenous spread to the kidney. Alternatively, a primary UTI may result in bloodstream infection. There is a higher incidence in male than female infants. The most common organism is *E. coli* but other gram-negative bacteria, especially *Klebsiella pneumoniae,* and enterococci are also causative agents.

2. Diagnosis. Culture of urine obtained by suprapubic bladder tap or bladder catheterization is essential for the diagnosis of UTI and should be part of the work-up for sepsis in all neonates. The newborn younger than 48 hours at risk for intrapartum sepsis is the only exception to this rule; UTI is uncommon with early-onset sepsis. A suprapubic bladder tap may be more reliable than bladder catheterization, because surface bacterial contamination or colonization of the prepuce and distal urethra may result in unreliable culture results. This can be done with ultrasound guidance if available. Gram stain of unspun urine may identify bacteria. A blood culture is part of the evaluation of a neonatal UTI. Perinatal maternal UTI may increase the risk for infection in the newborn.

3. Treatment. Presumptive therapy consists of ampicillin and an aminoglycoside until antibiotic sensitivities are obtained. A repeat urine culture should have no growth after 48 to 72 hours of therapy. Persistence of bacteriuria may indicate renal abscess, obstructive uropathy, or inappropriate therapy. The duration of therapy is 10 to 14 days. All infants with UTI should have ultrasonic examination of the urinary tract early in the course of treatment. A cystourethrogram is also performed. Until studies have ruled out an underlying anatomic defect of the renal and urogenital systems, or a diagnosed defect has been corrected, oral antibiotic prophylaxis (most often amoxicillin) should be started after the initial 10- to 14-day intravenous treatment course.

D. Pneumonia

1. Perinatal disease. The diagnosis of pneumonia in the immediate postpartum period can be difficult because of the frequency of other causes of respiratory distress, including hyaline membrane disease, retained fetal lung fluid, amniotic fluid aspiration, and meconium aspiration. In each of these cases, the radiographic findings can be identical to those seen with bacterial pneumonia. The diagnosis is best made by determining the risk factors for infection versus those for the other conditions, and observing the clinical course. For example, an infant with transient tachypnea after being delivered by cesarean section, with membranes intact and no other identified risk factors for infection, may not require antibiotic therapy unless symptoms persist and the likely diagnosis of retained fetal lung fluid becomes less certain. With greater than mild respiratory distress, or when symptoms are progressing or not improving, material for appropriate cultures should be obtained and antibiotic therapy considered. When doubt exists, it is best to initiate therapy, and later discontinue antibiotics if the clinical course is most consistent with a noninfectious etiology, cultures are negative, and subsequent radiographs do not support pneumonia.

The microbiology of perinatally acquired pneumonia parallels that of sepsis and meningitis, and the choice and doses of antibiotics are the same (see Table 23-9). Blood culture–negative pneumonia is generally treated with parenteral ampicillin and gentamicin for 10 days. A follow-up chest radiograph is important to demonstrate resolution of focal abnormalities. If this is not seen by the completion of antibiotic therapy, further evaluation may be needed to exclude other causes of parenchymal lung opacifications (e.g., bronchogenic cyst or pulmonary sequestration).

2. **Ureaplasma urealyticum.** This organism is frequently isolated from the vagina of pregnant women and is associated with chorioamnionitis, premature delivery, spontaneous abortion and stillbirth, and sepsis, pneumonia, and meningitis in the newborn. Despite a relatively high rate of colonization, there appears to be no clear increased risk of respiratory disease in full-term infants. However, there appears to be an association between the development of chronic lung disease and *U. urealyticum* infection in low-birth-weight infants. There are few data available on the efficacy of antibiotic therapy for newborn infection. It remains to be shown whether treatment of low-birth-weight infants decreases the incidence of chronic lung disease [11].

E. **Osteomyelitis.** This is an uncommon infection in the neonatal period. It may result from sepsis, direct inoculation in association with heel sticks and scalp electrodes, or extension from soft-tissue infections.

1. **Microbiology and diagnosis.** The most common organisms are *S. aureus*, GBS, gram-negative bacteria, *N. gonorrhoeae*, and *Candida* species. There is a good correlation between the most common causes of bacteremia in the newborn and the frequency of bone infections caused by a particular organism. Any bone can be involved, but most frequently infection occurs in the femur, humerus, tibia, radius, and maxilla. Multiple simultaneous foci of infection can occur. Symptoms supporting the diagnosis include apparent pain on motion, localized erythema and/or swelling, and an apparent paralysis. Samples of blood, urine, and CSF should be obtained for culture, and any soft-tissue lesions such as skin pustules or an abscess should be aspirated for Gram stain and culture. Plain film radiographs, and Gram stain and culture of material obtained by needle aspiration of the involved bone and soft tissues are valuable in establishing the diagnosis.

2. **Treatment.** Therapy is initiated with oxacillin and gentamicin until an organism is identified and antibiotic sensitivities are determined. The duration of therapy is 3 to 4 weeks after systemic and local signs have resolved. Any local purulent collection should be drained.

F. **Septic arthritis.** This can occur by direct seeding associated with bacteremia, by extension of infection from adjacent bone, or following local trauma. In general, the etiologic agents are similar to those seen with osteomyelitis, reflecting the association with bacteremia or spread from involved bone in the neonate. Open surgical drainage is recommended for diagnosis and relief of pressure in some joints (e.g., hip, shoulder), but needle aspiration may be sufficient for others (e.g., knee, wrist). Antibiotic therapy is the same as for osteomyelitis. Immobilization of joints is recommended until local signs have resolved and physiotherapy can be initiated.

G. **Otitis media.** The incidence of otitis media in the neonate is not known, but several risk factors for neonatal disease have been identified. These include nasotracheal intubation for more than 7 days, cleft palate, and other risk factors for sepsis including prematurity. Systemic cultures should be obtained. The most commonly identified agents are *S. aureus* and gram-negative enteric bacteria. Tympanocentesis may be indicated if a clinical response is not observed within 48 hours of therapy with broad-spectrum antibiotics.

III. **Fungal infections**
    A. **Mucocutaneous candidiasis.** Fungal infections in the well, immunocompetent term infant are generally limited to mucocutaneous disease. The of-

fending organism is *Candida albicans.* Oral candidiasis (thrush) is usually responsive to nystatin oral suspension (100,000 units/ml). One milliliter is delivered to each side of the mouth every 6 hours and is continued for several days after the mouth clears of lesions. Alternative therapy is gentian violet 1%, which may be very effective with as few as one or two applications, but may be safely used over longer periods for refractory lesions. Candida diaper dermatitis is treated with nystatin ointment or powder (100,000 units/gm) applied with each diaper change. Although mucocutaneous candidiasis most commonly occurs postnatally, rare intrauterine infections have been reported. Intrauterine infection occurs via the ascending route and can result in mucocutaneous or disseminated disease.

B. Disseminated candidiasis. Systemic candidiasis has emerged as a serious nosocomial infection occurring in very-low-birth-weight infants. As many as 3% of very-low-birth-weight infants develop systemic candidiasis. Risk factors may include prolonged use of antibiotics, parenteral hyperalimentation and intravenous fat emulsions, assisted ventilation, and the use of contaminated monitoring equipment. Several species of *Candida* have been isolated from infected neonates, including *C. albicans, C. tropicalis, C. parapsilosis, C. pseudotropicalis,* and *C. lusitaniae.* When an infectious process is suspected, but bacterial pathogens are not identified, and there is no response to antibiotic therapy, fungal disease should be considered.

Candida sepsis may result in meningitis, arthritis, endophthalmitis, endocarditis, and obstructive uropathy. Blood cultures are important but may be negative. CSF cultures are also important, and urine cultures may be valuable in identifying the infant with candidemia. Other aids include microscopic examination of urine and the buffy coat of blood, the determination of serum candida antigen, ophthalmologic examination, and renal ultrasonography. Treatment consists of intravenous amphotericin B. The addition of 5-fluorocytosine (5-FC) may be beneficial, particularly with CNS involvement. Given the fulminant nature of systemic *Candida* infection, a rapid increase in daily dosing from 0.5 mg/kg to 1.0 mg/kg over 48 to 72 hours is often used (see Appendix). The total dose is approximately 25 to 30 mg, but higher doses may be needed to treat unusual tissue involvement such as obstructive uropathy or endocarditis. It should be noted that there are limited data on amphotericin B pharmacology and toxicity in neonates; renal function and serum electrolytes should be monitored closely. Combination therapy with 5-FC is generally used with meningeal involvement, but single-drug therapy with amphotericin B has been successful [8]. The dose of 5-FC is 50 to 100 mg/kg once each day with monitoring of serum levels (should be <100 μg/ml). Liver function tests and CBC counts must also be routinely performed to monitor for drug toxicity.

Some experts initiate combination therapy if blood cultures remain positive for 5 days with optimal therapy, but the average duration of positive blood cultures with amphotericin B therapy is generally longer than this (up to 10 days). Fluconazole 6 mg/kg per day intravenously or orally may be an effective alternative to amphotericin B but studies are limited in neonates. For difficult-to-eradicate infections, liposomal amphotericin B provides a possible method of delivering up to 5 mg/kg per day of drug and has been used successfully in a small number of neonates.

C. Malassezia furfur. This organism is recognized as a cause of neonatal sepsis in the intensive care setting. In the neonatal special care nursery, 33 to 66% of infants may be colonized with this organism. Infections occur primarily in preterm infants receiving intravenous fat emulsions. The most common clinical presentation is apnea and bradycardia, although fever, thrombocytopenia, leukocytosis, and pulmonary infiltrates can occur. Treatment primarily consists of removal of the catheter used for lipid infusions. The need for antifungal agents is uncertain since symptoms usually resolve after catheter removal. Amphotericin B is active against *M. furfur* and may be used if clinical symptoms persist or are severe. *M. furfur* infection should be considered in preterm infants who are receiving intravenous lipid and show signs of sepsis but for whom cultures fail to identify an organism. Yeast forms may be identified by Gram stain of the buffy coat from peripheral blood, but special culture techniques may be required to isolate the organism.

IV. **Anaerobic infections.** Anaerobes make up a significant portion of the vaginal flora and are a well-known cause of maternal infection. Many anaerobes have low virulence and are spontaneously cleaned from the maternal and neonatal bloodstreams. Most episodes of clinically significant anaerobic bacteremia are associated with either in utero infection, gastrointestinal disease (bowel perforation, NEC), or cord or wound infection. Sometimes there are local infections from skin trauma (scalp monitors, forceps abrasions). While it is uncommon to have significant neonatal anaerobic bacteremia (<1% of cases of neonatal sepsis), when it is present in a sick infant, it is often associated with severe disease. The pathogens associated with significant neonatal anaerobic infection are *Bacteroides fragilis, Peptostreptococcus* organisms, *Clostridium perfringens,* and occasionally, *Fusobacterium* species. These infections are often complicated by other aerobic bacteria infection occurring at the same time. Infections with an anaerobic bacteria from either chorioamnionitis, congenital pneumonia, or bowel perforation during the first few days of life are often due to gram-positive, penicillin G–susceptible organisms. After this time, the clinical setting is usually neonatal gastrointestinal disease (NEC, bowel perforation), and the organisms are often gram-negative penicillin G–resistant organisms.

A. **Treatment.** Ampicillin is effective for most anaerobic infections but is ineffective against *B. fragilis.* Third-generation cephalosporins and vancomycin will not be effective against *B. fragilis.* Clindamycin is usually effective against *B. fragilis.* It may not penetrate the CSF well, and some resistant strains exist. Chloramphenicol is effective against *B. fragilis* and penetrates the CSF well. We usually treat intestinal perforation with ampicillin, gentamicin, and clindamycin. In cases of congenital pneumonia, considerations of anaerobic infection would suggest the need to include agents for *B. fragilis* in the antibiotic coverage.

B. **Tetanus** caused by *Clostridium tetani* is among the most severe anaerobic neonatal infections. It is seen in infants born to unimmunized women. It often arises from infection of the umbilical stump related to poor hygiene. It is rare in the United States. Diagnosis is made by history of an infected wound or cord followed by clinical signs in an infant born to an unimmunized mother. Laboratory tests are often not helpful.

Treatment of tetanus includes administration of antitoxin (tetanus immune globulin 500 units intramuscularly), immunization with tetanus toxoid, parenteral penicillin G (100,000 to 200,000 units/kg per day for 10 to 14 days), and surgical care of the cord or wound. For general sedation, although multiple drugs have been used, barbiturates afford good sedation as well as decrease muscle spasms. Diazepam is also used for muscle spasms. Phenothiazines also may be used, but tachyphylaxis to this drug may develop. In extreme cases, muscle relaxation with neuromuscular blocking agents may be necessary if ventilation is compromised. Finally, neonatal infection with tetanus does not provide long-term immunity. These infants should therefore not be omitted from active immunization programs. Immunization of pregnant women will prevent neonatal tetanus.

References
1. American College of Obstetrics and Gynecology Committee Opinion. *Prevention of Early Onset Group B Strep Disease in Newborns.* Technical Bulletin No. 173. Washington, D.C.: American Academy of Obstetrics and Gynecology, 1996.
2. American Academy of Pediatrics. *Report of Committee on Infectious Diseases* (24th Ed.). Elk Grove, Ill.: American Academy of Pediatrics, 1997.

3. Centers for Disease Control. Prevention of perinatal group B strep disease: A public health perspective. *MMWR* 45(RR7), 1996.
4. Cowles, T. A. Perinatal infections. In A. A. Fanaroff, et al. (Eds.). *Neonatal-Perinatal Medicine* (6th Ed.), Chap. 21. St. Louis: Mosby-Year Book, 1977.
5. Feigin, R. D., and Cherry, J. D. *Textbook of Pediatric Infectious Diseases* (3d Ed.). Philadelphia: Saunders, 1992.
6. Guerina, N. G., et al. Neonatal Nosocomial Infections: Prevention and Management. In S. L. Kaplan (Ed.), *Current Therapy in Pediatric Infectious Disease* (3d Ed.). St. Louis: B.C. Decker (Mosby-Year Book), 1993. P. 406.
7. Philip, A. G. S. Early diagnosis of neonatal sepsis. *Pediatrics* 65:1036, 1980.
8. Remington, J. S., and Klein, J. O. *Infectious Diseases of the Fetus and Newborn Infant* (4th Ed.). Philadelphia: Saunders, 1995.
9. Rouse, D. J., et al. Strategies for the prevention of early-onset neonatal group B streptococcal sepsis: A decision analysis. *Obstet. Gynecol.* 83:483, 1994.
10. Shigeoka, A. O., et al. Blood transfusion in group B streptococcal sepsis. *Lancet* 1:636, 1978.
11. Stoll, B. J., Weisman, L. E. Infections in perinatology. *Clin. Perinatol.* 24:1, 1997.
12. AAP Committee on Infectious Diseases. Respiratory syncytial virus immune globulin intravenous: indications for use. Pediatrics 99(4):645, 1997.
13. Pizzo, P., Wilfert, C. M. *Pediatric AIDS* (2nd Ed.). Baltimore: Williams & Wilkins, 1994.

Tuberculosis
John P. Cloherty

I. **Tuberculosis (TB)** is somewhat uncommon in the United States, however, in recent years there has been an increase in reported cases of TB from 22,517 cases in 1988 to 25,701 cases in 1990 [2,7].

In the past TB was a disease of older Americans, it is now becoming more prominent among younger adults. This is especially true in urban, low income, and non-white racial groups. Foreign-born persons make up 25% of new cases. The highest rates of infection are found in first-generation immigrants from high-risk countries, Hispanics, Blacks, Asians, American Indians, and Alaskan natives [2,9].

The increase in the incidence of TB between 1988 and 1990 has been greatest in the 25- to 44-year-old age group (44%) followed by the 5- to 14-year-old age group (39.8%) and then the under-5 age group (18.6%).

There are many reasons for the rise of TB in young adults and children. These are the HIV epidemic, recent immigration to the United States from areas with a high prevalence of TB and the usual factors which have always been associated with TB, poor nutrition, poverty, and poor living conditions.

Homeless persons, shelter dwellers, migrant workers, residents of institutions or prisons, as well as some health care workers are at increased risk. If women of child-bearing age have an increased incidence of TB and they live in an environment where TB is prevalent, there will be more cases of TB in infants and young children [7]. TB should be considered in patients with the preceding risk factors. The highest risk group for mortality from TB is in patients under age 5. Untreated TB in the newborn is almost always fatal.

II. **Diagnosis**

A. **Maternal tuberculosis.** As in nonpregnant adults, the tubercle bacilli is contracted in pregnant women by inhalation. Most cases are asymptomatic or have minimal disease. Identification and treatment of pregnant women with TB is the most efficient method of preventing TB in the newborn. Skin testing should be done on all pregnant women who are suspected to be exposed to a person with TB; have increased susceptibility to acquire TB because of HIV infection, diabetes, gastrectomy; live in a high prevalence area (for example, low socioeconomic population, new immigrant); or work in a profession with a high probability of exposure (for example, hospital, prison, agency for the homeless, nursing home). Pregnancy does not affect the response to a tuberculin skin test, and there have been no adverse effects on women or their babies from tuberculin testing.

1. **PPD** [6,7]. Finding a positive purified protein derivative (PPD) reaction in an asymptomatic woman is the most common method of diagnosing TB in pregnancy in the United States. If there is a conversion reaction to PPD in a pregnant woman, a careful history should be taken, emphasizing the above risk factors. A history of previous treatment should be sought and documented.

2. Chest radiography is helpful in defining the extent of the disease, but it exposes the fetus to radiation and is not reliable in identification of extrapulmonary disease. Only if the tuberculin skin test is positive should a chest radiograph be obtained to determine if there is active disease. The fetus should be shielded from the x-ray.

3. **Maternal symptoms.** Symptomatic women may present with cough, weight loss, fever, malaise, fatigue, or hemoptysis. Other manifestations may be mastitis, miliary tuberculosis, tuberculosis meningitis, and the later manifestation of tuberculosis of the skin, joints, kidney, and bone. Lymphohematogenous spread and endometritis are important in the pathogenesis of infection in the fetus and newborn. Finding a peritoneal fibrinous exudate at cesarean section or an infected placenta may lead to the diagnosis of tuberculosis in the mother and newborn. Sputum samples should be obtained for smear, culture, and sensitivity. There should be a search for extrapulmonary TB, and, if indicated, biopsies should be taken for examination and culture. If the history and clinical symptoms suggest TB in the absence of a positive skin test, material (sputum, nodes, biopsy) should be taken to confirm the diagnosis and treatment should be considered [3]. Untreated TB is a far greater risk to the pregnant woman and her fetus than the risks of treatment. Tuberculosis during pregnancy is not an indication for a therapeutic abortion. There is no significant increase in malformations in infants born to mothers who had tuberculosis and were treated for it. Since the use of antituberculosis chemotherapy, there is no increased risk to the pregnant mother from adequately treated tuberculosis as compared with nonpregnant women.

B. **Tuberculosis of the fetus or newborn**

1. **Pathogenesis.** Congenital tuberculosis is rare. Women with only pulmonary infection usually do not infect their offspring until after birth. In utero infection may occur by various mechanisms [5].

   a. The placenta may be infected by tubercular bacillemia with severe fetal involvement and fetal death.

   b. Placental TB may spread to the fetus by the umbilical vein. The primary complex may be in the fetal liver, gastrointestinal tract, or mesenteric nodes. A placental tubercle may rupture causing tubercular amnionitis and possible fetal aspiration with a primary complex in the fetal lung.

   c. The infant may aspirate infected secretions at the time of birth.

   d. Postnatal exposure may occur from an infected mother or other individuals such as infected family members or health care workers.

2. **Signs and symptoms.** The timing and type of neonatal symptomatology will depend on the **duration, mechanism, and the location** of the infection in the infant. The symptoms may start at birth or not until 8 weeks of age. The mean time of onset is 2–4 weeks. Respiratory distress, fever, hepatic and splenic enlargement, irritability, poor feeding, lethargy, lymphadenopathy, skin papules, failure to thrive, jaundice, biliary obstruction, ear discharge, and central nervous system signs may be seen. There may be few auscultatory findings even with a very abnormal chest x-ray. The chest x-ray may be normal. Calcification of the liver or spleen is seen rarely.

A PPD tuberculin skin test (5 units) should be performed on any infant suspected of having congenital or perinatally acquired tuberculosis. However, it may not be positive unless the infection has been present for 4–6 months. Acid-fast stains and cultures should be performed on blood, urine, gastric fluid, tracheal aspirates, and CSF. Tissue from lymph nodes, liver, lung, bone marrow, and the placenta may reveal organisms on pathologic examination and culture. Skin lesions should be examined pathologically and cultured, but may not contain organisms. Drug sensitivities should be performed on any organism grown from these cultures. If the mother has had recent active tuberculosis or develops an active lesion in the postpartum period, there should be aggressive investigation of the history and epidemiology and physical and laboratory examination of the infant. If all direct smears are negative and the infant is ill, antituberculosis therapy should be started until the diagnosis is ruled out.

III. Management [1–3,6,7,9]

   A. Mother. If active tuberculosis (positive culture, clinical or radiologic findings compatible with the presumptive diagnosis of active TB) is diagnosed during pregnancy, chemotherapy is necessary to protect the mother and the fetus.

   Isoniazid (INH) and rifampin (RIF) are given for 9 months. If drug resistance is suspected, ethambutol is added until sensitivities are known. When sensitivities are known, one of the drugs can be discontinued after 1 to 2 months. If ethambutol is discontinued because the bacteria is sensitive to INH and RIF, treatment is continued for 6 to 9 months. If the mother is HIV positive, she should be treated for 12 months. If INH or RIF is the discontinued drug, treatment with the other drugs is continued for 18 months. INH, RIF, and ethambutol have not been shown to be teratogenic. Streptomycin has teratogenic effects, causing vestibular damage and deafness. The benefit of ethambutol and rifampin therapy for active TB outweighs any potential risk to the fetus. There are no data on the effects of pyrazinamide in pregnancy so it should be avoided if possible. Cycloserine and enthanamide should be avoided in pregnancy. Mothers infected with organisms that are resistant to many drugs may need treatment with medications that are usually contraindicated in pregnancy or have unknown fetal effects. This will leave the mother and physician difficult choices about treatment and continuation of the pregnancy. If drug resistance is present, an expert in the management of tuberculosis should be consulted. Pyridoxine should be added during treatment in pregnancy.

   Asymptomatic pregnant women with a negative x-ray and a positive skin test who have never been treated should receive therapy with INH for 9 months starting in the 2nd trimester if they have recently been in contact with an infectious person or are HIV positive or immunosuppressed. If a mother has HIV infection, a PPD skin test with redness and induration of 5 mm or greater is an indication for treatment of tuberculosis. This is true even if the mother has had bacillus Calmette-Guérin (BCG) in the past [2,6]. If there is a positive skin test, a negative chest x-ray and no recent exposure, HIV positivity, or immunosuppression, therapy can be delayed until after pregnancy. Table 23-10 is an outline of the usual management of tuberculosis in pregnant women. INH is excreted in breast milk in amounts that would not cause toxicity yet in amounts inadequate for treatment or prophylaxis of the infant [1,2].

   B. Congenital or neonatal TB [1,2,4–8]. Women who have only pulmonary TB usually do not infect their offspring until after delivery. In utero infections while rare can occur (see **II.B**). If an infant is suspected of having congenital TB, a Mantoux test (5TU-PPD), chest x-ray, lumbar puncture, and all cultures should be done (see **II.B**). The child should then be started on therapy regardless of the skin test results (see Table 23-11). Treatment should initially include INH, RIF, and pyrazinamide until the drug sensitivity of the

Table 23-10. Diagnosis and treatment of tuberculosis in the pregnant woman

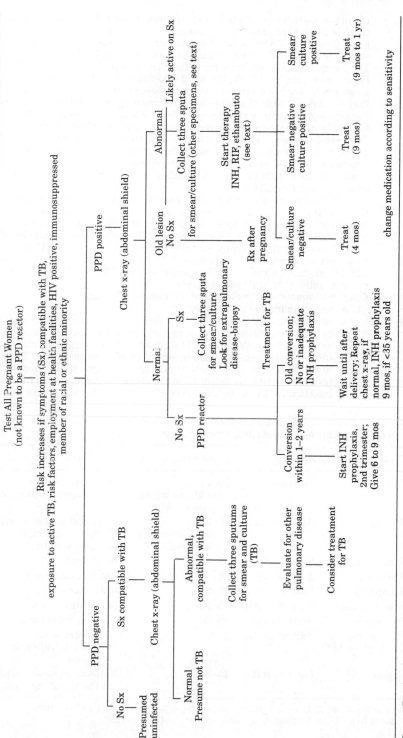

Test All Pregnant Women
(not known to be a PPD reactor)

Risk increases if symptoms (Sx) compatible with TB,
exposure to active TB, risk factors, employment at health facilities, HIV positive, immunosuppressed
member of racial or ethnic minority

PPD negative

- No Sx — Presumed uninfected
- Sx compatible with TB — Chest x-ray (abdominal shield)
  - Normal — Presume not TB
  - Abnormal, compatible with TB — Collect three sputums for smear and culture (TB) — Evaluate for other pulmonary disease — Consider treatment for TB

PPD positive — Chest x-ray (abdominal shield)

- Normal
  - No Sx — PPD reactor
    - Conversion within 1–2 years — Start INH prophylaxis, 2nd trimester; Give 6 to 9 mos
    - Old conversion; No or inadequate INH prophylaxis — Wait until after delivery; Repeat chest x-ray, if normal, INH prophylaxis 9 mos, if <35 years old
  - Sx — Collect three sputa for smear/culture Look for extrapulmonary disease-biopsy — Treatment for TB

- Old lesion No Sx — Rx after pregnancy
  - Smear/culture negative — Treat (4 mos)

- Abnormal — Likely active on Sx — Collect three sputa for smear/culture (other specimens, see text) — Start therapy INH, RIF, ethambutol (see text)
  - Smear negative culture positive — Treat (9 mos)
  - Smear/culture positive — Treat (9 mos to 1 yr)

change medication according to sensitivity

Source: Reprinted with permission, from Jacobs, R. F., and Abernathy, R. S. Management of tuberculosis in pregnancy and the newborn. *Clin. Perinatol.* 15:310, 1988.

infant's or mother's isolate is known. If there is a possibility that drug resistance is present (prior therapy to mother, recent immigrant, increased prevalence of resistant TB in the area), treatment with streptomycin or kanamycin should be considered after consultation with an expert in the management of TB. (Streptomycin is available from the Pfizer Streptomycin Program, Pfizer Pharmaceuticals, New York, NY, tel: 1-800-254-4445.) Since neonates are at greater risk to develop extrapulmonary tuberculosis (meningitis, miliary TB) they are initially treated as in tuberculosis meningitis with INH, RIF, pyrazinamide and sometimes streptomycin for 1–2 months followed by INH and RIF daily or twice weekly for 9–12 months, once sensitivities are known. Treatment of congenital TB must include two bactericidal drugs to which the organism is sensitive. Various combinations have been used [1,6,7]. The decision to use streptomycin should be made with great care because of the side effects and the fact that it may not significantly change the outcome except in drug resistant TB [1,2,6].

Drug susceptibility patterns from the mother are usually the same as those in the infant. Tuberculous meningitis requires 2 months of daily treatment with INH, RIF, pyrazinamide, and streptomycin followed by INH or RIF daily or twice weekly for 10 months. Dexamethasone should be considered as adjunctive therapy for tuberculous meningitis [1]. HIV-infected newborns need special treatment [1,2,7]. Syrup preparation of INH and RIF are unstable. Crushed tablets must be used. INH or RIF (Rifadin IV) are available as IM or IV preparations.

  C. **Other management of the infant of the mother with tuberculosis**
    1. **Active infections in the mother**
      a. **Hematogenous spread** (miliary disease, bone disease, meningitis, endometrial disease, etc., in mother) or untreated pulmonary disease in mother. Perform PPD skin test, chest x-ray, and culture on infant. If the baby appears infected, treat as in congenital TB (see **III.B**). If there are no clinical or radiographic signs of infection in the infant, separate the infant from the mother if the mother is felt to be infectious at the time of delivery. If the mother is judged to be nonin-

Table 23-11. Antituberculosis drugs for perinatal infection

Drug	Activity	Dosage (mg/kg/day)	Side effects
INH	Bactericidal	10–15 (or 20–40 mg/kg twice weekly)	Peripheral neuritis, convulsions, hepatoxic
Rifampin	Bactericidal	10–20 (or 10–20 mg/kg twice weekly)	Orange coloration of body fluids, hepatotoxic, nausea, vomiting
Pyrazinamide	Bactericidal	30–40	Hepatotoxic
Streptomycin	Bactericidal	20–40	Ototoxic, nephrotoxic
Ethambutol	Bacteriostatic	15–25	Optic neuritis
Ethionamide*	Bacteriostatic	15–20	Hepatotoxic
Cycloserine*	Bacteriostatic	15–20	CNS manifestations
Para-amino-salicylic acid*	Bacteriostatic	150	Gastrointestinal, hepatotoxic, allergic reactions
Capreomycin*	Bacteriostatic	15–30	Ototoxic, nephrotoxic, pain at the site of injection

Source: Rosenfeld, E. A., et al. Tuberculosis in infancy in 1990's. *PCNA* 40:1087, 1993.
*Should be used only for therapy of multidrug-resistant strains [1,9].

fectious (negative sputum smear, stable chest x-ray) the infant and mother can be united. The infant is given daily INH for at least 6 months. HIV positive children should be treated for one year. The PPD should be repeated at 4–6 weeks, 3 months, and 6 months of age. If it turns positive, INH should be given for 1 year. Other family members should be investigated for disease. If the skin test and the chest x-ray are negative, INH may be stopped depending on the status of the mother and other contacts. BCG should be considered if compliance is a problem (see V) [2,8].

b. **The mother has active disease, is on treatment, yet is suspected of being contagious.** The baby is separated from the mother until the mother is felt to be noncontagious and is known to be complying with therapy and the infant is on treatment. The baby is treated with INH and skin tested as in **a**. The household is carefully investigated. BCG vaccine should be considered for the infant if there is concern about compliance and because it may have some protective effect in this situation (see V).

c. **The mother with newly diagnosed, untreated minimal disease or disease that has been treated for over 2 weeks and who is felt to be noncontagious.** The infant should receive INH. The family and extended family should be carefully investigated. The mother can breast-feed. The infant should have a chest x-ray at 4–6 weeks of age. A PPD skin test should be performed at 4–6 weeks, 3 months, and 6 months of age. If the PPD is negative at 4 months of age and there is no active disease in the family, INH can be discontinued in the infant. Separation of the infant from the mother is not necessary if compliance with the treatment plan is ensured. If there is noncompliance, the mother has acid-fast bacillus (AFB)-positive sputum, other family members have active disease, or supervision is not possible the infant should be separated from contagious family members. BCG vaccine should be considered in a setting where compliance is doubtful.

2. **No active infection in the mother**
   a. **Mother with inactive infection, receiving treatment, with negative sputum and stable chest x-ray.** The infant is at some risk even if the mother's sputum is negative.
      (1) The mother should have a chest x-ray at 3 and 6 months postpartum and continued maternal treatment assured.
      (2) Other family members should be investigated.
      (3) The infant should be skin tested (5TU-PPD) at 4 months of age.
      (4) The infant should be treated with INH for 4 months.
      (5) At 4 months of age, if the infant has a negative skin test, the mother is AFB smear and culture negative, and contacts are not infectious, INH can be stopped.
      (6) The skin test on the infant should be repeated at 6, 9, and 12 months of age.
      (7) If the skin test has over 5 mm induration, the baby should have a chest x-ray, be investigated for TB and INH continued for 12 months.
      (8) BCG vaccine should be considered.
   b. **Mother with history of adequate treatment.** The mother should have a chest x-ray at 3 and 6 months postpartum, since there is some possibility that exacerbation may occur during pregnancy.
      (1) The infant is not separated from the mother. PPD skin tests are performed on the baby every 3 months for 1 year; after that, tests are performed yearly.
      (2) BCG vaccine and isoniazid are not given to the infant.
      (3) The family is investigated for evidence of infection.
   c. **Mother with positive result on testing with PPD tuberculin only.** The mother's sputum and chest x-ray are negative. There is some debate

as to whether the mother should be treated during pregnancy or whether treatment should commence only after delivery, because there is an increased risk of hepatitis associated with isoniazid therapy during pregnancy. The current recommendation is to avoid isoniazid therapy in pregnant women if possible. Generally, the woman is treated during pregnancy if she is a known recent converter (within the previous 2 years), has had recent contact with an infectious person, or if there is any suggestion of immunosuppression (HIV, steroids). INH is started during the second trimester [1,2].

(1) The infant is not separated from the mother.

(2) The infant is usually not given BCG vaccine, but it may be indicated if follow-up is poor.

(3) Isoniazid is usually not given. The baby is tested with PPD tuberculin every 3 months for 1 year. If the result is positive, the baby should be treated for 1 year.

IV. Newborns exposed to tuberculosis in the nursery. The documented risk is low, but there is a possibility of spread from infected infants or personnel. If the exposure is considered to be significant, the infant should be tested with 5 units of PPD and, if negative, treated with isoniazid 10 mg/kg per day for 3 months. The skin test should then be repeated; if it is still negative, therapy can be stopped. Nursery personnel should be tested with PPD yearly.

V. Bacillis Calmette-Guérin (BCG) vaccine [1,2]. BCG vaccines are live, attenuated strains of *Mycobacterium bovis*. These vaccines have been manufactured from many substrains of *M. bovis* that have been subcultured for years in many different laboratories. The last test of efficacy done in the United States was in 1955. There have been many culture passages since then. Some recent trials show efficacy; some do not. It does appear to have some protective effect against the development of tuberculosis and may make the disease less serious in those who contract it. The vaccine is considered for TB-free children who are at unavoidable risk of exposure and for whom other methods of prevention and control including INH preventive therapy have failed or are not feasible. BCG vaccine should be considered (1) for individuals, especially infants, who are tuberculin skin test negative and who live in a household with exposure to untreated or ineffectively treated patients with contagious tuberculosis or are exposed to persons with TB resistant to INH and rifampin and (2) for groups in which an excessive rate of new infection occurs and the usual surveillance and treatment have failed or are not feasible. BCG is often given to infants in whom there is a risk of exposure, preventive treatment might not be carried out, and there is uncertainty about the stability of the home situation. BCG may be given to infants from birth to 2 months of age. It is not necessary to skin test these infants. After 2 months, BCG is given only to individuals with negative skin tests. PPD should be repeated 2–3 months after vaccinations. If the PPD is negative, the vaccine should be readministered. The package insert should be read, and the instructions for administration should be followed carefully. In normal individuals, side effects or complications from BCG are rare. Complications reported are severe and include prolonged ulceration at the vaccination site, lymphadenitis, osteomyelitis, and lupoid reactions. In immunodeficient patients, disseminated BCG and death may occur. "If the risk of TB is low, BCG should not be given to children with known or suspected HIV infection. In populations where the risk of TB is high, the World Health Organization (WHO) has recommended that **asymptomatic** HIV infected children receive BCG at birth or shortly thereafter" [2]. Patients with burns or generalized skin infection should not receive BCG. INH may decrease the effectiveness of BCG. INH has **documented efficacy** and should not be withheld in order to give BCG, which has doubtful efficacy.

References
1. American Academy of Pediatrics: Chemotherapy for tuberculosis in infants and children. *Pediatrics* 89:161, 1992.

2. American Academy of Pediatrics. *Tuberculosis Redbook: Report of the Committee on Infectious Diseases* (24th Ed.). Elk Grove, Ill,: AAP, 1997, p. 541.
3. Davidson, P. T. Managing TB in pregnancy. *Lancet* 346:199, 1995.
4. Hageman, J., et al. Congenital tuberculosis. *Pediatrics* 66:980, 1980.
5. Mofenson, L. M., et al. TB transmission study. *Arch. Int. Med.* 155:1066, 1995.
6. Penn, R. L., and Betts, R. F., Tuberculosis: Basic concepts, chap. 9. In R. E. Reese and R. F. Betts (Eds.), *A Practical Approach to Infectious Diseases* (3rd Ed.). Little, Brown and Co., Boston, 1991.
7. Rosenfeld, E. A., et al. Tuberculosis in infancy in the 1990's. *PCNA* 40:1097, 1993.
8. Smith, M. H. D., and Teele, D. U. Tuberculosis. In: J. S. Remington and J. O. Klein (Eds), *Infectious Diseases of the Fetus and Newborn Infant* (4th Ed.). Philadelphia: W.B. Saunders, 1995.
9. Vellejo, J. G. Clinical features: Diagnosis and treatment of tuberculosis in infants. *Pediatrics* 94:1, 1994.

Syphilis [1,2]
John P. Cloherty

I. Epidemiology

The incidence of cases of primary and secondary syphilis reported in the United States increased from 13.7/100,000 in 1981 to 20.3/100,000 in 1990. It was 17.3/100,000 in 1991 and 13.7/100,000 in 1992. In blacks the incidence was 52.6/100,000 in 1985 and 121.8/100,000 in 1989. It is estimated that only one-third of cases are reported. These increases are mostly among teenagers and in heterosexuals. The number of cases of congenital syphilis reported to the Centers for Disease Control was 264 in 1985, 4408 in 1991, and 3850 in 1992. In most cases of congenital syphilis the maternal infection has been recently acquired or at least within 5 years of the pregnancy [3]. The more recent the maternal infection, the more likely the infant will be affected. Although transmission is thought to occur more commonly in the last two trimesters, the spirochete of syphilis can cross the placenta at any time during pregnancy, as shown by the recovery of spirochetes from the tissue of two fetuses of 9 and 10 weeks' gestation [4].

A. Congenital syphilis. The major factors contributing to the occurrence of congenital syphilis are as follows:

1. No prenatal care
2. Prenatal care—negative serologic test for syphilis (STS) in first trimester, but test not repeated
3. No STS test performed
4. Negative maternal STS at delivery in a mother who had syphilis but had not yet converted her blood test
5. Laboratory error
6. Delay in treatment
7. Prenatal treatment failures
8. Insufficient data

B. High-risk factors. Epidemiologic factors suggesting high risk for exposure are as follows [3]:

1. Inadequate prenatal care
2. Unwed mother
3. Teenaged mother
4. Drug abuse in mother or sexual partner
5. Sexual promiscuity
6. Sexual contact with someone known to have a sexually transmitted disease (STD)
7. Past history of a STD
8. Disadvantaged minority group
9. Poverty

10. Homelessness
11. HIV infection
    The majority of congenital syphilis cases reported in Massachusetts between 1986 and 1989 were associated with late or no prenatal care. Many were associated with drug abuse.

II. Diagnosis of syphilis [1,6]

A. Mother

1. Clinical signs. Syphilis is a chronic, often latent infection with some clinically recognizable stages. The incubation period is usually 3 weeks but ranges from 3 to 90 days.

   a. Primary syphilis is manifest by a chancre which may be in any area such as vagina, anus, or mouth. It is often accompanied by lymphadenopathy.

   b. Secondary syphilis occurs 3–6 weeks after the appearance of the chancre, often after the chancre is resolved. Sometimes the existence of the primary chancre is not noticed. The symptoms and signs may be rash, sore throat, fever, headache, adenopathy, myalgia, alopecia, condylomata lata, and painless ulcers of mucous membranes. These symptoms resolve without treatment with some patients developing recurrence of the manifestations of secondary syphilis.

   c. Latent syphilis—nonclinical symptoms but positive serologic tests.

   d. Late or tertiary syphilis: lymphocytic meningitis, meningovascular syphilis, dementia, posterior column disease (tabes dorsalis), cardiovascular syphilis, destructive lesions of the skin or bone.

2. Laboratory testing. All pregnant women should have serologic testing for syphilis (STS) at the first prenatal visit. A second STS should be performed at about **28 weeks' gestation.** Some states recommend this second test only for communities and populations with a high prevalence of syphilis or for high-risk patients. Women who are at high risk or if the results of testing are unknown should have serologic screening at delivery. Infants should not be discharged from the hospital until negative maternal serologic status or adequate therapy has been documented. In women at very high risk, consideration should be given to repeating serologic testing 1 month postpartum to capture the rare patient who had early primary infection at delivery and had not developed a positive blood test [2,5,6].

3. Serologic tests. The spirochete has a glycosaminoglycan layer, three sheathed flagella at each end, six major proteins in the outer membrane, and a double wall that contains cardiolipin. Some of the cardiolipin comes from damaged host tissues. Antibodies to the cardiolipin are the antigen for the non-treponemal serologic tests such as the VDRL and RPR.

   a. Nontreponemal tests [1,3,6]: RPR (rapid plasma reagin), VDRL (Venereal Disease Research Laboratory), ART (automated reagin test).

       These tests measure antibody directed against lipiodol antigen from *Treponema pallidum* and/or its interaction with host tissues. These antibodies correlate with ongoing tissue damage, give quantitative results, are helpful indicators of disease activity, and are useful for follow-up after treatment. Titers usually rise with each new infection and fall after treatment. Nontreponemal tests may be falsely negative, i.e., nonreactive, in early primary, latent acquired, and late congenital syphilis. Seventy-five percent of symptomatic cases of primary syphilis, 100% of cases of secondary syphilis, and 75% of cases of latent and tertiary syphilis will have a positive RPR or VDRL. In secondary syphilis, the VDRL or RPR is usually positive in a titer >1:16. If this is the first attack of primary syphilis, the RPR/VDRL will become nonreactive 1 year after treatment. Patients with secondary syphilis will usually become negative in 2 years. Those with early latent syphilis <1 year's duration will usually become negative within 4 years. After the first attack of early latent syphilis of 1–2 years' duration, 75% of patients will become RPR/VDRL-negative in 5 years. Of those with late latent syphilis, 45% will become seronegative in 5 years. The rest will remain seropositive. A sustained fourfold decrease in titer of the nontreponemal test with treatment (1:16 to 1:4) demonstrates adequate therapy; a similar increase after treatment suggests reinfection.

One percent of the time, the positive RPR or VDRL is not caused by syphilis. This has been called a **biologic false-positive (BFP) reaction** and is probably related to tissue damage from various causes. **Acute BFP reactions** are those which resolve in 6 months and are usually associated with illnesses such as viral exanthems, vaccinations, hepatitis, mononucleosis, endocarditis, IV drug abuse, and mycoplasma or protozoa infections. These patients usually have low titers (1:8 or less) and normal treponemal tests. Rarely, BFP reactions are seen as a result of pregnancy. **Chronic BFP reactions** may be seen in chronic hepatitis, cirrhosis, tuberculosis, some very elderly patients, malignancy (if associated with excess γ-globulin), connective tissue disease, or autoimmune disease. Many patients with systemic lupus erythematosus will have a positive RPR or VDRL. The titer is usually 1:8 or less. While most patients with BFP reactions have negative treponemal tests, some patients with systemic lupus erythematosus or rheumatoid arthritis and chronic BFP also may have positive treponemal tests. Another problem with the nontreponemal tests is the occasional negative reaction due to the **prozone phenomenon;** that is, a negative reaction may occur when undiluted serum is used. Negative reactions also may occur in late syphilis. Any positive nontreponemal test should be confirmed with one of the treponemal tests. Nontreponemal tests can be used to differentiate Lyme disease from syphilis, as the VDRL is uniformly nonreactive in Lyme disease [1].

   b. **Treponemal antibody tests.** These tests detect an interaction between surface antigens of *T. pallidum* and serum immunoglobulins. The test often used is the **fluorescent treponemal antibody absorption test (FTA-Abs).** This test is difficult to do and in many states has been replaced by the **microhemaglutination assay for antibody to T. pallidum (MHA-TP),** which gives similar results.

   Ninety percent of patients with a primary syphilitic chancre will have a positive FTA-Abs test. All patients with secondary and late syphilis will have a positive FTA-Abs test. Once these tests are positive, they will remain positive for life. They will tell if an infection ever occurred, but not if an actual infection is present. Treponemal antibody titers do not correlate with disease activity and should be reported as positive or negative and should not be used to monitor disease activity. In some cases, where an antibody to DNA is present, such as systemic lupus erythematosus, rheumatoid arthritis, polyarteritis, and other autoimmune diseases, a positive FTA-Abs will be present in the absence of any present or previous infection with syphilis. Rarely, pregnancy per se will cause a positive test. A negative test excludes previous or past infection except in very early primary infection or past infection that was treated before the FTA-Abs test turned positive. Treponemal tests are also not 100% specific for syphilis; positive reactions occur in subjects with other spirochetal diseases such as yaws, pinta, leptospirosis, rat-bite fever, and Lyme disease.

B. **Infant** [1,2]
   1. **Infants should be evaluated for syphilis** if they were born to seropositive women who

    a. Were untreated or have poorly documented treatment
    b. Were treated during pregnancy, especially in the last month
    c. Were treated with a drug other than penicillin
    d. Did not have the expected drop in nontreponemal titers after treatment (fourfold drop)
    e. Were treated but did not have serologic evidence of cure
    f. Have the risk factors listed in **I.B**
    g. Serologic testing also should be performed at delivery in communities and populations at risk for congenital syphilis. Serologic tests can be nonreactive among infants infected late during their mother's pregnancy.

2. Clinical signs. Clinical signs in the infant may be a persistent rhinitis, snuffles, rash, hepatosplenomegaly, distended abdomen, lymphadenopathy, anemia, hemorrhage, disseminated intravascular coagulation, jaundice, ascites, hydrops, nephrosis, chorioretinitis, meningitis, osteochondritis, or periostitis. Stillbirth, prematurity, intrauterine growth retardation, and a large placenta may be seen. There is a delayed effect in the nervous system, teeth, and eyes. Clinical signs of central nervous system (CNS) infection rarely appear in the newborn, even though one-third to one-half of infected infants will have CNS involvement. Some infants will have postnatal failure to thrive.

3. Infant laboratory tests
    a. Dark-field examination of nasal discharge, spinal fluid, or scrapings from any cutaneous lesion. The use of monoclonal or polyclonal antibody on these specimens may be diagnostic.
    b. X-rays for evidence of periostitis or osteochondritis
    c. Cerebrospinal fluid (CSF) examination may reveal an increased mononuclear count, elevated protein level, and positive serology (VDRL or RPR). If the VDRL is positive in the CSF, it is considered diagnostic of neurosyphilis. It may be negative in the presence of neurosyphilis and cannot be used to absolutely rule out neurosyphilis. The FTA-Abs test is less specific (more false-positive results), but is very sensitive. When the FTA-Abs test is negative in the CSF, it is good evidence against neurosyphilis.
    In the neonatal period interpretation of CSF values may be difficult. Normal values of protein and WBC are higher in preterm infants. Values of 25 WBC/mm^3 and 150 mg protein/dL may be normal. There are other causes of elevated WBC and protein in the CSF besides syphilis. If syphilitic infection cannot be excluded the infant should be treated.
    d. Pathologic examination of the placenta, cord, and membranes including specific fluorescent antitreponemal antibody staining.
    e. Nontreponemal reagin serologic tests (RPR) with titer, as in **A.3.**
    f. FTA-Abs test with titer, as in **A.3.** Since the IgG portion of the antibody in the nontreponemal (RPR) and treponemal (FTA-Abs) tests is transported across the placenta, these tests will be positive even if the mother did not transmit the infection to her infant and whether she was adequately treated or not. Monthly determination of the nontreponemal tests with titer (RPR/VDRL with titer) will show a fall in titer to zero by 2–4 months if the antibody is passively acquired. If the baby was infected and made antibody, the titer will not fall or may rise. The tests may be negative at birth if the infection was acquired late in pregnancy. Repeating the test later will confirm the diagnosis.
    g. IgM-FTA-Abs test. This test uses fluorescent-labeled anti-human IgM to detect fluorescent treponemal IgM antibodies in the newborn blood. Since IgM antibody is usually not transmitted across the placenta, a positive test should indicate congenital syphilis. However, clinical studies have shown false-negative results in 20–40% of cases and false-positive reactions possibly related to rheumatoid

factor in 10% of cases. The test cannot be recommended at this time.

h. A new FTA-Abs 19S IgM assay is better than the FTA-Abs IgM test but is difficult to do. The IgM ELISA is being evaluated for the diagnosis of congenital syphilis.

i. Infants with clinically evident syphilis should have an ophthalmologic examination [2,3].

III. Prevention of congenital syphilis by treatment of infected pregnant women [1–3,5]. Pregnant women should have serologic screening for syphilis as described in **II.**

A. Treatment protocol for pregnant women
  1. Clinical disease in mother—treat.
  2. No clinical disease in mother
   a. Negative serologic test (RPR/VDRL)
    (1) No disease—no treatment. Repeat test in late pregnancy, as in **II.**
    (2) Early disease, symptomatic—treat.
    (3) Exposure to a person with infectious syphilis in the past 90 days—treat. It may be prudent to treat even if the exposure is before 90 days, if tests are not available and follow-up is doubtful.
   b. Known positive (VDRL/RPR)
    (1) Previous adequate treatment—observe and follow titers.
    (2) Untreated—treat.
    (3) Previous inadequate treatment or questionable treatment—treat.
   c. Possible false-positive reactions (VDRL/RPR)
    (1) If positive FTA-Abs/MHA-TP—treat (see **I**).
    (2) If negative FTA-Abs/MHA-TP—observe (see **II**).
   d. Known biologic false-positive reaction—observe.
   e. New positive
    (1) Treat mother and infant.
    (2) Previous adequate treatment—observe and follow titers.
    (3) Previous inadequate treatment—treat.
    (4) Untreated—treat.
   f. Err on the side of treatment when the diagnosis of syphilis cannot be excluded with reasonable certainty. In pregnancy, nontreponemal test titers may rise for nonspecific reasons.
   Patients who have adequate documentation of proper treatment for syphilis need not be retreated unless clinical, serologic, or epidemiologic evidence of reinfection exists, e.g., clinical lesions, a sustained (for ≥2 weeks) fourfold titer rise in a quantitative nontreponemal test, or a history of recent (within 90 days) sexual exposure to a person with early infectious syphilis. A person with recent venereal exposure to a person with syphilis has a 25–50% chance of acquiring syphilis and may have negative tests because she is in the early stage of infection. Some chancres may be difficult to see.

B. Specific recommendations for treatment of pregnant mothers who have syphilis. Penicillin is the drug of choice. The regimen should be that appropriate for the stage of syphilis [2,5].
  1. Primary and secondary syphilis. Benzathine penicillin G (Bicillin) in a total dose of 4.8 million units in two doses divided 1 week apart (2.4 million units IM weekly × 2) or procaine penicillin G 600,000 units IM daily for 15 days. If the patient is HIV-positive with either early or late syphilis, the dose is procaine penicillin G 1.2 million units IM daily for 15 days or 4.0 million units IV every 4 hours for 15 days. In HIV-positive patients, treatment may be extended for 3 weeks.
  2. Early latent syphilis (without neurosyphilis). Patients are seroreactive, have no sign of disease and are thought to have **acquired syphilis**

within one year. The dosage is the same as in primary and secondary syphilis.

3. **Late latent syphilis** over one year duration or syphilis of unknown duration (without neurosyphilis). Benzathine penicillin G (Bicillin) in a total dose of 7.2 million units given as 2.4 million units IM weekly for 3 weeks (2.4 million units IM weekly × 3) or procaine penicillin G 600,000 units IM daily for 15 days.

4. **Neurosyphilis**

12–24 million units aqueous penicillin G daily administered as 2–4 million units IV every 4 hours for 10–14 days. If this cannot be accomplished, an alternative regimen of 2.4 million units of procaine penicillin IM daily plus two Benecid 500 mg orally 4 times a day for 10–14 days. At the end of these therapies, benzathine penicillin 2.4 million units is given. None of these regimens has been studied, and some have been associated with treatment failure in neurosyphilis.

5. **Late syphilis**

Patient with gumma or cardiovascular syphilis. Benzathine penicillin G 7.2 million units total given as 3 doses of 2.4 million units IM weekly for 3 weeks.

6. If the pregnant woman with syphilis is **allergic to penicillin,** she can still be treated with penicillin. There are no proven alternatives to penicillin. The history of penicillin allergy should be reviewed, and the patient should be skin-tested against the major and minor determinants for penicillin allergy. If these tests are negative, penicillin can be given under medical supervision. If the tests are positive, the patient can be desensitized and then given penicillin. Desensitization should be done in consultation with an expert and in a facility where emergency treatment is available. The specific method of desensitization to penicillin is reviewed in ref. 2.

7. The Jarisch-Herxheimer reaction may occur after treatment for syphilis. Febrile reactions with fetal distress, premature labor, or stillbirth are rare but possible. Therapy is necessary and must be given.

8. **Other drugs** have been associated with treatment failure in the fetus and should not be used. Ceftriaxone may be accepted in pregnant penicillin allergic women who cannot be desensitized, although there is limited experience and the dose and duration of treatment are not clear; 10 days of full dosage should be used.

If a mother is treated for syphilis in pregnancy, monthly follow-up should be provided. The antibody response should be the same as for a nonpregnant patient. Retreatment is given if needed. All patients with syphilis should be evaluated for other sexually transmitted diseases, such as gonorrhea, chlamydia, herpes, and HIV infection.

IV. Treatment for the infant [1–3]

A. In untreated pregnant women, syphilis can be transmitted to the infant regardless of the duration of the maternal disease, but transmission is more common the first year after infection. The infection appears to be more easily transmitted after the fourth month of pregnancy but can occur anytime in pregnancy. The organisms reach the fetus by way of the placenta and umbilical vein. The liver is the primary site of infection, with secondary spread to the skin, mucous membranes, bones, and CNS. Direct contact of the infant with infectious lesions at or after birth can result in infection. See **II.B** for diagnosis in the newborn.

1. **Negative serologic test**

a. **No disease—no treatment.** If the mother is infected late in pregnancy, it is possible to have a serologic-negative mother and infant as well as an initially asymptomatic infant, since there is no clinically observed primary infection stage in newborns who have in utero infection. Repeat clinical exam and testing are necessary for diagnosis especially in high-risk populations.

> b. **Early disease—treat.**
> **(1)** Symptomatic—treat.
2. **Positive serologic test**
   a. **Symptomatic** (e.g., snuffles, rash, hydrops, hepatomegaly, roentgeno-graphic findings, abnormal cerebrospinal fluid)—treat.
   b. **Asymptomatic**
      (1) If the baby's titer is three or four times higher than the mother's, treat. Some infants with syphilis will have the same titer as the mother.
      (2) If FTA-Abs test is 3 to 4+, treat.
      (3) If disease is poorly documented or the mother inadequately treated or untreated, treat.
      (4) If unreliable mother or doubtful follow-up, treat.
      (5) If the mother's infection was treated with any drug but peni-cillin, treat.
      (6) If the mother had a recent sexual exposure to an infected per-son, treat.
      (7) If the mother was treated in the last month of pregnancy, treat.
      (8) If the mother has HIV and was treated for syphilis with less than neurosyphilis regimen, treat.
      (9) If the mother was treated before or during pregnancy with an appropriate regimen but did not have an adequate serologic re-sponse, treat.
      (10) If the tests in **II.B.3** suggest infection, treat.
      (11) If CSF VDRL is reactive or CSF exam suggests infection, treat.
      (12) If lab tests cannot exclude infection, treat.
3. If the baby's VDRL/RPR, FTA-Abs, or both are positive and if history and clinical examination and lab tests make infection unlikely, it is safe to repeat titers on VDRL/RPR and FTA-Abs at monthly intervals. Any significant rise in titer or development of clinical signs requires treat-ment. If the serology is not negative by 6 months of age, treat.
4. If there are **only transferred antibodies,** the baby should have a falling titer and be negative by 4–6 months.
5. A **cerebrospinal fluid examination** should be performed on all infants to be treated for congenital syphilis (see **II.B.3.c**).
6. Some would treat all newborns with a positive serologic test for syphilis because it may be difficult to document that the mother has had adequate treatment and falling serologic titers, a low titer may be present in latent maternal syphilis, infected newborns may have no clinical signs at birth, and follow-up/compliance may be difficult in the population at risk for congenital syphilis. If the mother has received an appropriate regimen of penicillin therapy more than 1 month before delivery, the infant's clinical and laboratory examination are normal, and follow-up is assured, some would follow the infant without treat-ment [1].
B. **Specific therapy for the infant under 4 weeks of age** [1,2]
   1. Infants who are felt to be infected but who have no evidence of CNS in-fection should be treated with **aqueous crystalline penicillin G** 100,000 to 150,000 units/kg per day IM or IV (divided every 12 hours for the first 7 days of life and divided every 8 hours after 7 days) for 10 to 14 days or **aqueous crystalline penicillin** 150,000 units/kg per day IM once daily for 10 to 14 days. If more than one day of therapy is missed the entire regimen should be repeated.
   2. Infants with CNS infection (CSF pleocytosis, elevated CSF protein, pos-itive CSF serology) should be treated with **aqueous crystalline peni-cillin** 150,000 units/kg per day IV or IM divided every 12 hours for the first 7 days of life and divided every 8 hours after 7 days for three weeks or **aqueous procaine penicillin** 50,000 units/kg per day IM for 3 weeks. Err on the side of higher doses and longer treatment.

3. If infants who have been evaluated appear to be at low risk for congenital syphilis but close follow-up is doubtful, then they should be given **benzathine penicillin G** 50,000 units/kg per day IM as a one-time dose. It should be recognized that there will be treatment failures with this dosage.

4. Some cases of persistent hepatitis have been seen in infants treated for congenital syphilis.

V. **Follow-up of infant** [1–3]

A. A seroreactive infant (or an infant whose mother was seroreactive at delivery) who was not treated for congenital syphilis should have follow-up examination at 1, 2, 3, 6, and 12 months. Nontreponemal antibody titers should decline by 3 months and be negative by 6 months if the infant was not infected and the positive titers were the result of passive transfer of antibody from the mother. If the titers are stable or increasing the child should be re-evaluated, including CSF exam and fully treated. For dosage in children over 1 month of age see refs. 1 and 2. Passively transferred antibodies may last 6 months and rarely one year. If antibodies are present at 6 months even at low titer evaluate and treat. Infants treated for congenital syphilis should have follow-up serologic tests with titers at 2, 4, 6, and 12 months. Any rise in titer is an indication for retreatment. The nontreponemal tests will become negative in 90% of adequately treated infants. Patients with persistent titers, even though low, should be considered for retreatment. The FTA-Abs test may remain positive even with adequate treatment.

B. Infants with neurosyphilis should have follow-up serologic titers at monthly intervals for 3 months and then be followed as those with syphilis. Spinal fluid should be examined every 6 months for 3 years or until the cell count is normal. If the infant is adequately treated, the cell count and protein will usually become normal in 6 months, and the nontreponemal titers will fall. The FTA-Abs test may remain positive. Any rise in titers or increase in cell count is an indication for retreatment. A positive VDRL in the CSF at 6 months is an indication for retreatment. If the cell count is abnormal in 2 years or a downward trend is not present at each exam, retreat.

VI. **Infection control.** Nasal secretions and open syphilitic lesions are very infectious. Secretions, blood, and bodily fluid precautions should be taken, and health care personnel should wear gloves when caring for the newborn at risk for congenital syphilis. The infant is not infectious 24 hours after penicillin therapy is begun. Those who had close contact with an infected infant or mother before precautions were taken should be examined and tested for infection. Treatment should be considered.

VII. Infants and their mothers at risk for or with syphilis should be evaluated for the presence of other disease such as herpes, gonorrhea, chlamydia, and HIV.

VIII. Assistance and guidance is available from the Centers for Disease Control and Prevention, Atlanta, Georgia, or state departments of health.

References

1. American Academy of Pediatrics. *Report of the Committee on Infectious Diseases (Redbook).* Elk Grove Village, Ill.: AAP, 24th ed. 1997, p. 504.

2. Centers for Disease Control. Sexually transmitted disease treatment guidelines. *MMWR* 42:1, 1993.

3. Evans, H. E., et al. Congenital syphilis. *Clin. Perinatol.* 21:149, 1994.

4. Harter, C., et al. Fetal syphilis in the first trimester. *Am. J. Obstet. Gynecol.* 124:705, 1976.

5. Massachusetts Department of Public Health. STD Division. STD Guidelines. Boston, Massachusetts, May 1994.

6. Rein, M. F. Sexually transmitted diseases. In: R. E. Reese and R. F. Betts (Eds.), *A Practical Approach to Infectious Diseases* (3rd Ed.). Boston: Little, Brown: 1991, Chap. 13.

7. Sanchez, P. J. Syphilis. In: F. D. Bang, J. R. Inglefinger, and E. R. Wald (Eds.), *Gellis and Kagans Current Pediatric Therapy.* Philadelphia: Saunders, 1993.

Lyme Disease
John P. Cloherty

I. **Lyme disease** (Lyme borreliosis) [1,3,9,11,14] is caused by the spirochete *Borrelia burgdorferi.* Lyme disease is the most common tick-borne disease in the United States. Most cases in the U.S. are clustered in the Northeast from Massachusetts to Maryland, the Midwest in Wisconsin and Minnesota or in California. There have been cases reported from all states, Canada, Europe, China, Japan, and Russia. The distribution of cases correlated with the distribution of known tick vectors *Ixodes scapularis* (previously known as *Ixodes dammini*) in the East and Midwest and *Ixodes pacificus* in the West. *Ixodes racinus* is the vector in Europe. White-footed mice and deer are important in the life cycle of the tick. Distribution of Lyme disease correlates with the distribution of these hosts. Humans are the most likely to be infected in June, July, and August. Clinical manifestations of Lyme disease are noted in Table 23-12.

Fetal infection with *B. burgdorferi* has been documented with maternal infection in pregnancy, but the transmission appears to occur at a low frequency. However, data are insufficient to establish the true risk of fetal disease. Transmission has been documented in both early and late gestation, but the relative risk of transmission and severity of fetal disease as a function of gestational age has not been established. Schlesinger et al. [10] and Weber et al. [13] described newborn infants with multiple organ involvement with *B. burgdorferi.* The first infant died on day 2 from congenital heart disease and was found to have spirochetes in the spleen, kidney, and bone marrow. The second infant died on day 1 with respiratory failure and complications of CNS dysfunction, and spirochetes were identified in the liver and brain. In both cases, maternal infection was believed to have occurred in the first trimester. A third case report described the identification of spirochetes in a stillborn infant to a woman with a history of clinical symptoms of Lyme disease [5].

The pregnancy outcomes of 19 women with Lyme disease in pregnancy have been reported [7]. Adverse fetal/newborn findings were present in 5 cases. Complications included prematurity, intrauterine fetal demise, cortical blindness, syndactyly, and rash. In one of the cases, erythema chronicum migrans and meningoencephalitis occurred in a woman at 37 weeks' gestation. The infant was delivered 7 days later and was asymptomatic in the immediate postpartum period. On day 5, the infant developed petechiae and a vesicular rash that resolved with IV penicillin G. Three of the cases with adverse outcomes occurred in women who received antibiotic therapy. In a second study, 17 women who developed Lyme disease in pregnancy were followed [2]. All these women received antibiotic therapy. There was one aborted fetus and syndactyly in a second infant who had no other abnormalities. It is unclear if all these outcomes are a consequence of *B. burgdorferi* infection or occurred by chance but it is clear that fetal infection can occur and cause adverse effects.

II. **Diagnosis.** Lyme disease may be diagnosed by the appearance of a typical rash (erythema chronicum migrans) in women living in or visiting an area where cases of Lyme disease have been previously reported. However, the spectrum of clinical symptoms may be quite variable (see Table 23-12). At this time, there have been too few cases of neonatal disease to predict the likely clinical findings in newborn infants with active infection. Serologic testing begins with ELISA or ELISA capture for specific IgM or IgG. If tests are borderline or a false positive is suspected, a Western blot can be done [11]. Sometimes in pregnancy, there is a false negative result [6]. If there is possible neurologic Lyme disease spinal fluid should be analyzed for IgG, IgM, and IgA antibody [11].

Table 23-12. Manifestations of Lyme disease by stage*

System[†]	Localized (stage 1)	Early infection Disseminated (stage 2)	Late infection (persistent [stage 3])
Skin	Erythema migrans	Secondary annular lesions, malar rash, diffuse erythema or urticaria, evanescent lesions, lymphocytoma	Acrodermatitis chronica atrophicans, localized sclerodermalike lesions
Musculoskeletal system		Migratory pain in joints, tendons, bursae, muscle, bone; brief arthritis attacks; myositis;[†] osteomyelitis;[‡] panniculitis[‡]	Prolonged arthritis attacks, chronic arthritis, peripheral enthesopathy, periostitis or joint subluxations below lesions of acrodermatitis
Neurologic system		Meningitis, cranial neuritis, Bell's palsy, motor or sensory radiculoneuritis, subtle encephalitis, mononeuritis multiplex, myelitis;[‡] chorea,[‡] cerebellar ataxia[‡]	Chronic encephalomyelitis, spastic paraparesis, ataxic gait, subtle mental disorders, chronic axonal polyradiculopathy, dementia[‡]
Lymphatic system	Regional lymphadenopathy	Regional or generalized lymphadenopathy, splenomegaly	
Heart		Atrioventricular nodal block, myopericarditis, pancarditis	
Eyes		Conjunctivitis, iritis,[‡] choroiditis,[‡] retinal hemorrhage or detachment,[‡] panophthalmitis[‡]	Keratitis
Liver		Mild or recurrent hepatitis	
Respiratory system		Nonexudative sore throat, nonproductive cough, adult respiratory distress syndrome[‡]	
Kidney		Microscopic hematuria or proteinuria	
Genitourinary system		Orchitis[‡]	
Constitutional symptoms	Minor	Severe malaise and fatigue	Fatigue

*The classification by stages provides a guideline for the expected timing of the illness's manifestations, but this may vary from case to case.
[†]Systems are listed from the most to the least commonly affected.
[‡]The inclusion of this manifestation is based on one or a few cases.

III. Treatment of mothers and the newborn [1,8,11,13,14]. Patients known to have Lyme disease or who are suspected of having Lyme disease during pregnancy should be treated. The treatment is the same as for nonpregnant persons except that tetracycline is contraindicated.
Localized early Lyme disease (see stage 1, Table 23-12). Amoxicillin 500 mg po TID for 21 days.

In **mild localized disease** in pregnant women with penicillin allergy, erythromycin 250 mg po QID for 21–30 days has been used, but it may be less effective than amoxicillin [8]. For this reason it might be more prudent to treat with ceftriaxone as in disseminated disease.

Disseminated early Lyme disease or any manifestations of late disease—penicillin G 20 million units/day IV for 14–21 days. In penicillin allergy ceftriaxone, 2 gm/daily/IV as one dose for 14–21 days is given. Ceftriaxone may be more effective than penicillin in late disease [4]. It is often used because the once a day dosage is convenient for outpatient or home therapy.

Prophylactic treatment of tick bites in endemic areas remains controversial in the nonpregnant patient. It is recommended that asymptomatic pregnant women with tick bites from an endemic area be treated as in mild early localized disease [14]. This is done because the effects of infection in a developing fetus may be permanent, and false negative serologic results are common in pregnancy. The relative risk of fetal transmission as a function of severity of maternal disease, chronicity of maternal disease, or choice of antibiotic and route of administration is not known. Similarly, data are lacking on the optimal therapy for the newborn infant with symptoms of acute Lyme disease. In the study by Markowitz et al. [7], a 38-week fetus born to a mother who developed acute Lyme disease 1 week prior to delivery developed petechiae and a vesicular rash that resolved with the intravenous administration of penicillin G for 10 days. If an infant is thought to have Lyme disease, treatment with penicillin or ceftriaxone intravenously should be given for 14–21 days after studies are taken from blood and spinal fluid. If a mother was treated for Lyme disease with erythromycin during pregnancy, consideration should be given to treatment of the infant with penicillin or ceftriaxone.

References

1. American Academy of Pediatrics. Lyme disease. *Report of the Committee of Infectious Disease (Redbook),* 24th ed. Elk Grove, Ill.: American Academy of Pediatrics, 1997, p. 329.
2. Ciesielski, C. A., et al. Prospective study of pregnancy outcome in women with Lyme disease. Interscience Conference on Antimicrobial Agents and Chemotherapy, New York, 1987 (Abstract No. 39).
3. Kaslow, R. A. Current perspective on Lyme disease. *JAMA.* 267:1381, 1992.
4. Luft, B. J., et al. A perspective on the treatment of Lyme borreliosis. *Rev. Infect. Dis.* 2:S1518, 1989.
5. MacDonald, A. B., et al. Stillbirth following maternal Lyme disease. *N.Y. J. Med.* 87:615, 1987.
6. MacDonald, A. B. Gestational Lyme borreliosis: Implications for the fetus. *Rheum. Dis. Clin. North Am.* 15:657, 1989.
7. Markowitz, L. E., et al. Lyme disease during pregnancy. *JAMA* 255:3394, 1986.
8. Medical Letter. Treatment of Lyme disease. *Med. Drug. Ther.* 31:794, 1989.
9. Ostrov, B. E., et al. Lyme disease difficulties in diagnosis and management. *PCNA* 38:535, 1991.
10. Schlesinger, P. A., et al. Maternal-fetal transmission of the Lyme disease spirochete. *Ann. Intern. Med.* 103:67, 1985.
11. Shodick, N.A., and Liang, M. H. Management of Lyme disease: *Med. Update, Brigham & Women's Hospital.* V (1):1, 1993.
12. Stechenberg, B. W. Lyme disease: The latest great imitator. *Pediatr. Infect. Dis. J.* 7:402, 1988.
13. Weber, K., et al. *B. burgdorferi* in a newborn despite oral penicillin for Lyme disease during pregnancy. *Pediatr. Infect. Dis. J.* 7:286, 1988.

14. Weil, H. F. C., et al. Lyme Disease: Tick borne borreliosis. In: R. E. Reese and R. F. Betts (Eds.), *A Practical Approach to Infectious Diseases.* Boston: Little, Brown: 1991, Chap. 23.

Toxoplasmosis
Nicholas G. Guerina

I. **Toxoplasma gondii** is an obligate, intracellular protozoan parasite which is well-recognized as an important human pathogen. This is particularly true for the fetus, newborn infant, and immunocompromised adults. Many animals may become infected, but the cat is the only definitive host. During an acute infection the cat may shed up to 10 million oocysts in the stool per day for up to 2 weeks [22]. These oocysts may remain viable in soil for many months depending upon climactic conditions. Susceptible farm animals become infected by ingesting the oocysts resulting in localization of viable organisms in muscle cysts. Principal modes of transmission to humans beyond the newborn period is by the ingestion of the cysts in undercooked meat, or by the direct ingestion of oocysts. Transmission following the transfusion of whole blood or leukocytes may occur, but the risk is unknown. Normal children and adults are susceptible to acute infection if they lack specific antibody to the organism. Both humoral and cell-mediated immunity are important in the control of infection. Following an acute parasitemia, the organism invades tissues where cysts are formed. The cysts persist in multiple organs, probably for life. Most often these are of little consequence to the normal host, but progressive localized, or reactivated disease may occur in a subset of patients.

II. **Diagnosis**

A number of methods may be employed in the diagnosis of congenital toxoplasma infection [22]. These include isolation or histologic demonstration of the organism, detection of toxoplasma antigens in tissues and body fluids, detection of toxoplasma nucleic acid by polymerase chain reaction (PCR), and serological tests. Of these, serological tests are most frequently used and are often critical in diagnosing acute maternal and congenital infections. In addition, the PCR appears to be very sensitive and specific in determining fetal infection.

A. **Sabin-Feldman dye test.** This test makes use of the uptake by toxoplasma tachyzoites of the dye methylene blue (organisms appear swollen and blue). The tachyzoite membranes lyse in the presence of complement and specific antibody (IgG and IgM) resulting in a thin, unstained appearance to the organisms. There is extensive experience with the use of this test as a screening test for toxoplasma infection, and it has been recommended as the test of choice for antenatal maternal screening [25]. Since both IgG and IgM are detected, additional serologic tests may be required to further delineate acute from remote infection.

B. **Enzyme-linked immunosorbent assay (ELISA).** This test has been adapted for the detection of toxoplasma-specific IgG, IgM, IgA, and IgE. The IgG test is readily available in most commercial laboratories but has limited utility in the determination of acute infection in both pregnant women and newborn infants. A double-sandwich toxoplasma-specific IgM-ELISA (DS-IgM-ELISA) has been developed which greatly aids in the diagnosis of congenital toxoplasma infection [25]. Maternal IgM may remain elevated from months to more than one year so the test may not help in determining recent maternal infection. Since IgM does not cross the placenta, however, the test may be very useful in determining congenital infection.

Enzyme-linked immunosorbent assays have also been developed for measuring toxoplasma-specific IgA and IgE [25]. The IgA-ELISA aids in the diagnosis of recent maternal infection; although IgA may remain elevated for at least 26 weeks, it rises very early in infection and high titers correlate with recent maternal disease. The IgE-ELISA is a more recently developed

test which appears to be sensitive and specific and may be particularly useful in the serologic diagnosis of congenital infection.
C. **Immunosorbent agglutination assay (ISAGA).** This test measures toxoplasma-specific antibody captured from sera by the agglutination of a particulate antigen preparation [25]. Assays for detecting IgM and IgE have been developed and both tests may be complementary to ELISA procedures in determining congenital infection.
D. **Differential agglutination test.** This test compares agglutination titers for sera against formalin-fixed tachyzoites (HS antigen) with those against acetone- or methanol-fixed tachyzoites (AC antigen) [25]. The different test preparations display antigens present at different times in infection so the relative titers with each preparation are indicative of acute versus remote infection.
E. **Polymerase chain reaction (PCR).** This test has recently been adapted for the identification of *T. gondii* in amniotic fluid specimens obtained on women with acquired toxoplasma in pregnancy [14]. Ultrasonographic screening and studies on fetal blood obtained by percutaneous umbilical blood sampling were also used as previously described [16]. Congenital infection was identified in 34 of 339 fetuses by ultrasound/fetal blood testing and all of these cases were also identified by amniotic fluid PCR. In addition, 3 infants who were missed by ultrasound/fetal blood testing were identified by PCR. There was only one false negative and no false positive PCR result.
III. **Epidemiology and clinical manifestations**
A. **Maternal infection (Table 23-13).** The prevalence of toxoplasma antibody varies with age and geographic location. In the United States, 50 to 85% of women of childbearing age are at risk for acute toxoplasmosis in pregnancy. Seroprevalence data from New York City has shown that approximately 16% of childbearing women ages 15 years to 19 years are seropositive [7], but the seroprevalence increases to approximately 50% for >35 years old. Universal screening of newborn infants for toxoplasma-specific IgM has been conducted for the past 8 years in Massachusetts [11]. The screening is carried out on filter paper dried-blood spot specimens which are routinely sent to Public Health State Laboratories for screening for metabolic and endocrine abnormalities in all newborn infants. Over a 1-year period, screening for toxoplasma-specific IgG was also conducted. Since maternal IgG readily crosses the placenta, the prevalence of specific IgG in the newborn reflects the overall seroprevalence in childbearing women. It was found that 17% of <90,000 newborn specimens tested had IgG to *T. gondii* indicating that 83% of mothers were at risk for acute infection. Data from the National Collaborative Perinatal Project (National Institutes of Health) showed a toxoplasma seroprevalence rate of 38.7% for 22,000 women in the United States, and the estimated incidence of acute maternal infection in pregnancy was 1.1 per 1000 [23].
  Symptoms of acute toxoplasma infection in pregnant women may be transient and nonspecific, and most cases go undiagnosed in the absence of universal antibody screening. When symptoms are present they usually are limited to lymphadenopathy and fatigue; adenopathy may persist for months and a single lymph node may be involved. Less commonly, a mononucleosis-like syndrome characterized by fever, malaise, sore throat, headache, myalgia, and an atypical lymphocytosis has been described.
B. **Congenital infection.** Previous estimates of the incidence of congenital toxoplasma infection in certain areas of the United States have been as high as 1/1000 to 2/1000 births, but more recent studies suggest a lower incidence [1,6,8,9]. For example, cord blood screening for toxoplasma-specific IgM showed a decreasing incidence from 2/1000 to 0.1/1000 births [15,22]. An incidence of approximately 0.1/1000 births was also found for infected newborn identified through a newborn screening program in Massachusetts over a 6.5-year period beginning in January 1986 [11].

Table 23-13. Toxoplasma antibody screening algorithm for the determination of women with acute infection or who are at risk for acute infection in pregnancy

a. Initial serology performed at <2 months' gestation

neg dye test	pos dye test neg IgM	pos dye test pos IgM
↓	↓	↓
No infection (at risk for acute infection in pregnancy)	Infection before conception (no risk to fetus)*	Possible acute infection
		↓
		Repeat dye test in 3 weeks
		|
		Stable or decreased titer: Probable infection near or before conception (No risk to fetus)
		↓
		Increased dye titer: Acute material infection (fetus at risk)

b. Initial serology performed later in gestation

neg dye titer	Presence of 2 of the following:
↓	Clinical symptoms[†]
No infection (at risk for acute infection before delivery)	High dye titer[‡] pos IgM
	↓
	pAcute maternal infection (fetus at risk)

*Seropositive immunocompromised patients (especially HIV positive mothers) may be at risk for reactivation of toxoplasma with subsequent fetal transmission.
[†]Lymphadenopathy consistent with acute toxoplasma infection.
[‡]If clinical/IgM criteria met, but dye test titer low, repeat testing should demonstrate an increased titer.
Source: Guerina, N. G. Congenital infection with *Toxoplasma gondii. Pediatr. Ann.* 23:138, 1994.

Vertical transmission of *T. gondii* from mother to fetus occurs at an average rate of 30 to 40%, but the rate varies with the gestational age at which acute maternal infection occurs [8]. The average transmission rate is 15 percent for the first trimester but increases to 60% for the third trimester; transmission appears to correlate well with placental blood flow and may approach 90% at term. The severity of fetal disease is inversely proportional to gestational age. In the absence of toxoplasma-specific chemotherapy, most fetuses infected in the first trimester die in utero or in the neonatal period, or have severe central nervous system and ophthalmologic disease. Conversely, most fetuses infected in the second trimester, and all infants infected in the third trimester, have mild or subclinical disease in the newborn period.

Infants with congenital toxoplasma infection may present with one of four recognized patterns (Table 23-14): (1) symptomatic neonatal disease, (2) symptomatic disease occurring in the first months of life, (3) sequelae or relapse in infancy, or later childhood, of previously undiagnosed infection, and (4) subclinical infection [1]. The principal clinical findings for infants presenting with severe disease were described in the classic report of Eichenwald [10]. These infants invariably had some degree of central nervous system (CNS) involvement and often had significant retinal disease. The infants appeared to fall into one group who primarily had marked CNS

Table 23-14. Frequencies for initial clinical and laboratory abnormalities in infants with congenital toxoplasma infection from the Chicago Collaborative Treatment Trial* and the New England Regional Newborn Screening Program[†]

Clinical/laboratory finding	No. infants with specific finding (%)	
	Chicago study	New England study
Generalized abnormalities		
Fever	4/35 (11)	0/54 (0)
Respiratory illness	8/35 (23)	0/54 (0)
Splenomegaly	20/35 (57)	0/54 (0)
Hepatomegaly	18/35 (51)	1/54 (2)
Jaundice	23/35 (66)	1/54 (2)
Thrombocytopenia	14/35 (40)	0/54 (0)
Neurologic abnormalities		
Intracranial calcifications	25/35 (71)	13/50 (26)
Elevated CSF protein	19/33 (56)	11/35 (31)
Hydrocephalus	15/35 (43)	4/50 (8)
Seizures[‡]	6/35 (17)	1/54 (2)
Microcephaly	5/35 (14)	1/54 (2)
Motor deficit	21/35 (60)	7/54 (13)
Ophthalmologic abnormalities		
Peripheral retinal scars only	3/35 (9)	2/54 (4)
Macular lesions	21/35 (60)	11/54 (20)
Visual impairment[‡]	15/35 (43)	11/54 (20)

*From McAuley et al. *Clin. Infect. Dis.* 18(1):38, 1994; includes only infants ≤2 months of age at initial presentation.
[†]From Guerina et al. *N. Engl. J. Med.* 330:1858, 1994.
[‡]Abnormality at or shortly after initial presentation.
Source: Guerina N. G. Management strategies for infectious diseases in pregnancy. *Semin. Perinatol.* 18:305, 1994.

and retinal disease or one group with generalized clinical and laboratory abnormalities in addition to retinal disease and somewhat less prominent CNS findings. Infants with primary neurologic disease typically had intracranial calcifications, abnormal cerebrospinal fluid (CSF) profiles, chorioretinitis, and convulsions. Infants with signs and symptoms of generalized disease had hepatosplenomegaly, lymphadenopathy, jaundice and anemia, in addition to CSF abnormalities and chorioretinitis. More recently, McAuley et al. [20] reported the clinical presentations and treatment outcomes for infants with congenital toxoplasma infection followed in the Chicago collaborative treatment trial. Thirty-five of the infants were diagnosed at ≤2 months of age, and nearly all of them were diagnosed because of clinical findings indicating they had symptomatic congenital infection. These infants had clinical findings comparable to those described by Eichenwald [10] except that there was considerable overlap in the clinical presentations of generalized and neurologic disease.

It is important to note that 80 to 90% of infants with congenital toxoplasma do not have overt signs of infection at birth [1,2,11,22]. Nevertheless, these infants may have retinal and CNS abnormalities when further testing is performed. In addition, these infants remain at risk for severe long-term ophthalmologic and neurologic sequelae. In the New England Regional Newborn Screening program, filter paper dried-blood spot specimens are screened for toxoplasma-specific IgM [11]. Confirmation IgM and IgG tests are performed on a repeat blood sample from each infant with a positive screening test, and on a serum sample from each infant's mother. Infants with confirmed infection have an ophthalmologic examination, intracranial imaging (head CT scan), and cerebrospinal fluid (CSF) examination performed. Over a 6.5-year period starting January 1986, 52 of 635,000 infants screened were identified with congenital toxoplasma, and 50 of these infants were identified solely through newborn screening; all 50 were term, had normal routine physical examinations and were discharged home for routine newborn follow-up. After congenital infection was confirmed by follow-up serologic testing, additional studies revealed abnormalities of either the CNS or retina in 19 of 48 (40%) infants examined. Table 23-14 summarizes the clinical and laboratory findings for infants with congenital toxoplasma infection identified through the New England Newborn Screening Program compared with those from the Chicago collaborative treatment trial. Since infants from the New England Newborn Screening Program were identified by state-wide universal serologic screening, the clinical presentations of this group more accurately reflect the expected incidence of abnormalities.

   1. **Sequelae of congenital toxoplasma infection in the absence of extended chemotherapy.** Several prospective studies have been conducted to determine the frequency of adverse outcomes in infants with subclinical congenital toxoplasma infection. Koppe et al. [17,18] prospectively followed 11 infants with congenital toxoplasma infection and found that 9 (82%) developed chorioretinitis over a 20-year follow-up period. Four of these infants developed severe visual impairment and 3 had unilateral blindness. These infants either received no treatment (7 infants) or treatment was limited to a 3-week course of pyrimethamine and sulfadiazine (4 infants). Wilson et al. [24] reported similar results for 23 infants with congenital toxoplasma infection. Thirteen of these infants had no clinical evidence of disease at birth and were diagnosed solely by the presence of toxoplasma-specific IgM in cord blood specimens. As in the Koppe et al. study, infants received either no treatment or a brief course (one month) of pyrimethamine and sulfadiazine. On follow-up over several years, 11 (85%) children developed chorioretinitis, including 3 with unilateral blindness.

   Although the patients followed by Koppe et al. [17,18] were reported to have had normal school performance (based on parental reporting), the children described by Wilson et al. [24] were found to develop significant neurologic complications; of the 13 infants with subclinical infection identified through cord blood serologic screening, one child developed psychomotor retardation, microcephaly, and seizures, two children had delayed psychomotor development (reported to eventually become normal), and 2 children had persistent cerebellar dysfunction. Three children developed sensorineural hearing loss. The mean IQ for all 13 children was 88 ± 23 with two children reported to be severely affected with IQ values of 36 and 62. Furthermore, 6 children who had a mean IQ score of 97 on initial testing had a significant drop in their mean score to 74 when retested 5.5 years later. Neurologic complications were also reported in the study by Sever et al. [23]. In their follow-up over a 7-year period of mother–infant pairs in the Collaborative Perinatal Project, deafness occurred in infants born to mothers with toxoplasma-specific IgG. In addition, infants born to mothers with toxoplasma-specific titers suggestive of acute infection in pregnancy had a 60% increase in the incidence of microcephaly, and a 30% increase in the occurrence of low IQ scores (<70). These studies demonstrate the risk for long-term ophthalmologic and neurologic abnormalities in infants with congenital toxoplasma infection despite their initial clinical presentation.

IV. Treatment
   A. **Management of the at-risk and infected fetus.** The risk of vertical transmission of *T. gondii* from an acutely infected mother to her fetus may be significantly diminished by maternal treatment with spiramycin [9]. The drug

is currently available in the United States from Rhone-Poulenc (Montreal, Quebec) on an Investigational new drug (IND) number issued by the Food and Drug Administration (FDA). The dose is 1 gm every 8 hours. Although this drug reduces the incidence of vertical transmission, the severity of disease when fetal infection occurs may not be altered [9]. Thus, when acute maternal infection is determined it is important to evaluate the fetus for possible infection, in addition to initiating maternal spiramycin therapy. Daffos et al. [6] evaluated an antenatal screening and treatment program in which women were screened for acute infection by serial antibody assays. When a woman seroconverted, indicating acute infection, she was started on spiramycin, and fetal infection was assessed by amniotic fluid culture, fetal blood studies (percutaneous umbilical blood sampling for culture, specific IgM, total IgM, and blood chemistries), and fetal ultrasound surveys. When fetal infection was confirmed either abortion was carried out consistent with French law (first/second trimester), or maternal treatment was changed to combination anti-toxoplasma chemotherapy; the therapeutic regimen was pyrimethamine plus sulfonamide alternating every 3 weeks with spiramycin beginning at the 24th week of gestation. Folinic acid was also added to help prevent the potentially toxic side effects of pyrimethamine. Of 746 documented maternal infections, 42 cases of congenital infections were observed, 39 of which were identified by the antenatal screening tests. Twenty-four pregnancies were terminated. The remaining 15 pregnancies were carried to term and at 3 months follow-up 13/15 remain asymptomatic. The other 2 infants were diagnosed with chorioretinitis. A more recent study reported the outcome of infants with congenital toxoplasma born to mothers diagnosed with acute infection by seroconversion between 8 and 26 weeks' gestation [3]. One hundred and sixty-three women were diagnosed and treated with spiramycin. The fetuses of these women were evaluated for evidence of infection by cordocentesis and serial ultrasounds, and 23 of the women were treated with pyrimethamine and sulfadiazine. Three fetuses died and 27 of 162 liveborn infants had confirmed congenital infection. Ten of the infected infants had clinical signs of infection with intracranial calcifications (5 infants), moderate ventricular dilation (2 infants), and peripheral chorioretinitis (7 infants). All 27 infants are reported to be free from symptoms at 15 to 71 months of age. The investigators conclude that pregnancy termination may not be necessary for acquired toxoplasma in the first and second trimester, provided anti-toxoplasma chemotherapy is given and repeated fetal ultrasounds remain normal.

The benefits of antenatal screening for acute maternal toxoplasma infection seem apparent, but universal testing has been controversial in the United States. The major concerns have included the cost of serial tests in a relatively low incidence population, and the reliability of commercially available screening assays. These are not insurmountable obstacles and universal maternal screening should probably be performed. One possible algorithm for initial screening is shown in Table 23-13. Wong and Remington [25] have recommended antenatal maternal screening for pregnant women in the United States using the Sabin-Feldman dye test (or equivalent assay) at ≤12 weeks with retesting at 20 to 22 weeks and again near term. The dye test is available through the Toxoplasma Laboratory of the Palo Alto Research Foundation, Palo Alto, CA. Commercial laboratories offer other serologic tests but sensitivity and specificity vary and inconsistent results are sometimes obtained. If the dye test is not readily available, maternal toxoplasma-specific IgG ELISA and double-sandwich IgM ELISA may be requested. A positive IgG and negative IgM indicates remote infection (no risk to fetus if mother does not have immunodeficiency). If the IgM test is positive on the initial screen additional testing may be required to help determine the likelihood of a recent infection (e.g., IgM-ISAGA, IgA ELISA). If seroconversion is documented during pregnancy acute maternal infection should be assumed and infectious disease consultation obtained. It may be necessary to confirm titers through a reference laboratory (e.g., Palo Alto Research Foundation) before spiramycin therapy can be initiated. Testing for fetal infection (e.g., amniotic fluid PCR) should be attempted in all women with confirmed acute toxoplasma in pregnancy, provided testing can be done with minimal risks. **In confirmed cases of fetal infection, or in cases where testing cannot be performed but acute maternal disease occurred in the second trimester, pyrimethamine, folinic acid, and sulfadiazine should be given beginning at 24 weeks' gestation.** This regimen may be altered with spiramycin every 3 weeks.

B. **Treatment and follow-up of the infected newborn infant (Table 23-15).** Since many infants who develop long-term complications have no overt disease at birth, postnatal sequelae appear to result, at least in part, from ongoing insult or reactivated disease after delivery. Current treatment options do not eradicate *T. gondii* from infected hosts so investigators have attempted to control the infection in young infants by extended anti-toxoplasma drug regimens. The benefits of extended therapy was first suggested by the studies by Couvreur and colleagues [4,5] who prospectively followed infants diagnosed with congenital toxoplasma infection by postnatal serology. Follow-up on a portion of these infants over several years showed an 8% incidence of new-onset retinal disease in untreated infants compared with no new retinal lesions in treated infants. There also appeared to be an inverse relationship between the duration of therapy and the incidence of disease.

More recent studies have further demonstrated the benefit of extended therapy for both symptomatic and subclinical congenital infection. In the Chicago collaborative treatment trial [20] a total of 44 infected infants were followed during a 10-year period from 1981 to 1991. As noted previously, the majority of infants in this study were identified because they had clinical symptoms suspicious for congenital infection. Many of these infants had significant clinical and laboratory abnormalities on initial presentation (see Table 23-14). A total of 37 infants were entered into a 1-year treatment program, 35 of whom were ≤2 months of age when therapy was initiated. Most of the infants received sulfadiazine 50 mg/kg twice a day and pyrimethamine 1 mg/kg each day for 2 months followed by 1 mg/kg every other day for the remaining 10 months. Folinic acid (leucovorin) 5 mg to 10 mg 3 times each week was given to help prevent side effects of pyrimethamine. Ophthalmologic follow-up revealed new retinal lesions in 8% of treated infants (mean age 3.4 years) compared with 29% of untreated controls (mean age 5.6 years). Twenty-one (57%) of the 37 treated infants had motor abnormalities or seizures on initial evaluation, but on follow-up only 8 (24%) of 34 infants tested had significant neurologic complications. In contrast, there was no improvement in the neurologic status of untreated infants. In this study the untreated "controls" were a small number of infants who were referred beyond the treatment enrollment period, and thus they do not represent a randomized control population. They also were older with a longer period of follow-up. Nevertheless, these results were encouraging and demonstrate that even infants with significant disease from in utero infection may benefit from treatment. The most pronounced risk factors associated with poor outcomes were a delay in initiation of treatment (delay in diagnosis), prolonged concomitant neonatal hypoxemia and hypoglycemia, prolonged uncorrected hydrocephalus, and severe visual impairment. Of 19 infants without hydrocephalus nearly all were developmentally normal (IQ scores 85 to 140) whereas severe disabilities occurred in 8 of 10 infants who had hydrocephalus at birth, and 2 of 8 infants who were diagnosed with hydrocephalus in the first months of life.

Infants followed in the New England Newborn Screening Program [11] were also treated with a 1-year course of combination anti-toxoplasma chemotherapy. Most infants were treated with sulfadiazine/pyrimetha-

Table 23-15. Suggested evaluation and treatment program for infants with congenital toxoplasma infection*

Initial evaluation
  Complete physical examination
  Cranial CT scan
  CSF protein, glucose, cell count
  Complete eye examination by a pediatric ophthalmologist
  Complete blood count, liver function tests (especially ALT, bilirubin)
  Serum glucose-6-phosphate dehydrogenase screen (prior to initiating
    sulfadiazine)
  Urine culture for cytomegalovirus
  Pediatric neurology assessment if apparent symptomatic CNS disease
Follow-up evaluation:
  Complete blood counts to monitor for drug toxicity:*
    1–2 times/week while on daily pyrimethamine
    1–2 times/month while on every other day pyrimethamine
  Complete pediatric examination, including neurodevelopmental assessment
    every month
  Pediatric ophthalmology examination every 3 months until 18 months of life,
    then yearly thereafter.†
  Pediatric neurology examination every 3–6 months until 1 year of age‡
  Serum IgG and IgM determinations every 3 months until 18 months of age
Treatment regimen:
  Pyrimethamine 1 mg/kg daily for 2–6 months, then 1 mg/kg every other day to
    complete 1 year of therapy
  Sulfadiazine 100 mg/kg in 2 divided doses each day for 1 year
  Folinic acid (leukovorin) 10 mg 3 times/week with dose increased as needed for
    pyrimethamine toxicity

*Counts should be done at the more frequent interval if there is an intercurrent illness or any occurrence of neutropenia. Folinic acid (leucovorin) dose should be increased if the absolute neutrophil count (ANC) falls below 1000, and pyrimethamine should be temporarily withheld if the ANC falls below 500. Persistent neutropenia despite withholding of pyrimethamine may be caused by sulfadiazine. Measurement of serum ALT and creatinine, and obtaining a urinalysis every 3 months may be useful in monitoring for side effects of sulfadiazine.
†Frequency of examinations adjusted as needed if retinal disease present.
‡Frequency and duration of pediatric neurology follow-up determined by the presence of neurologic abnormalities.
Source: Guerina, N.G. Congenital infection with *Toxoplasma gondii. Pediatr. Ann.* 23:138, 1994.

mine/folinic acid as in the Chicago study except the pyrimethamine dose was 1 mg/kg every other day, and during the final 6 months pyrimethamine administration was given every other month. Thirty-nine infants had ophthalmologic follow-up from 1 to 6 years (number of person-years of follow-up: 115 years total and 3 years median). In 9 infants who had retinal disease at birth, only one had new retinal lesions noted on follow-up (small peripheral scars first noted at 6 years of age). New retinal lesions were found in 3 other infants who initially had no evidence of disease at birth, but only one of these infants had a clinically significant lesion; a macular scar with unilateral visual impairment. Thus, a total of 4 of 39 (10%) of infants had new retinal disease. Only one of 46 infants had a persistent neurologic deficit (hemiplegia attributable to a cerebral lesion present at birth). Because of the expected high incidence of long-term sequelae in untreated infants, no controls were used in this study. Nevertheless, the excellent clinical outcomes for these children indicate a likely benefit for extended therapy.

Table 23-15 outlines treatment guidelines for infants diagnosed with congenital toxoplasma infection. The principal side effect of therapy is neutropenia which primarily results from pyrimethamine treatment. For this reason close monitoring of blood counts is required. In the Chicago collaborative treatment trial 21 (58%) of 36 infants developed neutropenia, usually in conjunction with a viral illness [20]. The incidence in the New England study [11] was lower, possibly due to the greater interval used for pyrimethamine dosing. Neutropenia less commonly can result from sulfadiazine. In general, increasing the dose of folinic acid (leucovorin) can reverse the neutropenia associated with pyrimethamine, but temporary cessation of therapy or dose modification may be required. Recent published information on pyrimethamine levels in infants indicate that the serum half-life is approximately 33 hours with steady-state levels being nearly twice as high with daily dosing compared to every other day dosing [21]. Both dosing regimens produced serum and CSF levels in the concentration range that is active against *T. gondii* in vitro, but CSF levels were only 10 to 25% of serum levels. Based upon this information, as well as the minimal and reversible side effects which have been reported thus far, it is reasonable to maximize levels with daily pyrimethamine dosing for some initial period of treatment.

V. Prevention

The best way to prevent congenital toxoplasma is by preventing acute maternal infection in pregnancy. At present, this requires the appropriate education of pregnant women about simple procedures which may minimize exposure [22]. These include the following:

A. Cats
1. Keep indoors
2. Empty litter every day (avoid if pregnant or wear gloves)
3. Feed only dry, canned, or cooked food

B. Meat
1. Avoid eating undercooked meat in pregnancy
2. Wear gloves when handling, or wash hands thoroughly after handling
3. Keep cutting boards, utensils thoroughly cleaned

C. Vegetables
1. Wear gloves when gardening
2. Wash vegetables thoroughly before eating
3. Wear gloves when handling, or wash hands thoroughly after handling

Other, potentially more preventive measures are being investigated, including vaccine development for immunization of cats and possibly intermediate hosts. Recent reviews on toxoplasmosis are found in references 12, 19, and 22.

References

1. Alford, C. A., Jr., et al. Subclinical central nervous system disease of neonates: A prospective study of infants born with increased levels of IgM. *J. Pediatr.* 75:1167, 1969.
2. Alford, C. A., Jr., et al. Congenital toxoplasmosis: Clinical, laboratory and therapeutic considerations, with special reference to subclinical disease. *Bull. N.Y. Acad. Med.* 50:160, 1974.
3. Berrebi, A., et al. Termination of pregnancy for maternal toxoplasmosis. *Lancet* 344:36, 1994.
4. Couvreur, J., et al. Etude d'une serie homogene de 210 cases de toxoplasmose congenitale chez des nourrissons ages de 0 a 11 mois et depistes de facon prospective. *Ann. Pediatr. (Paris).* 31:815, 1984.
5. Couvreur, J., et al. Le prognostic oculaire de la toxoplasmose congenitale: Role du traitement. *Ann. Pediatr. (Paris).* 31(10):855, 1984.
6. Daffos, F., et al. Prenatal management of 746 pregnancies at risk for congenital toxoplasmosis. *N. Engl. J. Med.* 318:271, 1988.
7. Desmonts, G., et al. Toxoplasmosis in pregnancy and its transmission to the fetus. *Bull. N.Y. Acad. Med.* 50:146, 1974.
8. Desmonts, G., et al. Congenital toxoplasmosis: A prospective study of the offspring of 542 women who acquired toxoplasmosis during pregnancy. Pathophys-

iology of congenital disease. In O. Thalhammer, K. Baumgarten, and A. Pollak (Eds.). *Perinatal Medicine, 6th European Congress.* Stuttgart: Georg Thieme Publishers, 1979, p. 51.

9. Desmonts, G., et al. Immunoglobulin M-immunosorbent agglutination assay for diagnosis of infectious diseases: Diagnosis of acute congenital and acquired toxoplasma infections. *J. Clin. Microbiol.* 14(5):486, 1981.

10. Eichenwald, H. A study in congenital toxoplasmosis. In J. C. Siim (Ed.). *Human Toxoplasmosis.* Copenhagen: Williams & Wilkins, 1959, p. 41.

11. Guerina, N. G., et al. Neonatal serologic screening and early treatment of congenital *Toxoplasma gondii* infection. *N. Engl. J. Med.* 330:1858, 1994.

12. Guerina, N. G. Congenital infection with *Toxoplasma gondii. Pediatr. Ann.* 23:138, 1994.

13. Guerina, N. G. Management strategies for infectious diseases in pregnancy. *Semin. Perinatol.* 18:305, 1994.

14. Hohlfeld, P., et al. Prenatal diagnosis of congenital toxoplasmosis with a polymerase-chain-reaction test on amniotic fluid. *N. Engl. J. Med.* 331:695, 1994.

15. Hunter, K., et al. Prenatal screening of pregnant women for infections caused by cytomegalovirus, Epstein-Barr virus, herpesvirus, rubella, and *Toxoplasma gondii. Am. J. Obstet. Gynecol.* 145:269, 1983.

16. Kimball, A. C., et al. Congenital toxoplasmosis; a prospective study of 4,048 obstetric patients. *Am. J. Obstet. Gynecol.* 111:211, 1971.

17. Koppe, J. G., et al. Toxoplasmosis and pregnancy, with a long-term follow up of the children. *Eur. J. Obstet. Gynecol. Reprod. Biol.* 4:101, 1974.

18. Koppe, J. G., et al. Results of 20 year follow-up of congenital toxoplasmosis. *Lancet* 1:254, 1986.

19. Matsui, D. Prevention, diagnosis and treatment of fetal toxoplasmosis. *Clin. Perinatol.* 21:675, 1994.

20. McAuley, J., et al. Early and longitudinal evaluations of treated infants and children and untreated historical patients with congenital toxoplasmosis: The Chicago collaborative treatment trial. *Clin. Infect. Dis.* 18(1):38, 1994.

21. McLeod, R., et al. Levels of pyrimethamine in sera and cerebrospinal and ventricular fluids from infants treated for congenital toxoplasmosis. *Antimicrob. Agents Chemother.* 36(5):1040, 1992.

22. Remington, J. S., et al. Toxoplasmosis. In J. S. Remington, and J. O. Klein, (Eds.). *Infectious Diseases of the Fetus and Newborn Infant* (4th Ed.). Philadelphia: Saunders, 1994, p. 140.

23. Sever, J. L., et al. Toxoplasmosis: Maternal and pediatric findings in 23,000 pregnancies. *Pediatrics* 82(2):181, 1988.

24. Wilson, C. B., et al. Development of adverse sequelae in children born with subclinical congenital toxoplasma infection. *Pediatrics* 66:767, 1980.

25. Wong, S. Y., et al. Toxoplasmosis in pregnancy. *Clin. Infect. Dis.* 18:853, 1994.

24. RESPIRATORY DISORDERS

Respiratory Distress Syndrome/Hyaline Membrane Disease
Helen G. Liley and Ann R. Stark

The primary cause of respiratory distress syndrome (RDS) is inadequate pulmonary surfactant. The manifestations of the disease are caused by the consequent diffuse alveolar atelectasis, edema, and cell injury. Subsequently, serum proteins that inhibit surfactant function leak into the alveoli. The increased water content, immature mechanisms for clearance of lung liquid, lack of alveolar–capillary apposition, and low surface area for gas exchange typical of the immature lung also contribute to the disease. Significant advances made in the management of RDS include the development of prenatal diagnosis to identify infants at risk, prevention of the disease by prenatal administration of glucocorticoids, improvements in perinatal care, advances in respiratory support, and surfactant replacement therapy. As a result, the mortality from RDS has decreased. However, the survival of increasing numbers of extremely immature infants has provided new challenges, and RDS remains an important contributing cause of neonatal mortality and morbidity.

I. **Identification**
   A. **Perinatal risk factors**
      1. **Factors that affect the state of lung development at birth** include prematurity, maternal diabetes, and genetic factors (white race, history of RDS in siblings, male sex). Thoracic malformations that cause lung hypoplasia, such as diaphragmatic hernia, may also increase the risk for surfactant deficiency. Deficiency of surfactant protein B due to defects in its gene causes severe, usually lethal, congenital alveolar proteinosis that in its early stages can resemble RDS.
      2. **Factors that may acutely impair surfactant production, release, or function** include perinatal asphyxia in premature infants (e.g., secondary to antepartum hemorrhage or in some second-born twins) and cesarean section without labor. Infants delivered before labor commences do not benefit from the adrenergic and steroid hormones released during labor, which increase surfactant production and release.
   B. **Prenatal prediction** (see Chap. 1, Tests for Pulmonary Surfactant)
      1. Prenatal prediction of lung maturity can be made by tests of amniotic fluid. Prenatal prediction of risk for RDS is important because it will contribute to decisions regarding transfer of the mother to a perinatal center, administration of glucocorticoids to accelerate fetal lung maturation, and administration of artificial surfactant.
      2. We recommend maternal glucocorticoid treatment if delivery of an infant with severe RDS seems imminent. In general, this applies to pregnancies shorter than 34 weeks regardless of gender or race, or those in which lung immaturity is shown by amniotic fluid analysis and when delivery can be postponed to allow the glucocorticoid to take effect. Optimal benefit begins 24 hours after initiation of treatment and continues for 7 days, although treatment for less than 24 hours also improves outcome. Contraindications to glucocorticoid treatment include amnionitis or other indications for immediate delivery. Maternal glucocorticoid therapy induces surfactant production and also accelerates maturation of the lungs and other fetal tissues and organs, resulting in lower incidence of RDS, bronchopulmonary dysplasia, patent ductus arteriosus, and intraventricular hemorrhage. & NEC

C. **Postnatal diagnosis.** The premature infant with RDS will have clinical signs shortly after birth. These include tachypnea, retractions, flaring of the nasal alae, grunting, and cyanosis. The classic radiographic appearance is of low-volume lungs with a diffuse reticulogranular pattern and air bronchograms.

II. **Management.** The keys to the management of infants with RDS are (1) to prevent hypoxia and acidosis (this allows normal tissue metabolism, optimizes surfactant production, and prevents right-to-left shunting), (2) to optimize fluid management (avoiding hypovolemia and shock, on the one hand, and edema, particularly pulmonary edema, on the other), (3) to reduce metabolic demands, (4) to prevent worsening atelectasis and pulmonary edema, and (5) to minimize lung injury due to barotrauma or oxygen.

A. **Surfactant replacement therapy** has been shown in numerous recent clinical trials to be successful in ameliorating RDS. These trials have examined the effects of surfactant preparations delivered through the endotracheal tube either within minutes of birth (prevention studies) or after the symptoms and signs of RDS are present (treatment or "rescue" studies). Surfactants of human, bovine, or porcine origin and two synthetic preparations have been studied. In general, these studies have shown improvement in oxygenation and decreased need for ventilator support lasting hours to days after treatment and, in many of the larger studies, decreased incidence of air leaks and death. Survanta, a bovine surfactant extract, and Exosurf Neonatal, a synthetic surfactant consisting of dipalmitoyl phosphatidylcholine and emulsifying and dispersing agents, are currently available in the United States; other surfactant preparations are under investigation.

1. **Timing.** Research in animals suggests that preventive treatment of surfactant deficiency, before lung injury occurs, results in better distribution and less lung injury than supplementation once respiratory failure is severe. Taken together, human studies comparing prevention and rescue strategies do not consistently support one approach over the other. However, a large multinational study showed a small but statistically significant reduction in pneumothorax and in death or chronic oxygen dependency if "rescue" treatment was begun before 2 hours rather than after 3 hours of age. In general, we administer artificial surfactant as soon as the diagnosis of RDS is made, after adequate oxygenation, ventilation, perfusion, and monitoring have been established. Prophylactic therapy is justifiable in very premature infants who have a high incidence of RDS, in centers that have several skilled staff available to attend each delivery, so that resuscitation is not delayed by surfactant administration. Local conditions such as equipment to provide warmed, humidified, blended air/O_2 and full monitoring facilities in the delivery room will also influence the decision.

2. **The response to surfactant therapy** varies from baby to baby. The causes of this variability include timing of treatment, and patient factors such as other concurrent illnesses and degree of lung immaturity. Delayed resuscitation, insufficient lung inflation, and excessive fluid administration may negate the benefits of surfactant therapy. Animal and human studies indicate that the combined use of prenatal corticosteroids followed by postnatal surfactant when indicated improves neonatal outcome more than postnatal surfactant therapy alone.

In infants with RDS, **repeated surfactant treatments** over 24 hours after the first dose appear to be more effective than a single dose. However, there is no clear benefit to more than 2 doses of Exosurf or 4 of Survanta. Whether all infants should be retreated, or only those who meet certain criteria for severity of illness at the recommended intervals for retreatment (6 hours for Survanta, 12 for Exosurf), is unresolved. We generally retreat infants who still require mechanical ventilation with mean airway pressures above 7 to 8 cm H_2O and FiO_2 over 0.30.

3. **Administration.** The Survanta dose is 100 mg phospholipid per kilogram (4 ml/kg). It is administered during brief disconnection from the ventilator, in quarter doses via a feeding tube that is cut to a length slightly greater than that of the endotracheal tube. The baby is ventilated for at least 30 seconds, or until stable between quarter doses. Changes in positioning of the infant during administration are intended to facilitate distribution. Recent studies suggest that other strategies of administration, such as omitting the position changes, do not result in loss of efficacy, although delivery that is too slow does. Careful observation is necessary during treatment. Desaturation, bradycardia, and apnea are frequent adverse effects. Administration should be adjusted according to the infant's tolerance. Apnea commonly occurs at slow ventilation rates, so the rate should be at least 30 per minute during administration. In addition, some infants respond rapidly and need careful adjustment of ventilator settings to prevent hypotension or pneumothorax secondary to sudden improvement in compliance. Others become transiently hypoxic during treatment and require additional oxygen.

4. **Complications.** Pulmonary hemorrhage is an infrequent adverse event after surfactant therapy. It most commonly occurs in extremely low-birth-weight infants, in males, and in infants who have clinical evidence of patent ductus arteriosus. The risk is decreased by prenatal glucocorticoid therapy and by early postnatal treatment of PDA with indomethacin.

Surfactant treatment has not consistently reduced the incidence of intraventricular hemorrhage, necrotizing enterocolitis, and retinopathy of prematurity. Although these disorders tend to be associated with severe RDS, they are primarily caused by immaturity of other organs. Likewise, most studies have not demonstrated reduction in the incidence of chronic lung disease (CLD), particularly in the smallest infants, who are at the highest risk. However, the reduction in mortality attributable to surfactant therapy has not typically been associated with a large increase in rates of CLD, suggesting that surfactant therapy prevents CLD in some infants. The effect of surfactant treatment is probably smaller in mitigating CLD than that of prenatal glucocorticoid therapy.

B. **Oxygen**
1. **Delivery of oxygen** should be sufficient to maintain arterial tensions at 50 to 80 mm Hg. This range is generally sufficient to meet metabolic demands. Higher than necessary FiO_2 levels should be avoided because of the danger of potentiating the development of lung injury and retinopathy of prematurity. The oxygen is warmed, humidified, and delivered through an air-oxygen blender that allows precise control over the oxygen concentration. For infants with acute RDS, oxygen is ordered by concentration to be delivered to the infant's airway, not by flow, and oxygen concentration is checked at least hourly. When ventilation with an anesthesia bag is required during suctioning of the airway, during insertion of an endotracheal tube, or for an apneic spell, the oxygen concentration should be similar to that before bagging to avoid hyperoxia and should be adjusted in response to continuous monitoring.

2. **Blood gas monitoring** (see Blood Gas Monitoring). During the acute stages of illness, frequent sampling may be required to maintain arterial blood gases within appropriate ranges. Arterial blood gases (P_aO_2, P_aCO_2, and pH) should be measured 15 to 20 minutes after changes in respiratory therapy, such as alteration in the FiO_2, ventilator pressures, or rate. We use indwelling arterial catheters for this purpose. To monitor trends in oxygenation continuously, we use pulse oximeters. In more stable infants, capillary blood from warmed heels may be adequate for monitoring PCO_2 and pH.

C. **Continuous positive airway pressure (CPAP)**
1. **Indications.** We begin CPAP therapy in infants with RDS who have mild respiratory distress, require an FiO_2 below 0.4 to maintain a P_aO_2 of 50 to

80 mm Hg, and have P_aCO_2 less than 50 mm Hg. Early CPAP therapy may reduce the need for mechanical ventilation and the incidence of long-term pulmonary morbidity. In each infant, however, the relative benefits of endotracheal intubation and mechanical ventilation in order to administer artificial surfactant should be weighed. In infants with RDS, CPAP probably helps to prevent atelectasis and may mitigate lung edema and preserve the functional properties of surfactant. P_aO_2 therefore rises. P_aCO_2 may fall if the CPAP enables the infant to inspire on a more compliant portion of his or her pressure–volume curve. However, minute ventilation may decrease on CPAP, particularly if the distending pressure is too great. We obtain a chest radiograph before or soon after starting CPAP to confirm the diagnosis of RDS and to exclude disorders in which this type of therapy should be approached with caution, such as air leak.

2. **Methods of administering CPAP.** We usually begin CPAP via nasal prongs or nasopharyngeal tube using a continuous flow ventilator. We generally start at 5 to 7 cm H_2O pressure, using a flow high enough to avoid rebreathing (5 to 10 L/min), then adjust the pressure in increments of 1 to 2 cm H_2O to a maximum of 8 cm H_2O, observing the baby's respiratory rate and effort and monitoring oxygen saturation. A nasogastric tube is always placed to decompress swallowed air.

3. **Problems encountered with CPAP**
   a. CPAP may interfere with venous return to the heart and thus cardiac output. Positive pressure may be transmitted to the pulmonary vascular bed, raising pulmonary vascular resistance and thereby promoting right-to-left shunting. The risk of these phenomena increases as lung compliance increases, as with resolving RDS. In this circumstance, reduction of the CPAP may improve oxygenation.
   b. Hypercarbia may indicate that CPAP is too high and tidal volume is thereby reduced.
   c. The use of nasal prongs or nasopharyngeal tubes may be unsuccessful if crying or mouth opening prevents adequate transmission of pressure or if the infant's abdomen becomes distended despite insertion of a nasogastric tube. In these situations, endotracheal intubation is often necessary.

4. **Weaning.** As the infant improves, one should begin by reducing the FiO_2 in decrements of 0.05. Generally, when FiO_2 is less than 0.40, CPAP can be reduced in decrements of 1 to 2 cm H_2O, checking blood gases after each adjustment. Physical examination will provide evidence of respiratory effort during weaning, and chest radiographs may help estimate lung volume. Lowering of the distending pressure should be attempted with caution if the lung volumes appear low and alveolar atelectasis persists. We generally discontinue CPAP at about 4 to 6 cm H_2O. The ambient oxygen is then adjusted appropriately.

D. **Mechanical ventilation** (see Mechanical Ventilation, below)
   1. The initiation of ventilator therapy is influenced by the decision to administer surfactant (see **II.A**). Indications are a P_aCO_2 greater than 50 mm Hg or rapidly rising, a P_aO_2 less than 50 mm Hg or oxygen saturation less than 90% with an FiO_2 above 0.50, or severe apnea. The actual levels of P_aO_2 and P_aCO_2 necessitating intervention depend on the course of the disease and the size of the infant. For example, a high P_aCO_2 early in the course of RDS will generally indicate the need for ventilator support, while the same P_aCO_2 when the infant is recovering might be managed, after careful evaluation, by observation and repeated sampling before any intervention is made.
   2. **Ventilators.** A continuous-flow, pressure-limited, time-cycled ventilator is useful for ventilating newborns because pressure waveforms, inspiratory and expiratory duration, and pressure can be varied independently and because the flow of gas permits unobstructed spontaneous breathing.

High-frequency oscillatory ventilation may be useful to minimize lung injury in very small and/or sick infants and to manage infants in whom air leak syndromes complicate RDS.

a. **Initial settings.** We generally start mechanical ventilation with a peak inspiratory pressure of 20 to 25 cm H_2O, positive end-expiratory pressure (PEEP) of 4 to 6 cm H_2O, frequency of 20 to 30 breaths per minute, inspiratory duration of 0.4 to 0.5 second, and the previously required FiO_2 (usually 0.50 to 1.00). It is useful to ventilate the infant first by hand, using an anesthesia bag and manometer to determine the actual pressures required. The infant should be observed for color, chest motion, and respiratory effort, and the examiner should listen for breath sounds and observe changes in oxygen saturation. Adjustments in ventilator settings may be required on the basis of these observations or arterial blood gas results.

b. **Adjustments** (see Mechanical Ventilation). P_aCO_2 should be maintained in the range of 45 to 55 mm Hg. Acidosis may exacerbate RDS. Thus, if relative hypercapnia is accepted to minimize lung injury, meticulous control of any metabolic acidosis (e.g., by support of cardiac output) is necessary. Rising P_aCO_2 levels may indicate the onset of complications, including atelectasis, air leak, or symptomatic patent ductus arteriosus. Methods to decrease P_aCO_2 will increase minute ventilation by affecting respiratory rate or tidal volume or both. Thus, P_aCO_2 is lowered by increasing peak inspiratory pressure, decreasing PEEP, increasing expiratory time, or increasing respiratory rate. Determining the appropriate maneuver requires some experience and careful assessment of the baby. P_aO_2 usually rises in response to increases in FiO_2 or mean airway pressure (increases in peak inspiratory pressure, PEEP, or inspiratory time). Infants who remain hypoxemic despite these measures sometimes improve when narcotic sedatives or muscle relaxants, such as pancuronium, are given. Some infants have pulmonary hypertension resulting in right-to-left shunting through fetal pathways; in these infants, interventions to reduce pulmonary vascular resistance may improve oxygenation (see Persistent Pulmonary Hypertension of the Newborn, below). More commonly, premature infants remain hypoxemic because of shunting through atelectatic lung and respond to measures that improve lung inflation.

3. **Care of the infant** receiving ventilator therapy includes scrupulous attention to vital signs and clinical condition. FiO_2 and ventilator settings must be checked frequently. Blood gas levels should be checked at least every 4 to 6 hours during the acute illness, or more frequently if the infant's condition is changing rapidly, and 15 to 20 minutes following changes in ventilator settings. The effect of modest changes in FiO_2 can be assessed using an oximeter. Airway secretions may require periodic suctioning.

4. **Danger signs**
   a. If an infant receiving CPAP or mechanical ventilation deteriorates, the following should be suspected:
      (1) Blocked or dislodged endotracheal tube
      (2) Malfunctioning ventilator
      (3) Pneumothorax
   b. **Remedial action.** The infant should be removed from the ventilator and ventilated with an anesthesia bag, which should be immediately available at the bedside. An appropriate suction catheter is passed to determine patency of the tube, and the tube position is checked by auscultation of breath sounds or by laryngoscopy. If there is any doubt, the tube should be removed and the infant should be ventilated by bag and mask pending replacement of the tube. The ventilator should be checked to ensure that FiO_2 settings are appropriate. The

baby's chest is auscultated and transilluminated to check for pneumothorax (see Air Leak, below). If pneumothorax is suspected, chest radiographs should be obtained, but if the infant's condition is critical, immediate aspiration by needle is both diagnostic and therapeutic. Hypotension secondary to hemorrhage, capillary leak, or myocardial dysfunction also can complicate RDS and should be treated by blood volume expansion or pressors or both. Pneumopericardium and pulmonary or intraventricular hemorrhage also can cause a sudden deterioration. Immediate attention to treatable conditions is appropriate.

5. **Weaning.** As the infant shows signs of improvement, weaning from the ventilator should be attempted. The following steps are examples and should be varied depending on the infant's blood gases, physical examination, and responses.

   a. **Steps of weaning**

      (1) Reduce inspiratory pressure to 20 cm H_2O and PEEP to 5 cm H_2O in decrements of 1 to 2 cm H_2O.

      (2) Reduce FiO_2 to 0.30 to 0.40, by decrements of 0.05.

      (3) Lower the ventilator rate by 2 to 4 breaths per minute to 6 to 10 breaths per minute, as the infant's spontaneous breathing increases.

      (4) The settings at which mechanical ventilation can be successfully discontinued will vary with the size, condition, respiratory drive, and individual pulmonary mechanics of the infant. Infants weighing less than 2 kg are usually best weaned to ventilator rates of about 10 breaths per minute and then extubated if they are stable on FiO_2 less than 0.30 and peak inspiratory pressure less than 18 cm H_2O. Larger infants may tolerate extubation from higher settings. We frequently use CPAP via nasal prongs or nasopharyngeal tube to stabilize lung volumes after extubation.

   b. **Failure to wean** may result from a number of causes, of which the following is a partial list.

      (1) Pulmonary edema may be present owing to capillary leak during acute stages of the illness or may develop secondary to patency of the ductus arteriosus.

      (2) Recovery of the lung from RDS is not uniform, and segmental or lobar atelectasis, edema, or interstitial emphysema may delay weaning.

      (3) As the infant's lungs become more compliant, the inspiratory and expiratory times may have to be increased to allow optimal inflation and deflation of the lungs.

      (4) Other reasons include onset of chronic lung disease and of apnea of prematurity. We frequently begin aminophylline therapy before extubation in infants weighing less than 1250 gm to improve respiratory drive and prevent apnea (see also Apnea, below). Glottic or subglottic edema resulting in obstruction may respond to inhaled racemic epinephrine or systemic glucocorticoids.

E. **Supportive therapy**

   1. **Temperature** (see Chap. 12). Temperature control is crucial in all low-birth-weight infants, especially in those with respiratory disease. If the infant's temperature is too high or low, metabolic demands increase considerably. If oxygen uptake is limited by RDS, the increased demand cannot be met. An incubator or a radiant warmer must be used to maintain a neutral thermal environment for the infant.

   2. **Fluids and nutrition** (see Chaps. 9, 10)

      a. Infants with RDS initially require intravascular administration of fluids. We generally start fluid therapy at 70 to 80 ml/kg per day, using dextrose 10% in water. Very immature infants in whom poor glucose tolerance and massive transcutaneous losses are expected are usually started at 90 to 110 ml/kg per day. Phototherapy, skin trauma, and radiant warmers increase insensible losses. Excessive fluid administration may cause pulmonary edema and increases the risk for a symptomatic patent ductus arteriosus (PDA). The key to fluid management is careful monitoring of serum electrolytes and body weight, and frequent adjustments in fluids as indicated. Urine output and specific gravity also should be monitored but may not reliably reflect the state of hydration; fluid retention is common in infants with RDS. Conversely, extremely immature infants often lack renal concentration efficiency and have enormous evaporative losses.

  b. By the second day, we usually add sodium (3 mEq/kg/day), potassium (2 mEq/kg/day), and calcium (100 to 200 mg/kg/day) to the fluids. Sodium acetate or bicarbonate can be used instead of sodium chloride if metabolic acidosis is present. If it seems unlikely that adequate oral nutrition will be achieved within several days, we generally start adding an amino acid solution and intravenous fat solution by the second or third day.

  c. In most infants with RDS, spontaneous diuresis occurs on the second to fourth day, preceding improvement in pulmonary function. Although furosemide may help stimulate water secretion, its use has been associated with increased incidence of symptomatic PDA. If diuresis and improvement in lung disease do not occur by 1 to 2 weeks of age, this may signify the onset of chronic lung disease. In these infants, diuretics often improve pulmonary function.

3. **Circulation** is assessed by monitoring the heart rate, blood pressure, and peripheral perfusion. Judicious use of blood or volume expanders may be necessary, and pressors may be used to support the circulation. We often use dopamine (starting at 2.5 to 5 µg/kg/minute) to improve perfusion and urine output and to prevent metabolic acidosis. After the first 12 to 24 hours, hypotension and poor perfusion can also result from a large left-to-right shunt through a PDA, so careful assessment is warranted. The volume of blood drawn should be monitored and, in very-low-birth-weight infants who are sick with RDS, generally should be replaced by packed red cell transfusion when the hematocrit falls below 35 to 40%.

4. **Possible infection.** Since pneumonia can duplicate the clinical signs and radiographic appearance of RDS, we obtain blood cultures and complete blood counts with differential from all infants with RDS and treat with broad-spectrum antibiotics (ampicillin and gentamicin) for at least 48 hours.

F. **Acute complications**
  1. **Air leak** (see Air Leak, below). Pneumothorax, pneumomediastinum, pneumopericardium, or interstitial emphysema should be suspected when an infant with RDS deteriorates, typically with hypotension, apnea, bradycardia, or persistent acidosis.
  2. **Infections** (see Chap. 23) may accompany RDS and may present in a variety of ways. Also, instrumentation, such as catheters or respiratory equipment, provides access for organisms to invade the immunologically immature preterm infant. Whenever there is suspicion of infection, cultures should be obtained and antibiotics administered promptly.
  3. **Intracranial hemorrhage** (see Chap. 27). Infants with severe RDS are at increased risk for intracranial hemorrhage and should be monitored with cranial ultrasound examinations.
  4. **Patent ductus arteriosus (PDA)** (see Chap. 25) frequently complicates RDS. PDA typically presents as pulmonary vascular pressures begin to fall. If untreated, it may result in increasing left-to-right shunt and ultimately congestive heart failure, manifested by respiratory relapse and cardiomegaly. The systemic consequences of the shunt may include low mean blood pressure, metabolic acidosis, decreased urine output, and

worsening jaundice due to impaired organ perfusion. Infants with untreated PDA are at increased risk for intraventricular hemorrhage. We generally treat infants, especially those weighing less than 1500 gm, with intravenous indomethacin if they develop any signs of a symptomatic PDA, such as a systolic or continuous murmur, hyperdynamic precordium, bounding pulses, or widened pulse pressure. In infants who weigh less than 1000 gm, we treat with indomethacin when a PDA first becomes clinically apparent (i.e., presence of ductal murmur without the signs or symptoms of a large left-to-right shunt). We reserve surgical ligation for infants in whom indomethacin is contraindicated (e.g., those with renal failure or necrotizing enterocolitis) or those in whom one or more courses of indomethacin have failed. In larger infants who are improving steadily despite PDA and who have no evidence of heart failure, mild fluid restriction and time may result in closure.

G. **Long-term complications**
   1. **Chronic lung disease** (see below) occurs in 5 to 30% of survivors of respirator therapy for RDS.
   2. **Retinopathy of prematurity (ROP)** (see Chap. 35). Premature infants are at risk for ROP. Oxygen therapy should be monitored closely, and all very-low-birth-weight infants should have ophthalmologic examinations.
   3. **Neurologic impairment** is estimated to occur in 10 to 15% of the survivors of RDS. Contributing factors include circumstances of premature delivery, the immaturity of the infants at birth, and the accompanying risk for neurologic events such as intraventricular hemorrhage and periventricular leukomalacia. Prevention of perinatal asphyxia and careful attention to oxygenation, perfusion, nutrition, and metabolic demands may improve outcome.

References

Jobe, A. H. Pulmonary surfactant therapy. *N. Engl. J. Med.* 328:861, 1993.

Merritt, T. A., Soll, R. F., Hallman, M. Overview of exogenous surfactants. *J. Intens. Care Med.* 8:205, 1995.

NIH Consensus Development Panel on the effect of corticosteroids for fetal maturation on perinatal outcomes. *JAMA* 273:413, 1995.

Mechanical Ventilation
Eric C. Eichenwald

I. **General principles.** Mechanical ventilation is an invasive life-support procedure with many effects on the cardiopulmonary system. The goal is to optimize both gas exchange and clinical status at minimum FiO_2 and ventilator pressures. The ventilator strategy employed to accomplish this goal depends, in part, on the infant's disease process. In addition, recent advances in technology have brought more options for ventilatory therapy of newborns.

II. **Types of ventilatory support**
   A. **Continuous positive airway pressure (CPAP)**
      1. **CPAP** is usually administered by means of a ventilator. Any system used to deliver CPAP should allow continuous monitoring of the delivered pressure, and be equipped with safety alarms to indicate when the pressure is above or below the desired level.
      2. **General characteristics.** A continuous flow of heated, humidified gas is circulated past the infant's airway at a set pressure of 3 to 8 cm H_2O, maintaining an elevated end-expiratory lung volume while the infant breathes spontaneously. The air–oxygen mixture and airway pressure can be adjusted. CPAP is usually delivered by means of nasal prongs or nasopharyngeal tube. Prolonged endotracheal CPAP is not used because the high resistance of the endotracheal tube increases the work of

breathing, especially in small infants. Positive-pressure hoods and continuous-mask CPAP are not recommended.

3. **Advantages**
   a. CPAP is less invasive than mechanical ventilation and causes less barotrauma.
   b. When used early in infants with RDS, it can help prevent alveolar and airway collapse, which might result in deterioration of P_aO_2.
   c. CPAP decreases the frequency of obstructive and mixed apneic spells in some infants.

4. **Disadvantages**
   a. CPAP does not improve ventilation and may worsen it.
   b. CPAP provides inadequate respiratory support in the face of severe changes in pulmonary compliance and resistance.
   c. Maintaining nasal or nasopharyngeal CPAP in large, active infants may be technically difficult.
   d. Swallowed air can elevate the diaphragm and must be removed by a gastric tube.

5. **Indications**
   a. Early treatment of mild RDS
   b. Moderately frequent apneic spells
   c. After recent extubation
   d. Weaning chronically ventilator-dependent infants

B. **Pressure-limited, time-cycled, continuous-flow ventilators** are used most frequently in newborns with respiratory failure.

1. **General characteristics.** A continuous flow of heated and humidified gas is circulated past the infant's airway; the gas is a selected mixture of air with oxygen. Maximum inspiratory pressure (Pi) and positive end-expiratory pressure (PEEP) are selected. Respiratory timing (rate and duration of inspiration and expiration) is selected.

2. **Advantages**
   a. The continuous flow of fresh gas allows the infant to make spontaneous respiratory efforts between ventilator breaths (intermittent mandatory ventilation, IMV).
   b. Good control is maintained over respiratory pressures.
   c. Inspiratory and expiratory time can be independently controlled.
   d. The system is relatively simple and inexpensive.

3. **Disadvantages**
   a. Tidal volume is poorly controlled.
   b. The system does not respond to changes in respiratory system compliance.
   c. Spontaneously breathing infants who breathe out of phase with too many IMV breaths ("bucking" or "fighting" the ventilator) may receive inadequate ventilation and are at increased risk for air leak.

4. **Indications.** Useful in any form of lung disease in infants.

C. **Synchronized and patient-triggered (assist/control, or pressure support) ventilators** are adaptations of conventional pressure-limited ventilators used for newborns.

1. **General characteristics.** These ventilators combine the features of pressure-limited, time-cycled, continuous-flow ventilators with an airway pressure, air flow, or respiratory movement sensor. By measuring inspiratory flow or movement, these ventilators deliver intermittent positive-pressure breaths at a fixed rate in synchrony with the baby's inspiratory efforts ("synchronized IMV," or SIMV). During apnea, SIMV ventilators continue to deliver the set IMV rate. In patient-triggered ventilation, a positive pressure breath is delivered with **every** inspiratory effort. As a result, the ventilator delivers more frequent positive pressure breaths, usually allowing a decrease in the peak inspiratory pressure needed for adequate gas exchange. During apnea, the ventilator in patient-triggered mode delivers an operator-selected IMV ("control") rate. Ventilators

equipped with a flow sensor can also be used to monitor delivered tidal volume continuously by integration of the flow signal.

2. Advantages

   a. Synchronizing the delivery of positive-pressure breaths with the infant's inspiratory effort reduces the phenomenon of breathing out of phase with IMV breaths ("fighting" the ventilator). This may decrease the need for sedative medications and aid in weaning mechanically ventilated infants.

   b. Pronounced asynchrony with ventilator breaths during conventional IMV has been associated with the development of air leak and intraventricular hemorrhage. Whether the use of SIMV or assist/control ventilation reduces these complications is not known.

3. Disadvantages

   a. Under certain conditions, the ventilators may inappropriately trigger a breath because of artifactual signals, or fail to trigger because of problems with the sensor.

   b. Few data are available on the effects of patient-triggered ventilation in newborns. Pressure support ventilation may not be appropriate for small premature infants with irregular respiratory patterns and frequent apnea because of the potential for significant variability in ventilation.

   c. It is more expensive and complicated to use than a conventional pressure-limited device.

4. Indications. SIMV can be used when a conventional pressure-limited ventilator is indicated. If available, it may be the preferable mode of ventilator therapy in infants who are breathing spontaneously while on IMV. The indications for assist/control ventilation have not been established.

D. Volume-cycled ventilators are rarely used in newborn infants, although recent advances in technology have renewed interest in this mode of ventilation in selected situations. Only volume-cycled ventilators specifically designed for newborns should be used.

1. General characteristics. Volume-cycled ventilators are similar to pressure-limited ventilators except that the operator selects the volume delivered, rather than the peak inspiratory pressure.

2. Advantages. The pressure automatically varies with respiratory system compliance to deliver the selected tidal volume, theoretically minimizing variability in minute ventilation.

3. Disadvantages

   a. The system is complicated and requires more skill to operate.

   b. Because tidal volumes in infants are small, most of the tidal volume selected is lost in the ventilator circuit or from air leaks around uncuffed endotracheal tubes. A separate in-line tidal volume monitor may be helpful.

   c. It is more expensive than a pressure-limited device.

4. Indications. May be useful if lung compliance is rapidly changing.

E. The high-frequency ventilator (HFV) is an important adjunct to conventional mechanical ventilation in newborns. The recommended uses and the ventilatory strategies employed with high frequency ventilators continue to evolve with clinical experience. Three types of high-frequency ventilators are approved for use in newborns: a high-frequency oscillator (HFO), a high-frequency flow interrupter (HFFI), and a high-frequency jet ventilator (HFJ).

1. General characteristics. Available HFVs are similar despite considerable differences in design. All HFVs are capable of delivering extremely rapid rates (300 to 1500 breaths per minute, 5 to 25 Hz; 1 Hz = 60 breaths per minute) with tidal volumes equal to or smaller than anatomical dead space. These ventilators apply continuous distending pressure to maintain an elevated lung volume; small tidal volumes are superimposed at a rapid rate. HFJ ventilators are paired with a conventional pressure-limited device, which is used to deliver intermittent "sigh" breaths to help prevent atelectasis. "Sigh" breaths are not used with HFO ventilation. Expiration is passive (i.e., dependent on chest wall and lung recoil) with HFFI and HFJ machines, while it is active with HFO. The mechanisms of gas exchange with HFV are incompletely understood.

2. **Advantages**
   a. HFVs can achieve adequate ventilation while avoiding the large swings in lung volume required by conventional ventilators and associated with lung injury. Because of this, they may be useful in pulmonary air leak syndromes (pulmonary interstitial emphysema, pneumothorax).
   b. HFV allows the use of a high MAP for alveolar recruitment and resultant improvement in ventilation–perfusion matching. This may be advantageous in infants with severe respiratory failure requiring high MAP to maintain adequate oxygenation on a conventional mechanical ventilator.

3. **Disadvantages.** Despite theoretical advantages of HFV, no significant benefit of this method has been demonstrated in routine clinical use over more conventional ventilators. These ventilators are more complex and expensive, and there is less long-term clinical experience. The initial studies with HFO suggested an increased risk of significant intraventricular hemorrhage, although this complication has not been observed in recent clinical trials. Studies comparing the different types of HFVs are unavailable; thus, the relative advantages or disadvantages of HFO, HFFI, and HFJ, if any, are not characterized.

4. **Indications.** HFVs are primarily used as a rescue therapy for infants failing conventional ventilation. Both HFJ and HFO ventilators have been shown to be superior to conventional ventilation in infants with air leak syndromes, especially pulmonary interstitial emphysema. The Sensormedics 3100/3100A, a high-frequency oscillator, is the only HFV approved by the FDA for early intervention, rather than rescue therapy, in newborns with respiratory failure.

F. **Negative pressure.** These infant versions of the adult "iron lung" are rarely used because nursing access is limited by the negative-pressure cylinder and because the neck seal makes them feasible only for large babies. Their use is restricted to older infants with neuromuscular problems who can thus be ventilated without an endotracheal tube.

III. **Indications for respiratory support.** See Chap. 36 for intubation procedures and proper selection of endotracheal tube sizes.

A. **Indications for continuous positive airway pressure (CPAP) in the preterm infant with RDS include**
   1. FiO_2 above 0.30 by hood with clinical distress
   2. FiO_2 above 0.40 by hood
   3. Clinically significant retractions after recent extubation
   4. Infants with RDS who require FiO_2 above 0.30 to 0.35 on CPAP should generally be intubated, ventilated, and given exogenous surfactant therapy.

B. **Relative indications for mechanical ventilation in any infant include**
   1. Frequent intermittent apnea unresponsive to drug therapy
   2. Early treatment when use of mechanical ventilation is anticipated because of deteriorating gas exchange
   3. Relieving "work of breathing" in an infant with signs of respiratory difficulty
   4. Initiation of exogenous surfactant therapy in infants with RDS

C. **Absolute indications for mechanical ventilation**
   1. Prolonged apnea
   2. P_aO_2 below 50 mm Hg on FiO_2 above 0.80. This indication may not apply to the infant with cyanotic congenital heart disease.

3. P_aCO_2 above 60 mm Hg with persistent acidemia
4. General anesthesia

IV. How ventilator changes affect blood gases

A. Oxygenation (Table 24-1)

1. FiO$_2$. The goal is to maintain adequate tissue oxygen delivery. Generally, this can be accomplished by achieving a P_aO_2 of 50 to 80 mm Hg. This results in a hemoglobin saturation of 89 to 95% [see Fig. 24-1 (oxyhemoglobin curve)]. Increasing inspired oxygen is the simplest and most direct means of improving oxygenation. In premature infants, the risk of retinopathy and pulmonary oxygen toxicity argue for minimizing P_aO_2. For infants with other conditions, the optimum P_aO_2 may be higher. Direct pulmonary oxygen toxicity begins to occur at FiO$_2$ values greater than 0.60 to 0.70.

2. Mean airway pressure (MAP)

a. MAP is the average area under the curve of the pressure waveform. Many ventilators now display MAP or can be equipped with a device to do so. MAP is increased by increases in PEEP, inspiratory pressure (Pi), inspiratory time (Ti), rate, and flow rate. All these changes lead to higher P_aO_2, but each has different effects on P_aCO_2. For a given rise in MAP, increasing PEEP gives the greatest improvement in P_aO_2. Other ways to raise MAP are to increase Pi and prolong Ti.

b. Optimum MAP results from a balance between optimizing P_aO_2, minimizing direct oxygen toxicity, minimizing barotrauma, achieving adequate ventilation, and minimizing adverse cardiovascular effects. Barotrauma is probably most closely related to peak-to-peak swings in lung volume, although changes in airway pressure are also implicated.

c. MAP as low as 5 cm H_2O may be sufficient in infants with normal lungs, whereas 20 cm H_2O or more may be necessary in severe RDS.

Table 24-1. Ventilator manipulations to increase oxygenation

Parameter	Advantage	Disadvantage
↑ FiO$_2$	Minimizes barotrauma Easily administered	Fails to affect $\dot{V}/\dot{Q}$ matching Direct toxicity, especially >0.60
↑ Pi	Critical opening pressure Improves $\dot{V}/\dot{Q}$	Barotrauma: air leak, BPD
↑ PEEP	Maintains FRC/prevents collapse	Shifts to stiffer compliance curve
	Splints obstructed airways	Obstructs venous return
	Regularizes respiration	Increases expiratory work and CO_2 Increases dead space
↑ Ti	Increases MAP without increasing Pi "Critical opening time"	Necessitates slower rates, higher Pi Lower minute ventilation for given Pi-PEEP combination
↑ Flow	Square wave—maximizes MAP	Greater shear force, more barotrauma Greater resistance at greater flows
↑ Rate	Increases MAP while using lower Pi	Inadvertent PEEP with high rates or long-term constants

Note: All manipulations (except FiO$_2$) result in higher mean airway pressure (MAP).

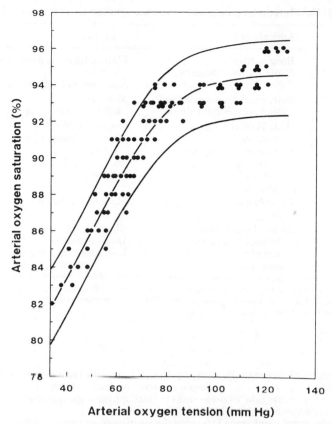

Fig. 24-1. Comparison of paired measurements of oxygen saturation by pulse oximetry and of oxygen tension by indwelling umbilical artery oxygen electrode. The lines represent ±2 standard deviations. (Modified from A. Wasunna and A. G. Whitelaw, Pulse oximetry in preterm infants. *Arch. Dis. Child.* 62:957, 1987.)

Excessive MAP may impede venous return and adversely affect cardiac output.

3. **Ventilation** (Table 24-2)

   a. **CO_2 elimination** depends on **minute ventilation.** Since minute ventilation is the product of respiratory rate and tidal volume, increases in ventilator rate will lower P_aCO_2. Increases in tidal volume can be achieved by increasing the Pi on pressure-cycled ventilators or by increasing volume on volume-limited machines. Because tidal volume is a function of the difference between Pi and PEEP, a reduction in PEEP also improves ventilation. At very low tidal volumes, the volume of dead space becomes important and may lead to CO_2 retention.

   b. **Optimal P_aCO_2** varies according to disease state. For very immature infants or infants with air leak, a P_aCO_2 of 50 to 60 mm Hg may be tolerated to minimize barotrauma, provided pH is greater than 7.25. When hyperventilation is used to reduce pulmonary vascular resistance, a P_aCO_2 as low as 30 mm Hg is occasionally required.

V. **Disease states**

Table 24-2. Ventilator manipulations to increase ventilation and decrease P_aCO_2

Parameter	Advantage	Disadvantage
↑ Rate	Easy to titrate Minimizes barotrauma	Maintains same dead space/tidal volume May lead to inadvertent PEEP
↑ Pi	Better bulk flow (improved dead space/tidal volume)	More barotrauma Shifts to stiffer compliance curve
↓ PEEP	Widens compression pressure Decreases dead space Decreases expiratory load Shifts to steeper compliance curve	Decreases MAP Decreases oxygenation/alveolar collapse Stops splinting obstructed/closed airways
↑ Flow	Permits shorter Ti, longer Te	More barotrauma
↑ Te	Allows longer time for passive expiration in face of prolonged time constant	Shortens Ti Decreases MAP Decreases oxygenation

Key: MAP = mean airway pressure; ↑ = increase; ↓ = decrease; Ti = inspiratory time; Te = expiratory time; Pi = peak inspiratory pressure; PEEP = positive end-expiratory pressure; FiO_2 = fraction of oxygen in inspired gas.

A. Effects of diseases. Respiratory failure can result from numerous illnesses through a variety of pathophysiologic mechanisms. Optimal ventilatory strategy must take into account the pathophysiology, expected time course, and particular vulnerabilities of the patient.

B. Pulmonary mechanics influence the ventilator strategy selected.

    1. Compliance is the stiffness or distensibility of the lung and chest wall, i.e., the change in volume (ΔV) produced by a change in pressure (ΔP), or $\Delta V/\Delta P$. It is decreased with surfactant deficiency, excess lung water, and lung fibrosis. It is also decreased when the lungs are hyperexpanded.

    2. Resistance is the impediment to airflow due to friction between gas and airways (airway resistance) and between tissues of the lungs and chest wall (viscous tissue resistance). Almost half of airway resistance is in the upper airways, including the endotracheal tube when in use. Resistance is high in diseases characterized by airway obstruction, such as meconium aspiration and bronchopulmonary dysplasia (BPD). Resistance can change rapidly if, for example, secretions partially occlude the endotracheal tube.

    3. Time constant is the product of compliance and resistance. This is a measure of the time it takes to equilibrate pressure between the proximal airway and the alveoli. Expiratory time constants are somewhat longer than inspiratory ones. When time constants are long, as in meconium aspiration, care must be taken to set ventilator inspiratory times and rates that permit adequate inspiration to deliver the required tidal volume and adequate expiration to avoid inadvertent PEEP.

    4. Functional residual capacity (FRC) is a measure of the volume of the lungs at end-expiration. FRC is decreased in diseases that permit alveolar collapse, particularly surfactant deficiency.

    5. Ventilation-perfusion matching (V/Q). Diseases that reduce alveolar surface area (through atelectasis, inflammatory exudates, or obstruction) permit intrapulmonary shunting of desaturated blood. The opposite occurs in persistent pulmonary hypertension, when extrapulmonary shunting diverts blood flow away from the ventilated lung. Both mechanisms result in systemic recirculation of desaturated blood.

  6. **Work of breathing** is especially important in the smallest infants and those with chronic lung disease, whose high airway resistance, decreased lung compliance, compliant chest wall, and weak musculature may overwhelm their metabolic energy requirements and impede growth.

C. **Specific disease states.** Several of the more common neonatal disease processes are described below and are presented in Table 24-3 along with the optimal ventilatory strategies. Before initiating ventilatory support, however, clinicians must evaluate for mechanical causes of distress, including pneumothorax or airway obstruction.

  1. **Respiratory distress syndrome (RDS)** (see Respiratory Distress Syndrome/Hyaline Membrane Disease, above)

    a. **Pathophysiology.** RDS is caused by surfactant deficiency, which results in a severe decrease in compliance (stiff lung). This causes diffuse alveolar collapse with $\dot{V}/\dot{Q}$ mismatching and increased work of breathing.

    b. **Surfactant replacement.** The availability of exogenous surfactant therapy for the treatment of RDS has changed ventilatory management of the disease. We recommend intubation and initiation of mechanical ventilation early in the course of the disease in order to provide surfactant therapy promptly. The distinctive time course of escalation, plateau, and weaning in classic RDS has changed with the use of exogenous surfactant therapy. Ventilatory strategy should anticipate the increased risk of pneumothorax as compliance increases and time constants lengthen, especially with the rapid improvements that can be seen after surfactant therapy. In all approaches, a P_aCO_2 value higher than the physiologic value is acceptable to minimize barotrauma.

    c. **Ventilatory strategy**

      (1) **CPAP.** In mildly affected infants who may not require intubation and surfactant administration, CPAP is used to prevent further atelectasis. CPAP is initiated at 5 to 6 cm H_2O, and increased to a maximum of 7 to 8 cm H_2O. CPAP is titrated by clinical assessment of retractions and respiratory rate and by observation of O_2 saturation.

      (2) **Mechanical ventilation** is used when $\dot{V}/\dot{Q}$ mismatching is so severe that increased FiO_2 and CPAP are inadequate or in infants who tire from the increased work of breathing. Our preferred approach maintains MAP with a relatively long Ti (0.4 to 0.5 second) and, consequently, a slow rate. Rarely, a longer Ti is required to provide adequate oxygenation. This ventilatory approach requires a moderate Pi to provide adequate minute ventilation and to maintain alveolar recruitment.

      (3) **Pi and PEEP.** Pi, applied to recruit alveoli, is initially estimated by good chest excursion and is usually 20 to 25 cm H_2O. PEEP is set at 4 to 5 cm H_2O and may go up to 6 cm H_2O. Higher PEEP may interfere with cardiac output and should be avoided.

      (4) **Flow.** Flow rates of 7 to 12 liters per minute are needed to provide a relatively square pressure wave form. Higher flows may be required at very high Pi (>35 cm H_2O).

      (5) **Rates** are generally set initially at 20 to 40 breaths per minute, and adjusted by blood gas results.

      (6) **Weaning.** When the patient becomes stable, FiO_2 and Pi are weaned first, alternating with rate, in response to assessment of chest excursion, oxygen saturation, and blood gas results. Extubation should be accomplished when ventilator rates are 10 to 12

Table 24-3. Neonatal pulmonary physiology by disease state

Disease	Compliance ml/cm H_2O	Resistance cm H_2O/ml/s	Time Constant (s)	FRC (ml/kg)	$\dot{V}/\dot{Q}$ Matching	Work
Normal term	4–6	20–40	0.25	30 ml/kg	—	—
RDS	↓↓	—	↓↓	↓	↓/↓↓	↑
Meconium aspiration	—/↓	↑/↑↑	↑	↑↑	↓↓	↑
BPD	↑/↓	↑↑	↑	↑↑	↓↓/↓↓	↑↑
Air leak	↓↓	—/↑	—/↑	↑↑	↓/↓↓	↑↑
VLBW apnea	↓	—	↓↓	—/↓	↓/—	—/↑

Key: ↑ = increase; ↓ = decrease; — = little or no change; / = either/or.

breaths per minute. Aminophylline may be used to facilitate spontaneous breathing prior to extubation and may increase the success rate of extubation in very-low-birth-weight infants.

(7) **Advantages and disadvantages.** This ventilatory strategy maximizes alveolar recruitment, but with a potential for greater barotrauma secondary to the higher Pi.

(8) **Alternative ventilatory strategies.** An alternative approach to mechanical ventilation in RDS relies on high rates to maintain MAP while reducing Pi to minimize barotrauma. Rates of 60 to 80 breaths per minute are used, with Ti as low as 0.2 to 0.3 second. Inadvertent PEEP is not encountered because the time constant in RDS may be as short as 0.05 second. Pi is set as low as 12 to 18 cm H_2O, with PEEP of 4 to 5 cm H_2O. Initial settings are based on auscultation of good breath sounds and are increased as needed to maintain adequate minute ventilation and oxygenation. In general, pressure is weaned first, while the rate remains high, or by 10% drops in rate alternating with pressure, as tolerated. This ventilator strategy may minimize barotrauma due to Pi, with the disadvantage of less alveolar recruitment and consequent need for higher FiO_2 to maintain adequate oxygen saturation.

High-frequency ventilation may be initiated after conventional ventilation fails to maintain adequate gas exchange. High-frequency ventilation should be used only by clinicians familiar with its use. We consider the use of HFV when the MAP required for adequate gas exchange exceeds 10 to 11 cm H_2O in small infants and 12 cm H_2O in larger infants, or if air leak occurs. Strategies differ depending on whether HFJ, HFO, or HFFI is used. We prefer HFOV over other available HFV because of its ease of use and applicability in a wide range of pulmonary diseases and infant weights.

a. **High-frequency jet ventilation.** HFJ requires reintubation with a special triple-lumen endotracheal tube, with a distal airway pressure port, a jet side port, and a standard connection for the conventional ventilator. The smallest triple-lumen endotracheal tube currently available (2.5 mm inside diameter) has an outside diameter equal to a standard 3.0-mm endotracheal tube. A special adapter for a standard endotracheal tube that is now available avoids the need for reintubation.

(1) **Pi and PEEP.** Peak pressures on the jet ventilator are initially set approximately 20% lower than on those being used with conventional ventilation, and adjusted to provide adequate chest vibration assessed clinically and by blood gas determinations. Pi, PEEP, and FiO_2 are adjusted as needed to maintain oxygenation. CO_2 elimination is dependent on the pressure difference (Pi −PEEP). Because of the lower peak pressures required to ventilate, PEEP may be increased to 8 to 10 cm H_2O if needed to improve oxygenation.

(2) **Rate.** The frequency is usually set at 420 breaths per minute, with an inspiratory jet valve on-time of 0.02 second.

(3) **Conventional ventilator settings.** Once the HFJ is properly adjusted, the conventional ventilator rate is decreased to 2 to 10 per minute to help maintain alveolar recruitment, with Pi set at 3 to 4 cm H_2O lower than the jet Pi.

(4) **Weaning** from HFJ ventilation is accomplished by decreasing the jet Pi in response to blood gas determinations and the FiO_2. PEEP is weaned as tolerated if pressures higher than 4 to 5 cm H_2O are used. Frequency and jet valve on-time are generally not adjusted.

(5) Similar strategies outlined for the HFJ apply in use of the HFFI.

b. **High-frequency oscillatory ventilation.** With HFO, operator-selected parameters include MAP, frequency, and piston amplitude.

(1) **Mean airway pressure.** In RDS, the initial MAP selected is usually 2 to 5 cm H_2O **higher** than that being used on the conventional ventilator to enhance alveolar recruitment. MAP used with

HFO is titrated to O_2 requirement and to provide adequate lung expansion on chest x-ray. Care must be exercised to avoid lung hyperinflation, which might adversely affect oxygen delivery by reducing cardiac output.

(2) **Frequency** is usually set at 10 to 15 Hz. Inspiratory time is set at 33%.

(3) **Amplitude.** Changes in piston amplitude primarily affect ventilation. It is set to provide adequate chest vibration, assessed clinically and through blood gas determinations.

(4) **Flow** rates of 8 to 15 liters per minute are usually adequate.

(5) **Weaning.** In general, FiO_2 is weaned first, followed by MAP in decrements of 1 to 2 cm H_2O once the FiO_2 falls below 0.6. Piston amplitude is adjusted by frequent assessment of chest vibration and blood gas determinations. Frequency is usually not adjusted. In both HFJ and HFO, we usually wean to extubation after transfer back to conventional ventilation, although infants can be extubated directly from HFV.

2. **Meconium aspiration syndrome (MAS)** (see Meconium Aspiration, below)

a. **Pathophysiology.** MAS results from aspiration of meconium-stained amniotic fluid. The severity of the syndrome is related to the associated asphyxial insult and the amount aspirated. The aspirated meconium causes acute airway obstruction, marked airway resistance, scattered atelectasis with V/Q mismatching, and hyperexpansion due to obstructive ball-valve effects. The obstructive phase is followed by an inflammatory phase 12 to 24 hours later that results in further alveolar involvement. Aspiration of other fluids (such as blood or amniotic fluid) has similar but milder effects.

b. **Ventilatory strategy.** Because of the ball-valve effects, the application of positive pressure may result in pneumothorax or another air leak, so initiating mechanical ventilation requires careful consideration of the risks and benefits. Low levels of PEEP (4 to 5 cm H_2O) are helpful in splinting open partially obstructed airways and equalizing V/Q matching. Higher levels may lead to hyperinflation. If airway resistance is high and compliance is normal, a slow-rate, moderate-pressure strategy is needed. If pneumonitis is more prominent, more rapid rates can be used. Rapid rates may be required in the hyperventilation strategy employed for persistent pulmonary hypertension of the newborn (PPHN) that may be associated with MAS, but care must be taken to avoid inadvertent PEEP. Sedation or muscle relaxation may be used to minimize the risks of air leak in severe MAS because of the high transpulmonary pressures these large infants can generate when "fighting" the ventilator and the ball-valve hyperexpansion caused by their disease. Use of synchronized IMV may be helpful. Weaning may be rapid if the illness is predominantly primarily related to airway obstruction or prolonged if complicated by barotrauma and severe inflammation.

High-frequency ventilation has also been successfully used in infants with MAS who are failing conventional ventilation or who have suffered air leak. The strategies are similar to those described above. During HFO, slower frequencies (6 to 10 Hz) may be useful to improve oxygenation in severe cases. The use of exogenous surfactant therapy in MAS remains investigational.

3. **Bronchopulmonary dysplasia (BPD)** (see Chronic Lung Disease, below)

a. **Pathophysiology.** BPD results from injury to the alveoli and airways. Bleb formation may lead to poor recoil. Fibrosis and excess lung water may cause stiffer compliance. Airways may be narrowed and fibrotic or hyperreactive. The upper airways may be overdistended and conduct airflow poorly. BPD is marked by shifting focal atelectasis, hyperinflation with V/Q mismatching, chronic and acute increases in airway resistance, and a significant increase in the work of breathing.

b. **Ventilatory strategy.** The optimal strategy is to wean infants off the ventilator as soon as possible to prevent further barotrauma and oxygen toxicity. If this is not feasible, ventilator settings should be minimized to permit tissue repair and long-term growth. Low rates (10 to 15 breaths per minute) and longer Ti (0.5 to 0.7 second) may be used to maintain FRC. Higher pressures are sometimes required (20 to 30 cm H_2O) because of the stiff lungs, although the high resistance prevents transfer of most of this to the alveoli. Acute decompensations can result from bronchospasm and interstitial fluid accumulation. These must be treated with adjustment of Pi, bronchodilators, and diuretics. Good oxygenation should be maintained (saturations of 90 to 92%), but higher P_aCO_2 values can be permitted (55 to 65 mm Hg), provided the pH is normal. Weaning is a slow and difficult process, decreasing rate by 1 to 2 breaths per minute every day when tolerated. Fortunately, with improved medical and ventilatory care of these infants, it is rare for infants with BPD to require tracheostomy for chronic ventilation.

4. **Air leak** (see Air Leak, below)
   a. **Pathophysiology.** Pneumothorax and pulmonary interstitial emphysema (PIE) are the two most common air leak syndromes. Pneumothorax results when air ruptures into the pleural space. In PIE, the interstitial air seriously reduces tissue compliance as well as recoil. In addition, peribronchial and perivascular air may compress the airways and vascular supply, causing "air block."
   b. **Ventilator strategy.** Since air is driven into the interstitium throughout the ventilatory cycle, the primary goal is to reduce MAP through any of its components (Pi, Ti, PEEP) and to rely on increased FiO_2 to provide oxygenation. This strategy holds for all air leak syndromes. If dropping the MAP is not tolerated, other techniques may be tried. Because the time constants for interstitial air are much longer than those for the alveoli, we sometimes use very rapid conventional rates (up to 80 breaths per minute), which may preferentially ventilate the alveoli.

   High-frequency ventilation is an important alternative therapy for severe air leak and, if available, may be the ventilatory treatment of choice. HFV strategies for air leak differ from those used in diffuse alveolar disease. As described for conventional ventilation, the ventilatory goal in air leak syndromes is to decrease MAP, relying on FiO_2 to provide oxygenation. With HFJ and HFFI, PEEP is maintained at lower levels (2 to 4 cm H_2O), and few to no sigh breaths provided. With HFO, the MAP initially used is the **same** as that being used on the conventional ventilator, and the frequency set at 15 Hz. While weaning, MAP is decreased progressively, tolerating higher FiO_2 in the attempt to limit the MAP exposure.

5. **Apnea** (see Apnea, below)
   a. **Pathophysiology.** Occasionally, apnea is severe enough to warrant ventilatory support, even in the absence of pulmonary disease. This may result from apnea of prematurity, during or following general anesthesia, or from neuromuscular paralysis.
   b. **Ventilator strategy.** For infants completely dependent on the ventilator, the goal should be to provide "physiologic" ventilation using moderate PEEP (3 to 4 cm H_2O), lower gas flow, and normal rates (30 to 40 breaths per minute), with Pi adjusted to prevent hyperventilation (10 to 18 cm H_2O). Prolonged Ti is unnecessary. For infants requiring a ventilator because of intermittent but prolonged apnea, low rates (10 to 12 breaths per minute) may be sufficient.

VI. **Adjuncts to mechanical ventilation**
   A. **Sedation** can be used when agitation or distress is associated with excessive lability of oxygenation and hypoxemia. Although this problem is more common in the neonate receiving long-term ventilation, acutely ill newborns may occasionally benefit from sedation. Morphine (0.1 to 0.2 mg/kg)

or fentanyl (1 to 3 μg/kg) can be used but may cause neurologic depression. Prolonged use may lead to dependence. Lorazepam (0.05 to 0.1 mg/kg per dose given every 4 to 6 hours) has been used in more mature infants in more chronic situations because of its long duration of action. Nonpharmacologic methods, such as limiting environmental light and noise as well as providing behavioral supports for the preterm infant, may help decrease agitation and limit the need for sedative medications. As discussed above, synchronized IMV or ventilation may also help diminish agitation and ventilatory lability.

B. **Muscle relaxation** with pancuronium bromide (0.1 mg/kg per dose, repeated as needed) may be indicated in some infants who continue to breathe out of phase with the ventilator after attempts at finding appropriate settings and sedation have failed. High FiO_2 requirement (over 0.75) or peak inspiratory pressure (over 30 cm H_2O) are also relative indications for muscle relaxation. Although unequivocal data are not available, gas exchange may be improved in some infants following muscle relaxation, and the occurrence of chronic lung disease may be reduced. Prolonged muscle relaxation leads to fluid retention and may result in deterioration in compliance. Sedation is routinely administered to infants receiving muscle relaxants.

C. **Blood gas monitoring** (see Blood Gas Monitoring, below). All infants receiving mechanical ventilation require continuous monitoring of oxygen saturation or TcO_2 and intermittent blood gas measurements.

VII. **Complications and sequelae.** As a complex and invasive technology, mechanical ventilation can result in numerous adverse outcomes, both iatrogenic and unavoidable.

A. **Barotrauma and oxygen toxicity**
  1. **Bronchopulmonary dysplasia (BPD)** is related to increased airway pressure and changes in lung volume, although oxygen toxicity, anatomic and physiologic immaturity, and individual susceptibility also contribute.
  2. **Air leak** is directly related to increased airway pressure, occurring frequently at MAPs in excess of 14 cm H_2O.

B. **Mechanical**
  1. **Obstruction** of endotracheal tubes may result in hypoxemia and respiratory acidosis.
  2. **Equipment malfunction,** particularly disconnection, is not uncommon and requires functioning alarm systems and vigilance.

C. **Complications of invasive monitoring**
  1. **Peripheral arterial occlusion with infarction (see Chap. 25)**
  2. **Aortic thrombosis** from umbilical arterial catheters, occasionally leading to renal impairment and hypertension.
  3. **Emboli** from flushed catheters, particularly to the lower extremities, the splanchnic bed, or even the brain.

D. **Anatomic**
  1. **Subglottic stenosis**
  2. **Palatal grooves** from prolonged orotracheal intubation
  3. **Vocal cord damage**

References

1. Carlo, W. Assisted Ventilation. In: M.H. Klaus and A.A. Fanaroff (eds.). *Care of the High Risk Neonate,* 4th ed. Philadelphia: W.B. Saunders, 1993.
2. Clark, R.H. High-frequency ventilation. *J. Pediatr.* 124:661, 1994.

Extracorporeal Membrane Oxygenation
Mark Levy and James Fackler

I. **Background.** Extracorporeal membrane oxygenation (ECMO) is a life support technique used for profound cardiorespiratory failure in infants who fail to respond to conventional therapy (Table 24-4). The efficacy of extracorporeal life

Table 24-4. ECMO survival rate by diagnosis*

	Treated no.	Survived no. (%)
MAS	4519	4239 (94)
PPHN	1730	1421 (82)
CDH	2627	1546 (59)
RDS	1199	1010 (84)
Sepsis	1971	1507 (76)

MAS = meconium aspiration syndrome; PPHN = persistent pulmonary hypertension in the newborn; CDH = congenital diaphragmatic hernia; RDS = respiratory distress syndrome.
*Unpublished data from Extracorporeal Life Support Organization, Ann Arbor, Michigan, 1997.

support (ECLS) is supported by two prospective randomized trials of newborns with respiratory failure associated with persistent pulmonary hypertension. Continued excellent results with ECMO have solidified its role in the treatment of respiratory failure in newborns. Emerging technologies (e.g., high-frequency oscillatory ventilation and inhaled nitric oxide), however, already seem to diminish the need for ECMO.

II. Physiology

A. Theory. While the lungs are inadequate, ECMO provides effective gas exchange, including oxygenation and removal of carbon dioxide. ECMO allows "lung rest"; the lungs are protected from further injury due to barotrauma or oxygen, since lower ventilator settings can be used.

B. Method. Extracorporeal life support (ECLS) is provided by draining blood from the venous circulation, adding oxygen, and removing carbon dioxide via an artificial lung (membrane oxygenator). Blood is returned to either the venous or the arterial circulation.

C. Veno-arterial ECMO. In veno-arterial ECMO, the oxygenated blood is returned to the systemic circulation. Partial cardiac bypass is created in that the circuit blood returned to the patient is mixed with blood from the patient's own cardiac output. The total cardiac output (CO) is thus the sum of the native cardiac output and the output (pump flow) generated by the circuit:

$$CO_{total} = CO_{native} + CO_{circuit}$$

Increasing the bypass flow decreases the cardiac preload and results in a decrease in the ventricular stroke volume and ventricular output. The total cardiac output, however, remains unchanged. Assuming there is no myocardial damage, these changes in native contractility and cardiac output resolve after cessation of ECMO.

D. Veno-venous ECMO. Oxygenated blood from the circuit in veno-venous bypass is returned to the right atrium, where it mixes with blood returning from the systemic circulation. Thus, the oxygen content of mixed venous blood increases while the carbon dioxide content is reduced. Some of this blood is recirculated in the ECMO circuit, and the rest goes to the right ventricle, through the pulmonary vascular bed, to the left side of the heart, and into the systemic circulation. Since the volume of blood removed from the venous circulation for ECLS is equal to the volume returned, the preload and thus the native cardiac output remain unchanged during veno-venous ECMO. ECMO flow rate, therefore, has no effect on cardiac output during veno-venous ECMO.

E. Oxygen delivery. Oxygen delivery is the product of cardiac output and arterial oxygen content. During extracorporeal life support, many factors contribute to the delivery of oxygen. They include gas exchange in the membrane oxygenator, rate of flow through the ECMO circuit, gas exchange from the infant's lung, and cardiac output from the infant's heart. The P_aO_2 and S_aO_2 in the systemic circulation measured by arterial blood gas are a function of total gas exchange. Membrane and pulmonary gas exchange, as well as ECMO flow rate and native cardiac output, contribute to arterial oxygen saturation. At a constant ECLS flow rate and sweep gas, an improvement in the P_aO_2 signifies an improvement in pulmonary gas exchange. Alternatively, a deterioration in P_aO_2 may signify increased pulmonary blood flow without improvement in oxygen diffusion.

F. CO_2 removal. Carbon dioxide removal is extremely efficient in the membrane lung. The amount of CO_2 removed is dependent on the PCO_2 of blood circulating in the membrane, the surface area of the membrane, and the ventilating gas flow (sweep gas flow) through the membrane lung. In ECLS, blood and sweep gas flow in opposite directions, setting up a counter-current exchange of CO_2 in the membrane. The PCO_2 of the blood decreases as it travels through the membrane. The exchange of CO_2 occurs maximally in the blood inlet region and decreases as it reaches the outlet. As physiologic pulmonary function and tidal volume improve, the P_aCO_2 decrease. The sweep gas can be adjusted by adding CO_2 to the sweep or decreasing sweep flow rate in order to prevent respiratory alkalosis.

G. Renal perfusion. Blood flow through an ECMO circuit is maintained by a nonpulsatile pump. In veno-arterial ECMO, as flow through the ECMO circuit increases, more and more blood is directed to the circuit. With increasing flows, the patient's heart contributes less to the total cardiac output. The pulse pressure eventually becomes dampened with increased flows and can flatten when maximal bypass is reached. At least one side effect of this nonpulsatile flow is an increase in renin production by the kidney. Although the mean arterial pressure may be normal, the kidneys produce renin in response. This can result in renal insufficiency. Hemodynamics during venovenous ECMO are unchanged and therefore have no effect on the systemic pulsatile flow.

H. Blood–prosthetic interaction. During ECLS, blood is in continuous contact with the prosthetic surface of the ECMO circuit. This blood–prosthetic surface interaction results in activation of both the complement and clotting cascades and the production of fibrin, lymphokines, and cytokines. Flow through the circuit has a tendency toward clot formation. This is a result of fibrinogen binding to the circuit surface and activation of the clotting cascade. Once activated, fibrin formation results in the accumulation of platelets and the formation of a clot, which can trap red cells.

I. Heparin/ACT. Heparin is used to inhibit the intrinsic clotting cascade and to prevent fibrin formation. Heparin infusion is adjusted according to blood activated clotting time (ACT). The ACT is maintained in the range of 180 to 200 seconds. Unfortunately, in an effort to prevent clot formation, heparin infusion may result in bleeding. Bleeding is the most significant complication of ECMO.

J. Free radicals and cytokines. Before beginning ECLS, patients are generally hypoxemic. The characteristic changes that occur after initiation of ECLS are consistent with hypoxia and shock followed by reperfusion. These changes include the production of oxygen free radicals and other cytokines. The effect of these substances on the outcome of ECMO patients is not understood.

K. Edema. Total body water and extracellular fluid increase during ECMO and resolve with its discontinuation. The resolution of lung "whiteout" that occurs during ECMO correlates with improvement in pulmonary gas exchange and discontinuation of ECLS. These findings result from the reperfusion injury that occurs when ECLS support is begun for an infant in shock. This reperfusion injury results in pulmonary edema and diffuse capillary leak syndromes.

III. Indications

A. Indications. The indications for neonatal ECLS are (1) reversible respiratory failure and (2) a predicted mortality rate with conventional therapy great enough to warrant the risks of ECMO. Defining the appropriate mortality rate is difficult, however, and varies with the primary disease. In two studies, an alveolar–arterial oxygen gradient (A–a)DO$_2$ greater than 600 torr for 12 hours was associated with 94% mortality and an (A–a)DO$_2$ greater than 610 torr for 8 hours was associated with 79% mortality.

B. Oxygen index (OI) is calculated as:

$$OI = \frac{MAP \times FiO_2}{P_aO_2} \times 100$$

where MAP equals mean airway pressure, the FiO$_2$ equals inspired oxygen concentration, and P$_a$O$_2$ equals partial pressure of arterial oxygen. We generally use an OI greater than 40 for 2 hours with conventional ventilation and an OI greater than 60 for 2 hours with high-frequency oscillatory ventilation as criteria for ECMO. A relative criterion to initiate ECMO is failure to respond to treatment, including the inability to wean from high MAP over a prolonged period, failure to wean inspired oxygen concentration to 0.60 or less, profound hypotension, or a precipitous deterioration in the patient's condition.

C. Contraindications. The relative contraindications for ECMO in newborns include ten or more days of mechanical ventilation, grade II intraventricular hemorrhage, body weight less than 2 kg, or gestational age less than 34 weeks. The absolute contraindications for ECLS include significant intraventricular or parenchymal hemorrhage or 2 or more weeks of mechanical ventilation.

IV. Management strategies

A. Basic. When a patient has met a center's criteria for ECMO, consent is obtained and cannulation of the blood vessels is performed. If the infant's condition allows, we perform head ultrasound examination and echocardiogram to exclude large intracranial hemorrhages and congenital heart defects that require surgical intervention.

B. Circuit priming. The appropriate circuit for a neonate is assembled using a 0.8 m² membrane oxygenator. The circuit is first primed with carbon dioxide, evacuated, and then primed with saline. At this point the circuit can be stored for use in 48 to 72 hours. After debubbling the circuit prior to use, albumin is added. The saline/albumin prime is then displaced with 400 cc of packed red blood cells, 150 cc of fresh frozen plasma, Tham, heparin, and calcium gluconate. Circuit pH, ionized calcium, and potassium are checked before ECMO is started. Once the patient is receiving ECMO, 2 units of concentrated platelets are given.

C. Cannulation. Anesthesia is given using narcotics, benzodiazepines, and paralytic agents. We try to use veno-venous ECMO whenever possible. A 14 French double-lumen cannula (DLC) is used for v-v ECMO. Patients who require multiple inotropic infusions for blood pressure support, or cardiopulmonary resuscitation (CPR), require v-a ECMO. A jugular vein not large enough to accommodate a 14F cannula may also preclude the use of v-v ECMO. In order to maximize venous drainage in v-a ECMO, the largest venous cannula that the jugular vein can accommodate is used. Similarly, the largest arterial cannula is used for the carotid artery to maximize flow capability and to prevent high postmembrane pressures.

D. Circuit upkeep. Circuits are examined twice daily for clots. The circuit tubing is shifted in the roller pump at 120 hours of ECLS. Circuit changes are made only if one of the following indications is met: (1) excessive clotting in the circuit, (2) elevation of the premembrane pressure, indicating membrane clotting and failure, (3) membrane failure proved by inadequate change from pre- to postmembrane PO$_2$ and PCO$_2$, (4) excessive platelet consumption not attributable to the patient, (5) an uncorrectable coagulopathy that is thought to be caused by the circuit/membrane, and (6) circuit disaster. If a circuit needs to be changed, a new circuit is primed, the patient is cycled off of ECLS, the old circuit is cut away, and the new circuit is connected, with care being taken to keep air out of the system.

E. **Blood product evaluation.** Heparin is used in all patients to prevent clot formation. The whole blood activated clotting time (ACT) is used to monitor heparin infusion and avoid hemorrhagic complications. We optimize other factors and keep ACT at 180 to 200 seconds. Prothrombin time is maintained at less than 17 seconds using fresh frozen plasma, fibrinogen is kept above 200 mg/dl using cryoprecipitate, and the platelet count is maintained above 150,000 using concentrated platelets. The hematocrit is kept above 38% to facilitate oxygen delivery.

F. **Aminocaproic acid (Amicar)** lowers the incidence of hemorrhagic complications associated with ECMO, including intracranial and postoperative hemorrhage. Patients who are considered to be at high risk for bleeding complications are given Amicar. They include infants who (1) are in the perioperative period, (2) are less than 35 weeks' gestational age, (3) have sepsis, (4) have prolonged hypoxia or acidosis before ECMO, or (5) have grade I or II intraventricular hemorrhage. A loading dose of Amicar (100 mg/kg) is given, followed by a 30 mg/kg/hour infusion. After 72 hours of Amicar, the patient is assessed for further risks of bleeding complications. If these risks still exist, Amicar is continued and the circuit is changed at 120 hours. Otherwise, the Amicar infusion is discontinued.

G. **Medications.** Standard medications for ECMO patients in addition to heparin include broad-spectrum antibiotics, inotropes for blood pressure support (primarily v-v ECMO), narcotic analgesics, and sedatives. In order to maximize mobilization of extracellular fluid, we try to avoid muscle relaxation.

H. **Nutrition.** Nutrition is provided with parenteral alimentation. A total of 80 to 100 ml/kg/day of fluid is generally given, excluding blood products. To prevent lipid accumulation and embolism in the circuit, no more than 1 g/kg/day of lipid is given.

I. **Fluid management.** In order to maximize diuresis during ECLS, patients are given loop diuretics and low-dose dopamine. Hemofiltration is used in parallel with the circuit when excessive extracellular fluid is noted, while maintaining a urine output of at least 1 ml/kg/hour.

J. **Neurologic evaluation.** Head ultrasound examinations are performed within 24 hours following cannulation, and every other day while the patient is receiving ECMO. Small intracranial hemorrhages are managed by optimizing clotting factors and using Amicar. Larger intracranial hemorrhages may force premature discontinuation of ECMO.

K. **Ventilator management.** While receiving ECMO, patients are maintained on "resting" ventilator settings with peak inspiratory pressure (PIP) = 25 cm H_2O, positive end-expiratory pressure (PEEP) = 5 cm H_2O, rate = 10, and FiO_2 = 0.4. Use of higher PEEP (12 to 14 cm H_2O) during ECMO, as advocated by others, may help prevent deterioration of pulmonary function and result in more rapid lung recovery. During ECMO, lung function is assessed as follows: (1) As lungs improve CO_2 removal and oxygen content of the native cardiac output improve, resulting in improving P_aO_2 and P_aCO_2. Sweep gases can be adjusted accordingly. (2) Chest radiographs show gradual resolution of pulmonary edema. (3) As pulmonary edema resolves, expired tidal volumes improve.

L. **Cycling and decannulation.** When expired tidal volumes reach approximately 5 to 7 cc/kg (in the nonparalyzed patient), attempts are made at cycling by temporarily clamping the ECMO circuit and obtaining blood gas determinations. Comparisons to previous cycling attempts are used to assess a patient's progress. Our criteria for decannulation are as follows: PIP = 30 cm H_2O, rate 25 breaths/minute, and FiO_2 = 0.35: P_aO_2 over 60 mm Hg, P_aCO_2 = 40 to 50 mm Hg, pH <7.50.

When these criteria are used, patients rarely require recannulation. At the time of decannulation from v-a ECMO, we attempt to reconstruct the common carotid artery. The jugular vein is routinely ligated. Two units of concentrated platelets are given following decannulation.

V. Follow-up
- **A. Pulmonary.** One study found that 25% of former ECMO patients required hospitalization within the first year because of pulmonary complications. This compares to a hospitalization rate of 10 to 36% in newborns with similar lung disease treated conventionally. In contrast, healthy infants with no previous history of respiratory disease have a 20 to 25% incidence of lower respiratory tract infections during the first 2 years of life with less than 1% requiring hospitalization.
- **B. Neurodevelopment.** Developmental outcome following ECMO appears to improve with age and does not differ from that of newborns with similar lung disease treated conventionally. A follow-up study found normal cognitive development in 90% of school-age children, 70% of preschoolers, and 57% of infants. Other studies of ECMO graduates have likewise shown a 79 to 90% incidence of normal cognitive development. In comparison, 25 to 60% of neonates with similar lung disease treated conventionally showed adverse neurologic outcomes. Neurodevelopmental morbidity included seizures, cerebral palsy, and mild developmental delay.
- **C. Hearing.** Sensorineuronal hearing loss occurs in 4 to 21% of infants treated with ECMO. Hearing loss occurred in 20 to 52% of infants with PPHN who received conventional therapy. Hearing loss in PPHN has been attributed to hyperventilation with resultant cerebral vasoconstriction and decreased cerebral perfusion. The use of furosemide and gentamicin may also contribute.
- **D. Intracranial hemorrhage.** Intracranial hemorrhage is a major factor in the morbidity and mortality following ECLS. In one study of 42 infants requiring ECLS, 12% had major hemorrhage and 17% had minor hemorrhage. The ELSO registry reports a 12% incidence of infarction. One study reports a higher incidence of right-sided brain lesions followed veno-arterial ECMO as a result of right common carotid artery ligation, although this has not been seen by others.

Reference
1. Kanto, W. P. A decade of experience with neonatal extracorporeal membrane oxygenation. *J. Pediatr.* 124:335, 1994.

Blood Gas Monitoring and Pulmonary Function Tests
Douglas K. Richardson and Eric C. Eichenwald

- **I. General principles.** The purpose of blood gas monitoring is to ensure adequate gas exchange while avoiding the risks of hypoxia or hyperoxia and excessive or inadequate ventilation. All sick infants with cardiopulmonary disorders should be monitored. The two major modes of monitoring are invasive blood gas analysis and noninvasive monitoring. Clinical circumstances, including severity and anticipated duration of lung disease, degree of instability, and availability of arterial access, will determine the appropriate combination of monitoring.
- **II. Blood gas analysis.** Arterial blood gases (ABGs) are the gold standard for assessing the adequacy of oxygen delivery, ventilation, and pH. All noninvasive methods should be correlated with ABGs.
  - **A. Sampling.** Blood samples are usually obtained from indwelling arterial catheters. ABGs should be obtained every 1 to 6 hours when acute respiratory support is required and less frequently with stable chronic respiratory illness. ABGs represent the major source of iatrogenic blood loss and need for transfusions. Percutaneous arterial puncture is preferred when sampling is infrequent or the course is expected to be short. Noxious stimuli, including arterial puncture, cause variable drops in measured P_aO_2, espe-

cially in chronically ill infants with little pulmonary reserve. This may influence the interpretation of the results. Sampling from venous catheters provides useful information on PCO_2 and pH only. Venous blood pH values are usually 0.02 to 0.04 lower, and PCO_2 is usually 6 to 10 mm Hg higher than paired arterial samples, but they vary depending on cardiac output and metabolic demands. Warmed capillary samples (CBGs) can be used to assess PCO_2 and pH. Capillary samples are unreliable in assessing oxygenation and may not always accurately reflect P_aCO_2.

B. **Measurements.** Blood gas analyzers make direct readings of PO_2, PCO_2, and pH. The bicarbonate and oxygen saturation are generally calculated from standard nomograms. Direct measurement of oxygen saturation is possible but requires 0.5 ml more blood and a co-oximeter.

C. **Interpretation.** Extreme hypothermia or hyperthermia may lead to over- or underestimates (respectively) of arterial oxygenation. Since heparin solutions equilibrate with room air, excessive heparinization of sample syringes may have the same effect as air bubbles, raising PO_2 and lowering PCO_2.

III. **Noninvasive monitoring.** Although ABGs are the gold standard, they have several drawbacks: (1) they require invasive catheters or painful and technically difficult arterial punctures, (2) they are not continuous, and (3) they are expensive in terms of both the cost of sample analyses and the clinical costs of iatrogenic anemia and transfusions. The continuous nature of noninvasive monitoring has made evident the inaccuracies of samples obtained by skin puncture. Continuous monitoring is especially useful in evaluating the clinical significance of apnea and acute changes such as pneumothorax, and it provides immediate feedback after changes in ventilator settings. It can be done at little risk to the patient. The long-term benefits of such monitoring are presumed but remain unproven.

IV. **Noninvasive oxygen monitoring.** The two technologies for monitoring oxygenation are pulse oximetry ($StcO_2$) and transcutaneous oxygen tension monitors ($PtcO_2$).

A. **Pulse oximetry**

1. **General characteristics.** Oximeters depend on the fact that reduced hemoglobin absorbs more red than infrared light, and oxygenated hemoglobin absorbs more infrared than red. The oximeter probe consists of a light-emitting diode and a photodetector placed on opposite sides of a narrow part of the body. The diode emits equal intensities of red and infrared light into the tissue, and the photodetector senses the ratio of red to infrared light. The proportion of oxygenated to reduced hemoglobin is calculated and displayed. Since a ratio rather than an absolute value is measured, no calibration is required. The instrument is programmed to look only at pulsatile increases in oxygenated hemoglobin and thus depends on detection of a reasonable pulse. The correlations between transcutaneous estimates ($StcO_2$) and measured arterial saturations (S_aO_2) are 0.90 to 0.95. The PaO_2 at any given SaO_2 is a function of the oxyhemoglobin dissociation curve (see Fig. 24-1). Because SaO_2 increases little as the P_aO_2 increases at the flat upper end of the curve, oximetry poorly distinguishes high normal oxygen tensions (80 to 100 mm Hg) from dangerously hyperoxic ones (200 to 400 mm Hg). This poor discrimination at the upper end of the curve is accentuated by any shifts in the curve itself. Both higher concentrations of adult hemoglobin and acidosis shift the dissociation curve to the right. A shift to the right means less saturation at a given P_aO_2. Increases in P_aCO_2, temperature, and concentration of 2,3-diphosphoglycerate (2,3-DPG) also shift the dissociation curve to the right.

a. **Calibration and maintenance.** The photosensors do not need calibration. However, comparison of P_aO_2 by ABG with transcutaneous saturation ($StcO_2$) allows the O_2 dissociation curve to be estimated for the individual infant. Different models of oximeters use different sensors and saturation computation programs that may result in different baseline saturation readings. For example, Ohmeda Biox oximeters register saturations 2% lower than Nellcor N-100 oximeters. Interference by bright lights can be helped by shielding, but motion artifacts can be a problem in active infants.

b. Limits and interpretation. Because of the unpredictable location of the upper end of the O_2 dissociation curve, a measured $StcO_2$ of 97% might correspond to a P_aO_2 ranging from 90 to 135 mm Hg, given the ± 2% limits of accuracy of an oximeter. This limit in precision is compounded by significant differences among makes and models of oximeters. In preterm infants with predominantly fetal hemoglobin, saturations of 86 to 92% correspond to P_aO_2 values of 37 to 97 mm Hg. Thus, for a premature baby receiving oxygen or ventilatory support, P_aO_2 should be monitored when the $StcO_2$ is greater than 90%. At the lower end of the curve, the effects of shifts in the curve are more evident in saturation than in P_aO_2. For example, at a P_aO_2 of 45 mm Hg, saturation may decrease from about 88% at pH 7.4 (which is satisfactory) to about 80% at pH 7.25 (which may be inadequate for tissue oxygenation). In general, saturation above 88% is adequate, and below 80% is inadequate. $StcO_2$ between 80 and 88% may be adequate if the P_aO_2 is greater than 45 mm Hg. These values assume normal cardiac output and hemoglobin concentration. Although monitoring saturation is useful at lower levels, it must be remembered that partial pressure determines the rate of oxygen transferred to the tissues and also muscle tone in the wall of the ductus arteriosus and pulmonary arterioles.

2. Advantages
  a. Saturation is the basic physiologic determinant of tissue oxygen delivery.
  b. No warm-up or equilibration time.
  c. Immediate readouts permit spot monitoring and shared equipment.
  d. Pulse-by-pulse detection of rapid or transient changes in saturation (e.g., apneic spells).
  e. Substantially lower maintenance and technician costs.

3. Disadvantages
  a. Risk of hyperoxia at saturations between 94 and 100%.
  b. Variability in hemoglobin saturation curve during the first weeks makes estimates of P_aO_2 unpredictable. This variability is affected by pH and relative amounts of adult and fetal hemoglobin.
  c. Motion and light artifacts frequently disrupt monitoring.
  d. Not usable in cases of severe hypotension or marked edema.
  e. Does not take clinical impact of anemia into account.
  f. May provoke evaluation of transient, clinically insignificant desaturations.
  g. Skin burns from sensors have been reported.
  h. Supplementary O_2 may be weaned too slowly because high P_aO_2 is not recognized.

B. Transcutaneous oxygenation ($PtcO_2$)
  1. General characteristics. $PtcO_2$ monitoring uses a sensor that is applied to the skin on an occlusive contact medium. The sensor is heated to produce localized hyperemia, which maximizes capillary blood flow under the sensor. Tissue oxygen then diffuses across the epidermis to the sensor membrane. A 10- to 15-minute equilibration time after sensor application is needed before the readings become reliable. Transcutaneous oxygen sensors have been generally supplanted by pulse oximetry for continuous monitoring, although they can be used to perform noninvasive hyperoxia tests to evaluate infants suspected to have cyanotic congenital heart disease (see Chap. 25).

V. Noninvasive PCO_2 monitoring. The role of noninvasive PCO_2 monitoring is less well established. This is because hyper- and hypocapnia are usually associated with acute changes in oxygenation. Noninvasive PCO_2 monitoring is useful to follow trends when unexpected changes in baseline PCO_2 may occur. Such clinical situations include rapid weaning in RDS, hyperventilation for persistent pulmonary hypertension, decompensation in established BPD, transition to high-frequency ventilation, and possibly high risk of pneumothorax. We employ these devices infrequently. Two technologies available are transcutaneous PCO_2 ($PtcCO_2$) and capnography to estimate end-tidal PCO_2 ($PetCO_2$).

A. Transcutaneous PCO_2 ($PtcCO_2$)

  1. General characteristics. $PtcCO_2$ monitors use a pH-sensitive glass electrode. When applied occlusively to the skin, the heated sensor causes vasodilation of the underlying capillary bed. Tissue CO_2 equilibrates across the epidermis and membrane. Combined O_2/CO_2 sensors are available.

    a. Maintenance and calibration. Reported correlations are 0.90 to 0.93, agreeing with P_aCO_2 ± 4 mm Hg. Sensors require 10 to 15 minutes of equilibration before providing stable readings. The heated sensor causes more dissolved CO_2 to come out of solution and also raises the local tissue metabolic rate. Both effects result in a higher PCO_2 reading. At 44°C, the increase is a factor of 1.37 times. It is proportionally lower at lower temperatures, but accuracy and response time are worse. Most monitors have an electronic means of reducing the displayed $PtcCO_2$ by this factor. Before use, sensors must be calibrated against a standard CO_2 gas mixture, and they tend to drift during use. Electrodes are costly and fragile, and replacement membranes are needed periodically. Sensor sites must be rotated every 2 to 6 hours to avoid burns.

    b. Interpretation and limits. The $PtcCO_2$ sensor is conceptually similar to the more familiar $PtcO_2$ electrode. Both are dependent on adequate tissue blood flow and are adversely affected by hypotension and tissue edema, although the $PtcCO_2$ is less affected. Rising $PtcCO_2$ and falling $PtcO_2$ should raise concerns about perfusion. Both sensors have relatively slow response times in vivo (30 to 90 seconds). Both require 5 to 15 minutes' equilibration. Both are less accurate in older infants with thicker skin.

  2. Advantages. $PtcCO_2$ can be used in any situation where continuous monitoring is indicated and can be used on nonintubated infants. It may be particularly useful when initiating and adjusting high-frequency ventilation or for close monitoring after extubation.

  3. Disadvantages. $PtcCO_2$ monitoring often fails to provide additional information beyond that readily available from intermittent blood gas analysis, and it is expensive and labor-intensive. Its slow response time makes it less useful for detecting acute rises in P_aCO_2. It is not useful for intermittent monitoring of chronic BPD because of unpredictable variations in baseline.

B. Capnography (end-tidal CO_2, $PetCO_2$)

  1. General characteristics. Capnographs use infrared spectroscopy or mass spectrometry readings of expired gas to analyze CO_2 content. This technique depends on the achievement of an end-tidal CO_2 plateau from which to estimate alveolar CO_2. It is therefore rate- and flow-dependent. In newborns, the relatively high respiratory rates and low tidal volumes (relative to the bias flow of fresh gas) and marked ventilation–perfusion mismatching mean that a stable $PetCO_2$ is often not achieved. This results in inconsistent underestimates of P_aCO_2, especially in sicker infants. Correlation coefficients with P_aCO_2 are 0.69 to 0.92. Newer systems with lower dead space and mainstream sensors may make this method practical for future use.

  2. Advantages. $PetCO_2$ may provide intermittent trend monitoring for larger intubated infants with chronic lung disease. It can also be used qualitatively at the nostrils of nonintubated infants to detect air flow obstruction and apnea.

  3. Disadvantages. The additional dead space introduced by the airway adapter can cause CO_2 retention of as much as 6 to 10 mm Hg. $PetCO_2$ cannot be employed during high-frequency ventilation.

VI. Other devices. The noninvasive technologies have been employed invasively in arterial catheters: **oxygen electrode catheters** and **oximetric catheters.** Both techniques share all the advantages and disadvantages. They provide accurate direct arterial readings with rapid response times. Both require invasive monitoring. In both there is a significant rate of catheter tip occlusion. Such occlusions seem more frequent than with conventional catheters, presumably because of the smaller lumen. Catheters are very expensive, cannot be reused, and require in vivo calibration.

VII. Tidal volume measurements. Several monitors are available for tidal volume measurements in neonates. The monitors measure flow with either a pneumotachometer or a hot wire anemometer; flow is integrated to give volume. Many neonatal ventilators now incorporate this technology, and they provide continuous information on inspiratory and expiratory tidal volume and minute ventilation. These monitors can help the clinician assess optimal settings for PEEP and PIP in individual patients by measuring the effect of changes in ventilator settings on delivered tidal volume and minute ventilation. We have found tidal volume measurements to be useful additional information in the mechanical ventilation of critically ill neonates, particularly in weaning strategy. The technology is limited, however, by the accuracy of the measurements, which can be affected by the infant's head position, variable leak around the endotracheal tube, or changes in ventilator circuit resistance from water or secretions in tubing.

VIII. Pulmonary function tests (PFTs). Several bedside, automated and computerized systems for the measurement of pulmonary mechanics in newborn infants are now commercially available. These systems have simplified the measurement of pulmonary mechanics in infants. Many centers have incorporated pulmonary function testing into the daily management of mechanically ventilated infants. However, routine use of PFT measurements in this population has not been demonstrated to affect clinical management or outcome. In addition, the data generated by these automated systems must be interpreted with caution because of potential errors resulting from artifacts.

A. Techniques. Obtaining useful data on pulmonary mechanics requires the measurement of **flow and airway and/or esophageal pressure.** Flow may be measured with a pneumotachograph with a differential pressure transducer, or with a hot wire anemometer. Tidal volume can then be determined from integration of the flow signal. Airway pressure is usually measured with a pressure transducer connected to a side port of the endotracheal tube in the intubated patient, or to a face mask in the nonintubated patient. Esophageal pressure, needed to calculate lung compliance and resistance, may be obtained with an esophageal balloon or a fluid-filled catheter. Several technical considerations may affect esophageal pressure measurements, including positioning of the catheter in the esophagus and the frequency response of the system.

B. Measurements. By using the measurement techniques described above, **tidal volume and static and/or dynamic compliance** and **resistance** of the respiratory system may be derived. Several different techniques to calculate compliance and resistance may be used, depending on the capabilities of the measurement system utilized.

The accuracy and reproducibility of PFT measurements may be affected by several variables. They include the lung volume at which the measurements are obtained, sleep state, the position of the infant (e.g., prone or supine), and the timing of the measurements in relationship to endotracheal suctioning or a feeding. In order for daily measurements to be comparable, they must be performed at the same ventilator settings. In addition, it is essential to understand the assumptions and calculation methods used by the computerized systems to interpret the accuracy of pulmonary mechanics data displayed for the clinician.

C. Clinical applications. Most investigators have demonstrated considerable interpatient as well as intrapatient variability in PFT measurements using these bedside systems. This variability limits the interpretation of PFT data and reduces its effectiveness as a prognostic tool. We have found PFT measurements to occasionally be useful in selected clinical situations, including the evaluation of airway obstruction and the assessment of the effectiveness of specific drug therapy. The clinical utility of more routine applications of this technology remains unproven.

References

1. Gerhardt, T.O., and Bancalari, E. Measurement and monitoring of pulmonary function. *Clin. Perinatol.* 18:581, 1991.
2. Hay, W.W. Jr., Thilo, E., Curlander, J.B. Pulse oximetry in neonatal medicine. *Clin. Perinatol.* 18:441, 1991.
3. Poets, C.F., Southall, D.P. Noninvasive monitoring of oxygenation in infants and children: practical considerations and areas of concern. *Pediatrics* 93:737, 1994.

Air Leak: Pneumothorax, Pulmonary Interstitial Emphysema, Pneumomediastinum, Pneumopericardium
Gary A. Silverman

I. **Background**
  A. **Incidence and risk factors.** Risk factors for air leak in premature infants include respiratory distress syndrome (RDS), mechanical ventilation, and pneumonia. Surfactant therapy has markedly decreased the incidence of pneumothorax. Risk factors in term infants are aspiration of meconium, blood, or amniotic fluid; pneumonia; congenital malformations; and mechanical ventilation.
  B. **Pathogenesis.** Air leak syndromes arise via a common mechanism. Transpulmonary pressures that exceed the tensile strength of the noncartilagenous terminal airways and alveolar saccules can damage the respiratory epithelium. Loss of epithelial integrity permits air to enter the interstitium, causing pulmonary interstitial emphysema. Persistent elevation in transpulmonary pressure facilitates the dissection of air toward the visceral pleura and/or the hilum via the peribronchial and perivascular spaces. In rare circumstances, air can enter the pulmonary veins and result in an air embolus. Rupture of the pleural surface allows the adventitial air to decompress into the pleural space, causing pneumothorax. Following a path of least resistance, air can dissect from the hilum and into the mediastinum, resulting in pneumomediastinum, or into the pericardium, resulting in pneumopericardium. Air in the mediastinum can decompress into the pleural space, the fascial planes of the neck and skin (subcutaneous emphysema), or the retroperitoneum. In turn, retroperitoneal air can rupture into the peritoneum (pneumoperitoneum) or dissect into the scrotum or labial folds.
    1. Elevations in transpulmonary pressure can occur during the infant's first breaths when negative inspiratory pressure can approach 100 cm H_2O. Uneven ventilation due to atelectasis, surfactant deficiency, pulmonary hemorrhage, or retained fetal lung fluid can increase transpulmonary pressure. In turn, this leads to alveolar overdistention and rupture. Similarly, aspiration of blood, amniotic fluid, or meconium can facilitate alveolar overdistention by a check-valve mechanism.
    2. In the presence of underlying pulmonary conditions, positive pressure ventilation increases the risk of air leak. The high airway pressure required to achieve adequate oxygenation and ventilation in infants with poor pulmonary compliance (e.g., pulmonary hypoplasia, RDS, pulmonary edema) further increases this risk. Excessive transpulmonary pressures can occur when ventilator pressures are not decreased as pulmonary compliance improves. This situation sometimes occurs in infants

with RDS who improve rapidly after surfactant treatment. Mechanically ventilated preterm infants who make expiratory efforts against ventilator breaths are also at increased risk for pneumothorax.

3. Direct trauma to the airways can also cause air leak. Laryngoscopes, endotracheal tubes, suction catheters, and malpositioned feeding tubes can damage the lining of the airways and provide a portal for air entry.

II. Types of air leaks

  A. Pneumothorax. Spontaneous pneumothoraces have been observed in 0.07% of otherwise healthy appearing neonates. One in 10 of these infants is symptomatic. The high inspiratory pressures and uneven ventilation that occur in the initial stages of lung inflation may contribute to this phenomenon. Since some infants with spontaneous pneumothorax have urinary tract abnormalities, we consider an abdominal ultrasound examination in this circumstance.

Pneumothorax is more common in newborns treated with mechanical ventilation for underlying pulmonary disease. Prior to the availability of surfactant therapy, right-sided pneumothoraces were twice as frequent as left-sided, and bilateral pneumothoraces occurred in approximately 15 to 20% of cases.

Clinical signs of pneumothorax range from insidious changes in vital signs to the complete cardiovascular collapse that frequently accompanies a tension pneumothorax. As intrathoracic pressure rises, there is decreased lung volume, mediastinal shift, compression of the large intrathoracic veins, and increased pulmonary vascular resistance. The net effect is an increase in central venous pressure, a decrease in preload, and, ultimately, diminished cardiac output. Clinicians should suspect a pneumothorax in mechanically ventilated infants who develop unexplained alterations in hemodynamics, pulmonary compliance, or oxygenation and ventilation.

    1. Diagnosis

      a. Physical examination

        (1) Signs of respiratory distress include tachypnea, grunting, flaring, and retractions.

        (2) Cyanosis.

        (3) Chest asymmetry with expansion of the affected side.

        (4) Episodes of apnea and bradycardia.

        (5) Shift in the point of maximum cardiac impulse.

        (6) Diminished or distant breath sounds on the affected side.

        (7) Alterations in vital signs. With smaller collections of extrapulmonary air, compensatory increases may occur in heart rate and blood pressure. As the amount of air in the pleural space increases, however, central venous pressure rises and severe hypotension, bradycardia, apnea, hypoxia, and hypercapnia may occur.

      b. Arterial blood gases. Changes in arterial blood gas measurements are nonspecific and demonstrate a decreased PO_2 and increased PCO_2 (and decreased pH).

      c. Chest radiographs. Anteroposterior (AP) views can show a hyperlucent hemithorax, a separation of the visceral from the parietal pleura, flattening of the diaphragm, and mediastinal shift. Smaller collections of intrapleural air can be detected beneath the anterior chest wall by obtaining a cross-table lateral view. The lateral decubitus view, with the side of suspected pneumothorax up, may be helpful in detecting a small pneumothorax and may help differentiate skin folds, congenital lobar emphysema, cystic adenomatoid malformations, and surface blebs that occasionally give the appearance of intrapleural air.

      d. Transillumination with a high-intensity fiberoptic light source may demonstrate a pneumothorax. This technique is less sensitive in infants with chest-wall edema or severe PIE, or in extremely small infants with thin chest walls. We often obtain a baseline transillumination in infants at high risk for air leak.

   e. Needle aspiration. In a rapidly deteriorating clinical situation, thoracentesis may confirm the diagnosis and be therapeutic (see **2.b**).

2. Treatment

   a. Conservative therapy. Close observation may be adequate for infants who have no underlying lung disease or complicating therapy (such as mechanical ventilation), are in no respiratory distress, and have no continuous air leak. The extrapulmonary air will usually resolve in 24 to 48 hours. Although some of these infants may require a small increase in their ambient O_2 concentration, we do not routinely administer 100% oxygen.

   b. Needle aspiration. Thoracentesis with a "butterfly" needle can be used to treat a symptomatic pneumothorax. Needle aspiration may be curative in infants not receiving mechanical ventilation and is frequently a temporizing measure in mechanically ventilated infants. In infants with severe hemodynamic compromise, thoracentesis may be a life-saving procedure.

      (1) Attach a 23- or 25-gauge butterfly needle to a 10- to 20-cc syringe previously fitted with a three-way stopcock.

      (2) Identify the second intercostal space in the midclavicular line, and prepare the overlying skin with an antibacterial solution.

      (3) Insert the needle firmly into the intercostal space and pass it just above the top of the third rib. This will minimize the chance of lacerating an intercostal artery, as these vessels are located on the inferior surface of the ribs. As the needle is inserted, apply continuous suction with the syringe. A rapid flow of air into the syringe occurs when the needle enters the pleural space. Once the pleural space has been entered, stop advancing the needle. This will reduce the risk of puncturing the lung while the remaining air is evacuated.

      (4) A continuous air leak can be aspirated while a chest tube is being inserted (see **c**). Otherwise, withdraw the needle after the air flow has ceased.

   c. Chest tube drainage. Chest tube drainage is generally needed to evacuate pneumothoraces that develop in infants receiving positive pressure ventilation. Frequently, these air leaks are continuous and will result in severe hemodynamic compromise if left untreated.

      (1) Insertion of a chest tube

         (a) Select a chest tube of the appropriate size. No. 10 (smaller) and no. 12 (larger) French catheters are adequate for most infants.

         (b) Prepare the chest area with an antibacterial solution. Infiltrate the subcutaneous tissues overlying the sixth rib at the anterior axillary line with a 1% lidocaine solution. We administer a narcotic to the patient if vital signs are stable.

         (c) In the anterior axillary line, parallel to the sixth rib, make a small incision (1.0 to 1.5 cm) through the skin. Incisions of breast tissue should be avoided by locating the position of the nipple and surrounding tissue.

         (d) With a small curved hemostat, dissect the subcutaneous tissue overlying the rib. Make a subcutaneous track to the third or fourth interspace. Care should be taken to avoid the nipple area, the pectoralis muscle, and the axillary artery.

         (e) Enter the pleural space with the closed hemostat. Guide the tip over the top of the rib to avoid trauma to the intercostal artery. Push the hemostat through the intercostal muscles and parietal pleura. Spread the tips to widen the opening. We rarely use trochars to enter the pleural cavity, since the use of these instruments may increase the risk of lung perforation.

(f) Grasp the end of the chest tube with the tips of the curved hemostat. The chest tube and the hemostat should be in a parallel orientation. Advance the hemostat and chest tube through the skin incision and into the pleural opening. After the pleural space has been entered, direct the chest tube anteriorly by rotating the curved points of the hemostat. Release the hemostat and advance the chest tube a few centimeters. Be certain that the side ports of the chest tube are in the pleural space.

(g) The chest tube will "steam up" once it has been placed into the pleural space.

(h) Direct the chest tube to the location of the pleural air. The anterior pleural space is generally most effective for infants in the supine position.

(i) Palpate the chest wall around the entry site to confirm that the chest tube is not in the subcutaneous tissues.

(j) Using 3-0 or 4-0 silk, close the skin incision. We place a purse-string suture around the tube or a single interrupted suture on either side of the tube. Secure the chest tube by wrapping and then tying the skin suture tails around the tube. A second loop may be placed around the chest tube at a position 2 to 4 cm from the skin surface.

(k) Cover the insertion site with petrolatum gauze and a small, clear, plastic, adhesive surgical dressing. We avoid extensive taping or large dressings, as they interfere with chest examination and may delay the discovery of a displaced chest tube.

(l) Attach the chest tube to a Heimlich valve (for transport) or an underwater drainage system such as a Pleur-evac. Apply negative pressure (10 to 20 cm H_2O) to the underwater drainage system.

(m) AP and lateral chest radiographs are obtained to confirm tube position and ascertain drainage of the pleural air.

(n) Radiographs may reveal chest tubes that are ineffective in evacuating extrapulmonary air. The most common cause of failure is tube placement in the posterior pleural space or the subcutaneous tissue. Other causes for ineffective drainage are tubes that perforate the lung, diaphragm, or mediastinum. Extrapulmonary air not in the pleural space, such as a pneumomediastinum or a subpleural pulmonary pseudocyst, will not be drained by a chest tube. Complications of chest tube insertion include hemorrhage, lung perforation, cardiac tamponade, and phrenic nerve injury.

(2) **Removal of a chest tube.** When the infant's lung disease has improved and the chest tube has not drained air for 24 to 48 hours, we discontinue suction and leave the tube under water seal. If radiographic examination shows no reaccumulation of extrapulmonary air in the next 12 to 24 hours, the chest tube is removed. To reduce the chance of introducing air into the pleural space, cover the chest wound with a small occlusive dressing while removing the tube. Remove the chest tube during expiration in spontaneously breathing infants and during inspiration in mechanically ventilated infants.

d. **Persistent pneumothorax** refractory to routine measures may improve with high-frequency oscillation; some infants require ECMO (see **B.2**). We sometimes place catheters under ultrasound or fluoroscopic guidance to drain air collections that are inaccessible by standard techniques.

3. Complications of pneumothorax

a. Profound **ventilatory and circulatory compromise** can occur and, if untreated, result in death.

b. Intraventricular hemorrhage may result, possibly secondary to a combination of fluctuating cerebrovascular pressures, impaired venous return, hypercapnia, hypoxia, and acidosis.

c. Inappropriate antidiuretic hormone secretion may occur.

B. Pulmonary interstitial emphysema (PIE).

PIE occurs most often in mechanically ventilated, preterm infants with RDS. Interstitial air can be localized or can spread to involve significant portions of one or both lungs. Interstitial air can dissect toward the hilum and the pleural surface via the adventitial connective tissue surrounding the lymphatics and pulmonary vessels. This can compromise lymphatic drainage and pulmonary blood flow. Furthermore, PIE alters pulmonary mechanics by decreasing compliance, increasing residual volume and dead space, and enhancing ventilation/perfusion mismatch. Rupture of interstitial air into the pleural space and mediastinum can result in pneumothorax and pneumomediastinum, respectively.

1. Diagnosis

a. PIE frequently develops in the first 48 hours of life.

b. PIE may be accompanied by hypotension, bradycardia, hypercarbia, hypoxia, and acidosis.

c. PIE has two radiographic patterns: cystlike and linear. Linear lucencies radiate from the lung hilum. Occasionally, large cystlike blebs give the appearance of a pneumothorax.

2. Treatment

a. If possible, attempt to decrease mean airway pressure by lowering peak inspiratory pressure, PEEP, and inspiratory time. We generally use high-frequency oscillatory ventilation in infants with PIE to avoid large swings in lung volume.

b. Unilateral PIE may improve if the infant is positioned with the affected lung dependent. Chest physiotherapy and endotracheal suctioning should be minimized. Severe localized PIE that has failed to improve with conservative management may require collapse of the affected lung by selective bronchial intubation or occlusion or, rarely, surgical resection.

3. Complications

a. PIE may precede more severe complications such as pneumothorax, pneumopericardium, or an air embolus.

C. Pneumomediastinum.

Mediastinal air can develop when pulmonary interstitial air dissects into the mediastinum or when direct trauma occurs to the airways or the posterior pharynx.

1. Diagnosis

a. Physical examination. Heart sounds may appear distant.

b. Chest radiograph. An AP radiograph may demonstrate air outlining the thymus. This results in the characteristic "spinnaker sail" sign.

2. Treatment

a. Pneumomediastinum is of little clinical importance, and specific drainage procedures are usually unnecessary. Rarely, cardiorespiratory compromise may develop if the air is under tension and does not decompress into the pleural space, the retroperitoneum, or the soft tissues of the neck. This situation may require mediastinostomy drainage.

b. If the infant is mechanically ventilated, reduce mean airway pressure if possible.

3. Complications

a. Observe for other air leaks.

D. Pneumopericardium.

Pneumopericardium is the least common form of air leak in newborns but the most common cause of cardiac tamponade. Asymp-

tomatic pneumopericardium is occasionally detected as an incidental finding on a chest radiograph. Most cases occur in preterm infants with RDS
treated with mechanical ventilation. The mortality rate for critically ill infants who develop pneumopericardium is 70 to 80%.

1. **Diagnosis.** Pneumopericardium should be considered in mechanically
   ventilated newborn infants who develop acute or subacute hemodynamic
   compromise.
   a. **Physical examination.** Although infants may initially have tachycardia and decreased pulse pressure, hypotension, bradycardia, and
      cyanosis may ensue rapidly. Auscultation reveals muffled or distant
      heart sounds. A pericardial knock (Hamman sign) or a characteristic
      millwheel-like murmur *(bruit de moulin)* may be present.
   b. **Chest radiograph.** Anteroposterior views show air surrounding the
      heart. Air under the inferior surface of the heart is diagnostic.
   c. **Transillumination.** A high-intensity fiberoptic light source may illuminate the substernal region. Flickering of the light with the heart
      rate may help differentiate pneumopericardium from pneumomediastinum or a medial pneumothorax.
   d. **ECG.** Decreased voltages, manifest by a shrinking QRS complex, are
      consistent with pneumopericardium.
2. **Treatment**
   a. **Conservative management.** Asymptomatic infants not receiving positive pressure ventilation can be managed expectantly. Vital signs are
      closely monitored (especially changes in pulse pressure), and frequent
      chest radiographs are obtained until the pneumopericardium resolves.
   b. **Needle aspiration.** Cardiac tamponade is a life-threatening event
      that requires immediate pericardiocentesis.
      (1) Prepare the subxiphoid area with antibacterial solution.
      (2) Attach a 20- to 22-gauge intravenous catheter with an inner needle to a short piece of IV extension tubing that, in turn, is connected to a three-way stopcock and a 20-cc syringe. In the subxiphoid space, insert the catheter at a 30° to 45° angle and
          toward the infant's left shoulder. Aspirate with the syringe as
          the catheter is advanced. Once air is aspirated, stop advancing
          the catheter. Slide the plastic catheter over the needle and into
          the pericardial space. Remove the needle, reattach the IV tubing
          to the hub of the plastic catheter, evacuate the remaining air,
          and withdraw the catheter. If air leak persists, prepare for pericardial tube placement. If blood is aspirated, immediately withdraw the catheter to avoid lacerating the ventricular wall. The
          complications of pericardiocentesis include hemopericardium
          and laceration of the right ventricle or left anterior descending
          coronary artery.
   c. **Continuous pericardial drainage.** Because pneumopericardium often
      progresses to cardiac tamponade and may recur following aspiration,
      a pericardial tube may be needed for continuous drainage. We manage
      the pericardial tube like a chest tube, although less negative pressure
      (-5 to -10 cm H_2O) is used for suction.
3. **Complications.** Ventilated infants who have a pneumopericardium
   drained by needle aspiration frequently (80%) have a recurrence. Recurrent pneumopericardium can occur days after apparent resolution of the
   initial event.

E. **Other types of air leaks**
1. **Pneumoperitoneum.** Intraperitoneal air may result from extrapulmonary air that decompresses into the abdominal cavity. Usually the
   pneumoperitoneum is of little clinical importance, but it must be differentiated from intraperitoneal air resulting from a perforated viscus.
   Rarely, pneumoperitoneum can impair diaphragmatic excursion and

compromise ventilation. In these cases, continuous drainage may be necessary.
2. **Subcutaneous emphysema.** Subcutaneous air can be detected by palpation of crepitus in the face, neck, or supraclavicular region. Large collections of air in the neck, although usually of no clinical significance, can partially occlude or obstruct the compressible, cartilaginous trachea of the premature infant.
3. **Systemic air embolism.** An air embolism is a rare but usually fatal complication of pulmonary air leak. Air may enter the vasculature either by disruption of the pulmonary venous system or by inadvertent injection through an intravascular catheter. The presence of air bubbles in blood withdrawn from an umbilical artery catheter can be diagnostic.

Persistent Pulmonary Hypertension of the Newborn
Linda J. Van Marter

I. **Definition. Persistent pulmonary hypertension of the newborn (PPHN)** is caused by a sustained elevation in **pulmonary vascular resistance (PVR)** after birth, preventing transition to the normal extrauterine circulatory pattern. The disorder is most common in full-term or postterm infants and occurs at a rate of 1 to 2 per 1000 live births. Improved ventilator management and treatment with extracorporeal membrane oxygenation (ECMO) have reduced the high mortality rate. Morbidity in survivors includes chronic pulmonary disease, neurodevelopmental disabilities, and intracranial hemorrhage or infarction.

The normal transitional circulation is characterized by a rapid fall in PVR with the first breath and a rapid rise in **systemic vascular resistance (SVR)** with the clamping of umbilical arterial flow to the placenta. These hemodynamic changes cause functional closure of the foramen ovale. The associated rise in arterial oxygen content results in constriction of the ductus arteriosus. These changes bring about the separation of the pulmonary and systemic circulations from parallel to series circuits. When PVR exceeds SVR, as a result of abnormal neonatal transition or other causes, right-to-left shunting occurs through the foramen ovale or ductus arteriosus, often resulting in severe hypoxemia.

II. **Epidemiologic associations.** The determinants of PPHN are not completely understood. The perinatal risk factors associated with PPHN include meconium-stained amniotic fluid and maternal conditions such as fever, anemia, and pulmonary disease. In a recent case-control interview study of antenatal risk factors for PPHN conducted at our institution, multivariate analyses showed associations between PPHN and maternal diabetes mellitus, urinary tract infection during pregnancy, aspirin and nonsteroidal antiinflammatory drug consumption during pregnancy, and fewer years of maternal education. Neonatal conditions linked with PPHN include the following:

A. **Intrauterine or perinatal asphyxia** is the most commonly associated diagnosis. Prolonged fetal stress may result in remodeling and abnormal muscularization of the smallest pulmonary arteries. Furthermore, acute asphyxia at birth may induce persistent pulmonary vasospasm. Chronic hypoxemia may be associated with intrauterine growth restriction and more complex neonatal pathophysiology.

B. **Pulmonary parenchymal disease,** including respiratory distress syndrome (RDS), pneumonia, and aspiration syndromes, especially meconium aspiration, can cause hypoxic pulmonary vasospasm or may be associated with the characteristic pulmonary vascular remodeling. The pulmonary vascular responses to hypoxemia, asphyxia, and sepsis appear to be enhanced by factors related to advanced gestational age.

C. **Abnormalities of pulmonary development,** including vascular malalignment and parenchymal hypoplasia, may be associated.

D. **Myocardial dysfunction** has been associated with perinatal asphyxia, myocarditis, metabolic aberrations such as hypoglycemia and hypocalcemia, and hyperviscosity. Intrauterine constriction of the ductus arteriosus results in increased PVR and possibly right ventricular (RV) failure.

E. **Congenital heart disease,** including both left- and right-sided obstructive lesions, may be associated with right-to-left shunting with or without elevated PVR.

F. **Pneumonia and/or sepsis** of bacterial or viral origin can initiate PPHN. The underlying mechanism may be endotoxin-mediated myocardial depression or pulmonary vasospasm associated with high levels of thromboxanes and leukotrienes. In addition to more common etiologic agents, unusual organisms, including *Ureaplasma* species and echovirus 11, occasionally have been linked with PPHN.

III. **Pathology and pathophysiology**

A. **Pulmonary vascular remodeling** has been seen in autopsy studies of infants who died with idiopathic PPHN and in some with PPHN associated with meconium aspiration. Abnormal muscularization of the normally nonmuscular intraacinar arteries, with increased medial thickness of the larger muscular arteries, results in a decreased cross-sectional area of the pulmonary vascular bed and elevated PVR. The cause of the vascular abnormalities usually is not known but may be mediated by chronic intrauterine hypoxemia. Vascular changes also may occur following fetal exposure to nonsteroidal antiinflammatory agents (prostaglandin synthetase inhibitors), which presumably cause constriction of the fetal ductus arteriosus and secondary pulmonary hypertension due to accumulation of vasoconstricting metabolites. Finally, humoral growth factors released by hypoxia-damaged endothelial cells may promote vasoconstriction and muscular overgrowth. Whether the abnormal muscle in these cases causes irreversible vascular obstruction or increases the vasoreactivity is not known.

B. **Pulmonary hypoplasia** usually affects both alveolar and pulmonary arterial development. It may be seen as an isolated anomaly or with congenital diaphragmatic hernia (see Chap. 33), oligohydramnios syndrome, renal agenesis (i.e., Potter's syndrome), or abnormalities associated with decreased fetal breathing.

C. **Pulmonary vasospasm** is suspected in infants with reversible PPHN. In addition to the underlying disease process, both the stage of the disease and the maturity of the host seem to play a role in determining the mediators and the response. Hypoxia induces profound pulmonary vasoconstriction, which is exaggerated by acidemia. Neural and humoral vasoactive substances may contribute to the pathogenesis of PPHN, the response to hypoxemia, or both. These include factors associated with platelet activation and production of arachidonic acid metabolites. Thromboxanes (A_2 and its metabolite, B_2) and leukotrienes (C_4 and D_4) may be mediators of the increased PVR seen with sepsis and hypoxemia, respectively.

D. **Myocardial dysfunction with elevated PVR**

1. **RV dysfunction** can be caused by intrauterine closure of the ductus arteriosus, which results in altered fetal hemodynamics, postnatal pulmonary hypertension, RV failure, and a right-to-left shunt at the atrial level. RV failure resulting in altered diastolic compliance can cause right-to-left atrial shunting even in the absence of elevated PVR.

2. **Left ventricular (LV) dysfunction** causes pulmonary venous hypertension and reflex pulmonary arterial hypertension, often to suprasystemic levels. Right-to-left shunting by means of the ductus arteriosus can occur subsequently. This problem must be differentiated from the other causes of PPHN, as treatment is aimed at improving LV function rather than at lowering elevated PVR.

E. **Mechanical factors** that can influence PVR include cardiac output and blood viscosity. Low cardiac output recruits fewer arteriolar channels and may raise PVR by this mechanism as well as by its primary effect of lowering mixed venous oxygen content. Hyperviscosity, often associated with polycythemia, may reduce flow in the pulmonary microvasculature. Pulmonary microthrombi have been seen at autopsy in some infants with intractable PPHN with and without thrombocytopenia.

IV. Diagnosis. PPHN must be suspected in any profoundly cyanotic newborn.

A. Differential diagnoses that are most common include uncomplicated pulmonary disease, sepsis, and congenital heart disease.

B. The physical examination is generally less remarkable for PPHN than for signs of the associated diagnoses. The precordial impulse may be prominent. The second heart sound is usually single or narrowly split and accentuated. In infants with perinatal asphyxia, a systolic murmur consistent with tricuspid regurgitation may be heard at the right or left lower sternal border.

C. A difference between simultaneous **preductal and postductal arterial blood gas (ABG)** values or transcutaneous oxygen monitors can be used to document a ductal right-to-left shunt. A gradient in **oxygen saturation** of at least 10% in the absence of structural heart disease suggests PPHN. The absence of a significant ductal shunt does not exclude pulmonary hypertension associated with an isolated atrial right-to-left hemodynamic shunt.

D. The **chest radiograph** usually appears normal or shows associated pulmonary parenchymal disease or air leak. The cardiothymic silhouette is normal or borderline enlarged; pulmonary blood flow is normal or may appear reduced.

E. The **ECG** may show RV predominance and be normal for age, or it may show signs of myocardial ischemia or infarction. It is sometimes helpful in suggesting structural heart disease.

F. An **echocardiographic study** should be performed in all infants with unexplained cyanosis, to exclude structural heart defects. Color Doppler examination can confirm the presence of intracardiac or ductal shunting. Additional echocardiographic markers of pulmonary hypertension, such as septal position that is flattened or bowed to the left, can be seen. Pulmonary artery pressure can be estimated using continuous-wave Doppler sampling of the velocity of a tricuspid regurgitation jet, if present.

G. Diagnostic pitfalls are not uncommon in the evaluation of patients with PPHN. The following diagnoses must be carefully considered:

1. **Structural cardiovascular abnormalities** associated with right-to-left ductal or atrial shunting include the following:
   a. **Obstruction to pulmonary venous return**—infradiaphragmatic total anomalous pulmonary venous return, hypoplastic left heart, cor triatriatum, congenital mitral stenosis
   b. **Myopathic LV disease**—endocardial fibroelastosis, Pompe's disease
   c. **Obstruction to LV outflow:** critical aortic stenosis, supravalvar aortic stenosis, interrupted aortic arch, coarctation of the aorta
   d. **Obligatory left-to-right shunt**—endocardial cushion defect, arteriovenous malformation, hemitruncus, coronary arteriovenous fistula
   e. **Miscellaneous disorders**—Ebstein's anomaly, transposition of the great arteries

2. Left or right **ventricular dysfunction** may be associated with right-to-left shunting. **LV dysfunction,** due to ischemia or obstruction caused by myopathic LV disease or obstruction to LV outflow, may present with a right-to-left ductal shunt. **RV dysfunction** may be associated with right-to-left atrial shunting as a result of decreased diastolic compliance and elevated end-diastolic pressure. These diagnoses must be differentiated from PPHN caused by pulmonary vascular abnormalities.

H. Signs favoring primary cardiac disease over PPHN include cardiomegaly, weak pulses, pulse differential between upper and lower extremities, pulmonary edema, grade 3+ murmur, and persistent arterial oxygen tension (P_aO_2) at or less than 40 mm Hg.

V. Management. The cyanotic newborn must be considered a medical emergency. Immediate, appropriate intervention is critical in reversing the instability or rapid downhill spiral often associated with PPHN. Correction of hypoxemia and acidosis is especially important. Key principles for management include (1) rapid response to clinical decompensation and (2) conservative weaning of therapeutic measures that have proved effective; weaning should be done in small steps and only after a substantial period of stability.

A. 100% oxygen should be administered by hood to any near-term or full-term cyanotic newborn. Because hypoxemia is one of the most powerful stimuli to pulmonary vasoconstriction, oxygen therapy may greatly reduce elevated PVR. After 10 minutes, the effects of oxygen therapy should be evaluated with a postductal ABG analysis. If the postductal P_aO_2 is less than 100 mm Hg in 100% oxygen, or oxygen saturation is less than 90%, simultaneous preductal and postductal ABG analyses or noninvasive measurements of oxygenation are performed to assess transductal shunting. Continuous noninvasive monitoring is useful to follow rapid changes in oxygenation. Placement of two sensors, one on the upper right extremity and the other on a lower extremity, can be used to monitor the effect of therapy on the gradient caused by a transductal shunt.

B. Intubation and mechanical ventilation should be instituted when hypoxemia is persistent despite maximal administration of oxygen by hood or when P_aO_2 is borderline after prolonged supplementation with 100% oxygen. Contrasting approaches to mechanical ventilation have been used (see **VI**). Our practice is to maintain adequate oxygenation and mild hyperventilation, initially attempting to keep the P_aO_2 greater than 80 mm Hg and arterial carbon dioxide tension (P_aCO_2) at 35 to 40 mm Hg. When the infant is more stable, usually at 12 to 48 hours, we maintain oxygen saturation greater than 90% and allow PCO_2 to rise. The nature of the underlying pulmonary parenchymal abnormality, if any, and the infant's clinical lability or stability are important factors to consider when choosing the specific strategy for respiratory support.

1. In the absence of alveolar disease, high mean airway pressure may impede cardiac output and elevate PVR. We use a strategy of rapid, low-pressure, short-inspiratory-time mechanical ventilation designed to minimize mean airway pressure. Typical ventilator settings are rate, 30 to 60 breaths per minute; peak inspiratory pressure (PIP), 20 to 25 cm H_2O; positive end-expiratory pressure (PEEP), 2 to 4 cm H_2O; and inspiratory duration, 0.2 to 0.4 second. High gas flow (20 to 30 liters per minute) may be required, and large-diameter ventilator tubing is used to maintain PEEP at low levels in the presence of high flow rates.

2. When PPHN complicates parenchymal pulmonary disease, mechanical ventilation with slower rates, longer inspiratory times, and PEEP of 4 to 6 cm H_2O may be required to provide adequate ventilation and oxygenation. We often use **high-frequency oscillatory ventilation** in infants with PPHN associated with severe pulmonary parenchymal disease.

3. Because infants with PPHN are often large and vigorously resist mechanical ventilation, and because catecholamine release stimulates pulmonary alpha-adrenergic receptors, thereby raising PVR, we frequently use a **narcotic analgesic. Fentanyl** (3 to 8 µg/kg per hour) is a potent, short-acting narcotic that reduces the extreme variability in oxygenation due to vasospasm, by blunting sympathetic output from the central nervous system. For extreme agitation or profound hypoxemia, we use **neuromuscular blockade** with **pancuronium** (0.1 mg/kg) to achieve muscle relaxation.

C. ECMO has been used as a lifesaving therapy for infants with PPHN who fail conventional management (see Extracorporeal Membrane Oxygenation). In a randomized clinical trial conducted at our institution, 28 of 29 ECMO-treated critically ill infants with PPHN survived. Four of 10 similarly ill infants died with maximal conventional medical therapy. In term or near-term infants meeting ECMO criteria, high-frequency oscillatory ventilation can reduce the need for ECMO treatment.

D. After adequate oxygenation, **correction of acidosis** is the most important aspect of the treatment of PPHN. The pH/P$_a$CO$_2$-related decrease in PVR is due to the physiologic effect of alkalosis rather than to hypocarbia. Alkalosis can be achieved by hyperventilation, correction of hypoperfusion acidosis, metabolic therapy with sodium bicarbonate, or all three, and may result in a marked reduction in PVR. For infants with PPHN we maintain pH in the range of 7.40 to 7.55 with sodium bicarbonate.

E. **Other metabolic abnormalities** can contribute to right-to-left shunting on the basis of poor cardiac output. Maintenance of a **neutral thermal environment** reduces the infant's energy demands. Correction of **hypoglycemia** and **hypocalcemia** is important to provide adequate substrates for myocardial function.

F. **Adequate cardiac output** is necessary to maximize mixed venous oxygen content. Likewise, achieving **optimal systemic blood pressure** may reduce or eliminate right-to-left hemodynamic shunts. Because pulmonary hypertension may result in pulmonary blood pressure at or near normal systemic blood pressures, we attempt to raise systemic blood pressure to levels of 60 to 80 mm Hg (systolic) and 50 to 60 mm Hg (mean). Volume resuscitation and cardiotonic agents are necessary to achieve adequate cardiac output and/or systemic blood pressure in many infants with PPHN (see Chap. 17).

G. **Intravascular volume** support with colloids such as albumin (5%), fresh-frozen plasma, or packed red blood cells may be necessary in the infant with pathophysiologic conditions associated with intravascular volume depletion (i.e., hemorrhage, hydrops, capillary leak) or decreased SVR (i.e., septic shock) or in whom SVR has been lowered by pharmacologic agents (i.e., sedative narcotics).

H. **Polycythemia**, associated with hyperviscosity, mechanically increases PVR and can lead to a release of vasoactive substances by platelet activation. On the other hand, a sufficient red blood cell mass is necessary for adequate oxygen-carrying capacity. Partial exchange transfusion is considered to reduce the hematocrit to 50 to 55% in the infant with PPHN whose central hematocrit exceeds 65% (see Chap. 26).

I. **Pharmacologic therapy** is directed at the simultaneous goals of optimizing cardiac output, enhancing systemic blood pressure, and reducing PVR. As no parenteral selective pulmonary vasodilator has been identified, the relative effects of the available agents must be considered in choosing the most appropriate agent (see Chap. 17). Pharmacologic intervention should be reserved for infants in whom hyperoxia and alkalosis have been attempted and for whom continuous monitoring of oxygenation and systemic arterial pressure is possible. Consideration of associated and differential diagnoses and the known or hypothetical pathogenesis of the right-to-left shunt may prove helpful in selecting the best agent or combination of agents for a particular infant.

1. **Dopamine** is often used in moderate (3 to 5 μg/kg per minute) to high (6 to 20 μg/kg per minute) doses for support of systemic blood pressure and improved cardiac output by means of alpha- and beta-adrenergic receptor stimulation. Dopamine in low doses (1 to 2 μg/kg per minute) also has a salutary effect of increasing renal blood flow. **Dobutamine,** a synthetic catecholamine with a chemical structure similar to that of isoproterenol, has an inotropic more than a chronotropic effect on the heart through beta-1-adrenergic stimulation. Dopamine may increase PVR, especially at higher infusion rates (>10 μg/kg per minute). At similar infusion rates, dobutamine may enhance peripheral vasodilation, especially in the setting of other predisposing conditions (e.g., "warm shock").

2. **Epinephrine** (0.03 to 0.10 μg/kg per minute) has both alpha- and beta-adrenergic effects; therefore, it is primarily useful in raising systemic blood pressure by enhanced cardiac output and profound peripheral vasoconstriction. Alpha-receptor stimulation may result in pulmonary vasoconstriction and elevated PVR as well as reduced renal and mesenteric blood flow.

3. **Tolazoline (Priscoline),** an alpha-adrenergic antagonist, histaminic agonist, and direct vasodilator, has been used to treat PPHN with mixed results. Complications include systemic hypotension, gastrointestinal hemorrhage, and renal insufficiency. We no longer use tolazoline.

4. **Prostaglandins E$_1$ (PGE$_1$), I$_2$ (PGI$_2$), and D$_2$ (PGD$_2$)** have been used in a few therapeutic trials but are not used clinically. PGE$_2$ has **not** been shown to be beneficial. Similarly, trials of PGD$_2$ and PGI$_2$ (prostacyclin), one of the most potent vasodilators known, had variable results. The use of other vasoactive pharmacologic agents, including leukotriene inhibitors, amrinone, calcium channel blockers, and magnesium sulfate, requires further study.

5. **A promising new therapy** is treatment with the investigational drug inhaled **nitric oxide (NO).** Nitric oxide is a naturally occurring substance produced by endothelial cells. The NO diffuses into neighboring smooth muscle cells, where it increases intracellular cyclic guanosine monophosphate (cGMP) and relaxes the actin-myosin complex leading to vasodilation. Inhaled NO administered by conventional or high-frequency ventilation in doses of 5 to 80 parts per million selectively decreases PVR. As it is bound by hemoglobin, it causes little systemic vasodilation. Inhaled NO improves oxygenation in some infants with PPHN and reduces the need for ECMO. Infants receiving NO must be monitored for the possible side effect of methemoglobinemia. Because not all infants with PPHN respond to inhaled NO and some may deteriorate rapidly, we recommend treatment of critically ill infants at a center where ECMO is readily accessible.

VI. **Controversies regarding the therapy** for PPHN reflect significant interinstitutional variability in the therapeutic approaches to PPHN. **Hyperventilation and hyperoxia** have been considered conventional therapy for PPHN, as improvement in oxygenation, decline in PVR, or both often follow the achievement of respiratory alkalosis. Successful treatment, however, has occurred without the use of hyperventilation. This approach accomplishes alkalosis with bicarbonate infusion and minimizes barotrauma by permitting normocarbia or hypercarbia.

References

1. Kinsella, J.P., Abman, S.H. Recent developments in the pathophysiology and treatment of persistent pulmonary hypertension of the newborn. *J. Pediatr.* 126:853, 1995.
2. Walsh-Sukys, M. Persistent pulmonary hypertension of the newborn. *Clin. Perinatol.* 20:127, 1993.

Transient Tachypnea of the Newborn
Mark E. Lawson

I. **Definition.** Transient tachypnea of the newborn (TTN) is also known as "wet lung" and type II respiratory distress syndrome (RDS). TTN is a common, mild, self-limited disorder, usually affecting near-term or term infants, and is characterized by tachypnea with mild retractions, and mild cyanosis, usually with an FiO$_2$ requirement of less than 0.40.

II. **Pathophysiology.** TTN represents a transient pulmonary edema that results from delayed resorption of fetal lung fluid by the pulmonary lymphatic system. In addition, it may result from any condition that elevates the central venous pressure with resultant delayed clearance of lung fluid via the thoracic duct. The increased fluid accumulates in the peribronchiolar lymphatics and bronchovascular spaces, interferes with forces promoting bronchiolar patency, and results in bronchiolar collapse and subsequent air trapping or hyperinflation. Hypoxemia results from continued perfusion of poorly ventilated alveoli, and hypercarbia results from mechanical interference with alveolar ventilation. The main effect of the excess lung fluid is decreased compliance. The infant develops tachypnea to counter the increased respiratory work caused by decreased lung compliance.

III. Risk factors. Premature or precipitous birth or operative delivery without labor may impair effective clearance of lung fluid, resulting in excess lung fluid. Delayed cord clamping or cord milking promotes a transfusion of blood from the placenta to the infant, resulting in transient elevation of the infant's central venous pressure. Other risk factors associated with TTN include macrosomia, male sex, excessive maternal sedation, prolonged labor, and obstetric circumstances necessitating intravenous administration of large volumes of fluids to the mother.

IV. Clinical presentation. The infant is usually near term or at term and develops tachypnea (>80 breaths per minute) within 2 to 6 hours after delivery. Premature infants may present with pulmonary edema from retained lung fluid, which may complicate surfactant deficiency and contribute to greater requirements for oxygen and ventilation. The infant with TTN usually has mild to moderate lung disease characterized by tachypnea, cyanosis, slight subcostal and intercostal retractions, increased anteroposterior diameter of the upper thorax, nasal flaring, and intermittent expiratory grunting. These infants usually have good air exchange without crackles or rhonchi. No other signs of cardiac, CNS, hematologic, or metabolic disease are demonstrable. These symptoms typically persist for 12 to 24 hours in infants with mild TTN, but may persist for longer than 72 hours in infants with severe TTN.

V. Diagnosis

  A. Laboratory studies

   1. Prenatal testing. RDS is unlikely if fetal lung testing demonstrates maturity.

   2. Postnatal testing

   a. Analysis of arterial blood gases on room air may show a mild respiratory acidosis, which usually resolves within 24 hours, and mild hypoxemia. Infants usually require an FiO_2 of less than 0.40 for adequate oxygenation and require no oxygen supplementation after 24 hours. Tachypnea associated with profound hypoxemia may be related to myocardial failure and/or increased pulmonary vascular resistance (see Persistent Pulmonary Hypertension of the Newborn).

   b. Complete blood cell count and differential will help rule out an infectious process.

   c. Chest x-ray study. Radiographic findings are as follows:

   (1) Prominent perihilar streaking that results from engorgement of periarterial lymphatics, and interstitial fluid accumulation along the bronchovascular spaces.

   (2) Mild to moderate cardiomegaly.

   (3) Coarse, fluffy densities may be present and represent liquid-filled alveoli. These densities usually clear within 24 hours and may help distinguish TTN from meconium aspiration or bacterial pneumonia.

   (4) Increased lung volume due to air trapping associated with bronchiolar collapse may be manifested by depression of the diaphragm and hyperaeration.

   (5) Fluid may be seen in the minor fissure, the pleural space, or both. Widening of the interlobar fissures and prominence of the right-lung minor fissure are occasional findings. These radiographic abnormalities usually resolve within 48 to 72 hours, with clearing evident within 12 to 18 hours of life. Increased pulmonary vascularity in the absence of significant cardiomegaly may be seen in a premature infant with patency of the ductus arteriosus or in a full-term infant with total anomalous pulmonary venous return.

   d. Hyperoxia test. A hyperoxia test to rule out cyanotic congenital heart disease should be considered in any infant with persistent hypoxemia.

VI. Differential diagnosis. TTN is a diagnosis of exclusion. Other causes of tachypnea must be excluded.
  A. Pneumonia/sepsis. The maternal history should be evaluated for sepsis risk factors. The infant may have laboratory evidence of infection, including neutropenia or an increased proportion of immature neutrophils noted on a white blood cell count and differential. Broad-spectrum antibiotics are given if there are maternal or infant sepsis risk factors, if there are laboratory findings suggestive of sepsis, or if the infant's respiratory symptoms do not improve within 6 to 8 hours.
  B. Cyanotic congenital heart disease. If suspected, this is evaluated initially with a hyperoxia test, ECG, four-extremity blood pressures, and a chest radiograph.
  C. RDS. The infant with RDS is premature or is at risk for pulmonary immaturity. The chest radiograph usually reveals low lung volumes, and shows the typical reticulogranular pattern with air bronchograms. The infant with RDS usually has a more significant oxygen requirement and degree of respiratory distress than does the infant with TTN. The prompt improvement in oxygenation associated with supplemental oxygen typifies the infant with TTN and further helps distinguish TTN from RDS.
  D. Central hyperventilation. This disorder is usually seen in term infants with birth asphyxia. They have tachypnea without retractions, expiratory grunting, or nasal flaring; minimal chest x-ray findings; and evidence of respiratory alkalosis on blood gas analysis.
VII. General management
  A. Oxygenation. Initial management consists of providing supplemental oxygenation to keep arterial oxygen saturation greater than 90%. If oxygen delivered by hood or nasal cannula is ineffective, consider using nasal continuous positive airway pressure. An FiO_2 of less than 0.40 is typically sufficient to support the infant while absorption of lung fluid occurs through pulmonary lymphatics. If the infant requires an FiO_2 of more than 0.60 or positive pressure ventilation to achieve adequate oxygenation, the diagnosis of TTN is unlikely, and another disease process should be considered.
  B. Feeding. Infants can be fed orally if the respiratory rate is less than 60 breaths per minute. If the respiratory rate is 60 to 80 breaths per minute, the infant can be fed via an orogastric feeding tube or intravenously.
  C. Diuretics. Although TTN symptoms are related to pulmonary edema, controlled studies have failed to find that furosemide is an effective therapy for this disorder.
VIII. Prognosis. TTN is a benign self-limited disease. Infants followed up for as long as 1 year had no recurrence of tachypnea or other evidence of pulmonary dysfunction.

Pulmonary Hemorrhage
Thomas M. Berger and Shoo Lee

  I. Definition. Pulmonary hemorrhage is defined pathologically as the presence of erythrocytes in air spaces, interstitial spaces, or both. Intraalveolar hemorrhages predominate in infants who survive for more than 24 hours. Confluent hemorrhages in at least two lobes of the lung have been termed **massive pulmonary hemorrhage (MPH)**. There is no uniformly accepted clinical definition of pulmonary hemorrhage.
 II. Epidemiology. Pulmonary hemorrhage of any degree has been observed in up to 68% of autopsied neonates and was thought to be the principal cause of death in 9% of such neonates. In the majority of infants, death occurred between days 2 and 4 after birth. MPH was observed in 1.7 to 28% of infants in large autopsy studies; it was only infrequently suspected before death. Overall incidence estimates range between 0.9 and 12 per 1000 live births, but may be

higher in risk groups such as premature infants and infants with severe intrauterine growth restriction.

III. **Pathogenesis.** The pathogenesis of pulmonary hemorrhage is unknown. Numerous retrospective autopsy surveys have statistically correlated pulmonary hemorrhage with several conditions, including prematurity, intrauterine growth restriction, intrauterine and intrapartum asphyxia, infection, congenital heart disease, oxygen toxicity, Rhesus isoimmunization, twin gestation, male sex, neonatal tetanus, breech delivery, and maternal smoking. The observation of a low hematocrit and the presence of relatively smaller protein molecules in the lung effluents compared to blood in patients with pulmonary hemorrhage suggests that the lung effluents in most infants were hemorrhagic edema fluid rather than whole blood. Acute left ventricular failure, often caused by hypoxia and acidosis, may lead to increased pulmonary capillary pressure, with rupture of some blood vessels and transudation from others. This may be the final pathway of many of the conditions associated with pulmonary hemorrhage. Factors that alter the integrity of the epithelial-endothelial barrier in the alveolus or that change the filtration pressure across these membranes could predispose infants to pulmonary hemorrhage (Fig. 24-2).

IV. **Pulmonary hemorrhage and exogenous surfactant.** It is controversial whether therapy with exogenous surfactant increases the risk of pulmonary hemorrhage. A meta-analysis of 11 surfactant trials that prospectively reported the clinical occurrence of pulmonary hemorrhage showed that exogenous surfactant overall increases the risk of pulmonary hemorrhage by about 50% [2]. This resulted mainly from a significant increase of pulmonary hemorrhages in trials in which synthetic surfactants were used as a prevention strategy. The adjusted odds ratios did not reach statistical significance for trials with synthetic surfactant rescue strategy, or for either strategy in natural surfactant trials. In an autopsy evaluation of pooled data from five synthetic surfactant trials, the incidence of pulmonary hemorrhage at autopsy was not different in infants treated with surfactant or air placebo. It has been suggested that the risk of pulmonary hemorrhage after surfactant therapy can be reduced by judicious use of fluids and by pharmacologic closure of the ductus arteriosus.

V. **Diagnosis.** The clinical diagnosis of pulmonary hemorrhage is made when sudden cardiorespiratory decompensation occurs, often on the second to fourth day after birth, and hemorrhagic fluid appears in the upper respiratory tract. It is noteworthy that only 19 to 42% of pulmonary hemorrhages observed at autopsy were diagnosed clinically, most likely because no blood can be suctioned from the airway when the hemorrhage is limited to the interstitial space. In these cases, respiratory deterioration is usually attributed to some other cause. Pulmonary hemorrhage is often accompanied by acute, though nonspecific, changes on chest radiograph with diffuse opacification of one or both lungs and the appearance of air bronchograms. Laboratory evaluation often reveals metabolic or mixed acidosis, a drop in the hematocrit, and sometimes evidence of coagulopathy. In most instances, the latter finding is probably a consequence rather than an initiating factor of the pulmonary hemorrhage.

VI. **Treatment.** Because the pathogenesis of this disorder is not well understood, the therapeutic approach remains nonspecific and supportive. No published trials are available evaluating the prevention or treatment of pulmonary hemorrhage.

Initially, the airways should be cleared of blood to allow adequate ventilation. Mechanical ventilation with 6 to 8 cm H_2O positive end-expiratory pressure helps to decrease the efflux of hemorrhagic fluid into the alveolar space. It is not clear whether high-frequency ventilation using high mean airway pressure is more effective than conventional positive pressure ventilation, and its use should be evaluated on an individual basis. Bicarbonate is administered to treat the metabolic acidosis. The cardiovascular system should be supported with infusions of fluid (blood, normal saline solution, or albumin) and pressors

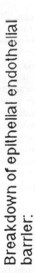

Breakdown of epithelial endothelial barrier:

- Ischemia/hypoxia
- oxygen toxicity
- Infection/DIC
- mechanical ventilation
- exogenous surfactant (?)

Increased capillary filtration pressure:

- Increased capillary pressure
- decreased oncotic pressure
- decreased surface tension

Acute left ventricular failure

Massive pulmonary hemorrhage

Fig. 24-2. Proposed mechanism of pulmonary hemorrhage. (DIC = disseminated intravascular coagulopathy. A = alveolus, C = capillary.)

to maintain adequate tissue perfusion. An echocardiographic evaluation should be considered to assess left ventricular function and the need for inotropic support. The presence of a hemodynamically significant patent ductus arteriosus may require pharmacologic closure with indomethacin unless contraindicated by coagulopathy. If coagulopathy is present or develops, aggressive correction with fresh-frozen plasma or cryoprecipitate is indicated.

VII. **Prognosis.** Prior to the introduction of positive pressure ventilation, pulmonary hemorrhage was uniformly fatal. The early reports of survivors emphasized the benefit of intermittent positive pressure ventilation and the correction of acidosis and clotting disorders. A more thorough understanding of the pathogenesis of pulmonary hemorrhage is needed to allow the development of better therapeutic approaches, further improving the prognosis of affected patients.

References

1. Halliday, H.L. Other acute lung disorders. In J.C. Sinclair and M.B. Bracken (Eds.), *Effective Care of the Newborn Infant.* New York: Oxford University Press, 1992.
2. Raju, T.N.K., and Langenberg, P. Pulmonary hemorrhage and exogenous surfactant therapy: a meta-analysis. *J. Pediatr.* 123:603, 1993.

Apnea
Ann R. Stark

I. **Background**
 A. **Definition.** An **apneic spell** can be defined as a cessation of respiration accompanied by bradycardia (heart rate <100 beats per minute) or cyanosis. Bradycardia and cyanosis are usually present after 20 seconds of apnea, although they can occur more rapidly in the small premature infant. After 30 to 45 seconds, pallor and hypotonia are seen, and infants may be unresponsive to tactile stimulation.
 B. **Incidence.** Apneic spells occur frequently in premature infants. The incidence of apnea increases with decreasing gestational age. As many as 25% of all premature infants who weigh less than 1800 gm (about 34 weeks' gestational age) will have at least one apneic episode, while the majority of very small premature infants (under 30 weeks' gestational age) will have occasional apneic spells. These spells generally begin at 1 or 2 days of life; if they do not occur during the first 7 days, they are unlikely to occur later. Apneic spells persist for variable periods postnatally and generally cease by 37 weeks' postmenstrual age. In infants born before 28 weeks' gestation, however, apnea and bradycardia often persist beyond 39 weeks' postmenstrual age. Apneic spells occurring in infants at or near term are always abnormal and are nearly always associated with serious, identifiable causes, such as birth asphyxia, intracranial hemorrhage, seizures, or depression from medication. Failure to breathe at birth in the absence of drug depression or asphyxia is generally caused by irreversible structural abnormalities of the central nervous system.
II. **Pathogenesis.** Several mechanisms have been proposed to explain apnea in premature infants. Many clinical conditions also have been associated with apneic spells, and some may be causative.
 A. **Developmental immaturity** is a likely contributing factor, since apnea spells occur more frequently in immature infants.
  1. The occurrence of apnea may correlate with **brainstem neural function.** The frequency of apnea decreases over a period in which brainstem conduction time of the auditory evoked response shortens as postmenstrual age increases.
  2. Breathing in infants is strongly influenced by **sleep state.** Active or rapid-eye-movement (REM) sleep is marked by irregularity of tidal volume and respiratory frequency. REM sleep predominates in preterm in-

fants, and apneic spells occur more frequently in this state than in quiet sleep.

B. Chemoreceptor response

1. In preterm infants, **hypoxia** results in transient hyperventilation, followed by hypoventilation and sometimes apnea, in contrast to the response in adults. In addition, hypoxia makes the premature infant less responsive to increased levels of carbon dioxide. Thus, hypoxemia may be involved in the pathogenesis of some apneic spells. Clinical conditions in which both hypoxemia and apnea may occur include pneumonia, respiratory distress syndrome (RDS) (especially during weaning from ventilatory assistance), symptomatic patent ductus arteriosus, anemia, and hypovolemia.

2. The ventilatory response to increased **carbon dioxide** is decreased in preterm infants with apnea compared with a matched group without apnea, which suggests that abnormal respiratory control likely contributes to the pathogenesis of apnea.

C. Reflexes. Active reflexes invoked by stimulation of the posterior pharynx, lung inflation, fluid in the larynx, or chest wall distortion can precipitate apnea in infants. These reflexes may be involved in the apnea that is sometimes associated, for example, with vigorous use of suction catheters in the pharynx or with fluid in the upper airway during feeding.

D. Respiratory muscles. Ineffective ventilation may result from impaired coordination of the inspiratory muscles (diaphragm and intercostal muscles) and the muscles of the upper airway (larynx and pharynx).

1. Although many infants have **central apnea,** in which inspiratory efforts and airflow cease simultaneously, a frequently observed type of apnea is **mixed apnea,** in which a central pause is either preceded or followed by airway obstruction. Purely **obstructive apnea,** defined as absent airflow in the presence of inspiratory efforts, occurs less frequently. The site of this obstruction is the upper pharynx.

2. Passive neck flexion, pressure on the lower rim of a face mask, and submental pressure (all encountered during nursery procedures) can obstruct the airway in infants and lead to apnea, especially in a small premature infant. Spontaneously occurring airway obstruction is seen more frequently when preterm infants assume a position of neck flexion.

III. Monitoring and evaluation. All infants less than 35 weeks' gestational age should be monitored for apneic spells for at least the first week of life because of the risk of apneic spells in this group. Monitoring should continue until no significant apneic episode has been detected for at least 5 days. Since impedance apnea monitors may not distinguish respiratory efforts during airway obstruction from normal breaths, heart rate should be monitored in addition to, or instead of, respiration. Even with careful monitoring, some prolonged spells of apnea and bradycardia may not be recognized.

A. When a monitor alarm sounds, one should remember to respond to the infant, not the monitor, checking for bradycardia, cyanosis, and airway obstruction.

B. Most apneic spells in premature infants respond to tactile stimulation. Infants who fail to respond to stimulation should be ventilated during the spell with bag and mask, generally with an FiO_2 of under 0.40 or equal to the FiO_2 prior to the spell to avoid marked elevations in arterial oxygen tension (PO_2).

C. After the first apneic spell, the infant should be evaluated for a possible underlying cause (Table 24-5); if a cause is identified, specific treatment can then be initiated. One should be particularly alert to the possibility of a precipitating cause in infants who are more than 34 weeks' gestational age. Evaluation should include a history and physical examination, arterial blood gas measurement with continuous transcutaneous oxygen saturation monitoring, complete blood count, and measurement of blood glucose, calcium, and electrolyte levels.

Table 24-5. Evaluation of an infant with apnea

Potential cause	Associated history or signs	Evaluation
Infection	Feeding intolerance, lethargy, temperature instability	Complete blood count, cultures if appropriate
Impaired oxygenation	Cyanosis, tachypnea, respiratory distress	Continuous oxygen monitoring, arterial blood gas measurement, chest x-ray examination
Metabolic disorders	Jitteriness, poor feeding, lethargy, CNS depression, irritability	Glucose, calcium, electrolytes
Drugs	CNS depression, hypotonia, maternal history	Magnesium, screen for toxic substances in urine
Temperature instability	Lethargy	Monitor temperature of patient and environment
Intracranial pathology	Abnormal neurologic examination, seizures	Cranial ultrasound examination
Gastroesophageal reflux	Difficulty with feeds	Specific observation, contrast UGI study

UGI = upper gastrointestinal.

IV. Treatment. When spells of apnea are repeated and prolonged (i.e., more than two to three times per hour) or when they require frequent bag and mask ventilation, treatment should be initiated in order of increasing invasiveness and risk.

   A. Specific therapy should be directed at an underlying cause, if one is identified. If intermittent hypoxemia is identified by oxygen saturation monitoring, supplemental oxygen is provided to maintain oxygen saturation at about 90%.

   B. Care should be taken to avoid reflexes that may trigger apnea. Suctioning of the pharynx should be done carefully, and oral feedings should be avoided. In addition, positions of extreme flexion or extension of the neck should be avoided, to reduce the likelihood of airway obstruction.

   C. Decreasing the environmental temperature to the low end of the neutral thermal environment range may lessen the number of spells. Avoiding swings in environmental temperature may prevent apnea.

   D. Whether blood transfusion reduces the frequency of apneic spells in some infants is controversial. We generally give a transfusion of packed red blood cells if the hematocrit is less than 25 to 30% and the infant has episodes of apnea and bradycardia that are frequent or severe while methylxanthine levels are therapeutic (see Chap. 26).

   E. Nasal continuous positive airway pressure (CPAP) at low levels (3 to 4 cm H_2O) can reduce the number of mixed and obstructive apneic spells. The additional airway care required and the difficulty with feeding often associated with use of nasal CPAP limit its usefulness.

   F. Drug therapy with methylxanthines can markedly reduce the number of apneic spells.

      1. If apneic spells are severe and rapid onset of action is desired, a loading dose of 5 to 7 mg of aminophylline per kilogram intravenously will rapidly achieve the steady-state concentration. The loading dose is followed by a maintenance dose of intravenous **aminophylline** or oral **theophylline** given in a dose of 1.5 to 2.0 mg/kg every 6 to 8 hours. The steady-state level can be measured 0.5 to 1 hour after any succeeding intravenous dose or 1 to 2 hours after any succeeding oral dose.

  a. There is no agreement on the appropriate serum level of theophylline, since efficacy for therapy of apnea does not necessarily correlate with the level achieved. We generally maintain levels at 7 to 12 μg/ml, although lower levels (3 to 4 μg/ml) achieved with lower doses of theophylline (2 mg/kg per day) may be effective.

  b. Dose adjustments are made if a therapeutic effect is not achieved or toxicity is observed.

  (1) If the level is too low, an additional dose of 1 mg of aminophylline per kilogram is given to raise the serum level by 1 to 2 μg/ml; the maintenance dose is increased by 10 to 25%, and the level is rechecked.

  (2) If the level is too high, the next dose is withheld and the maintenance dose is decreased by 10 to 25%.

  c. Theophylline is generally discontinued at 34 to 36 weeks' postmenstrual age if no apneic spells occur for 5 to 7 days.

  d. Mechanisms by which theophylline may decrease apnea include (1) respiratory center stimulation; (2) antagonism of adenosine, a neurotransmitter that can cause respiratory depression; and (3) improvement of diaphragmatic contractility.

  e. **Toxicity of theophylline** is related to serum level. Clinical manifestations of toxicity usually begin with tachycardia, followed by jitteriness, irritability, signs of gastrointestinal dysfunction, including abdominal distention, feeding intolerance, or vomiting. Seizures may occur at extremely high drug levels. Metabolic changes, including increased glucose and insulin levels, occur following a theophylline loading dose in some infants. Because some theophylline may be converted to caffeine in premature infants, the level of theophylline alone may not reflect the total xanthine load. Despite the theoretical risks related to decreased cerebral blood flow, retarded neuronal growth, and inhibition of constriction of the ductus arteriosus, no long-term sequelae have been demonstrated following xanthine treatment in infants.

2. **Caffeine citrate** also can be used to decrease the frequency of apneic spells. A suggested dosage schedule involves a loading dose of 20 mg of caffeine citrate (10-mg caffeine base) per kilogram orally or intravenously, followed by maintenance doses of 2.5 to 5.0 mg/kg daily (caffeine base) in one dose beginning 24 hours after the loading dose.

  a. Caffeine serum levels are maintained at 5 to 20 μg/ml.

  b. Caffeine may be less toxic than theophylline, as side effects are not generally seen until blood levels are much higher than therapeutic levels. There may be no change in heart rate in infants treated with caffeine, in contrast to the tachycardia often associated with theophylline therapy.

3. If theophylline therapy fails to reduce the frequency of apneic spells, infusion of the respiratory stimulant **doxapram** may be effective in reducing apnea. Toxic manifestations include hyperactivity, jitteriness, seizures, hyperglycemia, mild liver dysfunction, and hypertension; these abnormalities resolve when the drug is discontinued. In addition, benzyl alcohol is used as a preservative. For these reasons, we do not use doxapram.

  G. If all the previously mentioned interventions fail, **mechanical ventilation** may be required.

V. **Persistent apnea.** In some infants, especially those born at less than 28 weeks' gestation, apneic spells may persist at 37 to 40 weeks' postmenstrual age, when the infant may be otherwise ready for discharge home from the nursery. There is no consensus yet on the appropriate management of these infants, but efforts are directed at reducing the risk of apneic spells so that the child can be cared for at home.

A. Recordings of impedance pneumography and ECGs for 12 to 24 hours ("pneumograms") can be used to document the occurrence of apnea and bradycardia during that time period, but they do not predict the risk of sudden infant death syndrome (SIDS).

B. The infant should be reevaluated to detect a cause of the apnea. Attention should be paid to possible neurologic problems and to feeding problems such as reflux. Possible anatomic causes of airway obstruction should be investigated.

C. Continued use of theophylline may be helpful in infants whose spells recur when the drug is discontinued. Attempts to withdraw the drug can be made at intervals of approximately 2 months while the child is closely monitored.

D. Some infants are cared for with cardiorespiratory monitoring at home, although few data are available on its effectiveness. Routine home monitoring of asymptomatic preterm infants is not indicated.

E. Extensive psychosocial support must be provided for the parents, who should be skilled in CPR and in the use of a monitor, if one is provided.

VI. Strategies to prevent SIDS. Although the peak incidence of SIDS occurs after the newborn period, parents frequently express concern about their child's risk. Although SIDS occurs more frequently in premature or low-birth-weight infants, a history of apnea of prematurity does not increase this risk. We encourage strategies that may reduce the risk of SIDS.

A. Sleeping position. Prone sleeping position increases the risk of SIDS, and sleeping on the back or side reduces the risk. In general, babies should be placed on their back or side to sleep. The exceptions include preterm infants with respiratory disease, infants with symptomatic gastroesophageal reflux, and infants with craniofacial abnormalities or evidence of upper airway obstruction. For these infants, soft bedding should be avoided.

B. Smoking. Infants exposed to maternal smoking during pregnancy and postnatally have a higher risk of SIDS. Smoking should be avoided by parents, and infants should not be exposed to smoke.

C. Overheating. Infants exposed to excessively high room temperatures or overheating from excess wrapping have an increased risk of SIDS. Caregivers should avoid practices that result in overheating.

D. Breast-feeding. Infants who were never breast-fed have a higher risk of SIDS than do breast-fed infants. We encourage breast-feeding for many reasons (see Chap. 11).

References

1. Consensus statement: National Institutes of Health Consensus Development Conference on Infantile Apnea and Home Monitoring, Sept. 29 to Oct. 1, 1986. *Pediatrics* 79:292, 1987.
2. Hunt, C.E. (Ed.). Apnea and SIDS: Epidemiology of the sudden infant death syndrome: Maternal, neonatal, and postneonatal risk factors. *Clin. Perinatol.* 19: 701, 1992.
3. Rigatto, H. Maturation of breathing control in the fetus and newborn infant. In: R.C. Beckerman, R.T. Brouillete, and C.E. Hunt (Eds.), *Respiratory Control Disorders in Infants and Children.* Baltimore: Williams & Wilkins, 1992, pp. 61–75.
4. Willinger, M., Hoffman, H.J., and Hartford, R.B. Infant sleep position and risk for sudden infant death syndrome: Report of meeting held January 13 and 14, 1994, National Institutes of Health, Bethesda, MD. *Pediatrics* 93:814, 1994.

Chronic Lung Disease
Richard B. Parad and Thomas M. Berger

I. Definition. Infants are considered to have **chronic lung disease (CLD)** if they continue to require supplemental oxygen to maintain adequate oxygenation after 28 days of life and if their lung parenchyma appear abnormal on chest radiographs. This definition predicts the outcome for infants whose gestational age is more than 30 weeks. For infants weighing less than 1500 gm, the need for supplemental oxygen after 36 weeks' postconceptional age has a 63% positive predictive value for development of long-term pulmonary problems.

II. **Epidemiology.** Low-birth-weight infants are most susceptible to developing CLD. Differences in populations, clinical practices, and definitions account for a wide variation in the CLD incidence among centers. The risk for CLD is decreased in blacks, girls, and infants born to mothers who received antenatal glucocorticoid therapy.

III. **Pathogenesis**

A. **Acute lung injury** is caused by prolonged oxygen exposure and barotrauma from mechanical ventilation. Cellular and interstitial injury results in the release of mediators that cause secondary changes in alveolar permeability and recruit inflammatory cells into interstitial and alveolar spaces; this in turn causes leakage of water and protein. Airway and vascular tone may be altered. Proteolytic and oxidant injury may interfere with alveolar development and cause emphysematous changes. Sloughed cells and accumulated secretions not cleared adequately by the damaged mucociliary transport system cause inhomogeneous peripheral airway obstruction that leads to alternating areas of collapse and hyperinflation and proximal airway dilation.

B. In the **chronic phase** of lung injury, the interstitium may be altered by fibrosis and cellular hyperplasia that has resulted from excessive release of growth factors and mediators. Interstitial fluid clearance is disrupted, resulting in pulmonary fluid retention. Airways develop increased muscularization and hyperreactivity. The physiologic effects are decreased lung compliance, increased airway resistance, and impaired gas exchange with resulting ventilation-perfusion mismatching and air trapping.

C. **Factors that may contribute to the development of CLD** include the following:

1. Inadequate antioxidant enzyme activity (superoxide dismutase, catalase, glutathione peroxidase) or deficiency of free-radical sinks (vitamin E, glutathione, ceruloplasmin), or both, may predispose the lung to oxygen toxicity. Similarly, inadequate antiprotease protection may predispose the lung to injury from the unchecked proteases released by recruited inflammatory cells.

2. Excessive early intravenous fluid administration and persistent left-to-right shunt through the patent ductus arteriosus (PDA). Although prophylactic PDA ligation did not prevent CLD, persistent left-to-right shunt could still be a contributing factor.

3. An increase in vasopressin and a decrease in atrial natriuretic peptide release may alter pulmonary and systemic fluid balance in the setting of obstructive lung disease.

4. Familial airway hyperreactivity.

5. Increased inositol clearance, leading to diminished plasma inositol levels and decreased surfactant synthesis or impaired surfactant metabolism.

6. In utero or perinatal acquisition of organisms may contribute to either CLD etiology or modification of the CLD course: *Ureaplasma urealyticum* has been associated with CLD in premature infants, although it remains unclear whether a causal relationship exists. *Chlamydia trachomatis* and cytomegalovirus can cause gradually developing pneumonitis.

IV. **Clinical presentation**

A. **Physical examination** may reveal tachypnea, retractions, and rales on auscultation.

B. **Arterial blood gas (ABG)** analysis shows hypoxemia and hypercarbia with eventual metabolic compensation for the respiratory acidosis.

C. **The chest x-ray** appearance changes as the disease progresses. **Stage I** has the same appearance as RDS, **stage II** shows diffuse haziness with increased density and normal to low lung volumes, **stage III** shows streaky densities with bubbly lucencies and early hyperinflation, and **stage IV** shows hyperinflation with larger hyperlucent areas interspersed with thicker, streaky densities. Not all infants progress to stage IV, and some progress directly from stage I to stage III. Chest x-ray abnormalities often persist into childhood [4].

D. Cardiac evaluation. Nonpulmonary causes of respiratory failure should be excluded. **ECG** can show persistent or progressive right ventricular hypertrophy as cor pulmonale develops. Left ventricular hypertrophy may develop with systemic hypertension. **Two-dimensional echocardiography** may be useful in excluding left-to-right shunts (see Chap. 25).

E. Pulmonary function testing, if done, will show increased respiratory system resistance (Rrs), decreased dynamic compliance (Crs).

F. Pathologic changes are detectable by the first few days of life. By the end of the first week, necrotizing bronchiolitis, obstruction of small airway lumens by debris and edema, and areas of peribronchial and interstitial fibrosis are present. Emphysematous changes and significant impairment in alveolar development result in diminished surface area for gas exchange. Changes in both large airways (glandular hyperplasia) and small airways (smooth muscle hyperplasia) likely form the histologic basis for reactive airway disease. Pulmonary vascular changes associated with pulmonary hypertension may be seen.

V. Inpatient treatment. The goals of treatment are to minimize further lung injury, maximize nutrition, and diminish oxygen consumption.

A. Mechanical ventilation

1. **Acute phase.** Ventilator adjustments are made to minimize airway pressures while providing adequate gas exchange (see Mechanical Ventilation). Although prophylactic use of high-frequency oscillatory ventilation prevented CLD in baboons, evidence for its effectiveness in preventing CLD in human infants is still lacking. In most circumstances, we avoid hyperventilation (keeping P_aCO_2 at 45 to 55 mm Hg, with pH >7.25) and maintain oxygen saturation (S_aO_2) at 90 to 95% (arterial oxygen tension $[P_aO_2]$ 60 to 80 mm Hg).

2. **Chronic phase.** Once baseline ventilator settings are established with an arterial carbon dioxide tension (P_aCO_2) not higher than 65 mm Hg, we delay decreasing the ventilator rate until a pattern of steady weight gain is established.

B. Supplemental oxygen is supplied to maintain the P_aO_2 above 55 mm Hg at all times. The S_aO_2 should be individually correlated with P_aO_2 and generally will have to be maintained between 90 and 95% to reach this goal. When less than 30% oxygen by hood is required, we supply oxygen by nasal cannula. If saturation cannot be maintained on less than 1 liter per minute of flow, hood oxygen should be restored. If the flowmeter is accurate at low rates, flow of 100% oxygen is gradually decreased to maintain S_aO_2. Otherwise, the flow is decreased to the lowest marking on the flowmeter, as tolerated, and then oxygen concentration is decreased. Hypopharyngeal FiO_2 can be estimated from that delivered by nasal cannula (Fig. 24-3). S_aO_2 should remain above 90% during sleep, feedings, and active periods before supplemental oxygen is discontinued.

C. Surfactant. While surfactant replacement therapy has been reported to decrease the combined outcome of CLD or death at 28 days of life, there has been little or no impact on the overall incidence of CLD alone. Meta-analysis of randomized trials of surfactant replacement therapy indicated that the type of surfactant and the dosing strategy adopted may be important. In this analysis, the prophylactic use of natural surfactant decreased the incidence of CLD by 10.9% (95% confidence interval, −18.6 to −3.1) [2].

D. Aggressive early management of a hemodynamically significant **PDA** is recommended (see Chap. 25).

E. Monitoring (see Blood Gas Monitoring and Pulmonary Function Tests)

1. **ABG** analysis is used to monitor gas exchange and confirm noninvasive monitoring values.

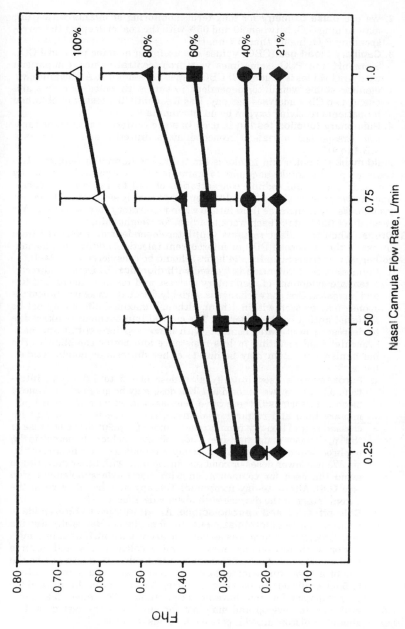

Fig. 24-3. Approximate conversion from nasal cannula flow FiO_2 to hypopharyngeal FiO_2 (FhO_2). (From Vain, N. E., Prudent, L. M., Stevens, D. P., et al., Regulation of oxygen concentration delivered to infants via nasal cannulas. *Am. J. Dis. Child.* 143:1459, 1989. By permission.)

2. We use **pulse oximetry** for long-term monitoring of infants with CLD, maintaining S_aO_2 between 90 and 95% with the goal of keeping the corresponding P_aO_2 higher than 55 mm Hg.

3. **Capillary blood gas** (CBG) values are useful to monitor pH and PCO_2. Since pH and PCO_2 sometimes vary from central values, comparison with ABG values is prudent. If CBG values are similar to ABG values, we monitor stable, ventilator-dependent infants with pulse oximetry and one or two CBG analyses per day; less frequent CBG tests are obtained for patients receiving oxygen by nasal cannula.

4. **Pulmonary function testing** is used in some centers to document functional responses to trials of bronchodilators, diuretics, and steroids (see **V.G.1 to 4**).

F. **Fluid management.** Fluid intake is limited to the minimum required. Initially, we provide intake adequate to maintain urine output at least 1 ml/kg per hour and serum sodium concentration of 140 to 145 mEq/L. Subsequently, we provide 130 to 150 ml/kg per day to supply sufficient calories for growth. We try to increase fluid intake when respiratory status is stable. We recalculate fluid intake each week to adjust for weight gain.

G. **Drugs.** When the infant remains ventilator-dependent on restricted fluid intake in the absence of PDA or intercurrent infection, additional pharmacotherapeutic trials (usually >24 hours) should be considered (Fig. 24-4).

1. Pulmonary fluid retention is treated with **diuretics.** Diuretics indirectly attenuate symptoms of respiratory distress and result in decreased Rrs and increased Crs; gas exchange is variably affected. An acute clinical response may be seen within 1 hour, although maximal effect may not be achieved until 1 week of therapy. The clinical improvement is likely due to decreased lung water content, with decreased interstitial and peribronchial fluid resulting in less resistance and better compliance. The mechanisms of action may be due to either diuresis or nondiuretic effects.

   a. **Furosemide** is used initially at a dose of 0.5 to 1.0 mg/kg intravenously one to two times daily. The dose may be given at the time of blood transfusions if these have been associated with increased pulmonary fluid and respiratory distress. Immature infants are at increased risk of toxicity from larger or more frequent doses because of the prolonged drug half-life. Side effects include hypercalciuria, nephrocalcinosis ototoxicity, electrolyte imbalance, and nephrolithiasis. We use lower doses or combine furosemide with other diuretics to avoid the need for compensation with electrolyte supplementation (see **G.6**). Alternate-day furosemide therapy may be effective in the chronic stage of the disease with fewer side effects.

   b. **Chlorothiazide and spironolactone.** An alternative to furosemide is treatment with **chlorothiazide** (20 to 40 mg/kg per day orally, divided bid). Chlorothiazide decreases calcium excretion and, if used in combination with furosemide, may minimize calcium loss and reverse nephrocalcinosis due to furosemide. The combination also allows the use of a lower furosemide dose. We occasionally add spironolactone (2.5 mg orally qd) for potassium sparing. The effects of this drug alone on pulmonary function have not been studied. This effect takes several days to develop and may last for days after the last dose. Use should be discontinued if potassium levels increase.

2. **Bronchodilators.** Acute obstructive episodes or chronically increased resistance may be related to increased airway tone or bronchospasm and may respond to bronchodilator therapy. Even early use (second week of life) of bronchodilators in infants with developing CLD may be beneficial.

   a. Administration of nebulized **beta-adrenergic agonists (BAAs)** results in decreased Rrs and increased Crs. Tachycardia is the major limiting side effect. Newer agents have increased beta-2 specificity with less beta-1 toxicity. We use **albuterol** 0.5% solution (5 mg/ml) 0.02 to 0.04

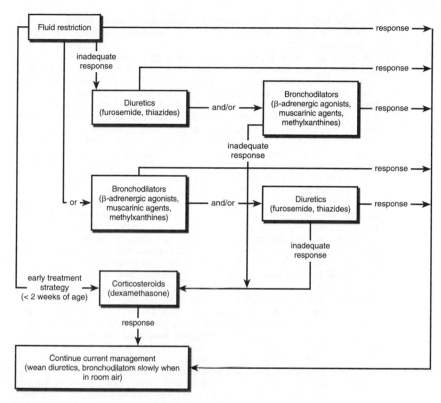

Fig. 24-4. Management flow chart.

ml/kg (up to 0.1 ml total), nebulized in 2 ml of normal saline solution every 6 to 8 hours. In ventilated infants, the nebulizer or a metered-dose inhaler (MDI) with a spacer device is placed in line with the ventilator near the endotracheal tube. In infants receiving both theophylline and BAA, we may alternate doses to avoid acute tachycardia. The combination of oral and aerosolized albuterol may decrease airway reactivity better than aerosol alone. Albuterol syrup (0.3 mg/kg per day p.o. or p.g. divided t.i.d.) given between aerosols can be tried in refractory infants.

  b. **Muscarinic agents.** Nebulized ipratropium bromide (25 μg/kg per dose) increases Crs and decreases Rrs and may have an additive effect with BAAs. BAAs and muscarinic agents can be concurrently nebulized.

  c. **Theophylline.** In addition to bronchodilation, infants with CLD may benefit from multiple actions of this drug, including diuresis, improved diaphragm contractility, inotropy, respiratory drive stimulation, and increased surfactant production. Improvements in mechanics have been demonstrated with low serum levels (5 to 10 μg/ml); however, increased levels used to treat reactive airway disease (12 to 18 μg/ml) may be needed for maximal response. For enteral administration, the intravenous preparation given enterally may induce fewer GI side effects than syrup. Theophylline combined with diuretics produces a better response than either alone. Side effects include tachycardia, irritability, feeding intolerance, gastroesophageal reflux (GER), tremors, and lowered seizure threshold. Caffeine may have a comparable effect.

3. **Cromolyn** acts on both airway and pulmonary vascular tone. Therapeutic and prophylactic treatment of reactive airways has been demonstrated with nebulized cromolyn (10 to 20 mg q6–8h). We add this drug in infants who respond to bronchodilator therapy but remain symptomatic.

4. **Steroids.** Treatment with glucocorticoids in infants who remain ventilator-dependent for 2 to 3 weeks results in increased Crs, decreased Rrs, and diminished oxygen requirement, resulting in earlier extubation. In spite of this, treatment with glucocorticoids does not seem to have a substantial impact on long-term outcomes, such as duration of supplemental oxygen requirement, length of hospital stay, or mortality. The data on 1-year neurodevelopmental outcome are inconsistent. The benefits of earlier administration (at <2 weeks of life) have not been adequately studied. The mechanism of action may be related to diminished inflammation and fibrosis or increased functional surfactant. **Dexamethasone** (0.5 mg/kg per day intravenously divided q12h for 3 days, followed by slow taper over 5 to 6 weeks) may be indicated in infants with chest x-ray findings evolving toward CLD who have failed ventilator weaning on conventional therapy by the age of 2 to 3 weeks. Doses may be given orally. We sometimes begin earlier treatment in extremely low-birth-weight infants who require substantial ventilator and oxygen support at one week of age. The duration of treatment (2 to 6 weeks) depends on the response and on complications. Treatment as early as the first 24 hours is currently under investigation. Common acute complications include glucose intolerance, systemic hypertension, and transient catabolic state. Total neutrophil counts, band counts, and platelet counts increase during steroid treatment. Hypertrophic cardiomyopathy can occur, but it is transient and does not appear to affect cardiac function. Cases of gastroduodenal perforation and gastric ulcerations have been reported. Adrenal suppression is transient. While metabolic parameters indicate that dexamethasone acutely induces protein catabolism, later growth, development, and bone age do not appear affected. The data on the effectiveness and safety of inhaled glucocorticoids in ventilated infants are incomplete.

Postextubation airway edema, with stridorous obstruction (see **VI.A**) leading to respiratory failure, may be attenuated with dexamethasone, 0.3 mg/kg per dose every 12 hours starting 8 to 12 hours before the next extubation. Edema also may be acutely diminished with nebulized racemic epinephrine.

5. **Sedatives.** Sedation and, when necessary, analgesia are used for physical or autonomic signs of pain or discomfort. These responses may interfere with the ability to ventilate and oxygenate. Chloral hydrate, phenobarbital, short-acting benzodiazepines, or morphine sulfate are used.

6. **Electrolyte supplements.** Hyponatremia, hypokalemia, and hypochloremia with secondary hypercarbia are common side effects of chronic diuretic therapy that are corrected by lowering the diuretic dose or adding NaCl and KCl supplements. Adequate sodium intake should be provided. Serum sodium level can fall below 130 mEq/L before intervention is required. Although hypochloremia may occur with compensated respiratory acidosis, low serum chloride concentration from diuretic-induced loss and inadequate intake can cause metabolic alkalosis and P_aCO_2 elevation. Hypochloremia may also contribute to poor growth. Chloride deficit can be corrected with potassium chloride. Monitoring should be carried out at regular intervals until equilibrium is reached.

H. **Chest physiotherapy and suctioning** may diminish expiratory resistance. Damaged mucociliary clearance mechanisms and inability to cough during intubation result in obstruction of airways by secretions and debris. Vibration and percussion loosen peripheral plugs and secretions and move them

centrally for clearance by suctioning. Normal saline solution distributed by positive pressure ventilation may loosen this material for easier removal.
I. **Nutrition** (see Chap. 10)
   1. In CLD, metabolic rate and energy expenditure are elevated while caloric intake is poor. Providing more calories by the administration of lipids instead of carbohydrates lowers the respiratory quotient, thus diminishing CO_2 production. To optimize growth, wasteful energy expenditure must be minimized and caloric intake maximized. Prolonged parenteral nutrition is often required. As enteral feeding is started, we feed by orogastric or nasogastric tube and limit oral feeding to avoid tiring the infant.
   2. **Vitamin, trace element, and other dietary supplementation.** Vitamin E and antioxidant enzymes diminish oxidant toxicity, although vitamin E supplementation does not prevent CLD. Vitamin A may promote epithelial repair and minimize fibrosis. Selenium, zinc, and copper are trace elements vital to antioxidant enzyme function, and inadequate intake may interfere with protection. It is uncertain whether vitamin A supplementation reduces incidence of CLD.
J. **Blood transfusions.** We generally maintain hematocrit about 30–35% (hemoglobin 8–10 gm/dl) during oxygen dependence. Fluid-sensitive patients may benefit from furosemide given immediately following the transfusion. Improved oxygen delivery may allow better reserves for growth in the infant with increased metabolic demands.
K. **Behavioral factors.** As with all sick infants, care is best provided with individualized attention to behavioral and environmental factors (see Chap. 14).
VI. **Associated complications**
A. **Upper airway obstruction.** Trauma to the nasal septum, larynx, trachea, or bronchi is common after prolonged or repeated intubation and suctioning. Abnormalities include laryngotracheobronchomalacia, granulomas, vocal cord paresis, edema, ulceration with pseudomembranes, subglottic stenosis, and congenital structural anomalies. Stridor may develop when postextubation edema is superimposed on underlying stenosis. Abnormalities are not excluded by the absence of stridor and may be asymptomatic, becoming symptomatic at the time of a viral upper respiratory tract infection. Flexible fiberoptic bronchoscopy should be used to evaluate stridor, hoarseness, persistent wheezing, recurrent obstruction, or repeated extubation failure.
B. **Cor pulmonale.** Pulmonary hypertension may have reversible and fixed components. Chronic hypoxemia leads to hypoxic vasoconstriction, pulmonary hypertension, and eventual right ventricular hypertrophy and failure. Decrease in cross-sectional perfusion area and abnormal muscularization of more peripheral vessels have been documented. Left ventricular function also can be affected. The ECG should be followed. Supplemental oxygen is used to maintain the P_aO_2 above 55 mm Hg. Further studies may be required to define the dysfunction and evaluate therapy. Pulmonary vasodilators including hydralazine and nifedipine have variable efficacy and should only be tried during pulmonary artery pressure and P_aO_2 monitoring. Echocardiographic studies can exclude structural heart disease, assess left ventricular function, and estimate pulmonary vascular resistance and right ventricular function.
C. **Systemic hypertension,** sometimes with left ventricular hypertrophy, may develop in CLD infants receiving prolonged O_2 therapy.
D. **Systemic-to-pulmonary shunting.** Left-to-right shunt through collateral vessels (e.g., bronchial arteries) can occur in CLD. The risk factors include chest tube placement, thoracic surgery, and pleural inflammation. When left-to-right shunt is suspected and echocardiography fails to show intracardiac or PDA shunting, collaterals may be demonstrated by angiography. Occlusion of large vessels has been associated with clinical improvement.
E. **Metabolic imbalance secondary to diuretics** (see V.G.1 and 6)

F. Infection. Because these chronically ill and malnourished infants are at increased risk, episodes of pulmonary and systemic decompensation should be evaluated for infection. Monitoring by Gram stain of tracheal aspirates may help distinguish endotracheal tube colonization from tracheobronchitis or pneumonia (presence of organisms and neutrophils). Viral and fungal infections should be considered when fevers or pneumonia develop. In infants with more severe clinical courses, we frequently culture tracheal aspirates for possible infection with *Ureaplasma* sp. and *Mycoplasma hominis* and may treat with erythromycin if these organisms are identified.

G. CNS dysfunction. A neurologic syndrome presenting with extrapyramidal signs has been described in infants with CLD.

H. Hearing loss. Ototoxic drugs (furosemide, gentamicin) and ischemic or hypoxemic CNS injury increase the risk for sensorineural hearing loss. Screening with auditory brainstem responses is recommended at discharge (see Chap. 35, Hearing Loss in Neonatal Intensive Care Unit Graduates).

I. Retinopathy of prematurity (ROP) (see Chap. 35, Retinopathy of Prematurity). Very-low-birth-weight infants with CLD are at highest risk for developing ROP. It is unclear whether the use of systemic steroids affects the incidence or severity of ROP. The use of phenylephrine-containing eyedrops prior to eye examinations can cause an increase in airway resistance in some infants with CLD.

J. Nephrocalcinosis is frequently documented on ultrasound examination and has been linked to the use of furosemide and possibly steroids. Hematuria and passage of stones may occur. Most infants are asymptomatic, with eventual spontaneous resolution, but renal function should be followed up (see **V.E.1**, see Chap. 31).

K. Prematurity, inadequate calcium and phosphorus retention, and prolonged immobilization can lead to **osteoporosis.** Calcium loss due to furosemide and corticosteroids also may contribute. Supplementation with vitamin D, calcium, and phosphorus should be optimized (see Chap. 29).

L. GER. We try to document and treat GER when reflux or aspiration may contribute to pulmonary decompensation, apnea, or feeding intolerance with poor growth.

M. The incidence of **inguinal hernia** is increased by the presence of the patent processus vaginalis in very-low-birth-weight infants, particularly boys with CLD. If the hernia is reducible, surgical correction should be delayed until respiratory status is improved. Spinal rather than general anesthesia avoids reintubation and postoperative apnea.

N. Early **growth failure** may result from inadequate intake and excessive energy expenditure and may persist after clinical resolution of pulmonary disease. Premature withdrawal of supplemental oxygen may contribute to slowing of growth.

VII. Discharge planning. The timing of discharge depends on the availability of home care support systems and parental readiness (see Chap. 16).

A. Weight gain and oxygen therapy. Supplemental oxygen should be weaned when the S_aO_2 is maintained above 94%, no significant periods of desaturations occur during feedings and/or sleep, good weight gain has been established, and respiratory status is stable (see **V.B** and **VI.N**). We prefer to delay discharge until oxygen has been discontinued. However, if long-term oxygen supplementation seems likely in an infant who is stable, is growing, and has capable caretakers, we offer the option of home oxygen therapy.

B. Teaching. The involvement of parents in caregiving is vital to the smooth transition from hospital to home care. Parents should be taught CPR and early signs of decompensation. Teaching about equipment use, medication administration, and nutritional guidelines should begin when discharge planning is initiated.

C. Baseline values. Baseline values of vital signs, daily weight gain, discharge weight and head circumference, blood gases, S_aO_2, hematocrit, electrolytes, and the baseline appearance of the chest x-ray and ECG must be documented at discharge. This information is useful to evaluate subsequent changes in clinical status. An eye examination and hearing screening should be performed prior to discharge.

VIII. Outpatient therapy

    A. Oxygen. Supplementary oxygen can be delivered by tanks or oxygen concentrator. Portable tanks allow mobility. Weaning is based on periodic assessment of S_aO_2.

    B. Medications. Infants receiving diuretics require monitoring of electrolytes. When the infant is stable, we allow the infant to outgrow the diuretic dose by 50% before discontinuing the drug. Bronchodilators are tapered when respiratory status in room air is stable. Nebulized medications are tapered last. Discontinued medications should remain available for early use when symptoms recur.

    C. Immunizations. In addition to standard immunizations, infants with CLD should receive pneumococcal and influenza vaccines. Prophylactic use of respiratory syncytial virus immune globulin can decrease the number and severity of lower respiratory tract infections caused by this organism (see Chap. 23).

    D. Nutrition. Weight gain is a sensitive indicator of well-being and should be closely monitored. Caloric supplementation is often required to maintain good growth after discharge.

    E. Passive smoke exposure. Because smoking in the home increases respiratory tract illness in children, parents of CLD infants should be discouraged from smoking and should minimize the child's exposure to smoke-containing environments.

IX. Outcome

    A. Mortality. Mortality is estimated at 10 to 20% during the first year of life. The risk increases with duration of oxygen exposure and level of ventilatory support. Death is frequently caused by infection. The risk of sudden unexpected death may be increased, but the cause is unclear.

    B. Long-term morbidity

        1. Pulmonary. Tachypnea, retractions, dyspnea, cough, and wheezing can be seen for months to years in seriously affected children. Although complete clinical recovery can occur, underlying pulmonary function, gas exchange, and chest x-ray abnormalities may persist beyond adolescence. The impact of persistent minor abnormalities of function and growth on long-term morbidity and mortality is not known. Reactive airway disease occurs more frequently, and infants with CLD are at increased risk for bronchiolitis and pneumonia. The rehospitalization rate for respiratory illness during the first 2 years of life is approximately twice that of matched control infants.

        2. Neurodevelopmental delay/neurologic deficits. CLD does not appear to be an independent predictor of adverse neurologic outcome. Early behavioral differences do exist, however, between very-low-birth-weight infants with CLD and RDS controls. Later outcome varies widely; one-third to two-thirds of infants with CLD are normal by 2 years, and subsequent improvement may occur in some of the remaining infants. Our experience suggests specific motor coordination delays and visual-perceptual impairment, rather than overall lower IQ, may occur, with resulting mean Bayley scores 1 standard deviation below the normal mean by ages 4 to 6 years.

        3. Growth failure. The degree of long-term growth delay is inversely proportional to birth weight and probably is influenced by the severity and duration of CLD. Weight is most affected, and head circumference is least affected. Delayed growth occurs in one-third to two-thirds of these infants at 2 years. One-third of our school-age population is 3 standard deviations below the mean for height and weight.

References

1. Davis, J.M., et al. Drug therapy for bronchopulmonary dysplasia. *Pediatr. Pulmonol.* 8:117, 1990.

2. Ehrenkrantz, R.A., and Mercurio, M.R. Bronchopulmonary dysplasia. In J.C. Sinclair and M.B. Bracken (Eds.), *Effective Care of the Newborn Infant*. New York: Oxford University Press, 1992, pp. 399–424.
3. Holtzman, R.B., and Frank, L. (Guest Eds.). *Clin. Perinatol.* 19, 1992 (entire issue).
4. Northway, W.H., Rosan, R.C., Porter, D.Y. Pulmonary disease following respirator therapy of hyaline-membrane disease. *N. Engl. J. Med.* 276:357, 1967.

Meconium Aspiration
Eric C. Eichenwald

I. **Background**
   A. **Cause.** Acute or chronic hypoxia can result in the passage of meconium in utero. In this setting, gasping by the fetus or newly born infant can then cause aspiration of amniotic fluid contaminated by meconium. Meconium aspiration before or during birth can obstruct airways, interfere with gas exchange, and cause severe respiratory distress (Fig. 24-5).
   B. **Incidence.** Meconium-stained amniotic fluid complicates delivery in approximately 9 to 15% of live births. Passage of meconium in utero rarely occurs prior to 37 weeks' gestation but may occur in more than 30% of pregnancies that continue past 42 weeks' gestation. Infants born with meconium-stained amniotic fluid frequently have had antepartum or intrapartum asphyxia. In Gregory's 1974 series [1], 46% of infants born through meconium-stained amniotic fluid had Apgar scores lower than 6 at 1 minute and 19% had Apgar scores lower than 6 at 5 minutes. The timing of the insult may be suggested by the color of the fluid; yellow meconium is usually old, while green meconium suggests a more recent insult.
   C. If the amniotic fluid is meconium-stained, about half the infants will have meconium in their tracheas as shown by direct suction. Meconium can be present in the trachea without any evidence of meconium in the mouth or larynx. The amount and thickness of meconium appear to be directly related to the severity of the respiratory symptoms and signs. Suctioning of the mouth and oropharynx before delivery of the shoulders, and direct suctioning of meconium from the trachea, favorably affect the clinical course. Two-thirds of Gregory's patients [1] from whom meconium was suctioned had no respiratory difficulties, although half had abnormal findings on chest x-ray films. Symptomatic meconium aspiration pneumonia is more common and may be more severe in meconium-stained infants who do not have tracheal suctioning performed. Adequate airway management, however, cannot prevent meconium aspiration altogether, since meconium may be aspirated by the fetus prior to delivery (see Chap. 4).
II. **Prevention of passage of meconium in utero.** Mothers who are at risk for uteroplacental insufficiency include those with toxemia or increased blood pressure, heavy smokers, those with chronic respiratory or cardiovascular disease, those with poor uterine growth, and those who are beyond their estimated day of confinement. These women should be carefully monitored during pregnancy, and the fetal heart rate should be monitored during labor, with fetal scalp blood samples obtained for pH determination when indicated.
   The use of transcervical amnioinfusion with normal saline solution in women whose labor is complicated by thick meconium and oligohydramnios may reduce the incidence of fetal distress and meconium aspiration. Prophylactic amnioinfusion for the prevention of meconium aspiration remains a subject of active investigation.
III. **Management of infants delivered through meconium-stained fluid**
   A. When thick, particulate, "pea soup" meconium is present, the obstetrician should attempt to clear the infant's nose and oropharynx before the chest is delivered. This can be done with a bulb syringe followed by passage of a De Lee suction catheter through the nose to the oropharynx.

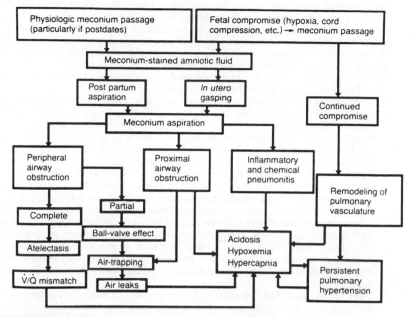

Fig. 24-5. Pathophysiology of meconium aspiration. (From T. Wiswell and R.C. Bent, Meconium staining and the meconium aspiration syndrome: Unresolved issues. *Pediatr. Clin. North Am.* 40:955, 1993. By permission.)

B. The infant should then be handed to the anesthesiologist or pediatrician, who intubates the trachea under direct laryngoscopy, if possible before inspiratory efforts have been initiated. A 3.0- or 3.5-mm internal-diameter endotracheal tube is used in term infants. After intubation, the tube is attached to wall suction at a pressure of 80 to 100 mm Hg by means of a plastic adapter (Neotech Meconium Aspirator, Neotech Products, Chatsworth, CA). Continuous suction is applied as the tube is being withdrawn; the procedure is repeated until the trachea is cleared. Visualization of the cords without suctioning is **not** adequate because significant meconium may be present below the cords. Positive pressure ventilation should be avoided until after the trachea is suctioned.

Direct tracheal suctioning is also indicated for infants delivered through thin or moderately meconium-stained fluid if fetal distress has been documented or if the infant is depressed at birth. Optimal management of the **vigorous** infant with thin or moderate meconium staining remains controversial. If the meconium is thin, the pediatrician should rapidly **evaluate** the infant and **decide** whether intubation and suctioning are required. In questionable cases, it is safer to intubate and suction, as meconium aspiration can occur in infants delivered through thinly stained amniotic fluid.

C. The infant's general condition must not be ignored in compulsive attempts to clear the trachea. This procedure should be accomplished rapidly, and ventilation with oxygen should be initiated before significant bradycardia occurs. Because a few inspiratory efforts by the infant will move the meconium from the trachea to the smaller airways, exhaustive attempts to remove it are unwise.

IV. Management of meconium aspiration. Infants who are depressed at birth and have had meconium suctioned from the trachea are at risk for meconium aspiration pneumonia and should be observed closely for respiratory distress. Chest x-ray examination may help determine which infants are most likely to develop respiratory distress, although a significant number of infants without respiratory distress will have an abnormal-appearing chest film. Chest physiotherapy and suctioning of the oropharynx may be useful to help remove meconium from the airways in infants who develop respiratory symptoms. Monitoring of oxygen saturation during this period aids assessment of the severity of the infant's condition and allows for prevention of hypoxemia.

A. Drug therapy. Differentiating between bacterial pneumonia and meconium aspiration by clinical course and chest x-ray findings may be difficult. Thus, the use of broad-spectrum antibiotics (e.g., ampicillin and gentamicin) is usually indicated in infants when an infiltrate is seen on chest x-ray studies. Blood cultures should be obtained to identify bacterial disease, if present. There is no evidence that steroids are beneficial.

B. Routine care. The thermal environment of all infants at risk for meconium aspiration pneumonia should be watched closely. Blood glucose and calcium levels should be assessed and corrected if necessary. In addition, severely depressed infants may have significant metabolic acidosis that should be corrected with bicarbonate. These infants may also require specific therapy for hypotension and poor cardiac output, including temporary support with colloid infusion or cardiotonic medications such as dopamine. Fluids should be restricted as much as possible to prevent cerebral and pulmonary edema. Renal function should be continuously monitored (see Chap. 27, Perinatal Asphyxia).

C. Obstruction. In infants with significant meconium aspiration, mechanical obstruction of both large and small airways can occur, as well as chemical pneumonitis (see Fig. 24-5). This results in severe arterial hypoxemia, partly secondary to right-to-left shunting through an atelectatic lung and partly due to the inflammatory change.

D. Management of hypoxemia should be accomplished by increasing the inspired oxygen concentration and by monitoring blood gases and pH. Usually an indwelling arterial catheter is required for blood sampling and infusion. It is crucial to provide sufficient oxygen, because repeated hypoxic insults may contribute to pulmonary artery hypertension. If FiO_2 requirements exceed 0.40, a trial of continuous positive airway pressure (CPAP) may be considered. CPAP is often helpful, and the appropriate pressures must be individualized for each infant. In some instances, CPAP may aggravate air trapping and should be instituted with caution if hyperinflation is apparent clinically or radiographically.

E. Mechanical ventilation. Hypercapnia may become a problem in infants with very severe disease. For severe carbon dioxide retention (P_aCO_2 >60 mm Hg) or for persistent hypoxemia (P_aO_2 <50 mm Hg), mechanical ventilation is indicated. In these infants, higher inspiratory pressures (about 30 to 35 cm H_2O) are more often required than in infants with respiratory distress syndrome; the positive end-expiratory pressure (PEEP) selected (usually 2 to 6 cm H_2O) should depend on the individual's response. Adequate expiratory time should be permitted to prevent air trapping behind partly obstructed airways. Useful starting points are an inspiratory time of 0.4 to 0.5 second at a rate of 20 to 25 breaths per minute. Some infants may respond better to conventional ventilation at more rapid rates with inspiratory times as short as 0.2 second. **High-frequency ventilation** with high-frequency jet or oscillatory ventilators may be successful in infants with severe meconium aspiration who fail to improve with conventional ventilation, and in those who develop air leak syndromes. Clinical improvement in oxygenation after exogenous bovine surfactant therapy in severely ill infants with meconium aspiration syndrome has been reported. We do not routinely use surfactant to treat infants with meconium aspiration syndrome.

F. Air leak. There is a 10 to 20% incidence of pneumothorax or pneumomediastinum associated with meconium aspiration, which may increase when mechanical ventilation is required. Thus, a high index of suspicion for air leak is required. Equipment should be available to evacuate a pneumothorax promptly (see Air Leak).

G. Pulmonary hypertension often accompanies meconium aspiration, and specific measures should be taken to ascertain the degree to which it is contributing to the infant's hypoxemia (see Persistent Pulmonary Hypertension of the Newborn).

Reference

1. Gregory, G.A. Meconium aspiration in infants—A prospective study. *J. Pediatr.* 85:848, 1974.

25. CARDIAC DISORDERS

Stephanie Burns Wechsler and Gil Wernovsky

I. **Introduction.** At the turn of the century Dr. William Osler wrote in his textbook of medicine that congenital heart disease was of "limited clinical interest as in a large proportion of cases the anomaly is not compatible with life, and in others, nothing can be done to remedy the defect or even relieve the symptoms." However, in the 55 years since Gross first successfully ligated a patent ductus arteriosus in a 7-year-old girl at Children's Hospital in Boston (with a 17-day postoperative stay, 12 of which were for "general interest in the case"), the outlook for children with congenital heart disease has changed dramatically for the better. This remarkable progress has been due to synergistic advances in pediatric and fetal cardiology, cardiac surgery, neonatology, cardiac anesthesia, intensive care, and nursing.

For critical lesions, the ultimate prognosis depends in part on a timely and accurate assessment of the structural anomaly and the evaluation and resuscitation of secondary organ damage. It is thus crucial that pediatricians and neonatologists be able to rapidly evaluate and participate in the initial medical management of neonates with congenital heart disease. A multidisciplinary approach involving several subspecialty services is frequently required, especially since one-fifth of patients with severe congenital heart disease may be premature or weigh less than 2500 gm at birth [19]. Although neonates (as a group) may have a slightly higher surgical mortality than older infants [19], the secondary effects of the unoperated lesion on the heart, lung, and brain may be quite severe, and may result in chronic congestive heart failure, failure to thrive, frequent infections, irreversible pulmonary vascular changes, delayed cognitive development, or focal neurologic deficits. For these reasons, at Children's Hospital in Boston primary surgical correction is carried out whenever possible in the neonatal period [8,9]. This chapter is intended as a practical guide for the initial evaluation and management, by pediatricians and neonatologists, of neonates and infants suspected of having congenital heart disease. For detailed discussion of the individual lesions, the clinician should consult current textbooks of pediatric cardiology and cardiac surgery [8,18, 20,24].

II. **Prevalence and survival.** The prevalence of structural heart disease in the first year of life confirmed by noninvasive imaging is 4 per 1000 live births. Including all patients diagnosed with congenital heart disease, including those diagnosed solely by clinical means, the prevalence is 8 per 1000 live births. The prevalence has been relatively constant over the years and in different areas around the world. Table 25-1 summarizes and compares prevalence data from several large population-based studies. Data from the New England Regional Infant Cardiac Program suggest that approximately 3 per 1000 live births have heart disease that results in death or requires cardiac catheterization or surgery during the first year of life [19]. The majority of these infants with congenital heart disease are identified by the end of the neonatal period [19]. Frequencies for the most common congenital heart lesions presenting in the first weeks of life are presented in Table 25-2. Recent advances in diagnostic imaging, cardiac surgery, and intensive care have reduced the operative risks for many complex lesions; the hospital mortality following all forms of neonatal cardiac surgery has significantly decreased in the past decade (Fig. 25-1).

III. **Clinical presentations of congenital heart disease in the neonate.** The timing of presentation and accompanying symptomatology depends on (i) the nature and severity of the anatomic defect, (ii) the in utero effects (if any) of the struc-

Table 25-1. Congenital heart disease in defined populations

	Baltimore-Washington Infant Study	New England Regional Infant Cardiac Program	Carlgren	Dickinson et al.	Laursen	Totals	Approximate no. of affected infants per live births (rounded to nearest 500)
Years of study	1981–1982	1969–1977	1941–1950	1960–1969	1963–1973	—	—
Reference population	Resident births, Maryland and Washington, DC metropolitan area	Resident births, 6 New England states	Resident births, Gothenburg, Sweden	Resident births, Liverpool, England	Live births, Denmark	—	—
Birth cohort: length of follow-up	1 yr	1 yr	7–16 yr	3–12 yr	Birth–15 yr	—	—
No. of congenital heart disease cases	664	2251	369	884	5249	9417	—
No. of live births	179,697	1,528,686	58,105	160,480	Approx. 855,000	Approx. 2,781,968	—
Prevalence per 1000 live births							
Conotruncal and major septation defects							
Transposition of great arteries	0.211	0.215	0.379	0.270	0.290	0.273	1 : 3500
Tetralogy of Fallot	0.262	0.214	0.310	0.320	0.360	0.293	1 : 3500
Truncus arteriosus	0.056	0.034	0.069	0.060	0.090	0.062	1 : 16,000
Endocardial cushion defects	0.362	0.118	0.172	0.130	0.150	0.186	1 : 5500
Total anomalous pulmonary venous return	0.083	0.058	0.052	0.070	—	0.066	1 : 15,000

Atresias							
Tricuspid atresia	0.039	0.057	0.086	0.090	0.050	0.064	1 : 15,500
Pulmonary atresia	0.083	0.071	0.069	0.040	0.040	0.061	1 : 16,500
Hypoplastic left heart syndrome	0.267	0.164	0.103	0.160	0.180	0.175	1 : 5500
Valve and vessel lesions							
Pulmonic stenosis	0.189	0.073	0.275	0.420	0.360	0.263	1 : 4000
Aortic stenosis	0.111	0.041	0.344	0.280	0.290	0.213	1 : 4500
Coarctation of aorta	0.239	0.185	0.620	0.350	0.430	0.365	1 : 2500
Septal defects							
Ventricular septal defect	0.863	0.379	1.699	1.80	1.480	1.244	1 : 1000
Atrial septal defect	0.317	0.073	0.241	0.320	0.580	0.306	1 : 3000
Patent ductus arteriosus	0.089	0.138	0.602	0.650	0.770	0.450	1 : 2000
Rate of confirmed congenital heart disease	3.70	2.03	4.00	3.75	4.30	3.560	

Source: Modified from C. Ferencz et al., Congenital heart disease: Prevalence at livebirth; The Baltimore-Washington Infant Study. *Am. J. Epidemiol.* 121:31, 1984.

Table 25-2. Frequency distribution of cardiac defects based on age at diagnosis

Age at diagnosis:	0–6 days (n = 1603)	7–13 days (n = 311)	14–28 days (n = 306)
	D-TGA (15%)	Coarctation (20%)	VSD (18%)
	HLHS (12%)	VSD (14%)	TOF (17%)
	TOF (8%)	HLHS (9%)	Coarctation (12%)
	Coarctation (7%)	D-TGA (8%)	D-TGA (10%)
	VSD (6%)	TOF (7%)	PDA (5%)
	Other (52%)	Other (42%)	Other (38%)

D-TGA = D-transposition of the great arteries; HLHS = hypoplastic left heart syndrome; TOF = tetralogy of Fallot; VSD = ventricular septal defect.
Source: From D. C. Fyler, and P. Lang, Neonatal Heart Disease. In G. A. Avery (Ed.), *Neonatology: Pathophysiology and Management of the Newborn.* Philadelphia: Lippincott, 1981.

tural lesion, and (iii) the alterations in cardiovascular physiology secondary to the effects of the transitional circulation: **closure of the ductus arteriosus** and the **fall in pulmonary vascular resistance.** This chapter focuses primarily on cardiovascular abnormalities with critical effects in the neonatal period.

In the first few weeks of life, the many heterogeneous forms of heart disease present in a surprisingly limited number of ways (in no particular order nor mutually exclusive): (i) cyanosis, (ii) congestive heart failure (with the most extreme presentation being cardiovascular collapse or shock), (iii) an asymptomatic heart murmur, and (iv) arrhythmia. With increasing frequency, neonates with congenital heart disease have been diagnosed prior to delivery by fetal echocardiography [3] and thus are born with a presumptive diagnosis into an expectant team of physicians and nurses. In the majority of neonates, however, congenital heart disease is not suspected until after birth. Not infrequently the

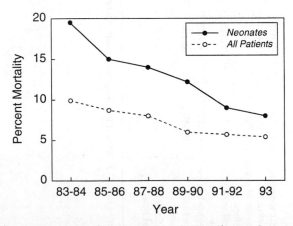

Fig. 25-1. Hospital mortality for all patients (dashed line) and neonates (<28 days, solid line) in the cardiac intensive care unit at Children's Hospital, Boston. This represents all patients admitted, including those receiving palliative therapy (e.g., Norwood operation), corrective surgery, or no surgery. Note a continued decrease in overall and neonatal mortality in the past decade.

clinician is diverted away from a diagnosis of heart disease because of the report of "normal" findings on prenatal ultrasonography performed for screening purposes. Finally, the diagnosis of "heart disease" should never divert the clinician from a complete noncardiac evaluation with a thorough search for additional or secondary medical problems—occasionally the neonate with complex congenital heart disease and hypoxemia has inadequate attention paid to an initial and continued assessment of an adequate airway and ventilation.

A. Cyanosis
   1. **Clinical findings.** Cyanosis (bluish tinge of the skin and mucous membranes) is one of the most common presenting signs of congenital heart disease in the neonate. Although cyanosis usually indicates underlying hypoxemia (diminished level of arterial oxygen saturation), there are a few instances when cyanosis is associated with a normal arterial oxygen saturation (see **III.A.2**). Depending on the underlying skin complexion, clinically apparent cyanosis is usually not visible until there is more than 3 gm of **desaturated** hemoglobin per deciliter in the arterial system. Thus, the degree of visible cyanosis depends on both the severity of hypoxemia (which determines the percent oxygen saturation) and the hemoglobin concentration. For example, consider two infants with similar degrees of hypoxemia—each having an arterial oxygen saturation of 85%. The polycythemic newborn (hemoglobin of 22 gm/dl) will have 3.3 gm (15% of 22) of desaturated hemoglobin per deciliter and be more easily appreciated to be cyanotic than will the anemic (hemoglobin of 10 gm/dl) infant who will only have 1.5 gm (15% of 10) of desaturated hemoglobin per deciliter. An additional note: True central cyanosis should be a generalized finding (i.e., not acrocyanosis, blueness of the hands and feet only, which is a normal finding in a neonate).
   2. **Differential diagnosis.** Differentiation of cardiac from respiratory causes of cyanosis in the neonatal intensive care unit (NICU) is a common problem. Pulmonary disorders frequently are the cause of cyanosis in the newborn due to **intrapulmonary** right-to-left shunting. Primary lung disease (e.g., pneumonia, hyaline membrane disease, pulmonary arteriovenous malformations), pneumothorax, airway obstruction, extrinsic compression of the lungs (e.g., congenital diaphragmatic hernia, pleural effusions), and central nervous system abnormalities may produce varying degrees of hypoxemia manifesting as cyanosis in the neonate. For a more complete differential diagnosis of pulmonary causes of cyanosis in the neonate, see Chap. 24. Finally, clinical cyanosis may occur in an infant without hypoxemia in the setting of methemoglobinemia or pronounced polycythemia. Table 25-3 summarizes the differential diagnosis of cyanosis in the neonate.
      Cyanosis due to congenital heart disease can be broadly grouped into those lesions with (i) decreased pulmonary blood flow and intracardiac right-to-left shunting and (ii) normal to increased pulmonary blood flow with intracardiac mixing (complete or incomplete) of the systemic and pulmonary venous return. Specific lesions and lesion-specific management are covered in more detail in sec. **V.**

B. Congestive heart failure
   1. **Clinical findings.** Congestive heart failure in the neonate (or in a patient of any age) is a **clinical** diagnosis made on the basis of the existence of certain signs and symptoms rather than on radiographic or laboratory findings (though these may be supportive evidence for the diagnosis). Signs and symptoms of congestive heart failure occur when the heart is unable to meet the metabolic demands of the tissues. Clinical findings are frequently due to homeostatic mechanisms attempting to compensate for this imbalance. In early stages, the neonate may be tachypneic and tachycardiac with an increased respiratory effort, rales, hepatomegaly, and delayed capillary refill. In contrast to adults, edema is rarely seen. Diaphoresis, feeding difficulties, and growth failure may be

Table 25-3. Differential diagnosis of cyanosis in the neonate

Primary cardiac lesions
  Decreased pulmonary blood flow, intracardiac right-to-left shunt
    Critical pulmonary stenosis
    Tricuspid atresia
    Pulmonary atresia/intact ventricular septum
    Tetralogy of Fallot
    Ebstein's anomaly
    Total anomalous pulmonary venous connection with obstruction
  Normal or increased pulmonary blood flow, intracardiac mixing
    Hypoplastic left heart syndrome
    Transposition of the great arteries
    Truncus arteriosus
    Tetralogy of Fallot/pulmonary atresia
    Complete common atrioventricular canal
    Total anomalous pulmonary venous connection without obstruction
    Other single-ventricle complexes
Pulmonary lesions (intrapulmonary right-to-left shunt) (see Chap. 24)
  Primary parenchymal lung disease
    Aspiration syndromes (e.g., meconium and blood)
    Respiratory distress syndrome
    Pneumonia
  Airway obstruction
    Choanal stenosis or atresia
    Pierre Robin syndrome
    Tracheal stenosis
    Pulmonary sling
    Absent pulmonary valve syndrome[a]
  Extrinsic compression of the lungs
    Pneumothorax
    Pulmonary interstitial or lobar emphysema
    Chylothorax or other pleural effusions
    Congenital diaphragmatic hernia
    Thoracic dystrophies or dysplasia
  Hypoventilation
    Central nervous system lesions
    Neuromuscular diseases
    Sedation
    Sepsis
  Pulmonary arteriovenous malformations
Persistent pulmonary hypertension (see Chap. 24)
Cyanosis with normal PO_2
  Methemoglobinemia
  Polycythemia[b]

[a]Typically associated with tetralogy of Fallot with intracardiac shunt as well.
[b]In the case of polycythemia, these infants have plethora and venous congestion in the distal extremities, which gives the appearance of distal cyanosis; these infants actually are not hypoxemic (see text).

present. Finally, congestive heart failure may present acutely with cardiorespiratory collapse, particularly in "left-sided" lesions (see **V.A**). Hydrops fetalis is an extreme form of intrauterine congestive heart failure.

  2. **Differential diagnosis.** The age when congestive heart failure develops depends on the hemodynamics of the responsible lesion. When heart failure develops in the first weeks of life, the differential diagnosis includes (i) a structural lesion causing severe pressure and/or volume overload,

(ii) a primary myocardial lesion causing myocardial dysfunction, and (iii) arrhythmia. Table 25-4 summarizes the differential diagnosis of congestive heart failure in the neonate.

C. **Heart murmur.** Heart murmurs are commonly heard when one is examining a newborn. In fact, hemodynamically benign heart murmurs may be heard in 60% and transient murmurs of a patent ductus arteriosus are heard in 14% of healthy term infants. Murmurs from transient mitral or tricuspid regurgitation following perinatal asphyxia are noted in the early perinatal period, and typically resolve within 1 to 2 weeks of life [6].

Pathologic murmurs tend to appear at characteristic ages. Stenotic (systolic ejection murmurs) and atrioventricular valvar insufficiency (systolic regurgitant) murmurs tend to be noted very shortly after birth. In contrast, murmurs due to left-to-right shunt lesions (systolic regurgitant ventricular septal defect murmur or continuous patent ductus arteriosus murmur) may not be heard until the second to fourth week of life, when the pulmonary vascular resistance has decreased and the left-to-right shunt increases. Thus the **age of the patient** when the murmur is first noted and the **character of the murmur** provide important clues to the nature of the malformation.

D. **Arrhythmias.** See sec. **VIII** for a detailed description of identification and management of the neonate with an arrhythmia.

Table 25-4. Differential diagnosis of congestive heart failure in the neonate

---

Pressure overload
  Aortic stenosis
  Coarctation of the aorta
Volume overload
  Left-to-right shunt at level of great vessels
    Patent ductus arteriosus
    Aorticopulmonary window
    Truncus arteriosus
    Tetralogy of Fallot, pulmonary atresia with multiple aorticopulmonary
      collaterals
  Left-to-right shunt at level of ventricles
    Ventricular septal defect
    Common atrioventricular canal
    Single ventricle without pulmonary stenosis (includes hypoplastic left heart
      syndrome)
  Arteriovenous malformations
Combined pressure and volume overload
  Interrupted aortic arch
  Ventricular septal defect and coarctation
  Coarctation of the aorta with ventricular septal defect
  Aortic stenosis with ventricular septal defect
Myocardial dysfunction
  Primary
    Cardiomyopathies
      Inborn errors of metabolism
      Idiopathic
    Myocarditis
  Secondary
    Sustained tachyarrhythmias
    Perinatal asphyxia
    Sepsis
    Severe intrauterine valvar obstruction (e.g., aortic stenosis)
    Premature closure of the ductus arteriosus

E. Fetal echocardiography. It is increasingly common for infants to be born with a diagnosis of probable congenital heart disease, owing to the widespread use of obstetric ultrasound and fetal echocardiography. This may be quite valuable to the team of physicians caring for the mother and baby and for guiding plans for prenatal care, the site and timing of delivery, as well as immediate perinatal care of the infant. The recommended timing for fetal echocardiography is 18 to 22 weeks' gestation, although reasonable images can be obtained as early as 16 weeks, and transvaginal ultrasound is being investigated for diagnostic purposes in fetuses in the first trimester. Indications for fetal echocardiography are summarized in Table 25-5. Most severe forms of congenital heart disease can be accurately diagnosed by fetal echocardiography [2]. However, coarctation of the aorta, small ventricular and atrial septal defects, total anomalous pulmonary venous return, and mild aortic or pulmonary stenosis are abnormalities that may be missed by fetal echocardiography [3]. In general, in complex congenital heart disease, the main abnormality is noted; however, the full extent of cardiac malformation may be better determined on postnatal examinations.

Finally, fetal tachyarrhythmias or bradyarrhythmias (intermittent or persistent) may be detected on routine obstetric screening ultrasound ex-

Table 25-5. Indications for fetal echocardiography

Fetal risk factors
  Extracardiac anomalies
    Chromosomal
    Anatomic
  Fetal cardiac arrhythmia
    Irregular rhythm
    Tachycardia (>200 beats/min)
    Bradycardia (nonperiodic)
  Nonimmune hydrops fetalis
  Suspected cardiac anomaly on level 1 scan
Maternal risk factors
  Congenital heart disease
  Cardiac teratogen exposure
    Lithium carbonate
    Amphetamines
    Alcohol
    Anticonvulsants
      Phenytoin
      Trimethadione
      Carbamazepine
      Valproate
    Isotretinoin
  Maternal metabolic disorders
    Diabetes mellitus
    Phenylketonuria
  Polyhydramnios
Familial risk factors
  Congenital heart disease
    Previous sibling
    Paternal
  Syndromes (examples)
    Noonan
    Tuberous sclerosis

Source: From A. H. Friedman, J. A. Copel, and C. S. Kleinman, Fetal echocardiography and fetal cardiology: Indications, diagnosis and management. *Semin. Perinatol.* 17(2): 76, 1993.

aminations; this should prompt more complete fetal echocardiography to rule out associated structural heart disease and further define the arrhythmia.

IV. **Evaluation of the neonate with suspected congenital heart disease.** As noted above, the suspicion of congenital heart disease in the neonate typically follows one of a few clinical scenarios. Circulatory collapse is, unfortunately, not an uncommon means of presentation for the neonate with congenital heart disease. It must be emphasized that **emergency treatment of shock precedes definitive anatomic diagnosis.** Although sepsis may be suspected and treated, the signs of low cardiac output should always alert the examining physician to the likely possibility of congenital heart disease.

A. **Initial evaluation**

1. **Physical examination.** A complete physical examination provides important clues to the anatomic diagnosis. Inexperienced examiners frequently focus solely on the presence or absence of cardiac murmurs, but much more additional information should be obtained during a complete examination. Mottling of the skin and an ashen gray color are important clues to severe cardiovascular compromise and incipient shock. While observing the infant, the physician should pay particular attention to the pattern of respiration including the work of breathing and use of accessory muscles.

Prior to auscultation, palpation of the distal extremities with attention to temperature and capillary refill is imperative. The cool neonate with delayed capillary refill should always be evaluated for the possibility of severe congenital heart disease. While palpating the distal extremities, one should note the presence and character of the distal pulses. Diminished or absent distal pulses are highly suggestive of obstruction of the aortic arch. Palpation of the precordium may provide an important clue to the presence of congenital heart disease. The presence of a precordial thrill usually indicates at least moderate pulmonary or aortic outflow obstruction, though a restrictive ventricular septal defect with low right ventricular pressure may present with a similar finding. A hyperdynamic precordium suggests a sizable left-to-right shunt.

During auscultation, the examiner should first pay particular attention to the heart rate, noting its regularity or variability. The heart sounds, particularly the second heart sound, can be helpful clues to the ultimate diagnosis as well. A split second heart sound is a particularly important marker of the existence of two semilunar valves. Differentiating an S_3 from an S_4 heart sound is challenging in a tachycardiac newborn; however, a gallop rhythm of either type is unusual and suggests the possibility of a significant left-to-right shunt or myocardial dysfunction. Ejection clicks suggest pulmonary or aortic valvar stenosis.

The presence and intensity of systolic murmurs can be very helpful in suggesting the type and severity of the underlying anatomic diagnosis; systolic murmurs are usually due to (i) semilunar valve or outflow tract stenosis, (ii) atrioventricular valve regurgitation, or (iii) shunting through a septal defect or patent ductus arteriosus. Diastolic murmurs are **always** indicative of cardiovascular pathology. For a more complete description of auscultation of the heart, refer to one of the cardiology texts mentioned in sec. I.

A careful search for other anomalies is essential, since congenital heart disease is accompanied by at least one extracardiac malformation 25% of the time [20]. Table 25-6 summarizes some malformation and chromosomal syndromes commonly associated with congenital heart disease.

2. **Four-extremity blood pressure.** Blood pressure (usually with an automated Dynamapp) should be measured in both arms and both legs. A systolic pressure that is more than 10 mm Hg higher in the upper body compared to the lower body is abnormal and suggests coarctation of the

Table 25-6. Common chromosomal anomalies, syndromes, and associations associated with congenital heart disease

	Incidence or mode of inheritance	Extracardiac features	Cardiac features
CHROMOSOMAL ANOMALIES			
Trisomy 13 (Patau's syndrome)	1/7000–8000	Facies (midfacial hypoplasia, cleft lip and palate, microphthalmia coloboma, low-set ears); brain anomalies (microcephaly, holoprosencephaly); aplasia cutis congenita of scalp; polydactyly	≥80% have cardiac defects, VSD most common
Trisomy 18 (Edwards' syndrome)	1/7000 (female-male = 3 : 1)	SGA; facies (dolicocephaly, prominent occiput, short palpebral fissures, low-set posteriorly rotated ears, small mandible); short sternum; rocker-bottom feet; overlapping fingers with "clenched fists"	≥95% have cardiac defects, VSD most common (sometimes multiple); redundant valvar tissue with regurgitation often affecting more than one valve (polyvalvar disease)
Trisomy 21 (Down syndrome)	1/650	Facies (brachycephaly, flattened occiput, midfacial hypoplasia, mandibular prognathism, upslanting palpebral fissures, epicanthal folds, Brushfield spots, large tongue); simian creases, clinodactyly with short fifth finger; pronounced hypotonia	40–50% have cardiac defects, CAVC, VSD most common, also TOF, ASD, PDA; complex congenital heart disease is very rare
Monosomy X (Turner's syndrome)	1/2500	Lymphedema of hands, feet; short stature; short webbed neck; facies (triangular with downslanting palpebral fissures, low-set ears); shield chest	25–45% have cardiac defects, coarctation, bicuspid aortic valve most common

	Inheritance	Clinical features	Cardiac involvement
SYNDROMES OF SINGLE-GENE DEFECTS			
Noonan's syndrome	AD	Facies (hypertelorism, epicanthal folds, downslanting palpebral fissures, ptosis); low-set ears; short webbed neck with hairline; shield chest; cryptorchidism in males	≥50% have cardiac defect, usually valvar pulmonary stenosis, also ASD, hypertrophic CM
Holt-Oram syndrome	AD	Spectrum of upper limb and shoulder girdle anomalies	≥50% have cardiac defect, usually ASD or VSD
Ellis-van Creveld syndrome	AR	Short distal extremities, polydactyly; hypoplastic nails; dental anomalies	Approximately 50% have cardiac defect, usually ASD or common atrium
SYNDROMES OF UNKNOWN ETIOLOGY			
Alagille syndrome	Probably single-gene defect; AR	Cholestasis; facies (micrognathism, broad forehead, deep-set eyes); vertebral anomalies	Peripheral pulmonic stenosis most common
Thrombocytopenia–absent radius (TAR) syndrome	Probably single-gene defect; AR	Thrombocytopenia; absent or hypoplastic radii	Approximately 33% have cardiac defect, usually TOF and VSD
Williams syndrome	Contiguous gene deletion syndrome	SGA, FTT; facies ("elfin" with short palpebral fissures, periorbital fullness or puffiness, flat nasal bridge, stellate iris, long philtrum, prominent lips); friendly personality; characteristic mental deficiency (motor more reduced than verbal performance)	50–70% have cardiac defect, most commonly supravalvar aortic stenosis; other arterial stenoses also occur, including PPS, CoA, renal artery and coronary artery stenoses
DiGeorge syndrome	Contiguous gene deletion syndrome (chromosome 22q)	Thymic hypoplasia/aplasia; parathyroid hypoplasia/aplasia; cleft palate or velopharyngeal incompetence	IAA and conotruncal malformations including truncus, TOF

Table 25-6. *Continued*

	Incidence or mode of inheritance	Extracardiac features	Cardiac features
ASSOCIATIONS			
VACTERL	0.16/1000	Vertebral defects; anal atresia; TE fistula; radial and renal anomalies; limb defects	Approximately 50% have cardiac defect, most commonly VSD
CHARGE		Coloboma; choanal atresia; growth and mental deficiency; genital hypoplasia (in males); ear anomalies and/or deafness	50–70% have cardiac defect, most commonly conotruncal anomalies (TOF, DORV, truncus arteriosus)

VSD = ventricular septal defect; SGA = small for gestational age; CAVC = complete atrioventricular canal; TOF = tetralogy of Fallot; ASD = atrial septal defect; PDA = patent ductus arteriosus; AD = autosomal dominant; AR = autosomal recessive; CM = cardiomyopathy; FTT = failure to thrive; PPS = peripheral pulmonary stenosis; CoA = coarctation of the aorta; TEF = tracheoesophageal fistula; DORV = double outlet right ventricle; IAA = interrupted aortic arch.

aorta, aortic arch hypoplasia, or interrupted aortic arch. It should be noted that a systolic blood pressure gradient is quite specific for an arch abnormality but not as sensitive; a systolic blood pressure gradient will not be present in the neonate with an arch abnormality in whom the ductus arteriosus is patent and nonrestrictive. Thus, the lack of a systolic blood pressure gradient in a newborn does **not** conclusively rule out coarctation or other arch abnormalities, but the presence of a systolic pressure gradient is diagnostic of an aortic arch abnormality.

3. **Chest x-ray.** Frontal and lateral views (if possible) of the chest should be obtained. In infants, particularly newborns, the size of the heart may be difficult to determine owing to an overlying thymus. Nevertheless, useful information can be gained from the chest x-ray study. In addition to heart size, notation should be made of visceral and cardiac situs (dextrocardia and situs inversus are frequently accompanied by congenital heart disease). The aortic arch side (right or left) can frequently be determined; a right-sided aortic arch is associated with congenital heart disease in more than 90% of patients [18]. Dark or poorly perfused lung fields suggest decreased pulmonary blood flow while diffusely opaque lung fields may represent increased pulmonary blood flow or significant left atrial hypertension.

4. **Electrocardiogram (ECG).** The neonatal ECG reflects the hemodynamic relationships that existed in utero; thus the normal ECG is notable for right ventricular predominance. As many forms of congenital heart disease have minimal prenatal hemodynamic effects, the ECG is frequently "normal for age" despite significant structural pathology (e.g., transposition of the great arteries, tetralogy of Fallot). Throughout the neonatal period, infancy, and childhood, the ECG will evolve due to the expected changes in physiology and the resulting changes in chamber size and thickness that occur. Since the majority of findings on a neonate's ECG would be abnormal in an older child or adult, it is essential to refer to age-specific charts of normal values for most ECG parameters. Refer to Table 25-7 for normal ECG values in term and premature neonates.

   For interpretation of an ECG, the following determinations should be made: (i) rate and rhythm; (ii) P, QRS, and T axes; (iii) intracardiac conduction intervals; (iv) evidence for chamber enlargement or hypertrophy; (v) evidence for pericardial disease, ischemia, infarction, or metabolic abnormalities; and whether the ECG pattern fits with the clinical picture. When the ECG is abnormal, one should also suspect incorrect lead placement; a simple confirmation of lead placement may be done by comparing QRS complexes in limb lead I and precordial lead V_6—each should have a similar morphology if the limb leads have been properly placed. The ECG of the premature infant is somewhat different from that of the term infant (Table 25-8).

5. **Hyperoxia test.** For **all** neonates with suspected critical congenital heart disease (not just those who are cyanotic), a hyperoxia test should be performed. **This single test is perhaps the most sensitive and specific tool in the initial evaluation of the neonate.**

   To investigate the possibility of a fixed, intracardiac right-to-left shunt, the arterial oxygen tension should be measured in room air (if tolerated) followed by repeat measurements with the patient receiving 100% inspired oxygen (the "hyperoxia test"). If possible, the arterial partial pressure of oxygen (pO_2) should be measured directly via arterial puncture, though properly applied transcutaneous oxygen monitor (TCOM) values for pO_2 are also acceptable. **Pulse oximetry cannot be used** for documentation; in a neonate given 100% inspired oxygen, a value of 100% oxygen saturation may be obtained with an arterial pO_2 of 80 mm Hg (abnormal) or 680 mm Hg (normal, see **III.A.1**).

   Measurements should be made (by arterial blood gas or TCOM) at **both** preductal and postductal sites and the exact site of pO_2 measure-

Table 25-7. ECG standards in newborns

	Age (days)			
Measure	0–1	1–3	3–7	7–30
Term infants				
Heart rate (beats/min)	122 (99–147)	123 (97–148)	128 (100–160)	148 (114–177)
QRS axis (degrees)	135 (91–185)	134 (93–188)	133 (92–185)	108 (78–152)
PR interval, II (sec)	0.11 (0.08–0.14)	0.11 (0.09–0.13)	0.10 (0.08–0.13)	0.10 (0.08–0.13)
QRS duration (sec)	0.05 (0.03–0.07)	0.05 (0.03–0.06)	0.05 (0.03–0.06)	0.05 (0.03–0.08)
V_1, R amplitude (mm)	13.5 (6.5–23.7)	14.8 (7.0–24.2)	12.8 (5.5–21.5)	10.5 (4.5–18.1)
V_1, S amplitude (mm)	8.5 (1.0–18.5)	9.5 (1.5–19.0)	6.8 (1.0–15.0)	4.0 (0.5–9.7)
V_6, R amplitude (mm)	4.5 (0.5–9.5)	4.8 (0.5–9.5)	5.1 (1.0–10.5)	7.6 (2.6–13.5)
V_6, S amplitude (mm)	3.5 (0.2–7.9)	3.2 (0.2–7.6)	3.7 (0.2–8.0)	3.2 (0.2–8.2)
Preterm infants				
Heart rate (beats/min)	141 (109–173)	150 (127–182)	164 (134–200)	170 (133–200)
QRS axis (degrees)	127 (75–194)	121 (75–195)	117 (75–165)	80 (17–171)
PR interval (sec)	0.10 (0.09–0.10)	0.10 (0.09–1.10)	0.10 (0.09–0.10)	0.10 (0.09–0.10)
QRS duration (sec)	0.04	0.04	0.04	0.04
V_1, R amplitude (mm)	6.5 (2.0–12.6)	7.4 (2.6–14.9)	8.7 (3.8–16.8)	13.0 (6.2–21.6)
V_1, S amplitude (mm)	6.8 (0.06–17.6)	6.5 (1.0–16.0)	6.8 (0.0–15.0)	6.2 (1.2–14.0)
V_6, R amplitude (mm)	11.4 (3.5–21.3)	11.9 (5.0–20.8)	12.3 (4.0–20.5)	15.0 (8.3–21.0)
V_6, S amplitude (mm)	15.0 (2.5–26.5)	13.5 (2.6–26.0)	14.0 (3.0–25.0)	14.0 (3.1–26.3)

Sources: Term infant values from A. Davignon et al., *Pediatr. Cardiol.* 1: 123, 1979–1980; preterm infant values from V. V. Streenivasan et al., *Am. J. Cardiol.* 31: 57, 1973.

Table 25-8. ECG findings in premature infants (compared to term infants)

Rate
  Slightly higher resting rate with greater activity-related and circadian variation
  (sinus bradycardia to 70, with sleep not uncommon)
Intracardiac conduction
  PR and QRS duration slightly shorter
  Maximum QT_c <0.44 second (longer than for term infants, QT_c <0.40 second)
QRS complex
  QRS axis in frontal plane more leftward with decreasing gestational age
  QRS amplitude lower (possibly due to less ventricular mass)
  Less right ventricular predominance in precordial chest leads

Source: Reproduced with permission from C. Thomaidis, G. Varlamis, and S. Karamperis, *Acta Paediatr. Scand.* 77: 653, 1988.

ment **must** be recorded, since some congenital malformations with desaturated blood flow entering the descending aorta through the ductus arteriosus may result in "differential cyanosis" (as seen with persistent pulmonary hypertension of the newborn). A markedly higher oxygen content in the upper versus the lower part of the body can be an important diagnostic clue to such lesions, including all forms of critical aortic arch obstruction or left ventricular outflow obstruction. There are also the rare cases of "reverse differential cyanosis" with elevated **lower**-body saturation and lower upper-body saturation. This occurs only in children with transposition of the great arteries with an abnormal pulmonary artery to aortic shunt due to coarctation, interruption of the aortic arch, or suprasystemic pulmonary vascular resistance ("persistent fetal circulation").

When a patient breathes 100% oxygen, an arterial pO_2 of more than **250 mm Hg** in both upper and lower extremities virtually eliminates critical structural cyanotic heart disease (a "passed" hyperoxia test). An arterial pO_2 of less than 100 mm Hg in the absence of clear-cut lung disease (a "failed" hyperoxia test) is most likely due to intracardiac right-to-left shunting and is virtually diagnostic of cyanotic congenital heart disease. Patients who have an arterial pO_2 between 100 and 250 **may** have structural heart disease with complete intracardiac mixing and greatly increased pulmonary blood flow, as is occasionally seen with single-ventricle complexes such as hypoplastic left heart syndrome. **The neonate who "fails" a hyperoxia test is very likely to have congenital heart disease involving ductal-dependent systemic or pulmonary blood flow, and should receive prostaglandin E_1 (PGE_1) until anatomic definition can be accomplished** (see IV.B.2).

B. **Stabilization and transport.** On the basis of the initial evaluation, if an infant has been identified as likely to have congenital heart disease, further medical management must be planned as well as details arranged for a definitive anatomic diagnosis to be made. This may involve transport of the neonate to another medical center where a pediatric cardiologist is available.

  1. **Initial resuscitation.** For the neonate who presents with evidence of decreased cardiac output or shock, initial attention is devoted to the basics of advanced life support. A stable airway as well as adequate ventilation must be established and maintained. Reliable vascular access is essential, usually including an arterial line. In the neonate, this can be accomplished most reliably via the umbilical vessels. Volume resuscitation, inotropic support, and correction of metabolic acidosis are required with the goal of improving cardiac output and tissue perfusion. (See Chap. 17.)

2. **Prostaglandin E₁ (PGE₁).** The neonate who "fails" a hyperoxia test (or has an equivocal result in addition to other signs or symptoms of congenital heart disease) and the neonate who presents in shock within the first 3 weeks of life are highly likely to have congenital heart disease. These neonates are very likely to have congenital lesions that include anatomic features with ductal-dependent systemic or pulmonary blood flow, or in whom a patent ductus arteriosus will aid in intercirculatory mixing; thus PGE₁ infusion to maintain ductal patency is indicated.

PGE₁, administered as a continuous intravenous infusion, has important side effects that must be anticipated. PGE₁ causes **apnea** in 10 to 12% of neonates, usually within the first 6 hours of administration. Thus the infant who will be transferred to another institution while receiving PGE₁ should be intubated for maintenance of a stable airway prior to leaving the referring hospital. Infants who do not require transport may not require intubation but continuous cardiorespiratory monitoring is essential. PGE₁ should be given in a setting where ventilatory support is available. In addition, PGE₁ typically causes peripheral vasodilation and subsequent hypotension in many infants. A separate intravenous line should be secured for volume administration in any infant receiving PGE₁, especially those who require transport.

Other adverse reactions to PGE₁ include fever (14%), cutaneous flushing (10%), bradycardia (7%), seizures (4%), tachycardia (3%), cardiac arrest (1%), and edema (1%). Specific information regarding dose and administration of PGE₁ is in sec. **VII.A.**

We cannot overemphasize the need to begin PGE₁ in **any** neonate in whom congenital heart disease is strongly suspected (i.e., a failed hyperoxia test and/or severe, acute congestive heart failure). In the neonate with ductal-dependent pulmonary blood flow, oxygen saturation will typically improve and the pulmonary blood flow will remain secure until an anatomic diagnosis and plans for surgery are made. In neonates with transposition of the great arteries, maintenance of a patent ductus improves intercirculatory mixing. Most importantly, **neonates who present in shock in the first few weeks of life have duct-dependent systemic blood flow until proved otherwise;** resuscitation will not be successful unless the ductus is opened. In these cases, it is appropriate to begin an infusion of PGE₁ even **before** a precise anatomic diagnosis can be made by echocardiography.

It is prudent to remeasure arterial blood gases and reassess perfusion, vital signs, and acid–base status within 15 to 30 minutes of starting a PGE₁ infusion. Rarely, patients may become more unstable after beginning PGE₁. This is usually due to lesions with obstruction to left atrial return (hypoplastic left heart syndrome with restrictive patent foramen ovale, subdiaphragmatic total anomalous pulmonary venous return, mitral atresia with restrictive patent foramen ovale, transposition of the great arteries with intact ventricular septum and restrictive patent foramen ovale). In these lesions, deterioration with PGE₁ treatment is often a helpful diagnostic finding, and **urgent** plans for echocardiography and possible interventional catheterization or surgery should be made.

3. **Inotropic agents.** Continuous infusions of inotropic agents, usually the sympathomimetic amines, can improve myocardial performance as well as perfusion of vital organs and the periphery. Care should be taken to replete intravascular volume before institution of vasoactive agents. **Dopamine** is a precursor of norepinephrine and stimulates beta-1, dopaminergic, and alpha-adrenergic receptors in a dose-dependent manner. Dopamine can be expected to increase mean arterial pressure, improve ventricular function, and improve urine output with a low incidence of side effects at doses less than 10 μg/kg per minute. **Dobutamine** is an analogue of dopamine, with predominantly beta-1 effects and rela-

tively weak beta-2- and alpha-receptor–stimulating activity. In comparison with dopamine, dobutamine lacks renal vasodilating properties, has less chronotropic effect (in adult patients), and does not depend on norepinephrine release from peripheral nerves for its effect. There are few published data available concerning the use of dobutamine in neonates, although clinical experience has been favorable. A combination of low-dose dopamine (up to 5 μg/kg per minute) and dobutamine may be used to minimize the potential peripheral vasoconstriction induced by high doses of dopamine while maximizing the dopaminergic effects on the renal circulation. See sec. **VII.B** for details of administration of inotropic agents, and additional pharmacologic agents.

4. **Transport.** After initial stabilization, the neonate with suspected congenital heart disease often needs to be transferred to an institution that can provide subspecialty care in pediatric cardiology and cardiac surgery. A successful transport actually involves two transitions of care for the neonate: (a) from the referring hospital staff to the transport team and (b) from the transport team staff to the accepting hospital staff. The need for accurate, detailed, and complete communication of information between all these teams cannot be overemphasized. If possible, the pediatric cardiologist who will be caring for the patient should be included in the discussion of care while the neonate is still at the referring hospital.

Reliable **vascular access** should be secured for the neonate receiving continuous infusions of PGE_1 or inotropic agents. Umbilical lines placed for resuscitation and stabilization should be left in place for transport; the neonate with congenital heart disease may potentially require cardiac catheterization via this route. (see ch. 13)

Particular attention should be paid to the patient's **airway and respiratory effort** before transport. In general, all neonates receiving a PGE_1 infusion should be intubated for transport (see **IV.B.2**). Neonates with probable or definite congenital heart disease most likely will require surgical treatment or interventional catheterization management during the hospitalization; thus it is likely that they will be intubated at some point. Since there is real risk in **not** intubating these infants, as a general rule, all should be intubated for transport unless there is a compelling reason not to do so. All intubated patients should have gastric decompression by nasogastric or orogastric tube.

Acid–base status and oxygen delivery should be checked with an arterial blood gas analysis prior to transport. Although most noncardiac patients are transported receiving supplemental oxygen at or near 100%, this is often **not** the inspired oxygen concentration of choice for the neonate with congenital heart disease (see **V** for details of lesion-specific care). This management decision for transport is particularly important for infants with duct-dependent systemic blood flow and complete intracardiac mixing with single-ventricle physiology, and emphasizes the need to consult with a pediatric cardiologist **prior** to transport to achieve optimal intratransport patient care.

Finally, it is important to remember in neonates that hypotension is a late finding in shock; thus other signs of incipient decompensation such as persistent tachycardia and poor tissue perfusion are important to note and treat before transport. Before the patient leaves the referring hospital, the current hemodynamic status (distal perfusive, heart rate, systemic blood pressure, acid–base status, etc.) should be reassessed and relayed to the receiving hospital team.

C. **Confirmation of the diagnosis**
1. **Echocardiography.** Two-dimensional echocardiography, supplemented with Doppler and color Doppler imaging, provides information about the structure and function of the heart and great vessels in a timely fashion. While not an invasive test per se, complete echocardiography on a newborn suspected of having congenital heart disease may take an hour or

more to perform, and thus may not be well tolerated by a sick or premature newborn. Temperature instability due to exposure during this extended time of examination may be a problem in the neonate. Extension of the neck for suprasternal notch views of the aortic arch may be problematic, particularly in the neonate with respiratory distress or with a tenuous airway. Thus, in sick neonates close monitoring by a medical staff person **other** than the one performing the echocardiographic examination is recommended.

2. **Cardiac catheterization**
   a. **Indications** (Table 25-9). It is rarely necessary to perform a cardiac catheterization for anatomic definition of intracardiac structures (though catheterization is still necessary for definition of the distal pulmonary arteries, aortic-pulmonary collaterals, and certain types of coronary artery anomalies) or for physiologic assessment, as Doppler technology has assumed an increasingly important role in this regard. Increasingly, catheterization is performed for catheter-directed therapy of congenital lesions [27]. See Fig. 25-2 for normal newborn oxygen saturation and pressure measurements obtained during cardiac catheterization.
   b. **Interventional catheterization.** Since the first balloon dilation of the pulmonary artery reported by Kan in 1982, balloon valvuloplasty has become the procedure of choice for many types of valvar lesions, even extending to critical lesions in the neonate [27]. At Children's Hospital, Boston, balloon valvuloplasty is considered the initial treatment of choice for both pulmonary and aortic stenosis, with a greater than 90% immediate success rate in the neonate [14,16]. The application of balloon dilation of native coarctation of the aorta is controversial (see below).
   c. **Preparation for catheterization.** Catheterization in the neonate is not without its attendant risks; in one survey, the risk of a major complication in newborns and young infants was 12% [13]. With appropriate anticipatory care, complications can be minimized. In addition to basic medical stabilization (see **IV.B**), specific attention to airway management is crucial. Sedation and analgesia are necessary, but will

Table 25-9. Indications for neonatal catheterization

Interventions
   Therapeutic*
      Balloon atrial septostomy
      Balloon pulmonary valvuloplasty
      Balloon aortic valvuloplasty
      Balloon angioplasty of native coarctation of the aorta
      Coil embolization of abnormal vascular communications
   Diagnostic
   Endomyocardial biopsy
Anatomic definition (not visualized by echocardiography)
   Coronary arteries
      Pulmonary atresia/intact ventricular septum
      Transposition of the great arteries
      Tetralogy of Fallot
   Aortic to pulmonary artery collateral vessels
      Tetralogy of Fallot
   Distal pulmonary artery anatomy
Hemodynamic measurements

*All of these interventions have alternative surgical options and are controversial based on institutional experience (see text).

Normal Newborn

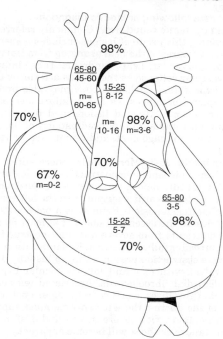

Fig. 25-2. Typical hemodynamic measurements obtained at cardiac catheterization in a newborn, term infant without congenital or acquired heart disease. In this (and subsequent diagrams), oxygen saturations are shown as percentages, and typical hemodynamic pressure measurements in mm Hg are shown. In this example, the transition from fetal to infant physiology is complete; the pulmonary vascular resistance has fallen, the ductus arteriosus has closed, and there is no significant shunt at the foramen ovale. M = mean value.

depress the respiratory drive in the neonate. When a neonate is catheterized, intubation and mechanical ventilation should be strongly considered, especially if an intervention is contemplated. In our institution, a separate staff person **not performing the catheterization** is present during the study, dedicated to the supervision of the infant's overall hemodynamic and respiratory status, including periodic evaluation of the patient's body temperature, acid–base status, serum glucose, and blood loss. All infants undergoing interventional catheterization should have 10 to 25 ml of packed red blood cells per kilogram typed and crossmatched **in the catheterization laboratory** during the procedure. Intravenous lines are recommended in the upper extremities or head (since the lower body will be draped and inaccessible during the procedure), to provide unobstructed access for medications, volume infusions, etc. Finally, the neonate may have the catheterization performed via umbilical vessels that were previously utilized for the administration of fluid, glucose, PGE_1, inotropic agents, or blood. Thus a peripheral line should be started and medications changed to that site prior to transfer of the neonate to the cardiac catheterization laboratory.

V. "Lesion-specific" care following anatomic diagnosis

A. Duct-dependent systemic blood flow. Commonly referred to as **left-sided obstructive lesions,** this group of lesions includes a spectrum of hypoplasia of left-sided structures of the heart ranging from isolated coarctation of the aorta to hypoplastic left heart syndrome. These infants typically present in cardiovascular collapse as the ductus arteriosus closes, with resultant systemic hypoperfusion; though they may also present more insidiously with symptoms of congestive heart failure (see **III.B**). Although all infants with significant left-sided lesions and duct-dependent systemic blood flow require prostaglandin-induced patency of the ductus arteriosus as part of the initial management, additional care varies somewhat with each lesion [33].

1. Aortic stenosis (Fig. 25-3). Morphologic abnormalities of the aortic valve may range from a bicuspid, nonobstructive functionally normal valve to a unicuspid, markedly deformed and severely obstructive valve, which greatly limits systemic cardiac output from the left ventricle. By convention, "severe" aortic stenosis is defined as a peak systolic gradient from the left ventricle to the ascending aorta of at least 60 mm Hg. "Critical" aortic stenosis results from severe anatomic obstruction with accompanying left ventricular failure or shock. Patients with critical aortic stenosis have severe obstruction present in utero (usually due to a unicuspid, "platelike" valve), with resultant left ventricular hypertrophy and frequently, endocardial fibroelastosis. Associated left-sided abnormalities such as mitral valve disease and coarctation are not uncommon. Following closure of the ductus, the left ventricle must supply all of the systemic cardiac output. With severe myocardial dysfunction, clinical congestive heart failure or shock will become apparent.

Initial management of the severely affected infant includes treatment of shock, stable vascular access, airway management and mechanical ventilation, sedation and muscle paralysis, inotropic support, and administration of PGE$_1$. Positive end-expiratory pressure is helpful to overcome pulmonary venous desaturation from pulmonary edema secondary to left atrial hypertension. For a patient with critical aortic stenosis to benefit from a PGE$_1$ infusion, there must be a small patent foramen ovale to allow effective systemic blood flow (pulmonary venous return) to cross the atrial septum and ultimately enter the systemic vascular bed through the ductus. Inspired oxygen should be limited to an FiO$_2$ of 0.5 to 0.6 unless severe hypoxemia is present.

Following anatomic definition of left ventricular size, the mitral valve, and the aortic arch by echocardiography, cardiac catheterization or aortic valvotomy should be performed as soon as possible. With either type of therapy, patient outcome will depend largely on (i) the degree of relief of the obstruction, (ii) the degree of aortic regurgitation, (iii) associated cardiac lesions (especially left ventricular size), and (iv) the severity of end-organ dysfunction secondary to the initial presentation (e.g., necrotizing enterocolitis or renal failure). All patients with critical aortic stenosis will require lifelong follow-up, as stenosis frequently recurs. Multiple procedures in childhood are common.

2. Coarctation of the aorta (Fig. 25-4) is an anatomic narrowing of the descending aorta, most commonly at the site of insertion of the ductus arteriosus (i.e., "juxtaductal"). Additional cardiac abnormalities are common, including bicuspid aortic valve (which occurs in 80% of patients) and ventricular septal defect (which occurs in 40% of patients). In addition, hypoplasia or obstruction of other left-sided structures including the mitral valve, the left ventricle, and the aortic valve is not uncommon and must be evaluated during the initial echocardiographic evaluation.

Valvar Aortic Stenosis

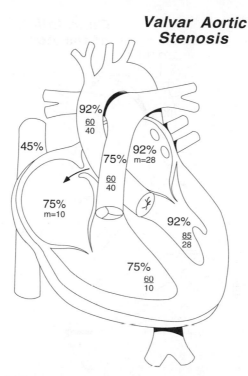

Fig. 25-3. Critical valvar aortic stenosis with a closed ductus arteriosus. Typical anatomic and hemodynamic findings include: (a) a morphologically abnormal, stenotic valve; (b) poststenotic dilatation of the ascending aorta; (c) elevated left ventricular end diastolic pressure and left atrial pressures contributing to pulmonary edema (mild pulmonary venous and arterial desaturation); (d) a left-to-right shunt at the atrial level (note increase in oxygen saturation from superior vena cava to right atrium); (e) pulmonary artery hypertension (also secondary to the elevated left atrial pressure); (f) only a modest (25-mm Hg) gradient across valve. The low measured gradient (despite severe anatomic obstruction) across the aortic valve is due to a severely limited cardiac output, as evidenced by the low mixed venous oxygen saturation (45%) in the superior vena cava.

In utero, systemic blood flow to the lower body is via the patent ductus arteriosus. Following ductal closure, in the newborn with a critical coarctation, the left ventricle must suddenly generate adequate pressure and volume to pump the entire cardiac output past a significant point of obstruction. This sudden pressure load may be poorly tolerated by the neonatal myocardium and the neonate may become rapidly and critically ill because of lower body hypoperfusion.

As in critical aortic stenosis, initial management of the severely affected infant includes treatment of shock, stable vascular access, airway management and mechanical ventilation, moderate supplemental oxygen, sedation and muscle paralysis, inotropic support, and administration of PGE_1. Positive end-expiratory pressure is helpful to overcome pulmonary venous desaturation from pulmonary edema secondary to left

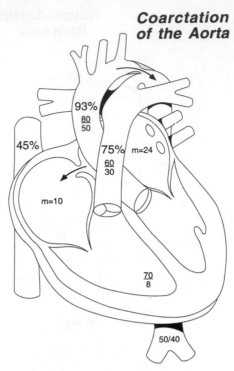

Coarctation of the Aorta

Fig. 25-4. Coarctation of the aorta in a critically ill neonate with a nearly closed ductus arteriosus. Typical anatomic and hemodynamic findings include: (a) "juxtaductal" site of the coarctation; (b) a bicommissural aortic valve (seen in 80% of patients with coarctation); (c) narrow pulse pressure in the descending aorta and lower body; (d) a bidirectional shunt at the ductus arteriosus. As in critical aortic stenosis (see Fig. 25-3) there is an elevated left atrial pressure, pulmonary edema, a left-to-right shunt at the atrial level, pulmonary artery hypertension and only a moderate (30-mm Hg) gradient across the arch obstruction. The low measured gradient (despite severe anatomic obstruction) across the aortic arch is due to low cardiac output.

atrial hypertension. In some infants, PGE_1 is unsuccessful in opening the ductus.

In infants with symptomatic coarctation, surgical repair is performed as soon as the infant has been resuscitated and medically stabilized. Usually the procedure is performed through a left lateral thoracotomy. In infants with symptomatic coarctation and a large, coexisting ventricular septal defect, consideration should be given to repairing both defects in the initial procedure via a median sternotomy. Balloon dilation of native coarctation is not routinely done at our institution because of the high incidence of restenosis and aneurysm formation, especially given the safe and effective surgical alternative.

3. **Interrupted aortic arch** (Fig. 25-5) consists of complete atresia of a segment of the aortic arch. There are three anatomic subtypes of interrupted aortic arch based on the location of the interruption: distal to the left subclavian artery (type A), between the left subclavian artery and

Interrupted Aortic Arch

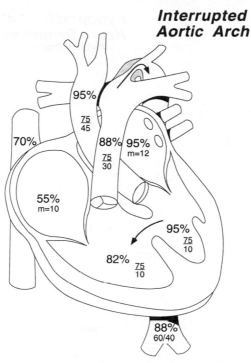

Fig. 25-5. Interrupted aortic arch with restrictive patent ductus arteriosus. Typical anatomic and hemodynamic findings include: (a) atresia of a segment of the aortic arch between the left subclavian artery and the left common carotid (the most common type of interrupted aortic arch—"type B"); (b) a posterior malalignment of the conal septum resulting in a large ventricular septal defect and a narrow subaortic area; (c) a bicuspid aortic valve occurs in 60% of patients; (d) systemic pressure in the right ventricle and pulmonary artery (due to the large, nonrestrictive ventricular septal defect); (e) increased oxygen saturation in the pulmonary artery due to left-to-right shunting at the ventricular level; (f) "differential cyanosis" with a lower oxygen saturation in the descending aorta due to a right-to-left shunt at the patent ductus. Note the lower blood pressure in the descending aorta due to constriction of the ductus; opening the ductus with PGE₁ results in equal upper and lower extremity blood pressures, but continued "differential cyanosis."

the left carotid artery (type B), and between the innominate artery and the left carotid artery (type C). Type B is the most common variety. Over 99% of these patients have a ventricular septal defect; abnormalities of the aortic valve and narrowed subaortic regions are associated anomalies.

Infants with interrupted aortic arch are completely dependent on a patent ductus arteriosus for lower body blood flow; thus they become critically ill when the ductus closes. Immediate management is similar to that described for coarctation (see **V.A.2**); PGE₁ infusion is essential. All other resuscitative measures will be ineffective if blood flow to the lower body is not restored. Oxygen saturation should be measured in the upper body; pulse oximetry readings in the lower body are reflective of

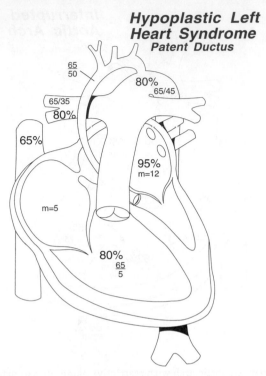

Hypoplastic Left Heart Syndrome
Patent Ductus

Fig. 25-6A. Hypoplastic left heart syndrome in a 24-hour-old patient with falling pulmonary vascular resistance and a nonrestrictive ductus arteriosus. Typical anatomic and hemodynamic findings include: (a) atresia or hypoplasia of the left ventricle, mitral and aortic valves; (b) a diminutive ascending aorta and transverse aortic arch, usually with an associated coarctation; (c) coronary blood flow is usually *retrograde* from the ductus arteriosus through the tiny ascending aorta; (d) systemic arterial oxygen saturation (in FiO_2 of 0.21) of 80%, reflecting relatively balanced systemic and pulmonary blood flows—the pulmonary artery and aortic saturations are equal (see text); (e) pulmonary hypertension secondary to the nonrestrictive ductus arteriosus; (f) minimal left atrial hypertension; (g) normal systemic cardiac output (note superior vena cava oxygen saturation of 65%) and blood pressure (65/45).

the pulmonary artery oxygen saturation, and are typically lower than that distributed to the central nervous system and coronary arteries. High concentrations of inspired oxygen may result in low pulmonary vascular resistance, a large left-to-right shunt, and a "run-off" during diastole from the lower body into the pulmonary circulation. Inspired oxygen levels should therefore be minimized, aiming for normal (95%) oxygen saturations in the **upper** body.

Surgical reconstruction should be performed as soon as metabolic acidosis (if present) has resolved, end-organ dysfunction is improving, and the patient is hemodynamically stable. The repair typically entails a corrective approach via a median sternotomy, with arch reconstruction (usually an end-to-end anastomosis) and closure of the ventricular septal defect. Arch reconstruction and a pulmonary artery band (via a lateral

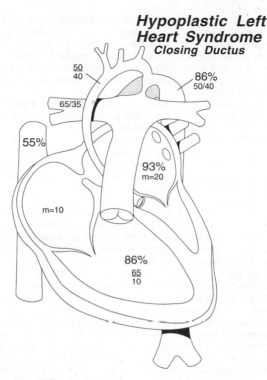

Hypoplastic Left Heart Syndrome
Closing Ductus

Fig. 25-6B. Acute circulatory collapse following constriction of the ductus arteriosus in hypoplastic left heart syndrome. These neonates are typically in shock with poor perfusion, tachycardia, acidosis and in respiratory distress. The anatomic features are similar to those in Fig. 25-6A, with the exception of the narrowed ductus arteriosus. Note (a) the low cardiac output (as evidenced by the low mixed venous oxygen saturation in the superior vena cava of 55%); (b) narrow pulse pressure; (c) elevated atrial and ventricular end-diastolic pressure—elevated left atrial pressure may cause pulmonary edema (note left atrial saturation of 93%); (d) significantly increased pulmonary blood flow, as reflected in an arterial oxygen saturation (in FiO_2 of 0.21) of 86%.

thoracotomy) are generally not recommended and typically reserved for patients with multiple ventricular septal defects.

4. **Hypoplastic left heart syndrome** (Fig. 25-6) represents a heterogeneous group of anatomic abnormalities in which there is a small or absent left ventricle with hypoplastic or atretic mitral and aortic valves. Prior to surgery, the right ventricle supplies both the pulmonary and the systemic blood flow (via the patent ductus arteriosus); the proportion of cardiac output going to either circuit is dependent on the relative resistances of these vascular beds.

   As the pulmonary vascular resistance begins to fall (see Fig. 25-6A), blood flow is preferentially directed to the pulmonary circulation at the expense of the systemic circulation. As systemic blood flow decreases, stroke volume and heart rate increase as a mechanism to preserve systemic cardiac output. The right ventricle becomes progressively volume-overloaded with mildly elevated end-diastolic and left atrial pressures. The infant may be tachypneic or in respiratory distress, and hepatomegaly may be present. The greater proportion of pulmonary venous return in the mixed ventricular blood results in a near-normal systemic arterial oxygen saturation (80%), and visible cyanosis may be mild or absent. Not infrequently, these infants are discharged from the nursery as normal newborns.

At this point the continued fall in pulmonary vascular resistance results in a progressive increase in pulmonary blood flow and a relative decrease in systemic cardiac output. As the total right ventricular output is limited by heart rate and stroke volume, there is the onset of clinically apparent congestive heart failure, right ventricular dilation and dysfunction, progressive tricuspid regurgitation, poor peripheral perfusion with metabolic acidosis, decreased urine output, and pulmonary edema. Arterial oxygen saturation approaches 90%.

Alternatively, a sudden deterioration takes place with rapidly progressive congestive heart failure and shock as the ductus arteriosus constricts (see Fig. 25-6B). There is decreased systemic perfusion and increased pulmonary blood flow, which is largely independent of the pulmonary vascular resistance. The peripheral pulses are weak to absent. Renal, hepatic, coronary, and central nervous system perfusion is compromised, possibly resulting in acute tubular necrosis, necrotizing enterocolitis, or cerebral infarction or hemorrhage. A vicious cycle may also result from inadequate retrograde perfusion of the ascending aorta (coronary blood supply), with further myocardial dysfunction and continued compromise of coronary blood flow. The pulmonary to systemic flow ratio approaches infinity as systemic blood flow nears zero. Thus, one has the paradoxical presentation of profound metabolic acidosis in the setting of a relatively high pO_2 (70 to 100 mm Hg).

The arterial blood gas may represent the single best indicator of hemodynamic stability. Low arterial saturation (75 to 80%) with normal pH indicates an acceptable balance of systemic and pulmonary blood flow with adequate peripheral perfusion, while elevated oxygen saturation (>90%) with acidosis represents significantly increased pulmonary and decreased systemic flow with probable myocardial dysfunction and secondary effects on other organ systems.

Resuscitation of these neonates involves pharmacologic maintenance of ductal patency with PGE_1 and ventilatory maneuvers to **increase** pulmonary resistance. In our experience, a mild respiratory acidosis (e.g., pH 7.35) is appropriate for most of these infants. It is important to note that hyperventilation or supplemental oxygen is usually of no significant benefit and may be harmful by causing excessive pulmonary vasodilation and pulmonary blood flow at the expense of the systemic blood flow.

Hypotension in these infants is more frequently caused by increased pulmonary blood flow (at the expense of systemic flow) rather than intrinsic myocardial dysfunction. Although small to moderate doses of inotropic agents are frequently beneficial, large doses of inotropic agents may have a deleterious effect, depending on the relative effects on the systemic and pulmonary vascular beds. Preferential selective elevations of systemic vascular tone will secondarily increase pulmonary blood flow, and careful monitoring of mean arterial blood pressure and arterial oxygen saturation is warranted.

Similar to the patient with critical aortic stenosis, in order for the neonate with hypoplastic left heart syndrome to benefit from a PGE_1 infusion, there must be at least a small patent foramen ovale to allow effective systemic blood flow (pulmonary venous return) to cross the atrial septum and ultimately enter the systemic vascular bed through the ductus. An infant with hypoplastic left heart syndrome and a severely restrictive or absent patent foramen ovale will be critically ill with profound cyanosis (oxygen saturation <60 to 65%), and will not improve after the institution of PGE_1 treatment. In these neonates, emergent balloon dilation of the atrial septum may be necessary.

After a period of medical stabilization and support to allow recovery of ischemic organ system injury (particularly of the kidneys, liver, central nervous system, and the heart itself), surgical relief of left-sided obstruction is required. Surgical intervention involves either staged reconstruction (with a neonatal Norwood procedure followed by a Fontan operation later in childhood) or neonatal cardiac transplantation. Recent results from both reconstructive surgery and transplantation demonstrate a vastly improved outlook for infants born with this previously 100% fatal condition [8].

B. Duct-dependent pulmonary blood flow. This underlying physiology is shared by a diverse group of lesions with the common finding of restricted pulmonary blood flow due to severe pulmonary stenosis or complete pulmonary atresia. Closure of the ductus arteriosus results in marked cyanosis.

1. **Pulmonary stenosis** with obstruction to pulmonary blood flow may occur at several levels: (i) within the body of the right ventricle; (ii) at the pulmonary valve (Fig. 25-7); and (iii) in the peripheral pulmonary arteries. Valvar pulmonary stenosis with an intact ventricular septum is the second most common form of congenital heart disease, though "critical" obstruction occurs more rarely. Grading of the degree of pulmonary stenosis is similar to that of aortic stenosis (see **V.A.1**), with severe pulmonary stenosis defined as a peak systolic gradient from the right ventricle to the pulmonary artery of 60 mm Hg or more. By convention, critical pulmonary stenosis is defined as severe valvar obstruction with associated hypoxemia due to a right-to-left shunt at the foramen ovale. Critical pulmonary stenosis may be associated with hypoplasia of the right ventricle or tricuspid valve and significant right ventricular hypertrophy. The pressure in the right ventricle is often higher than the left ventricular pressure (i.e., suprasystemic) in order to eject blood past the severe narrowing. Due to the long-standing (in utero) increased right ventricular pressure, there is typically a hypertrophied, noncompliant right ventricle with a resultant increase in right atrial filling pressure. When right atrial pressure exceeds left atrial pressure, a right-to-left shunt at the foramen ovale results in cyanosis and hypoxemia. There may be associated right ventricular dysfunction or tricuspid regurgitation.

   After initial stabilization of the patient and definitive diagnosis by echocardiography, transcatheter balloon valvotomy is the treatment of choice for this lesion at our institution [14,20,27], though surgical valvotomy may be utilized in specific cases. Despite successful relief of the obstruction during catheterization, cyanosis is usually not completely relieved, but rather resolves gradually over the first weeks of life as the right ventricle becomes more compliant and tricuspid regurgitation lessens. Successful balloon valvuloplasty is associated with excellent clinical results among patients, with the need for repeat procedures quite low.

2. **Pulmonary atresia with intact ventricular septum ("hypoplastic right heart syndrome,"** Fig. 25-8) is comparable to hypoplastic left heart syndrome in that there is atresia of the pulmonary valve with varying degrees of right ventricular and tricuspid valve hypoplasia. Perhaps the most important associated anomaly is the presence of coronary artery–myocardial–right ventricular sinusoidal connections. The coronary arteries may be quite abnormal, including areas of stenoses or complete atresia. Myocardial perfusion may therefore depend on a hypertensive right ventricle to supply the distal coronary arteries; surgical relief of the pulmonary atresia (with a right ventricle–pulmonary artery connection) may lead to myocardial infarction and death. The presence of si-

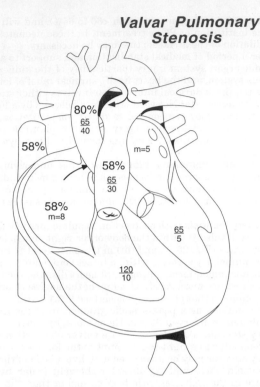

Valvar Pulmonary Stenosis

Fig. 25-7. Critical valvar pulmonary stenosis in a neonate with a nonrestrictive patent ductus arteriosus while receiving PGE₁. Typical anatomic and hemodynamic findings include: (a) thickened, stenotic pulmonary valve; (b) poststenotic dilatation of the main pulmonary artery with normal-sized branch pulmonary arteries; (c) right ventricular hypertrophy with suprasystemic pressure; (d) a right-to-left shunt at the atrial level via the patent foramen ovale with systemic desaturation (80%); (e) suprasystemic RV pressure with a 55-mm Hg peak systolic ejection gradient; (f) systemic pulmonary artery pressure (due to the nonrestrictive patent ductus).

nusoidal connections between the right ventricle and the coronary arteries is associated with poorer long-term survival in all studies [20]. Because there is no outlet of the right ventricle, there is typically suprasystemic pressure in the right ventricle and some tricuspid regurgitation. There is an obligatory right-to-left shunt at the atrial level and pulmonary blood flow is entirely dependent on a patent ductus arteriosus.

Although the cornerstone of initial management is PGE₁ infusion to maintain ductal patency, a more permanent and reliable form of pulmonary blood flow must be surgically created for the infant to survive. Surgical management is often preceded by catheterization to define the coronary artery anatomy. In patients without significant coronary abnormalities, pulmonary blood flow is established by creating an outflow for the right ventricle by pulmonary valvotomy or right ventricular outflow tract augmentation, or both. Usually at the time of this procedure, a systemic-to-pulmonary artery shunt (most often a Blalock-Taussig shunt) is constructed to also augment pulmonary blood flow. In patients with

PA/IVS

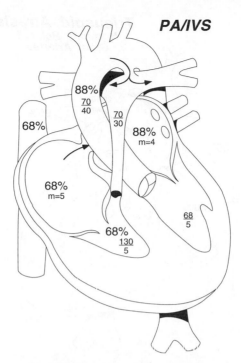

Fig. 25-8. Pulmonary atresia with intact ventricular septum (PA/IVS) in a neonate with a nonrestrictive patent ductus arteriosus while receiving PGE₁. Typical anatomic and hemodynamic findings include. (a) hypertrophied, hypoplastic right ventricle; (b) hypoplastic tricuspid valve and pulmonary annulus; (c) atresia of the pulmonary valve with no antegrade flow; (d) suprasystemic right ventricular pressure; (e) pulmonary blood flow via the patent ductus; (f) right-to-left shunt at the atrial level with systemic desaturation. Many patients have significant coronary abnormalities with sinusoidal or fistulous connections to the hypertensive right ventricle or significant coronary stenoses (not shown).

"right ventricular–dependent" coronary arteries, a systemic-to-pulmonary artery shunt is the typical procedure performed in the neonate.
3. **Tricuspid atresia** (Fig. 25-9) involves complete absence of the tricuspid valve and thus no direct communication from the right atrium to the right ventricle. The right ventricle may be severely hypoplastic or completely absent. More than 90% of patients have an associated ventricular septal defect, allowing blood to pass from the left ventricle to the right ventricular outflow and pulmonary arteries. The majority of patients have some form of additional pulmonary stenosis. In 70% of patients the great arteries are normally aligned with the ventricle; however, in the remaining 30% the great arteries are transposed. An atrial level communication is necessary for blood to exit the right atrium; there is an obligatory right-to-left shunt at this level. In patients with normally related great arteries, pulmonary blood flow is derived from the right ventricle (through its connection with the left ventricle via a ventricular septal defect). If the right ventricle is severely diminutive, the pulmonary blood

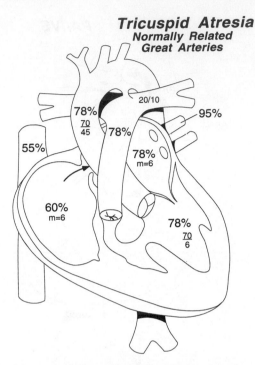

Tricuspid Atresia
Normally Related Great Arteries

Fig. 25-9. Tricuspid atresia with normally related great arteries and a small patent ductus arteriosus. Typical anatomic and hemodynamic findings include: (a) atresia of the tricuspid valve; (b) hypoplasia of the right ventricle; (c) restriction to pulmonary blood flow at two levels: a (usually) small ventricular septal defect and a stenotic pulmonary valve; (d) all systemic venous return must pass through the patent foramen ovale to reach the left ventricle; (e) complete mixing at the left atrial level, with systemic oxygen saturation of 78% (in FiO_2 of 0.21), suggesting balanced systemic and pulmonary blood flow ("single ventricle physiology"—see text).

flow may be duct-dependent; closure of the ductus leads to profound hypoxemia and acidosis.

Immediate medical management is primarily aimed at maintenance of adequate pulmonary blood flow. In the usual case of severe pulmonary stenosis and limited pulmonary blood flow, PGE_1 infusion maintains pulmonary blood flow via the ductus arteriosus. Surgical creation of a more permanent source of pulmonary blood flow (usually a Blalock-Taussig shunt) is undertaken as soon as possible. More complex cases (e.g., with transposition) may require more extensive palliative procedures [8].

4. **Tetralogy of Fallot** (Fig. 25-10) consists of right ventricular outflow obstruction, a ventricular septal defect (of the anterior malalignment variety), "overriding" of the aorta over the ventricular septum, and hypertrophy of the right ventricle. There is a wide spectrum of anatomic variation encompassing these findings, depending particularly on the site and severity of the right ventricular outflow obstruction. The severely cyanotic neonate with tetralogy most likely has severe right ventricular outflow tract obstruction and a large right-to-left shunt at the ventricular

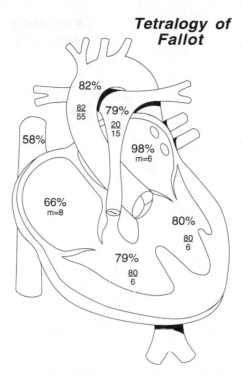

Fig. 25-10. Tetralogy of Fallot. Typical anatomic and hemodynamic findings include: (a) an anteriorly displaced infundibular septum, resulting in subpulmonary stenosis, a large ventricular septal defect and overriding of the aorta over the muscular septum; (b) hypoplasia of the pulmonary valve, main and brain pulmonary arteries; (c) equal right and left ventricular pressures; (d) a right-to-left shunt at ventricular level, with a systemic oxygen saturation of 82%.

level via the large ventricular septal defect. Pulmonary blood flow may be duct-dependent.

Immediate medical management involves establishing adequate pulmonary blood flow, usually with PGE_1 infusion, though some have attempted balloon dilation of the right ventricular outflow tract. Detailed anatomic definition, particularly regarding coronary artery anatomy, the presence of additional ventricular septal defects, and the sources of pulmonary blood flow (systemic to pulmonary collateral vessels), is necessary prior to surgical intervention. If echocardiography is not able to fully show these details, then diagnostic catheterization is performed. The optimal timing of surgical management of the **asymptomatic** child with tetralogy of Fallot remains controversial, though many are recommending repair within the first 6 to 9 months of life. The **symptomatic** (i.e., severely cyanotic) neonate should have operative intervention. Complete repair is generally performed at our institution, though a systemic-to-pulmonary artery shunt is sometimes employed in infants with multiple ventricular septal defects or in patients with origin of the left anterior descending coronary artery from the right coronary artery (in

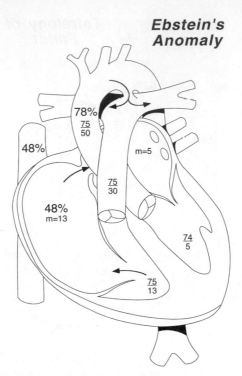

Ebstein's Anomaly

48%

78%
$\frac{75}{50}$

m=5

48%
m=13

$\frac{75}{30}$

$\frac{74}{5}$

$\frac{75}{13}$

Fig. 25-11A. Ebstein's anomaly (with large nonrestrictive ductus arteriosus). Typical anatomic and hemodynamic findings include: (a) inferior displacement of the tricuspid valve into the right ventricle, which may also cause subpulmonary obstruction; (b) diminutive muscular right ventricle; (c) marked enlargement of the right atrium due to "atrialized" portion of right ventricle as well as tricuspid regurgitation; (d) right-to-left shunting at the atrial level (note arterial oxygen saturation of 78%); (e) a left-to-right shunt and pulmonary hypertension secondary to a large patent ductus arteriosus supplying the pulmonary blood flow; (f) low cardiac output (note low mixed venous oxygen saturation in the superior vena cava).

    whom the left anterior descending crosses the right ventricular outflow tract).

5. **Ebstein's anomaly** (Fig. 25-11) is an uncommon but grave anatomic lesion when presenting in the neonatal period. Anatomically there is "downward displacement" of the tricuspid valve into the body of the right ventricle. The tricuspid valve is frequently regurgitant, resulting in marked right atrial enlargement and a large right-to-left shunt at the atrial level; there is little forward flow out the right ventricular outflow tract into the pulmonary circulation. The prognosis for neonates presenting with profound cyanosis due to Ebstein's anomaly is quite grave [20]. Surgical options are controversial and generally reserved for the severely symptomatic child. Further complicating the medical condition, Ebstein's anomaly is often associated with Wolff-Parkinson-White (WPW) syndrome and supraventricular tachycardia (SVT).

    Medical management is aimed at supporting the neonate through the initial period of transitional circulation. Because of elevated pulmonary

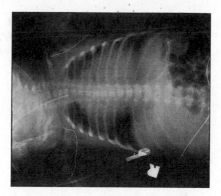

Fig. 25-11B. Chest radiograph in a neonate with severe Ebstein's anomaly and no significant pulmonary blood flow from the ductus arteriosus. The cardiomegaly is due to marked dilation of the right atrium. The pulmonary vascular markings are diminished due to the decreased pulmonary blood flow. Hypoplasia of the lungs are common due to the large heart causing a "space occupying lesion."

vascular resistance, pulmonary blood flow may be quite severely limited with profound hypoxemia and acidosis as a result. PGE_1 is used to maintain a patent ductus arteriosus; other measures to decrease pulmonary vascular resistance and promote antegrade pulmonary blood flow (such as a high level of supplemental oxygen and maintaining a mild respiratory alkalosis) are helpful. Recently, nitric oxide has been utilized with limited success (see Chap. 24). An important contributor to the high mortality rate in the neonate with severe Ebstein's anomaly is the associated pulmonary hypoplasia (due to the massively enlarged right side of the heart in utero).

C. Parallel circulation/transposition of the great arteries (Fig. 25-12). Transposition of the great arteries is defined as an aorta arising from the morphologically right ventricle and the pulmonary artery from the morphologically left ventricle. Approximately one-half of all patients with transposition have an associated ventricular septal defect.

In the usual arrangement this creates a situation of "parallel circulations," with systemic venous return being pumped via the aorta back to the systemic circulation, and pulmonary venous return being pumped via the pulmonary artery to the pulmonary circulation. Following separation from the placenta, neonates with transposition are dependent on mixing between the parallel systemic and pulmonary circulations in order for them to survive. In patients with an intact ventricular septum, this communication exists through the patent ductus arteriosus and the patent foramen ovale. These patients are usually clinically cyanotic within the first hours of life, leading to their early diagnosis. Infants with an associated ventricular septal defect typically have somewhat improved mixing between the systemic and pulmonary circulations and may not be as severely cyanotic.

In neonates with transposition of the great arteries and an intact ventricular septum, a very low arterial pO_2 (15 to 20 mm Hg), high pCO_2 (despite adequate chest motion and ventilation), and metabolic acidosis are markers for severely decreased effective pulmonary blood flow. These infants need urgent attention. The initial management of the severely hypoxemic pa-

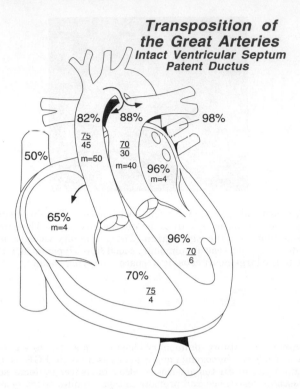

Fig. 25-12. Transposition of the great arteries with an intact ventricular septum, a large patent ductus arteriosus (on PGE$_1$) and atrial septal defect (status post balloon atrial septostomy). Note the following: (a) The aorta arises from the anatomic right ventricle, and the pulmonary artery from the anatomic left ventricle; (b) "transposition physiology," with a higher oxygen saturation in the pulmonary artery than in the aorta; (c) "mixing" between the parallel circulations (see text) at the atrial (after balloon atrial septostomy) and ductal levels; (d) shunting from the left atrium to the right atrium via the atrial septal defect (not shown) with equalization of atrial pressures; (e) shunting from the aorta to the pulmonary artery via the ductus arteriosus; (f) pulmonary hypertension due to a large ductus arteriosus.

tient with transposition includes (i) **ensurance of adequate mixing** between the two parallel circuits and (ii) **maximization of mixed venous oxygen saturation.**

In patients who do not respond with an increased arterial oxygen saturation to the opening of the ductus arteriosus with prostaglandin (usually these neonates have very restrictive atrial defects and/or pulmonary hypertension), **the foramen ovale should be emergently enlarged by balloon atrial septostomy.** Hyperventilation and treatment with sodium bicarbonate are important maneuvers to promote alkalosis, lower pulmonary vascular resistance, and increase pulmonary blood flow (which increases atrial mixing following septostomy).

In transposition of the great arteries, the majority of systemic blood flow is recirculated systemic venous return. In the presence of poor mixing (see above), much can be gained by increasing the mixed venous oxygen saturation, which is the **major determinant of systemic arterial oxygen satura-tion.** These maneuvers include (i) decreasing the whole-body oxygen con-sumption (muscle relaxants, sedation, mechanical ventilation) and (ii) im-proving oxygen delivery (increase cardiac output with inotropic agents, increase oxygen carrying capacity by treating anemia) [31]. Coexisting causes of pulmonary venous desaturation (e.g., pneumothorax) should also be sought and treated. Increasing the FiO_2 to 100% will have little effect on the arterial pO_2, unless it serves to lower pulmonary vascular resistance and increase pulmonary blood flow.

In the current era, definitive management is surgical correction with an arterial switch operation in the early neonatal period [8,31]. If severe hy-poxemia persists despite medical management, mechanical support with extracorporeal membrane oxygenation or an urgent arterial switch opera-tion [12] may be indicated.

D. Lesions with complete intracardiac mixing

1. **Truncus arteriosus** (Fig. 25-13) consists of a single great artery arising from the heart that gives rise to (in order) the coronary arteries, the pul-monary arteries, and the brachiocephalic arteries. The truncal valve is often anatomically abnormal (only 50% are tricuspid), and is frequently thickened, stenotic, or regurgitant. A coexisting ventricular septal defect is present in more than 98% of patients. The aortic arch is right-sided in approximately one-third of infants; other arch anomalies such as hy-poplasia, coarctation, and interruption are seen in 10% of patients. Ex-tracardiac anomalies are present in 20 to 40% of patients. DiGeorge syn-drome has been noted in as many as one-third of patients with truncus in some series.

   The overwhelming majority of infants with truncus arteriosus pres-ent with symptoms of congestive heart failure in the first weeks of life. The infants may be somewhat cyanotic, but congestive heart failure symptoms and signs are usually dominant. The pulmonary blood flow is increased, with significant pulmonary hypertension common. The nat-ural history of truncus arteriosus is quite bleak. Left unrepaired, only 15 to 30% of patients survive the first year of life. Furthermore, in sur-vivors of the immediate neonatal period, the occurrence of accelerated irreversible pulmonary vascular disease is common, making surgical repair in the neonatal period (or as soon as the diagnosis is made) the treatment of choice. "Medical management" of heart failure should be considered a temporizing measure until surgical correction can be ac-complished.

2. **Total anomalous pulmonary venous connection** (Fig. 25-14) occurs when all pulmonary veins drain into the systemic venous system with complete mixing of pulmonary and systemic venous return, usually in the right atrium. The systemic blood flow is thus dependent on an obli-gate shunt through the patent foramen ovale into the left side of the heart. The anomalous connections of the pulmonary veins may be (a) supracardiac (usually into the right superior vena cava or to the innomi-nate vein via a persistent vertical vein), (b) cardiac (usually to the right atrium or coronary sinus), (c) subdiaphragmatic (usually into the portal system), or (d) mixed.

   In patients with total connection below the diaphragm, the pathway is frequently obstructed, resulting in severely limited pulmonary blood flow, pulmonary hypertension, and profound cyanosis. This form of total anomalous pulmonary venous connection is a surgical emergency, with minimal beneficial effects from medical management. Although PGE_1 will maintain ductal patency, the limitation of pulmonary blood flow in these patients is **not** due to limited antegrade flow into the pulmonary circuit, but rather to outflow obstruction at the pulmonary veins. In the current era of prostaglandin, ventilatory support, and advanced medical intensive care, obstructed total anomalous pulmonary venous connection

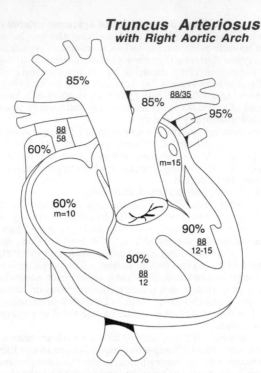

Fig. 25-13. Truncus arteriosus (with right aortic arch). Typical anatomic and hemo-dynamic findings include: (a) a single artery arises from the conotruncus giving rise to coronary arteries (not shown), pulmonary arteries, and brachiocephalic vessels; (b) abnormal truncal valve (quadricuspid shown) with stenosis and/or regurgitation common; (c) right-sided aortic arch (occurs in approximately 30% of cases); (d) large conoventricular ventricular septal defect; (e) pulmonary artery hypertension with a large left-to-right shunt (note superior vena caval oxygen saturation of 60% and pulmonary artery oxygen saturation of 85%); (f) complete mixing (of the systemic and pulmonary venous return) occurs at the great vessel level.

represents one of the few remaining lesions that requires emergent, "middle of the night" surgical intervention. Early recognition of the problem (see Fig. 25-14B) and prompt surgical intervention (surgical anastomosis of the pulmonary venous confluence to the left atrium) are necessary for the infant to survive. Patients with a mild degree of obstruction typically have minimal symptoms, with many neonates escaping recognition until later in infancy.

3. **Complex single ventricles.** There are multiple complex anomalies that share the common physiology of complete mixing of the systemic and pulmonary venous return, frequently with anomalous connections of the systemic and/or pulmonary veins, and with obstruction to one of the great vessels (usually the pulmonary artery) [33]. In cases with associated polysplenia or asplenia, the term "heterotaxy syndrome" is frequently applied. It is beyond the scope of this chapter to define this heterogeneous group of patients, though all will fail a hyperoxia test, most have significantly abnormal ECGs, and the diagnosis of complex congen-

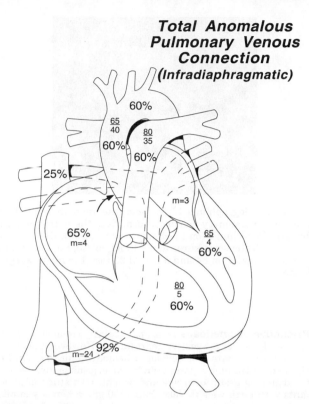

Total Anomalous Pulmonary Venous Connection
(Infradiaphragmatic)

Fig. 25-14A. Infradiaphragmatic total anomalous pulmonary venous connection. Note the following: (a) pulmonary venous confluence does not connect with the left atrium, but descends to connect with the portal circulation below the diaphragm. This connection is frequently severely obstructed as shown; (b) obstruction to pulmonary venous return results in significantly elevated pulmonary venous pressures, decreased pulmonary blood flow, pulmonary edema and pulmonary venous desaturation (92%); (c) systemic to suprasystemic pressure in the pulmonary artery (in the absence of a patent ductus arteriosus, pulmonary artery pressures may exceed systemic pressures when severe pulmonary venous obstruction is present); (d) all systemic blood flow must be derived via a right-to-left shunt at the foramen ovale; (e) nearly equal oxygen saturations in all chambers of the heart (i.e., complete mixing at right atrial level), with severe hypoxemia (systemic oxygen saturation 60%) and low cardiac output (mixed venous oxygen saturation 25%).

ital heart disease is rarely in doubt (even before anatomic confirmation with echocardiography). As there is complete mixing of venous return and essentially a single pumping chamber, initial management is similar to that described above for hypoplastic left heart syndrome (see **V.A.4**).

E. **Left-to-right shunt lesions.** For the most part, infants with pure left-to-right shunt lesions are not diagnosed because of severe systemic illness, but rather because of the finding of a murmur or symptoms of congestive heart failure, usually occurring in the late neonatal period or beyond. The lesion of this group most likely to require attention in the neonatal nursery is that of a patent ductus arteriosus.

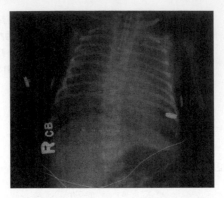

Fig. 25-14B. Chest radiograph in a 16-hour-old neonate with severe infradiaphragmatic obstruction to pulmonary venous return. Note the pulmonary edema, small heart and hyperinflated lungs (on mechanical ventilation). Despite high inflating and positive end-expiratory pressures and an FiO_2 of 1.0, the arterial blood gas revealed a pH of 7.02, a pCO_2 of 84 and a pO_2 of 23 torr. Emergent surgical management is indicated.

1. **Patent ductus arteriosus** is not particularly common in term newborns and rarely causes congestive heart failure. However, the frequency that a premature neonate will develop a hemodynamically significant left-to-right shunt through a patent ductus arteriosus is inversely proportional to advancing gestational age and weight. In a study of almost 1700 infants with birth weights less than 1750 gm, a hemodynamically significant patent ductus arteriosus was noted in 42% of infants with birth weights less than 1000 gm, 21% of infants with birth weights between 1000 and 1500 gm, and only 7% of those with birth weights between 1500 and 1750 gm [17].

   The typical presentation of a patent ductus arteriosus begins with a harsh systolic ejection murmur heard over the entire precordium, but loudest at the left upper sternal border and left infraclavicular areas. As the pulmonary vascular resistance decreases, the intensity of the murmur increases and later becomes continuous (i.e., extends through the second heart sound). The peripheral pulses increase in amplitude ("bounding pulses"), the pulse pressure widens to more than 25 mm Hg, the precordial impulse becomes hyperdynamic, and the patient's respiratory status deteriorates (manifesting as tachypnea or apnea, carbon dioxide retention, and an increasing mechanical ventilation requirement). Serial chest x-ray films show an increase in heart size and the lungs may appear more radiopaque.

   It is important to remember that this typical progression of clinical signs is not specific only for a hemodynamically significant patent ductus arteriosus. Other lesions may produce bounding pulses, a hyperdynamic precordium, and cardiac enlargement (e.g., an arteriovenous fistula or an aorticopulmonary window). Generally, however, the clinical assessment of a premature infant with the typical findings of a hemodynamically significant ductus is adequate to guide therapeutic decisions. If the diagnosis is in doubt, echocardiography will clarify the anatomic diagnosis.

   Initial medical management includes increased ventilatory support, fluid restriction, and diuretic therapy. Indications for closure of a patent ductus arteriosus vary from institution to institution. In general, we recommend treatment for mechanically ventilated premature infants weighing less than 1000 gm when a patent ductus first becomes apparent, regardless of the presence of signs or symptoms of a significant left-to-right shunt. In this group of premature infants, approximately 80% will go on to develop a large hemodynamically significant left-to-right shunt. **Early treatment in infants weighing less than 1000 gm has been associated with a decreased requirement for surgical patent ductus arteriosus ligation, as well as decreased neonatal morbidity.** For infants larger than 1000 gm, we recommend treatment with indomethacin only after cardiovascular or respiratory signs of a hemodynamically significant ductus develop [28]. Indomethacin is effective in approximately 80% of symptomatic patients [21]. Birth weight does not affect the efficacy of indomethacin, and there is no increase in complications associated with surgery after unsuccessful indomethacin therapy [21].

Adverse reactions to indomethacin include transient oliguria, electrolyte abnormalities, decreased platelet function, and hypoglycemia. Contraindications to the use of indomethacin are listed in Table 25-10. The presence of an intraventricular hemorrhage (IVH) is not a contraindication to indomethacin therapy; however, its routine use is not recommended in infants in the first few days of life who have an active or evolving IVH. See sec. **VII.F** and Table 25-11 for dosing information.

Several randomized controlled studies examined the effect of **prophylactic** indomethacin treatment during the first 24 hours of life to prevent the development of symptomatic patent ductus arteriosus in mechanically ventilated infants who weigh less than 1500 gm (28,33). Most studies demonstrated that prophylactic indomethacin decreases the incidence of a hemodynamically significant patent ductus arteriosus in these infants. However, despite differences in the development of symptomatic patent ductus arteriosus, no significant differences between the prophylactically treated and untreated groups have been observed in relation to total duration of oxygen therapy or ventilatory support, or in the incidence of bronchopulmonary dysplasia. The lack of demonstrable changes in short- and long-term outcomes, as well as the observation that only approximately 40% of very-low-birth-weight babies develop a symptomatic patent ductus arteriosus, suggest that **routine prophylactic use of indomethacin is controversial.** Finally, although the risk of pulmonary hemorrhage **may** be increased in infants with a patent ductus receiving artificial surfactant therapy, routine prophylactic administration of indomethacin to all infants receiving surfactant is not supported by the available evidence.

If signs and symptoms of a patent ductus arteriosus recur after the first course of indomethacin, a second course should be given after

Table 25-10. Contraindications for indomethacin in infants with patent ductus arteriosus

---

BUN $\geq$30 mg/dl

Serum creatinine $\geq$1.8 mg/dl

Total urine output $\leq$0.6 ml/kg/hr over preceding 8 hours

Platelet count <60,000/μl

Stool blood test >3+ (or moderate to large)

Evidence of bleeding diathesis

Clinical or radiographic evidence of necrotizing enterocolitis

Evidence of enlarging intraventricular hemorrhage

Source: Adapted from W. M. Gersony et al., *J. Pediatr.* 102: 895, 1983.

Table 25-11. Dose of intravenous indomethacin in premature infants with patent ductus arteriosus

	Dose (12–18-hour intervals)	
Age	Initial	Second and third
>48 hours	0.2 mg/kg	0.1 mg/kg
2–7 days	0.2 mg/kg	0.2 mg/kg
>7 days	0.2 mg/kg	0.25 mg/kg

echocardiographic confirmation of the diagnosis. In addition, we recommend that in infants with relative contraindications to the use of indomethacin, including diminished renal function, bowel symptomatology, or thrombocytopenia, the clinical diagnosis be confirmed by echocardiography prior to indomethacin use. If symptoms recur after a second course of therapy, it is unlikely that further indomethacin doses will close the ductus. If medical management fails to close the ductus, surgical ligation should be seriously considered. Although ligation through a left lateral thoracotomy remains the standard surgical approach, recent reports of minimally invasive, video-assisted thoracoscopic techniques show promise in selected newborns [7].

2. **Complete atrioventricular canal** (Fig. 25-15) consists of a combination of defects in the (i) endocardial portion of the atrial septum, (ii) the inlet portion of the ventricular septum, and (iii) a common, single atrioventricular valve. Because of the large net left-to-right shunt, which increases as the pulmonary vascular resistance falls, these infants typically present early in life with congestive heart failure. There may be some degree of cyanosis as well, particularly in the immediate neonatal period before the pulmonary vascular resistance has fallen. In the absence of associated right ventricular outflow tract obstruction, pulmonary artery pressures are at systemic levels; pulmonary vascular resistance is frequently elevated, particularly in patients with trisomy 21.

Nearly 70% of infants with complete atrioventricular canal have trisomy 21; notation of the phenotypic findings of Down syndrome often lead to evaluation of the patient for possible congenital heart disease (see Table 25-6). In the immediate neonatal period, these infants may have an equivocal hyperoxia test since there may be some right-to-left shunting through the large intracardiac connections. Symptoms of congestive failure ensue during the first weeks of life as the pulmonary vascular resistance falls and the patient develops a marked left-to-right shunt. These patients have a characteristic ECG finding of a "superior axis" (Fig. 25-16), which can be very useful in screening for the presence of congenital heart disease in an infant with trisomy 21.

The majority of patients with complete atrioventricular canal will require medical treatment with digoxin and diuretics for symptomatic congestive heart failure, though prolonged medical therapy in patients with failure to thrive and symptomatic heart failure is not warranted. Complete surgical repair is undertaken electively in the first year of life, with earlier repair in symptomatic patients. In our experience, corrective surgery for complete atrioventricular canal can be performed successfully in early infancy with good results [8].

3. **Ventricular septal defect** is the most common cause of congestive heart failure after the initial neonatal period. Moderate to large ventricular septal defects become hemodynamically significant as the pulmonary vascular resistance decreases and pulmonary blood flow increases owing to a left-to-right shunt across the defect. As this usually takes 2 to 4

Complete Common Atrioventricular Canal

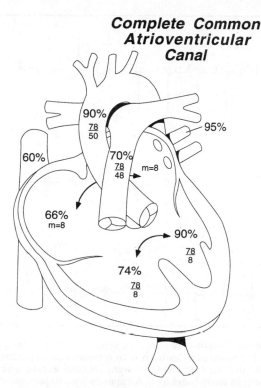

Fig. 25-15. Complete common atrioventricular canal. Typical anatomic and hemo dynamic findings include: (a) large atrial and ventricular septal defects of the endocardial cushion type; (b) single, atrioventricular valve; (c) pulmonary artery hypertension (due to large ventricular septal defect); (d) bidirectional shunting (with mild hypoxemia) at atrial and ventricular level when pulmonary vascular resistance is elevated in the initial neonatal period. With subsequent fall in pulmonary vascular resistance, the shunt becomes predominantly left to right with symptoms of congestive heart failure.

weeks to develop, term neonates with ventricular septal defect and symptoms of congestive heart failure should be investigated for coexisting anatomic abnormalities, such as left ventricular outflow tract obstruction, coarctation of the aorta, and patent ductus arteriosus. Premature infants, who have a lower initial pulmonary vascular resistance, may develop clinical symptoms of heart failure earlier or require longer mechanical ventilation compared with term infants.

Ventricular septal defects may occur anywhere in the ventricular septum and are usually classified by their location (Fig. 25-17). Defects in the membranous septum are the most common type. The diagnosis of ventricular septal defect is usually initially suspected on physical examination of the infant; echocardiography confirms the diagnosis and localizes the defect in the ventricular septum. Because a large number (as many as 50% depending on the anatomic type) of ventricular septal defects may close spontaneously in the first months of life, surgery is usually deferred beyond the neonatal period. In large series, only 15% of all

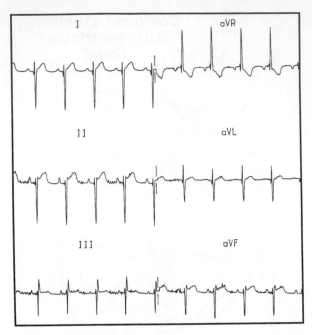

Fig. 25-16. Superior ("northwest") axis as seen on the electrocardiogram (only frontal plane leads shown) in a newborn with complete atrioventricular canal. Note the initial upward deflection of the QRS complex (and subsequent predominantly negative deflection) in leads I and aVF. A superior axis (0 to −180 degrees) is present in 95% of patients with endocardial cushion defects.

patients with ventricular septal defects ever become clinically symptomatic. Medical management of congestive heart failure includes digoxin, diuretics, and caloric supplementation. Growth failure is the most common symptom of congestive heart failure not fully compensated by medical management. When it occurs, failure to thrive is an indication for surgical repair of the defect [20].

F. **Cardiac surgery in the neonate.** In the past, because of the perceived high risk of open heart surgery early in life, critically ill neonates were mostly subjected to palliative procedures or prolonged medical management. The unrepaired circulation and residual hemodynamic abnormalities frequently resulted in secondary problems to the heart, lungs, and brain, as well as more nonspecific problems of failure to thrive, frequent hospitalizations, and infections [15,19]. In addition, there are difficult to quantitate psychological burdens to the family of a chronically ill infant.

Low birth weight should not be considered an absolute contraindication for surgical repair. In a recent series, prolonged medical therapy in low-birth-weight infants to achieve further weight gain in the presence of a significant hemodynamic burden did not appear to improve the survival rate, and prolonged intensive care management was associated with nosocomial complications [10]. We believe that the symptomatic neonate with congenital heart disease should undergo repair as early as possible, to prevent the secondary sequelae of the congenital lesion on the heart, lungs, and brain [9].

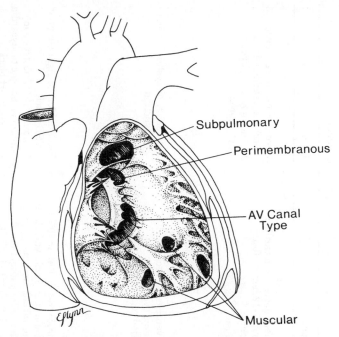

Fig. 25-17. Diagram of types of ventricular septal defects as viewed from the right ventricle. From ref. 20 with permission.

Improvements in surgical techniques, cardiopulmonary bypass, and intensive care of the neonate and infant have resulted in significant improvements in surgical mortality and quality of life in the survivors [8,9] (see Table 25-12 and general texts of cardiac surgery [8,24]).

VI. Acquired heart disease

A. Myocarditis may occur in the neonate as an isolated illness or as a component of a generalized illness with associated hepatitis or encephalitis. Myocarditis is usually the result of a viral infection (coxsackie, rubella, and varicella viruses are most common), though other infectious agents such as bacteria and fungi as well as noninfectious conditions such as autoimmune diseases also can cause myocarditis. Although the clinical presentation (and in some instances endomyocardial biopsy) makes the diagnosis, specific identification of the etiologic agent is currently not made in most cases. However, recent improvements in molecular biology techniques (polymerase chain reactions for viral-specific RNA) will most likely improve the frequency of accurate identification of viral pathogens [32].

The infant with acute myocarditis presents with signs and symptoms of congestive heart failure (see **III.B.1**) or arrhythmia (see **VIII**). The course of the illness is frequently fulminant and fatal; however, full recovery of ventricular function may occur if the infant can be supported and survive the acute illness [11,29]. Supplemental oxygen, diuretics, inotropic agents, afterload reduction, and mechanical ventilation are frequently used for supportive care. In severe cases, mechanical support of the myocardium with extracorporeal membrane oxygenation or ventricular assist can be considered [11]. Care should be used when administering digoxin, due to the potential for the potentiation of arrhythmias or complete heart block.

Table 25-12. Common neonatal operations and their early sequelae

Lesion	Surgical repair (eponym)	Early postoperative sequelae	
		Common	Rare
Corrective procedures			
TGA	Arterial switch procedure (Jatene) 1. Division and reanastomosis of PA and aorta to anatomically correct ventricle 2. Translocation of coronary arteries 3. Closure of septal defects if present	Transient decrease in cardiac output 6–12 hours after surgery	Coronary ostial stenosis or occlusion/sudden death Hemidiaphragm paresis Chylothorax
	Atrial switch procedure (Senning or Mustard) 1. Intraatrial baffling of systemic venous return to LV (to PA) and pulmonary venous return to RV (to AO) 2. Closure of septal defects if present	Supraventricular tachycardia Sick sinus syndrome Tricuspid regurgitation	Pulmonary or systemic venous obstruction
TOF	1. Patch closure of VSD via ventriculotomy or right atrium 2. Enlargement of RVOT with infundibular patch 3. ±Pulmonary valvotomy 4. ±Transannular RV to PA patch 5. ±RV to PA conduit	Pulmonary regurgitation (if transannular patch, valvotomy, or nonvalved conduit) Transient RV dysfunction Right-to-left shunt via PFO, usually resolves 1–2 days postoperatively as RV function improves	Residual left-to-right shunt at VSD patch Residual RVOT obstruction Junctional ectopic tachycardia Complete heart block

COA	Subclavian flap (Waldhaussen), or Resection with end-to-end anastomosis, or Patch augmentation	Systemic hypertension Absent left-arm pulse (if Waldhaussen)	Ileus Hemidiaphragm paresis Vocal cord paresis Chylothorax
PDA	Ligation (±division) of PDA using open thoracotomy and direct visualization or video-assisted thoracoscopic visualization	—	Hemidiaphragm paresis Vocal cord paresis Chylothorax Interruption of left PA or descending aorta
TAPVC	1. Reanastomosis of pulmonary venous confluence to posterior aspect of left atrium 2. Division of connecting vein	Pulmonary hypertension Transient low cardiac output	Residual pulmonary venous obstruction
Truncus arteriosus	1. Closure of VSD; baffling LV to truncus (neoaorta) 2. Removal of PAs from truncus 3. Conduit placement from RV to PAs	Reactive pulmonary hypertension Transient RV dysfunction with right-to-left shunt via PFO Hypocalcemia (DiGeorge syndrome)	Truncal valve stenosis or regurgitation Residual VSD Complete heart block

Table 25-12. *Continued*

Lesion	Surgical repair (eponym)	Early postoperative sequelae	
		Common	Rare
Palliative procedures			
HLHS*	Stage I (Norwood) 1. Connection of main PA to aorta with reconstruction of aortic arch 2. Systemic-to-pulmonary shunt 3. Atrial septectomy	Low systemic cardiac output due to excessive pulmonary blood flow	Aortic arch obstruction Restrictive atrial septal defect
Complex lesions with decreased pulmonary blood flow*	Systemic-to-pulmonary shunt (using prosthetic tube = modified Blalock-Taussig shunt; using subclavian artery = classic Blalock-Taussig shunt)	Excessive pulmonary blood flow and mild congestive heart failure	Hemidiaphragm paresis Vocal cord paralysis Chylothorax Seroma
Complex lesions with excessive pulmonary blood flow*	PA band (prosthetic or Silastic constriction of main PA)	—	PA distortion Aneurysm of main PA

TGA = transposition of the great arteries; LV = left ventricle; PA = pulmonary artery; RV = right ventricle; AO = aorta; TOF = tetralogy of Fallot; VSD = ventricular septal defect; RVOT = right ventricular outflow tract; PFO = patent foramen ovale; COA = coarctation of the aorta; PDA = patent ductus arteriosus; TAPVC = total anomalous pulmonary venous connection; HLHS = hypoplastic left heart syndrome.

*In patients with a single ventricle, the goal is to separate pulmonary and systemic venous return, rerouting systemic venous blood directly to pulmonary arteries (Fontan operation) though this is done in late infancy or early childhood.

Source: Adapted from G. Wernovsky, L. C. Erickson, and D. L. Wessel, Cardiac Emergencies. In H. L. May (Ed.), *Emergency Medicine*. Boston: Little, Brown, 1992.

B. Transient myocardial ischemia with myocardial dysfunction may occur in any neonate with a history of perinatal asphyxia (see Chap. 27, Perinatal Asphyxia). Myocardial dysfunction may be associated with maternal autoimmune disease such as systemic lupus erythematosus. A tricuspid or mitral regurgitant murmur is often heard. A serum creatine kinase MB fraction greater than 5 to 10% may be helpful in determining the presence of myocardial damage. Supportive treatment is dictated by the severity of myocardial dysfunction.

C. Hypertrophic and dilated cardiomyopathies represent a rare and multifactorial complex of diseases, the complete discussion of which is beyond the scope of this chapter. The differential diagnosis includes primary diseases (e.g., metabolic and storage disorders, "idiopathic") and secondary diseases (e.g., end-stage infection, ischemia, endocrine, neuromuscular, nutrition, drugs). The reader is referred to more general texts [18,20] and review articles [22,23,32].

The most common hypertrophic cardiomyopathy presenting in neonates is that seen in infants born to diabetic mothers (see Chap. 2, Diabetes Mellitus). Echocardiographically and hemodynamically, these infants are indistinguishable from patients with the familial form of hypertrophic cardiomyopathy. They are different in one important respect: Their cardiomyopathy will completely resolve in 6 to 12 months. Noting a systolic ejection murmur, with or without congestive heart failure, in the infant of a diabetic mother should raise the question of congenital heart disease including hypertrophic cardiomyopathy. Treatment is supportive, addressing the infant's particular symptoms of congestive heart failure. Propranolol has been used successfully in some patients with severe obstruction. Most patients require no specific care and no long-term cardiac follow-up.

VII. Pharmacology of cardiac drugs

A. PGE$_1$ has been used since the late 1970s to pharmacologically maintain patency of the ductus arteriosus in patients with duct-dependent systemic or pulmonary blood flow. Most cyanotic and congestive lesions will benefit from distal blood flow. Some lesions will be made worse with prostaglandins. These include total anomalous pulmonary venous return with obstruction (see **V.D.2**), mitral atresia, and transposition of the great arteries with intact ventricular and atrial septum (see **V.C**). Because apnea may be a side effect, we first *intubate* the patient. Also, because vasodilation and hypotension are side effects, one should be prepared to administer fluids and pressors to maintain blood pressure. PGE$_1$ must be administered as a continuous parenteral infusion. The usual starting dose is 0.05 to 0.10 µg/kg per minute. Once a therapeutic effect has been achieved, the dose may often be decreased to as low as 0.025 µg/kg per minute without loss of therapeutic effect. The response to PGE$_1$ is often immediate if patency of the ductus is important for the hemodynamic state of the infant. Failure to respond to PGE$_1$ may mean that the initial diagnosis was incorrect, the ductus is unresponsive to PGE$_1$ (usually only in an older infant), or the ductus is absent. The infusion site has no significant effect on the ductal response to PGE$_1$. Adverse reactions to PGE$_1$ include apnea (10 to 12%), fever (14%), seizures (4%), cutaneous flushing (10%), bradycardia (7%), tachycardia (3%), cardiac arrest (1%), and edema (1%). See Table 25-13 for recommended mixing and dosing protocol for PGE$_1$.

B. Sympathomimetic amine infusions (see Chap. 17) are the mainstay of pharmacologic therapies aimed at improving cardiac output and are discussed in detail elsewhere. Catecholamines, endogenous (dopamine, epinephrine) or synthetic (dobutamine, isoproterenol), achieve an effect by stimulating myocardial and vascular adrenergic receptors. These agents must be given as a continuous parenteral infusion. They may be given in combination to the critically ill neonate in an effort to maximize the positive effects of each agent while minimizing the negative effects. While re-

Table 25-13. Suggested preparation of prostaglandin E$_1$

Add 1 ampule (500 μg) to:	Concentration (μg/ml)	ml/hr × weight (kg), needed to infuse 0.1 μg/kg/min
250 ml	2	3.0
100 ml*	5	1.2
50 ml	10	0.6

*Usually the most convenient dilution, provides one-fourth of maintenance fluid requirement. Usually mix in dextrose-containing solution for newborns.
Source: Adapted from G. Wernovsky, L. C. Erickson, and D. L. Wessel, Cardiac Emergencies. In H. L. May (Ed.), *Emergency Medicine.* Boston: Little, Brown, 1992.

ceiving catecholamine infusions, patients should be closely monitored, usually with an ECG monitor and an arterial catheter. Prior to beginning sympathomimetic amine infusions, intravascular volume should be repleted if necessary, though this may further compromise a congenital lesion with coexisting volume overload. Adverse reactions to catecholamine infusions include tachycardia (which increases myocardial oxygen consumption), atrial and ventricular arrhythmias, and increased afterload due to peripheral vasoconstriction (which may decrease cardiac output). See Table 25-14 for recommended mixing and dosing of the sympathomimetic amines.
C. **Afterload-reducing agents**
1. **Phosphodiesterase inhibitors** such as **amrinone** and **milrinone** are bipyridine compounds that selectively inhibit cyclic nucleotide phosphodiesterase. These new nonglycosidic and nonsympathomimetic agents exert their effect on cardiac performance by increasing cyclic adenosine monophosphate (cAMP) in the myocardial and vascular muscle, but do so independently of beta receptors. cAMP promotes improved contraction via calcium regulation through two mechanisms: (a) activation of protein kinase (which catalyzes the transfer of phosphate groups from ATP), leading to faster calcium entry through the calcium channels, and (b) ac-

Table 25-14. Sympathomimetic amines

Drug	Usual dose (μg/kg/min)	Effect
Dopamine	1–5	↑ urine output, ↑ HR (slightly), ↑ contractility
	6–10	↑ HR, ↑ contractility, ↑ BP
	11–20	↑ HR, ↑ contractility, ↑ SVR, ↑ BP
Dobutamine	1–20	↑ HR (slightly), ↑ contractility, ↓ SVR
Epinephrine	0.05–0.50	↑ HR, ↑ contractility, ↑ SVR, ↑ BP
Isoproterenol	0.05–1.00	↑ HR, ↑ contractility, ↓ SVR, ↓ PVR

These infusions may be mixed in intravenous solutions containing dextrose and/or saline. For neonates, dextrose-containing solutions with or without salt should usually be chosen. Calculation for convenient preparation of IV infusions:

$$6 \times \frac{\text{desired dose (μg/kg/min)} \times \text{weight (kg)}}{\text{desired rate (ml/hr)}} = \frac{\text{mg drug}}{100 \text{ ml fluid}}$$

HR = heart rate; BP = blood pressure; SVR = systemic vascular resistance; PVR = pulmonary vascular resistance.

tivation of calcium pumps in the sarcoplasmic reticulum, resulting in release of calcium.

There are three major effects of phosphodiesterase inhibitors: (a) increased inotropy, with increased contractility and cardiac output as a result of a cAMP-mediated increase in transsarcolemmal calcium flux; (b) vasodilatation, with an increase in arteriolar and venous capacitance as a result of a cAMP-mediated increase in uptake of calcium and decrease in calcium available for contraction; and (c) increased lusitropy, or improved relaxation properties during diastole. There appear to be differences between the immature and adult myocardium in the handling of amrinone. One study [26] suggested that neonates and infants require a higher loading dose (3.0 to 4.5 mg/kg) than do adults to achieve adequate serum levels. Clinical experience with amrinone suggests that a continuous infusion to 5 to 15 μg/kg per minute is effective.

Indications include low cardiac output with myocardial dysfunction and elevated systemic vascular resistance not accompanied by severe hypotension. Side effects have been minimal and are typically the need for volume infusions (5 to 10 ml/kg) following bolus (>2 mg/kg) administration, and occasional thrombocytopenia following prolonged (>7 to 10 days) use.

The use of amrinone after cardiac surgery in the pediatric patient population can increase cardiac index and decrease systemic vascular resistance without a significant increase in heart rate. Despite successful application of amrinone treatment in adults and children with myocardial failure, some have avoided its use because of concerns of potential side effects and its relatively long biologic half-life. However, following successful clinical trials [25], amrinone has now become the second-line drug (after dopamine) in the treatment of low cardiac output in neonates, infants, and children following cardiopulmonary bypass in our institution.

2. **Other vasodilators** improve low cardiac output principally by decreasing impedance to ventricular ejection; these effects are especially helpful after cardiac surgery in children and in adults when systemic vascular resistance is particularly elevated.

Sodium nitroprusside is the most widely used afterload-reducing agent. It acts as a nitric oxide donor, increasing intracellular cyclic guanosine monophosphate (cGMP), which effects relaxation of vascular smooth muscle in both arterioles and veins. The overall effect is a decrease in atrial filling pressure and systemic vascular resistance with a concomitant increase in cardiac output. The vasodilatory effects of nitroprusside occur within minutes of intravenous administration. The principal metabolites of sodium nitroprusside are thiocyanate and cyanide; thiocyanate toxicity is unusual in children with normal hepatic and renal function, and cyanide and thiocyanate concentrations in children may not be correlated with clinical signs of toxicity. Although one study in neonates with low cardiac output showed that there was an increase in urine output and improvement in perfusion with institution of nitroprusside [4], another study in neonates with respiratory distress syndrome noted a significant drop in blood pressure [5].

Many other agents have been used as arterial and venous vasodilators to treat hypertension, reduce ventricular afterload and systemic vascular resistance, and improve cardiac output. A second nitrovasodilator, **nitroglycerin,** principally a **venous dilator,** also has rapid onset of action and a short half-life (about 2 minutes). Tolerance may develop after several days of continuous infusion. Nitroglycerin is used extensively in adult cardiac units for patients with ischemic heart disease; experience in pediatric patients is more limited. **Hydralazine** is more typically used for acute hypertension; its relatively long half-life limits its use in postoperative patients with labile hemodynamics. The angiotensin-converting enzyme inhibitor **enalapril** similarly has a relatively long half-life (2 to 4 hours), which limits its use in the acute setting. **Beta blockers** (e.g., propranolol, esmolol, labetolol), although excellent in reducing blood pressure, may have deleterious effects on ventricular function. **Calcium channel blockers** (e.g., verapamil) may cause acute and severe hypotension and bradycardia in the neonate and should **rarely be used.** All intravenous vasodilators must be used cautiously in patients with moderate to severe lung disease; their use has been associated with increased intrapulmonary shunting and acute reductions of arterial pO_2.

D. **Digoxin** remains the cornerstone of treatment for congestive heart failure. Term infants can begin initial treatment (a "digitalizing dose") with a total dose of 30 μg/kg in 24 hours; premature infants can usually be effectively digitalized with a total dose of 20 μg/kg in 24 hours. One-half of this **total digitalizing dose (TDD)** may be given intravenously, intramuscularly, or orally, followed by one-fourth of the TDD every 8 to 12 hours for the remaining two doses. An initial maintenance dose of one-fourth to one-third of the TDD (range, 5 to 10 μg/kg per day) may then be adjusted according to the patient's clinical response, renal function, and tolerance for the drug (Table 25-15). Alternatively, infants with mild symptoms, primary myocardial disease, renal dysfunction, or the potential for atrioventricular block may be digitalized using only the maintenance dose (omitting the loading dose).

Digoxin toxicity most commonly manifests with gastrointestinal upset, somnolence, and sinus bradycardia. More severe digoxin toxicity may cause high-grade atrioventricular block and ventricular ectopy. Infants suspected of having digoxin toxicity should have their digoxin level measured and further doses withheld. The therapeutic level is approximately 2.0 ng/ml, with probable toxicity occurring at levels over 4.0 ng/ml. In infants particularly, however, digoxin levels do not always correlate well with therapeutic efficacy or with toxicity.

Digoxin toxicity in neonates is usually manageable by withholding further doses until the signs of toxicity resolve and by correcting electrolyte abnormalities (such as hypokalemia) that can potentiate toxic effects. Severe ventricular arrhythmias associated with digoxin toxicity may be managed with phenytoin, 2 to 4 mg/kg over 5 minutes, or lidocaine, 1 mg/kg loading dose, followed by an infusion at 1 to 2 mg/kg per hour. Atrioventricular block is usually unresponsive to atropine. Severe bradycardia may be refractory to these therapies and require temporary cardiac pacing.

The use of a digoxin-specific antibody Fab fragment preparation (Digibind, Burroughs Wellcome) is reserved for patients with evidence of severe digoxin intoxication and clinical symptoms of refractory arrhythmia or atrioventricular block; in these patients it is quite effective [34]. Calculation of the Digibind dose in milligrams is as follows: (Serum digoxin concentration in nanograms per milliliter $\times$ 5.6 $\times$ body weight in kilograms/1000) $\times$ 64. The dose is given as a one-time intravenous infusion. A second dose of Digibind may be given in patients who continue to have clinical evidence of residual digoxin toxicity. Skin testing for hypersensitivity is recommended prior to the first dose.

E. **Diuretics** are frequently used in patients with congestive heart failure, usually in combination with digoxin. **Furosemide,** 1 to 2 mg/kg per dose, usu-

Table 25-15. Digoxin dosage

	Total digitalizing dose	Maintenance*
Premature infants	20 μg/kg	5 μg/kg/day
Term infants	30 μg/kg	3–10 μg/kg/day

*Usually the maintenance dose is divided into equal twice-daily doses 12 hours apart.

ally results in a brisk diuresis within an hour of administration. If no response is noted in an hour, a second dose (double the first dose) may be given. Chronic use of furosemide may produce urinary tract stones as a result of its calciuric effects. A more potent diuretic effect may be achieved using a combination of a thiazide and a "loop" diuretic. Combination diuretic therapy may be complicated by hyponatremia and hypokalemia. Oral or intravenous potassium supplementation (3 to 4 mEq/kg per day) or an aldosterone antagonist usually should accompany the thiazide or loop diuretics to avoid excessive potassium wasting. It is important to carefully monitor serum potassium and sodium levels when beginning or changing the dose of diuretic medications. When changing from an effective parenteral to oral dose of furosemide, the dose should be increased by 50 to 80%. Furosemide may increase the nephrotoxicity and ototoxicity of concurrently used aminoglycoside antibiotics. Detailed discussion of alternative diuretics (e.g., chlorothiazide, spironolactone, ethacrynic acid) is found elsewhere in the text.

F. Indomethacin (see Tables 25-10 and 25-11 and V.E.1). The dosage of indomethacin needs to be adjusted for postnatal age secondary to increased drug clearance with advancing postnatal age. Individual infants may require further adjustment of the dosage depending on maturity of renal function. Indomethacin is provided as 1 mg of lyophilized powder per vial. The manufacturer recommends reconstitution of the drug with **no more** than 1 or 2 ml of normal saline solution or sterile water. Once reconstituted, the drug should be used immediately. Additional dilution or delay in use of the reconstituted drug may result in precipitation of the drug out of solution. Administration should be by slow intravenous push over approximately 5 minutes.

We recommend that infants being treated with indomethacin not be fed by mouth prior to therapy, and feeding held for at least 12 hours after the last dose of the drug because of possible effects on intestinal blood flow. Concurrent use of a low-dose dopamine infusion in the range of 1 to 2 µg/kg per minute may help alleviate the decreased urine output often observed during indomethacin treatment. Dopamine infusions can be either used prophylactically prior to the initiation of therapy or added once effects on urine output are observed.

In general, all three doses of indomethacin should be given even if symptoms disappear during the course of therapy. If significant concerns of potential complications of indomethacin therapy are present, it is recommended that a minimum of two doses be administered.

VIII. Arrhythmias
A. Initial evaluation. For evaluation of any infant with an arrhythmia, it is essential to simultaneously assess the electrophysiology and hemodynamic status. If the baby is poorly perfused or hypotensive, reliable intravenous access should be secured and a level of resuscitation employed appropriate for the degree of illness. As always, **emergency treatment of shock should precede definitive diagnosis.** It should be emphasized, however, that there is **rarely** a situation in which it is justified to omit a 12-lead ECG from the evaluation of an infant with an arrhythmia, the exceptions being ventricular fibrillation or torsade de pointes with accompanying hemodynamic instability. These arrhythmias frequently require immediate defibrillation but are extremely rare arrhythmias in neonates and young infants.

In nearly all circumstances, appropriate therapy (short and long term) depends on an accurate electrophysiologic diagnosis. Determination of the mechanism of a rhythm disturbance is most often made from a 12-lead ECG in the abnormal rhythm, comparing the tracing to the patient's normal 12-lead ECG of sinus rhythm. While rhythm strips generated from a cardiac monitor can be helpful supportive evidence of the final diagnosis, they are typically **not** diagnostic and should **not** be the only documentation of arrhythmia if at all possible.

The three broad categories for arrhythmias in neonates are (i) tachyarrhythmias, (ii) bradyarrhythmias, and (iii) irregular rhythms. An algorithm for approaching the differential diagnosis of **narrow complex tachyarrhythmias** can be consulted (Fig. 25-18) in most cases. For analysis of the ECG for the mechanism of arrhythmia, a stepwise approach should be taken in three main areas: **rate** (variability, too fast or too slow), **rhythm** (regular or irregular, paroxysmal or gradual), and **QRS morphology**.

B. **Differential diagnosis and initial management**
   1. **Narrow-QRS-complex tachycardias** (see Fig. 25-18)
      a. **Supraventricular tachycardias (SVTs)** are the most common symptomatic arrhythmias in all children including neonates. SVTs usually have (i) a rate greater than 200 beats per minute, frequently "fixed" with no beat-to-beat variation in rate; (ii) rapid onset and termination (in reentrant rhythms); and (iii) normal ventricular complexes on the surface ECG. The infant may initially be asymptomatic, but later may become irritable, and refuse feedings. Congestive heart failure usually does not develop prior to 24 hours of continuous SVT; however, heart failure is seen in 20% of patients after 36 hours and in 50% after 48 hours.

      SVT in the neonate is almost always "reentrant," either involving an accessory atrioventricular pathway and the atrioventricular (AV) node or due to atrial flutter. About half of these patients will manifest

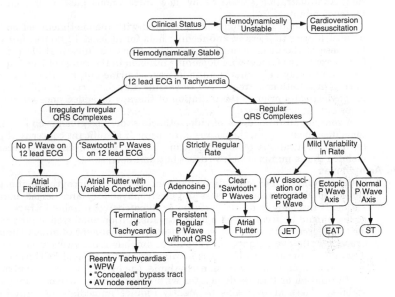

Fig. 25-18. Bedside differential diagnosis of narrow complex tachycardias in neonates, the most common type of arrhythmia in this age group. Note that, regardless of the mechanism of tachycardia, if the patient is hemodynamically unstable immediate measures to resuscitate the infant including cardioversion are required. Also, treatment with adenosine is helpful therapeutically as well as diagnostically. In general, tachycardias which terminate (even briefly) after adenosine are of the reentry type. JET = junctional ectopic tachycardia, EAT = ectopic atrial tachycardia, ST = sinus tachycardia, WPW = Wolff-Parkinson-White syndrome. Algorithm for analysis of arrhythmias in neonates.

preexcitation (delta wave) on the ECG when not in tachycardia (Wolff-Parkinson-White [WPW] syndrome, Fig. 25-19). In rarer cases, the reentrant circuit may be within the atrium itself (atrial flutter) or within the AV node (AV node reentrant tachycardia). Patients with SVTs may have associated structural heart disease; evaluation for structural heart disease should be considered in all neonates with SVTs. Another rare cause of SVTs in a neonate is ectopic atrial tachycardia, in which the distinguishing features are an abnormal P-wave axis, normal QRS axis, and significant variability in the overall rate.

Long-term medical therapy for SVTs in the neonate is based on the underlying electrophysiologic diagnosis. *Digoxin* is the initial therapy in patients without congestive heart failure and without demonstrable WPW syndrome. Parenteral digitalization is described in sec. **VII.D.** During digitalization, vagal maneuvers (facial/malar ice wrapped in a towel to elicit the "diving reflex") may be tried in stable neonates. Direct pressure over the eyes should be avoided. Parenteral digitalization usually abolishes the arrhythmia within 10 hours. If digoxin successfully maintains the patient in sinus rhythm, it typically is continued for 6 to 12 months. Although digoxin has long been the mainstay of treatment for SVTs, reliance on this drug acutely has decreased, as more efficacious and faster-acting agents have become available.

Digoxin should probably be avoided in chronic management of WPW syndrome because of its potential for enhancing antegrade conduction across the accessory pathway. *Propranolol* may be used as the initial and chronic drug therapy for patients with SVTs due to the WPW syndrome, to avoid the potential facilitation of antegrade (atrioventricular) conduction through the accessory pathway, which is sometimes seen with digoxin. Treatment with *propranolol* may be associated with *apnea* and *hypoglycemia;* thus neonates started on propranolol, especially premature infants, should be observed with a continuous cardiac monitor and have serial serum glucose checks for several days.

The addition or substitution of other antiarrhythmic drugs such as sotalol, flecainide, quinidine, and amiodarone alone or in combination may be necessary and should be done only in consultation with a pediatric cardiologist. In neonates, *verapamil* should **only rarely be used** because it has been associated with *sudden death* in babies.

In utero SVT may be suspected when a very rapid fetal heart rate is noted by the obstetrician during prenatal care. The diagnosis can be

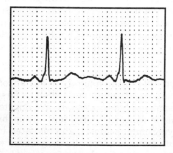

Fig. 25-19. Wolff-Parkinson-White syndrome. Note the characteristic "slurred" initial QRS deflection and short PR interval.

confirmed by fetal echocardiography. At that time, an initial search for congenital heart disease and fetal hydrops can be made (see Chaps. 1, 18). In utero treatment of the immature fetus with SVTs can be accomplished by treatment of the mother with antiarrhythmic drugs that cross the placenta. Digoxin, propranolol, procainamide, quinidine, and verapamil have been successful therapies. Failure to control fetal SVT in the presence of fetal hydrops is an indication for delivery. Cesarean delivery of an infant in persistent SVT may be necessary, as the fetal heart rate will not be a reliable indicator of fetal distress.

    b. Sinus tachycardia in the neonate is defined as a persistent heart rate greater than 2 standard deviations above the mean for age, with normal ECG complexes including a normal P-wave morphology and axis. Sinus tachycardia is common and occurs particularly in response to systemic events such as anemia, stress, fever, high levels of circulating catecholamines, hypovolemia, and xanthine (e.g., aminophylline) toxicity. An important clue to the existence of sinus tachycardia, in addition to its normal ECG morphology, is that the rate is not fixed but rather will vary by 10 to 20% over time. Medical management consists of identifying and treating the underlying cause.

2. Wide-complex tachycardias

    a. Ventricular tachycardia in the neonate is relatively rare and is usually associated with severe medical illnesses including hypoxemia, shock, electrolyte disturbances, digoxin toxicity, and catecholamine toxicity. It rarely is due to an abnormality of the electrical conducting system of the heart such as prolonged QT_c syndrome and intramyocardial tumors. Wide and frequently bizarre QRS complexes with a rapid rate are diagnostic; though this ECG pattern may be simulated by SVTs in patients with WPW syndrome, in whom there is antegrade conduction through the anomalous pathway (SVT with "aberration"). Ventricular tachycardia is a potentially unstable rhythm, commonly with hemodynamic consequences. The underlying cause should be rapidly sought and treated. The hemodynamically stable patient should be treated with a *lidocaine* bolus, 1 to 2 mg/kg, followed by a lidocaine infusion, 20 to 50 μg/kg per minute. Direct current cardioversion (starting dose to 1 to 2 watt-seconds/kg or 5 to 10 watt-seconds) should be used if the patient is hemodynamically compromised, though will frequently be ineffective in the presence of acidosis. Severe acidosis (pH < 7.2) should be treated with hyperventilation or sodium bicarbonate, or both, prior to cardioversion. Phenytoin, 2 to 4 mg/kg, may be effective if the arrhythmia is due to digoxin toxicity (see **VII.D**).

    b. Ventricular fibrillation in the neonate is almost always an agonal (preterminal) arrhythmia. There is a coarse irregular pattern on ECG with no identifiable QRS complexes. There are no peripheral pulses or heart sounds on examination. Cardiopulmonary resuscitation should be instituted and defibrillation (starting dose, 1 to 2 watt-seconds/kg or 5 to 10 watt-seconds) performed. A bolus of lidocaine, 1 mg/kg, followed by a lidocaine infusion should be started. Once the infant has been resuscitated, the underlying problems should be evaluated and treated.

3. Bradycardia

    a. Sinus bradycardia in the neonate is not uncommon, especially during sleep or during vagal maneuvers, such as bowel movements. If the infant's perfusion and blood pressure are normal, transient bradycardia is not of major concern. Persistent sinus bradycardia may be secondary to hypoxemia, acidosis, and elevated intracranial pressure. Finally, a stable sinus bradycardia may occur with digoxin toxicity, hypothyroidism, or sinus node dysfunction (usually a complication of cardiac surgery).

    b. Heart block

(1) First-degree atrioventricular block occurs when the PR interval is longer than 0.15 second. In the neonate, first-degree atrioventricular block may be due to a nonspecific conduction disturbance, medications (e.g., digoxin), myocarditis, hypothyroidism, or associated with certain types of congenital heart disease (e.g., complete atrioventricular canal or ventricular inversion). No specific treatment is generally indicated.

(2) Second-degree atrioventricular block refers to intermittent failure of conduction of the atrial impulse to the ventricles. Two types have been described: (i) Mobitz I (Wenckebach's phenomenon) and (ii) Mobitz II (intermittent failure to conduct P waves, with a constant PR interval). Second-degree atrioventricular block may occur with SVT, digitalis toxicity, or a nonspecific conduction disturbance. No specific treatment is usually necessary other than diagnosis and treatment of the underlying cause.

(3) Complete heart block (CHB) refers to **complete** absence of conduction of any atrial activity to the ventricles. CHB typically has a slow, constant ventricular rate that is independent of the atrial rate. CHB is frequently detected in utero as fetal bradycardia. Although CHB may be secondary to surgical trauma, **congenital** CHB falls into two main categories. The most common causes include (i) anatomic defects (ventricular inversion and complete atrioventricular canal) and (ii) fetal exposure to maternal antibodies related to systemic lupus erythematosus. The presence of CHB without structural heart disease should alert the clinician to investigate the mother for connective tissue disease.

Symptoms related to CHB are related to both the severity of the associated cardiac malformation (when present) and the degree of bradycardia. Fortunately, the fetus with CHB adapts well by increasing stroke volume, and will usually come to term without difficulty. Infants with isolated congenital CHB usually have a heart rate faster than 50 beats per minute, are asymptomatic, and grow normally.

4. Irregular rhythms

a. Premature atrial contractions (PACs, Fig. 25-20) are common in neonates, are usually benign, and do not require specific therapy. Most PACs result in a normal QRS morphology (see Fig. 25-20A), thus easily distinguishing them from premature ventricular contractions (PVCs). If the PAC occurs while the AV node is partially repolarized, an aberrantly conducted ventricular depolarization pattern may be observed on the surface ECG (see Fig. 25-20B). If the premature beat occurs when the AV node is refractory (i.e., early in the cardiac cycle, occurring soon after the normal sinus beat), the impulse will not be conducted to the ventricle ("blocked") and may thus give the appearance of a marked sinus bradycardia (see Fig. 25-20C).

b. PVCs are "wide-QRS-complex" beats that occur when a ventricular focus stimulates a spontaneous beat prior to the normally conducted sinus beat. Isolated PVCs are not uncommon in the normal neonate and do not generally require treatment. Although PVCs frequently occur sporadically, they occasionally are grouped, such as every other beat (bigeminy, Fig. 25-21A), every third beat (trigeminy), etc. These more frequent PVCs are typically no more worrisome than isolated PVCs, though their higher frequency usually prompts a more extensive diagnostic work-up. PVCs can be caused by digoxin toxicity, hypoxemia, electrolyte disturbances, and catecholamine or xanthine toxicity. PVCs occurring in groups of two or more (i.e., couplets, triplets, etc.; see Fig. 25-21B) are pathologic and "high grade"; they may be a marker for myocarditis or myocardial dysfunction and further evaluation should be strongly considered.

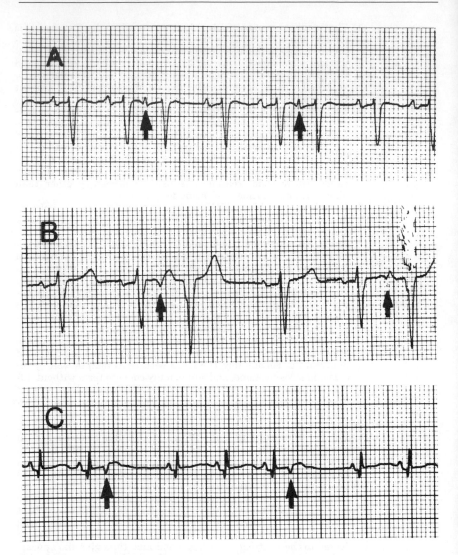

Fig. 25-20. Atrial premature beats (arrows) causing: **(A)** early ventricular depolarization with a normal QRS complex; **(B)** early ventricular depolarization with "aberration" of the QRS complex; **(C)** block at the atrioventricular node. From ref. 20 with permission.

C. **Emergency treatment of arrhythmia in the hemodynamically compromised patient.** With all therapies described below, it is important to have easily accessible resuscitation equipment available before proceeding with these antiarrhythmic interventions.

1. **Tachycardias**

   a. **Adenosine.** A relatively new pharmacologic agent for termination of SVT, adenosine has become the drug of choice for acute management.

A.

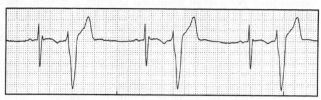

B.

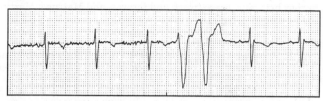

Fig. 25-21. Ventricular premature beats. **(A)** Ventricular premature beats alternating with normal sinus beats (ventricular bigeminy) are usually not indicative of significant pathology. **(B)** Paired ventricular premature beats ("couplet") are a potentially more serious rhythm and require further investigation.

Adenosine transiently blocks AV node conduction, allowing termination of rapid reentrant rhythms involving the AV node. It must be given by very rapid intravenous push since its half-life is 10 seconds or less. Owing to this short half-life, adenosine is a relatively safe medication; however, it has been reported to cause transient atrioventricular block severe enough to require pacing (albeit briefly) so it should be used with caution and in consultation with a pediatric cardiologist. Adenosine, by virtue of its acute action on the AV node, is frequently **diagnostic** as well. Patients who respond with abrupt termination of the SVT have reentrant tachycardias involving the AV node; those with SVT due to atrial flutter will have acute atrioventricular block and easily visible flutter waves with reappearance of SVT in 10 to 15 seconds.

   b. **Cardioversion.** In the hemodynamically unstable patient, the **first** line of therapy is synchronized direct current cardioversion. The energy should start at 1 watt-second and be increased by a factor of two if unsuccessful. Care should be taken to avoid skin burns and arcing of the current outside the body by only using electrical transmission gel with the paddles. The paddle position should be anterior-posterior if possible.

   c. **Transesophageal pacing.** When available, esophageal overdrive pacing is a very effective maneuver for terminating tachyarrhythmias. The close proximity of the left atrium to the distal esophagus allows electrical impulses generated in the esophagus to be transmitted to atrial tissue; burst pacing may then terminate reentrant tachyarrhythmias.

2. **Bradycardias.** Therapeutic options for treating a symptomatic bradyarrhythmia are somewhat more limited. A transvenous pacemaker is a temporary measure in severely symptomatic neonates while preparing

for placement of permanent epicardial pacemaker leads; however, transvenous pacing in a small neonate is technically difficult and frequently requires fluoroscopy. A number of transcutaneous pacemakers are available but long-term use must be avoided due to cutaneous burns. An isoproterenol infusion may temporarily increase the ventricular rate and cardiac output in an infant with congestive heart failure. The treatment of choice for sinus node dysfunction is transesophageal pacing at an appropriate rate, but this can only be accomplished with intact atrioventricular conduction and is not effective in patients with CHB. For the infant with transient bradycardia (due to increased vagal tone), intravenous atropine may be used.

Acknowledgments: The authors would like to thank Emily Flynn McIntosh for her help with the artwork and figures, and Matthew Martin and Tannis Bolton for secretarial assistance.

References

1. Aisenberg, R. B., et al. Developmental delay in infants with congenital heart disease: Correlation with hypoxemia and congestive heart failure. *Pediatr. Cardiol.* 3:133, 1982.
2. Allan, L. D., et al. Prospective diagnosis of 1,006 consecutive cases of congenital heart disease in the fetus. *J. Am. Coll. Cardiol.* 23:1452, 1994.
3. Benacerraf, B. R., et al. Fetal echocardiography. *Radiol. Clin. North Am.* 28:131, 1990.
4. Benitz, W. E., et al. Use of sodium nitroprusside in neonates: Efficacy and safety. *J. Pediatr.* 106:102, 1985.
5. Beverly, D. W., et al. Early use of sodium nitroprusside in respiratory distress syndrome. *Arch. Dis. Child.* 54:403, 1979.
6. Braudo, M., et al. Auscultation of the heart in the early neonatal period. *Am. J. Dis. Child.* 101:575, 1961.
7. Burke, R. P., et al. Video-assisted thoracoscopic surgery for congenital heart disease. *J. Thorac. Cardiovasc. Surg.* 109(3):499–507, 1995.
8. Castaneda, A. R., et al. *Cardiac Surgery of the Neonate and Infant.* Philadelphia: Saunders, 1994.
9. Castaneda, A. R., et al. The neonate with critical congenital heart disease: Repair—a surgical challenge. *J. Thorac. Cardiovasc. Surg.* 98:869, 1989.
10. Chang, A. C., et al. Management and outcome of low birth weight neonates with congenital heart disease. *J. Pediatr.* 124:461, 1994.
11. Chang, A. C., et al. Left heart support with a ventricular assist device in an infant with acute myocarditis. *Crit. Care Med.* 20:712, 1992.
12. Chang, A. C., et al. Management of the neonate with transposition of the great arteries and persistent pulmonary hypertension. *Am. J. Cardiol.* 68:1253, 1991.
13. Cohn, H. E., et al. Complications and mortality associated with cardiac catheterization in infants under one year: A prospective study. *Pediatr. Cardiol.* 6:123, 1985.
14. Colli, A. M., et al. Balloon dilation of critical valvar pulmonary stenosis in the first month of life. *J. Am. Coll. Cardiol.* 34(1):23, 1995.
15. DeMaso, D. R., et al. Psychological functioning in children with cyanotic heart defects. *J. Dev. Behav. Pediatr.* 11:289, 1990.
16. Egito, E. S. T., et al. Percutaneous balloon valvuloplasty as initial treatment for neonatal critical aortic stenosis: Long-term results. *J. Am. Coll. Cardiol.* 1994.
17. Ellison, R. C., et al. Evaluation of the preterm infant for patent ductus arteriosus. *Pediatrics* 71:364, 1983.
18. Emmanouilides, G. C., et al. (Eds.). *Moss and Adams' Heart Disease in Infants, Children, and Adolescents, Including the Fetus and Young Adult* (5th Ed.). Baltimore: Williams & Wilkins, 1994.
19. Fyler, D. C. Report of the New England Regional Infant Cardiac Program. *Pediatrics* 65(Suppl.):377, 1980.
20. Fyler, D. C. *Nadas' Pediatric Cardiology.* Philadelphia: Hanley & Belfus, 1992.

21. Gersony, W. M., et al. Effects of indomethacin in premature infants with patent ductus arteriosus: Results of a national collaborative study. *J. Pediatr.* 102:895, 1983.
22. Griffin, M. L., et al. Dilated cardiomyopathy in infants and children. *J. Am. Coll. Cardiol.* 11:139, 1988.
23. Hohn, A. R., et al. Myocarditis in children. *Pediatr. Rev.* 9(3):83, 1987.
24. Kirklin, J. W., et al. *Cardiac Surgery* (2d Ed.). New York: Churchill Livingstone, 1993.
25. Lang, P., et al. Hemodynamic Effects of Amrinone in Infants after Cardiac Surgery. In G. Crupi, L. Parenzan, and R. H. Anderson (Eds.), *Perspectives in Pediatric Cardiology.* Vol. 2, *Pediatric Cardiac Surgery,* part 2. Mount Kisco, NY: Futura, 1989. Pp. 292–295.
26. Lawless, S., et al. Amrinone pharmacokinetics in neonates and infants. *J. Clin. Pharmacol.* 28:283, 1988.
27. Lock, J. E., et al. *Diagnostic and Interventional Catheterization in Congenital Heart Disease.* Boston: Martinus Nijhoff, 1987.
28. Mahony, L., et al. Prophylactic indomethacin therapy for patent ductus arteriosus in very-low-birth-weight infants. *N. Engl. J. Med.* 306:506, 1982.
29. Matitiau, A., et al. Infantile dilated cardiomyopathy: Relation of outcome to left ventricular mechanics, hemodynamics and histology at the time of presentation. *Circulation* 91(5):1613, 1994.
30. Newburger, J. W., et al. Cognitive function and age at repair of transposition of the great arteries in children. *N. Engl. J. Med.* 310:1495, 1984.
31. Paul, M. H., et al. Transposition of the Great Arteries. In G. C. Emmanouilides, et al. (Eds.), *Moss and Adams' Heart Disease in Infants, Children, and Adolescents, Including the Fetus and Young Adult* (5th Ed.). Baltimore: Williams & Wilkins, 1994, 1154–1224.
32. Towbin, J. A. Molecular genetic aspects of cardiomyopathy. *Biochem. Med. Metab. Biol.* 49:285, 1993.
33. Wernovsky, G., et al. Intensive Care. In G. C. Emmanouilides, et al. (Eds.), *Moss and Adams' Heart Disease in Infants, Children, and Adolescents, Including the Fetus and Young Adult* (5th Ed.). Baltimore: Williams & Wilkins, 1994, 398–439.
34. Woolf, A. D., et al. The use of digoxin-specific Fab fragments for severe digitalis intoxication in children. *N. Engl. J. Med.* 326:1739, 1992.

26. HEMATOLOGIC PROBLEMS

Anemia
Helen A. Christou and David H. Rowitch

I. **Hematologic physiology of the newborn** [2,3,6,10,11]. Significant changes occur in the red blood cell (RBC) mass of an infant during the neonatal period and ensuing months. The evaluation of anemia must take into account this developmental process, as well as the infant's physiologic needs.
   A. **Normal development: The physiologic anemia of infancy** [2]
      1. In utero, the fetal aortic oxygen saturation is 45%; erythropoietin levels are high, RBC production is rapid, and reticulocyte values are 3 to 7%.
      2. After birth, the oxygen saturation is 95%, and erythropoietin is undetectable. RBC production by day 7 is less than one-tenth the level in utero. Reticulocyte counts are low, and the hemoglobin level falls (Table 26-1).
      3. Despite dropping hemoglobin levels, the ratio of hemoglobin A to hemoglobin F increases, and the levels of 2,3-diphosphoglycerate (2,3-DPG) (which interacts with hemoglobin A to decrease its affinity for oxygen, thus enhancing oxygen release to the tissues) are high. As a result, oxygen delivery to the tissues actually increases. This physiologic "anemia" is not a functional anemia in that oxygen delivery to the tissues is adequate. Iron from degraded red blood cells is stored.
      4. At 8 to 12 weeks, hemoglobin levels reach their nadir (Table 26-2), oxygen delivery to the tissues is impaired, erythropoietin production is stimulated, and RBC production increases.
      5. Infants who have received transfusions in the neonatal period have lower nadirs than normal because of their higher percentage of hemoglobin A [2].
      6. During this period of active erythropoiesis, iron stores are rapidly utilized. The reticuloendothelial system has adequate iron for 15 to 20 weeks in term infants. After this time, the hemoglobin level decreases if iron is not supplied.
   B. **Anemia of prematurity** is an exaggeration of the normal physiologic anemia (see Tables 26-1 and 26-2).
      1. RBC mass is decreased at birth, although the hemoglobin level is the same as in the term infant.
      2. The hemoglobin nadir is reached earlier than in the term infant because of the following:
         a. RBC survival is decreased in comparison with the term infant.
         b. There is a relatively more rapid rate of growth in premature babies than in term infants. For example, a premature infant gaining 150 gm per week requires approximately a 12-ml-per-week increase in total blood volume.
         c. Vitamin E deficiency is common in small premature infants, unless the vitamin is supplied exogenously.
      3. The hemoglobin nadir in premature babies is lower than in term infants because erythropoietin is produced by the term infant at a hemoglobin level of 10 to 11 gm/dl but is produced by the premature infant at a hemoglobin level of 7 to 9 gm/dl. This reflects the lower oxygen requirements in healthy preterm infants rather than a defect in erythropoietin production [2].
      4. Iron administration before the age of 10 to 14 weeks does not increase the nadir of the hemoglobin level or diminish its rate of reduction. However, this iron is stored for later use.

Table 26-1. Hemoglobin changes in babies in the first year of life

Week	Term babies	Hemoglobin level Premature babies (1200–2500 gm)	Small premature babies (< 1200 gm)
0	17.0	16.4	16.0
1	18.8	16.0	14.8
3	15.9	13.5	13.4
6	12.7	10.7	9.7
10	11.4	9.8	8.5
20	12.0	10.4	9.0
50	12.0	11.5	11.0

Source: From B. Glader and J. L. Naiman. Erythrocyte Disorders in Infancy. In H. W. Taeusch, R. A. Ballard, and M. E. Avery (Eds.), *Diseases of the Newborn*. Philadelphia: Saunders, 1991.

5. Once the nadir is reached, RBC production is stimulated, and iron stores are rapidly depleted because less iron is stored in the premature infant than in the term infant.

II. **Etiology of anemia in the neonate** [9]

A. Blood loss is manifested by a decreased or normal hematocrit, increased or normal reticulocyte count, and a normal bilirubin level (unless the hemorrhage is retained) [10,11]. If blood loss is recent (e.g., at delivery), the hematocrit and reticulocyte count may be normal and the infant may be in shock. The hematocrit will fall later as a result of hemodilution. If the bleeding is chronic, the hematocrit will be low, the reticulocyte count up, and the baby normovolemic.

1. **Obstetric causes of blood loss,** including malformations of placenta and cord:

a. Abruptio placentae

b. Placenta previa

c. Incision of placenta at cesarean section

d. Rupture of anomalous vessels (e.g., vasa previa, velamentous insertion of cord, or rupture of communicating vessels in a multilobed placenta)

e. Hematoma of cord caused by varices or aneurysm

f. Rupture of cord (more common in short cords and in dysmature cords)

2. **Occult blood loss**

a. **Fetomaternal bleeding** may be chronic or acute. It occurs in 8% of all pregnancies, and in 1% of pregnancies the volume may be as large as 40 ml. The diagnosis of this problem is by Kleihauer-Betke stain of

Table 26-2. Hemoglobin nadir in babies in the first year of life

Maturity of baby at birth	Hemoglobin level at nadir	Time of nadir
Term babies	9.5–11.0	6–12 wk
Premature babies (1200–2500 gm)	8.0–10.0	5–10 wk
Small premature babies (< 1200 gm)	6.5–9.0	4–8 wk

Source: From B. Glader and J. L. Naiman. Erythrocyte Disorders in Infancy. In H. W. Taeusch, R. A. Ballard, and M. E. Avery (Eds.), *Diseases of the Newborn*. Philadelphia: Saunders, 1991.

maternal smear for fetal cells [3]. Many conditions may predispose to this type of bleeding:

 (1) Placental malformations—chorioangioma or choriocarcinoma

 (2) Obstetric procedures—traumatic amniocentesis, external cephalic version, internal cephalic version, breech delivery

 (3) Spontaneous fetomaternal bleeding

b. Fetoplacental bleeding

 (1) Chorioangioma or choriocarcinoma with placental hematoma

 (2) Cesarean section, with infant held above the placenta

 (3) Tight nuchal cord or occult cord prolapse

c. Twin-to-twin transfusion

3. Bleeding in the neonatal period may be due to the following causes:

 a. Intracranial bleeding associated with

  (1) Prematurity

  (2) Second twin

  (3) Breech delivery

  (4) Rapid delivery

  (5) Hypoxia

 b. Massive cephalhematoma, subgaleal hemorrhage, or hemorrhagic caput succedaneum

 c. Retroperitoneal bleeding

 d. Ruptured liver or spleen

 e. Adrenal or renal hemorrhage

 f. Gastrointestinal bleeding

  (1) Peptic ulcer

  (2) Enterocolitis

  (3) Nasogastric catheter

  (4) Maternal blood swallowed from delivery or breast should be ruled out by the Apt test (see Bleeding).

 g. Bleeding from umbilicus

4. Iatrogenic causes. Excessive blood loss may result from blood sampling with inadequate replacement.

B. Hemolysis is manifested by a decreased hematocrit, increased reticulocyte count, and an increased bilirubin level [2,3].

1. Immune hemolysis (see Chap. 18)

 a. Rh incompatibility

 b. ABO incompatibility

 c. Minor blood group incompatibility (e.g., c, E, Kell, Duffy)

 d. Maternal disease (e.g., lupus), autoimmune hemolytic disease, rheumatoid arthritis (positive direct Coombs' test in mother and newborn, no antibody to common red cell antigen Rh, AB, etc.), or drugs (e.g., penicillin antibodies in mother or infant, child on penicillin [4]).

2. Hereditary RBC disorders

 a. RBC membrane defects such as spherocytosis, elliptocytosis, or stomatocytosis

 b. Metabolic defects—glucose-6-phosphate dehydrogenase (G6PD) deficiency (significant neonatal hemolysis due to G6PD deficiency is usually seen only in Mediterranean or Asian G6PD-deficient males; blacks in the United States have a 10% incidence of G6PD deficiency but rarely have significant neonatal problems unless an infection or drug is operative), pyruvate-kinase deficiency, 5'-nucleotidase deficiency, and glucose-phosphate isomerase deficiency.

 c. Hemoglobinopathies

  (1) Alpha- and gamma-thalassemia syndromes

  (2) Alpha- and gamma-chain structural abnormalities

3. Acquired hemolysis

 a. Infection—bacterial or viral

 b. Disseminated intravascular coagulation

 c. Vitamin E deficiency and other nutritional anemias [2]

     d. Microangiopathic hemolytic anemia—cavernous hemangioma, renal artery stenosis, and severe coarctation of the aorta

C. Diminished RBC production is manifested by a decreased hematocrit, decreased reticulocyte count, and normal bilirubin level (see Chap. 18).

1. **Diamond-Blackfan syndrome**
2. **Congenital leukemia** or other tumor
3. **Infections,** especially rubella and parvovirus (see Chap. 23)
4. **Osteopetrosis,** leading to inadequate erythropoiesis
5. **Drug-induced RBC suppression**
6. **Physiologic anemia or anemia of prematurity** (see I.A and B)

III. Diagnostic approach to anemia in the newborn (Table 26-3)

A. The **family history** should include questions about anemia, jaundice, gallstones, and splenectomy.

B. The **obstetric history** should be evaluated.

C. The **physical examination** may reveal an associated abnormality and provide clues to the **origin** of the anemia.

1. **Acute blood loss** leads to shock, with cyanosis, poor perfusion, and acidosis.
2. **Chronic blood loss** produces pallor, but the infant may exhibit only mild symptoms of respiratory distress or irritability.
3. **Chronic hemolysis** is associated with pallor, jaundice, and hepatosplenomegaly.

D. **Complete blood cell count.** Capillary blood samples are 3.7 to 2.7% higher than venous hematocrits. Warming the foot reduced the difference from 3.9 to 1.9% [2,3].

E. **Reticulocyte count** (elevated with chronic blood loss and hemolysis, depressed with infection and production defect)

F. **Blood smear** (see Table 26-3)

G. **Coombs' test and bilirubin level**

H. **Apt test** (see Bleeding) on gastrointestinal blood of uncertain origin

I. **Kleihauer-Betke preparation** of the mother's blood. A 50-ml loss of fetal blood into the maternal circulation will show up as 1% fetal cells in the maternal circulation [3].

J. **Ultrasound of abdomen and head**

K. **Test on parents**—complete blood cell count, smear, RBC indices, RBC enzymes (G6PD, pyruvate kinase)

L. **Studies for infection** (TORCH infection; see Chap. 23)

M. **Bone marrow** (rarely used except in cases of bone marrow failure from hypoplasia or tumor)

IV. Therapy

A. **Transfusion** (see Blood Products Used in the Newborn)

1. **Indications for transfusion.** The decision to transfuse must be made in consideration of the infant's condition and physiologic needs [13].

a. Infants with significant respiratory disease or congenital heart disease (e.g., large left-to-right shunt) may need their hematocrit maintained above 40%. Transfusion with adult RBCs provides the added benefit of lowered oxygen affinity, which augments oxygen delivery to tissues. Blood should be fresh (3 to 7 days old) to ensure adequate 2,3-DPG levels.

b. Healthy, asymptomatic newborns will self-correct a mild anemia, provided that iron intake is adequate.

c. Infants with ABO incompatibility who do not have an exchange transfusion may have protracted hemolysis and may require a transfusion several weeks after birth. If they do not have enough hemolysis to require treatment with phototherapy, they will usually not become anemic enough to need a transfusion.

d. Premature babies may be quite comfortable with hemoglobin levels of 6.5 to 7.0 mg/dl. The level itself is not an indication for transfusion. Sick infants (e.g., with sepsis, pneumonia, or bronchopulmonary dys-

Table 26-3. Classification of anemia in the newborn

Reticulocytes	Bilirubin	Coombs' test	RBC morphology	Diagnostic possibilities
Normal or ↓	Normal	Negative	Normal	Physiologic anemia of infancy or prematurity; congenital hypoplastic anemia; other causes of decreased production
Normal or ↑	Normal	Negative	Normal	Acute hemorrhage (fetomaternal, placental, umbilical cord, or internal hemorrhage)
			Hypochromic microcytes	Chronic fetomaternal hemorrhage
↑	↑	Positive	Spherocytes	Immune hemolysis (blood group incompatibility or maternal autoantibody)
Normal or ↑	↑	Negative	Spherocytes	Hereditary spherocytosis
			Elliptocytes	Hereditary elliptocytosis
			Hypochromic microcytes	Alpha- or gamma-thalassemia syndrome
			Spiculated RBCs	Pyruvate-kinase deficiency
			Schistocytes and RBC fragments	Disseminated intravascular coagulation; other microangiopathic processes
			Bite cells (Heinz bodies with supravital stain)	Glucose-6-phosphate dehydrogenase deficiency
			Normal	Infections; enclosed hemorrhage (cephalohematoma)

RBC = red blood cell; ↓ = decreased; ↑ = increased.
Source: Adapted from the work of Dr. Bertil Glader, Director of Division of Hematology-Oncology, Children's Hospital at Stanford, CA.

plasia) may require increased oxygen-carrying capacities and therefore need transfusion. Growing premature infants also may manifest a need for transfusion by exhibiting poor weight gain, apnea, tachypnea, or poor feeding [13]. Transfusion guidelines are shown in Table 26-4.

In our units when we instituted the practice of requiring parental permission for elective transfusion, the transfusion rate dropped markedly for premature infants.

2. **Blood products and methods of transfusion** (see Blood Products Used in the Newborn and ref. 2)

   a. **Packed RBCs.** The volume of transfusion may be calculated as follows:

   $$\frac{\text{Weight in kg} \times \text{blood volume per kilogram} \times (\text{hematocrit desired} - \text{hematocrit observed})}{\text{Hematocrit of blood to be given}}$$

   The average newborn blood volume is 80 ml/kg; the hematocrit of packed RBCs is 60 to 90% and should be checked prior to transfusion. We generally transfuse 15–20 ml/kg; larger volumes may need to be divided.

   b. **Whole blood** is indicated when there is acute blood loss.

Table 26-4. RBC transfusion guidelines for premature infants

Consider RBC transfusions in the following conditions:
1. For infants requiring significant mechanical ventilation, defined as FiO_2 >40%, and/or pressor support if the central hematocrit is ≤40% (hemoglobin ≤11 gm/dL).
2. For infants requiring minimal mechanical ventilation, with FiO_2 ≤35%, if the central hematocrit is ≤35% (hemoglobin ≤10 gm/dL).
3. For infants on supplemental oxygen who are not requiring mechanical ventilation, if the central hematocrit is ≤25% (hemoglobin ≤8 gm/dL), and one or more of the following is present:
   - ≥24 hours of tachycardia (heart rate >180) or tachypnea (RR >80)
   - An increased oxygen requirement from the previous 48 hours, defined as ≥4-fold increase in nasal cannula flow (i.e., 0.25 L/min to 1 L/min) or an increase in nasal CPAP ≥20% from the previous 48 hours (i.e., 5 cm to 6 cm H_2O)
   - Weight gain <10 gm/kg/day over the previous 4 days while receiving ≥100 kcal/kg/day
   - An increase in the number or severity of apnea and bradycardia (in general ≥10 spells, or ≥3 spells requiring bag mask ventilation, however, absolute number is up to individual interpretation)
   - Undergoing surgery
4. For infants **without any symptoms,** if the central hematocrit is ≤20% (hemoglobin <7 gm/dL) and the absolute reticulocyte count is <3%.
5. For infants with a cumulative blood loss of 10% or more of blood volume in 72 hour period when infant has significant cardiorespiratory illness if further blood sampling is anticipated. Stable infants are not transfused only to replace blood lost through phlebotomy. If an erythrocyte transfusion is not given, "blood out" may be replaced cc for cc with 0.9% saline when 10–15 ml of blood per kg body weight is reached, in order to avoid hypovolemia. In addition to the saline used for the above indication, clinicians may administer additional albumin, fresh frozen plasma, platelet transfusions, or WBC transfusions, as they deem clinically indicated.

Whenever possible, RBC transfusions should be 15 to 20 cc/kg, divided in 2 aliquots if necessary.

c. **Exchange transfusion** with packed RBCs may be required for severely anemic infants, when routine transfusion of the volume of packed RBCs necessary to correct the anemia would result in circulatory overload (see Chap. 18).

d. **Irradiated** (5000 rads) [12] or **frozen RBCs** may be used if there is concern about the immunocompetence of the infant, and are recommended in premature infants weighing less than 1200 gm. Premature infants may be unable to reject foreign lymphocytes in transfused blood. We use irradiated blood for all neonatal transfusions. **Leukocyte depletion** with third-generation transfusion filters has substantially reduced the risk of exposure to foreign lymphocytes and cytomegalovirus (CMV) [1,10]. Frozen RBCs probably reduce the incidence of transfusion-related infection. In the past we used only blood from CMV-negative donors for neonatal transfusion. We now use blood treated by prestorage leukodestruction as approved by the American Association of Blood Banks for prevention of CMV infection.

e. **Directed-donor transfusion** is requested by many families. Irradiation of directed-donor cells is especially important, given the HLA compatibility among first-degree relatives and the enhanced potential for foreign lymphocyte engraftment.

B. **Prophylaxis**

1. **Term infants** should be sent home from the hospital on iron-fortified formula (2 mg/kg per day) if they are not breast-feeding [5].

2. **Premature infants** (preventing or ameliorating the anemia of prematurity). The following is a description of our usual nutritional management of premature infants from the point of view of providing RBC substrates and preventing additional destruction:

a. **Iron** supplementation in the preterm infant prevents late iron deficiency [7]. We routinely supplement iron in premature infants at a dose of 2 to 4 mg of elemental iron per kilogram per day once full enteral feeding is achieved (see Chap. 10).

b. **Mother's milk** or formulas similar to mother's milk in that they are low in linoleic acid are used to maintain a low content of polyunsaturated fatty acids in the RBCs [6].

c. **Vitamin E** (15 to 25 IU of water-soluble form) is given daily until the baby is 38 to 40 weeks' postconceptional age (this is usually stopped at discharge from the hospital).

d. These infants should be followed carefully, and additional iron supplementation may be required.

e. Methods and hazards of transfusion are in this chapter, Blood Products Used in the Newborn.

f. **Recombinant human erythropoietin** offers promise in ameliorating the anemia of prematurity [8,13,14]. While studies in which we participated showed that recombinant human erythropoietin may decrease the frequency and volume of RBC transfusions administered to premature infants, we have not yet used it as a routine procedure [2,8,13–16].

References

1. Andreu, G. Role of leucocyte depletion in the prevention of transfusion-induced cytomegalovirus infection. *Sem. in Hematol.* 28(Suppl. 5):26, 1991.
2. Bifano, E. M., and Ehrenkranz, Z. (Eds.). Perinatal hematology. *Clin. Perinatol.* 23(3), 1995.
3. Blanchette, V., et al. Hematology. In G. B. Avery (Ed.), *Neonatology* (4th Ed.). Philadelphia: Lippincott, 1994. Chap. 45;952.
4. Clayton, E. M., et al. Penicillin antibody as a cause of positive direct antiglobulin tests. *Am. J. Clin. Pathol.* 44:648, 1965.
5. Committee on Nutrition AAP. Iron-fortified infant formulas. *Pediatrics* 84:1114, 1989.

6. Glader, B., and Naiman, J. L. Erythrocyte Disorders in Infancy. In H. W. Taeusch, R. A. Ballard, and M. E. Avery (Eds.), *Diseases of the Newborn.* Philadelphia: Saunders, 1991.

7. Hall, R. T., et al. Feeding iron-fortified premature formula during initial hospitalization to infants less than 1800 grams birthweight. *Pediatrics* 92:409, 1993.

8. Maier, R. F., et al. The effect of epoietin beta (recombinant human erythropoietin) on the need for transfusion in very low-birth-weight infants. European Multicentre Erythropoietin Study Group. *N. Engl. J. Med.* 330:1173, 1994.

9. Molteni, R. A. Prenatal blood loss. *Pediatr. Rev.* 12:47, 1990.

10. Nathan, D. G., and Oski, F. A. *Hematology of Infancy and Childhood.* Philadelphia: Saunders, 1992.

11. Oski, F. A., and Naiman, J. L. *Hematologic Problems in the Newborn* (3rd Ed.). Philadelphia: Saunders, 1982.

12. Parkman, R., et al. Graft-versus-host disease after intrauterine and exchange transfusions for hemolytic disease of the newborn. *N. Engl. J. Med.* 290:359, 1974.

13. Ross, M. P., et al. A randomized trial to develop criteria for administering erythrocyte transfusions to anemic preterm infants 1 to 3 months of age. *J. Perinatol.* 9:246, 1989.

14. Shannon, K. M., et al. Recombinant human erythropoietin stimulates erythropoiesis and reduces erythrocyte transfusions in preterm infants. *Pediatrics* 95:1, 1995.

15. Straus, R. G. Erythropoietin and neonatal anemia (Editorial). *N. Engl. J. Med.* 330:1227, 1994.

16. Willmas, J. A. Erythropoietin—Not yet a standard treatment for anemia of prematurity. *Pediatrics* 95:9, 1995.

Bleeding
Allen M. Goorin and John P. Cloherty

The hemostatic mechanism in the neonate differs from that in the older child. In neonates there is decreased activity of certain clotting factors, impaired platelet function, and suboptimal defense against clot formation. References 4, 6, 9, and 10 are reviews of this subject.

I. Etiology
A. Deficient clotting factors
1. **Transitory deficiencies** of the vitamin K-dependent factors II, VII, IX, and X and protein C are characteristics of the newborn period and may be accentuated by the following:
   a. The administration of total parenteral alimentation or antibiotics or the lack of administration of vitamin K to premature infants.
   b. **Term infants** may develop vitamin K deficiency by day 2 or 3 if they are not supplemented with vitamin K parenterally, because of negligible stores and inadequate intake.
   c. **The mother** may have received certain drugs during pregnancy that can cause bleeding in the first 24 hours of the infant's life.
      (1) Phenytoin (Dilantin), phenobarbital, and salicylates interfere with the vitamin K effect on synthesis of clotting factors.
      (2) Coumadin compounds given to the mother interfere with the synthesis of vitamin K–dependent clotting factors by the livers of both the mother and the fetus, and the bleeding may **not** be immediately reversed by administration of vitamin K.
2. **Disturbances of clotting** may be related to associated diseases such as **disseminated intravascular coagulation (DIC)** due to infection, shock, anoxia, necrotizing enterocolitis, renal vein thrombosis, or the use of vascular catheters. Any significant liver disease may interfere with the production of clotting factors by the liver.

   a. Extracorporeal membrane oxygenation in neonates (ECMO). Thirteen
      of 135 patients on ECMO required surgical procedures related to com-
      plications of bleeding [2]. The administration of aminocaproic acid, an
      inhibitor of fibrinolysis, appears to decrease the incidence of intracra-
      nial and other hemorrhagic complications [12] (see Chap. 24).
 3. Inherited abnormalities of clotting factors
   a. Sex-linked recessive (expressed in males)
      (1) Factor VIII clotting activity and factor VIII procoagulant antigen
          are decreased in the fetus with classic hemophilia.
      (2) Christmas disease is due to an inherited quantitative deficiency of
          plasma thromboplastin component (PTC) (factor IX).
   b. Autosomal dominant (expressed in boys and girls with one parent
      affected)
      (1) Von Willebrand's disease involves decreased levels of factor VIII
          and platelet dysfunction due to decreased platelet adhesiveness.
      (2) Dysfibrinogenemia is due to fibrinogen (factor I) dysfunction.
      (3) Factor XI [plasma thromboplastin antecedent (PTA)] deficiency
          (see **c.4**).
   c. Autosomal recessive (occurs in both boys and girls; the parents are
      carriers)
      (1) Deficiencies of factors V, VII, X, XII, and XIII. (Factor XIII defi-
          ciency appears to be inherited as an X-linked trait in some kin-
          dreds.)
      (2) Prothrombin (factor II) or fibrinogen (factor I) deficiency.
      (3) Dysprothrombinemia due to an abnormal factor II.
      (4) Factor XI or PTA deficiency is incompletely recessive and is often
          classified as autosomal dominant, since heterozygotes will have
          some minor bleeding problems.
      (5) Variants of von Willebrand's disease.
 B. **Platelet problems** (see Thrombocytopenia)
 1. **Qualitative disorders** include hereditary conditions [e.g., Glanzmann's
    disease (thromboasthenia)] and disorders that result from the mother's
    use of aspirin.
 2. **Quantitative disorders** include immune disorders, infective dissemi-
    nated intravascular coagulation, congenital megakaryocytic hypoplasia,
    leukemia, inherited thrombocytopenia, giant hemangiomas, hyperviscos-
    ity, renal vein thrombosis, and necrotizing enterocolitis (see Thrombocy-
    topenia).
 C. **Other causes of bleeding** include **vascular problems** such as central ner-
    vous system hemorrhage, pulmonary hemorrhage, A-V malformations, and
    hemangiomas.
 D. **Miscellaneous problems**
 1. **Trauma** (see Chap. 20)
   a. Rupture of spleen or liver associated with breech delivery
   b. Retroperitoneal or intraperitoneal bleeding may present as scrotal ec-
      chymosis
   c. Subdural hematoma, cephalhematoma, or subgaleal hemorrhage (the
      latter may be associated with vacuum extraction)
 2. **Liver dysfunction**
II. **Diagnostic workup of the bleeding infant**
 A. The **history** includes (a) family history of excessive bleeding or clotting, (b)
    maternal medications (aspirin, phenytoin), (c) information about the preg-
    nancy and the birth, (d) maternal history of a previous birth of an infant
    with a bleeding disorder, and (e) any illness, medication, anomalies, or pro-
    cedures done to the infant.
 B. **Examination.** The crucial decision in diagnosing and managing the bleeding
    infant is determining whether the infant is sick or well (Table 26-5).
 1. **Sick infant.** Consider DIC, infection, or liver disease (vascular injury in-
    duced by hypoxia may lead to DIC).

Table 26-5. Differential diagnosis of bleeding in the neonate

Clinical evaluation	Laboratory studies			Likely diagnosis
	Platelets	PT	PTT	
"Sick"	D−	I+	I+	DIC
	D−	N	N	Platelet consumption (infection, necrotizing enterocolitis, renal vein thrombosis)
	N	I+	I+	Liver disease
	N	N	N	Compromised vascular integrity (associated with hypoxia, prematurity, acidosis, hyperosmolality)
"Healthy"	D−	N	N	Immune thrombocytopenia, occult infection, thrombosis, bone marrow hypoplasia (rare) or bone marrow infiltrative disease
	N	I+	I+	Hemorrhagic disease of newborn (vitamin K deficiency)
	N	N	I+	Hereditary clotting factor deficiencies
	N	N	N	Bleeding due to local factors (trauma, anatomic abnormalities); qualitative platelet abnormalities (rare); factor XIII deficiency (rare)

Key: PT = prothrombin time; PTT = partial thromboplastin time; D− = decreased; I+ = increased; DIC = disseminated intravascular coagulation; N = normal.
Source: Modified from B. E. Glader and M. D. Amylon. Bleeding Disorders in the Newborn Infant. In H. W. Taeusch, R. A. Ballard, and M. E. Avery (Eds.), *Diseases of the Newborn.* Philadelphia: Saunders, 1991.

2. **Well infant.** Consider vitamin K deficiency, isolated clotting factor deficiencies, or immune thrombocytopenia.
3. **Petechiae, small superficial ecchymosis, or mucosal bleeding** suggest a platelet problem.
4. **Large bruises** suggest deficiency of clotting factors, DIC, liver disease, or vitamin K deficiency.
5. **Enlarged spleen** suggests congenital infection or erythroblastosis.
6. **Jaundice** suggests infection or liver disease.
7. **Abnormal retinal findings** suggest infection (see Chap. 23).
C. **Laboratory tests** (Table 26-6)
   1. **The Apt test** is used to rule out maternal blood. If the child is well and only gastrointestinal bleeding is noted, an Apt test is performed on gastric aspirate or stool to rule out the presence of maternal blood swallowed during labor or delivery or from a bleeding breast. A breast pump can be used to collect milk to confirm the presence of blood in the milk, or the infant's stomach can be aspirated before and after breast-feeding.
      a. **Procedure.** Mix 1 part bloody stool or vomitus with 5 parts water; centrifuge it and separate the clear pink supernatant (hemolysate); add 1 ml of sodium hydroxide 1% to 4 ml of hemolysate.
      b. **Result.** Hemoglobin A (HbA) changes from pink to yellow brown (maternal blood); HbF stays pink (fetal blood).
   2. **Blood smear** is used to determine the number, size, and kind of platelets and the presence of fragmented red blood cells as seen in DIC. Large platelets are young platelets and imply an immune cause of thrombocytopenia.
   3. **Platelet count.** The platelet count from the smear equals the number of platelets from 10 oil-immersion fields times 1000. A platelet count also should be performed on the mother if the infant's count is decreased. Sig-

Table 26-6. Normal values for laboratory screening tests in the neonate

Laboratory test	Premature infant having received vitamin K	Term infant having received vitamin K	Child over 1 to 2 months of age
Platelet count/μl	150,000–400,000	150,000–400,000	150,000–400,000
Platelets on peripheral blood smear	10–20/Platelets/oil-immersion field, including 1 or 2 small clumps	Same as premature infant	Same as premature infant
PT (sec.)*	14–22	13–20	12–14
PTT (sec.)*	35–55	30–45	25–35
Fibrinogen (mg/dl)	150–300	150–300	150–300

Key: PT = prothrombin time; PTT = partial thromboplastin time.
*Normal values may vary from laboratory to laboratory, depending on the particular reagent employed. In full-term infants who have received vitamin K, the PT and PTT values generally fall within the normal "adult" range by several days (PT) to several weeks (PTT) of age. Small premature infants (under 1500 gm) tend to have longer PT and PTT than larger babies. In infants with hematocrit levels greater than 60%, the ratio of blood to anticoagulant (sodium citrate 3.8%) in tubes should be 19 : 1 rather than the usual ratio of 9 : 1; otherwise, spurious results will be obtained, since the amount of anticoagulant solution is calculated for a specific volume of plasma. Blood drawn from heparinized catheters should not be used. The best results are obtained when blood from a clean venipuncture is allowed to drip directly into the tube from the needle or scalp vein set. Factor levels II, VII, IX, and X are decreased. Three-day-old full-term baby not receiving vitamin K has levels similar to a premature baby. Factor XI and XII levels are lower in preterm infants than in term infants and account for prolonged PTT. Fibrinogen, factor V, and factor VII are normal in premature and term infants. Factor XIII is variable.
Source: Data from normal laboratory values at the Hematology Laboratory, The Children's Hospital, Boston; J. B. Alpers and M. T. Lafonet (Eds.), *Laboratory Handbook*. Boston: The Children's Hospital, 1984.

nificant bleeding from thrombocytopenia is usually associated with platelet counts under 20,000 to 30,000/μl.

4. **Prothrombin time (PT)** is a test of (1) the extrinsic clotting system, (2) the activation of factor X by factor VII, and (3) factors VI, X, V, and II and fibrinogen.

5. **Partial thromboplastin time (PTT)** is a test of the intrinsic clotting system and of the activation of factor X by factors XII, XI, IX, and VIII. PTT is also a test of the final coagulation pathway (factors V and II and fibrinogen).

6. **Fibrinogen** can be measured on the same sample used for PTT. It may be decreased in liver disease.

7. **Fibrin split products (FSP)** are degradation products of fibrin and fibrinogen found in the sera of patients with DIC and in patients with liver disease who have problems clearing FSP. Improper collection of blood will result in increased FSP in the sample.

8. ***d*-Dimer test.** This replaces the FSP in some laboratories. *d*-Dimers are formed from the action of plasmin on the fibrin clot, generating derivatives of cross-linked fibrin containing *d*-dimer. Normal levels are less than 0.5 μg/ml. Levels are higher in DIC, deep vein thrombosis, and pulmonary embolism.

9. **Bleeding time.** This test measures platelet quantity and quality, as well as vascular integrity. It is useful to diagnose von Willebrand's disease and functional platelet disorders. The template bleeding time is 3.4 ±1.3 minutes for preterm infants.

III. Treatment of neonates with abnormal bleeding parameters who have not had clinical bleeding: In one study, preterm infants with respiratory distress syndrome (RDS) or term infants with asphyxia were treated for abnormal bleeding parameters (without DIC) to correct the hemostatic defect. Although the treatment was successful in correcting the defect, no change in mortality was seen in comparison with controls [11].

In general, we treat clinically ill infants or infants weighing less than 1500 gm with fresh-frozen plasma (10 ml/kg) if the PT or PTT or both are greater than two times normal or with platelets (1 unit) (see **IV.C**) if the platelet count is under 20,000/µl (see Thrombocytopenia and Blood Products Used in the Newborn).

IV. Treatment of bleeding

A. Vitamin K₁ oxide (Aquamephyton). An intravenous dose of 1 mg is administered in case the infant was not given vitamin K at birth. Infants receiving total parenteral nutrition and infants receiving antibiotics for more than 2 weeks should be given 0.5 mg of vitamin K_1 IM or IV weekly to prevent vitamin K depletion. Vitamin K should be given before transfusion therapy is begun, since it takes several hours to work and should not be forgotten.

B. Fresh-frozen plasma (see Blood Products Used in the Newborn) (10 ml/kg) is given intravenously for active bleeding and is repeated every 8 to 12 hours as needed. This is used because it replaces the clotting factors immediately.

C. Platelets (see Thrombocytopenia). If there is no increased platelet destruction (as a result of DIC, immune platelet problem, or sepsis), 1 unit of platelets given to a 3-kg infant will raise the platelet count to 50,000 to 100,000/µl. If no new platelets are made or transfused, the platelet count will drop slowly over 3 to 5 days. If available, platelets from the mother or from a known platelet-compatible donor should be used if the infant has an alloimmune platelet disorder. The blood of the donor should be matched for Rh factor and type and washed, since red blood cells will be mixed in the platelet concentrates. In our nurseries, platelets are irradiated before transfusion.

D. Fresh whole blood (see Blood Products Used in the Newborn). The baby is given 10 ml/kg; more is given as needed. Fresh blood should be used for exchange transfusion, since it removes antibodies and provides fresh platelets and clotting factors.

E. Clotting factor concentrates (see Blood Products Used in the Newborn). When there is a known deficiency of factor VIII or IX, the plasma concentration needs to be raised to 20% of normal to stop serious bleeding. 10 ml/kg of fresh-frozen plasma will do this. If a higher plasma concentration is desired, factor concentrates or cryoprecipitate must be used to avoid volume overload.

F. Diagnosis and treatment should be aimed at the underlying cause (e.g., infection, liver rupture, catheter, or enterocolitis).

G. Treatment of specific disorders

1. **Disseminated intravascular coagulation (DIC).** The baby usually appears sick and may have petechiae, gastrointestinal hemorrhage, oozing from venipunctures, infection, asphyxia, or hypoxia. The platelet count is decreased, and PT and PTT are increased. Fragmented red blood cells (RBCs) are seen on the blood smear. Fibrinogen is decreased, and FSPs or d-dimers are increased. Treatment involves the following steps:

a. The underlying cause should be treated (e.g., sepsis, necrotizing enterocolitis, herpes).

b. Vitamin K_1, 1.0 mg IV, is given.

c. Platelets and fresh-frozen plasma are given as needed to keep the platelet count over 50,000/µl and to stop the bleeding.

d. If the bleeding persists, one of the following steps should be taken, depending on the availability of blood, platelets, or fresh-frozen plasma:

    (1) Exchange transfusion with fresh citrated whole blood or packed cells mixed with fresh-frozen plasma

    (2) Transfusion with platelets and fresh-frozen plasma

    (3) Administration of cryoprecipitate (10ml/kg)

  e. If DIC is associated with thrombosis of large vessels, heparin is given as a bolus of 25 to 35 units/kg, followed by 10 to 15 units/kg per hour as a continuous infusion. Platelets and plasma are continued after the heparin has been started. Platelet counts should be kept at or above 50,000/μl. The aim of heparin treatment is to keep the PTT at 1.5 to 2 times normal. See Major Arterial and Venous Thrombosis Management for treatment of thrombosis.

2. **Hemorrhagic disease of the newborn (HDN)** occurs in 1 of every 200 to 400 neonates not given vitamin K prophylaxis.

  a. In the healthy infant, hemorrhagic disease of the newborn may occur when the infant is not given vitamin K. The infant may have been born in a busy delivery room, at home, or transferred from elsewhere. Bleeding and bruising may occur after the infant is 48 hours old. The platelet level is normal, and PT and PTT are prolonged. If there is active bleeding, 10 ml/kg of fresh-frozen plasma and an IV dose of 1 mg of vitamin K are given.

  b. If the mother has been treated with phenytoin (Dilantin), primidone (Mysoline), methsuximide (Celontin), or phenobarbital, the infant may be vitamin K deficient and bleed during the first 24 hours. The mother should be given vitamin K 24 hours prior to delivery (10 mg of vitamin K_1 IM). The newborn should have PT, PTT, and platelet counts monitored if any signs of bleeding occur. The usual dose of vitamin K_1 (1 mg) should be given to the baby post partum and repeated in 24 hours. Repeated infusions of fresh-frozen plasma are given if any bleeding occurs.

  c. **Delayed hemorrhagic disease** of the newborn can occur at 4 to 12 weeks of age. This may happen in breast-fed infants who are not receiving supplementation. Infants who are undergoing treatment with broad-spectrum antibiotics or infants with malabsorption (liver disease, cystic fibrosis) are at greater risk of hemorrhagic disease. Vitamin K_1, 1 mg/week orally for the first 3 months of life, may prevent late hemologic disease of the newborn. An oral preparation like that used in Europe has not yet been approved in the USA. Although blood tests show that breast-fed infants are at potential risk for HDN, HDN has not been reported in infants who received intramuscular vitamin K at birth (see comments from Fanaroff [3]). Concerns about an increased risk of childhood cancer after neonatal administration of vitamin K have proved unfounded [5,7,8].

References
1. Andrew, M. The homeostatic system in the infant. In: D. G. Nathan and F. A. Oski (Eds.), *Hematology of Infancy and Childhood,* 4th ed. Philadelphia: W. B. Saunders, 1993.
2. Atkinson, J. B., et al. Major surgical intervention during extracorporeal membrane oxygenation. *J. Pediatr. Surg.* 27(9):1197, 1992.
3. Fanaroff, A. A. *Yearbook of Neonatal and Perinatal Medicine.* St. Louis: Mosby, 1994; 330.
4. Glader, B. E., et al. Hemostatic disorders in the newborn. In: H. W. Taeusch, R. A. Ballard, and M. E. Avery (Eds.), *Shaffer and Avery's Disease of the Newborn,* 6th ed. Philadelphia: W. B. Saunders, 1991.
5. Green, F. R. Vitamin K deficiency and hemorrhage in infancy. *Clin. Perinatol.* 22:759, 1995.
6. Hawiger, J., Handin, R. I., Soff, G. A., Rosenberg, R. D., Beardsley, D. S., and Montgomery, R. R. Hemostasis. In: D. G. Nathan and F. A. Oski (Eds.), *Hematology of Infancy and Childhood,* 4th ed. Philadelphia: W. B. Saunders, 1993.

7. Klaus, M. H. Editorial comment. In: *Yearbook of Neonatal and Perinatal Medicine.* St. Louis: C. V. Mosby, 1994; 380.

8. Klebanoff, M. A., et al. The risk of childhood cancer after neonatal exposure to vitamin K. *N. Engl. J. Med.* 329:905, 1993.

9. Oski, F. A., et al. *Hematologic Problems in the Newborn,* 3rd ed. Philadelphia: W. B. Saunders, 1982.

10. Pramanik, A. K. Bleeding disorders in neonates. *Pediatr. Rev.* 13:163, 1992.

11. Turner, T. Treatment of premature infants with abnormal clotting parameters. *Br. J. Hematol.* 47:65, 1981.

12. Wilson, J. M., et al. Aminocaproic acid decreases the incidence of intracranial hemorrhage and other hemorrhagic complications in ECMO. *J. Pediatr. Surg.* 28:536, 1993.

Polycythemia
Allen M. Goorin

As the central (venous) hematocrit rises, there is increased viscosity and decreased blood flow; when the hematocrit increases to more than 60%, there is a fall in oxygen transport [6] (Fig. 26-1). Newborns have erythrocytes that are less deformable than the erythrocytes of adults. As viscosity increases, there is impairment of tissue oxygenation and decreased glucose in plasma, and a tendency to form microthrombi. If these events occur in the cerebral cortex, kidneys, or adrenal glands, significant damage may result. Hypoxia and acidosis increase viscosity and deformity further. Poor perfusion increases the possibility of thrombosis.

I. Definitions
A. Polycythemia: venous hematocrit of over 65% [5], a venous hematocrit over 64% or more at 2 hours of age [14], an umbilical venous or arterial hematocrit over 63% or more [14]. The mean venous hematocrit of term infants is 53 in cord blood, 60 at 2 hours of age, 57 at 6 hours of age, and 52 at 12 to 18 hours of age [14].

B. Hyperviscosity is defined as greater than 14.6 centipoise at a shear rate of 11.5 sec^{-1} as measured by a viscometer [13]. The relationship of hematocrit and viscosity is nearly linear below a hematocrit of 60%, but viscosity increases exponentially at a hematocrit of 70% or greater (Fig. 26-1) [6,12].

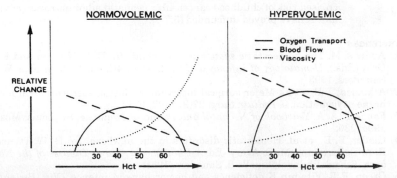

Fig. 26-1. Effect of hematocrit on viscosity, blood flow, and oxygen transport. (Adapted from B. Glader and J. L. Naiman. Erythrocyte disorders in infancy. In: H. W. Taeusch, R. A. Ballard, and M. E. Avery (Eds.). *Diseases of the newborn.* Philadelphia: Saunders, 1991; 823.

Other factors may alter viscosity. These include plasma proteins, especially fibrinogen, and local blood flow [14]. The hyperviscosity syndrome is usually seen only in infants with venous hematocrits above 60.

II. Incidence. The incidence of polycythemia in newborns is increased in babies who are small for gestational age and in postterm babies; on average it is 0.4 to 5% [10,14,15].

III. Causes of polycythemia [14]

   A. Placental red cell transfusion

      1. Delayed cord clamping may occur either intentionally or in unattended deliveries.

        a. When the cord is clamped within 1 minute after birth, the blood volume of the infant is 83.4 ml/kg.

        b. When the cord is clamped 2 minutes after delivery, the blood volume of the infant is 93 ml/kg.

        c. In newborns with polycythemia, blood volume per kilogram of body weight varies inversely in relation to birth weight (Fig. 26-2).

      2. Cord stripping (thus pushing more blood into the infant).

      3. Holding the baby below the mother at delivery.

      4. Maternal-to-fetal transfusion is diagnosed with the Kleihauer-Betke stain technique of acid elution to detect maternal cells in the newborn circulation (see Anemia).

      5. Twin-to-twin transfusion (see Chap. 7).

      6. Forceful uterine contractions before cord clamping.

   B. Placental insufficiency (increased fetal erythropoiesis secondary to chronic intrauterine hypoxia)

      1. Small-for-gestational-age infants

      2. Maternal hypertension syndromes (toxemia, renal disease, etc.)

      3. Postmature infants

      4. Infants born to mothers with chronic hypoxia (heart disease, pulmonary disease)

      5. Pregnancy at high altitude

      6. Maternal smoking

   C. Other conditions

      1. Infants of diabetic mothers (increased erythropoiesis)

      2. Some large-for-gestational-age babies

      3. Infants with congenital adrenal hyperplasia, Beckwith-Wiedemann syndrome, neonatal thyrotoxicosis, congenital hypothyroidism, trisomy 21, trisomy 13, trisomy 18

      4. Drugs (maternal use of propranolol)

      5. Dehydration of infant

IV. Clinical findings: Most infants with polycythemia are asymptomatic. Clinical symptoms, syndromes, and laboratory abnormalities that have been described in association with polycythemia include the following:

   A. CNS: poor feeding, lethargy, hypotonia, apnea, seizures, cerebral venous thrombosis

   B. Cardiorespiratory: cyanosis, tachypnea, heart murmurs, congestive heart failure, cardiomegaly, elevated pulmonary vascular resistance, prominent vascular markings on chest x-ray

   C. Renal: renal vein thrombosis, hematuria, proteinuria

   D. Other: other thrombosis, thrombocytopenia, poor feeding, increased jaundice, persistent hypoglycemia, testicular infarcts, necrotizing enterocolitis, priapism, disseminated intravascular coagulation

   All of these symptoms may be associated with polycythemia/hyperviscosity but may not be caused by it. They are common symptoms in many neonatal disorders.

V. Screening: The routine screening of all newborns for polycythemia/hyperviscosity is being advocated by some authors [16]. The timing and site of blood sampling alter the hematocrit value [12, 13]. We do not routinely screen well term newborns for this syndrome, since there are few data showing that treatment of asymptomatic patients with partial exchange transfusion is beneficial in the long term [1,5,14].

VI. **Diagnosis:** The capillary blood or peripheral venous hematocrit level should be determined in any baby who appears plethoric, who has any predisposing cause of polycythemia, who has any of the symptoms mentioned in IV, or who is not well for any reason.

   A. Depending on local perfusion, the **capillary blood hematocrit** will be 5 to 20% higher than the central hematocrit [14]. Warming the heel prior to drawing blood for a capillary hematocrit determination will give a better correlation with the peripheral venous or central hematocrit. If the capillary blood hematocrit is above 65%, the peripheral venous hematocrit should be determined. The hematocrit should be measured with an automated hematology analyzer. Most of the old studies of hematocrits were done with spun hematocrits, which may give falsely high levels [14].

   B. Few hospitals are equipped to measure blood viscosity. If the equipment is available the test should be done, because some infants with venous hematocrits under 65% will have hyperviscous blood [15].

VII. **Management**

   A. Any child with symptoms that could be due to hyperviscosity should have a partial exchange transfusion if the peripheral **venous hematocrit** is more than 65%.

   B. **Asymptomatic infants** with a peripheral venous hematocrit between 60 and 70% can usually be managed by increasing fluid intake and repeating the hematocrit in 4 to 6 hours.

   C. Most neonatologists perform an exchange transfusion when the peripheral venous hematocrit is more than 70% in the absence of symptoms, but this is controversial [1,2,5,10,11].

   D. The following formula can be used to calculate the exchange with albumin 5% or normal saline that will bring the hematocrit to 50%. In infants with polycythemia, the blood volume varies inversely with the birth weight (see Fig. 26-2). We usually take the blood from the umbilical vein and replace it with albumin 5% or normal saline in a peripheral vein. There are many methods of exchange (see Chap. 18).

   Volume of exchange (in ml)

   $$= \frac{\text{observed hematocrit} - \text{desired hematocrit} \times \text{body weight (kg)} \times 80 \text{ ml}}{\text{observed hematocrit}}$$

   Example: A 3-kg infant, hematocrit 75%, blood volume 80 ml/kg—to bring hematocrit to 50%:

   $$\text{Volume of exchange (in ml)} = \frac{(80 \text{ ml} \times 3 \text{ kg}) \times (75 - 50)}{75}$$

   $$= \frac{240 \text{ ml} \times 25}{75}$$

   $$= 80\text{-ml exchange}$$

   The total volume exchanged is usually 15 to 20 ml/kg of body weight. This will depend on the observed hematocrit. (Blood volume may be up to 100 ml/kg in polycythemic infants.)

VIII. **Outcome**

   A. Infants with polycythemia and hyperviscosity who have decreased cerebral blood flow velocity and increased vascular resistance develop normal cerebral blood flow following partial exchange transfusion [10]. They also have improvement in systemic blood flow and oxygen transport [1,11,13,14].

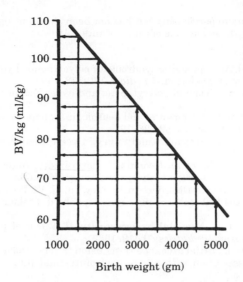

Fig. 26-2. Nomogram designed for clinical use, correlating blood volume per kilogram with birth weight in polycythemic neonates. BV, blood volume. From J. S. Rawlings, et al. Estimated blood volumes in polycythemic neonates as a function of birth weight. *J. Pediatr.* 101:594, 1982.

B. The long-term neurologic outcome in infants with asymptomatic polycythemia/hyperviscosity, whether treated or untreated, remains controversial.

  1. One trial with small numbers of randomized patients has shown decreased IQ scores in school-aged children who had neonatal hyperviscosity syndrome, whether or not the newborns were treated [3,5].

  2. Another retrospective study, with small numbers of patients, showed no difference in the neurologic outcome of patients with asymptomatic neonatal polycythemia, whether they were treated or not [9].

  3. Some earlier preliminary prospective studies favored treatment [2,7].

  4. A small prospective study showed no difference at follow-up between control infants and those with hyperviscosity, between those with symptomatic and asymptomatic hyperviscosity, and no difference between asymptomatic infants treated with partial exchange transfusion and those who were observed. Analysis revealed that other perinatal risk factors and race, rather than polycythemia or partial exchange transfusion, significantly influenced the long-term outcome [1,14].

  5. An increased incidence of necrotizing enterocolitis following partial exchange transfusions by umbilical vein has been reported [2,4]. Enterocolitis was not seen in one retrospective analysis of 185 term polycythemic babies given partial exchange transfusions with removal of blood from the umbilical vein and reinfusion of a commercial plasma substitute through peripheral veins [8].

  6. A large prospective, randomized clinical trial comparing partial exchange transfusion with symptomatic care (increased fluid intake, etc.) equally balanced for risk factors and the etiologies of the polycythemia will be necessary to give guidelines for treatment of the asymptomatic newborn with polycythemia/hyperviscosity.

  7. Partial exchange transfusion will lower hematocrit, decrease viscosity, and reverse many of the physiologic abnormalities associated with polycythemia/hyperviscosity but has not been shown to significantly change the long-term outcome of these infants [14].

References

1. Bada, H., et al. Asymptomatic syndrome of polycythemic hyperviscosity: Effect of partial plasma transfusion. *J. Pediatr.* 120:578, 1992.
2. Black, V. D., et al. Neonatal polycythemia and hyperviscosity. *Ped. Clin. N. Am.* 5:1137, 1982.
3. Black, V. D., et al. Developmental and neurologic sequelae in neonatal hyperviscosity syndrome. *Pediatrics* 69:426, 1982.
4. Black, V. D., et al. Gastrointestinal injury in polycythemic term infants. *Pediatrics* 76:225, 1985.
5. Delaney-Black, V. D., et al. Neonatal hyperviscosity: Association with lower achievement and IQ scores at school age. *Pediatrics* 83:662, 1989.
6. Glader, B. Erythrocyte Disorders in Infancy. In: H. W. Taeusch, R. A. Ballard, M. E. Avery (Eds.). *Diseases of the Newborn,* 6th ed. Philadelphia: W. B. Saunders, 1991.
7. Goldberg, K., et al. Neonatal hyperviscosity. II. Effect of partial plasma exchange transfusion. *Pediatrics* 69:419, 1982.
8. Hein, H. A., et al. Partial exchange transfusion in term, polycythemic neonates: Absence of association with severe gastrointestinal injury. *Pediatrics* 80:75, 1987.
9. Host, A., et al. Late prognosis in untreated neonatal polycythemia with minor or no symptoms. *Acta Paediatr. Scand.* 71:629, 1982.
10. Oski, F. A., and Naiman, J. L. *Hematologic Problems in the Newborn,* 3rd ed. Philadelphia: W. B. Saunders, 1982, 87–96.
11. Phibbs, R. H., et al. Hematologic problems. In: M. H. Klaus and A. A. Fanaroff (Eds.). *Care of the High Risk Neonate.* Philadelphia: W. B. Saunders, 1993, 421.
12. Ramamurthy, R. S. J., et al. Postnatal alteration in hematocrit and viscosity in normal and polycythemic infants. *J. Pediatr.* 110:929, 1987.
13. Swernam, S. M., et al. Hemodynamic consequences of neonatal polycythemia. *J. Pediatr.* 110:443, 1987.
14. Wexner, E. J. Neonatal polycythemia and hyperviscosity. *Clin. Perinatol.* 22:693, 1995.
15. Wirth, F. H., et al. Neonatal hyperviscosity I. Incidence. *J. Pediatr.* 63:833, 1979.
16. Wiswell, T. E., et al. Neonatal polycythemia: Frequency of clinical manifestations and other associated findings. *Pediatrics* 78:26, 1986.

Thrombocytopenia
Jed B. Gorlin and Allen M. Goorin

Neonatal thrombocytopenia is a platelet count of less than 150,000/mm³. The causes include increased consumption or decreased production (rare). Consumption may be caused by antibodies, mechanical problems, or intravascular coagulation. The incidence in the general neonatal population is small (approximately 0.1% of cord bloods had counts <50,000), and most neonates with thrombocytopenia have only a modest reduction in platelet counts (50,000–100,000). These are generally self resolved [5]. More serious reductions, under 20,000, or 50,000 with bleeding, warrant evaluation and intervention.

In contrast, thrombocytopenia in the neonatal intensive care unit is quite common. Indeed, in one prospective study, thrombocytopenia developed in 22% of 807 NICU admissions. The etiology in about 80% of cases is generally consumptive. This is particularly true for sick infants, in whom thrombocytopenia may represent just part of a spectrum of consumptive coagulopathy [18]. The most severe sequelae of severe thrombocytopenia, such as intracranial hemorrhage, are associated with alloimmunization or are related to the degree of prematurity.

Thrombocytopenia may precede delivery. A recent retrospective review observed an incidence of approximately 5% of thrombocytopenia in fetal blood samplings.

Congenital infections or chromosomal disorders accounted for almost half of these (reflecting the indications for the fetal blood sampling itself). Antibody-mediated causes included both maternal autoimmune and alloimmune conditions [11].

I. **Diagnosis** (Fig. 26-3)
  A. **Maternal history.** There may be a history of thrombocytopenia, bleeding before or during pregnancy, a previous splenectomy, drug use, or infection. A history of pre- or postnatal bleeding in a previous pregnancy is important.
  B. **Infant.** The baby may seem healthy or may appear sick. There may be petechiae or large bruises, hepatosplenomegaly, jaundice, limb enlargement, hemangioma, or bruits [3].
  C. **Laboratory studies**
    1. **Mother:** needs to have a platelet count and platelet typing (if the maternal count is normal).
    2. **Baby:** complete blood count (CBC), platelet count, prothrombin time (PT), and partial thromboplastin time (PTT).
II. **Therapy**
  A. **Platelet transfusion**
    1. **Indications**
      a. When bleeding or platelets <20,000: There have been few prospective controlled trials of the best time to transfuse platelets in neonates. One attempt randomized sick preterm infants to conventional therapy (typically keeping platelets >50,000) vs. maintaining platelets >150,000 with 1 to 3 transfusions) over the first week of life. There was no difference in the rate of intracranial hemorrhage in either group [2].
      b. This confirms that routine platelet transfusion does not help in severe prematurity, but it does not address the minimum number to which platelet counts should be allowed to fall.
    2. **Source.** Use a random donor, except for the infant with alloimmune thrombocytopenia. In this case, use the mother's platelets after appropriate testing (washed to remove the alloantibody) or platelets from a platelet antigen–compatible donor.
    3. **Quantity.** One unit of platelets per 3 kg raises the platelet count by 50,000 to 100,000/ml, unless there is peripheral destruction of the platelets.

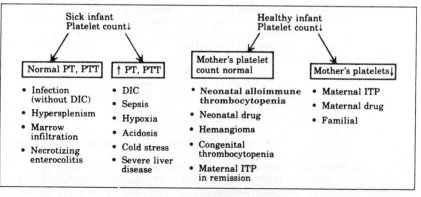

Fig. 26-3. Clinical status in neonatal thrombocytopenia with features that determine a quick differential diagnosis. PT, prothrombin time; PTT, partial thromboplastin time; DIC, disseminated intravascular coagulation; ITP, immune thrombocytopenic purpura; ↑, increase; ↓, decrease.

4. **Frequency.** The normal half-life of platelets is 4 to 5 days; it is shorter if there is increased platelet consumption.
5. **Route.** Give platelets intravenously through a peripheral vein. **Never give platelets through an arterial line or into the liver (umbilical line) because thrombosis may occur.**
6. Irradiate **platelet transfusions** if using a relative as donor, if the infant is premature (<1200 gm) or suspected to be immunocompromised. We irradiate **all** platelet transfusions for newborns.

B. **Steroid therapy** in bleeding infants. Prednisone 2 mg/kg per day may reduce bleeding.

C. In an emergency, whole blood may be used for exchange transfusion.

III. **Thrombocytopenia with decreased platelet survival**

A. **Immune**

In immune thrombocytopenias (ITP), maternal antibody crosses the placenta, resulting in destruction of neonatal platelets. Considerable amounts of antibody may cross, resulting in thrombocytopenias that persist for several weeks. It is called an AUTOAntibody when the antibody is directed against an antigen on the mother's own platelets shared in common with the baby's platelets. ALLOAntibodies are antibodies directed against antigens on the baby's platelets (and, perforce, paternal platelets) but not present on maternal platelets.

1. **Auto-maternal ITP**

These include various autoimmune syndromes such as systemic lupus erythematosus (SLE).

a. **Clinical picture:** the baby usually has mild to moderate thrombocytopenia (20,000 to 50,000) and is healthy, but has petechiae or bruising. There may be increased bruising at the vitamin K injection site or bleeding at circumcision or heel stick sites. The mother usually has thrombocytopenia or a history of ITP.

b. **Pathophysiology:** Maternal autoantibodies cross the placenta and bind to neonatal platelets. A normal maternal platelet count does not rule out this cause, as the maternal count may reflect compensated increased destruction. Although it is rare, one center had 11 mothers with normal platelet counts, in whom alloimmune differences were excluded, who delivered 17 infants with severe thrombocytopenia. In 10 of these 11, the center was able to identify a maternal autoanti–GP1b antibody and subsequently demonstrate compensated maternal thrombocytolysis or hypersplenism [20]. This may be more common if the mother has had a splenectomy. Elicit a **maternal history** of thrombocytopenia or symptoms of autoimmune syndromes. Maternal thrombocytopenia at delivery is common (about 7% of women at delivery have platelet counts <150,000). Almost all infants born to women with thrombocytopenia are either unaffected or have mild to moderate reductions that are self-resolving. Only one of 756 of infants born to women with incidental thrombocytopenia, 5 of 1414 with hypertension and 4 of 46 with ITP had cord blood platelet counts less than 50,000, and all of them were over 20,000 and without sequelae [5]. Identification of autoantibody on maternal platelets is not sufficient to diagnose an autoimmune cause. There was elevated platelet-associated IgG (not directed against Gp1b) in the serum of about 1/3 of mothers of infants with documented anti–HPAa1 alloimmune thrombocytopenia [14].

c. **Treatment** of autoimmune thrombocytopenia

(1) **Prenatal management:** Even if the mother has true ITP, it appears that fetal hemorrhage in utero is very rare (compared with the small but definite risk of such hemorrhage in alloimmune thrombocytopenia [5,7]). One uncontrolled study [10] showed a 3.6-fold increase in neonatal platelet counts following **steroid** administration to mothers with ITP and positive antiplatelet antibodies.

Prednisone, 10 to 20 mg qd, was given for 10 to 14 days prior to delivery. A small prospective randomized trial of low-dose betamethasone (1.5 mg orally per day from day 259 to day 273 and 1 mg until delivery) failed to prevent thrombocytopenia in newborns [9]. These discrepant data need further study before steroid administration becomes routine practice. **Intravenous IGG** given prenatally to the mother with ITP has not been clearly shown to affect the fetal platelet count. **Percutaneous umbilical blood sampling (PUBS)** is beginning to be used as a safe, accurate, and direct method of obtaining the fetal platelet counts. In experienced hands, the mortality from this procedure is less than 1% [7]. This may still be too great a risk for cases of maternal ITP (see Chap. 1, Assessment and Prenatal Diagnosis). There may be little correlation between fetal and maternal platelet counts. Mothers who have had recent platelet counts under 80,000, who are on steroids, or who have had a splenectomy are at increased risk to have a child with significant thrombocytopenia. Since a **cesarean section** reduces trauma to the infant, it would decrease the risk of bleeding in the occasional infant who is severely thrombocytopenic. The issue of when to do cesarean section in mothers known to have ITP is controversial. The maternal mortality from cesarean sections in most centers is the same as from vaginal deliveries. Our usual management of these cases is to allow vaginal delivery to progress until a fetal scalp platelet count can be done. If the fetal scalp platelet count is over 50,000 and labor is progressing normally, the infant is delivered vaginally. If these criteria are not met, then a cesarean section is done. One should remember that obstetricians would like a maternal platelet count of 50,000 to 100,000 before they are willing to operate, and anesthesiologists are often unwilling to give epidural anesthesia to mothers with platelet counts under 100,000. The use of steroids, IGG, PUBS, or cesarean sections in the prenatal management of maternal ITP is controversial and requires cooperation between the obstetrician, neonatalogist, hemotologist, and family. These therapies are not usually required in maternal ITP [3,13].

    (2) Postnatal treatment of infants affected by maternal ITP may include platelet transfusion, steroids, IGG, or exchange transfusion (treatment is as in Bleeding, **III, IV**).

2. Alloimmune thrombocytopenia

    Maternal serum that shows antibodies that react against the father's but not against the mother's own platelets demonstrates an alloantibody. Of 19 fetuses known to be at risk for alloimmune thrombocytopenia (typically because of severely affected siblings from a prior delivery) 6 had platelet counts under 20,000 and three suffered intracranial bleeding episodes, two of which were antenatal [5]. Hence, alloimmune thrombocytopenia, although uncommon, when present may result in severe hemorrhagic complications in utero. We have seen one mother who had recurrent episodes of severe fetal hemorrhage. A majority of cases are secondary to antiHPA1 (P1^{A-1}) antibody; however, there are also numerous other antigens as targets (Table 26-7) [8].

    a. Clinical picture. The baby appears healthy but has petechiae, bruising, bleeding, and a low platelet count (often <20,000). The mother has a normal platelet count; it may be her first pregnancy, or she may have a history of a previously affected pregnancy. There may be a history of alloimmune thrombocytopenia in children born to the mother's sisters.

    b. Pathophysiology: Approximately 97% of Caucasians are HPA-1a+ and, hence about 3% of pregnancies involve an HPA-1a negative mother carrying an HPA-1a positive fetus. Roughly one in 1000 to

Table 26-7.   Platelet-specific alloantigen systems

New HPA nomenclature	Original designations	Caucasian phenotype frequency	Clinical alloimmune syndromes described
HPA-1a	Zw^a, P1^{A1}	0.97	NAIT, PTP, PTR, PAT, TAT
HPA-1b	Zw^b, P1^{A2}	0.27	NAIT, PTP, PTR
HPA-2a	Ko^b	0.992	
HPA-2b	Ko^a, Sib^a	0.169	NAIT, PTR
HPA-3a	Bak^a, Lek^a	0.85	NAIT, PTP
HPA-3b	Bak^b, Lek^b	0.66	NAIT, PTP, PTR
HPA-4a	Pen^a, Yuk^b	>0.999	NAIT, PTP
HPA-4b	Pen^b, Yuk^a	<0.0001	NAIT
HPA-5a	Br^b, Zav^b	0.99	NAIT
HPA-5b	Br^a, Zav^a, Hc^a	0.21	NAIT, PTP, PTR, PAT
HPA-6b	Tu^a, Ca	<0.007	NAIT
HPA-7b	Mo^a	<0.002	NAIT
HPA-8b	Sr^a	<0.01	NAIT
	P1^{E1}	0.999	—
	P1^{E2}	0.05	NAIT
	Gov^a	0.81	NAIT, PTP
	Gov^b	0.74	
	Va^a	<0.004	NAIT
	Nak^a GPIV isoantibody	0.9966	PTR

NAIT = neonatal alloimmune thrombocytopenia; PTP = post-transfusion purpura; PTR = platelet transfusion refractoriness; PAT = passive alloimmune thrombocytopenia; TAT = transplant-associated thrombocytopenia; HPA = human platelet antigen.
From Burrows, R. F., and Kelton, J. G. Prenatal thrombocytopenia. *Clin. Perinatol.* 22:779, 1995.

5000 deliveries are affected; therefore, 3% of pregnancies at risk are actually affected [5,6]. There is a link between maternal production of alloantibodies and HLA type DR-3; there may be other factors that also regulate maternal antibody formation [4]. Virtually all identified platelet antigens have been implicated in neonatal alloimmune thrombocytopenia [16]. In one series of 295 patients with suspected neonatal alloimmune thrombocytopenia referred to a platelet serology reference laboratory, only 36% were found to have platelet specific antibody. Two-thirds of them were anti-HPA-1a directed, and 4% anti-HPA-3a [19]. Twenty-four percent revealed only HLA antibodies, although the presence of an anti-HLA antibody does not prove that the antibody resulted in the thrombocytopenia.

   c. **Diagnostic evaluation:** DNA techniques that define platelet-specific polymorphisms add to the diagnostic armamentarium but do not eliminate the usefulness of serological techniques [15]. The identification of numerous polymorphisms, including those in Table 26-7, makes the role of a centralized platelet serology laboratory paramount [17]. The Blood Center of Southeastern Wisconsin (1-800-245-3117), Tom Kickler (Johns Hopkins, Baltimore, Maryland), and Scott Murphy (Temple University, Philadelphia, Pennsylvania) have excellent labs providing outside diagnostic services. Proper identification of the cause of the thrombocytopenia may be more important for the proper management of future pregnancies than for acute treatment of the thrombocytopenic infant. In cases of paternal heterozygosity, amniocentesis will identify the platelet antigen genotype of the fetus [8]. Although controversial, the antenatal treatment of alloimmune thrombocytopenia with PUBS (percutaneous umbilical cord blood sampling) and administration of IVIG to the mother may affect the natural history of a disorder associated with intracranial hemorrhage during the third trimester [6,8,14].

Infusion of maternal compatible platelets at the time of cordocentesis may decrease the incidence of hemorrhage during the procedure.

DNA testing is performed on 1 to 5 ml of the mother's and the infant's (or, alternatively, the father's) blood. Serologic testing typically requires testing of both maternal and paternal platelets, as testing of the affected infant's platelets generally proves impossible because of thrombocytopenia. Again, not all infants of HPA-a1 (P1A1)-negative women with documented anti-HPA-a1 (P1A1) Ab are thrombocytopenic; use caution when interpreting treatment results of such "high-risk" women [4].

d. **Treatment**

(1) **Prenatal treatment**

Intravenous gammaglobulin, steroids, prenatal (by PUBS) platelet transfusion, fetal scalp platelet counts in labor, and elective cesarean section should be considered as management tools on a case-by-case basis with cooperation between the obstetrician, neonatologist, and hematologist. If the fetal platelet count is over 50,000/ml as measured by PUBS or fetal scalp platelet count, we allow **vaginal delivery** if presentation and labor are normal. If these criteria are not met, a **cesarean section** is done.

(2) **Postnatal treatment** (see II)

(a) **Platelet transfusion**

If the diagnosis is known to be alloimmune neonatal thrombocytopenia, the mother's platelets are collected 24 hours prior to delivery. If the baby has a platelet count of less than 20,000/ml, or if the baby shows any signs of bleeding, the mother's platelets (P1A1 negative) are transfused into the baby. The mother's serum will have P1A1 positive antibody, which potentially can react with the newborn's platelets. Using washed maternal platelets resuspended in plasma will avoid this complication. If there is an emergency secondary to bleeding in the newborn, and the mother's platelets have not been previously collected, either the mother's whole blood or platelets from a previously typed P1A1 negative platelet donor can be used. Random platelets should be used if there is serious bleeding and P1A1 negative platelets are not available. To avoid the possibility that the infant will develop **graft-versus-host (GVH) disease**, the blood products should be irradiated (see Blood Products Used in the Newborn).

Apheresis services are generally not necessary, as a single unit of antigen negative platelets should give a 50,000 to 100,000 boost. By collecting the platelet-rich plasma from the mother and reinfusing the red blood cells to the mother, there can be multiple collections over the ensuing several days. While an apheresis unit could be obtained and aliquoted to achieve a platelet supply for up to 5 days of transfusions, it is unclear that this benefits the patient [13].

(b) **Gamma-globulin (IGG)**

There has been successful postnatal use of intravenous IGG 0.4 gm/kg per day for 2 to 5 days [1,7].

(c) **Prednisone**

Usually, 2 mg/kg per day is given to newborns with continued low platelet counts or continued bleeding [7].

(3) Treatment of additional children
It is important to make the diagnosis for other children and to refer the family to a high-risk center for additional pregnancies. Sisters of P1^A1-negative mothers should have platelet typing done to anticipate problems. If they are P1^A1-negative and their husbands are P1^A1-positive, anticipatory planning is indicated. Three platelet serology laboratories are The Blood Center of Southeastern Wisconsin (1-800-245-3117), Tom Kickler (Johns Hopkins, Baltimore, Maryland), and Scott Murphy's lab (Temple University, Philadelphia, Pennsylvania).

(4) Outcome
Roughly 20% of all infants with identified cases of neonatal alloimmune thrombocytopenia (NAIT) have intracranial hemorrhages. As many as half occur antenatally. We have seen two fetal deaths with bleeding associated with fetal alloimmune thrombocytopenia. Obtain a **cranial ultrasound study** after delivery to document any intracranial bleeding, since intracranial hemorrhages are sometimes clinically silent.

3. Drug-induced
Although a long list of drugs is associated with neonatal thrombocytopenia, it is unclear how many of them are the true cause. If the mother has an antibody that results in thrombocytopenia by immune mechanisms, the infant may become thrombocytopenic if given the same medication. (Treatment is as in Bleeding, **III, IV**)

B. Peripheral consumption of platelets
1. Disseminated intravascular coagulation (DIC) (see Bleeding)
  a. Clinical picture: The infant appears sick and has thrombocytopenia, a prolonged PT, and a prolonged PTT. There is a decrease in fibrinogen, and an increase in split products or in d-dimers.
  b. Therapy
    (1) Treat the underlying disorder (e.g., sepsis, acidosis, hypoxia, or hypothermia). Give vitamin K and replace clotting factors and platelets.
    (2) Perform exchange transfusion with fresh whole blood for patients with active bleeding that does not respond to repeated plasma and platelet transfusions.
2. Giant hemangioma (Kasabach-Merritt syndrome) [3]
  a. Clinical picture: The baby appears healthy and has a large hemangioma and thrombocytopenia.
  b. Therapy involves platelet transfusion, clotting factors, and prednisone. Most hemangiomas involute by 1 to 2 years of age, so attempt medical management. We and others have had good results treating some of these hemangiomas with alpha interferon. Embolization or surgery is sometimes necessary.
3. Necrotizing enterocolitis (see Chap. 32)
  a. Clinical picture: thrombocytopenia with necrotizing enterocolitis.
  b. Therapy: Treat the underlying disorder and give platelet transfusions as necessary.
4. Type IIB Von Willebrand's disease may present as thrombocytopenia secondary to platelet aggregation in newborns [10].
C. Direct toxic injury to platelets
1. Sepsis may be of bacterial or viral origin. Therapy involves treatment of the underlying disorder. Platelet transfusion is necessary if there is bleeding.
  a. Thrombocytopenia as an early sign of sepsis in newborns is nonspecific, although high mean platelet volume and high platelet distribution widths correlated with late sepsis.
  b. There is some evidence that an immune mechanism may be involved in the thrombocytopenia of neonatal sepsis.

2. **Drug injury:** Thiazides, tolbutamide, hydralazine, and aspirin have been implicated. Therapy involves the removal of the offending drug, and platelet transfusion if there is bleeding. **Maternal ingestion** of aspirin during pregnancy should be avoided. If ingestion occurs within 1 week of delivery, 90% of newborns will have bleeding tendencies. Maternal use of aspirin has been associated with a reduced mean birth weight of the offspring, prolongation of gestation and labor, increased blood loss at delivery, and increased perinatal mortality [3].

3. **Neonatal cold injury:** Massive pulmonary hemorrhage secondary to hyperaggregation of platelets has been associated with infants who die while being rewarmed.

D. **Hypersplenism**
1. **Clinical picture:** The baby has an enlarged spleen and thrombocytopenia; there may or may not be hemolytic anemia. The condition is associated with congenital hepatitis, congenital viral infection, and portal vein thrombosis.
2. **Therapy:** Treat the underlying disorder. Administer platelet transfusion if there is bleeding. Splenectomy is the last resort for uncontrollable bleeding.

E. **Familial shortened platelet survival** results from intrinsic problems with platelets. Production also may be abnormal.
1. **Wiskott-Aldrich syndrome** is manifested by the presence of abnormal, small platelets.
2. **May-Hegglin anomaly** is an autosomal dominant disorder in which the infant has giant, bizarre platelets with Doehle bodies, abnormal platelet survival, and impaired production of platelets.
3. **Bernard-Soulier syndrome** is demonstrated by large platelets with granules clumped to appear as a nucleus.

IV. **Thrombocytopenia with normal platelet survival and decreased platelet production.**
A. **Toxic injury to megakaryocytes** due to bacterial or viral infections or drug-induced injury.
B. **Congenital thrombocytopenias** due to syndrome of thrombocytopenia with absent radii, Fanconi's anemia, familial thrombocytopenias, or marrow aplasia, which may be isolated or general.
C. **Marrow infiltration** due to neonatal leukemia, congenital neuroblastoma, or storage disease.

V. **Thrombocytopenia associated with erythroblastosis fetalis:** The mechanism may possibly involve platelet trapping in the liver and spleen, anoxia with secondary intravascular coagulation, or associated antiplatelet antibodies.

VI. **Thrombocytopenia after exchange or other transfusion:** Blood more than 24 hours old has few viable platelets.

VII. The management of a high-risk fetus requires orchestration of interventional obstetricians, reference lab, and comprehensive blood bank services. A review of platelet problems in the newborn is found in ref. 3.

References

1. Amato, M., et al. Treatment of neonatal thrombocytopenia. *J. Pediatr.* 107:650, 1985.
2. Andrew, M., et al. A randomized, controlled trial of platelet transfusions in thrombocytopenic premature infants. *Pediatrics* 123:285, 1993.
3. Beardsley, D. S. Platelet abnormalities in infancy and childhood. In: D. G. Nathan and F. A. Oski (Eds.). *Hematology of Infancy and Childhood,* 4th ed. Philadelphia: W. B. Saunders, 1992.
4. Blanchette, V. S., et al. Alloimmunization to the P1A1 platelet antigen: Results of a prospective study. *Br. J. Haematol.* 74:209, 1990.
5. Burrows, R. F. Fetal thrombocytopenia and its relation to maternal thrombocytopenia. *N. Engl. J. Med.* 329:1463, 1993.
6. Burrows R. F., et al. Perinatal thrombocytopenia. *Clin. Perinatol.* 22:779, 1995.

7. Bussel, J. B., et al. Recommendations for the evaluation and treatment of neonatal autoimmune and alloimmune thrombocytopenia. *Thrombosis Haemostasis* 65:631, 1991.

8. Bussel J. B., et al. Fetal alloimmune thrombocytopenia. *N. Engl. J. Med.* 337:23, 1997.

9. Christiaens, G. C., et al. Idiopathic thrombocytopenic purpura in pregnancy: A randomized trial on the effect of antenatal low dose corticosteroids on neonatal platelet counts. *Br. J. Obstet. Gynaecol.* 97:893, 1990.

10. DeCarolis, S., et al. Immune thrombocytopenic purpura and percutaneous umbilical blood sampling: An open question. *Fetal Diagnos. Ther.* 8:154, 1993.

11. Hohlfeld, P., et al. Fetal thrombocytopenia: A retrospective survey of 5,194 fetal blood samplings. *Blood* 84:1851, 1994.

12. Karpatkin, M. Platelet counts in infants of women with autoimmune thrombocytopenia: Effect of steroid administration to the mother. *N. Engl. J. Med.* 305:936, 1981.

13. Kaplan, C., et al. Fetal and neonatal alloimmune thrombocytopenia: Current trends in diagnosis and therapy. *Transfusion Med.* 2:265, 1992.

14. Kickler, T. S. Elevated platelet-associated IgG in PLA1-negative mothers following sensitization to the PLA-1 antigen during pregnancy. *Vox Sanguinus* 63:210, 1992.

15. McFarland, J. G., et al. Prenatal diagnosis of neonatal alloimmune thrombocytopenia using allele-specific oligonucleotide probes. *Blood* 78:2276, 1991.

16. Menell, J. S., et al. Antenatal management of the thrombocytopenias. *Clin. Perinatol.* 21:591, 1994.

17. Pao, M., et al. Importance of platelet serologic testing for defining the cause of neonatal thrombocytopenia. *Am. J. Pediatr. Hematol. Oncol.* 13:71, 1991.

18. Schmidt, B. K. Coagulation screening in high risk neonates: A prospective cohort study. *Arch. Dis. Child.* 67:1196, 1992.

19. Schnell, M., et al. Serologic investigation of 295 cases of suspected neonatal alloimmune thrombocytopenia. *Transfusion* 34:16S-abstracts64, 1994.

20. Tchernia, G., et al. Neonatal thrombocytopenia and hidden maternal autoimmunity. *Br. J. Haematol.* 84:457, 1993.

Blood Products Used in the Newborn [9,19,23,30]
Sherwin V. Kevy

I. Products and components

A. Whole blood. Three different anticoagulants are available: citrate-phosphate-dextrose (CPD), CPD with adenine (CPD A-1), and CPD with a nutrient solution (one of which contains adenine and mannitol, the other adenine and additional glucose). Heparinized blood is no longer available.

1. Contents of 1 unit of whole blood [23,28]

a. Total volume is 510 ml; red cell volume is 210 ml, and plasma volume is 300 ml.

b. Sodium citrate, 1.66 gm; dextrose, 1.61 gm; citric acid, 206 mg; and sodium biphosphate, 140 mg per 500 ml (total volume).

c. Sodium, 25 mEq; potassium, 15 mEq; and plasma acid, 80 mEq.

d. Plasma pH and plasma potassium values are as follows:

	CPD				CPD A-1			
Day:	0	7	14	21	0	7	14	21
pH:	7.20	7.00	6.90	6.87	7.35	7.25	6.95	6.90
Plasma K+ (mEq/L):	4	10	21	27	4	9	18	25

e. Red blood cell contents:
   (1) Hemoglobin A (HbA) only (we exclude donors with sickle-cell trait because of the potential for extreme hypoxia in neonates)
   (2) 2,3-Diphosphoglycerate (2,3-DPG) levels (in CPD blood):

Day:	0	7	14	21
μmol/gm Hb:	13.2	14.1	9.8	3.2

   Units stored at room temperature for 8 hours in order to prepare platelets and fresh frozen plasma lose 25% of their 2,3-DPG content. Adenine-fortified anticoagulants have 10% less 2,3-DPG than CPD solution during storage.
f. **Coagulation factor activity:** Storage longer than 24 hours ablates half the coagulation factor activity. 10 to 20 ml/kg of whole blood <24 hours old will provide enough plasma to restore a normal prothrombin time (PT) and partial thromboplastin time (PTT) in the absence of consumption or severe liver failure.
g. Normal immunoglobulins.
h. Fresh, nonrefrigerated whole blood (used within 6 hours) contains clotting factors, active platelets, and a functional white blood count (WBC) of 6000 to 10,000/mm^{3}L [11,12]. Parents must sign a special release, since it is not possible to complete transmissible disease testing. It is safest to use a previously tested donor who is confirmed to be CMV-negative at this donation.

2. **Production from components of a whole-blood unit** for exchange transfusion
   a. May be used when fresh blood is not available, but the clinician requests very young red cells or active plasma factors.
   b. Mix packed red blood cells and fresh-frozen plasma (FFP).

   Example: Creation of a unit with a hematocrit (Hct) of 50%:

   $$\text{Volume of packed cells} = \frac{\text{total exchange volume} \times 0.5 \text{ (desired Hct)}}{0.7 \text{ (Hct of packed cells)}}$$

   Volume of FFP = total exchange volume − packed cell volume

   c. Beware of increased acid load from FFP made with the anticoagulant [acid-citrate-dextrose (ACD) plasma pH = 6.6].
   d. There is no platelet activity in old or reconstituted blood unless platelets are added.

3. **Indications** for whole blood transfusion in the neonate
   a. Exchange for neonatal hyperbilirubinemia
      (1) Uncomplicated simple transfusions (10–15 ml/kg by slow infusion) in term infant: up to 14-day-old whole blood
      (2) Premature or sick newborn: as fresh as possible
   b. Exchange for sepsis, respiratory distress syndrome (RDS), toxic substances: as fresh as possible (<6 hours old, nonrefrigerated for sepsis to preserve white cell function) [11,12]
   c. When anemia is present with **a** or **b**, one may wish to elevate the hematocrit in the unit by removing plasma. To create a whole-blood unit with a hematocrit of 50%:

   Plasma to be removed

   $$= \text{total volume of the unit} - \frac{0.4 \times \text{total volume of the unit}}{0.5}$$

   d. Treatment of acute blood loss and shock. (*Note:* Whole blood is not a useful product to increase hematocrit sharply; for this purpose, use packed red cells.

4. **Amount of infusion**
   a. **Shock or blood loss:** Estimate amount of blood loss and infuse at maximum rate (usually 10 to 20 ml/kg/hour), monitoring vital signs and slowing infusion when vital signs begin to improve. Monitoring the mean arterial pressure or central venous pressure is essential. In the tiny premature infant, hypocalcemia or hypoglycemia can result from rapid infusion of whole blood or fresh frozen plasma (see Chap. 29).
   b. For **exchange transfusion** see Chap. 18.
5. **Preparation of product**
   a. Whole blood is drawn into quad or quint packs so that the unit can be split to create several red blood cell or whole blood infusions. This can be enhanced by utilizing a sterile docking device to further limit donor exposure.
   b. Group, type, direct antiglobulin test, and antibody screening are performed on the mother and baby. We do not accept samples drawn outside our hospital for antibody screening, typing, and cross-matching.
   c. Type-specific red blood cell product is used unless
      (1) Type-specific product is unavailable (use type O Rh-negative)
      (2) ABO incompatibility is present (use type O Rh-negative or positive; depends on baby).
      (3) Maternal or infant direct antiglobulin test or screening is positive (e.g., Rh sensitization; use compatible blood) (see Chap. 18)
   d. Special product is available (e.g., cytomegalovirus-negative) in all blood types by screening for the CMV antibody or by leukodepletion [4,14,26].
   e. Major and minor cross-matching is performed against maternal or infant serum or both [28]. Cross-matching need not be repeated up to age 4 months since infants rarely make alloantibodies, provided that the patient has not had exchange transfusion or multiple plasma infusions [28]. In neonates receiving long-term red blood cell and plasma infusions, weekly screening may be performed to search for antibody development [28].
   f. Blood is drawn up through a 150-μm macroaggregate filter prior to infusion [9,28].
B. **Fresh-frozen plasma (collected in ACD, CPD, CPD A-1)**
   1. **Contents**
      a. Volume: 250 ml; smaller aliquots can be aseptically prepared with a sterile connection device (SCD) (Haemonetics, Terumo).
      b. Electrolyte concentration: sodium, 160 to 170 mEq/L; potassium, 3.5 to 5.5 mEq/L; pH, 6.6 to 6.75.
      c. Clotting factors.
      d. Plasma proteins, including colloid (e.g., albumin) and antibodies.
      e. White cells, 30 to 50/μL.
   2. **Indications**
      a. Replacement of clotting factors (see Bleeding).
      b. Volume expansion (see Chap. 17).
   3. **Amount of infusion**
      a. To replace clotting factors, 10 to 20 ml/kg will normalize the PT and PTT if chronic consumption [e.g., bleeding, disseminated intravascular coagulation (DIC)] is not present and there is no evidence of a congenital coagulation defect. Active bleeding from clotting factor deficiency may require treatment every 8 or 12 hours.
      b. **Volume expansion:** Usually use 5 to 10 ml/kg given over at least 1/2 hour (see Chap. 17).
   4. **Preparation of product**
      a. Use type-specific product or AB-negative.

b. No cross-matching is necessary.

c. Filter through a macroaggregate (150 to 170 μm) filter.

C. Packed red blood cells (PRBC)

1. Contents of 1 unit of packed red blood cells

a. Volume: 300 ml, hematocrit 70%; red cell volume, 210 ml, and plasma volume, 90 ml. The unit can be aseptically subdivided using a multiple pack system or a sterile connection device.

b. Sodium, 15 mEq; potassium, 4 mEq; and plasma acid, 25 mEq.

c. White cells, 6000 to 10,000/mm³.

d. No immunoglobulin or clotting factors.

2. Indications

a. Replacement of phlebotomy losses

b. Improvement of oxygen-carrying capacity in patients with pulmonary or cardiac disease

c. Chronic anemia when there is no expectation that therapy other than transfusion would increase red blood cell mass before life-threatening effects of anemia (e.g., congestive heart failure) supervene (see Anemia)

3. Amount of infusion

a. Volume of packed red blood cells to be infused is determined by the following equation:

PRBC volume to be infused =

$$\frac{\text{Patient's blood volume} \times (\text{hematocrit desired} - \text{hematocrit observed})}{\text{hematocrit of packed cells (usually 0.7)}}$$

In most circumstances, this volume is about 10 ml/kg.

b. In patients without congestive heart failure, maximum rate of infusion is 10 ml/kg per hour.

c. In patients with impending heart failure, do not exceed 2 ml/kg per hour. Intravenous furosemide (0.25 to 0.50 mg/kg) may be given during the transfusion to prevent worsening heart failure. Careful attention must be paid to vital signs under either circumstance.

d. Patients in overt heart failure or with unstable vital signs may benefit from partial exchange transfusion with packed red blood cells to increase the hematocrit while maintaining isovolemia.

4. Special red blood cell products

a. In general, these products are used for patients in whom low WBC levels and decreased plasma protein levels in blood will be valuable. Situations of concern for neonates are the following:

(1) Nonhemolytic transfusion reactions (see **F.2**).

(2) Prevention of cytomegalovirus infection (see **F.5.c**) (see Chap. 23).

b. Washed packed red blood cells: 70% hematocrit in normal saline; 92% reduction in WBCs, and significant dilution of plasma proteins.

c. Filters are now available that will remove more than 99.9% of the WBCs. They do retain a 10- to 15-ml volume of packed red blood cells or whole blood in the filter [14,20,23,28].

d. Frozen washed red blood cells: volume, 200 ml; hematocrit, 70%; sodium, 9 mEq; potassium, 1 to 2 mEq; pH, 6.8; 95% reduction in WBCs and no plasma proteins; most expensive of all.

5. Preparation of product (see **A.5**)

D. Platelets (see Thrombocytopenia)

1. Contents of 1 unit of platelets

a. Total volume of a standard platelet unit is 50 ml (platelets, 5×10^{10}; this can be concentrated 5 to 20 ml prior to infusion; plasma volume, 6 ml; pH, 6.35 to 6.85).

b. CPD (see **A.1.b**)

c. White cells, 10^7 μl

2. **Indications for the neonate**
   a. Absolute thrombocytopenia (platelet count <50,000/mm³) **with bleeding.** The aim should be to raise the platelet count to approximately 100,000/mm³.
   b. Absolute thrombocytopenia **without bleeding.** The use of prophylactic platelet transfusion is controversial. Since spontaneous bleeding can occur with a platelet count less than 20,000 to 30,000/mm³, we currently recommend transfusion at this point. Prophylactic platelet transfusion is indicated when the platelet count is under 50,000/mm³ in sepsis, DIC, or necrotizing enterocolitis [19].
   c. Thrombocytopenia secondary to massive transfusion or exchange transfusion

3. **Amount of infusion**
   a. If no ongoing consumption, 0.1 unit/kg raises the platelet count by 30,000/mm³ if the platelet unit is less than 5 days old.
   b. Failure to achieve this increment suggests consumption (sepsis, DIC, bleeding), maternal idiopathic thrombocytopenic purpura (ITP), neonatal isoimmune thrombocytopenia, splenomegaly, or injured platelets (prolonged storage, washed processed platelets).

4. **Preparation for patient**
   a. A single donor is used to produce 1 unit of platelets. The unit can be concentrated to a volume of 15 to 20 ml. In the case of neonatal isoimmune thrombocytopenia, maternal platelets are concentrated and resuspended in appropriate plasma to reduce infusion of maternal antibody-laden plasma [19]. Compatible platelets from any source may be used (see Thrombocytopenia).
   b. Patient should be given type-specific or group O platelets in plasma compatible with the patient.
   c. Washing and resuspending platelets may slightly decrease platelet function, survival, or both.
   d. Platelets are drawn up through a macroaggregate filter and **must always be given** through a peripheral **venous** line to avoid serious embolic phenomena. *(Do not use arterial lines to infuse platelets.)*
   e. Platelets should be irradiated to 1500 to 3200 rads to avoid graft-versus-host (GVH) disease [6,10,15,21,24].

E. **Granulocyte transfusion**
   1. **Contents of granulocyte transfusion** depends on collection technique. Continuous-flow apheresis (most common) yields a 450-ml unit containing approximately 2×10^{10} granulocytes per unit with a hematocrit of 5 to 15% and the equivalent of 4 units of platelets in CPD or ACD. In most instances this product also contains some hydroxy ethyl starch. The neonate will use only a portion of the unit.
   2. **Indications (controversial):** severe neutropenia (600/PMNsL absolute neutrophil count or the criteria of Manroe [22]) without expectation of rapid bone marrow recovery and with clinical evidence of sepsis [12] (see Chap. 23).
   3. **Amount of infusion**
      a. If tolerated, 10- to 15-ml/kg infusions can be administered every 12 hours [11,12,17,20,29]. Beware of pulmonary symptoms with granulocyte concentrates.
      b. Between 20 and 30 ml/kg may be given by partial exchange transfusion, but beware of decreasing the child's hematocrit by dilution.
      c. Whole blood (nonrefrigerated) used within 6 hours of collection can be used for a two-volume exchange transfusion. This will significantly raise the neutrophil count and also provide platelets, clotting factors, and immunoglobulins [11,12]. Obtain special releases as previously indicated.
   4. **Preparation of product for patient**

a. In the event that type-specific products are unavailable, a product containing type O-negative red cells and compatible plasma may be used.

b. Major cross-matching of baby and maternal sera against red blood cells in granulocyte unit; minor cross-matching of donor unit plasma against baby red blood cells.

c. Irradiate to 1500 to 3200 rads to prevent GVH disease [6,10,15,21].

F. Blood product transfusion reactions

1. **Acute hemolytic transfusion reactions (rare)**

   a. Caused by incompatibility, usually of donor red cells with patient's plasma, owing to passive transfer of maternal antibody. The neonate will not produce its own isoagglutinins (anti-A, anti-B) until the age of 4 to 6 months.

   b. In neonates one may observe changes in vital signs and red urine only, since there will be no report of chills or back pain. Sudden fall in hematocrit, documentation of hemoglobinemia, and demonstration of incompatibility in the blood bank confirm the diagnosis.

   c. Treatment

   (1) Restore hematocrit with compatible red blood cells.

   (2) Administer volume to maintain blood pressure.

   (3) If vital signs permit, a dose of furosemide (0.5 to 1.0 mg/kg) should be given to enhance urine flow and prevent renal failure.

   (4) If shock occurs, use dopamine at a dose of 0.2 to 0.5 mcg per minute.

   (5) In the presence of DIC or refractory shock, fresh whole blood exchange transfusion may be attempted.

2. **Nonhemolytic transfusion reactions**

   a. Caused by allergic or nonspecific response to protein antigens or WBC fragments.

   b. Clinical diagnosis depends on small changes in vital signs, loss of temperature control, wheezing, rash, and demonstration of compatibility in the blood bank.

   c. Treatment consists of prevention of future reactions by using plasma and WBC-poor products.

3. **Ancillary effects of transfusion**

   a. Hypothermia may occur if cool blood is infused into small babies. Blood should be placed through a blood warmer for very small babies or babies with temperature control problems.

   b. Overheating of blood in warmers can lead to a syndrome of hyperthermia and the effects of heat damage to red blood cells (hemoglobinuria, hemoglobinemia, hyperbilirubinemia, and anemia).

   c. Rapid infusion (<30 minutes) of blood products, especially FFP, has been associated with sudden deterioration of vital signs and should be reserved for urgent situations only.

   d. Hypoglycemia may occur in babies receiving hyperalimentation if the hyperalimentation is interrupted during a prolonged transfusion (>30 minutes); therefore, the baby's blood glucose level should be monitored carefully. If a drop in blood sugar occurs, either the transfusion can be interrupted intermittently for glucose infusion or a separate constant glucose drip can be given simultaneously (see Chap. 29).

   e. Hypocalcemia is a well-known complication, because calcium is bound by citrate in blood. For treatment see Chap. 29.

4. **Graft-versus-host disease (GVH)** [6,10,15,21,24]

   a. GVH disease can occur with any cellular blood product but is proportional to the number of white cells in the product. There are numerous reports of GVH occurring in immunocompetent patients, primarily those undergoing open-heart or vascular surgery. Investigations have determined that the donor lymphocytes were compatible with the recipient's HLA haplotype. We irradiate all directed cell products, including red blood cells. The latter should be irradiated just prior to the actual transfusion because of the increased potassium leak of irradiated red blood cells.

  b. GVH disease can probably occur in any neonate (even a full-term neonate) receiving granulocytes or platelets.

  c. GVH disease has been reported in babies undergoing intrauterine transfusion [24].

  d. There is no report to date of GVH disease occurring in any normal full-term neonate from red blood cell products. This is theoretically possible for high-risk premature infants and for severely ill full-term infants. Since irradiation does not have a deleterious effect on red blood cells, these are routinely irradiated to 3200 rads immediately prior to transfusion.

5. Infection (see Chap. 23)

  a. The magnitude and significance of transfusion-transmitted viruses has led to profound changes in both attitudes and practice in transfusion therapy [14,28].

  b. Blood bank laboratories currently screen for syphilis, hepatitis B surface antigen, hepatitis C antibody, surrogate testing for non-A, non-B hepatitis (alanine aminotransferase level and hepatitis B core antibody), HIV 1-2 antibody (AIDS), HTLV-1 antibody (human lymphotropic virus type 1, and HIV p24 antigen). The donor medical history includes questions relating to AIDS and other transmissible viral diseases. High-risk groups are eliminated by direct questioning and a confidential donor exclusion form. American Association of Blood Banks standards include rejection of donors with recent minor viral or bacterial infections as well as parasitic and endemic infections (e.g., malaria). In creating a neonatal donor program, one should be particularly careful to use only volunteers with carefully taken donor histories. Recent data, supported by our own experience, indicate that directed donors have no higher incidence of positive viral markers than occurs in a first-time donor population [14].

  c. Cytomegalovirus (CMV) is a serious potential nosocomial infection in the neonate [2,3,4,14,26,27]. The risk of CMV acquisition is proportional to the number of WBCs containing CMV virions in blood or blood product. Different approaches may be adopted to handle the threat of this disease in babies receiving transfusion:

  (1) Use of WBC-poor blood products exclusively, regardless of donor CMV status.

  (2) Identification of CMV antibody–negative units.

  (3) Exposure of high-risk babies to as few units as possible by using quint packs.

  (4) Review of our transfused neonatal population indicates that more than 90% are very premature or acutely ill. We therefore have found it prudent to provide CMV antibody–negative or leukodepleted blood products in all instances of neonatal transfusion.

  d. Following the implementation of HBsAg testing and elimination of paid donors, **hepatitis B** accounted for approximately 10% of posttransfusion hepatitis. Anti-HBc testing initially introduced as a surrogate test to reduce the incidence of non-A, non-B hepatitis (NANB/HCV) has been retained because of studies linking it to the transmission of hepatitis B. Currently, several hundred cases of acute hepatitis B following transfusion are reported annually despite HBsAg and anti-HBc testing. The period between hepatitis B exposure and the emergence of serum HBsAg is only 1 to 6 weeks [18].

  Prospective monitoring of transfusion recipients for extended intervals (longer than 9 months) is required to determine the incidence of posttransfusion hepatitis. The etiological agent of NANB was identified and labeled **hepatitis C (HCV)** in 1989. The incidence of NANB-HCV declined from 4.9% in patients who received 1 to 10 exposures before the testing for HCV was implemented to 1.9% afterwards. Among those receiving 11 to 20 donor exposures, the incidence decreased from 16.3% before testing to 3.3% afterwards. In March 1992 the second-generation anti-HCV test was introduced. Preliminary clinical trials indicated that the second-generation test was twice as effective in detecting anti-HCV–positive donors and detected anti-HCV in patients with posttransfusion hepatitis 13.7 weeks after transfusion, compared with 20.6 weeks with the first-generation test [1,5].

    e. **HIV:** With implementation of the anti-HIV assay in 1985, there was an initial expectation that the blood supply would become essentially risk-free. Reports of transmission of HIV by screened blood have appeared [13]. The continued focus on careful donor histories, confidential unit exclusion techniques, and the introduction of the combination HIV 1-2 test has reduced the risk in the general donor population to 1 in 493,000 in units such as ours, which exclusively transfuse CMV-negative blood to neonates. This has an additional protective effect, since 94 to 100% of AIDS patients, excluding those with hemophilia, are positive for the CMV antibody [8,13,25]. The addition of HIV P24 antigen screening is expected to cut the risk of HIV infection to 1 in 616,000.

    f. Try to limit the number of donors who will give blood products to any one newborn. At admission, identify infants who are likely to receive multiple transfusions (infants with birth weights under 750 gm, very sick infants who will have large blood losses) and give multiple transfusions from a single donor unit if possible [8].

    g. We use direct donor transfusions for many of our neonatal transfusions. The donor may give as often as once a week. The donor may give small amounts so this is possible. All the usual screening is done.

References

1. Aach, R. D., et al. Hepatitis C virus infection in post-transfusion hepatitis. *N. Engl. J. Med.* 325:1325, 1991.
2. Adler, S. P. Cytomegalovirus infections in neonates acquired by blood transfusions. *Pediatr. Infect. Dis. J.* 2:114, 1983.
3. Adler, S. P., et al. Molecular epidemiology of cytomegalovirus in a nursery: Lack of evidence for nosocomial transmission. *J. Pediatr.* 108:117, 1986.
4. Adler, S. P., et al. Prevention of transfusion-associated cytomegalovirus infection in very low-birthweight infants using frozen blood and donors seronegative for cytomegalovirus. *Transfusion* 24:333, 1984.
5. Alter, H. J. New kit on the block: Evaluation assays for detection of antibody to the hepatitis C virus. [editorial; comment] *Hepatology* 15:350, 1992.
6. Anderson, K. C., et al. Transfusion-associated graft-versus-host disease [published erratum appears in *N. Engl. J. Med.* 1990 N 8; 323:1360][see comments]. [review] *N. Engl. J. Med.* 323:315, 1990.
7. Andrew, M., et al. Development of the human coagulation system in the healthy premature infant. *Blood* 72:1651, 1988.
8. Bifano, E. M., et al. Minimizing donor blood exposure in the neonatal intensive care unit. *Clin. Perinatol.* 22:657, 1995.
9. Butch, S. *Transfusion Techniques in Hemotherapy of the Infant and Premature.* Arlington, Va.: American Association of Blood Banks, 1983.
10. Button, L. N., et al. The effects of irradiation on blood components. *Transfusion* 21:419, 1981.
11. Christensen, R. D., et al. The leukocyte left shift in clinical and experimental neonatal sepsis. *J. Pediatr.* 98:101, 1981.
12. Christensen, R. D., et al. Granulocyte transfusions in neonates with bacterial infection, neutropenia, and depletion of mature marrow neutrophils. *Pediatrics* 70:1, 1982.

13. Donahue, J. G. Transmission of HIV by transfusion of screened blood. [letter] *N. Engl. J. Med.* 323:1709, 1990.
14. Dodd, R. Y. The risk of transfusion-transmitted disease. *N. Engl. J. Med.* 327:419, 1992.
15. Drobyski, W., et al. Third-party-mediated graft rejection and graft-versus-host disease after T-cell-depleted bone marrow transplantation, as demonstrated by hypervariable DNA probes and HLA-DR polymorphism. *Blood* 74:2285, 1989.
16. Fisher, M. C. Transfusion-associated acquired immunodeficiency syndrome—what is the risk? *Pediatrics* 79:157, 1987.
17. Hill, H. R. Biochemical, structural, and functional abnormalities of polymorphonuclear leukocytes in the neonate. [review] *Pediatr. Res.* 22:375, 1987.
18. Hoofnagle, H. Posttransfusion hepatitis B. *Transfusion* 30:384, 1990.
19. Kevy, S. V. *The Use of Platelets, Plasma, and Plasma Derivatives in the Newborn in Hemotherapy of the Infant and Premature.* Arlington, Va.: American Association of Blood Banks, 1983.
20. Lane, T. A. Leukocyte reduction in blood component therapy. [review] *Ann. Intern. Med.* 117:151, 1992.
21. Leitman, S. F. *Posttranfusion Graft-Versus-Host Disease in Special Considerations in Transfusing the Immunocompromised Patient.* Arlington, Va.: American Association of Blood Banks, 1985.
22. Manroe, B. L. The neonatal blood count in health and disease. I. Reference values for neutrophilic cells. *J. Pediatr.* 95:89, 1979.
23. Mollison, P. L., Engelfriet, B. L., and Contreras, M. *Blood Transfusion in Clinical Medicine.* Oxford: Blackwell Scientific, 1993.
24. Parkman, R., et al. Graft-versus-host disease after intrauterine and exchange transfusions for hemolytic disease of the newborn. *N. Engl. J. Med.* 290:359, 1974.
25. Peterson, L. R. Serological characterization of HIV PCR positive pre seroconversion specimens. *Transfusion* 32:46S, 1992.
26. Preiksaitis, J. K. Indications for the use of cytomegalovirus-seronegative blood products. [review] *Trans. Med. Rev.* 5:1, 1991.
27. Stevens, C. E., et al. Hepatitis B virus antibody in blood donors and the occurrence of non-A, non-B hepatitis in transfusion recipients. An analysis of the transfusion-transmitted viruses study. *Ann. Intern. Med.* 101:733, 1984.
28. Walker, R. H. (Ed.). *Technical Manual of the American Association of Blood Banks.* Arlington, Va: AABB, 1990.
29. Wilson, C. B. Immunologic basis for increased susceptibility of the neonate to infection. [review] *J. Pediatr.* 108:1, 1986.
30. Wolfe, L., et al. Blood transfusion for the neonatal patient. *Hum. Pathol.* 14:256, 1983.

Major Arterial and Venous Thrombosis
Yao Sun

I. **Risk factors:** The presence of an **indwelling vascular catheter** is the single greatest risk factor for arterial or venous thrombosis.
  A. **Hematologic factors:** The highest incidence of thrombosis in otherwise healthy patients occurs in the neonatal period. Both thrombogenic and fibrinolytic pathways are altered in the neonate. Generally, these alterations are balanced, and healthy neonates do not clinically demonstrate hypercoagulable states or a bleeding diathesis. In sick or premature infants, or in cases of inherited hematologic disorders, changes in hemostatic protein levels may tip the balance toward thrombogenesis or coagulopathy [5,6,10, 18,25].
    1. Compared with adults, neonates have decreased levels of protein C, protein S, plasminogen, and anti–thrombin III. Decreased levels of these factors generally increase the risk of thrombus formation.

2. Platelets aggregate more easily in neonates.
3. Prostacyclin-regenerating activity in neonates is decreased.
4. Although rare, inherited deficiencies of inhibitory proteins (e.g., protein C, protein S, anti–thrombin III, APC mutation in factor V) may predispose an infant to thrombus formation.
5. Maternal lupus and antiphospholipid antibodies that cross the placental circulation may also cause thrombus formation.

B. Clinical factors [5,6,10]

1. **Surgery or catheterization:** Infants undergoing surgery that involves the vascular system (e.g., in congenital heart disease) are at increased risk for thrombotic complications. Diagnostic or interventional catheterizations also increase the risk for thrombus formation.
   a. **Vascular disruption and endothelial damage** during surgery or catheterization activates platelet aggregation and initiates the reactions that will lead to a fibrin clot. Thrombus formation may exceed fibrinolytic activity and lead to obstruction of the vascular space.
   b. **Foreign bodies** such as artificial vascular grafts, conduits, and embolization material are more thrombogenic than normal vascular endothelium.

2. **Other clinical conditions** have been associated with an increased incidence of thrombosis. These conditions include asphyxia, polycythemia, congenital heart disease, and maternal diabetes.
   a. **Prematurity** is associated with changes in coagulation factors, including decreased levels of anti–thrombin III.
   b. **Neonatal illness,** such as respiratory distress syndrome, has been associated with decreased levels of protein C.

II. Aortic or major arterial thrombosis [9]

A. Diagnosis of aortic thrombus: The formation of an aortic thrombus should be suspected if clinical signs appear or the umbilical arterial catheter (UAC) is not functioning optimally. Thrombosis of peripheral arteries is usually diagnosed by clinical signs that include decreased perfusion, decreased pulses, pallor, and embolic phenomena that may manifest as skin lesions or petechiae.

1. **Mild clinical signs of aortic thrombosis**
   a. Hematuria
   b. Hypertension
   c. Intermittent lower extremity color change or decreased perfusion
   d. Hematuria in the absence of transfusions or hemolysis, or hematuria with RBCs on microscopic analysis

2. **Strong clinical signs of aortic thrombosis**
   a. Persistent lower extremity color change or decreased perfusion
   b. Blood pressure differential between upper and lower extremities
   c. Decrease or loss of lower extremity pulses
   d. Signs of peripheral thrombosis
   e. Oliguria in the face of adequate intravascular volume
   f. Signs of congestive heart failure

3. **Ultrasound:** If clinical signs of aortic/arterial thrombosis progress or cause clinical deterioration, ultrasound with Doppler flow imaging should be performed as soon as possible. This test is diagnostic in most cases.

4. **Contrast study:** If ultrasound is inconclusive, and a major arterial thrombus is still suspected, the arterial catheter should be left in place, and a radiographic contrast study should be performed (with careful attention to dye load if renal insufficiency is suspected).

B. Prevention

1. **Heparin** 0.5–1 unit/ml in all infusions (compatibility permitting) through arterial catheters [13,14].
2. **Placement of umbilical artery catheter:** high or low line placement is left to the discretion of the clinician [15]. **In infants weighing >1500 gm, consider placing a peripheral arterial line.**

3. **Monitor carefully for clinical evidence** of aortic thrombus formation when a UAC is present:
   a. Check for lower extremity color and perfusion.
   b. Check all urine for heme.
   c. Check upper extremity and lower extremity blood pressures 3 times daily.
   d. Watch for hypertension and decreased urine output.
   e. Suspect aortic thrombosis if CHF occurs or respiratory status worsens.
   f. If clinical signs of necrotizing enterocolitis occur, also consider the possibility of aortic thrombus.
4. **Monitor the UAC for optimal functioning.** Check for the waveform damping and difficulty flushing or withdrawing from the UAC.
C. **Management of thrombosis**
   1. **Surgery:** surgical thrombectomy is not indicated, since the mortality and morbidity far exceed that of current medical management.
   2. **Mild clinical signs:** for "minor" aortic thrombi with hematuria and hypertension as the only clinical signs, **the arterial catheter should be removed.** Ultrasound is not necessary if the clinical signs resolve [7].
   3. **Large but nonocclusive thrombus:** if the patient is clinically stable, and the thrombus is nonocclusive to blood flow (as demonstrated by ultrasound or contrast study), **the arterial catheter should be removed and heparin therapy should be considered** (see IV).
   4. **Occlusion of aorta/major tributary** or **severe clinical compromise** (e.g., renal failure, congestive heart failure, necrotizing enterocolitis (NEC), signs of peripheral ischemia)
      a. If the catheter is still present, **leave it in place and start local thrombolytic therapy through the catheter** (see IV). Local therapy through the catheter is theoretically safer than systemic therapy for patients at risk for hemorrhage at other sites (e.g., after surgery, previously documented intraventricular hemorrhage, infants <1500 gm).
      b. If the catheter has already been removed or cannot be used (i.e., is obstructed), **start systemic thrombolytic therapy.** In infants <1500 gm or with documented IVH, the risks of CNS hemorrhage must be weighed against the clinical compromise caused by the thrombus.
      c. If the catheter is in place but obstructed, remove it.
III. **Major venous thrombosis:** The most common cause of venous thrombosis is occlusion secondary to thrombosis of a central venous line (CVL), although spontaneous renal vein thrombosis occurs and thrombosis of other veins (inferior vena cava, adrenal, splenic, portal, and hepatic) has been reported [8, 20,23].
   A. **Prevention: Heparin** 0.5 unit/ml in all infusions (compatibility permitting) through CVLs.
   B. **Diagnosis**
      1. **Clinical signs**
         a. Thrombosis of vessels related to CVLs usually present first with problems infusing through or withdrawing from the line.
         b. Signs of venous obstruction include swelling of the extremities, possibly including the head and neck, and distended superficial veins.
         c. Renal vein thrombosis classically presents with a triad of an enlarged kidney (by palpation), hematuria, and thrombocytopenia (see Chap. 31).
         d. The onset of thrombocytopenia in the presence of a CVL also raises the suspicion of thrombosis.
      2. **Ultrasound:** In general, clinical suspicion of a venous thrombosis can be confirmed by ultrasound as the initial diagnostic study. In smaller infants or in low flow states, however, the ultrasound study may not provide sufficient information about the size of the thrombus.
      3. **Radiographic line study:** Using contrast material injected through a CVL may sometimes be useful if the ultrasound is not informative.

4. **Venography:** Venography through peripheral vessels in the upper extremities may sometimes be indicated when other diagnostic methods fail to demonstrate the extent and severity of thrombosis.

C. Management [2]

1. **Surgery:** surgical thrombectomy is not indicated.

2. **Nonfunctioning CVL:** if fluid can no longer be easily infused through the catheter, **remove the catheter** unless the CVL is absolutely necessary.

   a. If continued central access through this catheter is judged to be clinically necessary, **urokinase** (for blood-related blockage) or **HCl** (for chemical-related blockage) may be used in an attempt to clear a nonfunctioning CVL.

   (1) **Urokinase** 5000 units/ml comes in unit doses prepared expressly for clearance of catheters. Gently infuse 1 to 2 ml = 5000–10,000 units urokinase into the CVL if possible (if there is too much resistance, do not force the infusion in). Wait 2 to 4 hours, then attempt to withdraw fluid through the catheter. If the catheter still will not allow fluid aspiration, leave the urokinase in for another 8 hours, then attempt to withdraw again. If the catheter still has not been cleared, the previous steps may be repeated once.

   (2) **HCl** 0.1M, 1 to 2 cc may be instilled using the same techniques as for urokinase.

3. **Local obstruction:** If a small occlusive thrombosis is documented, a low-dose continuous infusion of urokinase should be started at 150 units/kg/hour if infusion through the CVL is still possible. If infusion is not possible, the CVL should be removed, and heparin therapy should be considered (see **IV**).

4. **Extensive venous thrombosis:** Consider leaving the catheter in place and attempting systemic thrombolytic therapy. Otherwise, remove the catheter and begin heparin therapy (see **IV**).

IV. Therapy guidelines [1–4,11,12,14,16,17,21,22,24,26,27]

A. Precautions

1. Avoid IM injections and arterial punctures during anticoagulation or thrombolytic therapy.

2. Avoid aspirin or other antiplatelet drugs during therapy.

3. Thrombolytic therapy should not be initiated in the presence of active bleeding or significant risk for local bleeding, and should be carefully considered if there is a history of recent surgery of any type (particularly neurosurgery).

4. Use minimal physical manipulation of patient (e.g., no physical therapy) during thrombolytic therapy.

5. Heparin and thrombolytic therapy should not be used concurrently.

6. Monitor clinical status carefully for signs of hemorrhage (including internal hemorrhage and intracranial hemorrhage).

7. Consider giving 10 ml/kg of fresh frozen plasma to any patient who needs anticoagulation (see **IV.D.3.d**).

B. Heparin therapy

1. **Loading dose** of 75 units/kg over 10 minutes followed by **continuous infusion** of 28 units/kg/hour (for infants <1 year).

2. Adjustment of the heparin infusion is based on clinical response and serial evaluation of the thrombus (preferably by ultrasonography). No validated therapeutic ranges exist for heparin therapy in neonates, although the recommendation is to maintain the partial thromboplastin time (PTT) at 60 to 85 seconds, or 2 to 3 times the control.

3. The heparin should be infused through a dedicated IV line that is not used for any other medications or fluids.

4. **Lab work:** prior to starting heparin, obtain complete blood count (CBC), prothrombin time (PT), and PTT. If appropriate, consider workup for thrombophilic state.

a. Check PT/PTT 4 hours after loading dose is finished and every 12 to 24 hours after. Adjust heparin infusion if necessary.
b. Follow CBC and PT/PTT at least daily when "therapeutic" PTT levels are reached.
5. **Duration of therapy:** may continue up to 10 to 14 days. Consider initiating coumadin therapy after 5 to 7 days (after consultation with hematology) if long-term anticoagulation is necessary.
6. **Reversal of anticoagulation:** termination of heparin infusion will usually suffice. In cases where rapid reversal is necessary, **protamine sulfate** given IV may be used as follows:
a. calculate the total amount of heparin given in the **last 2 hours**
b. give **protamine sulfate** according to the following dosage schedule:

Time (min) since last heparin dose	Protamine dose (mg/100 units heparin received)
<30	1
30–60	0.5–0.75
60–120	0.375–0.5
>120	0.25–0.375

C. **Preparation for thrombolytic therapy**
   1. Place sign at head of bed indicating thrombolytic therapy.
   2. Have topical thrombin available in unit refrigerator.
   3. Notify blood bank to insure availability of cryoprecipitate.
   4. Notify pharmacy to insure availability of amino caproic acid (Amicar).
   5. Obtain good venous access.
D. **Urokinase systemic dosing**
   1. **Load** with 4000 units/kg over 20 minutes, then administer **continuous infusion** of 4400 units/kg/hour.
   2. **Lab work:** Monitor thrombin time (TT), PT/PTT, fibrinogen every 6 to 12 hours to target thrombin time 1.5 times normal value (normal 10 to 12 seconds, target 15 to 18 seconds) and fibrinogen levels >100 mg/dl. Also monitor hematocrit every 12 to 24 hours.
      a. Expect fibrinogen to decrease by 20 to 50%.
      b. If there is no decrease in fibrinogen, obtain D-dimers or fibrin split products to show evidence that a thrombolytic state has been initiated.
   3. **Infusion adjustment**
      a. If the TT is still within normal range but there is clinical improvement or the ultrasound shows thrombus size decreasing, do not increase the urokinase dosing.
      b. Otherwise, may increase continuous infusion by 4000 units/kg/hour increments if TT does not approach target value (if there is no evidence of bleeding).
      c. Repeat ultrasonography in 12 to 24 hours to document stabilization or decrease in thrombus size. If there is no improvement, may increase continuous infusion as above.
      d. If there is no improvement in clinical condition or clot size as shown by ultrasonography, and fibrinogen levels remain high, **consider infusion of 10 ml/kg fresh frozen plasma (FFP)** in addition to urokinase. This may correct deficiencies of thrombolytic factors such as plasminogen, anti–thrombin III, and hereditary factor deficiencies.
E. **Urokinase local dosing through catheter**
   1. 150 units/kg/hour continuous infusion.
   2. Monitor TT, fibrinogen, hematocrit as above.

3. Repeat ultrasound in 12 to 24 hours, and increase infusion by 200 units/kg/hour if no improvement.
4. If there is no improvement and fibrinogen levels remain high, consider giving **FFP** (see **IV.D.3.d**) in addition to urokinase.
F. **Tissue plasminogen activator (TPA)** is an alternative to urokinase [1,19].
   1. Local dosing through catheter: 0.5 mg/kg bolus over 20 minutes, followed by continuous infusion at 0.1 to 0.5 mg/kg/hour.
      a. Monitor TT, PT/PTT, fibrinogen, and hematocrit every 6 to 12 hours (see **IV.D.2**).
      b. Adjust infusion rate for clinical effect (see **IV.D.3**). May increase the infusion rate by 0.1 mg/kg/hour (to a maximum of 0.5 mg/kg/hour) if no improvement in 12 to 24 hours.
      c. High dose "local infusion" of TPA is as likely to cause bleeding as "systemic infusion." If bleeding is a significant risk, use low dose.
   2. Systemic dosing: initial dose of 0.5 mg/kg/hour IV over 6 hours.
      a. Evaluation of clinical effect (e.g., increased perfusion or return of pulses for arterial clots, or decreased swelling for venous clots) and/or ultrasound should be performed after 6 hours. If response is inadequate, may continue infusion for another 12 to 24 hours, with continuing reevaluation of thrombus size and clinical response.
      b. Monitor TT, PT/PTT, fibrinogen, hematocrit (see **IV.D.2**).
   3. If no improvement and fibrinogen levels remain high, consider giving **FFP** (see **IV.D.3.d**) in addition to TPA.
G. **Bleeding during thombolytic therapy**
   1. For local sites, local pressure, topical thrombin, and supportive care.
   2. Severe bleeding: stop infusion, give **cryoprecipitate** (1 unit / 5 kg).
   3. In life-threatening bleeding, stop infusion, give **cryoprecipitate**, and infuse **amino caproic acid (Amicar)** (at the usual dose of 100 mg/kg IV every 6 hours); consult hematology before giving Amicar.
H. **Post-thrombolytic therapy:** Consider initiating heparin therapy, but without the initial loading dose (i.e., start continuous infusion dose). Consider discontinuing heparin if no reaccumulation of the thrombus occurs after 24 to 48 hours.

References

1. Anderson, B. J., Keeley, S. R., Johnson, N. D. Caval thrombolysis in neonates using low doses of recombinant human tissue-type plasminogen activator. *Anaesth. Intens. Care* 19:22, 1991.
2. Andrew, M. Thrombosis management protocols of The Hospital for Sick Children, Toronto, Canada and McMaster University Medical Center, Hamilton, Canada. (Personal communication.)
3. Andrew, M., Brooker, L., Leaker, M., et al. Fibrin clot lysis by thrombolytic agents is impaired in newborns due to a low plasminogen concentration. *Thromb. Haemost.* 68:325, 1992.
4. Bagnall, H. A., Gomperts, E., Atkinson, J. B. Continuous infusion of low-dose urokinase in the treatment of central venous catheter thrombosis in infants and children. *Pediatrics* 83:963, 1989.
5. Beardsley, D. S. Hemostasis in the perinatal period: Approach to the diagnosis of coagulation disorders. *Semin. Perinatol.* 15 Suppl 2:25, 1991.
6. Buchanan, G. R. Coagulation disorders in the neonate. *Pediatr. Clin. North Am.* 33:203, 1986.
7. Caplan, M. S., Cohn, R. A., et al. Favorable outcome of neonatal aortic thrombosis and renovascular hypertension. *J. Pediatr.* 155:291, 1989.
8. Carey, B. E. Major complications of central lines in neonates. *Neonatal Network* 7:17, 1989.
9. Chaikof, E. L., et al. Acute arterial thrombosis in the very young. *J. Vasc. Surg.* 16:428, 1992.
10. Corrigan, J. J., Jr. Neonatal thrombosis and the thrombolytic system: Pathophysiology and therapy. *Am. J. Pediatr. Hematol. Oncol.* 10:83, 1988.

11. Dillon, P. W., et al. Recombinant tissue plasminogen activator for neonatal and pediatric vascular thrombolytic therapy. *J. Pediatr. Surg.* 28:1264, 1993.
12. Giacoia, G. P. High-dose urokinase therapy in newborn infants with major vessel thrombosis. *Clin. Pediatr.* 32:231, 1993.
13. Horgan, M. J., et al. Effect of heparin infusates in umbilical arterial catheters on frequency of thrombotic complications. *J. Pediatr.* 111:774, 1987.
14. Jackson, J. C., et al. Efficacy of thromboresistant umbilical artery catheters in reducing aortic thrombosis and related complications. *J. Pediatr.* 110:102, 1987.
15. Kempley, S. T., et al. Randomized trial of umbilical arterial catheter position: Clinical outcome. *Acta Paediatr.* 82:173, 1993.
16. Kennedy, L. A., et al. Successful treatment of neonatal aortic thrombosis with tissue plasminogen activator. *J. Pediatr.* 166:798, 1990.
17. Kothari, S. S., et al. Thrombolytic therapy in infants and children. *Am. Heart J.* 127:651, 1994.
18. Lao, T. T. H., et al. Coagulation and anticoagulation systems in newborns—correlation with their mothers at delivery. *Gynecol. Obstet. Invest.* 29:181, 1990.
19. Levy, M., et al. Tissue plasminogen activator for the treatment of thromboembolism in infants and children. *J. Pediatr.* 118:467, 1991.
20. Mehta, S., et al. Incidence of thrombosis during central venous catheterization of newborns: A prospective study. *J. Pediatr. Surg.* 27:18, 1992.
21. Pritchard, S. L., et al. Low-dose fibrinolytic therapy in infants. *J. Pediatr.* 106:594, 1985.
22. Reznik, V. M., et al. Successful fibrinolytic treatment of arterial thrombosis and hypertension in a cocaine-exposed neonate. *Pediatrics* 84:735, 1989.
23. Ricci, M. A., et al. Renal venous thrombosis in infants and children. *Arch. Surg.* 125:1195, 1990.
24. Richardson, R., et al. Effective thrombolytic therapy of aortic thrombosis in the small premature infant. *J. Pediatr. Surg.* 23:1198, 1988.
25. Schmidt, B., et al. Neonatal thrombotic disease. *J. Pediatr.* 113:407, 1988.
26. Schmidt, B., et al. Report of scientific and standardization subcommittee on neonatal hemostasis. Diagnosis and treatment of neonatal thrombosis. *Thromb. Haemost.* 67:381, 1992.
27. Vailas, G. N., et al. Neonatal aortic thrombosis: Recent experience. *J. Pediatr.* 109:101, 1986.

27. NEUROLOGY

Neonatal Seizures
Karl C.K. Kuban and James Filiano

I. **Clinical patterns.** The usual well-organized tonic-clonic seizure patterns seen in older infants are not seen in the newborn because of the immaturity of the newborn brain. The predominance of oral and buccal phenomena (such as chewing, lip smacking, and sucking), as well as gaze abnormalities and apnea, may be related to the advanced development of the limbic structures and their connections to the brain stem and diencephalon in comparison with other forebrain structures.
   A. **Seizure patterns**
      1. **Focal clonic seizures.** In focal clonic seizures, the movements involve well-localized clonic jerking. These types of seizures are not associated with loss of consciousness. They are most often provoked by metabolic disturbances, but they may be associated with focal traumatic injury (i.e., cerebral contusion), subarachnoid hemorrhage (SAH), or focal infarct. The electroencephalogram (EEG) is most often unifocally abnormal. The prognosis is generally good.
      2. **Multifocal clonic seizures.** These seizures are characterized by random clonic movements of limbs similar to those seen in normal infants under 34 weeks' gestation. The EEG most often is multifocally abnormal.
      3. **Tonic seizures.** The movements are focal or generalized and may resemble the decerebrate or decorticate posturing seen in older children; the movements are most often associated with eye deviation and occasionally with clonic movements or apnea. This condition is more often seen in premature babies and is most often associated with diffuse central nervous system (CNS) disease or intraventricular hemorrhage (IVH). The prognosis is mixed but is generally poor. Most often, the EEG is multifocally abnormal, has a burst-suppression pattern, or has extremely attenuated amplitude. When tonic seizures occur on the heels of an apneic or hypoxic episode, the prognosis is better.
      4. **Myoclonic seizures.** The manifestations include synchronous single or multiple slow jerks of the upper or lower limbs (or both) and are associated with diffuse CNS pathology; the prognosis is poor. The EEG shows a burst-suppression pattern or focal sharp, transient waves and may evolve into hypsarrhythmia. Rapid multifocal polymyoclonus is not usually associated with an epileptiform EEG.
      5. **Subtle seizures** constitute 50% of seizures in newborns (both term and premature) and most often occur in infants who manifest the other seizure types described above. Subtle seizures may not be associated with an epileptiform or hypersynchronous EEG, may be subcortical in origin, and may not be ameliorated by anticonvulsant therapy. Examples of subtle seizures include the following:
         a. Tonic horizontal deviation, usually with jerking of the eyes.
         b. Repetitive blinking or fluttering of the eyelids.
         c. Oral and buccal movements: drooling, sucking, and yawning.
         d. Tonic posturing of a limb.
         e. Apnea (see Chap. 24, Apnea) due to seizure most often has either an accelerated or a normal heart rate when evaluated 20 seconds following its onset. The heart rate may slow subsequently as a result of sustained hypoxemia. Apnea due to other causes is often associated with bradycardia near the onset of the episode. Apnea without

associated epileptic movements is rarely the sole manifestation of seizure.

f. Rhythmic fluctuations in vital signs and degree of oxygenation in pharmacologically paralyzed infants. These observations, although suggestive, are not diagnostic of seizure, and establishment of the diagnosis requires an EEG.

g. Complex, purposeless movements, such as "swimming" or "bicycling" movements.

B. Jitteriness and clonus may be associated with hypocalcemia, hypoglycemia, neonatal encephalopathy, and drug withdrawal. However, the problem is most commonly seen in infants, particularly premature infants, who have none of these problems. Infants of diabetic mothers (IDMs) are frequently "jittery" with normal blood sugar and calcium levels. Jitteriness or clonus in infants may be confused with seizures. Characteristics of jitteriness and clonus that help to differentiate them from seizures are as follows:

1. Absence of abnormal gaze or eye movements.

2. Provocation by stimulation of the infant or by stretching a joint, in contrast to the usual spontaneous occurrence of seizures.

3. Cessation of movements with passive flexion or gentle restraint.

4. Absence of the fast and slow components that are characteristic of a clonic fit (tremor and clonus oscillate rhythmically).

5. Tremor and clonus with no associated EEG abnormality.

6. Repetitive jerks in seizures are at a rate of 2 or 3 per second, whereas clonus tends to be faster (5 to 6 per second).

7. Jitteriness and nonseizure clonus not accompanied by increased blood pressure, bradycardia, or tachycardia.

C. Use of EEG in diagnosis. The EEG is an adjunct to the clinical determination of seizures. As a result of the immaturity of the CNS, ictal and interictal abnormalities can take many, often nonspecific forms. Neonates commonly have abnormal movements of uncertain meaning. It is often difficult to determine which movements represent seizures and which do not. Routine EEGs may be inadequate to electrographically confirm suspected seizures. In difficult cases, several studies or continuous recordings with computer-scored methods are more reliable. The EEG may have sharp or, more rarely, spike forms, but it also may have rhythmic activity in the delta, theta, or alpha frequency as the EEG correlate of seizures. Focal and multifocal clonic seizures often, but not invariably, have focal and multifocal EEG abnormalities; subtle, tonic, and myoclonic seizures usually have a greater range of EEG correlates to include most of the forms mentioned previously. Apparent clinical seizures may not be correlated with EEG discharges for at least two reasons. First, many of the motor phenomena often thought to represent subtle seizures or complex motor patterns may reflect subcortical EEG-negative spells or behaviors that may be refractory to anticonvulsant therapy. Whether some or any of these clinical phenomena should be viewed as seizures is controversial. Second, neonates with severely damaged nervous systems may not be able to transmit electrical activity from deeper cerebral structures to the cortex, which is where surface EEG electrodes are most likely to pick up discharges. In such circumstances, the background EEG is usually blunted or flat, or shows a burst-suppression pattern. Conversely, epileptiform discharges seen on the EEG tracings do not necessarily guarantee the presence of clinical seizures. In a prospective study of 275 neonates, EEG seizure activity was found in 55, but only 12 had obvious simultaneous clinical signs. In 20 others there were some questionable (subtle) simultaneous clinical events, but clinical signs were completely absent in 23. In another study of 80 infants with abnormal movements, only 8 had EEG evidence of seizures during those movements. Nonetheless, we would advocate treating paralyzed neonates who have epileptiform discharges. In nonparalyzed babies, treatment should be administered to babies with clonic seizures. Although one cannot be certain that tonic, myoclonic, or subtle events are epileptic, if they occur in the absence of an acute metabolic disturbance, are associated with an epileptiform EEG, or interfere with the care of the neonate, we would advocate a trial of anticonvulsant treatment. A normal interictal EEG does not rule out seizures. Some diseases have such characteristic EEG patterns that the EEG may be a rapid way to make the diagnosis. The 5–7-Hz "comb-like" rhythm is a very characteristic pattern in **maple syrup urine disease**. Patients with **pyridoxine dependency** may have generalized 1–4-Hz sharp and slow wave activity, which, when present in a neonate without evidence of infection, is highly suggestive of the diagnosis, even if the patient has had some response to traditional anticonvulsants. In the presence of an inflammatory condition of the CSF, multifocal periodic pattern EEG is a good early indicator of **herpes encephalitis**.

II. **Etiology of seizures**
  A. **Perinatal causes** include neonatal encephalopathy, cerebral contusion, and intracranial hemorrhage (ICH). **Neonatal encephalopathy** designates cerebral dysfunction in the neonate, including seizures, when the etiology is not known. We specifically avoid the term **hypoxic-ischemic encephalopathy** unless there is very clear and direct evidence of prenatal ischemia or postnatal hypoxia and/or ischemia. Hypoxic-ischemic encephalopathy should never be a diagnosis of exclusion. Furthermore, even clear or direct evidence of compromised oxygen delivery to the fetus or the neonate does not preclude the presence of an underlying neurologic disorder that may have predisposed the fetus or neonate to the subsequent hypoxic or ischemic disturbance. The criteria traditionally used to identify past hypoxic-ischemic events, including abnormal fetal heart rate patterns, low Apgar scores, jitteriness, lethargy, and seizures, simply are not specific for hypoxic-ischemic events. In fact, hypoxic-ischemic events are an infrequent cause of any of these signs, and the vast majority of babies with these signs do not have long-term repercussions. Continued presumptive use of the term **hypoxic-Ischemic encephalopathy** impedes further search for other or underlying causes and tends to implicate the perinatal period as the time frame for the insult with little or no firm substantiation. Neonatal encephalopathy, cerebral contusion, and intracranial hemorrhage account for more than 40% of all neonatal seizures and a larger proportion in premature babies.
   1. **Neonatal encephalopathy** occurs in babies with severe fetal distress who are apneic at birth. It accounts for 24 to 40% of neonatal seizures. Seizures usually occur on the first day of life, most often beginning in the first 12 hours.
      a. **Ictal manifestations** of neonatal encephalopathy include subtle seizures, tonic seizures, and multifocal seizures. Seizures occur in 8% of such infants. Associated metabolic disorders may include hypoglycemia, hypocalcemia, inappropriate secretion of antidiuretic hormone (ADH) with hyponatremia, and diabetes insipidus.
      b. **Early seizures** associated with clear hypoxic or ischemic events are often difficult to control. Infants who require multiple medications have high morbidity and mortality (see Perinatal Asphyxia).
   2. **ICH and CNS trauma** may result from breech delivery or difficult forceps extraction. Trauma in these circumstances may cause cerebral contusion or hemorrhage, subdural hematoma, or subarachnoid bleeding and may be manifested by focal seizures and lateralized neurologic signs, often occurring after the first day of life. ICH is usually associated with prematurity and signs of neonatal encephalopathy (see Intracranial Hemorrhage, below).
      a. **Primary subarachnoid hemorrhage (SAH)** may occur in infants subjected to trauma but may occur without apparent trauma. It occurs more often in premature than in term infants. The majority of infants with SAH are asymptomatic. When seizures occur, however, they usually do so on the second day. The baby appears well between seizures, and 90% of these infants develop normally.

    b. Periventricular hemorrhage (PVH) usually occurs in premature infants, is likely to occur within 3 days of birth, and may present with tonic seizures. The seizures may be associated with rapid deterioration, respiratory arrest, and death. Most babies with PVH do not have seizures. It is not usually associated with trauma.

    c. Subdural hemorrhage (SDH) results from a tear of the falx, tentorium, or superficial cortical veins. It is most likely to occur in large babies and after breech deliveries. The seizures are associated with cerebral contusion or hemorrhage and may have focal features. The seizures occur on the first days of life. When considering this diagnosis, one should consider bleeding below the tentorium, which may not be seen on ultrasound and which may cause sudden, acute brain stem dysfunction.

    d. Choroid plexus hemorrhage occurs in full-term infants. Its triggers are unknown.

B. Metabolic problems. These seizures usually present as focal or multifocal clonic seizures (see Chap. 29).

  1. Hypoglycemia is defined as a blood glucose level of less than 40 mg/dl (see Chap. 29, Hypoglycemia). Most often, it occurs in IDMs, babies who are small for gestational age (SGA), premature babies, and infants in whom asphyxia or other stress occurs. Hypoglycemia is often associated with or is a complication of other causes of seizures, such as sepsis and meningitis. Neonatal hypoglycemia also occurs in hereditary fructose intolerance, Beckwith-Wiedemann syndrome, congenital glucagon deficiency, maternal ingestion of an oral hypoglycemic agent, the glycogenoses, and other metabolic disorders. The symptoms of hypoglycemia include hypotonia, apnea, stupor, jitteriness, and seizures. Seizures occur in the minority of babies with hypoglycemia. When they do occur, however, they usually imply long-standing hypoglycemia; as a result, such infants often have poor outcomes.

  2. Hypocalcemia is defined as a calcium level less than 7 mg/dl with an albumin level greater than 3.5 gm/dl (see Chap. 29, Hypocalcemia).

    a. Early hypocalcemia occurs in babies who are premature, babies in whom asphyxia or trauma has occurred, infants of mothers with hyperparathyroidism, and IDMs. Hypocalcemia is often accompanied by other causes of seizures, such as hypoglycemia, and may occur as part of neonatal encephalopathy. As a result, treatment with calcium may not stop the seizures. The prognosis reflects the prognosis of the underlying problem.

    b. Late hypocalcemia results from ingestion of formula with a suboptimal ratio of calcium to phosphorus, from abnormalities in vitamin D metabolism, or from renal disease. The symptoms include clonus, jitteriness, and hyperactive deep tendon reflexes. Seizures occur after the first week of life, are usually focal with a focally abnormal EEG, and respond to treatment with calcium. The prognosis for a normal outcome is excellent.

  3. Hypomagnesemia is defined as a magnesium level of less than 1.2 mg/dl (see Chap. 29, Hypocalcemia, Hypercalcemia, and Hypomagnesemia). It is most often associated with hypocalcemia, but it may occur in isolation.

  4. Hyponatremia may result from inappropriate ADH secretion, excessive renal salt loss, or excessive administration of hyponatremic fluids (see Chap. 9, Fluid and Electrolyte Management).

  5. Hypernatremia may be caused by dehydration, renal disease, or diabetes insipidus. It may be iatrogenic (see Chap. 9).

  6. Pyridoxine dependency

  7. Disorders of amino acid metabolism may cause seizures after the second day of life (see Chap. 29, Inborn Errors of Metabolism). Diagnosis is made by serum, urine, and CSF amino acid determinations. Acidosis with an elevated anion gap is common. Dietary and metabolic interventions may be helpful for many of these disorders (e.g., maple syrup urine disease, isovaleric acidemia, urea cycle disorders, methylmalonic acidemia, proprionic acidemia, congenital lactic acidosis, and biotin responsive disorders), and appropriate consultation is therefore indicated. The more common disorders associated with seizures include the following:

   a. Maple syrup urine disease. Seizures occur after institution of feeding and are associated with alteration of consciousness, poor feeding, and hypotonia occasionally alternating with opisthotonus or decerebration.

   b. Phenylketonuria. Seizures due to phenylketonuria are more likely to occur in the third or fourth week of life or later.

   c. Hyperglycinemia occurs in ketotic and nonketotic forms.

   d. Isovaleric acidemia presents with vomiting, anion gap acidosis, tremor, convulsions, coma, and a cheesy odor. Death occurs a few weeks after birth in half of the patients.

   e. Urea cycle disorders are usually associated with hyperammonemia.

   f. Beta-alanine abnormalities. This class of disorders is composed of two related disorders: hyperbeta-alaninemia and carnosinemia. They present with severe seizures early in neonatal life and result in progressive neurologic deterioration. Diagnosis is made by the presence of elevated serum levels of either beta-alanine or carnosine. Beta-aminoaciduria and gamma-aminobutyricaciduria may be present in hyperbeta-alaninemia.

8. **Organic acidemias.** Both methylmalonic acidemia and proprionic acidemia usually present with vomiting and stupor and are associated with acidosis, an elevated anion gap, hyperammonemia, and ketotic hyperglycinemia. Diagnosis is made by urine and serum organic acid screen.

   a. Methylmalonic acidemia. Some infants are vitamin B_{12} responsive.

   b. Propionic acidemia. Biotinidase deficiency may be associated with multiple carboxylase deficiency.

   c. Congenital lactic acidosis is caused by several inborn errors of metabolism, some of which respond to dietary therapy or pharmacologic dosages of thiamine.

   d. Glutaric aciduria type II. Hypoglycemia, hyperammonemia, a sweaty-foot odor, anemia, seizures, and death within 90 hours of life are common.

9. **Biotin-responsive disorders.** These disorders include deficiencies in biotinidase, holocarboxylase synthetase, or the multiple carboxylase complex. Metabolic acidosis, alopecia totalis, scaly eruption, hypotonia, an odor of cat urine, and elevated glycine and organic acid levels are common but not universal features. Diagnosis is made by blood or cultured fibroblast assay of the enzymes. Patients with these disorders are usually very responsive to pharmacy-grade biotin, 10 mg by mouth, daily.

10. **Fructose intolerance.** Seizures and other symptoms occur only if fructose-containing foods are ingested.

11. **Peroxisomal disorders** are a heterogeneous collection of disorders that include Zellweger's cerebrohepatorenal syndrome and neonatal adrenoleukodystrophy. Diagnosis is made by elevations of one or more of the following serum metabolites: very-long-chain fatty acids, plasmalogens, phytanic acid, and pipecolic acid. X-linked dominant and recessive forms have been identified. Babies with Zellweger's disease frequently have prepatellar calcifications revealed by x-ray.

12. **Mitochondrial disorders** are another heterogeneous collection of encephalopathies with multiorgan involvement caused by a variety of enzyme deficiencies involved in pyruvate metabolism and electron transport–respiratory chain metabolism. Some forms of Leigh's disease (subacute necrotizing encephalomyelopathy) and Alper's disease may be

so induced. Pyruvate, lactate, and alanine levels may be elevated in the serum and/or the CSF.

13. **Storage diseases:** G^m1- and G^m3-gangliosidoses

14. **Menkes' kinky hair disease.** Menkes' disease in the newborn is characterized by seizures, pili torti (kinky hair), connective-tissue defects, and hypothermia. Diagnosis is made by demonstration of decreased serum levels of copper and ceruloplasmin and the characteristic gross and microscopic appearance of the hair. This is an X-linked disorder of cellular copper distribution that is not improved by copper supplementation. In the neonate, the hair may not appear kinky, but if kinky hair is present, it has the characteristic sandy brown color.

15. **Molybdenum-cofactor deficiency** is an inborn error of metabolism that combines the finding seen in the individual enzyme defects of **sulphite oxidase deficiency** and **xanthine dehydrogenase deficiency** and which is missed on most metabolic screens. It can be detected when a sulphite strip test in a fresh urine sample reveals elevated urinary thiosulphate, or the urine and serum levels of uric acid are low, or the serum levels of xanthine and hypoxanthine are markedly elevated. Antenatal diagnosis is possible through chorionic villus sampling. Symptoms include eye lens dislocation (sulphite oxidase deficiency) and/or deposits of calculi in kidney and muscle (xanthine dehydrogenase), feeding difficulties, cortical atrophy, and thalamic calcifications.

C. **Infections may lead to seizures at any time** (see Chap. 23) and include the following causes:

1. **Bacterial meningitis,** including brain abscess

2. **Viral infections** (coxsackievirus, echovirus, rubella, cytomegalovirus, and herpesvirus). Sometimes a characteristic EEG pattern is present during herpes encephalitis.

3. **Toxoplasmosis**

4. **Syphilis**

5. **Human immunodeficiency virus** as a direct cause of seizures in the neonate, without opportunistic infection, has not been established.

D. **Developmental problems**

1. **Cerebral dysgenesis.** The absence of obvious morphologic disturbances on CT scan, head ultrasound, or MRI scan does not rule out microscopic forms of cerebral dysgenesis such as heterotopias and neuronal disorganization.

2. The **phakomatoses** include Sturge-Weber anomaly, neurofibromatosis, tuberous sclerosis, incontinentia pigmenti, and the organoid nevus syndrome (see Chap. 34).

E. **Drug-associated seizures**

1. **Narcotic and sedative withdrawals** are characterized by jitteriness, irritability, autonomic instability, and occasionally seizures (see Chap. 19). Seizures occur within 2 days with heroin withdrawal but may be delayed for 1 to 2 weeks with methadone or barbiturate withdrawal. Methadone withdrawal leads to seizures six times more often than heroin withdrawal does. Seizures and tremor have been associated with the direct effects of cocaine and methamphetamine intoxication and cocaine withdrawal. Infarcts can be associated with maternal cocaine use in pregnancy.

2. **Inadvertent administration of local anesthetic** into the fetal circulation either directly by scalp injection or indirectly by transplacental transmission during labor and delivery can lead to seizures that are usually tonic. The clinical picture includes hypotonia, bradycardia, fixed and dilated pupils, and complete external ophthalmoplegia. Such babies have an excellent prognosis if their conditions are properly diagnosed and managed.

3. **Theophylline** at toxic blood levels can lead to seizures.

4. **Propylene glycol,** a diluent in IV nutrition formulations and several medications, has been associated with seizures and other disorders in premature infants.

5. **Fluoxetine hydrochloride toxicity** can cause seizures in the perinatal infant when the drug is taken in excess by the pregnant or peripartum mother.

F. **Polycythemia/hyperviscosity** (see Chap. 26, Polycythemia). Lethargy and hypotonia are more common signs of this condition, although seizures can occur. Hypoglycemia is also a possible complication.

G. **Focal infarcts** from arterial or venous occlusion. These events may be provoked by deficiency in protein C or S, thrombocytosis, polycythemia, maternal lupus, maternal cocaine use, cardiac anomalies (including the myomata of tuberous sclerosis), and paradoxical emboli. Most focal infarcts have no recognized antecedents and are presumed to be emboli seeded from the placenta. Some deep venous stasis infarcts are not detectable except by MRI scan and present as idiopathic transient seizures or lethargy.

H. **Familial neonatal seizures** occur as an autosomal-dominant inherited trait. These seizures occur late in the first week of life. They generally do not continue after the perinatal period but may last several months.

I. **Hypertensive encephalopathy** may be associated with seizures in the newborn.

J. **Unknown causes** are involved in 3 to 25% of cases.

III. **Treatment.** Recurrent or continuous seizures may cause biochemical or physiologic effects that may lead to brain injury.
A. Optimize ventilation, cardiac output, blood pressure, serum electrolytes, and pH.
B. The underlying disease should be treated. Certain specific causes of seizures such as narcotic withdrawal (see Chap. 19, Drug Abuse and Withdrawal), metabolic abnormalities (see Chap. 29, Metabolic Abnormalities), and meningitis (see Chap. 23, Infections) need specific therapy. Diuresis and occasionally gastric lavage are required to remove inadvertently administered local anesthetic from symptomatic infants. Most of the therapy of neonatal seizures is symptomatic. To date, there is no evidence to confirm that high-dose phenobarbital is a useful therapy for the nonepileptic aspects of neonatal encephalopathy.
C. **Intravenous therapy.** A reliable intravenous line should be established, through an umbilical vein if necessary.
D. **Glucose** given prior to induced seizures in experimental animals appears to reduce mortality and brain damage; it also prevents the secondary fall in the blood glucose level seen in status epilepticus. Excessive glucose, however, promotes the accumulation of cerebral lactic acid, which also may be damaging to the brain. Thus, we advocate maintenance of the serum glucose level within physiologic bounds (70 to 120 mg/dl).
   1. If rapid screen with Dextrostix shows a low blood glucose level, it should be corrected, even if it is not the primary cause of the seizures. The treatment of hypoglycemia is described in Chap. 29.
   2. If the glucose levels remain low, treatment with glucagon or hydrocortisone should be considered even if signs are not present (see Chap. 29, Hypoglycemia and Hyperglycemia).
E. **Pyridoxine dependency** is diagnosed by giving pyridoxine 50 mg IV as a therapeutic trial (under EEG control, if possible). Seizures will cease within minutes if pyridoxine dependency or deficiency is causing them. Maintenance therapy in dependency calls for a dose of 10 to 100 mg of pyridoxine by mouth daily. In deficiency, the dose is 5 mg by mouth daily, and the EEG does not always normalize immediately when seizures cease during pyridoxine infusion. Rarely, pyridoxine therapy has been associated with hypotonia and apnea.
F. **Anticonvulsants.** If hypoglycemia or metabolic problems are not the evident cause of seizures, anticonvulsant medications should be administered.
   1. **Phenobarbital**
      a. **Ongoing seizures (acute administration).** Phenobarbital 15 to 20 mg/kg is given intravenously over several minutes for seizures. If the

seizures continue after 60 minutes, a second dose of phenobarbital (10 mg/kg) may be given, usually concomitantly with loading dosages of phenytoin (see **2**). Traditionally, loading dosages of phenytoin are recommended, but in refractory status epilepticus, one may elect to use **very-high-dose phenobarbital**. This can be administered in 10 mg/kg boluses every 30 minutes (usually totaling less than 60 mg/kg) until seizures cease. If the infant has intermittent seizures, without true status epilepticus, and has phenobarbital levels of 30 to 45 μg/ml, then **phenytoin** may be administered (see **2**). Cumulative loading doses of phenobarbital greater than 20 mg/kg require careful monitoring of blood pressure and respiratory status for the possible development of hypotension and, more rarely, apnea. Hypotension, usually due to peripheral vasodilation but occasionally due to myocardial depression in neonates with diseased hearts, may be treated with volume expansion. Rarely, dopamine may be necessary (see Chap. 17). Hypotension or apnea tends to occur more often with the simultaneous use of other anticonvulsants or CNS-depressant medications, especially benzodiazepines. A surprisingly high percentage of patients maintain spontaneous respiration even on very-high-dose phenobarbital, but some require intubation to protect the airway from pharyngeal hypotonia.

b. Interictal (acute administration). If an infant has had a seizure but is not currently having seizures, the intravenous administration of 15 to 20 mg/kg of phenobarbital will lead to therapeutic plasma levels.

c. Maintenance doses range from 3.5 to 4.5 mg/kg per day of phenobarbital, given as a single dose or divided in two doses given every 12 hours intravenously or by mouth. Serum phenobarbital levels tend to rise during the first 1 to 2 weeks with doses of 5 to 6 mg/kg per day. Phenobarbital half-life diminishes subsequently.

d. Therapeutic plasma levels range from 15 to 45 μg/ml, measured at least 1 hour after an intravenous dose or 2 to 4 hours after an oral dose. The goal is to maintain the lowest therapeutic level that controls seizures; this level is usually in the range of 15 to 30 μg/ml. Phenobarbital can cause sedation and hypotonia in neonates, and it may increase theophylline requirement in premature infants with apnea.

2. Phenytoin (Dilantin) 15 to 25 mg/kg is given intravenously, administered in normal saline at a rate not greater than 1 mg/kg per minute. Phenytoin is generally given if there has been no response to phenobarbital or if there is a critical need to monitor the level of consciousness. A maintenance dose of 4 to 8 mg/kg per day, divided into two or three doses, can be given intravenously. The therapeutic plasma level is 10 to 20 μg/ml, taken at least 1 hour after IV administration. Phenytoin is poorly absorbed from the gastrointestinal tract and/or the half-life is very short when administered during the newborn period.

3. Diazepam (Valium) is used only when immediate cessation of seizures is required (i.e., when seizures interfere with vital functions). Although diazepam has a rapid therapeutic onset, redistribution pharmacodynamics result in an anticonvulsant half-life measured in minutes. Its sedative-effect half-life, by contrast, exceeds 24 hours.

a. If diazepam is required, it should be administered after dilution of 0.2 ml (1 mg) of diazepam with 0.8 ml of normal saline. The titration of dosage is otherwise difficult.

b. The initial dose should be 0.1 to 0.3 mg/kg given slowly, IV, until the seizure stops.

c. Diazepam acts synergistically with phenobarbital to increase the risk of provoking respiratory arrest. Appropriate facilities for circulatory and ventilatory support should be available.

d. Diazepam contains sodium benzoate, which may interfere with the binding of bilirubin to albumin.

4. **Lorazepam (Ativan)** is an effective anticonvulsant when administered acutely. However, experience with lorazepam is limited. Its anticonvulsant effect lasts longer than that of diazepam. The current recommended dose is 0.05 mg/kg per dose IV over 2 to 5 minutes. The dose may be repeated. The complications generally are the same as those of diazepam. On occasion, lorazepam has been associated with the triggering of myoclonic jerks and repetitive clonic activity.

5. **Midazolam** can be used as an anticonvulsant at an initial dose of 0.02 to 0.4 mg/kg IM (maximum 5 mg); or 0.02 to 0.1 mg/kg IV followed by 0.06 to 0.4 mg/kg/hour.

6. **Paraldehyde** is used as adjunct therapy only after maximum therapeutic levels of phenobarbital and phenytoin are attained and if seizures have not been controlled. We rarely use this drug.

   a. Paraldehyde may be given rectally, 0.1 to 0.3 ml/kg diluted in a ratio of 1:1 or 2:1 with mineral oil, and no more frequently than three times daily.

   b. Excretion of paraldehyde is predominantly hepatic, but 7 to 18% is excreted by the lung. One of the important toxic effects provoked by paraldehyde is pulmonary hemorrhage.

   c. Paraldehyde also can provoke mucosal slough and circulatory collapse, particularly when old paraldehyde is used.

   d. Intravenous paraldehyde can be used, but it is corrosive to blood vessels and is apt to provoke circulatory instability. Some plastic bottles and tubing are dissolved by old paraldehyde. Paraldehyde can be administered in burettes and tubing made of polyethylene or polypropylene, but not polyvinyl. When the drug is used to terminate status epilepticus, it should be diluted into a 5% solution that is mixed with dextrose 5% in water. This solution is given at the rate of 50 to 150 mg/kg/hour. Paraldehyde may be tapered after seizures have ceased. Continuous infusion of paraldehyde should not be continued beyond 3 hours. Therapeutic levels are 10 to 16 mg/dl.

7. **Adjunctive anticonvulsants** have not been studied extensively in neonates and are approved, if at all, only for seizures that fail to respond well to other more standard therapies. **Pyridoxine** (vitamin B$_6$) in high doses (300 mg/kg/day) has been used with some success in infants with refractory infantile spasms. Such seizures are termed *pyridoxine-responsive seizures* and are distinct from the classic pyridoxine dependency, which responds to low doses of pyridoxine. It probably works by increasing the formation of endogenous gamma-aminobutyric acid (GABA), because it is the known cofactor for glutamic acid decarboxylase. Other anticonvulsants with which there is limited experience in the newborn include primidone (Mysoline), carbamazepine (5 to 10 mg/kg orally, twice daily), pentobarbital, and valproic acid given rectally.

8. The adequacy of therapy may be difficult to judge. Electrical seizures may be seen despite the absence of clinical seizures. We attempt to stop all clinical evidence of seizures, including blood pressure and heart rate changes in infants who are paralyzed. We use phenobarbital to attain levels of 40 µg/ml if necessary. Other drugs are used as indicated if clinical seizures continue. Do not attempt to stop all electrical epileptiform activity because of the side effects of doses required to do this.

G. **Follow-up anticonvulsant medications.** If possible, all medications except maintenance phenobarbital at 3.5 to 5 mg/kg per day should be discontinued before the infant is discharged. The other medications, except phenobarbital, are often stopped when intravenous therapy is stopped. Normal findings on examination, the absence of recurrent seizures, and a nonepileptiform EEG are indications for the discontinuation of all anticonvulsants. Occasionally, this may be done prior to discharge; more often, however, anticonvulsants are continued for the first 2 months of life. Decisions to treat longer are based on the risk of recurrence of seizures. Factors entering into this risk are the original cause of the seizure, the neurologic examination, and the EEG. Infants whose seizures were caused by a **transient metabolic disturbance** have little risk of recurrent seizures, infants whose seizures were caused by **hypoxic-ischemic encephalopathy** have a 30 to 50% risk of recurrent seizures, and infants whose seizures were caused by **malformations of the cerebral cortex** have a high incidence of recurrent seizures.

H. Other medications

1. **Calcium.** If hypocalcemia is the cause of the seizure, calcium gluconate 10%, 2 ml/kg (18 mg of elemental calcium per kilogram) mixed with an equal volume of water, is given intravenously over 3 minutes. The patient's condition is checked during the administration using an electrocardiogram (ECG) or cardiac monitor (see Chap. 29, Hypocalcemia, Hypercalcemia, and Hypermagnesemia).

   a. Calcium should not be mixed with sodium bicarbonate.

   b. If the infusion is too rapid, bradycardia can result.

   c. Calcium should not be given through the umbilical vein unless the catheter tip is in the inferior vena cava.

   d. To avoid tissue necrosis caused by extravasation, the peripheral veins should be observed directly when calcium is being rapidly infused.

   e. If hypocalcemia is the cause of the seizures, they will stop immediately after the calcium level in the blood is returned to normal; maintenance calcium should be given (see Chap. 29, Hypocalcemia, Hypercalcemia, and Hypermagnesemia).

   f. When the hypocalcemia is a secondary cause of seizures (as is most common), or when there is concurrent untreated hypomagnesemia, the seizures may continue after the administration of calcium.

2. **Magnesium.** Hypomagnesemia is treated with magnesium sulfate 50%, 0.2 ml/kg. Half of all hypocalcemic infants also have hypomagnesemia; failure to treat hypomagnesemia may cause a lack of clinical response to administration of calcium for hypocalcemia (see Chap. 29).

IV. Prognosis. At present, the overall prognosis in neonatal seizures is **death in 15%; neurologic sequelae** such as mental retardation, motor deficits, and seizures **in 30%;** and **normal outcome in 56%.** Chronic seizure disorder will develop in 15 to 20% of survivors. In the individual case, prognosis is estimated by the level of maturity, underlying etiology of the seizures, EEG, neurologic examination, and imaging studies of the brain such as ultrasound, CT, and MRI.

A. Prognosis by maturity. The prognosis of newborns with seizures is related to maturity regardless of etiology or other clinical factors. Earlier reports generally combined the outcome data of full-term and premature neonates. Recent reports, however, have considered these two groups separately. In one study, seizures developed in 22.7% of infants with a gestational age of 31 weeks or less, in 1.6% of infants between 32 and 36 weeks' gestation, and in 0.16% of infants born at 37 weeks' gestation or more. Neonatal mortality associated with seizures was 84% in infants with a gestational age of 31 weeks or less, 57% in infants between 32 and 36 weeks' gestation, and 17% in infants with a gestational age of 37 weeks or more. Other studies show the same relationship among seizures, mortality associated with seizures, and gestational age.

B. Prognosis by etiology. Seizures represent signs and not a disease state. The outcome, in general, reflects the seriousness of the disorder that provokes the seizures (Table 27-1).

C. Prognosis by seizure pattern. Certain patterns are associated with poor prognosis, as summarized in Table 27-2.

D. Prognosis by EEG. Both ictal and interictal EEG patterns have prognostic value. Table 27-3 reviews outcome data by EEG pattern. Prognostication on the basis of either clinical or EEG findings should generally be made from assessments performed 5 to 10 days after the initial evaluation. Abnormali-

Table 27-1. Prognosis of seizures by etiology*

Etiology	Normal outcome (%)
Subarachnoid hemorrhage	90
Uncertain	75
Early hypocalcemia	50
Late hypocalcemia	100
Hypoglycemia	33–71
Neonatal encephalopathy	31–50
Intraventricular hemorrhage	10
Meningitis	11–65
Dysgenesis	0

*This means prognosis for the etiology when **seizures** are a manifestation of the etiology.
Sources: Data from I. Bergman et al., Outcome in neonates with convulsions treated in an intensive care unit, *Ann. Neurol.* 14: 642, 1983; J. Dennis, Neonatal convulsions: Aetiology, late neonatal status and long-term outcome, *Dev. Med. Child Neurol.* 20: 143, 1978; T. K. McInerny and W. K. Schubert, Prognosis of neonatal seizures, *Am. J. Dis. Child.* 117: 261, 1969; and J. J. Volpe, Neonatal Seizures. In *Neurology of the Newborn.* Philadelphia: W. B. Saunders, 1995, pp. 172–207.

ties of background rhythm are more strongly associated with future clinical outcome than an epileptiform, maturationally delayed, or asymmetrical EEG. A **normal background EEG** is associated with an **under 10% incidence** of neurologic sequelae; **severe background abnormalities** such as burst-suppression pattern, electrical silence, or marked voltage suppression are associated with a **90% incidence** of neurologic sequelae; and **moderate background abnormalities** such as immaturity and voltage asymmetries are associated with a **50% incidence** of neurologic sequelae. The burst suppression pattern is an ominous sign, seen in many severe, global cerebral insults, but when it occurs in a treatable metabolic disorder, its prognosis is related to the degree of treatability of the disorder. When voltage suppressions are less than 20 seconds, the link to poor outcome is much less than when suppressions are greater than 20 seconds. In neonatal encephalopathy, if the background normalizes by the 7th day after birth, outcome is good; but if marked voltage suppression is present after the 7th day, or if mild voltage suppression is present after the 12th day, subsequent neurologic handicaps are more likely to be present. Other background abnor-

Table 27-2. Prognosis of seizures by seizure pattern: Normal outcome (%) by gestational age at birth

Seizure pattern	Full-term (%)	Premature (%)
Focal clonic	100*	33
Multifocal	33	33
Generalized	59	41
Tonic	50	36
Myoclonic	0	0
Subtle	57	44

*Probably not normal in cases of neonatal stroke.
Source: Data from I. Bergman et al., Outcome in neonates with convulsions treated in an intensive care unit, *Ann. Neurol.* 14: 542, 1983.

Table 27-3. Prognosis of seizures by ictal and interictal electroencephalogram patterns

Pattern	Normal (percent)*,†	Normal (%)‡,§		
		≤ 31 weeks	32–36 weeks	≥ 37 weeks
Ictal				
Normal background (focal discharge)	57			
Abnormal background (multifocal discharge)	24			
Alpha, beta, theta, or delta discharge	20	38	67	83
Repeated sharp waves (abnormal background)	21			
No discharge	0			
Interictal				
Normal	89	20	50	77
Unifocal discharge		33		80
Multifocal discharge		52	41	62
Flat	0			
Low amplitude	11			
Burst suppression	8	17	33	18
Focal status				0
Generalized status				
Persistent dysmaturity for age	33			

*Data from J. Dernis, Neonatal convulsions: Aetiology, late neonatal status and long-term outcome, *Dev. Med. Child Neurol.* 20: 143, 1978.

†Premature and full-term infants were grouped together in this study.

‡Data from I. Bergman et al., Outcome in neonates with convulsions treated in an intensive care unit, *Ann. Neurol.* 14: 642, 1983.

§Infants in this study were grouped together according to gestational age.

malities are less predictive of outcome, so that prediction based on a single EEG feature is hazardous. The prognostic value is increased substantially by the performance of serial studies. In one study, if the EEG background was normal in the acute phase of neonatal meningitis, the infants were neurologically normal by 34 months; if the background was markedly abnormal, and the infants had seizures or depressed consciousness during the illness, the infants had neurologic sequelae.

Positive temporal and Rolandic sharp waves are associated with a high incidence of nonhemorrhagic cerebral structural abnormalities, particularly in the white matter, and positive Rolandic sharp waves are particularly associated with subsequent periventricular leukomalacia.

E. Other prognostic features. The National Collaborative Perinatal Project found that in neonatal seizures, death, mental retardation, cerebral palsy, or epilepsy is related to the following factors: (1) Apgar scores less than or equal to 6 at 5 minutes, (2) the need for 5 minutes of positive-pressure ventilation following birth, (3) early onset of seizures, (4) seizures lasting longer than 30 minutes, (5) hypotonia at 5 minutes following birth, (6) 3 or more days with uncontrolled seizures, and (7) the presence of tonic or myoclonic seizures. Nonetheless, when evaluated at 7 years of age, 70% of surviving neonates with seizures had normal outcome. Other reports suggest that 20 to 30% of neonates with seizures will develop epilepsy. The prognostic importance of the duration of seizures and the presence of tonic seizure patterns has been confirmed. However, the importance of low Apgar scores to development of early seizures has not been supported. Poor outcome is associated with the need for more than one anticonvulsant. Most studies, unfortunately, have limited long-term follow-up.

Reference
Volpe, J. J. Neonatal seizures. In: J. J. Volpe (Ed.). *Neurology of the newborn,* 3rd ed. Philadelphia: W.B. Saunders, 1995.

Intracranial Hemorrhage
Karl C.K. Kuban

I. **Intracranial hemorrhage (ICH)** occurs in 20% to more than 40% of infants with birth weights under 1500 gm but is less common among more mature newborns. Bleeding within the skull can occur extracerebrally (1) into epidural, subdural, or subarachnoid spaces, (2) into parenchyma of the cerebrum or cerebellum, or (3) into ventricles from the subependymal germinal matrix or choroid plexus. The incidence, pathogenesis, presentation, diagnosis, management, and prognosis of these hemorrhages vary according to their location (Table 27-4); each type of hemorrhage will be considered separately.

A. **Subependymal hemorrhage-intraventricular hemorrhage (SEH-IVH)**
1. **Incidence.** Bleeding from the subependymal germinal matrix with or without subsequent rupture into a ventricle occurs in approximately 17 to 40% of infants born before 34 weeks' gestation. The incidence appears to have diminished over the past 5 to 10 years, so that most tertiary centers currently report an incidence of 17 to 25%. Although IVH can occur in the full-term neonate, it is rare, and the source of bleeding is usually the choroid plexus.

2. **Pathogenesis.** Germinal matrix or subependymal tissue overlies the head of the caudate nucleus; after 26 weeks' gestation it is comprised of glial cells, which subsequently migrate into the adjacent cerebrum. The supportive tissue of the germinal matrix then involutes and almost disappears by 34 weeks' gestation. The maximum rate of involution occurs between 26 and 32 weeks, the period of greatest risk for development of SEH-IVH.

Table 27-4.   Categories of neonatal intracranial hemorrhage

1. Subependymal hemorrhage—intraventricular hemorrhage (SEH-IVH)
2. Posterior fossa hemorrhage
   a. Cerebellar
   b. Subdural (SDH)
3. Anterior fossa hemorrhage
   a. Subdural
   b. Intraparenchymal
4. Subarachnoid hemorrhage (SAH)

The predisposing associations for development of SEH-IVH may be organized as intravascular inflow, intravascular outflow, and structural (both vascular and extravascular) factors (Table 27-5). The vasculature of the germinal matrix region lacks musculorum, is poorly supported by perivascular structures, and is an end bed to the only muscularized arterioles (striatal arteries) in the cerebrum before term. Loss of vascular autoregulation in these arterioles, leading to a pressure-passive state, makes the vessels just distal to them unusually vulnerable to rupture during surges in arterial blood flow. This is particularly true if there is resistance to egress of blood, as occurs with increases in venous pressure.

The intravascular factors associated with SEH-IVH include events that provoke surges in cerebral inflow or compromise the outflow of blood on the venous side of the matrix circulation. Surges of cerebral blood flow may occur with seizures, episodes of hypoxia, apnea, respiratory distress, rapid infusion of colloid, patent ductus arteriosus, extracorporeal membrane oxygenation, and possibly certain caretaking procedures such as tracheal suctioning. Increased venous pressure may be associated with respiratory distress syndrome, pneumothorax, congestive heart failure, certain ventilator parameters such as high continuous positive airway pressure, possibly labor and/or delivery, and possibly hyperviscosity. Large second-to-second fluctuations in cerebral blood flow velocity in the anterior cerebral arteries, as measured by Doppler ultrasonography, are significantly associated with the development of SEH-IVH. The large measured fluctuations may reflect alterations in arterial flow and/or the degree of respiratory distress and/or other confounding variables.

SEH-IVH most often begins as a small hemorrhage, usually petechial, between birth and 48 hours of life. Extravascular factors may act to promote bleeding or extension of bleeding. These factors include the presence of fibrinolytic enzymes within the germinal matrix region, thrombocytopenia, vitamin K deficiency, the administration of intravenous flush solutions containing benzyl alcohol as a preservative, and possibly the use of heparin. Occasionally, large hemorrhages develop abruptly.

3. **Clinical presentation.** Clinical symptoms and signs may occur as a result of blood volume loss or neurologic dysfunction (Table 27-6) and depend, in part, on how rapidly blood loss evolves. None of the signs is specific for SEH-IVH, although pallor, indicating blood loss, is most useful.

The clinical presentation depends on the size, site, and rapidity of the hemorrhage. IVH can present as a catastrophic event when blood loss is large and rapid. Presentation can be stuttering, with intermittent periods of stabilization when there is a slower evolution of blood loss. A clinically silent presentation may occur in up to 50% of cases, usually with smaller hemorrhages.

4. **Diagnosis.** Real-time gray-scale portable sector ultrasonography is the method of choice in evaluating infants for the presence of SEH-IVH.

Table 27-5. Possible etiologic factors associated with SEH-IVH in low-birth-weight infants

Intravascular inflow factors	Intravascular outflow factors	Vascular and extravascular structural factors
Impaired autoregulation	Respiratory distress	Normal regression of germinal matrix
Seizures	Pneumothorax	Relatively large blood flow to deep cerebral structures (in first half of third trimester)
Manipulation of the infant	Congestive heart failure	Hypoxic-ischemic injury to germinal matrix or its vessels
Infusion of hyperosmotic solutions	Continuous positive airway pressure	
Rapid colloid infusion	Acute angle of the internal cerebral vein	
Apnea		Presence of fibrinolytic enzymes
Large fluctuations in second-to-second cerebrovascular flow velocity	Labor/delivery	Poor structural support of germinal matrix vessels
		Abrupt termination of media in arteries proximal to germinal matrix
Presence of patent ductus arteriosus		
		Presence of a bleeding diathesis
Hypertension and use of ECMO		Use of benzyl alcohol as a preservative

Key: SEH-IVH = subependymal hemorrhage–intraventricular hemorrhage; ECMO = extracorporeal membrane oxygenation.

Clinical signs and symptoms, combined with the presence of hemorrhagic cerebrospinal fluid (CSF), were used to make the presumptive diagnosis before ultrasonic evaluation became available. Because of the high incidence of traumatic lumbar puncture in premature infants, a diagnosis made in this manner can only be presumptive. Although computerized tomographic (CT) scans define the pathologic anatomy of SEH-IVH extremely well, they require transport of the infant to the machine, and in most circumstances, the stress associated with transport is a relative contraindication to the test. Magnetic resonance imaging (MRI) is both a sensitive and a specific manner of identifying SEH-IVH after the first several days of life. The abnormal images persist for up to 3 months after the bleed. However, submitting newborns to MRI testing has the same disadvantages noted for CT scans and requires nonmetallic monitoring wires and equipment for the babies undergoing the test.

There is no universally accepted system for grading hemorrhages, although the systems reported by Papile and Levene are most often cited (Table 27-7). Since none of the grading systems is completely satisfactory, however, description of the ultrasonic characteristics of the hemor-

Table 27-6. Clinical presentation of SEH-IVH

Blood volume loss		
Signs of blood loss	Laboratory correlates of blood loss	Neurologic dysfunction
Shock	Metabolic acidosis	Bulging anterior fontanel
Pallor	Low hematocrit	Excessive somnolence
Respiratory distress	Hypoxemia, hypercarbia and respiratory acidosis	Hypotonia
		Weakness, seizures
Disseminated intravascular coagulation	Thrombocytopenia and prolongation of both PT and PTT	Temperature instability
Jaundice	Hyperbilirubinemia	Brain stem signs (apnea, lost extraocular movements, facial weakness)

Key: SEH-IVH = subependymal hemorrhage–intraventricular hemorrhage; PT = prothrombin time; PTT = partial thromboplastin time.

rhage is most useful. This description should include the following observations:

  a. Presence or absence of blood in the germinal matrix

  b. Laterality (or bilaterality) of the hemorrhage

  c. Presence or absence of blood in a ventricle, and its location and amount (small, moderate, large)

  d. Presence or absence of blood in cerebral parenchyma, with specification of location

  e. Presence or absence of ventricular dilatation

  f. Presence or absence of other echogenic abnormalities

    Echogenic areas of parenchyma, especially white matter, are most often identified in prematurely born babies with SEH-IVH. They may develop independently of hemorrhage. Parenchymal echoabnormalities correlate highly with subsequent motor and development deficits.

 5. **Timing of ultrasound examinations.** Ultrasound examination should be performed when clinical indications (abrupt fall in hematocrit, shock, bulging fontanel, change in level of consciousness, or change in respiratory support needs without other explanation) appear at any time in premature babies. Otherwise, **we perform routine ultrasound screens in infants with birth weight <1500 gm or gestational age <32 weeks. We also screen those ≤32 weeks who have risk factors for hypoxic-ischemic injury (e.g., RDS, NEC, pneumothorax, sepsis).** Screens are performed on days 0–2, 7–10, 21–28, and close to 40 weeks postconceptional age or before discharge. Screening for hydrocephalus also should be undertaken in babies with hemorrhage (see **7**).

 6. **Management**

  a. **Prevention.** Avoid rapid intravenous administration of osmotically active agents and unnecessary manipulations of the infant. Phenobarbital does not prevent the development of IVH. The use of indomethacin as a prophylactic agent against the development of IVH is controversial, may work differently in babies below and above 1000 gm in birth weight, and requires further clinical studies prior to recommendations for its routine use.

Table 27-7. Grading system for subependymal hemorrhage–intraventricular hemorrhage

First author	Assessment technique	Grading system	Definitions*
Papile[a]	CT	1	Isolated SEH
		2	IVH without ventricular dilatation
		3	IVH with ventricular dilatation
		4	IVH with parenchymal extension
Volpe[b]	US	I	SEH ± blood in less than 10% of ventricular system
		II	SEH + blood in 10–50% of ventricular area
		III	>50% filling ± distension of ventricles
Mantovani[c]	CT	1	SEH or IVH filling less than 10% of ventricles
		2	IVH filling from 10 to 50% of ventricles
		3	IVH filling 50% or greater of ventricles
Lazzara[d]	CT	Mild	SEH ± one-fourth of AP diameter of ventricles blood-filled
		Moderate	One-fourth to one-half of AP diameter of ventricles blood-filled
		Severe	One-half of AP diameter of ventricles blood-filled
Shankaran[e]	US	Mild	SEH ± small amount of blood in ventricle (normal-sized)
		Moderate	Intermediate amount of blood in enlarged ventricles
		Severe	Filling ventricles forming a cast or intracerebral extension of hemorrhage
Levene[f]	US	1	SEH ± with no inferior or lateral extension of blood beyond most lateral border of ventricles
		2	Downward extension into basal nuclei on at least one side or involvement of caudate to genu of ventricle posteriorly on parasagittal scan
		3	Large hemorrhage with any degree of extension laterally or superiorly into cerebral parenchyma

Key: CT = computerized tomography; SEH = subependymal hemorrhage; IVH = intraventricular hemorrhage; ± = with or without; AP = anteroposterior; US = ultrasound.
*Ventricles are lateral ventricles.
[a]Papile, L. A. *J. Pediatr.* 92: 529, 1978.
[b]Volpe, J. J. *Neurology of the Newborn*, 3rd ed. Philadelphia: W.B. Saunders, 1995, Chap. 11.
[c]Mantovani, J. F. *J. Pediatr.* 97: 278, 1980.
[d]Lazzara, A. *Pediatrics* 65: 30, 1980.
[e]Shankaran, S. *Pediatrics* 114: 109, 1989.
[f]Levene, M. I. *Arch. Dis. Child.* 57: 410, 1988.

The prophylactic use of pancuronium has been reported to reduce the risk of SEH-IVH in specific preselected populations. Before the routine use of pancuronium can be recommended, however, studies are needed to affirm the initial study's beneficial effects, to better define the population most likely to benefit from pancuronium, and to evaluate more fully the limitations and risks of paralysis when pancuronium is used prophylactically.

Prenatal treatment of the fetus with steroids to prevent RDS decreases the incidence of IVH. Other prophylactic agents that hold promise but require further study include vitamin E and ethamsylate, which are not recommended currently.

b. **Specific treatment.** The treatment of SEH-IVH is supportive and is directed at avoiding extension of the hemorrhage. No interventions have been shown conclusively to limit the extent of hemorrhage once it has occurred, although the recommendations for prevention of SEH-IVH (see **a**) are probably applicable. Avoid excessive suctioning and manipulations. Administer osmotically active agents slowly, including albumin, plasma, and blood. Vitamin K administration may be important for those infants who have evidence of abnormalities of coagulation (see Chap. 26, Bleeding). Treat seizures (see Neonatal Seizures, above) and hyperbilirubinemia associated with the breakdown of red blood cells from the hemorrhage (see Chap. 18). The use of ECMO is usually contraindicated. Infants with SEH-IVH may have low CSF glucose levels in the absence of infection.

In addition to acute cardiovascular and neurologic dysfunction, concomitant or continued cerebral injury may occur because of reduced cerebral perfusion pressure (mean arterial pressure minus intracranial pressure) or because of intermittent ischemia. Avoid hypotension (see Chap. 17). Marked elevations in ICP indicates that hydrocephalus likely has occurred.

7. **Complications: posthemorrhagic hydrocephalus (PHH)**
   a. **Definition.** Hydrocephalus should be differentiated from ventricular dilatation. It indicates either a state of progressively expanding ventricles or enlarged ventricles and increased ICP (an ICP >5 cm H_2O). In babies without elevations of venous pressure (e.g., CPAP, pneumothorax), a good estimate of intracranial pressure is the vertical distance, measured in centimeters, between the anterior fontanel and the heart, measured at the point where the anterior fontanel flattens as you manually tilt the baby up. Ventriculomegaly indicates a static increase in ventricular size without elevated ICP. Some infants may proceed from a state of ventriculomegaly to hydrocephalus after a stable period of 3 months or longer.
   b. **Clinical features.** Hydrocephalus can occur immediately following hemorrhage but usually evolves over the weeks following SEH-IVH. It occurs in approximately 25% of infants with SEH-IVH and is most readily identified by cranial ultrasound. Hydrocephalus is more likely to occur with large hemorrhages. A bulging anterior fontanel, a rapidly expanding head circumference, and brain stem signs, including "sunset eyes," are generally late signs. Milder clinical signs such as lethargy and weakness of the lower extremities are often too difficult to evaluate in the ill premature infant; therefore, a weekly ultrasonic evaluation until there is clear stabilization of ventricular size is a minimum requirement following the development of SEH-IVH. Infants with small hemorrhages, particularly if the hemorrhages are limited to the germinal matrix, may require only a few follow-up scans, whereas infants with ventricular expansion with large volumes of blood may need to be followed up for months.
   c. **Pathophysiology.** Hydrocephalus usually occurs because of a combination of factors, including obstruction of CSF outflow through the

fourth ventricle or at the base of the brain at the foramina of Luschka and Magendie and impairment of CSF resorption at the arachnoid granulations over the convexity of the brain. If there is complete obstruction of CSF flow at the fourth ventricle or at the base of the brain, the hydrocephalus is noncommunicating. This occurs more often when the hydrocephalus develops rapidly after a massive hemorrhage. Communicating hydrocephalus caused by impaired CSF resorption usually develops gradually.

d. **Management.** Static ventricular dilatation without elevated ICP does not require intervention. Hydrocephalus, however, requires intervention so that normal cerebral perfusion pressure (CPP) can be maintained and compression of both periventricular white matter and cerebral arteries, in particular the anterior cerebral arteries, can be avoided.

(1) The natural history of PHH is to (1) progress, occasionally after a period of stabilization, (2) come to an equilibrium of CSF production and efflux at some state of ventricular dilatation, or (3) recede toward normalcy. Since the long-term complication rate of ventricular shunts and their placement exceeds 50%, and since premature infants with PHH are fragile and thus poor surgical risks, avoidance or delay in the placement of shunts is often preferred.

Serial lumbar punctures with removal of at least 10 to 15 ml/kg of CSF are advocated as a means of transiently reducing ventricular pressure and size. This procedure often enables postponement of definitive shunting and may permit time for an individual patient's hydrocephalus to either come to equilibrium or recede. The success and required frequency of lumbar punctures should be evaluated by the results of opening pressures on lumbar puncture or by manual measurement of ICP over the anterior fontanel (see **a**) and by repetitive ultrasonic examination. Serial head circumference measures also may be useful. Lumbar puncture opening pressures of less than 80 mm of water for 3 consecutive days in the presence of a static ventricular size are highly predictive of successful management without the need for surgery. Lumbar puncture treatment may need to be continued for several weeks. Serial lumbar punctures will be effective only if the hydrocephalus is at least partially communicating. Serial lumbar punctures have been shown to be an ineffective means of preventing the development of hydrocephalus following SEH-IVH.

(2) Surgical intervention is required when hydrocephalus persists despite lumbar puncture treatment for as long as 3 or 4 weeks or with rapid development of raised ICP with florid clinical signs not responsive to lumbar puncture. Surgical intervention can occur in the form of a ventriculoperitoneal shunt, a temporary ventriculostomy with external drainage, or a ventricular drain tunneled to a subcutaneous reservoir or space. Temporary external ventriculostomy need not necessarily be followed by permanent shunt placement.

(3) Pharmacologic treatment of PHH with acetazolamide (20 to 100 mg/kg/day) divided into doses given every 6 hours), or furosemide (1 mg/kg/day, divided into doses given every 6 hours), may be used as an alternative initial form of therapy. It may be used as an adjunct to lumbar punctures, however, or when other forms of therapy fail and shunting is contraindicated. We usually start with acetazolamide 40 mg/kg per day, divided into doses given every 6 hours, and furosemide 1 mg/kg per day, divided into doses given every 12 hours. The dose of acetazolamide may be increased up to

100 mg/kg/day depending on effect. We have not used glycerol. Particular care should be given to blood pressure, fluid, acid–base, and electrolyte status when these agents are used. The administration of furosemide and acetazolamide may predispose to the development of hypercalciuria and nephrocalcinosis (see Chaps. 9; 29, Hypercalcemia; and 31). Infants treated with acetazolamide may need treatment with Polycitra (sodium bicarbonate and potassium bicarbonate) to correct electrolyte disturbances. The usual starting dose is 1 to 3 mEq/kg. The dose is then titrated according to response.

8. **Prognosis.** Since longitudinal studies of very-low-birth-weight infants with SEH-IVH were not feasible until high-resolution portable ultrasound units became available, the prognosis of babies with SEH-IVH is only currently becoming available. Approximately 30% of babies with SEH-IVH die in the newborn period, although not necessarily as a result of hemorrhage. Numerous long-term studies are in progress, and some series have been reported. For the most part, these series attempt to correlate the grade of SEH-IVH with degree of neurologic impairment. The limited data available are conflicting, however, and already have provoked considerable controversy. It is likely that associated tissue destruction of white matter is more important in determining the ultimate neurologic outcome than the hemorrhage per se.

Disparate views of the effects of SEH-IVH on outcome may be explained in part by differences in the populations studied, variable definitions of abnormality, the timing and nature of evaluations, the use of diverse grading systems, and probably, most importantly, the lack of consideration of other parenchymal injury such as periventricular leukomalacia (PVL).

In general, the more extensive the hemorrhage, the more likely it is that there will be motor or cognitive impairments. When there is major parenchymal hemorrhage or associated parenchymal damage with or without parenchymal hemorrhage, some form of motor impairment is common. Recent studies suggest that ventricular enlargement, either as a static state or as PHH and parenchymal abnormalities, is most highly predictive of compromised neurologic outcome.

It is uncertain whether minor abnormalities such as language delay, fine motor disability, learning impairments, and behavioral dysfunctions are related to SEH-IVH or concomitants of SEH-IVH. Some studies suggest that more subtle developmental and educational difficulties may occur in children who have smaller grades of SEH-IVH. If such disabilities are related to SEH-IVH, it is also uncertain whether the critical prognostic factor is (1) involvement of both germinal matrices or ventricles, (2) disturbances of white matter (e.g., unilateral white matter necrosis, PVL), (3) development of PHH, (4) cerebral perfusion alterations that may precede, occur with, or follow development of SEH-IVH, (5) associated medical diseases, (6) preexisting predisposition to such problems, or (7) a combination of factors. Delay in shunting also has been associated with poor outcome.

B. Posterior fossa hemorrhage

1. **Pathogenesis.** The presentation of hemorrhages into the cerebellum or the subdural space of the posterior fossa is often similar to that of space-occupying lesions in the posterior fossa. Such hemorrhages usually result from trauma in the full-term infant. In the premature infant, they either result from trauma or may develop as a cerebellar component of germinal matrix hemorrhage. Vertical molding, fronto-occipital elongation, and torsional forces acting on the head during delivery may provoke laceration of dural leaflets of either the tentorium cerebelli or the falx cerebri, through which vessels and sinuses course. Laceration may occur with either vertex or breech presentations. Breech presentation

also predisposes to occipital osteodiastasis, a depressed fracture of the occipital bone or bones, which may lead to direct laceration of the cerebellum or rupture of vessels in the subdural space.

2. **Clinical presentation.** When the accumulation of blood is rapid and large, as occurs with rupture of arterioles, large veins, or sinuses, the presentation follows shortly after birth and evolves rapidly. When the sources of hemorrhage are small veins, there may be few symptoms or signs for up to a week, at which time the hematoma either attains a critical size and imposes on brain stem structures or provokes hydrocephalus. Presenting signs may result from (1) the effects of blood volume loss, as with SEH-IVH (see Table 27-6), (2) neurologic dysfunction caused by increased ICP or, more often, by brain stem dysfunction. Seizures are less common. The signs of elevated ICP include a bulging anterior fontanel or increasing head circumference, lethargy, and irritability. Head circumference enlargement occurs late, particularly in premature babies. Brain stem signs involve abnormal respirations (including apnea), cranial nerve palsies, nystagmus, and dysconjugate gaze (including skew deviation of the eyes). Hypotonia and vomiting may occur as well.

3. **Diagnosis.** The diagnosis should be suspected on the basis of clinical signs and confirmed with a CT scan. Although ultrasound may be valuable in evaluating intracerebellar hematomas, ultrasonic imaging of structures adjacent to bone (e.g., the subdural space) may be inadequate.

4. **Management and prognosis.** Attend to blood volume and cardiovascular status. Excessive hyperbilirubinemia also may occur (see Chap. 18). Open surgical evacuation of the clot is the usual management for infants with neurologic signs. The prognosis for normal development is good if surgical evacuation of the hematoma is successful. It has been suggested that when the clinical picture is stable and no deterioration in neurologic function or unmanageable increase in ICP exists, supportive care, using serial CT examinations, should be utilized in the management of cerebellar hematoma instead of surgical intervention.

C. **Anterior fossa hemorrhage**

1. **Pathogenesis.** Intracerebral hematomas and convexity epidural or subdural hematomas can occur as a result of birth trauma. Intracerebral hematoma also can occur (1) into necrotic cerebral tissue, as occurs with periventricular leukomalacia (PVL) and arterial distribution infarction (stroke), (2) in association with germinal matrix hemorrhage, either contiguous or to separate from the matrix, (3) with exposure to cocaine, (4) with persistent pulmonary hypertension, (5) with hemophilia or other bleeding disorders, and (6) rarely as a result of arteriovenous malformation or aneurysmal rupture. Hemorrhages that occur in the cerebrum may be in the cortex, in white matter, in the thalamus, or in the caudate. **Arterial infarcts** may occur with coagulopathies (deficiency of protein C, S, or antithrombin III; thrombocytosis; the presence of passively transferred lupus and anticardiolipin antibody; hyperviscous state), cardiac lesions (myomas or clots), and exposure to cocaine. Approximately a third of babies born after 35 weeks' gestation who undergo extracorporeal membrane oxygenation suffer from parenchymal or subarachnoid hemorrhage or hemorrhagic infarction of brain parenchyma. **However, infarcts and/or hemorrhage in most babies do not have a clear predisposing cause.** Such infarcts and hemorrhages may represent emboli seeded from the degenerating placenta.

2. **Clinical presentation.** As with other ICHs in the newborn period, signs may result from blood loss (see Table 27-6) or neurologic dysfunction. With either subdural or intracerebral hematomas, focal neurologic signs predominate. These signs may be obvious or quite subtle and may in-

clude lethargy, irritability, focal seizures, hemiparesis, or gaze prefer-ence. Dysfunction of the sixth nerve may occur as a result of elevated ICP. When the hematoma is large, compression of the third cranial nerve may occur, leading to a dilated and poorly reactive pupil. A small sub-dural hematoma may be unrecognized clinically and can either resolve or evolve into a chronic subdural fluid collection and can be associated with the development of hydrocephalus.

3. **Diagnosis.** Consider the diagnosis whenever the patient has focal or lat-eralized signs, including seizures. Hemorrhagic or xanthochromic CSF or both are consistent with the diagnosis, particularly when there are clear signs of elevated ICP that include bulging anterior fontanel or brain stem dysfunction. Lumbar puncture should be deferred unless meningitis is a strong consideration. Definitive evaluation requires CT scan. Ultrasound is a sensitive imaging technique for deep intra-parenchymal or intraventricular hemorrhages. It is less sensitive at dis-cerning SDH, although it may demonstrate a distortion or shift of the ventricular system as indirect evidence of the more superficial space-occupying lesion.

4. **Management and prognosis.** In general, surgical intervention for sub-dural hematomas is not required unless there are signs of progressive increased ICP, progressive worsening of neurologic signs, or signs of her-niation. Surgery may take the form of a subdural tap or an open evacua-tion. There is no specific therapy for intracerebral hematomas. Seizures should be treated. Intracerebral hematoma often results in some form of subsequent motor impairment. The prognosis following SDH is variable, although it is generally favorable when the hemorrhage does not pro-voke either cardiovascular compromise or herniation. In addition, hy-drocephalus occasionally develops as a late sequela.

D. **Subarachnoid hemorrhage (SAH)** is a common form of ICH among new-borns. Usually, the hemorrhage is trivial and goes unrecognized. Hemor-rhagic or xanthochromic CSF may be the only indication of such a hemor-rhage. SAH should be distinguished from subarachnoid extension of blood from an SEH-IVH.

1. **Pathogenesis.** SAH is nearly always the result of the normal trauma associated with the birth process. A role for hypoxia has been debated. The source of blood is usually ruptured bridging veins of the subarach-noid space or ruptured small leptomeningeal vessels. Occasionally, SAH develops as a result of laceration of the tentorium cerebelli or falx cerebri and may, in this circumstance, be associated with subdural hemorrhage. SAH also can occur as an extension of a cerebral contu-sion.

2. **Clinical features.** As with other forms of ICH, clinical presentations can occur because of blood loss or neurologic dysfunction (see Table 27-6). Only rarely is the volume loss large enough to provoke catastrophic re-sults. More often, neurologic signs manifest as irritability or seizures. Hemiparesis is occasionally seen when there is associated cerebral con-tusion or hemorrhage.

3. **Diagnosis.** The history of seizures and the CSF findings suggest the di-agnosis. Distinguishing SAH from other forms of ICH may be difficult. With simple SAH, the interictal neurologic state is usually normal, which has led to the designation "well baby with seizures." The diagno-sis, however, must be confirmed with a CT scan. Ultrasonography is not a sensitive technique for identifying a small SAH.

4. **Management and prognosis.** Management of SAH usually requires only symptomatic therapy, such as an anticonvulsant for seizures (see Neonatal Seizures, above) and attention to blood volume and cardiovas-cular status. Hyperbilirubinemia should be treated. Occasionally, hydro-cephalus will develop if the hemorrhage is large. The vast majority of in-fants do well without recognized sequelae.

Reference

Volpe, J. J. (Ed.). *Neurology of the newborn*, 3rd ed. Philadelphia: Saunders, 1995.

Perinatal Asphyxia
Evan Y. Snyder and John P. Cloherty

I. **Definition.** **Perinatal asphyxia** is an insult to the fetus or newborn due to a **lack of oxygen** (hypoxia) and/or a **lack of perfusion** (ischemia) to various organs. It is associated with tissue lactic acidosis. If accompanied by hypoventilation, it also may be associated with hypercapnia. The effects of hypoxia and ischemia may not be identical, but they are difficult to separate clinically. Both factors probably contribute to asphyxial injury. Normal blood gas values in term newborns are shown in Table 27-8. The many facets of perinatal asphyxia were reviewed extensively in a recent multiauthored volume devoted to that topic [16].

II. **Incidence.** The incidence of perinatal asphyxia is about 1.0 to 1.5% in most centers and is usually related to gestational age and birth weight. It occurs in 9% of infants less than 36 weeks' gestational age and in 0.5% of infants more than 36 weeks' gestational age, accounting for 20% of perinatal deaths (or as high as 50% of deaths if stillborns are included). The incidence is higher in term infants of diabetic or toxemic mothers; these factors correlate less well in preterm infants. In both preterm and term infants, intrauterine growth retardation and breech presentation are associated with an increased incidence of asphyxia. Postmature infants are also at risk.

III. **Pathophysiology and etiology of asphyxia.** Ninety percent of asphyxial insults occur in the antepartum or intrapartum periods as a result of **placental insufficiency,** resulting in an inability to provide O_2 to and remove CO_2 and H^+ from the fetus. The remainder are postpartum, usually secondary to pulmonary, cardiovascular, or neurologic insufficiency.

During **normal labor** uterine contractions and some degree of cord compression result in reduced blood flow to the placenta, and hence decreased O_2 delivery to the fetus. Because there is a concomitant increase in O_2 consumption by both mother and fetus, fetal O_2 saturation falls. Maternal dehydration and maternal alkalosis from hyperventilation may further reduce placental blood flow; maternal hypoventilation may also contribute to decreased maternal and fetal O_2 saturation. These *normal* events cause *most* babies to be born with little O_2 reserve. Newborns, however, including their central nervous systems (CNS), are fairly resistant to asphyxic damage. Late decelerations are uncommon until the partial pressure of O_2 (PO_2) is less than 20 mm Hg and O_2 saturation is less than 31%; in the experimental monkey fetus, a decline in heart rate due to this degree of hypoxia can be maintained for several hours without producing encephalopathy [8].

Table 27-8. Normal blood gas values in term newborns

| | At birth | | | | At age | |
	Maternal artery	Umbilical vein	Umbilical artery	10 minutes	30 to 60 minutes (umbilical artery)	5 hours
PO_2	95	27.5	16	50	54	74
PCO_2	32	39	49	46	38	35
pH*	7.4	7.32	7.24	7.21	7.29	7.34

PO_2 = partial pressure of oxygen; PCO_2 = partial pressure of carbon dioxide.
*A scalp pH in labor of 7.25 or above is considered normal (see Chaps. 1, 4).

In addition to the normal factors mentioned above, any process that (1) impairs maternal oxygenation, (2) decreases blood flow from the mother to the placenta or from the placenta to the fetus, (3) impairs gas exchange across the placenta or at the fetal tissue, or (4) increases fetal O_2 requirement will exacerbate perinatal asphyxia. Such factors include maternal hypertension (either chronic or preeclampsic); maternal vascular disease; maternal diabetes; maternal drug use; maternal hypoxia from pulmonary, cardiac, or neurologic disease; maternal hypotension; maternal infection; placental infarction or fibrosis; placental abruption; cord accidents (prolapse, entanglement, true knot, compression); abnormalities of umbilical vessels; fetal anemia; fetal or placental hydrops; fetal infection; intrauterine growth retardation; and postmaturity.

In the presence of a hypoxic-ischemic challenge to the fetus, reflexes are initiated, causing shunting of blood to the brain, heart, and adrenals and away from the lungs, gut, liver, kidneys, spleen, bone, skeletal muscle, and skin ("diving reflex"). In mild hypoxia, there is a decreased heart rate, slight increase in blood pressure (BP) to maintain cerebral perfusion, increased central venous pressure (CVP), and little change in cardiac output. As asphyxia progresses with severe hypoxia and acidosis, there is a decreased heart rate, decreased cardiac output, and initially increased then falling BP as oxidative phosphorylation fails and energy reserves become depleted. During asphyxia, anaerobic metabolism produces lactic acid, which, because of poor perfusion, remains in local tissues. Systemic acidosis may actually be mild until perfusion is restored and these local acid stores are mobilized.

A. Perinatal assessment of risk includes awareness of preexistent maternal or fetal problems and assessment of changing placental and fetal conditions by ultrasound, biophysical profile, nonstress tests, and urinary estriol measurements (see Chap. 1, Assessment and Prenatal Diagnosis).

B. Perinatal management of high-risk pregnancies consists of fetal heart monitoring, evaluation of fetal scalp pH, when indicated, and awareness of the progress of labor and the presence of meconium. (While the value of any one of these parameters is uncertain, and even controversial [11], the presence of a constellation of abnormal findings may alert and allow proactive mobilization of the perinatal team for a newborn that may potentially require immediate intervention.) The pH is considered a better determinant of fetal oxygenation than PO_2; if a hypoxic-ischemic insult occurs intermittently, the PO_2 may improve transiently, whereas pH will fall progressively; pH less than 7.0 is good evidence of substantial and prolonged intrauterine asphyxia. (It should be remembered, however, that scalp and cord pH values may be profoundly affected by **maternal** acid–base status.) Abnormalities of fetal heart rate and rhythm plus heavy meconium staining may provide possible supporting evidence of asphyxia but provide no information concerning the severity or duration of the asphyxia. The decision to perform a cesarean section, to augment a vaginal delivery, or to allow labor to progress is the most difficult obstetric decision. Each medical center should have guidelines for intervention in cases of suspected fetal distress (see Chap. 1, Assessment and Prenatal Diagnosis).

IV. Delivery room management (see Chaps. 4, 17, and 24, Meconium Aspiration and Persistent Pulmonary Hypertension of the Newborn). An Apgar score of 3 or less prolonged for more than 5 minutes is generally regarded as evidence of asphyxia. However, a low Apgar score may *not* indicate asphyxia in *preterm* or *small-for-gestational-age* infants (see Chap. 4), who are more likely to be hypotonic, have cyanotic extremities, and have diminished responsiveness; a score of 6 to 7 may be maximal for a "normal" preterm infant. Infants below 30 weeks' gestation often have an Apgar score of 2 to 3 without asphyxia. Low Apgar scores may be present in **nonasphyxiated** infants with (1) depression from maternal anesthesia or analgesics, (2) trauma, (3) metabolic or infectious insults, (4) neuromuscular disorders, or (5) CNS, cardiac, or pulmonary malformations. Further, a low Apgar score, even when a marker of a depressed infant, does not indicate the mechanism for the depression, duration or severity of the specific insult, or the adaptive response of the fetus. A high Apgar score (>6 by 5 minutes), however, speaks compellingly **against** substantial peripartum asphyxia.

V. Postnatal management of asphyxia

A. The differential diagnosis of acute asphyxia in a newborn includes the effect of maternal drugs or anesthesia, acute blood loss, acute intracranial bleeding, CNS malformation, neuromuscular disease, cardiopulmonary disease, mechanical impediments to ventilation (airway obstruction, pneumothorax, hydrops, pleural effusion, ascites, diaphragmatic hernia), and infection (including septic shock and hypotension). These problems may be the cause of asphyxia or merely coincident with it. A common presentation is the postmature infant with asphyxia, meconium aspiration, persistent pulmonary hypertension, pneumothorax, and birth trauma. Another common presentation is the premature infant with asphyxia, hyaline membrane disease, and an intracranial bleed. **Intrauterine ischemia,** early in gestation, may present in the newborn as a hypoplastic organ (e.g., lung, gut) or extremity (e.g., sirenomelia), as hydranencephaly, or as a more subtle congenital abnormality of neurocytoarchitecture.

B. Target organs of perinatal asphyxia are the brain, heart, lungs, kidneys, liver, bowel, and bone marrow. In a study of asphyxiated newborns [13], 34% had no evidence of organ injury, 23% had an abnormality confined to one organ, 34% involved two organs, and 9% had three affected organs. The most frequent abnormalities involved the kidney (50%), followed by the CNS (28%), cardiovascular system (25%), and pulmonary (23%) system. Often, asphyxiated infants will succumb to dysfunctions of organs other than the CNS (e.g., persistent fetal circulation) while showing minimal evidence of hypoxic-ischemic brain injury. In such instances, the brain is spared at the expense of cardiac output to the affected organ. The degree of asphyxia required to cause permanent neurologic impairment is close to that which causes death from multisystem failure.

1. Hypoxic-ischemic brain injury

a. Pathophysiology. Hypoxic-ischemic brain injury [3,8,16,19] is the most important consequence of perinatal asphyxia. Brief **hypoxia** impairs cerebral oxidative metabolism leading to an increase in lactate, a fall in pH, and given the inefficiency of anaerobic glycolysis to generate ATP, a decrease in high-energy phosphate compounds (first phosphocreatine, then ATP) [3]. The hypoxic brain therefore increases its glucose utilization. Vascular dilation, caused by hypoxia, increases glucose availability for anaerobic glycolysis, but this leads to increased local lactic acid production. The worsening acidosis is ultimately associated with decreased glycolysis, loss of cerebrovascular autoregulation, and diminished cardiac function, which causes local **ischemia** and decreased glucose delivery to the very tissue that has increased its substrate utilization. Local glucose stores therefore become depleted, energy reserves fall further, and accumulated lactic acid remains unremoved. During prolonged hypoxia, cardiac output falls, cerebral blood flow (CBF) is compromised, and a combined **hypoxic-ischemic insult** produces further failure of oxidative phosphorylation and ATP production. Such energy failure impairs ion pumps with accumulation of Na^+, Cl^-, H_2O, and Ca^{2+} intracellularly and K^+ and excitatory amino acid neurotransmitters (e.g., glutamate, aspartate) extracellularly. The nature of asphyxial damage at the cellular level is presently the subject of intense investigation. Current theories [10] implicate these **excitotoxic amino acids,** which, through action at glutamate or N-methyl-D-aspartate (NMDA) receptors, open ion channels allowing Na^+ and Cl^- to enter a cell, inducing **immediate** neuronal death from the osmolar load. Furthermore, these excitotoxins, by means of direct activation of the NMDA channel (mediated by the phosphoinositol second messenger system) and/or activation of voltage-dependent Ca^{2+} channels, provoke excessive Ca^{2+} i which in turn leads to a **delayed** form of neuronal death by (1) activation of undesirable enzyme and second messenger systems (e.g., Ca^{2+}-dependent lipases and proteases), (2) perturbation of mitochondrial respiratory electron chain transport, (3) generation of free radicals and leukotrienes, and (4) depletion of energy stores. Reperfusion of previously ischemic tissue may also promote the formation of excess oxygen free radicals (e.g., superoxide ion, hydrogen peroxide, hydroxyl radical, singlet oxygen), which, when they overwhelm endogenous scavenger mechanisms, may damage cellular lipids, proteins, and nucleic acids and the blood-brain barrier. The degree of hypoxia necessary to produce permanent brain damage in the rat or monkey is close to that which is lethal.

Grossly, the following lesions may be seen after moderate or severe asphyxia:

(1) **Focal or multifocal cortical necrosis** (occasionally with cerebral edema) with resultant **cystic encephalomalacia and/or ulegyria** (**attenuation** of depths of sulci), due to loss of perfusion in one or several vascular beds (usually middle cerebral artery) and affecting all cellular elements

(2) **Watershed infarcts** in boundary zones between cerebral arteries (particularly following severe hypotension) (e.g., **periventricular leukomalacia** [PVL] in the preterm infant, which reflects poor perfusion of the vulnerable periventricular border zones in the centrum semiovale and produces predominantly white matter injury; bilateral **parasagittal** cortical and subcortical white matter injury of the term infant; and injury to parietooccipital cortex)

(3) **Selective neuronal necrosis** is injury at specific sites to specific cell types (neurons > glia) (e.g., CA1 region of the hippocampus, Purkinje cells of the cerebellum, brain stem nuclei)

(4) **Necrosis of thalamic nuclei and basal ganglia (status marmoratus),** a subtype of selective neuronal necrosis

The precise pathologic pattern seen in any case is not predictable. However, the longer the asphyxia, the more extensive the involvement. Insults due to **prolonged partial episodes of asphyxia** (e.g., from placental abruption) seem to cause diffuse cerebral (especially cortical) necrosis, while **acute total asphyxia** (e.g., from cord prolapse) seems to spare the cortex and affect primarily the brain stem, thalamus, and basal ganglia. In the former instance, seizures and paresis might be expected. In the latter instance, one might see disturbances of consciousness, respiration, heart rate, BP, and temperature control; disorders of tone and reflexes; and cranial nerve palsies. Most cases, however, represent a combination of the two patterns: partial prolonged asphyxia followed by a terminal acute asphyxial event. If diffuse cerebral necrosis and subsequent swelling is severe, increased intracranial pressure (ICP) could theoretically compromise CBF with further damage to the thalamus and brain stem. Recent data, however, indicate that swelling is an effect from *prior,* rather than a cause of *subsequent,* neural damage [5,9] [see **V.B.1.c.(7)**].

b. The **syndrome of hypoxic-ischemic encephalopathy (HIE)** [8,15,16, 18] has a **spectrum of clinical manifestations from mild to severe.** In its most dramatic form, the initial phase lasts about 12 hours after the insult and consists of signs of cerebral dysfunction. The infants are stuporous or comatose, have periodic breathing or irregular respiratory effort (a reflection of bihemispheric dysfunction), are hypotonic, and have lost most complex reflexes (Moro, suck, etc.). They may have roving eye movements while the pupillary responses are intact. Subtle, tonic, or multifocal-clonic seizures occur 6 to 24 hours after the insult in 50% of moderately to severely asphyxiated infants.

Between 12 and 24 hours there may be apnea requiring respiratory support, reflecting brain stem dysfunction. Severely affected infants have a progressive deterioration in CNS function over 24 to 72 hours following the insult, with coma, prolonged apnea, and further brain stem dysfunction (e.g., abnormalities of pupillary reactivity, loss of oculomotor and caloric responses, loss of bulbar function). "Brain death" (see **d**) may ensue between 24 and 72 hours later. In the most severely affected infants, for whom the incidence of death or significant permanent neurologic sequelae is greatest, other organ systems inevitably also display evidence of asphyxial damage. The most striking reduction in blood flow, due to shunting of cardiac output to vital organs, involves the kidneys, particularly the proximal tubule, resulting in acute tubular necrosis (ATN) (see Chap. 31). In fact, persistent **oliguria** (<1 ml/kg per hour for the first 36 hours) is significantly associated with severe HIE and a poor outcome (90% of cases). This suggests that when the asphyxic insult is severe enough to manifest as persistent oliguria, it is likely the brain also has suffered ischemic injury. As previously noted, **the degree of asphyxia required to cause permanent neurologic impairment is close to that which causes death from multisystem failure.** We also use the Sarnat clinical stages to estimate the severity of asphyxial insult to infants more than 36 weeks' gestational age [15] (Table 27-9). The sequential appearance and resolution of various transitory clinical signs and their duration over the first 2 postnatal weeks not only indicate the extent and permanence of neurologic impairment but also define clinical categories that have proved fairly accurate for early assessment of prognosis in neonates with HIE [15] (e.g., prognosis is good if a neonate does not progress to and/or remain in stage 3 and if total duration of stage 2 is less than 5 days) (see **VI**). Electrodiagnostic tests such as **electroencephalography (EEG)** and evoked potentials, in conjunction with these clinical signs, may assist in evaluating and classifying the severity of the damage (e.g., seizure foci, or even more significantly, *interictal and/or background activity*—suppressed?, normal?) [see **V.B.1.c.(7)** and **VI.C**]. **Ultrasonic examination** of the brain may reveal hemorrhage (useful in preterm infants) and, less well, the extent of edema (midline shift, ventricular compression). Cranial **computed tomography (CT)** is more useful in assessing the degree of edema, when performed early (2 to 4 days after the insult), and the extent of cerebral injury (encephalomalacia), when performed late (at least 2 to 4 weeks after the insult). There is a correlation between areas of hypodensity and later sequelae in term infants [8]. CT may not be as useful in predicting sequelae in premature infants because the excess water and lower myelin content of the premature brain obscures gray-white differentiation. (In this case, serial ultrasound studies may suffice for localizing, for example, periventricular echoes suggestive of PVL.) CT is useful as well for diagnosing cerebral dysgenesis and malformation and will provide information similar to an ultrasound regarding intracranial bleeding and hydrocephalus. While neonatal brain **magnetic resonance imaging (MRI)** may provide the best anatomic resolution of hypoxic-ischemic brain lesions and CNS architecture, and may ultimately be useful for long-term prognosis, it is presently unclear whether this information is sufficiently superior to the more accessible ultrasound, CT, or clinical examination in guiding management and assessment in the immediate neonatal period [4]. **Brain scan with isotope** may reveal areas without blood flow [8]. Several studies documented significant increases (>5 IU) in the serum **creatine kinase brain fraction (CK-BB)** at 4 and 10 hours of life (peaking between 6 and 10 days) in asphyxiated infants who ultimately died or developed neurologic sequelae;

CN CASE
1PRM

Table 27-9. Sarnat and Sarnat stages of hypoxic-ischemic encephalopathy (HIE)*

Stage	Stage 1 (mild)	Stage 2 (moderate)	Stage 3 (severe)
Level of consciousness	Hyperalert; irritable	Lethargic or obtunded	Stuporous, comatose
Neuromuscular control:	Uninhibited, overreactive	Diminished spontaneous movement	Diminished or absent spontaneous movement
Muscle tone	Normal	Mild hypotonia	Flaccid
Posture	Mild distal flexion	Strong distal flexion	Intermittent decerebration
Stretch reflexes	Overactive	Overactive, disinhibited	Decreased or absent
Segmental myoclonus	Present or absent	Present	Absent
Complex reflexes:	Normal	Suppressed	Absent
Suck	Weak	Weak or absent	Absent
Moro	Strong, low threshold	Weak, incomplete high threshold	Absent
Oculovestibular	Normal	Overactive	Weak or absent
Tonic neck	Slight	Strong	Absent
Autonomic function:	Generalized sympathetic	Generalized parasympathetic	Both systems depressed
Pupils	Mydriasis	Miosis	Midposition, often unequal; poor light reflex
Respirations	Spontaneous	Spontaneous; occasional apnea	Periodic; apnea
Heart rate	Tachycardia	Bradycardia	Variable
Bronchial and salivary secretions	Sparse	Profuse	Variable
Gastrointestinal motility	Normal or decreased	Increased diarrhea	Variable
Seizures	None	Common focal or multifocal (6 to 24 hours of age)	Uncommon (excluding decerebration)
Electroencephalographic findings	Normal (awake)	Early: generalized low-voltage, slowing (continuous delta and theta) Later: periodic pattern (awake); seizures focal or multifocal; 1.0 to 1.5 Hz spike and wave	Early: periodic pattern with isopotential phases Later: totally isopotential

Table 27-9. *Continued.*

Stage	Stage 1 (mild)	Stage 2 (moderate)	Stage 3 (severe)
Duration of symptoms	<24 hours	2 to 14 days	Hours to weeks
Outcome	About 100% normal	80% normal; abnormal if symptoms more than 5 to 7 days	About 50% die; remainder with severe sequelae

*The stages in this table are a continuum reflecting the spectrum of clinical states of infants over 36 weeks' gestational age.
Source: From H. B. Sarnat and M. S. Sarnat. Neonatal encephalopathy following fetal distress: A clinical and electroencephalographic study. *Arch. Neurol.* 33:696, 1976.

however, CK-BB also may rise after intraventricular hemorrhage (IVH). CK-BB serial determinations were inferior, however, to CT/EEG in prognostic reliability [2]. An elevated **neuron-specific enolase (NSE)** level in the cerebrospinal fluid (CSF) recently was advanced as a biochemical marker for early estimates of hypoxic-ischemic brain damage in asphyxiated full-term newborns [3]. While its specificity for CNS damage due to asphyxia remains to be determined, a *normal* CSF NSE (<25 ng/ml) at 12 to 72 hours of life may speak against the presence of a significant insult.

It should be emphasized that HIE is just one (and not the most common) of a number of etiologies in the differential diagnosis of neurologic dysfunction in the neonate, which also includes genetic and structural abnormalities, drugs and toxins, infection, inherited metabolic diseases, trauma, intracranial hemorrhage (ICH), and transient homeostatic derangements such as hypoglycemia, hypocalcemia, hypermagnesemia, hypomagnesemia, hypernatremia, and hypothermia. Asphyxia may be suspected and HIE reasonably included in the differential diagnosis of neonatal coma or neurologic dysfunction if the following have been documented: (1) 5- to 10-minute Apgar score (or more reliably, 15- to 20-minute Apgar score) less than 3, (2) fetal heart rate of less than 60, (3) prolonged (1 hour) antenatal acidosis, (4) neonatal seizure within the first 24 to 48 hours (though 50% of seizures are *not* asphyxial in character), (5) burst-suppression pattern on EEG, and (6) need for positive-pressure resuscitation for more than 1 minute or more than 5 minutes until the first cry. Whether **permanent** neurologic sequelae can be **attributed** to HIE is a completely different question and is addressed in **VI.**

  c. Management of hypoxic-ischemic brain injury. The initial management of hypoxic-ischemic damage in the delivery room is described in Chap. 4. Other specific management consists of supportive care to maintain temperature, perfusion, ventilation, and a normal metabolic state, including glucose, Ca^{2+}, and acid–base balance. Control of seizures is important.

    (1) O_2 levels should be kept in the **normal range** by monitoring transcutaneous or arterial PO_2 or percent O_2 saturation by pulse oximeter. Hypoxia should be treated with O_2 and/or ventilation. Hyperoxia also may cause a decrease in CBF or exacerbate free radical damage. Aminophylline may decrease CBF and should not be used in the initial management of apnea due to asphyxia.

    (2) CO_2 should be kept in the **normal range** because hypercapnia may cause cerebral vasodilation, which may cause more flow to uninjured areas with relative ischemia to damaged areas ("steal phenomenon") and extension of infarct size. The excess flow to uninjured areas may furthermore be associated with ICH because of loss of autoregulation of CBF (see Intracranial Hemorrhage). Excessive hypocapnia may decrease CBF. Hyperventilation is not recommended.

    (3) Perfusion. It is important to maintain cerebral perfusion pressure (CPP) within a narrow range. Too little can cause ischemic injury; too much can cause hemorrhage in the areas of damaged blood vessels, with germinal matrix hemorrhage and IVH in premature infants. Excessive reperfusion of infarcted tissue may cause the infarct to become hemorrhagic because of loss of vascular integrity. Abrupt changes in perfusion and rapid infusions of volume expanders or sodium bicarbonate may be associated with IVH [18]. Because cerebrovascular autoregulation is lost, cerebral perfusion entirely reflects systemic BP in a pressure-passive fashion. To maintain cerebral perfusion, a systemic mean arterial BP of at least 45 to 50 mm Hg is usually desirable for term infants, 35 to 40 mm Hg for infants weighing 1000 to 2000 gm, and 30 to 35 mm Hg for infants weighing less than 1000 gm [5,18]. Conversely, if hypertension develops and persists despite the discontinuation of pressors and the institution of adequate sedation, the systemic BP should **not** be lowered further, since it may be needed to maintain adequate CPP in the face of increased ICP. The following recommendations should be adhered to:

(a) Continuously monitor arterial BP. Continuously monitor CVP, if possible, to ensure there is adequate preload, i.e., that infant is *not* hypovolemic due to vasodilatation or third spacing.

(b) Keep systemic mean arterial BP at no lower than 45 to 50 mm Hg in term infants, 35 to 40 mm Hg in 1000- to 2000-gm infants, and 30 to 35 mm Hg in infants weighing less than 1000 gm. Keep CVP 5 to 8 mm Hg in term infants and 3 to 5 mm Hg in preterm infants.

(c) Minimize pushes of colloid or sodium bicarbonate, but regularly replace intravascular volume losses as needed to avoid lactic acidosis.

(d) Give volume replacement slowly.

(e) Minimize administered free H_2O (insensible losses plus urine output); however, if urine output is low, first ensure that intravascular volume is adequate (i.e., rule out *pre*renal etiology) before fluid restriction (see Chaps. 9, 31).

(f) Judicious use of pressors may help minimize the need for colloid in maintaining BP and perfusion (see Chap. 17).

(g) Monitor ICP if possible.

(4) **Glucose** (see Chap. 27, Neonatal Seizures, and Chap. 29). Blood glucose level should be kept at 75 to 100 mg/dl to provide adequate substrate for the brain. Higher levels may lead to elevation of brain lactate, damage to cellular integrity, increased edema, and further disturbances in vascular autoregulation [18]. Lower levels may potentiate excitotoxic amino acids and extend the infarct size. **Hypoglycemia**, due both to glycogen depletion secondary to catecholamine release and to an unexplained hyperinsulinemic state, is often seen in asphyxiated infants. An initial phase of *hyper*glycemia and hypoinsulinemia (5 to 10 minutes following an acute event due to a catecholamine surge which inhibits insulin release and stimulates glucagon release) may be followed within 2 to 3 hours by profound *hypo*glycemia. **Normal glucose infusion rates of 5 to 8 mg/kg per minute may not be sufficient to maintain normoglycemia; rates as high as 9 to 15 mg/kg per minute may be required for short periods.** Because hypoglycemia may be difficult to control without causing fluid overload, concentrated glucose infusions may be necessary by means of a central line (e.g., a "high" umbilical venous line with its tip in the right atrium). Since rapid glucose boluses should be avoided, serum glucose level should be monitored frequently and adjustments **anticipated**. Glucose infusions should be discontinued slowly to avoid rebound hypoglycemia. **Seizures** may result from hypoglycemia; therefore, if seizures do occur, the possibility of hypoglycemia should be ruled out or treated appropriately before reflexly instituting anticonvulsant therapy (see below). Seizures in such an instance would **not** be used for Sarnat clinical staging.

(5) **Temperature** should be kept in a **normal range**. While animal studies are promising, deep hypothermia has not yet proved to be "brain sparing" after asphyxia in humans [12].

(6) **Calcium** level should be kept in a normal range. **Hypocalcemia** is a common metabolic alteration in the neonatal postasphyxial

syndrome. A subnormal serum Ca^{2+} level will **not** forestall neuronal damage and may only serve to compromise cardiac contractility or cause seizures (see Chap. 29, Hypocalcemia, Hypercalcemia, and Hypermagnesemia).

(7) **Seizures.** Seizures should be controlled as described above in Neonatal Seizures. In neonatal HIE, they are typically focal or multifocal (myelinization and synaptogenesis not having developed sufficiently for generalization of seizures). Seizures occur in about 50% of infants with HIE in most series [15], characteristically on the first or second day, usually in stage 2, only rarely in stage 3, and almost never in stage 1 (see Sarnat and Sarnat stages, Table 27-9). They may be associated with an increased cerebral metabolic rate, which in the absence of adequate O_2 and perfusion may lead to a fall in blood glucose level, an increase in brain lactate level, and a fall in high-energy phosphate compounds. In infants not mechanically ventilated, seizures may be associated with hypoxemia and/or hypercapnia. Abrupt elevations in BP associated with seizures may contribute to ICH in preterm infants. When seizures are clinically apparent and of typical morphology, an EEG is not necessary to confirm the diagnosis (though data regarding *interictal background* activity may be useful for assessing the overall "well-being" of the brain). In infants paralyzed with pancuronium for mechanical ventilation, seizures may be manifested by abrupt changes in BP, heart rate, and oxygenation. An EEG should be obtained in these circumstances. Whether seizures alone, in the *absence* of metabolic or cardiopulmonary abnormalities, lead to brain injury is controversial. While one should have a low threshold for diagnosing seizures in the setting of HIE, it is no longer thought that asphyxiated infants should be treated prophylactically with anticonvulsants in the absence of clinical seizures (or electrical seizures on EEG in the case of an infant pharmacologically paralyzed). There is actually very little change in ICP during most electrographic seizures [5]. The clinical distinction between multifocal seizures and the "jitteriness" (actually a **rhythmic segmental myoclonus**) seen frequently in stage 1 and even stage 2 HIE is often difficult to make by observation alone. Taking hold of the clonic extremity and changing the tension on the muscle stretch receptor by slightly flexing or extending the joint immediately arrests clonus but does not alter true seizure activity, during which rhythmic convulsive movements continue to be felt in the examiner's hand [15]. When seizures are diagnosed, **phenobarbital** should be loaded slowly, **20 mg/kg intravenously to be followed by a maintenance dose of 3 to 5 mg/kg per day.** One should always be vigilant for respiratory depression and/or cardiovascular compromise with hypotension. If the infant is already mechanically ventilated, respiratory depression is not a concern. In non–intensive care unit (ICU) settings, one may divide the loading dose of phenobarbital or use phenytoin. Phenobarbital, especially at high levels, itself can cause lethargy, stupor, and occasionally brain stem signs. If seizures persist, **phenytoin may be administered slowly as a second drug (20 mg/kg intravenously as a loading dose followed by 4 to 8 mg/kg per day as a maintenance dose).** One should, of course, ascertain that metabolic derangements that may complicate asphyxia and cause seizures have been addressed (e.g., **hypoglycemia, hypocalcemia,** and **hyponatremia**) (see Chap. 29). **Pyridoxine-dependency seizures** and **local anesthetic toxicity** may mimic postasphyxic seizures and should be considered in the differential diagnosis. If seizures nevertheless

persist, a **benzodiazepam** (e.g., **lorazepam 0.05 to 0.10 mg/kg per dose intravenously**) may be given transiently as a third drug. If vascular access cannot be achieved in the non-ICU setting, rectal diazepam, valproate, or paraldehyde may provide a stopgap. (Intramuscular phenobarbital is absorbed too slowly and, because it may confound subsequent management, its use is discouraged.) Seizures in HIE are notoriously difficult to control and often resistant to even aggressive anticonvulsant therapy in the early stages (first 72 hours) of the syndrome. Once levels of conventional anticonvulsants are maximized (phenobarbital level to 40 mg/dl, phenytoin level to 20 mg/dl), unless there is cardiopulmonary compromise from the seizures, there is often little utility or desirability to eliminating every "twitch" or electrographic seizure. (There is a growing understanding that even status epilepticus will not extend extant cortical damage or heighten morbidity.) For unexplained reasons, even refractory seizures in HIE ultimately "burn themselves out" and cease after approximately 48 hours. **When the infant's condition has been stable for 3 to 4 days, all anticonvulsants are weaned except phenobarbital** (the level of which may be allowed to drop to 15 to 20 mg/dl if possible). If seizures have resolved, if neurologic findings are normal, and if the EEG is normal, anticonvulsants are stopped in the neonatal period (14 days of life). If this is not the case, anticonvulsants are continued for 1 to 3 months. If the neurologic findings are then normal with no recurrent seizures, phenobarbital is tapered over 4 weeks. If the neurologic results are not normal, the advisability of continued anticonvulsant therapy requires consideration of the initial cause of the seizures. The risk of subsequent epilepsy is 100% with seizures secondary to cerebral cortical dysgeneses but only 20 to 30% after seizures secondary to perinatal asphyxia and essentially nil after seizures secondary to transient metabolic disturbances. Infants with a higher risk of subsequent seizures are those with a persistent neurologic deficit (50% risk) and those with an abnormal EEG between seizures (40% risk). If the result of neurologic examination is not normal, an EEG is obtained; if there is no electrographic seizure activity, phenobarbital is tapered and discontinued over 4 weeks, even if the infant has abnormal neurologic signs.

(8) **Cerebral edema.** Devices applied to the anterior fontanel provide noninvasive methods for measuring ICP [5,9]. Cerebral edema may be minimized by avoiding fluid overload, although initial resuscitation of an asphyxiated infant and maintenance of cardiovascular stability and CPP (CPP = systemic mean arterial BP −ICP) should *always* take priority. Two processes may predispose to fluid overload in asphyxiated infants: (1) **syndrome of inappropriate secretion of antidiuretic hormone (SIADH)** (see Chap. 9) and (2) **ATN** (see Chap. 31). SIADH, often seen for 3 to 4 days after the insult, is manifested by **hyponatremia** and hypoosmolarity with excretion of an inappropriately concentrated and Na^+-containing urine (elevated urine specific gravity, osmolarity, and Na^+). SIADH should be monitored by daily determinations of serum and urinary Na^+ and osmolarity. Urine output may further be compromised by ATN resulting from shunting of cardiac output away from the kidneys. Persistent oliguria (<1 ml/kg per hour for the first 36 hours of life) can provide an index of the severity of asphyxia and risk for neurologic sequelae. **To avoid fluid overload and the exacerbation of cerebral edema, both SIADH and ATN should be managed by limitation of free H_2O administration only to replacement of insensible losses and urine output (u**

ally <60 ml/kg per day) (see Chap. 9). Before attributing oliguria to SIADH or ATN, rule out prerenal etiologies (hypovolemia, vasodilation) with a 10 to 20 ml/kg fluid challenge followed by a loop diuretic if there is no urine output.

(3) Cerebral edema and increased ICP (>10 mm Hg) are actually fairly **uncommon** concomitants of perinatal asphyxia [5]. When present, they more often reflect extensive prior cerebral necrosis rather than swelling of intact cells, and because they bespeak such extensive cell death, they have a uniformly bad prognosis. They peak 36 to 72 hours after the insult. They are more properly regarded as an **effect** rather than a cause of brain damage. For this reason, efforts specifically to reduce cerebral edema or ICP do not affect outcome; neither do ICP elevations reduce cerebral perfusion or introduce any acute functional neurologic disturbances [5]. Therefore, such interventions previously explored in the literature as antiedema agents (e.g., high-dose phenobarbital, steroids, mannitol, and other hypertonic solutions) are not employed at our institution. The infant's patent sutures and open fontanel are protective of any acute increases in ICP that might occur [5,8]. **Our major efforts are devoted to ensuring an adequate CPP through maintaining an adequate systemic mean arterial BP,** shown in recent studies to be a more important variable than ICP in ensuring adequate CBF [5]. **A simple beside estimate of ICP** can be made in infants (assuming no elevations of CVP such as occurs with pneumothorax or during treatment with continuous positive airway pressure) by measuring the vertical distance between the anterior fontanel and the heart, measured at the point that the midportion of the fontanel flattens as the baby is tilted up. Normal will be 50 mm H_2O or lower.

(9) Many **brain-sparing, cerebroprotective, and/or infarct-limiting interventions** have been proposed in recent years, many based on the postulated mechanisms of asphyxial damage described earlier **V.B.1.a)** (reviewed in ref. 12). Administration of high-dose barbiturates to decrease cerebral metabolism) and naloxone (for endogenous opioid blockade) has proved ineffective in humans despite their initial promise in animal models. Newer possibilities such as (a) antagonists of excitotoxic neurotransmitter receptors (e.g., NMDA receptor blockers), (b) free radical scavengers (e.g., superoxide dismutase, vitamin E), (c) Ca^{2+} channel blockers (e.g., nifedipine, nicardipine), (d) cyclooxygenase inhibitors (e.g., indomethacin), (e) hypothermia, (f) benzodiazepine receptor stimulation (e.g., midazolam), (g) enhancers of protein synthesis (e.g., dexamethasone), and (h) vasodilators (e.g., prostacyclin) all have a theoretical basis (see **V.B.1.a**), but have not yet undergone any systemic human trials [18].

d. **Brain death in the neonate.** In 1987, recommendations for determination of brain death in children and infants older than 7 days were proposed by an ad hoc task force committee [1]. The guidelines avoided specific recommendations in infants less than 7 days old, citing lack of published data. Though controversial, Ashwal et al. [2] recently argued that the current task force guidelines may be extended to include the term infant and the preterm infant more than 32 weeks' gestational age. The clinical diagnosis of brain death might, in their opinion, be made on the basis of (1) coma, manifested by lack of response to pain, light, or auditory stimulation; (2) apnea, confirmed by documentation of failure to breathe when partial pressure of CO_2 (PCO_2) is higher than 60 mm Hg (tested by 3 minutes without ventilator support while continuing 100% O_2 supplementation or for shorter periods if hypotension or bradycardia intervene); (3) absent bulbar movements and brain stem reflexes (including midposition or fully dilated pupils with no response to light or pain and with absent oculocephalic, caloric, corneal, gag, cough, rooting, and sucking reflexes), all normally elicitable by 33 weeks' gestation; and (4) flaccid tone and absence of spontaneous or induced movements (excluding activity mediated at the spinal cord level). If these clinical findings remain unchanged for 24 hours, electrocerebral silence, in the absence of a barbiturate level over 25 μg/ml, hypothermia (<24°C), or cerebral malformations (e.g., hydranencephaly, hydrocephalus), it is confirmatory of brain death. Further, if the initial EEG (done after 24 hours of life) shows electrocerebral silence and the infant remains brain-dead for 24 hours, a repeat study is not necessary. Absence of radionuclide uptake (a reliable estimate of CBF) contemporaneous with initial electrocerebral silence is also associated with brain death. Alternatively, if no radionuclide uptake is demonstrated initially (signifying CBF <2 ml/min/100 gm) and the infant remains clinically brain-dead for 24 hours, a diagnosis of brain death also can be made, even if some EEG activity persists. Sensitivity is increased in this regard by repeating the scan in 24 hours and reconfirming no uptake. Term infants clinically brain-dead for 2 days and preterm infants brain-dead for 3 days do not survive regardless of the EEG or CBF status, indicating that determination of brain death in the newborn might be made solely by using clinical criteria over this prolonged period of observation. Therefore, confirmatory neurodiagnostic studies are of value in potentially shortening the period of observation to 24 hours. Phenobarbital levels higher than 25 μg/ml may suppress EEG activity in this age group. The diagnosis of brain death must also be made in the appropriate clinical setting, wherein the cause of coma has been determined and all remediable or reversible conditions eliminated. In isolation, neither EEG alone nor radionuclide flow studies alone are sufficiently sensitive to diagnose brain death. Persistent EEG activity and/or prognostically small variations in radionuclide uptake do **not** obviate the diagnosis of brain death in the newborn. (Unlike in adults or older children, minimal radionuclide uptake may persist in brain-dead neonates, perhaps due to patent sutures, which may moderate acute increases in ICP, which would otherwise diminish CPP to a no-flow state.) Clinical correlation and/or coupled neurodiagnostic studies are necessary. These recommendations, Ashwal et al. contend [2], take into account all reported cases to date of possible misdiagnosis of brain death. Based on these, the combination of neurologic assessment, an EEG showing electrocerebral silence, and isotope estimation of CBF followed by 24 hours of observation seems valid, they suggest, in deciding that irreversible cessation of brain function has occurred in the preterm and term infant. At present, insufficient information is available to warrant the use of brain stem evoked response testing for confirmation of brain death in the newborn. In neonates, an additional clinical clue to brain death is a **fixed heart rate** without decelerations or accelerations. (See Chap. 22 and Table 22-1.)

2. **Cardiac effects of asphyxia** (see Chap. 25)
   a. **Diagnosis.** Infants with perinatal asphyxia may have **transient myocardial ischemia.** They develop respiratory distress and cyanosis shortly after birth. They will have signs of congestive heart failure, such as tachypnea, tachycardia, an enlarged liver, and a gallop rhythm. Many infants will have a systolic murmur at the lower left sternal border **(tricuspid regurgitation),** and some will have a murmur at the apex **(mitral regurgitation). Chest x-ray** studies will show cardiomegaly and sometimes pulmonary venous congestion. The **electrocardiogram (ECG)** may show ST depression in the mid-

precordium and T-wave inversion in the left precordium. A serum **creatine kinase plasma MB isoenzyme** fraction higher than 5 to 10% may be present in myocardial damage. The echocardiogram/ Doppler study will show normal cardiac structures but decreased left ventricular contractions, especially of the posterior wall, and perhaps persistent pulmonary hypertension. It is important to rule out Epstein's disease of the tricuspid valve, pulmonary stenosis, and pulmonary atresia with intact ventricular septum. The ventricular end-diastolic pressures are usually elevated because of poor ventricular function. Some infants will show tricuspid regurgitation with right-to-left shunting at the atrial level. In a recent study of moderately to severely asphyxiated newborns [13], left ventricular dysfunction occurred in less than 10% of infants, while right ventricular dysfunction was found in 30% of infants. Many of these infants will have meconium aspiration syndrome with persistent pulmonary hypertension (see Chap. 24). Of significance, the presence of a fixed heart rate without variation may raise suspicion of clinical brain death.

   b. Management of the cardiac effects of asphyxia. The treatment is adequate ventilation with correction of hypoxemia, acidosis, and hypoglycemia. Volume overload must be avoided. (Diuretics may be ineffective if there is concomitant renal failure.) These infants will require continuous monitoring of systemic mean arterial BP, CVP, mixed venous saturation, and urine output. Infants with cardiac collapse will require inotropic drugs such as **dopamine** and/or **dobutamine** (see Chap. 17). Some infants in great distress may require afterload reduction with a peripheral beta agonist (e.g., isoproterenol), a peripheral alpha blocker (e.g., phentolamine or tolazoline), or nitroprusside (see Chap. 25). The prognosis for the heart is good, with most surviving infants having normal cardiac findings in 3 weeks and a normal ECG in 3 months. If there is severe cardiogenic shock, the infant usually dies or has a severe insult to the brain or other vital organ.

3. Renal effects of asphyxia. The asphyxiated infant is at risk for **ATN** and for **SIADH. Urine output, urinalysis, urine specific gravity, and urine and serum osmolarity and electrolytes should be monitored. Measure**ment of serum and urine creatinine together with serum and urine Na+ allows calculation of the **fractional excretion of Na+ (FE^{Na})** and the **renal index** to help confirm a renal insult (see Chap. 31 for diagnosis and management of ATN). Measurement of urinary levels of **beta-2-microglobulin,** a low-molecular-weight protein freely filtered through the glomerulus and reabsorbed almost completely in the proximal tubule of even immature kidneys, may provide a sensitive indicator of subtle proximal tubular dysfunction. Renal size should be monitored by **ultrasound. Do****pamine infusion at 1.25 to 2.50** μg/kg per hour intravenously may aid **renal perfusion.** Oliguria should not be attributed to SIADH or ATN until prerenal etiologies such as hypovolemia or vasodilation have been ruled out (see Chaps. 9, 31).

4. Gastrointestinal effects of asphyxia. The asphyxiated infant is at risk for bowel ischemia and **necrotizing enterocolitis.** We usually do not feed **severely asphyxiated** infants for 5 to 7 days after the insult or until good bowel sounds are heard and stools are negative for blood and/or reducing substance (see Chap. 32).

5. Hematologic effects of asphyxia. Disseminated intravascular coagulation may be seen in asphyxiated infants because of damage to blood vessels. The liver may fail to make clotting factors, and the bone marrow may not produce platelets. Clotting factors (partial thromboplastin time [PTT] and prothrombin time [PT]), fibrinogen, and platelets should be monitored and replaced as needed (see Chap. 26).

6. **Liver.** The liver may be so damaged **(shock liver)** that it cannot provide its basic functions. **Liver function (transaminases [SGOT, SGPT], clotting factors [PT, PTT, fibrinogen], albumin,** and **bilirubin)** should be monitored, and serum **ammonia** level should be measured. Clotting factors should be provided as indicated. Serum **glucose** level should be kept at 75 to 100 mg/dl; glycogen stores have usually been depleted. Drugs that are detoxified by the liver must have their levels monitored closely. Total liver failure is usually a bad prognostic sign.

7. **Lung.** The pulmonary effects of asphyxia include **increased pulmonary vascular resistance, pulmonary hemorrhage, pulmonary edema** secondary to cardiac failure, and possibly failure of surfactant production with secondary hyaline membrane disease **(acute respiratory distress syndrome). Meconium aspiration** may be present. Treatment consists of oxygenation and ventilation (and possibly mild alkalinization). The method of ventilation may be different if the primary problem is hyaline membrane disease, persistent pulmonary hypertension, or meconium aspiration (see Chap. 24). **High-frequency ventilation** may play a role in some of these strategies (see Chap. 24). **Extracorporeal membrane oxygenation (ECMO)** may also provide a therapeutic modality in an asphyxiated infant whose CNS appears otherwise intact (see Chap. 24).

VI. **Prognosis of perinatal asphyxia** [16,18]. The degree of asphyxia necessary to cause permanent brain damage in experimental animals is quite close to that which causes death (<25 minutes of acute, total asphyxia). Survival with brain damage due to asphyxia is actually uncommon in this model, the extremes of death or intact survival being the most likely outcomes. Likewise, in humans, birth asphyxia severe enough to damage the fetal brain usually kills before or soon after birth. Approximately one-fourth of asphyxiated term newborns die. The remainder, however, even those with seizures, will overwhelmingly be normal. The only group with significant neurologic impairment are those who were **severely** asphyxiated yet narrowly escaped death, a relatively small group. Except in extreme cases where an infant is asphyxiated to near-lethal proportions, if an infant does not die from the asphyxia, the prognosis is quite favorable for normal neurologic status (including absence of mental retardation and epilepsy).

Given this, no infant will have undergone a perinatal asphyxial insult severe enough to cause permanent brain damage without **other organs** being equally severely affected. Thus a diagnosis of asphyxia severe enough to offer a poor prognosis must hinge on **assessment of other systems** in addition to the CNS. A corollary of this statement is that no neurologic abnormality diagnosed later in childhood (e.g., cerebral palsy) can be ascribed to perinatal asphyxia in the absence of evidence in the perinatal period of severe, **multisystemic** asphyxial insult. Conversely, even when perinatal asphyxia is confirmed, most etiologies of such asphyxia are due **not** to preventable intrapartum events or interventions but to **preexisting,** usually congenital, often subtle (cytoarchitectural) developmental malformations and dysgeneses, neurologic and otherwise (e.g., microscopic defects in neuronal migration or connectivity) [11].

A. **Outcome** [8,13–15]. Overall, full-term asphyxiated infants have a mortality of 10 to 20%. The incidence of neurologic sequelae in survivors is 20 to 45% (approximately 40% of these are minimal; 60% severe); i.e., the **majority will be normal.** Analyzed according to **Sarnat's stages** of severity [15] (see Table 27-9), virtually 100% of newborns with evidence of mild encephalopathy (stage 1) have normal neurologic outcome; 80% of those with moderate encephalopathy (stage 2) are normal neurologically (those who are abnormal exhibiting stage 2 signs over 7 days); and virtually all the children with severe encephalopathy (stage 3) die (one-half) or develop major neurologic sequelae (the other half) (e.g., cerebral palsy [CP], retardation, epilepsy, microcephaly). (Preterm infants may have a higher morbidity and mortality at less severe stages because of the high frequency of ICH and problems with other systems.) While the **risk** of CP in the asphyxiated newborn is elevated—5 to 10% versus 2 per 1000 in the general population of live births—the actual number is quite small in absolute terms. (Regarding the existence of school problems among the "neurologically and mentally normal" survivors of HIE, in one study [14], at 8 years of age, all "unimpaired" children from the "mild" HIE group and a majority [65 to 82%] of "unimpaired" children from the "moderate" HIE group were performing at expected grade level, indistinguishable from a matched peer group.)

The cardiac, renal, gastrointestinal, pulmonary, hepatic, and hematologic problems usually resolve if the infant survives.

B. Risk of CP [9,11]. Data from the National Collaborative Perinatal Project (NCPP) and the British National Child Development Study (BNCDS) suggest that perinatal factors of labor and delivery *contribute little to the incidence of mental retardation and seizure.* Only 3 to 13% of infants with CP had evidence of intrapartum asphyxia. In support of this assessment is the observation that despite improvements in perinatal care, the incidence of long-term neurologic sequelae has not decreased. The following previously implicated obstetric events **do not** correlate with CP: oxytocin administration, nuchal cord, midforceps use, and duration of labor. Factors found to be statistically associated with an increased risk for the development of CP were gestational age less than 32 weeks, fetal heart rate less than 60 beats per minute, breech presentation (although *not* breech delivery), chorioamnionitis, low placental weight, placental complications, and birth weight less than 2000 gm. Most of these factors, however, reflect preexistent, unpreventable sources of neurologic dysfunction that occur independent of asphyxia but that might also predispose to concomitant asphyxia at birth. (For example, it recently was postulated that an abnormal CNS may cause otherwise unexplained premature onset of labor and that a fetus with CNS abnormalities might not possess appropriate reflex cardiovascular responses to stress during labor and delivery to ensure proper fetal and placental perfusion [11].) No constant relationship between measures of fetal distress and subsequent long-term neurologic outcome has been demonstrated; that is, most infants with only **one** of the following predictors do **not** develop CP: meconium staining (98% do **not** develop CP), fetal heart rate less than 60 beats per minute (98% do **not** develop CP), pH less than 7.1 (no correlation with CP), more than 5 minutes to the first cry (98% do **not** develop CP), and 10-minute Apgar score less than 3 (83% do **not** develop CP). These clearly better reflect clinical status during the perinatal period than they do ultimate long-term outcome. Clustering perinatal events improves prediction of CP. For example, seizures alone were associated with CP in only 0.13%, but low Apgar score, signs of HIE, and seizures identified a small subgroup in whom the risk for CP was 55%. **Most CP, however, is not related to birth asphyxia, and most birth asphyxia does not cause CP.**

C. Indicators of poor outcome. While permanent brain damage from perinatal asphyxia is actually uncommon, are there reliable prognostic indicators of the small subgroup in which this does occur? Within the first 2 weeks of life it is very difficult to offer a prognosis for an individual infant because the present methods of prognostication are so unreliable. Unfavorable signs are (1) severe, prolonged asphyxia; (2) **Sarnat stage 3** encephalopathy; (3) seizures of early onset that are difficult to control *when accompanied by other signs of asphyxia in multiple systems;* (4) **elevated ICP** (>10 mm Hg); (5) persistence of abnormal neurologic signs at discharge (usually for more than 1 to 2 weeks), especially absence of the **Moro reflex**; (6) persistence of extensive hypodensities **(cystic encephalomalacia)** on CT [3,8] obtained at least 4 weeks after the insult; (7) abnormalities on brain scan [8]; (8) an elevated CK-BB level (>5 IU), although this measure is inferior to CT/EEG in prognostic reliability [6]; and (9) persistent oliguria (<1 ml/kg per hour for the first 36 hours of life). While a single early Apgar score correlates poorly with acid–base status, which itself correlates poorly with outcome, the **extended Apgar score** may help predict outcome. Term infants with Apgar scores of 0 to 3 at 10, 15, and 20 minutes have mortality rates of 18, 48, and 59%, respectively; in survivors, the CP rates are 5, 9, and 57%, respectively. It should be noted that many features of the Apgar score relate to cardiovascular integrity and *not* neurologic function. (Clearly, if an infant responds in the delivery room by 15 to 20 minutes, it has an excellent chance of being normal; conversely, only a small percentage of infants have a score less than 3 at 20 minutes and survive.) By electrodiagnostic criteria, the neonate with seizures was 50 to 70 times more likely to develop CP than one without seizures; however, more importantly, 70 to 80% of infants with neonatal seizures who survived had no CP. Of neonates, however, who required resuscitation (not merely intubation) after 5 minutes of life and subsequently developed seizures, one-half died and almost half the survivors had CP. Simply stated, **seizure without depression is not ominous, and depression without seizure is not ominous. Background EEG activity** is actually a better indicator of prognosis than ictal patterns per se. Term infants with normal or maturationally delayed interictal EEGs after seizures have an almost 86% probability of normal development at the age of 4 years. However, interictal background abnormalities such as burst-suppression, low-voltage, or electrocerebral inactivity are associated with poor outcome (30 to 75% likelihood). When EEG records are categorized as of mild, moderate, or marked severity, only markedly abnormal records predict subsequent morbidity or mortality; for example, 93% of neonates with extreme burst-suppression activity have a poor outcome. It should be noted that not all neonates who have seizures and later neurologic deficits have those seizures because of asphyxia; often there is concurrent evidence of a metabolic disorder, infection, or malformation that might predispose to both asphyxia *and* neurologic deficit. Evoked potentials have not yet proved to be reliable prognosticators. In vivo measurement of decreased ratios of high-energy phosphate compounds by phosphorus **magnetic resonance spectroscopy** may ultimately prove clinically useful as a prognostic tool [3]. In a prospective study [3] of neonates with significantly reduced ratios, 95% died or survived with serious multiple neurologic impairments and had diffuse echodensities on ultrasound. Monitoring CPP by Doppler in the asphyxiated infant may prove of benefit in prognostication. Despite initial enthusiasm that **MRI** (especially T1-weighted images) may prove better than CT regarding anatomic definition of ischemic lesions at an earlier stage, preliminary prospective studies [4] suggest that the high water content of the neonatal brain may still preclude such detection, indicating limited clinical usefulness presently in the immediate neonatal period. While still an experimental modality, in the future **near-infrared spectroscopy (NIRS)** (which detects the concentrations of various chromophores within biologic tissue whose light-absorbing properties in the near-infrared region of the spectrum vary with oxygenation) may provide noninvasive quantification of indices of cerebral oxygenation and hemodynamics. For example, in preliminary studies [10], elevated cerebral blood volume, assessed noninvasively by NIRS in asphyxiated full-term infants within the first 24 hours after birth, appeared to correlate with the clinical severity of the encephalopathy and with adverse outcome.

   In perinatal cardiac arrest, several studies indicated that if the heart beat is back within 5 minutes and if the baby is breathing regularly and spontaneously within 30 minutes, the prognosis is good. If this is not the case, the outcome is poor [17].
D. **Clinical manifestations of neurologic sequelae.** The precise neurologic sequelae one will see following a severe asphyxic insult will reflect the location, identity, and extent of the neural cellular population affected. **CP** is a nonprogressive motor and/or postural deficit of early onset. The specific types—**pyramidal**, i.e., **spastic quadriplegia** commonly associated with **mental retardation** and **epilepsy; spastic diplegia** (more common in "preemies") or **hemiplegia; and extrapyramidal** (including **dystonic** and **choreo-**

athetoid types)—are determined by the topography of brain injury. Mixed varieties exist. Focal or multifocal **cortical necrosis**, especially in the distribution of the middle cerebral artery, usually at the depths of sulci, may lead to **pyramidal CP** (unilateral or bilateral spastic hemiplegia or quadriplegia), **focal seizures**, and **mental retardation**, depending on the extent of the damage. A **boundary zone infarct** in a term newborn involving predominantly the parasagittal cortical regions (a watershed between the anterior, middle, and posterior cerebral arteries) may be recognized as weakness of the shoulder girdle and proximal upper extremities. **Auditory, visual-spatial**, or **language** difficulties probably reflect more extensive **parasagittal injury** more laterally and posteriorly in the border zones of the parietooccipital lobe. In the initially preterm infant, **spastic diplegia** probably represents an ischemic cystic lesion in watershed zones of the periventricular white matter at the angles of the ventricle superior to the germinal matrix **(PVL)**; concomitant **visual impairment** suggests involvement of the optic radiations as well. **Extrapyramidal CP** is probably the long-term clinical correlate of necrosis of the basal ganglia and thalamus **(status marmoratus).**

References

1. Ad Hoc Task Force. Guidelines for the determination of brain death in children. American Academy of Pediatrics Task Force on Brain Death in Children. *Pediatrics* 80:298, 1987.
2. Ashwal, S., et al. Brain death in the newborn [see comments]. *Pediatrics* 84:429, 1989.
3. Azzopardi, D., et al. Prognosis of newborn infants with hypoxic-ischemic brain injury assessed by phosphorus magnetic resonance spectroscopy. *Pediatr. Res.* 25:445, 1989.
4. Byrne, P., et al. Serial magnetic resonance imaging in neonatal hypoxic-ischemic encephalopathy. *J. Pediatr.* 117:694, 1990.
5. Clancy, R., et al. Continuous intracranial pressure monitoring and serial electroencephalographic recordings in severely asphyxiated term neonates. *Am. J. Dis. Child.* 142:740, 1988.
6. Fernandez, F., et al. Serum CPK-BB isoenzyme in the assessment of brain damage in asphyctic term infants. *Acta Paediatr. Scand.* 76:914, 1987.
7. Garcia-Alix, A., et al. Neuron-specific enolase and myelin basic protein: Relationship of cerebrospinal fluid concentrations to the neurologic condition of asphyxiated full-term infants. *Pediatrics* 93:234, 1994.
8. Hill, A., et al. Perinatal asphyxia: Clinical aspects [Review]. *Clin. Perinatol.* 16:435, 1989.
9. Kuban, K. C. K., et al. Cerebral palsy. *N. Engl. J. Med.* 330:188, 1994.
10. McDonald, J. W., et al. Physiological and pathophysiological roles of excitatory amino acids during central nervous system development [Review]. *Brain Res. Brain Res. Rev.* 15:41, 1990.
11. Painter, M. J. Fetal heart rate patterns, perinatal asphyxia, and brain injury [Review]. *Pediatr. Neurol.* 5:137, 1989.
12. Palmer, C., et al. Potential new therapies for perinatal cerebral hypoxia-ischemia [Review]. *Clin. Perinatol.* 20:411, 1993.
13. Perlman, J. M., et al. Acute systemic organ injury in term infants after asphyxia. *Am. J. Dis. Child.* 143:617, 1989.
14. Rosen, M. G., et al. The paradox of electronic fetal monitoring: More data may not enable us to predict or prevent infant neurologic morbidity [Review]. *Am. J. Obstet. Gynecol.* 168:745, 1993.
15. Sarnat, H. B., et al. Neonatal encephalopathy following fetal distress: A clinical and electroencephalographic study. *Arch. Neurol.* 33:696, 1976.
16. Shankaran, S. Perinatal asphyxia. *Clin. Perinatol.* 20:287, 1993.
17. Steiner, H., et al. Perinatal cardiac arrest. Quality of the survivors. *Arch. Dis. Child.* 50:696, 1975.
18. Vannucci, R. C. Current and potentially new management strategies for perinatal hypoxic–ischemic encephalopathy. *Pediatrics* 85:961, 1990.

19. Volpe, J. J. Hypoxic-Ischemic Encephalopathy. In J. J. Volpe, (Ed.), *Neurology of the newborn,* 2d ed. Philadelphia: Saunders, 1987, p. 209.

Neural Tube Defects
Lawrence C. Kaplan

I. Definitions and pathology. Neural tube defects constitute one of the most common groups of congenital malformations in newborns, often accounting for over one-third of all admissions of children with multiple congenital anomaly syndromes. They represent, however, a heterogeneous group of disorders based on such factors as embryologic timing and the involvement of specific elements of the neural tube and its derivatives. A recent review of neural tube defects can be found in ref. 2.

A. Types of neural tube defects
  1. Primary neural tube defects. These constitute approximately 95% of all neural tube defects. They are due to primary failure of closure of the neural tube or possibly disruption of an already closed neural tube between 18 and 28 days' gestation. The resulting abnormality usually consists of two anatomic lesions: an exposed (open or *operta*) neural placode along the midline of the back caudally, and rostrally, the Arnold-Chiari II malformation (malformation of pons and medulla, downward displacement of cerebellum, and fourth ventricle), with aqueductal stenosis and hydrocephalus [2]. The most severe are craniorachischisis and anencephaly. Anencephaly is always incompatible with life [5].

  a. Meningomyelocele. This is the most common primary neural tube defect. It involves a saccular outpouching of neural elements (neural placode), typically through a defect in the bone and the soft tissues of the posterior thoracic, lumbar, or sacral regions. Structural abnormalities often extend the length of the central nervous system and include hydromyelia, abnormalities of the corpora quadrigemina, the corpus callosum, third and lateral ventricles, and the gyral patterns of the cerebral hemispheres. Hydrocephalus occurs in 84% of these children; Arnold-Chiari II malformation occurs in approximately 90%. Dura and arachnoid are typically included in the sac (meningo-), which contains visible neural structures (myelo-), and the skin is usually discontinuous over the sac [4].

  b. Encephalocele. Occipitally, cervically, and more rarely frontally, this defect is an outpouching of dura with or without brain. It may vary in size from a few millimeters to many centimeters.

  c. Anencephaly. In the most severe form of this defect, the cranial vault and posterior occipital bone are defective, and derivatives of the neural tube are exposed, including both brain and bony tissue. The defect usually extends through the foramen magnum and involves the brain stem.

  2. Secondary neural tube defects. Five percent of all neural tube defects are secondary neural tube defects resulting from abnormal development of the caudal cell mass late or following primary neural tube closure. This leads to defects primarily in the lumbosacral spinal region. These heterogeneous lesions rarely are associated with hydrocephalus or the Arnold-Chiari II malformation, and the skin is typically intact over the defect [4].

  a. Meningocele. This is an outpouching of skin and dura without obvious involvement of the neural elements. These may be bone and contiguous soft-tissue abnormalities.

  b. Lipomeningocele. A lipomeningocele is a lipomatous mass usually in the lumbar or sacral region, occasionally off the midline, typically covered with full-thickness skin. Adipose tissue frequently extends through the defect into the spine and dura and adheres extensively to a distorted spinal cord or nerve roots.

   c. **Sacral agenesis/dysgenesis, diastematomyelia, myelocystocele.** These and others all may have varying degrees of bony involvement. While rarely as extensive as with primary neural tube defects, neurologic manifestations may be present representing distortion or abnormal development of peripheral nerve structures. These lesions may be inapparent on surface examination (occulta) of the child.

B. **Epidemiology.** In the United States, the overall frequency of neural tube defects is 1 in 2000 live births, and this appears to be decreasing. A well-established increased incidence is known among individuals living in parts of Ireland and Wales (4.2 to 12.5 per 1000), and carries over to descendants of these individuals who live elsewhere in the world. This also may be true for other ethnic groups, including Sikh Indians and certain groups in Egypt. The exact cause of failed neural tube closure remains unknown. Over 95% of all neural tube defects occur to couples with no known family history. Primary neural tube defects carry an increased empiric recurrence risk of 1 in 33 for couples with one affected pregnancy and 1 in 10 for those with two affected pregnancies. Affected individuals have a 1 in 25 risk of having one offspring with a primary neural tube defect. Sisters of women with an affected child have a 1 in 100 risk, and sisters of a man with an affected child have a 1 in 300 risk. Brothers of a parent with an affected child have a 1 in 500 risk. Secondary neural tube defects are generally sporadic and carry no increased recurrence risk. In counseling families for recurrence, however, it is critical to obtain a careful history of drug exposure and/or family history [3].

C. **Etiologies** proposed for both primary and secondary neural tube defects are heterogeneous. They include such **known** factors as maternal alcohol, aminopterin, or thalidomide ingestion; maternal diabetes; prenatal x-irradiation; and amniotic band disruption. **Suspected** factors and associations are maternal hyperthermia; hallucinogen, trimethadione, or valproate ingestion; and prenatal exposure to rubella. Both dominant and recessive mendelian inheritance have been documented, and neural tube defects can occur with trisomies 13 and 18, triploidy, and Meckel-Gruber syndrome (autosomal recessive, encephalocele, polydactyly, cystic dysplasia of kidneys), as well as other chromosome disorders. There is concordance for neural tube defect in monozygotic twins and an increased incidence with consanguinity. Both zinc and folic acid deficiencies have been proposed as possible etiologies.

D. **Prevention.** Controlled, randomized clinical studies of prenatal multivitamin administration to mothers with prior affected offspring suggest a lower recurrence risk than in control groups. There has been no demonstrated harm from folate administration, supporting the recommendation of folate supplementation starting prior to pregnancy for all women who have had one affected fetus [6]. However, the heterogeneity of neural tube defects in particular warrants caution in proposing single vitamins or multivitamins to prevent these congenital malformations. The Centers for Disease Control of the U.S. Public Health Service recommends that women of childbearing age who are capable of becoming pregnant should consume 0.4 mg of folic acid per day to reduce their risks of having a fetus affected with spina bifida or other neural tube defects [1].

II. **Diagnosis**
A. **Prenatal diagnosis.** The combination of maternal serum alpha-fetoprotein (AFP) determinations and prenatal ultrasound, especially when combined with AFP and acetylcholinesterase determinations on amniotic fluid where indicated, greatly improves the ability to make a prenatal diagnosis. Maternal serum AFP measurements in the second trimester (16 to 18 weeks) can diagnose 90% of fetuses with encephalocele and 80% of those with open meningomyelocele. The exact timing of the measurement is critical. Ultrasound assists in assessing ventricle size and other congenital anomalies,

and aids in confirming the suspected prenatal diagnosis. Determining the prognosis based on prenatal ultrasound remains difficult, except in obvious cases of encephalocele or anencephaly (see Chap. 1). Accurate readings of abnormal-appearing ultrasound scans in the presence of elevated levels of maternal serum AFP may obviate the need for amniocentesis altogether.

B. Postnatal diagnosis. Except for some secondary neural tube defects, most neural tube defects, especially meningomyelocele, are immediately obvious at birth. Occasionally some saccular masses, including sacrococcygeal teratomas, are confused with these. These are usually in the low sacrum.

III. Evaluation

A. History. Obtain a detailed family history. Ask about the occurrence of neural tube defects, and other congenital anomalies or malformation syndromes.

B. Physical examination. It is important to do a thorough physical examination, including a neurologic examination. The following are portions of the examination likely to reveal abnormal conditions:

1. **General newborn assessment.** Without exception, evaluate all newborns with neural tube defects for the presence of congenital heart disease, renal malformation, and structural defects of the airway, gastrointestinal tract, ribs, and hips. While rare in primary neural tube defects, these can be encountered in a subspecialty evaluation and should be considered before beginning surgical treatment or before discharge from the hospital [3]. In addition, plan an ophthalmologic examination and hearing evaluation during the hospitalization or following discharge.

2. **Back.** Inspect the defect and note if it is leaking cerebrospinal fluid (CSF). Use a sterile nonlatex rubber glove when touching a leaking sac (in most circumstances, only the neurosurgeon needs to touch the back). Note the location, shape, and size of the defect, and observe the size of the cutaneous defect or thin "parchment like" skin, although it has little relation to the size of the sac. Often the sac is deflated and has a wrinkled appearance. It is important to note the curvature of the spine and the presence of a bony gibbus underlying the defect. Occasionally, there is more than one meningomyelocele.

3. **Head.** Record the head circumference and plot daily throughout the first hospitalization. At birth, some infants will have macrocephaly due to hydrocephalus, and still more will develop hydrocephalus after closure of the defect on the back.

4. **Intracranial pressure (ICP).** Assess the ICP by palpating the anterior fontanel and tilting the head forward until the midportion of the anterior fontanel is flat. The fontanels may be quite large and the calvarial bones widely separated. (See Intracranial Hemorrhage.)

5. **Eyes.** Abnormalities in conjugate movement of the eyes are common and include esotropias, esophorias, and abducens paresis.

6. **Lower extremities.** Look for deformities and evidence of muscle weakness. Abnormalities in the lower extremities, some representing deformations, are common [3]. Look at thigh positions and skinfolds for evidence of congenital dislocation of the hips. Dislocation of the hips can be diagnosed clinically and by ultrasound (see Chap. 28).

7. **Neurologic examination.** Observe the child's spontaneous activity and response to sensory stimuli in all extremities. Predicting ambulation and muscle strength based on the "level" of the neurologic deficit can be misleading, and very often the anal reflex, or "wink," will be present at birth and absent postoperatively, owing to spinal shock and edema. Repeating neurologic examinations at periodic intervals is more helpful in predicting functional outcome than a single newborn examination. Similarly, sensory examination of the newborn can be misleading because of the potential absence of a motor response to pinprick. Carefully examine deep tendon reflexes (Table 27-10).

8. **Bladder and kidneys.** Observe bladder function, particularly for the possibility of inadequate emptying. Palpate the abdomen for evidence of

kidney enlargement. Observe the pattern of urination, and check the child's response to Credé's maneuver by monitoring residual urine in the bladder.

IV. Consultation. The care of infants with neural tube defects requires the coordinated efforts of a number of medical and surgical specialists as well as specialists in nursing, physical therapy, and social service. If follow-up is by a myelodysplasia team, follow their protocols. If not, the following specialties represent the areas needing careful assessment:

A. Specialty consultations

1. **Neurosurgery.** The initial care of the child with a neural tube defect is predominantly neurosurgical. The neurosurgeon is responsible for assessment and surgical closure of the defect, and for control and treatment of elevated ICP.

2. **Pediatrics.** A thorough evaluation before surgical procedures is important, particularly for detecting other abnormalities that might influence surgical risk.

3. **Clinical genetics.** Begin a complete dysmorphology evaluation and genetic counseling during the first hospitalization and follow up during outpatient visits.

4. **Urology.** Consult a urologist on the day of birth because of the risk of obstructive uropathy.

5. **Orthopedics.** The pediatric orthopedic surgeon is responsible for the initial assessment of musculoskeletal abnormalities and long-term management of ambulation, seating, and spine stability. Clubfeet, frequently encountered in the newborn period, should be assessed and may be managed during this hospitalization.

6. **Physical therapy.** Perform a thorough muscle examination as early as possible and involve physical therapists in planning for outpatient physical therapy programs.

7. **Social service.** Arrange for a social worker familiar with the special needs of children with neural tube defects to meet the parents as early as possible. Children with meningomyelocele may require a considerable amount of parents' time and resources, thereby placing considerable strain on parents and siblings.

B. Diagnostic tests. During the first hospitalization, the following tests should be done on most children with meningomyelocele. Scheduling these tests will vary depending on each situation.

1. **Radiographs**
   a. **Chest.** Rib deformities are common; cardiac malformations also may be identified.
   b. **Spine.** Abnormalities in vertebral bodies, absent or defective posterior arches, and evidence of kyphosis are common [3].
   c. **Hips.** Evidence of dysplasia of hips is common, and some children with neural tube defects are born with dislocated hips. As noted, ultrasound examination of the hips can be very helpful to the orthopedic surgeon (see Chap. 28).

2. **Serum creatinine** level should be measured if voiding patterns appear initially abnormal. Occasionally, potassium levels may be elevated in the nonvoiding newborn.

3. **Urodynamic study** should be done early in the hospitalization or shortly after discharge to document the status of the bladder and urinary sphincter function and innervation and to serve as a basis for comparison later in life.

4. **Intravenous pyelogram (IVP)** provides detailed information about urinary tract anatomy.

5. **Ultrasound of the urinary tract** is useful to assess possible hydronephrosis and/or structural abnormalities of the upper urinary tract.

Table 27-10. Correlation between segmental innervation; motor, sensory, and sphincter function; reflexes; and ambulation potential

Lesion	Segmental innervation	Cutaneous sensation	Motor function	Working muscles	Sphincter function	Reflex	Potential for ambulation
Cervical/ thoracic	Variable	Variable	None	None	—	—	Poor, even in full braces
Thoracolumbar	T12	Lower abdomen	None	None	—	—	Full braces, long-term ambulation unlikely
	L1	Groin	Weak hip flexion	Iliopsoas	—	—	
	L2	Anterior upper thigh	Strong hip flexion	Iliopsoas and sartorius	—	—	
Lumbar	L3	Anterior distal thigh and knee	Knee extension	Quadriceps	—	Knee jerk	May ambulate with braces and crutches
	L4	Medial leg	Knee flexion and hip abduction	Medial hamstrings	—	Knee jerk	
Lumbosacral	L5	Lateral leg and medial knee	Foot dorsiflexion and eversion	Anterior tibial and peroneals	—	Ankle jerk	Ambulate with or without short leg braces
	S1	Sole of foot	Foot plantar flexion	Gastrocnemius, soleus, and posterior tibial	—	Ankle jerk	
Sacral	S2	Posterior leg and thigh	Toe flexion	Flexor hallucis	Bladder and rectum	Anal wink	Ambulate without braces
	S3	Middle of buttock	—	—	Bladder and rectum	Anal wink	
	S4	Medial buttock	—	—	Bladder and rectum	Anal wink	

Source: From M. J. Noetzel, Myelomeningocele: Current concepts of management. *Clin. Perinatol.* 6:318, 1984.

6. Consider a **voiding cystourethrogram** if there is an abnormality seen on IVP or urodynamic study or in the setting of a rising serum creatinine level.

7. **Computed tomography (CT) of the head** is usually not necessary before repair of the defect on the back, but generally should be done soon thereafter, even if there is no clinical evidence of hydrocephalus. If ultrasonography is available and can accurately evaluate the presence of hydrocephalus, this may be a useful alternative to an initial CT. Magnetic resonance imaging (MRI) is particularly valuable in assessment of the posterior fossa and syringomyelia but should not necessarily replace CT or ultrasound in the initial assessment period.

V. **Selection of an approach to caring for children with neural tube defects**
   A. **Initial general approach.** Regardless of the management plan ultimately undertaken, every child with neural tube defects should receive well-planned and consistent care that respects his or her need for nutrition, comfort, and dignity and that honors the right of parents to participate in all decisions regarding care, including the right to withhold aggressive surgical management. Prognostic criteria, if considered, should guide discussion, **not** replace the dialogue that is necessary between parents and care providers. In our experience, discussing "quality of life" is not helpful unless it includes descriptions of possible outcomes in concrete and understandable terms based on clinical data. Parents almost always prefer to hear details in initial discussions, especially regarding cognitive and functional prognosis. An informed recommendation by a clinician central in the child's care can provide a basis for more frank dialogue but should be made as an entry into discussion.

   B. **Specific selection of care**
      1. **Supportive care.** This implies no surgical repair of the back or placement of a ventriculoperitoneal shunt but includes nurturing, feeding on demand, and consideration of the child's comfort. The child may die of infection of the open lesion not treated with antibiotics or of complications from hydrocephalus or other congenital malformations. If death appears inevitable, exercise care not to prolong undue suffering with such interventions as ventilator support and pressors. Survival without surgery may occur for months or even years. In children who stabilize (e.g., complete epithelialization of the spinal defect), periodic reassessment of treatment options and discussion with the family become critical. Acceptable options to consider may include placement of a ventriculoperitoneal shunt to arrest progressive hydrocephalus, referral for foster and adoptive care, and alternative feeding techniques.

      2. **Aggressive care.** The goal here is habilitation and planning intervention as completely as possible to prevent any further injury to the central nervous system or to prevent morbidity secondary to complications of bladder and bowel dysfunction and progressive orthopedic deformity.

      3. **Ethical considerations.** Many physicians, nurses, and other nonmedical personnel hold strong opinions on the treatment of infants born with neural tube defects. Certain concepts need to be considered, especially if selection criteria enter into discussions. Early surgery permits survival of increased numbers of patients with neural tube defects, and most centers cite advances in medical technology and certain societal changes as contributing factors to this. It is our practice to identify risk factors that will likely contribute to poor outcome, but not to base management decisions on any set protocol or scoring system. Consult a hospital ethics committee to guide decision making and to help establish a forum to discuss various opinions and treatment options.

VI. **Management**
   A. **Initial.** The very thin sac is often leaking at birth. Keep the newborn in the prone position, with a sterile saline-moistened gauze sponge placed over the defect. This reduces bacterial contamination and damage related to dehy-

dration. Administer intravenous antibiotics (ampicillin and gentamicin) to diminish the risk of meningitis, particularly that due to group B streptococci. Children with an open spinal defect can receive a massive inoculation directly into the nervous system at the time of vaginal delivery or even in utero if the placental membranes rupture early. Meningitis is a particularly devastating complication. Because of the potential for allergy to latex rubber and possible anaphylaxis, no latex equipment should be used.

B. Surgical treatment. The initial neurosurgical treatment of an open meningomyelocele consists of (1) closing the defect to prevent infection and (2) reducing the elevated ICP. The back should be closed on the first day of life or as soon thereafter as safely possible to minimize bacterial contamination and the risk of infection. Techniques are available to close rapidly even very large cutaneous defects without skin grafting. Intracranial hypertension can be initially controlled by continuous ventricular drainage. Typically, once the back is sealed, a ventriculoperitoneal shunt catheter can be placed. Some neurosurgeons may elect to insert the catheter at the time of back closure. If a shunt is to be placed as a second procedure after back closure, careful monitoring of head circumference should be done because ICP often increases following closure of the back in unshunted patients.

Children whose defect is covered with skin and whose nervous system is therefore not at risk of bacterial contamination can undergo elective repair. This may be done at the age of 1 month or much later.

C. Parents. Keep parents accurately informed of their child's condition. The involvement of multiple specialists heightens the importance of the identification of a primary care provider to coordinate the flow of information [3].

VII. Prognosis

A. Survival. Mostly because of various interventions, nearly all children with neural tube defects, even those severely affected, can survive for many years. The overall 1-year survival rate for children with meningomyelocele exceeds 96%, and the 10-year survival rate is 90% (computed by life-table technique). Most deaths occur in the most severely affected children, but sudden infant death syndrome (SIDS) is more common in children with meningomyelocele than in the general population. If there is the expectation of survival of a child born with spina bifida, then survival is high. On the contrary, withholding the medical care as part of the program of "selection" will result in lower survival.

B. Motor and intellectual outcome

1. **Motor outcome.** This depends more on the level of paralysis, motivation, and surgical intervention than it does on congenital hydrocephalus. There is a likelihood that there will be a delay in motor progress in most children with neural tube defects, but appropriate bracing, physical therapy interventions, and monitoring and treatment of **kyphosis** and scoliosis can mitigate this. Also, such factors as obesity, frequent hospitalizations, tethering of the spinal cord, and decubitus ulcers can contribute to motor delays [3]. Table 27-10 is a rough guide to motor, sensory, and sphincter function and ambulation potential.

2. **Intellectual outcome.** Three identifiable subgroups are at risk for mental retardation: those with severe hydrocephalus at birth, those who develop infection in the central nervous system early in life, and those whose intracranial hypertension is not properly controlled. True mental retardation is encountered most commonly in children who have high thoracic level lesions, a history of central nervous system infection, and hydrocephalus with less than 1 cm of cortical mantle. Formal developmental testing is critical, since visual/perceptual deficits and fine motor difficulties may interfere with intellectual functioning. In addition, complex partial seizures can contribute to impaired intellectual function and should be considered in children, especially school-age children who have lost cognitive milestones. Eighty-five percent of children whose spinal lesions are at L3 or lower usually complete twelfth grade or be-

yond. Overall, do not discount the developmental needs. These children require educational and social supports throughout life.

C. Morbidity. The numbers of hospitalizations, of days in the hospital, and of operations required are much lower for children with sacral level lesions and much higher for those with thoracic lesions. Of 132 children consecutively admitted to the Children's Hospital of Boston for whom outcome is known beyond the age of 2 years, 12% have a "normal" gait, 7% have an abnormal gait but require no braces, 38% require braces, and 16% are only able to sit. Eighty-six percent live at home with the parents, and 4.6% live in a skilled nursing facility. Of children over 4 years old, 18% have "normal" bladder function, 21% receive intermittent catheterization, 42% void by Credé's maneuver, and 19% have an ileal conduit. Parents of 45% of the children over 4 years old report bowel function to be acceptable, and 49% report chronic bowel dysfunction, including encopresis. Of children over 5 years old, 45% attend regular public schools, and 89% of these are believed to be at grade level. Approximately 5% of newborns with open neural tube defects develop symptoms related to the Arnold-Chiari II malformation. These pontomedullary symptoms include stridor, ophthalmoplegia, apnea, abnormal gag, and vomiting (often confused with gastroesophageal reflex). These symptoms may indicate shunt malfunction and frequently disappear without treatment. If they persist, especially in association with cyanosis, the prognosis is poor, with the risk of respiratory failure and death. Posterior fossa decompression and cervical laminectomy are surgical options but are often not successful.

References

1. Centers for Disease Control. Recommendations for the use of folic acid to reduce the number of spina bifida cases and other NTD. *JAMA* 269:1233, 1993.
2. Dias, M. S., et al. Spinal Dysraphism. In S. L. Weinstein (Ed.), *The Pediatric Spine: Principles and Practice.* New York: Raven, 1994.
3. Kaplan, L. C. Evaluation of the Child with Congenital Anomalies. In I. L. Rubin and A. C. Crocker (Eds.), *Developmental Disabilities: Medical Care for Children and Adults.* Philadelphia: Lea & Febiger, 1989.
4. McLaughlin, D. G., et al. Early Neural Development and the Embryogenesis of Dysraphism. In W. Chadduck (Ed.), *Pediatric Neurosurgery* (3d Ed.). Philadelphia: Saunders, 1994.
5. Volpe, J. J. Human Brain Development. In J. J. Volpe (Ed.), *Neurology of the Newborn,* 3rd Ed. Philadelphia: Saunders, 1995. p. 3.
6. Wald, N. Folic acid and the prevention of neural tube defects. *Ann. N.Y. Acad. Sci.* 678:112, 1993.

28. ORTHOPEDIC PROBLEMS

James R. Kasser

This chapter considers common musculoskeletal abnormalities that may be detected in the neonatal period. Consultation with an orthopedic surgeon is often required to provide definitive treatment after the initial evaluation.

I. **Torticollis**
  A. **Torticollis** is a disorder characterized by limited motion of the neck, asymmetry of the face and skull, and a tilted position of the head. It is usually caused by shortening of the **sternocleidomastoid (SCM) muscle** but may be secondary to muscle adaptation from an abnormal in utero position of the head and neck.
    1. The **etiology** of the shortened SCM muscle is unclear; in many infants it is due to an abnormal in utero position, and in some it may be due to stretching of the muscle at delivery. The result of the latter is a contracture of the muscle associated with fibrosis. One hypothesis is that the SCM abnormality is secondary to a compartment syndrome occurring at the time of delivery.
    2. **Clinical course.** The limitation of motion is minimum at birth, but increases over the first few weeks. At 10 to 20 days, in torticollis related to stretching, a mass is frequently found in the SCM muscle. This mass gradually disappears, and the muscle fibers are partially replaced by fibrous tissue, which contracts and limits head motion. Because of the limited rotation of the head, the infant rests on the ipsilateral side of the face in the prone position and on the contralateral side when supine. The pressure from resting on one side of the face and the opposite occipital bone contributes to the facial and skull asymmetry. The ipsilateral zygoma is depressed and the contralateral occiput flattened.
    3. **Treatment.** Most infants will respond favorably to positioning the head in the direction opposite to that produced by the tight muscle. Padded bricks or sandbags can be used to help maintain the position of the head until the child is able to move actively to free the head. Passive stretching by rotating the head to the ipsilateral side and tilting it toward the contralateral side also may help. The torticollis in most infants resolves by the age of 1 year. Patients who have asymmetry of the face and head and limited motion after 1 year should be considered for surgical release of the SCM muscle.
  B. **Torticollis with limited motion of the neck** may be due to a congenital abnormality of the cervical region of the spine. Some infants with this disorder also have a tight SCM muscle. These infants are likely to have significant limitation of motion at birth. Radiologic evaluation of the cervical region is necessary to make this diagnosis.
  C. **A third type of torticollis** is associated with congenital asymmetric contractures of the hip abductor and unilateral metatarsal adduction. The torticollis always subsides spontaneously. Since some infants with this type of torticollis have unilateral hip dysplasia, ultrasonography of the hips should be performed if examination reveals tightness in the hip abductors sufficient to cause a pelvic obliquity.

II. **Polydactyly**
  A. **Duplication of a digit** may range from a small cutaneous bulb to an almost perfectly formed digit. Treatment of this problem is variable. Syndromes associated with polydactyly include Laurence-Moon-Biedl syndrome, chon-

droectodermal dysplasia, Ellis-van Creveld syndrome, and trisomy 13. Polydactyly is generally thought to be inherited in an autosomal dominant fashion with variable penetrance.
  B. **Treatment**
    1. The small functionless skin bulb without bone or cartilage at the ulnar
       border of the hand or lateral border of the foot can be ligated and allowed
       to develop necrosis for 24 hours. The part distal to the suture should be
       removed. The residual stump should have an antiseptic applied twice a
       day to prevent infection. Do not tie off digits on the radial side of the
       hand (thumb) or the medial border of the foot.
    2. When duplicated digits contain bony parts, the decision about treatment
       is more difficult and should be delayed until the patient is evaluated by
       an orthopedist or hand surgeon.
III. **Fractured clavicle** (see Chap. 20)
  A. The **clavicle** is the site of the most common fracture associated with deliv-
     ery.
  B. **Diagnosis** is usually made soon after birth, when the infant does not move
     the arm on the affected side or cries when that arm is moved. There may be
     tenderness, swelling, or crepitance at the site. Occasionally, the bone is an-
     gulated. Diagnosis can be confirmed by radiographic examination. A "pain-
     less" fracture discovered by radiography of the chest is more likely a congen-
     ital pseudarthrosis (nonunion). Nearly all pseudarthroses occur on the right
     side.
  C. The **clinical course** is such that clavicle fractures heal without difficulty.
     Treatment consists of providing comfort for the infant. If the arm and shoul-
     der are left unprotected, motion occurs at the fracture site when the baby is
     handled. We usually pin the infant's sleeve to the shirt and put a sign on the
     baby to remind personnel to decrease motion of the clavicle. No reduction is
     necessary. If the fracture appears painful, a wrap to decrease motion of the
     arm is useful.
IV. **Congenital and infantile scoliosis**
  A. **Congenital scoliosis** is a lateral curvature of the spine secondary to a fail-
     ure either of formation of a vertebra or of segmentation. Scoliosis in the
     newborn may be difficult to detect; by bending the trunk laterally in the
     prone position, however, a difference in motion can usually be observed.
     Congenital scoliosis must be differentiated from **infantile scoliosis,** in
     which no vertebral anomaly is present. Infantile scoliosis often improves
     spontaneously, although the condition may be progressive in infants who
     have a spinal curvature of more than 20 degrees. If the scoliosis is progres-
     sive, treatment is indicated.
  B. **Clinical course.** Congenital scoliosis will increase in many patients. Bracing
     of congenital curves is usually not helpful. Surgical correction and fusion
     are frequently indicated before the curve becomes severe. Since many pa-
     tients with congenital curves have renal or other visceral abnormalities,
     studies should be done to detect these abnormalities.
V. **Congenital dislocation of the hip.** Most (but not all) hips that are dislocated at
   birth can be diagnosed by a careful physical examination (see Chap. 3). Ultrasound examination of the hip is useful for diagnosis in high-risk cases. X-ray
   examination will not lead to a diagnosis in the newborn because the femoral
   head is not calcified but will reveal an abnormal acetabular fossa seen with hip
   dysplasia. There are three types of congenital dislocations.
  A. The **classic congenitally dislocated hip** is diagnosed by the presence of Or-
     tolani's sign. The hip is unstable and dislocates on adduction and also on ex-
     tension of the femur but readily relocates when the femur is abducted in
     flexion. No asymmetry of the pelvis is seen. This type of dislocation is more
     common in females and is usually unilateral, but it may be bilateral. Hips
     that are unstable at birth often become stable after a few days. The infant
     with hips that are unstable after 5 days of life should be treated with a
     splint that keeps the hips flexed and abducted. The Pavlik harness has been

used effectively to treat this group of patients. Ultrasound is used to monitor the hip during treatment as well as to confirm the initial diagnosis.
   B. The **teratologic type of dislocation** occurs very early in pregnancy. The
femoral head does not relocate on flexion and abduction; that is, Ortolani's
sign is not present. If the dislocation is unilateral, there may be asymmetry
of the gluteal folds and asymmetric motion with limited abduction. In bilateral dislocation, the perineum is wide and the thighs give the appearance of
being shorter than normal. This may be easily overlooked, however, and requires an extremely careful physical examination. Treatment of the teratologic hip dislocation is by open reduction.
   C. The **third type of dislocation** occurs late, is unilateral, and is associated
with a **congenital abduction contracture** of the contralateral hip. The abduction contracture causes a pelvic obliquity. The pelvis is lower on the side
of the contracture, which is unfavorable for the contralateral hip, and the
acetabulum may not develop well. After the age of 6 weeks, infants with this
type of dislocation develop an apparent short leg and have asymmetric
gluteal folds. Some infants will develop a dysplastic acetabulum, which may
eventually allow the hip to subluxate. Treatment of the dysplasia is with the
Pavlik harness, but after the age of 8 months, other methods of treatment
may be necessary.
VI. **Genu recurvatum,** or hyperextension of the knee, is not a serious abnormality
and is easily recognized and treated. It must be differentiated, however, from
subluxation or dislocation of the knee, which also may present with hyperextension of the knee. The latter two abnormalities are more serious and require
more extensive treatment.
   A. **Congenital genu recurvatum** is secondary to in utero position with hyperextension of the knee. This can be treated successfully by repeated cast
changes, with progressive flexion of the knee until it reaches 90 degrees of
flexion. Minor degrees of recurvatum can be treated with passive stretching
exercises.
   B. All infants with **hyperextension of the knee** should have a radiographic examination to differentiate genu recurvatum from true dislocation of the
knee. In congenital genu recurvatum, the tibial and femoral epiphyses are
in proper alignment except for the hyperextension. In the subluxed knee
with dislocation, the tibia is completely anterior or anterolateral to the femur. The tibia is shifted forward in relation to the femur and is frequently
lateral as well. Congenital fibrosis of the quadriceps is frequently associated
with the subluxed and dislocated knee, and open reduction is essential, for
attempted treatment of the dislocated knee by stretching or by repeated
cast changes is hazardous and may result in epiphyseal plate damage.
VII. **Deformities of the feet**
   A. **Metatarsus adductus** is a condition in which the metatarsals rest in an ad-
ducted position, but the appearance does not always reveal the severity of
the condition. Whether or not treatment is necessary is determined by the
difference in the degree of structural change in the metatarsals and tar-
sometatarsal joint.
      1. Most infants with metatarsus adductus have positional deformities that
are probably caused by in utero position. The positional type of metatarsus adductus is flexible and the metatarsals can be passively corrected
into abduction with little difficulty. This condition does not need treatment.
      2. The **structural metatarsus adductus** has a relatively fixed adduction de-
formity of the forefoot and the metatarsals cannot be abducted passively.
The etiology has not been definitely identified but is probably related to
in utero position. This is seen more commonly in the firstborn infant and
in pregnancies with oligohydramnios. Most infants with the structural
types of metatarsus adductus have a valgus deformity of the hindfoot.
The structural deformity needs to be treated with manipulation and cast
immobilization until correction occurs. Although there is no urgency to

treat this condition, it is more easily corrected earlier than later and should be done before the child is of walking age.

B. **Calcaneovalgus deformities** result from an in utero position of the foot that holds the ankle dorsiflexed and abducted. At birth, the top of the foot lies up against the anterior surface of the leg. Structural changes in the bones do not seem to be present. The sequela to this deformity appears to be a valgus or pronated foot that is more severe than the typical pronated foot seen in toddlers. Whether this disorder is treated or not is variable, and no study supports either course. **Treatment** consists of either exercise or application of a short-leg cast that will keep the foot plantar flexed and inverted. If the foot cannot be plantar flexed to a neutral position, casts are indicated. Casts are changed appropriately for growth and maintained until plantar flexion and inversion are equal to those of the opposite foot. Generally, the foot is held in plaster for about 6 to 8 weeks. Feet that remain in the calcaneovalgus position for several months may be more likely to have significant residual **pes valgus;** a fixed or rigid calcaneovalgus deformity probably represents a congenital vertical talus.

C. **Congenital clubfoot** is a congenital deformity with a multifactorial etiology. A first-degree relative of a patient with this deformity has 20 times the risk of having a clubfoot than does the normal population. The risk in subsequent siblings is 3 to 5%. The more frequent occurrence in the firstborn and the association with oligohydramnios suggest an influence of in utero pressure as well. Sometimes clubfoot is part of a syndrome. Infants with neurologic dysfunction of the feet (spina bifida) often have clubfoot.

1. There are three and sometimes four components to the deformity. The foot is in equinus, cavus, and varus position, with a forefoot adduction; thus the clubfoot is a talipes equinocavovarus with metatarsal adduction. Each of these deformities is sufficiently rigid to prevent passive correction to a neutral position by the examiner. The degree of rigidity is variable in each patient.

2. **Treatment** should be started early, within a few days of birth. An effective method of treatment consists of manipulation and application of either tapes or plaster casts that are changed every few days. If conservative treatment does not successfully correct the deformities, surgical correction will be necessary.

References

1. Cooperman, D.R., Thompson, G.H. Neonatal Orthopaedics. In A.A. Fanatoff and R.J. Martin (Eds.), Neonatal Perinatal Medicine, 6th ed. St. Louis: Mosby, 1997; 1709.
2. Graham, J.M. Smith's Recognizable Patterns of Human Deformation, 2nd ed. Philadelphia: W.B. Saunders, 1988.
3. Jones, K.L. Smith's Recognizable Patterns of Human Malformation, 5th ed. Philadelphia: W.B. Saunders, 1997.

29. METABOLIC PROBLEMS

Hypoglycemia and Hyperglycemia [4]
Richard E. Wilker

Hypoglycemia is commonly seen in both the newborn nursery and the neonatal intensive care unit (NICU). It is important to anticipate this problem and evaluate babies with either risk factors for hypoglycemia or symptoms, because hypoglycemia is usually easily treatable and can occur in infants who appear well.
Hyperglycemia, however, is less likely to be seen in the newborn nursery and usually occurs in the NICU in babies with other associated problems.

I. **Hypoglycemia.** Glucose crosses the placenta by facilitated diffusion, and fetal glucose levels are approximately two-thirds of maternal levels. After the exogenous source of glucose is stopped by the severing of the umbilical cord, newborn glucose levels rapidly fall to a low point in the first 1 to 2 hours of life. The levels then will increase and stabilize at mean levels of 65 to 71 mg/dl by the age of 3 to 4 hours.

A. **Incidence.** Hypoglycemia is reported to occur in 8.1% of full-term large-for-gestational-age (LGA) infants and 14.7% of small-for-gestational-age (SGA) newborns [5].

B. **Definition.** Discussion of the incidence, effects, and treatment of hypoglycemia has been hampered by lack of agreement on its definition [2,3, 10]. Early definitions of normal neonatal glucose levels were derived from surveys of infants who were often not being fed or given other sources of glucose. The statistical definition of normal, values that are within 2 standard deviations of the mean, resulted in the acceptance of glucose levels in the range of 20 to 30 mg/dl. On the basis of more recent neurophysiologic [7], metabolic, and statistical studies [2,3], most neonatologists now attempt to maintain neonatal glucose levels at or above 40 mg/dl.

1. **The significance of hypoglycemia depends on the infant's gestational age, chronological age, and other risk factors in addition to a low blood glucose level** [2,3].

2. **The absence of overt symptoms at low glucose levels does not rule out central nervous system (CNS) injury. There is no evidence indicating that the premature or young infant is being protected from the effects of inadequate glucose delivery to the CNS.**

3. **There is no single value below which brain injury definitely occurs** [2,3,10].

4. **A glucose level less than 40 mg/dl at any time in any newborn deserves evaluation and treatment. Our goal is to maintain the glucose value above 40 mg/dl in the first day, and more than 40 to 50 mg/dl thereafter** [2,3].

C. **Etiology**
1. **Increased utilization of glucose: hyperinsulinism [9]**
a. **Diabetic mothers** (see Chap. 2, Diabetes Mellitus)
b. **Erythroblastosis** (hyperplastic islets of Langerhans) [2,3] (see Chaps. 18, Hyperbilirubinemia and 26, Thrombocytopenia)
c. **Islet-cell hyperplasia or hyperfunction**
d. **Beckwith-Weidemann syndrome** (macrosomia, mild microcephaly, omphalocele, macroglossia, hypoglycemia, and visceromegaly) [2,3]

e. Insulin-producing tumors (nesidioblastosis, islet-cell adenoma, or islet-cell dysmaturity)

f. Maternal tocolytic therapy with beta-sympathomimetic agents (terbutaline, isoxsuprine, albuterol [salbutamol])

g. Maternal chlorpropamide therapy (Diabinese); possibly maternal benzothiadiazides (chlorothiazide)

h. Malpositioned umbilical artery catheter used to infuse glucose in high concentration into the celiac and superior mesenteric arteries T11–12, stimulating insulin release from the pancreas

i. Abrupt cessation of high-glucose infusions

j. After exchange transfusion with blood containing a high glucose concentration

2. Decreased production/stores [2,3,9]

a. Prematurity. Incidence: premature SGA, 67%; premature LGA, 38%

b. Intrauterine growth retardation (IUGR). Incidence: premature SGA, 67%; postterm SGA, 18%

c. Inadequate caloric intake

3. Increased utilization and/or decreased production or other causes. Any baby with one of the following conditions should be evaluated for hypoglycemia; parenteral glucose may be necessary for the management of these infants.

a. Perinatal stress
  (1) Sepsis
  (2) Shock [2,3]
  (3) Asphyxia [2,3]
  (4) Hypothermia (increased utilization)

b. Exchange transfusion with heparinized blood that has a low glucose level in the absence of a glucose infusion; reactive hypoglycemia after exchange with relatively hyperglycemic citrate-phosphate-dextrose (CPD) blood [2,3]

c. Defects in carbohydrate metabolism (see Inborn Errors of Metabolism)
  (1) Glycogen storage disease [2,3]
  (2) Fructose intolerance [2,3]
  (3) Galactosemia [2,3]

d. Endocrine deficiency
  (1) Adrenal insufficiency [2,3]
  (2) Hypothalamic deficiency [2,3]
  (3) Congenital hypopituitarism [2,3]
  (4) Glucagon deficiency
  (5) Epinephrine deficiency

e. Defects in amino acid metabolism (see Inborn Errors of Metabolism) [9]
  (1) Maple syrup urine disease
  (2) Propionic acidemia
  (3) Methylmalonic acidemia
  (4) Tyrosinemia
  (5) Glutaric acidemia type II
  (6) Ethylmalonic adipic aciduria
  (7) Glutaricidemia

f. Polycythemia (possibly due to glucose utilization by the increased mass of red blood cells. The decreased amount of serum per drop of blood may cause a reading consistent with hypoglycemia on whole blood measurements, but may yield a normal glucose level on laboratory analysis of serum.) [3] (see Chap. 26, Polycythemia)

g. Maternal therapy with propranolol. Possible mechanisms include the following:
  (1) Prevention of sympathetic stimulation of glycogenolysis

(2) Prevention of recovery from insulin-induced decreases in free fatty acids and glycerol

(3) Inhibition of epinephrine-induced increases in free fatty acids and lactate after exercise [3]

D. Diagnosis

1. **Symptoms, nonspecific** [3]
   a. **Lethargy, apathy, and limpness**
   b. **Apnea**
   c. **Cyanosis**
   d. **Weak or high-pitched cry**
   e. **Seizures, coma**
   f. **Poor feeding, vomiting**
   g. **Tremors, jitteriness, or irritability**
   h. **Seizures**
   i. **Some infants may have no symptoms**

2. **Reagent strips.** Although in widespread use as a screening tool, reagent strips are of unproven reliability in documenting hypoglycemia in neonates.
   a. Reagent strips measure whole blood glucose, which is 15% lower than plasma levels.
   b. Reagent strips are subject to false-positive and false-negative results, even when used with a reflectance meter.
   c. A confirmatory laboratory glucose determination is required before one can diagnose hypoglycemia.
   d. If a reagent strip reveals a concentration less than 40 mg/dl, treatment should not be delayed while one is awaiting confirmation of hypoglycemia by laboratory analysis. If an infant has either symptoms that could be due to hypoglycemia and/or a low glucose level as measured by reagent strip, treatment should be initiated immediately after the confirmatory blood sample is obtained.

3. **Laboratory diagnosis.** Serial blood glucose level should be routinely measured in infants who have risk factors for hypoglycemia and in infants who have symptoms that could be due to hypoglycemia (see **I.C** and **I.D**).
   a. The optimal time for screening depends on the baby's risk factors.
      (1) Infants of diabetic mothers usually develop hypoglycemia in the first hours of life and should have frequent early measurements of blood glucose level (see Chap. 2, Diabetes Mellitus).
      (2) Preterm and SGA infants should have blood glucose measurements during the first 3 to 4 days of life.
      (3) Infants with **erythroblastosis fetalis** should have blood glucose levels measured after exchange transfusions with CPD blood.
   b. **Lab measurement.** The laboratory sample must be obtained and analyzed promptly to avoid the measurement being falsely lowered by glycolysis [2,3]. The glucose level can fall 18 mg/dl per hour in a blood sample that awaits analysis.

      Confirmation of the diagnosis of **symptomatic hypoglycemia** requires both of the following:
      (1) A laboratory-determined serum glucose level of less than 40 mg/dl at the time symptoms are present
      (2) Prompt resolution of the symptoms with the administration of intravenous glucose and correction of the hypoglycemia
   c. When the hypoglycemia or need for large glucose infusions lasts over 1 week, evaluation of some of the rare causes of hypoglycemia should be considered [11]. At that time an endocrine consultation may be helpful and measurements of the following should be considered:
      (1) Insulin

(2) Growth hormone
(3) Cortisol
(4) Adrenocorticotropic hormone (ACTH)
(5) Thyroxine (T$_4$)
(6) Glucagon
(7) Plasma amino acids
(8) Urine ketones
(9) Urine reducing substance
(10) Urine amino acids
(11) Urine organic acids

d. Some infants with glucose being infused through an umbilical artery line may have normal glucose levels in their feet but hypoglycemic levels in the hands and brain.

4. Differential diagnosis [3]. The symptoms mentioned in **I.D** can be due to many other causes with or without associated hypoglycemia. If symptoms persist after the glucose concentration is in the normal range, other etiologies should be considered. Some of these are as follows:

a. Adrenal insufficiency
b. Maternal drug use
c. Heart disease
d. Renal failure
e. Liver failure
f. CNS disease
g. Metabolic abnormalities [11]
   (1) Hypocalcemia
   (2) Hyponatremia or hypernatremia
   (3) Hypomagnesemia
   (4) Pyridoxine deficiency
h. Sepsis
i. Asphyxia

E. Management. Anticipation and prevention, when possible, are key to the management of hypoglycemia.

1. Well infants who are at risk for hypoglycemia (see **I.C**) should have their blood glucose levels measured. Infants of diabetic mothers should have glucose measured, and be treated, according to the protocol in Chap. 1. Other **asymptomatic** infants who are at risk for hypoglycemia should have blood glucose measured in the first 2 hours of life. In the first hour of life they should be **nursed** or given **formula.** This feeding should be repeated every 2 to 3 hours. The interval between measurement of glucose levels requires clinical judgment. If the glucose concentration is as low as 20 to 30 mg/dl, it should be measured 1 to 2 hours after feeding. While early feeding of glucose water will transiently raise the serum glucose level, there is often an associated rebound hypoglycemia, in infants with hyperinsulinemia within an hour or two of the glucose water feeding. The early introduction of milk feeding will often result in raising glucose levels to normal, maintaining normal stable levels, and avoiding problems with rebound hypoglycemia. Feeding of dextrose 5% or 10% may be used initially as long as the blood glucose level is followed closely and confirmed to be in the normal range, and the concentration of feedings is then increased to one-half strength or full strength. We sometimes find it useful to add **Polycose** (4 cal/oz) to feedings in infants who feed well but have marginal glucose levels.

2. Infants who cannot tolerate oral feeding, are symptomatic, or in whom oral feedings do not maintain normal glucose levels
   a. Administer intravenously 200 mg/kg of glucose over 1 minute:
      2 ml of dextrose 10% in water (10% D/W) per kilogram over 1 minute

10% D/W   10 gm/100 ml
                 1 gm/10 ml
                 200 mg/2 ml
Follow this by an infusion of glucose at a rate of:
8 mg of glucose/kg per minute
10% D/W at a rate of 110 ml/kg per day or 4.6 ml/kg/hour gives 8
mg/kg per minute of glucose (Fig. 29-1, glucose rate calculation)
Give this rate, 8 mg of glucose/kg per minute, and then taper off the
rate of infusion as permitted by blood glucose levels.
b. Recheck glucose level after 20 to 30 minutes and hourly until stable,
to determine if additional therapy is needed.
c. Glucose infusions for maintenance
   (1) For most infants, intravenous 10% D/W at daily maintenance
   rates will provide adequate glucose. The concentration of the
   dextrose fluids will depend on the daily water requirement. It
   is suggested that calculation of both glucose intake (i.e., milligrams of glucose per kilogram per minute) and water requirements be done each day. For example, on the first day the fluid
   requirement is 80 ml/kg per day, or 0.055 ml/kg per minute;
   therefore, 10% D/W provides 5.5 mg of glucose per kilogram per
   minute, and 15% D/W provides 8.12 mg of glucose per kilogram
   per minute.

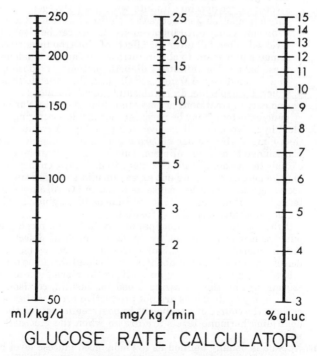

GLUCOSE RATE CALCULATOR

Use a straight edge to determine the volume required per 24 hours.

Fig. 29-1. Interconversion of glucose infusion units. (From M. H. Klaus and A. A.
Faranoff, eds. *Care of the high-risk neonate*, 2nd ed. Philadelphia: Saunders, 1979, p.
430.)

    (2) Some infants with hyperinsulinism and infants with IUGR will require 12 to 15 mg of dextrose per kilogram per minute (often as 15% D/W) [3].

    (3) The concentration of glucose and the rate of infusion are increased as necessary to maintain a normal blood glucose level. A central venous catheter may be necessary to give adequate glucose (15% to 20% D/W) in an acceptable fluid volume. Taper glucose to 4 to 6 mg/kg per minute, monitoring glucose levels; then wean slowly while oral feedings are advanced [3].

  d. Consider adding hydrocortisone, 10 mg/kg per day intravenously in two divided doses, if the infant requires more than 12 mg of glucose per kilogram per minute to maintain an adequate serum level [2]. Hydrocortisone reduces peripheral glucose utilization, increases gluconeogenesis, and increases the effects of glucagon. The hydrocortisone will usually result in stable and adequate glucose levels, and it can then be rapidly tapered over the course of a few days. Before administering hydrocortisone, obtain a blood sample for measurements of insulin and cortisol levels. Cortisol levels can be used to screen for the integrity of the hypothalamic-pituitary-adrenal axis.

  e. Unless there is a suspicion of a metabolic defect, feedings can be started and advanced as the clinical situation allows. As the feedings are advanced and the intravenous glucose infusion is tapered, it is important to continue to monitor glucose levels.

  f. Glucagon 0.1 mg/kg intramuscularly (maximum 1.0 mg) may be given to hypoglycemic infants with good glycogen stores but it is only a temporizing measure to mobilize glucose for 2 to 3 hours [3,5] in an emergency until intravenous glucose can be given. The glucose level will often fall after the effects of glucagon have worn off, and it remains important to obtain intravenous access to adequately treat these babies. For infants of diabetic mothers, the dose is 0.3 mg/kg (maximum dose is 1.0 mg) (see Chap. 2, Diabetes Mellitus).

  g. Other. Epinephrine, diazoxide, and growth hormone are used rarely and only in treatment of persistent hypoglycemia. Surgical subtotal pancreatectomy may be necessary for insulin-secreting tumors.

  3. Most hypoglycemia will resolve in 2 to 3 days. A requirement of more than 8 mg of glucose per kilogram per minute suggests increased utilization due to hyperinsulinism. This is usually transient as in infants of diabetic mothers. If it lasts more than 7 days, endocrine evaluation may be necessary to rule out excess insulin secretion from an insulin-secreting tumor or other cause as listed in **I.C.** A sample drawn to determine insulin level at the same time as blood glucose will document an inappropriate secretion of insulin.

    If the insulin level is not inappropriate for the blood glucose level, other causes of persistent hypoglycemia such as defects in carbohydrate metabolism (see **I.C.3.c**), endocrine deficiency (see **I.C.3.d**), and defects in amino acid metabolism (see **I.C.3.e**) should be considered.

    Evaluation will often require letting the blood glucose level get low (20 mg/dl) and then drawing blood for insulin, cortisol, and amino acids. Many evaluations are not productive because they are done too early in the course of a transient hypoglycemic state or the samples to determine hormone levels are drawn when the glucose level is normal.

II. Hyperglycemia is usually defined as a whole-blood glucose level higher than 125 mg/dl [3] or plasma glucose values higher than 145 mg/dl. This problem is commonly encountered in low-birth-weight premature infants receiving parenteral glucose but is also seen in other infants who are sick. The major clinical problems associated with hyperglycemia are hyperosmolarity and osmotic diuresis. Hyperosmolarity (each 18 mg/dl rise in blood glucose concentration increases serum osmolality 1 mOsm/L) of more than 300 mOsm/L usually leads to osmotic diuresis. Subsequent dehydration may occur rapidly in small premature infants. The hyperosmolar state, an increase of 25 to 40 mOsm or a glucose level of more than 450 to 720 mg/dl, can cause water to move from the intracellular compartment to the extracellular compartment. The resultant contraction of the intracellular volume of the brain may be a cause of intracranial hemorrhage.

A. Etiology

1. **Exogenous parenteral glucose** administration of more than 6.0 mg of glucose per kilogram per minute in normal term infants or of more than 6.6 mg of glucose per kilogram per minute in preterm infants weighing less than 1100 gm may be associated with hyperglycemia [7].

2. **Drugs.** The most common association is with steroids used for treatment of bronchopulmonary dysplasia. Other drugs associated with hyperglycemia are caffeine, theophylline, phenytoin, and diazoxide [6,7].

3. **Very-low-birth-weight** (<1000 gm), possibly due to variable insulin response, to persistent endogenous hepatic glucose production despite significant elevations in plasma insulin, or to insulin resistance that may in part be due to immature glycogenolysis enzyme systems [9]. Very-low-birth-weight infants will often have fluid requirements exceeding 200 ml/kg per day, and when this fluid is administered as dextrose 10%, the infant will be presented with an excessive glucose load.

4. **Sepsis,** possibly due to depressed insulin release, cytokines, or endotoxin, resulting in decreased glucose utilization. Stress hormones such as cortisol and catecholamines are elevated in sepsis. In an infant who has normal glucose levels and then becomes hyperglycemic without an excess glucose load, sepsis should be the prime consideration.

5. **"Stressed"** premature infants requiring mechanical ventilation, from persistent endogenous glucose production due to catecholamines and other "stress hormones." Insulin levels are usually appropriate for the glucose level [6,7,9].

6. **Hypoxia,** possibly due to increased glucose production in the absence of a change in peripheral utilization

7. **Surgical procedures.** Hyperglycemia in this setting is possibly due to the secretion of epinephrine, glucocorticoids, and glucagon as well as excess administration of glucose-containing intravenous fluids [6,9].

8. **Transient neonatal diabetes mellitus** [6]. In this rare disorder, infants present with hyperglycemia usually before the age of 15 days (range 2 days to 6 weeks). They characteristically are SGA term infants, they have no sex predilection, and a third have a family history of diabetes mellitus. They present with marked glycosuria, hyperglycemia (240 to 2300 mg/dl), polyuria, severe dehydration, acidosis, mild or absent ketonuria, reduced subcutaneous fat, and failure to thrive. Insulin values are either absolutely or relatively low for the corresponding blood glucose elevation. Treatment consists of rehydration, and the majority require insulin (regular 0.5 to 3.0 units/kg per day subcutaneously divided q6h or 0.01 to 0.10 unit/kg per hour by constant infusion). Start with the intravenous dose, and then switch to the subcutaneous dose. Monitor serum electrolytes, glucose, and acid–base balance. Repeated plasma insulin values are necessary to distinguish transient from permanent diabetes mellitus. The average length for insulin treatment is 65 days (range, 3 days to 18 months). Fifty percent of the cases are transient. Some transient cases will have a later recurrence. Some cases are permanent. Cases presenting after 3 weeks and in infants with HLA-DR3+DR4 haplotypes have a higher incidence of permanent diabetes. The transient nature of this disorder may be due to delayed or abnormal maturation of the B cell, transiently deficient or delayed in-

sulin secretion, or secretion of an abnormal insulin molecule [3]. Treatment with subcutaneous ultralente insulin appeared to make management easier in a recently described case [8].

9. **Diabetes due to pancreatic lesions** such as pancreatic aplasia, hypoplastic or absent pancreatic beta cells is usually seen in small for gestational age infants who may have other congenital defects. They usually present soon after birth and rarely survive.

10. **Transient hyperglycemia associated with ingestion of hyperosmolar formula.** Clinical presentation may mimic transient neonatal diabetes with glycosuria, hyperglycemia, and dehydration. A history of inappropriate formula dilution is key. Treatment consists of rehydration, discontinuation of the hyperosmolar formula, and appropriate instructions for mixing concentrated or powder formula. Insulin has been used briefly but cautiously.

B. **Treatment.** The primary goal is prevention and early detection of hyperglycemia by frequent monitoring of blood glucose levels and urine for glycosuria. If present, evaluation and possible intervention are indicated.

1. Blood is drawn for whatever tests are indicated.

2. Very-low-birth-weight premature infants (<800 gm) should start with an intravenous glucose concentration no higher than 5%. If hyperglycemia is documented, parenteral glucose intake is reduced to 4.0 to 6.0 mg of glucose per kilogram per minute by reducing the concentration or the rate (or both) of glucose infusion and monitoring the falling blood glucose level. Hypotonic fluids (solutions < dextrose 5%) should be avoided or used with caution.

   Decrease the glucose infusion by 2 mg/kg per minute every 4 to 6 hours [9] (see Fig. 29-1).

3. Many small infants will initially be unable to tolerate a certain glucose load (e.g., 6 mg/kg per minute) but will eventually develop tolerance if they are presented with just enough glucose to keep their glucose level high yet not enough to cause glycosuria.

4. Exogenous insulin therapy has been used when glucose values exceed 250 mg/dl despite efforts to lower the amount of glucose delivered or when prolonged restriction of parenterally administered glucose has substantially decreased total caloric intake and the infant is failing to thrive. Neonates may be extremely sensitive to the effects of insulin. It is desirable to decrease the glucose level gradually to avoid rapid fluid shifts. Very small doses of insulin are used and the actual amount delivered may be difficult to determine because some of the insulin is adsorbed on the glass or plastic surfaces of the intravenous tubing [1].

   a. **Continuous insulin infusion** (regular insulin, 100 units/ml) 0.01 to 0.10 unit/kg per hour. The rate is adjusted based on hourly glucose reagent strip results. Monitor potassium level. The tubing is flushed with insulin solution to saturate binding sites. Monitor for rebound hyperglycemia [4].

   b. **Subcutaneous insulin,** 0.10 to 0.20 unit/kg every 6 hours (rarely used except in neonatal diabetes). Monitor glucose level at 1, 2, and 4 hours and potassium level every 6 hours initially [9].

References

1. Binder, N. D., et al. Insulin infusion with parenteral nutrition in extremely low birth weight infants with hyperglycemia. *J. Pediatr.* 114:273, 1989.
2. Cornblath, M., et al. Hypoglycemia in the neonate. *J. Pediatr. Endocrinol.* 6:113, 1993.
3. Cornblath, M., et al. *Disorders of Carbohydrate Metabolism in Infancy* (3d Ed.). Cambridge, MA: Blackwell Scientific, 1991.

4. Cowett, R. M. Hypoglycemia and Hyperglycemia in the Newborn. In R. A. Polin and W. W. Fox (Eds.), *Fetal and Neonatal Physiology.* Philadelphia: Saunders, 1992, p. 406.
5. Holtrop, P. C. The frequency of hypoglycemia in full-term large and small for gestational age newborns. *Am. J. Perinatol.* 10:150, 1993.
6. Kalkon, S. C. Metabolic and endocrine disorders. In A. A. Fanaroff and R. J. Martin, (Eds.), *Neonatal–Perinatal Medicine,* 6th ed. St. Louis: Mosby, 1997, p. 1439.
7. Koh, T. H. H. G., et al. Neural dysfunction during hypoglycemia. *Arch. Dis. Child.* 63:1353, 1988.
8. Mitamara, R., et al. Ultralente insulin treatment of transient neonatal diabetes mellitus. *J. Pediatr.* 128:268, 1996.
9. Pildes, R. S., et al. Hypoglycemia and hyperglycemia in tiny infants. *Clin. Perinatol.* 13:351, 1986.
10. Schwartz, R. Neonatal hypoglycemia—Back to basics in diagnosis and treatment. *Diabetes* 40:71, 1991.
11. Scriver, C. R., et al. *The Metabolic Basics of Inherited Disease.* New York: McGraw-Hill, 1995.

Hypocalcemia, Hypercalcemia, and Hypermagnesemia*
Kenneth M. Huttner

Calcium is physiologically important in two general ways. First, **calcium salts in bone** provide structural integrity. Decreased skeletal calcium is a hallmark of neonatal metabolic bone disease (see Metabolic Bone Disease of Prematurity). Second, **calcium ions (Ca²⁺) in cellular and extracellular fluid (ECF)** are essential for many biochemical processes. Significant aberrations of serum calcium concentrations are observed frequently in the neonatal period. One must evaluate these alterations in light of the normal dynamic changes in serum calcium level that take place during the first week of life. Consequently, a given serum calcium level cannot be interpreted without knowing the newborn's postnatal age.

I. **Principles of mineral metabolism**
   A. **Laboratory measurement of serum calcium**
      1. There are three definable fractions of calcium in serum: (a) **ionized calcium** (about 50% of serum total calcium); (b) **calcium bound to serum proteins,** principally albumin (about 40%); and (c) **calcium complexed to serum anions,** mostly phosphates, citrate, and sulfates (about 10%). **Ionized calcium is the only biologically available form of calcium.**
      2. For routine clinical purposes, measurement of serum total calcium level usually is adequate. Some clinical laboratories can measure the ionized calcium level in microspecimens of anticoagulated blood collected anaerobically. Algorithms for correcting serum total calcium level for alterations in serum albumin concentration and/or pH or for calculating "free" calcium concentrations are not reliable compared with actual measurements of ionized calcium.
      3. Calcium concentration reported as milligrams per deciliter can be converted to molar units by dividing by 4 (e.g., 10 mg/dl converts to 2.5 mmol/L).
   B. **Hormonal regulation of calcium homeostasis** (Fig. 29-2). Regulation of serum and ECF ionized calcium concentration within a narrow range is critical for blood coagulation, neuromuscular excitability, cell membrane integrity and function, and cellular enzymatic and secretory activity. The principal calcitropic or calcium-regulating hormones are **parathyroid hormone (PTH)** and **1,25-dihydroxyvitamin D (1,25(OH)₂D₃).**

*This section represents a modification of the work of Lewis Rubin, M.D., published in the third edition of *Manual of Neonatal Care.*

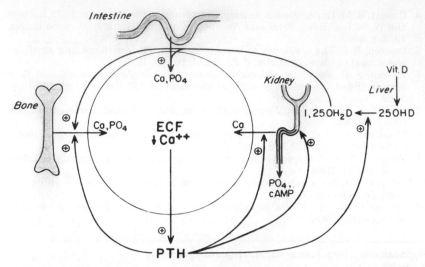

Fig. 29-2. Hormonal regulation of calcium and phosphate by PTH and 1,25(OH)$_2$D$_3$. Decreased Ca^{2+} stimulates PTH and 1,25 (OH)$_2$D secretion. Renal, gastrointestinal, and skeletal mechanisms will increase Ca^{2+}, inhibiting PTH secretion and closing the negative-feedback loop. (PTH = parathyroid hormone; 1,25(OH)$_2$D = 1,25-dihydroxyvitamin D; 25(OH)D = 25-hydroxyvitamin D; Ca^{2+} = ionized calcium; PO$_4$ = inorganic phosphate; ECF = extracellular fluid; cAMP = cyclic adenosine monophosphate.) (From E. M. Brown, *Contemp. Issues Nephrol.* 11:179, 1983.)

1. **PTH.** When ECF ionized calcium level declines, parathyroid cells secrete PTH. PTH mobilizes calcium from bone, increases calcium resorption in the renal tubule, and stimulates renal production of 1,25(OH)$_2$D$_3$. PTH also mobilizes phosphate from bone and produces significant phosphaturia. Therefore, **PTH secretion causes the serum calcium level to rise and the serum phosphorus level to be maintained or fall.** Newborns in the first 2 days of life may exhibit decreased renal responsiveness to PTH.

2. **1,25(OH)$_2$D$_3$ (calcitriol).** Inactive vitamin D is synthesized in skin exposed to sunlight and is also ingested in the diet. The liver then synthesizes **25(OH)D$_3$ (the major storage form of the hormone)** and the kidney synthesizes the **biologically active hormone, 1,25(OH)$_2$D$_3$.** 1,25(OH)$_2$D$_3$ increases intestinal calcium and phosphate absorption and mobilizes calcium and phosphate from bone.

3. **Calcitonin.** Calcitonin, secreted by thyroid C cells, **inhibits bone resorption and has an antihypercalcemic effect.** Its significance for calcium regulation in the human adult is controversial. Calcitonin may play a more important calcitropic role during fetal and/or neonatal development.

C. **Postnatal changes in serum calcium concentrations.** The flow of calcium ions from mother to fetus during the third trimester of gestation is associated with **fetal chronic hypercalcemia.** At birth, the umbilical serum calcium level is elevated (10 to 11 mg/dl). In healthy term babies, calcium concentrations decline for the first 24 to 48 hours; the nadir is usually 7.5 to 8.5 mg/dl. Thereafter, calcium concentrations progressively rise to the mean values observed in older children and adults. Serum calcium concentrations in the first 3 days of life are also positively correlated with gestational age.

II. **Hypocalcemia.** Neonatal **hypocalcemia** usually is defined as a total serum calcium concentration of less than 7.0 mg/dl and an ionized calcium concentration of less than 4.0 mg/dl.

A. **Etiology**

1. **Early-onset hypocalcemia (during the first 3 days)**

   a. **Preterm newborns** are born amid the third-trimester growth spurt. They are poorly adapted to the cessation of maternal calcium flow and at birth face a calcium crisis. About 50% of low-birth-weight infants and **nearly all** very-low-birth-weight (VLBW) infants exhibit total serum calcium levels of less than 7.0 mg/dl by day 2. This hypocalcemia appears to be an exaggeration of the normal term pattern; the nadir occurs by 12 to 24 hours, with little change until 72 hours. The pathogenesis is probably multifactorial. Preterm newborns do mount a PTH response, but target-organ responsiveness to PTH may be diminished. Even VLBW newborns can synthesize $1,25(OH)_2D_3$ if vitamin D stores are adequate. Hypercalcitoninemia may be important. High renal sodium excretion in preterm newborns may aggravate calciuric losses.

   b. **Infants of diabetic mothers (IDMs)** have a 25 to 50% incidence of hypocalcemia during the first 24 to 48 hours. The natural history may be similar to that of early neonatal hypocalcemia in preterm infants, or hypocalcemia may persist for several days. Hypercalcitoninemia, hypoparathyroidism, abnormal vitamin D metabolism, and hyperphosphatemia have been implicated, but none has been found consistently. The lower mean maternal and umbilical calcium and magnesium levels associated with diabetes may be important. The macrosomia associated with IDMs also may increase neonatal calcium demands, producing a more profound and prolonged hypocalcemia (see Chap. 2).

   c. **Birth asphyxia** is associated frequently with hypocalcemia and hyperphosphatemia, possibly related to renal insufficiency, acidosis, and/or impaired PTH secretion or responsiveness (see Chap. 27, Perinatal Asphyxia). Decreased calcium intake, increased endogenous phosphate load, and increased calcitonin concentrations may contribute.

2. **Late-onset hypocalcemia** usually presents at the end of the first week, but onset ranges from the first days to several weeks after birth. The classical syndrome was described in term infants fed **high-phosphate diets.** Contributing factors probably include neonatal immaturity of renal tubular phosphate excretion, hypoparathyroidism, hypomagnesemia, and vitamin D deficiency. Specific etiologies include the following:

   a. **Hypoparathyroidism (most common)**

      (1) **Idiopathic, transient**

      (2) **Congenital.** Parathyroids may be absent in **DiGeorge's sequence** (hypoplasia or absence of the third and fourth branchial pouch structures) as an isolated defect in the development of the parathyroid glands or as part of the Kenny-Coffey syndrome.

      (3) **Pseudohypoparathyroidism**

      (4) **Maternal hyperparathyroidism** induces transient neonatal hypoparathyroidism.

      (5) **Magnesium deficiency** (including inborn error of intestinal magnesium transport) impairs PTH secretion.

   b. **Vitamin D deficiency**

      (1) Secondary to **maternal vitamin D deficiency**

      (2) **Malabsorption**

      (3) Maternal anticonvulsant therapy during pregnancy increases catabolism of vitamin D.

      (4) Renal insufficiency may impair $1,25(OH)_2D_3$ production.

      (5) Nephrosis and **impaired enterohepatic circulation** accelerate losses of $25(OH)D_3$.

      (6) Hepatobiliary disease may decrease production of $25(OH)D_3$.

  c. Miscellaneous

      (1) Rapid or excessive skeletal mineral deposition **("hungry bones" syndrome)** may occur in small-for-gestational-age (SGA) infants or in infants with rickets or hypoparathyroidism who receive aggressive vitamin D therapy.

      (2) Hyperphosphatemia is associated with phosphate-rich diets, excessive phosphate administration, renal insufficiency, asphyxia, hypervitaminosis D, hypoparathyroidism, and rhabdomyolysis.

      (3) Hypoalbuminemia. Ionized calcium level is unchanged.

      (4) Alkalosis and **bicarbonate therapy**

      (5) Rapid infusion of **citrate-buffered blood** (exchange transfusion) chelates ionized calcium.

      (6) Lipid infusions may lower the ionized calcium level by enhancing calcium-albumin binding.

      (7) Furosemide produces marked hypercalciuria.

      (8) Shock or **sepsis**

      (9) Hypothyroidism infrequently is associated with hypocalcemia in patients with pseudohypoparathyroidism.

      (10) Rapid **albumin infusion** may lead to a transient increase in protein-bound and a decrease in ionized calcium.

      (11) Phototherapy may be associated with hypocalcemia by decreasing melatonin secretion and increasing bone uptake of calcium.

B. Evaluation

  1. Clinical manifestations

    a. Hypocalcemia increases cellular permeability to sodium ions and increases cell membrane excitability. The signs are usually nonspecific: apnea, seizures, jitteriness, increased extensor tone, clonus, hyperreflexia, and stridor (laryngospasm). Carpopedal spasm and Chvostek's sign are present less frequently.

    b. Early-onset hypocalcemia in preterm newborns is usually asymptomatic or clinically mild.

    c. Late-onset syndromes, in contrast, may present as hypocalcemic seizures.

  2. Laboratory evaluation

    a. Suggested schedule for monitoring calcium levels in infants at risk for developing hypocalcemia

      (1) Preterm infants (>1000 gm): at 24 and 48 hours of life

      (2) Preterm infants (<1000 gm): at 12, 24, and 48 hours

      (3) Sick or stressed infants: at 12, 24, and 48 hours, and then as indicated

      (4) Healthy preterm infants (>1500 gm) and healthy IDMs who begin milk feedings on the first day do not need to be monitored in the absence of signs or symptoms.

    b. An electrocardiographic $Q-T_c$ interval longer than 0.4 second (due to prolonged systole), when present, is a useful indicator of hypocalcemia and helpful in monitoring therapy.

$$Q-T_c = \text{corrected QT interval} = \frac{\text{measured QT (seconds)}}{\sqrt{R-R \text{ interval (secs)}}}$$

c. For other than straightforward early-onset hypocalcemia, measure calcium, ionized calcium, phosphorus, and magnesium levels. Assessment of albumin, urinary calcium, PTH, vitamin D_3 metabolite levels and renal function also may be helpful.

   (1) **Elevated serum phosphorus level** suggests phosphate loading, renal insufficiency, or hypoparathyroidism.

   (2) Magnesium level of 0.8 mg/dl or less strongly suggests **primary hypomagnesemia.**

   (3) Normal to moderately elevated $1,25(OH)_2D_3$ levels are consistent with hypoparathyroidism.

   (4) Absence of a thymic shadow on a chest radiograph may suggest DiGeorge's sequence.

   (5) Urinary calcium excretion of more than 4 mg/kg per day or a 24-hour urine calcium/creatinine ratio of more than 0.2 (mg/mg) is indicative of hypercalciuria in individuals with mature renal function. Hypercalciuria associated with hypocalcemia suggests a **deficiency of PTH.** In the premature infant, especially one receiving large amounts of supplemental calcium, these values may not be applicable.

C. **Management**

   1. **Treatment of hypocalcemia is associated with certain risks,** which are minimized by attention to details.

      a. Rapid intravenous infusion of calcium can cause sudden elevation of serum calcium level, leading to bradycardia or other dysrhythmias. Intravenous calcium should only be "pushed" for treatment of hypocalcemic crisis (e.g., with seizures).

      b. Infusion by means of the umbilical vein may result in hepatic necrosis if the catheter is lodged in a branch of the portal vein.

      c. Rapid infusion by means of the umbilical artery can cause arterial spasms and, at least experimentally, intestinal necrosis.

      d. Intravenous calcium solutions are incompatible with sodium bicarbonate, since calcium carbonate will precipitate.

      e. Intravenous infusion of calcium chloride may produce chloride loading and hyperchloremic acidosis in neonates.

      f. **Extravasation of calcium** solutions into subcutaneous tissues can cause severe necrosis and subcutaneous calcifications.

         (1) Scrupulous attention to the peripheral intravenous site is indicated when calcium-containing solutions are infused.

         (2) Extravasations have been treated successfully with **hyaluronidase** injection. Subcutaneous injection around the periphery of the extravasation is reported most commonly, although injection through the peripheral intravenous line has theoretical advantages in that it would deliver the hyaluronidase to the same tissue plane as the calcium.

         (3) The dose of hyaluronidase for injection is reported as 15 units (in 1 ml of normal saline solution) up to 300 units (in 2 ml). Treatment of extravasation within the first hour is preferable.

   2. **Calcium preparations.** We prefer calcium gluconate 10% solution for intravenous (and occasionally oral) use (Table 29-1). Calcium glubionate syrup (Neo-Calglucon) is a convenient oral preparation. However,

Table 29-1. Common calcium preparations

Preparation	Elemental calcium content (mg/ml)
Calcium gluconate (10% injection)	9.0
Calcium chloride (10% injection)	27.2
Calcium glubionate syrup	23.6

the high sugar content and osmolality may cause gastrointestinal irritation or diarrhea.

3. **Treatment of early-onset hypocalcemia**

   a. Hypocalcemic preterm infants who have no symptoms and are not ill from any other cause do not require specific treatment. The hypocalcemia should resolve spontaneously by day 3.

   b. If the serum calcium level drops to 6.5 mg/dl or less (usually VLBW newborns), we recommend beginning a continuous calcium infusion with the goal of producing a sustained serum calcium level (7 to 8 mg/dl). A convenient starting dose is 45 mg/kg per day (5 ml/kg per day of calcium gluconate 10%). Bolus infusions are ineffective and hazardous. Prophylaxis or treatment with pharmacologic doses of vitamin D is **not recommended**.

   c. It may be desirable to prevent the onset of hypocalcemia for newborns who exhibit cardiovascular compromise (e.g., severe respiratory distress syndrome, asphyxia, septic shock, persistent pulmonary hypertension of the newborn) and require cardiotonic drugs or blood pressure support. Use a continuous calcium infusion, preferably by means of a central catheter, to maintain a total calcium level higher than 7.0 mg/dl and an ionized calcium level higher than 4.0 mg/dl.

4. **Treatment of hypocalcemic crisis with seizures, apnea, or tetany.** Serum calcium level is usually less than 5.0 mg/dl.

   a. **Emergency calcium therapy** consists of 1 to 2 ml of calcium gluconate 10% per kilogram (9 to 18 mg of elemental calcium per kilogram) by intravenous infusion over 5 minutes.

      (1) Monitor heart rate and the infusion site.

      (2) Repeat the dose in 10 minutes if there is no clinical response.

      (3) Following the initial dose(s), maintenance calcium should be given parenterally or orally (see **II.C.3.b**).

   b. Symptomatic hypocalcemia unresponsive to calcium therapy may be due to **hypomagnesemia**.

      (1) The preferred preparation for treatment is magnesium sulfate. The 50% solution contains 500 mg, or 4 mEq/ml.

      (2) Correct severe hypomagnesemia (<1.2 mg/dl) with 0.1 to 0.2 ml of magnesium sulfate 50% per kilogram intravenously or intramuscularly. When administering intravenously, infuse slowly and monitor heart rate; intramuscular administration may cause local tissue necrosis. The dose may be repeated every 6 to 12 hours. Obtain serum magnesium levels before each dose.

      (3) Maintenance magnesium therapy consists of oral administration of magnesium sulfate 50% 100 mg, or 0.2 ml/kg per day. If there is significant malabsorption, the dose may be increased twofold to fivefold.

5. Treatment of specific hypocalcemic syndromes

   a. **Hypocalcemia associated with hyperphosphatemia**

      (1) **Classic late-onset neonatal hypocalcemia** is frequently preventable by ensuring adequacy of maternal vitamin D stores during pregnancy and avoiding high-phosphate diets in infants.

      (2) The goal of therapy is to **reduce renal phosphate load.** Reduce phosphate intake by feeding the infant human milk or a low-phosphorus formula (Similac PM 60/40 or SMA). Mineral contents of some infant diets are shown in Table 29-2.

      (3) Increase the calcium-phosphate ratio of the milk to 4:1 with oral calcium supplements (e.g., 0.5 ml of Neo-Calglucon per 30 ml of PM 60/40). This will inhibit intestinal absorption of phosphorus. Phosphate binders are generally not necessary.

Table 29-2. Mineral contents of common infant diets

Type of milk	Approximate mineral content	
	Calcium (mg/L)	Phosphorus (mg/L)
Human milk	280	140
Similac PM 60/40	380	190
SMA	425	290
Similac	510	390
Enfamil	470	320
Isomil	710	510
ProSobee	635	500
Human milk/HMF 24 cal*	1180	590
Similac Special Care 24	1460	730
Enfamil Premature 24	1340	670

*Human milk with fortifier to 24 kcal/oz.

    (4) Gradually wean calcium supplements over 2 to 4 weeks. Monitor serum calcium and phosphorus levels one to two times weekly.

  b. Hypoparathyroid infants are hyperphosphatemic. Use a low-phosphate diet with calcium supplementation (see **II.C.5.a.(1)–(4)**) and correct vitamin D deficiency if present.

  c. Vitamin D disorders

    (1) Vitamin D deficiency in neonates is usually treatable with initial doses up to 5000 units per day of oral vitamin D_2 (Drisdol, 8000 units/ml), although occasionally higher doses may be required. Wean slowly as the deficiency resolves. Frequent assay of serum calcium level is necessary to avoid rebound hypervitaminosis D.

    (2) Defects in vitamin D metabolism are treated with vitamin D analogues, for example, dihydrotachysterol (Hytakerol) and calcitriol (Rocaltrol). The shorter initiation of action and short half-life of these drugs lessen the risk of rebound hypercalcemia.

III. Hypercalcemia. Neonatal hypercalcemia (serum total calcium level >11.0 mg/dl, serum ionized calcium level >5.0 mg/dl) may be asymptomatic and discovered incidentally during routine screening. Alternatively, the presentation of severe hypercalcemia (>14.0 mg/dl) can be dramatic and life-threatening, requiring immediate medical intervention.

  A. Etiology. The physiologic mechanisms that prevent hypercalcemia are inhibition of PTH and $1,25(OH)_2D_3$ synthesis, which **reduces calcium mobilization from bone, absorption from intestine, and reclamation from kidney.** (The potential pathophysiologic role for calcitonin is unclear.) Elevated serum calcium concentration, therefore, implies inappropriately increased calcium efflux from one of these pools into the ECF.

    1. Increased bone resorption

      a. Hyperparathyroidism

        (1) Congenital hyperparathyroidism associated with maternal hypoparathyroidism usually resolves over several weeks. Decreased availability of maternal calcium for the fetus stimulates the fetal parathyroids.

        (2) Neonatal severe primary hyperparathyroidism (NSPHP). The parathyroids are refractory to regulation by calcium, producing marked hypercalcemia (frequently 15 to 30 mg/dl) and lack of response to subtotal parathyroidectomy. Milder forms of the disorder probably occur also. NSPHP occurs frequently in **familial hypocalciuric hypercalcemia** kindreds (see **III.A.3.b**) as the consequence of homozygosity for a gene encoding a mutated calcium sensor.

b. **Hyperthyroidism.** Thyroid hormone stimulates bone resorption and bone turnover.

c. **Hypervitaminosis A** accelerates bone resorption.

d. **Phosphate depletion** can cause hypercalcemia in preterm infants fed phosphate-poor diets, usually human milk, or undergoing parenteral nutrition. Low phosphate intake stimulates $1,25(OH)_2D_3$ production, which mobilizes phosphate and calcium from bone into the ECF.

e. **Hypophosphatasia,** an autosomal recessive bone dysplasia, produces severe bone demineralization and fractures.

2. **Increased intestinal absorption of calcium**

a. **Hypervitaminosis D** may result from excessive vitamin D ingestion by the mother (during pregnancy) or the neonate. Since vitamin D is extensively stored in fat, intoxication may persist for weeks to months (see Chap. 10 for nutritional requirements for vitamin D).

b. Variation in vitamin D content of **human milk fortifier** may lead to excessive vitamin D intake in premature infants fed breast milk supplemented to 24 kcal/oz.

3. **Decreased renal calcium clearance**

a. **Thiazide diuretics** can induce or exacerbate hypercalcemia, largely by hypocalciuric effects.

b. **Familial hypocalciuric hypercalcemia,** a clinically benign autosomal dominant disorder, can present in the neonatal period. The gene mutation is on chromosome 3q21-24. Mutations in the calcium sensor lead to a dual defect in parathyroid cells (causing parathyroid hyperplasia) and renal tubules (causing hypocalciuria).

4. **Uncertain mechanisms**

a. **Idiopathic neonatal/infantile hypercalcemia** occurs in the constellation of **Williams syndrome** (hypercalcemia, supravalvular aortic stenosis or other cardiac anomalies, "elfin" facies, psychomotor retardation) and in a familial pattern lacking the Williams phenotype. Increased calcium absorption has been demonstrated; increased vitamin D sensitivity and impaired calcitonin secretion are proposed, but controversial mechanisms (see Chap. 25).

b. **Subcutaneous fat necrosis** is a sequela of trauma or asphyxia. Only the more generalized necrosis seen in asphyxia is associated with significant hypercalcemia. Granulomatous (macrophage) inflammation of the necrotic lesions may be a source of unregulated $1,25(OH)_2D_3$ synthesis. The accompanying hypercalcemia may present several weeks postnatally.

c. **Acute renal failure,** usually during the diuretic or recovery phase

d. **Acute adrenal insufficiency**

e. **Blue diaper syndrome,** causes excretion of water-insoluble blue tryptophan metabolites (indacanuria). The pathogenesis of the hypercalcemia is uncertain.

B. **Evaluation**

1. The **clinical manifestations** of severe hypercalcemia (usually hyperparathyroidism) include hypotonia, encephalopathy (lethargy or irritability, occasionally seizures), hypertension, respiratory distress (due to hypotonia and demineralization and deformation of the rib cage), poor feeding, vomiting, constipation, polyuria, hepatosplenomegaly, anemia, and extraskeletal calcifications, including nephrocalcinosis. Mortality is high for untreated infants. Milder hypercalcemia may present as feeding difficulties or poor linear growth.

2. **History**
   a. Maternal history of hypercalcemia or hypocalcemia, parathyroid disorders, nephrocalcinosis, and unexplained fetal losses
   b. Maternal dietary and drug history (e.g., excessive vitamin A or D, thiazides)
   c. Family history of hypercalcemia or familial hypocalciuric hypercalcemia
   d. Medications (e.g., vitamin A or D, thiazides, antacids)
   e. Low-phosphate diet in preterm infants or excessive dietary calcium
3. **Physical examination**
   a. Small for dates (hyperparathyroidism, Williams syndrome)
   b. Craniotabes, fractures (hyperparathyroidism), or characteristic bone dysplasia (hypophosphatasia)
   c. "Elfin" facies (Williams syndrome)
   d. Cardiac murmur (supravalvular aortic stenosis and peripheral pulmonic stenosis associated with Williams syndrome)
   e. Indurated, bluish-red lesions (subcutaneous fat necrosis)
   f. Evidence of hyperthyroidism
   g. Blue discoloration of diaper
4. **Laboratory evaluation**
   a. The clinical history and **serum and urine mineral levels** (e.g., calcium, ionized calcium [if available], phosphorus, and urinary calcium/creatinine ratio [U_{Ca}/U_{Cr}]) should suggest a likely diagnosis.
      (1) Very elevated serum calcium level (>15 mg/dl) usually indicates primary hyperparathyroidism or in VLBW infants, phosphate depletion.
      (2) Low phosphorus level indicates phosphate depletion, hyperparathyroidism, or familial hypocalciuric hypercalcemia.
      (3) Very low U_{Ca}/U_{Cr} suggests familial hypocalciuric hypercalcemia.
   b. Specific **serum hormone levels** (immunoreactive PTH, 25(OH)D, 1,25(OH)$_2$D) will confirm the diagnostic impression.
   c. **Serum alkaline phosphatase level** increases with increased bone resorption. Very low activity suggests hypophosphatasia (confirmed by increased urinary phosphoethanolamine level).
   d. **Radiographs** of hand/wrist may suggest hyperparathyroidism (demineralization, subperiosteal resorption) or hypervitaminosis D (submetaphyseal rarefaction).
C. **Treatment**
1. **Emergency medical treatment** (symptomatic or calcium >14 mg/dl)
   a. **Volume expansion with isotonic saline solution.** Hydration and sodium promote urinary calcium excretion. If cardiac function is normal, infuse normal saline solution (10 to 20 ml/kg) over 15 to 30 minutes (monitoring blood glucose level), then about one to three times "maintenance" fluids using, for example, dextrose 5% in water (5% D/W) with 40 to 60 mEq/L sodium chloride and 20 mEq/L potassium chloride.
   b. **Furosemide** (1 mg/kg q6–8h intravenously) induces calciuria. Since potassium and magnesium may become depleted, monitor and supplement as necessary.
   c. **Inorganic phosphate** may lower serum calcium levels in **hypophosphatemic patients** by inhibiting bone resorption and promoting bone mineral accretion. Parenteral phosphate should be avoided in severely hypercalcemic patients (serum total calcium level >12 mg/dl) unless hypophosphatemia is severe (<1.5 mg/dl). **Extraskeletal calcification** may occur. Oral phosphate (e.g., Neutra-phos, 200 mg of phosphate per milliliter) is preferred. Initial dosage (orally, or in parenteral nutrition) is 3.0 to 5.0 mg/dl.
   d. **Glucocorticoids** are effective in hypervitaminosis A and D and subcutaneous fat necrosis by inhibiting both bone resorption and in-

testinal calcium absorption; they are ineffective in hyperparathyroidism. Administer cortisone, 10 mg/kg per day, or methylprednisolone, 2 mg/kg per day.

2. **Other therapies**
   a. **Low-calcium, low-vitamin D diets** are an effective adjunctive therapy for hypervitaminosis A or D, subcutaneous fat necrosis, and Williams syndrome. Prolonged use may induce rickets.
   b. **Calcitonin** is a potent inhibitor of bone resorption. The antihypercalcemic effect is transient but may be prolonged if glucocorticoids are used concomitantly. There is little reported experience in neonates.
   c. **Parathyroidectomy with autologous reimplantation** may be indicated for severe persistent neonatal hyperparathyroidism.

IV. **Hypermagnesemia**
   A. **Etiology.** Usually an exogenous magnesium load exceeding renal excretion capacity produces hypermagnesemia.
      1. Magnesium sulfate therapy for maternal preeclampsia or preterm labor
      2. Administration of magnesium-containing antacids to the newborn
      3. Excessive magnesium in parenteral nutrition
      4. Magnesium sulfate enemas (contraindicated in newborns)
      5. Saline enemas or glycerin suppositories may be used to initiate bowel movements.
   B. **Diagnosis**
      1. Elevated serum magnesium level (normal newborn range, 1.6 to 2.8 mg/dl)
      2. Hypermagnesemic signs are unusual in term infants if the serum magnesium level is less than 6.0 mg/dl. The common curariform effects include apnea, respiratory depression, lethargy, hypotonia, hyporeflexia, poor suck, decreased intestinal motility, and delayed passage of meconium.
      3. Administration of **aminoglycosides** to a hypermagnesemic infant can lead to an additive inhibition of cholinergic function and an **increased risk of respiratory compromise.** An alternative antibiotic should be considered in this setting (see Chap. 23).
   C. **Treatment**
      1. Often the only intervention necessary is removal of the source of exogenous magnesium.
      2. When hypermagnesemic symptoms are severe, an intravenous calcium infusion may reverse them. (Calcium acts as a magnesium antagonist.)
      3. Exchange transfusion, peritoneal dialysis, and hemodialysis are usually not necessary.
      4. Begin feedings only after suck and intestinal motility are established.
      5. Saline enemas or glycerin suppositories may be used to initiate bowel movements.

References

De Marini, S., et al. Disorders of calcium, phosphorus, and magnesium metabolism. In A. A. Fanaroff and R. J. Mouton (Eds.). *Neonatal–Perinatal Medicine,* 6th ed. St. Louis: Mosby, 1997.

Tsang, R. C. Calcium, phosphorus, and magnesium metabolism. In R. A. Polin and W. W. Fox (Eds.), *Fetal and Neonatal Physiology.* Philadelphia: Saunders, 1992.

Metabolic Bone Disease of Prematurity*
Kenneth M. Huttner

Metabolic bone disease occurs in more than 30% of infants weighing 1500 gm or less at birth and 50% of those weighing less than 1000 gm. **Osteopenia** ("washed out" or undermineralized bones) develops during the first postnatal weeks. Signs of

*This section represents a modification of the work of Lewis Rubin, M.D., published in the third edition of *Manual of Neonatal Care.*

rickets (epiphyseal dysplasia and skeletal deformities) usually become evident in 2 to 4 months or by term-corrected gestational age. The risk of bone disease is greatest for the sickest, most premature infants [2].

I. **Etiology**
  A. **Deficiency of calcium and phosphorus is the principal cause.** Demands for rapid growth in the third trimester are met by intrauterine mineral accretion rates of 120 to 150 mg of calcium and 60 to 120 mg of phosphorus per kilogram per day [3]. Poor mineral intake and absorption after birth result in undermineralized new and remodeled bone [1].
    1. **Diets** low in mineral content predispose preterm newborns to metabolic bone disease.
      a. Unsupplemented human milk
      b. Parenteral nutrition
      c. Formulas not designed for use in preterm infants (e.g., soy-based)
    2. **Furosemide** therapy causes renal calcium wasting.
    3. **Renal phosphorus wasting**
      a. Acquired tubular acidosis
      b. The Fanconi syndromes
      c. X-linked hypophosphatemic rickets may present in late infancy.
      d. Tumor osteomalacia. Many mesenchymal tumors, including **sclerosing hemangiomas**, produce humoral phosphaturic factors.
  B. **Vitamin D deficiency.** Human milk has a total antirachitic sterol content of only 25 to 50 IU/L, insufficient for maintaining normal 25-hydroxyvitamin D ($25(OH)D_3$) levels in preterm infants (400 to 1000 IU per day required). However, when vitamin D intake is adequate, even very-low-birth-weight newborns can synthesize 1,25-dihydroxyvitamin D ($1,25(OH)_2D_3$).
    1. **Maternal vitamin D deficiency** can cause **congenital rickets.**
    2. Inadequate vitamin D intake or absorption produces **nutritional rickets.**
    3. **Hepatobiliary rickets** results largely from vitamin D malabsorption.
    4. **Chronic renal failure** (renal osteodystrophy)
    5. Chronic use of phenytoin or phenobarbital increases 25(OH)D metabolism.
    6. Hereditary pseudo–vitamin D deficiency: type I (abnormality or absence of 1-alpha-hydroxylase activity) or type II (tissue resistance to $1,25(OH)_2D_3$).
II. **Diagnosis**
  A. **Clinical signs** include respiratory insufficiency or failure to wean from a ventilator, hypotonia, pain on handling due to pathologic fractures, decreased linear growth with sustained head growth, frontal bossing, enlarged anterior fontanel and widened cranial sutures, craniotabes (posterior flattening of the skull), "rachitic rosary" (swelling of costochondral junctions), Harrison's grooves (indentation of the ribs at the diaphragmatic insertions), and enlargement of wrists, knees, and ankles.
  B. **Radiographic signs** include widening of epiphyseal growth plates; cupping, fraying, and rarefaction of the metaphyses; subperiosteal new-bone formation; osteopenia, particularly of the skull, spine, scapula, and ribs; and occasionally osteoporosis or pathologic fractures.
  C. **Laboratory evaluation**
    1. **Serum calcium level** (low, normal, or slightly elevated) **and phosphorus level** (low to normal) generally are **not** good indicators of the presence or severity of metabolic bone disease.
    2. **Serum alkaline phosphatase level** (an indicator of osteoclast activity) often is correlated with disease severity (>1000 U/L in severe rickets). Note the following:
      a. **Normal neonatal range** may be up to four times the adult upper limit.
      b. Hepatobiliary disease also elevates alkaline phosphatase level.
      c. Solitary elevated alkaline phosphatase level rarely occurs in the absence of bone or liver disease (transient hyperphosphatasemia of infancy).

3. **25(OH)D$_3$ levels** are usually low to normal. Measures of 25(OH)D$_3$ are useful for establishing the sufficiency of vitamin D stores; levels are less than 6 ng/ml in severe vitamin D deficiency.

4. **Radiographs.** A loss of up to 40% of bone mineralization can occur without radiographic changes [1]. Chest films may show osteopenia and sometimes rachitic changes. Wrist or knee films and a skeletal series (pathologic fractures) can be useful.

5. Measurement of **bone mineral content** by photon densitometry remains investigational.

6. Reserve measurement of 1,25(OH)$_2$D$_3$ or PTH for complicated or refractory cases.

III. **Prevention and treatment**

A. **Dietary management** (see Chap. 10)

1. **Mineral-fortified human milk or "premature" formulas** are the appropriate diets for preterm infants; their use can prevent and treat metabolic bone disease of prematurity (see Table 29-2). Attempts at reproducing intrauterine mineral accretion rates may be unnecessary and potentially result in complications.

2. Use of other diets and specific supplementation with calcium gluconate or glubionate (see Table 29-1, to a total of 200 mg of elemental calcium per kilogram per day) and/or potassium phosphate (93 mg phosphate per milliliter, to a total of 100 mg/kg per day) is less desirable because of concern over medication error. The addition of both calcium and phosphorus supplements directly to standard formulas should be avoided, as it will lead to the formation of a precipitate.

B. **Ensure adequate vitamin D stores** by an intake of 150 to 400 IU per day (see Chap. 10).

1. **Vitamin D deficiency rickets** is usually treatable with initial doses of up to 5000 IU of vitamin D per day. Oral calcium supplements may be necessary during therapy, since serum calcium levels may drop precipitously as bone rapidly mineralizes.

2. Defects in vitamin D metabolism may respond better to dihydrotachysterol (DHT) or calcitriol (see Hypocalcemia, Hypercalcemia, and Hypermagnesemia).

C. Furosemide-induced renal calcium wasting can be lessened by adding a thiazide diuretic.

D. Avoid nonessential handling and vigorous chest physiotherapy in preterm infants with severely undermineralized bones.

E. Infants receiving mineral-modified human milk as "premature" formulas or extra vitamin D should have periodic monitoring of calcium, PO$_4$, and alkaline phosphatase levels to prevent hypercalcemia. (See Chap. 10, Nutrition.)

References

1. Koo, W. W. K., et al. Calcium, Magnesium, Phosphorus, and Vitamin D. In R. C. Tsang et al. (Eds.), *Nutritional Needs of the Preterm Infant: Scientific Basis and Practical Guidelines.* Baltimore: Williams & Wilkins, 1993. P. 135.

2. Tsang, R. C. Calcium, Phosphorus and Magnesium Metabolism. Section XXV. In R. A. Polin and W. W. Fox (Eds.), *Fetal and Neonatal Physiology.* Philadelphia: Saunders, 1995.

3. Ziegler, E. E., et al. Body composition of the reference fetus. *Growth* 40:329, 1976.

Inborn Errors of Metabolism

Gary A. Silverman, John P. Cloherty, Harvey L. Levy, and Mark S. Korson

I. **Clinical indications.** The following clinical situations may prompt one to consider an inborn error of metabolism. Reviews of this subject are found in references 9, 13, 16, 23, and 28. The primary reference for this subject is reference 31.

A. **A history of unexplained neonatal deaths** or any family history of deaths in infancy, mental retardation, developmental disability, or intolerance to certain foods should alert one to the possibility of metabolic disease. Since most inborn errors of metabolism are inherited in an autosomal recessive manner, there is often no family history. Symptoms are usually caused by accumulation of a substrate proximal to a metabolic block, deficiency of a product of the blocked metabolic pathway, or both. The symptoms may be mild or severe depending on the defect, the severity of the mutation in a specific patient, and environmental factors that may destabilize a patient, such as diet or infections.

B. **Neonatal signs and symptoms** of weight loss, poor feeding, vomiting, dehydration, diarrhea, lethargy, hypotonia, hypertonia, coma, seizures, hiccoughs, rapid respirations, apnea, jaundice, hepatomegaly, cardiomyopathy, unusual urine color, unusual odor of sweat or urine, coarse facial features, and abnormalities of the skin, hair, eyes, joints, or bones. **Acute symptoms** may be indistinguishable from those of sepsis, cardiorespiratory failure, or central nervous system (CNS) disease. **Chronic symptoms** are failure to thrive, neurologic deficits or degeneration, and developmental delay.

C. Onset of the preceding signs and symptoms after an interval of good health, especially in a full-term baby who has no risk factors, or onset of symptoms after a change in diet. Less commonly, an infant may show signs from birth, e.g., hepatomegaly and hypotonia in Zellweger syndrome.

D. Persistence or progression of these signs and symptoms with no evidence of infection, CNS hemorrhage, or other congenital or acquired defects

E. Lack of relief of signs and symptoms with the usual therapy for such conditions as sepsis and respiratory distress syndrome

F. Primary metabolic acidosis with increased anion gap, primary respiratory alkalosis, hyperammonemia, hypoglycemia, lactic acidosis, ketonuria, non–glucose-reducing substances in the urine, abnormal results of liver function tests [serum glutamic-oxaloacetic transaminase (SGOT), serum glutamic-pyruvic transaminase (SGPT), prothrombin time (PT), and partial thromboplastin time (PTT)], and hyperbilirubinemia (conjugated or unconjugated).

G. Other causes of these symptoms such as sepsis, CNS bleeding, or blood loss should be considered. Ultrasound or CT of the head may show brain edema in metabolic disease (e.g., with prolonged hyperammonemia). An EEG may be abnormal but not show a specific pattern. Some patterns such as burst-suppression, which often suggest a poor prognosis after asphyxia, may be reversible in metabolic disease. A seizure pattern is frequently multifocal.

II. **Clinical problems associated with metabolic disease in the newborn**
  A. **Feeding difficulties or vomiting** is associated with many metabolic diseases (nonspecifically) but is prominent with the following:
    1. **Protein intolerance,** such as the organic acidemias or defects in the urea cycle.
    2. **Carbohydrate intolerance,** such as galactosemia (lactose) or, rarely, hereditary fructose intolerance (fructose, sucrose).
    3. The **adrenogenital syndrome** (see Chap. 30)
  B. **Hepatomegaly** is prominent in the following conditions:
    1. **Disorders of carbohydrate metabolism,** such as galactosemia, hereditary fructose intolerance, or glycogen storage diseases
    2. **Disorders of amino acid metabolism,** such as
      a. Tyrosinemia, type I
      b. Alpha-1-antitrypsin deficiency
      c. Organic acidemias in association with acidosis, with or without hyperammonemia
      d. Urea cycle disorders in association with hyperammonemia

    3. Lysosomal disorders such as Wolman disease and, on occasion, mucolipidosis type II and GM_1 gangliosidosis.

    4. Peroxisomal disorders such as Zellweger syndrome and neonatal adrenoleukodystrophy

    5. Disorders of carnitine metabolism and fatty acid oxidation, e.g., carnitine palmitoyl transferase (CPT) deficiency

    6. Mitochondrial disorders, e.g., defects in the respiratory chain

C. Dysmorphic facial features are often seen in the following conditions:

    1. Peroxisomal disorders (Zellweger syndrome, neonatal adrenoleukodystrophy, rhizomelic chondrodysplasia punctata)

    2. Pyruvate dehydrogenase complex deficiency (see **J.7.b**)

    3. Glutaric acidemia, type II (multiple acyl-CoA dehydrogenase deficiency)

    4. Carnitine palmitoyltransferase II deficiency

    5. Lysosomal storage diseases (e.g., mucolipidosis II, I cell disease)

D. Seizures may be seen in the following disorders with or without hypoglycemia, hypocalcemia, or acidosis. Any infant with seizures should be investigated for hypoglycemia, hypocalcemia, and hypomagnesemia as well as the other causes of seizures (see Chap. 27, Neonatal Seizures).

    1. Disorders of carbohydrate metabolism, such as

      a. Glycogen storage disease, type I

      b. Galactosemia

      c. Hereditary fructose intolerance (not seen until an infant is several months old)

    2. Disorders of amino acid metabolism, such as

      a. Organic acidemias such as maple syrup urine disease, propionic acidemia, methylmalonic acidemia, isovaleric acidemia

      b. Nonketotic hyperglycinemia

      c. Urea cycle disorders

    3. Pyridoxine dependency (see Chap. 27)

    4. Molybdenum cofactor deficiency

    5. Disorders of peroxisomes, such as

      a. Zellweger syndrome

      b. Neonatal adrenoleukodystrophy

    6. Vitamin D–resistant rickets (see Chap. 29)

      a. Hypocalcemic seizures, after 1 week of age

    7. Mitochondrial disorders (glutaric acidemia, type II)

E. Neurologic features: encephalopathy with altered (fluctuating hypotonia and hypertonia) tone and reflexes (with or without seizures)

    1. Nonketotic hyperglycemia

    2. Hypophosphatasia

    3. Organic acid disorders

    4. Urea cycle defects

    5. Peroxisomal disorders such as Zellweger cerebrohepatorenal syndrome and neonatal adrenoleukodystrophy (see Chap. 27, Neonatal Seizures).

    6. Mitochondrial disorders (glutaric acidemia, type II)

F. Neonatal cardiomyopathy and failure may be seen in the mitochondrial disorders associated with lactic acidosis, glycogen storage disease type IX, systemic carnitine deficiency, glutaric acidemia type II, and galactosemia.

G. Jaundice (see Chap. 18)

    1. Elevated indirect bilirubin

      a. Inborn errors of red blood cell metabolism, such as pyruvate-kinase deficiency or glucose-6-phosphate dehydrogenase (G-6-PD) deficiency.

      b. Galactosemia (early)

      c. Crigler-Najjar syndrome

      d. Gilbert syndrome

      e. Hypothyroidism

  f. Tyrosinemia, type I (early)
 2. Elevated direct bilirubin
  a. Rotor syndrome
  b. Dubin-Johnson syndrome
  c. Galactosemia (late)
  d. Hereditary fructose intolerance (after a few months of age)
  e. Alpha-1-antitrypsin deficiency
  f. Tyrosinemia, type I, like galactosemia; early presentation is often associated with indirect hyperbilirubinemia, later presentation with direct hyperbilirubinemia.
H. Hepatic dysfunction as manifested by jaundice, hepatomegaly, coagulopathy, hepatocellular dysfunction, elevated liver enzymes, hypoglycemia, or hyperammonemia
 1. Galactosemia
 2. Tyrosinemia, type I
 3. Niemann-Pick disease, type C
 4. Glycogen storage disease, type I and type IV (liver disease late)
 5. Neonatal hemochromatosis [11]
 6. Disorders of bile acid acid synthesis (e.g., 3-oxosteroid-5B-reductase deficiency)
 7. Organic acidemias, urea cycle disorders, and fatty acid B-oxidation defects during acute metabolic crisis are often associated with abnormal liver function test results.
 8. Mitochondrial disease (e.g., cytochrome c oxidase deficiency)
I. Hypoglycemia
 1. Galactosemia
 2. Hereditary fructose intolerance
 3. Glycogen storage disease (e.g., type I)
 4. Hyperglycerolemia
 5. Organic acidemias
 6. Tyrosinemia, type I
 7. Systemic carnitine deficiency
 8. Glutaric acidemia, type II
 9. Any illness with significant liver dysfunction
J. Metabolic acidosis with increased anion gap
 1. Organic acidemias
  a. Multiple carboxylase deficiency (early onset)
   (1) Metabolic acidosis
   (2) Lactic acidosis without ketosis
   (3) Patients often die shortly after birth; responsive to biotin supplementation
  b. Late-onset biotinidase deficiency (also known as multiple carboxylase); rarely occurs in newborn period, usually after several months of life.
   (1) Metabolic acidosis without ketosis
   (2) Biotinidase assay: deficiency is screened for in newborn screening programs in some states
   (3) treated with biotin
 2. Fatty acid oxidation disorder
 3. Glycogen storage disease (e.g., type I)
 4. Hereditary fructose intolerance
 5. Renal tubular acidosis (see Chap. 31) (normal anion gap, urine pH >5)
 6. Glutaric acidemia, type II
 7. Mitochondrial disorders presenting in the newborn with lactic acidemia
  a. Pyruvate carboxylase deficiency
   (1) Seizures
   (2) Failure to thrive
   (3) Neurologic delay
   (4) Metabolic acidosis

(5) Elevated lactate, pyruvate, alanine, beta-hydroxybutyrate, and acetoacetate in blood and urine
(6) Some infants are hypoglycemic.
(7) Treatment is acute: treatment of acidosis with prevention of acidosis and hypoglycemia through a regular exogenous supply of glucose.
(8) Biotin is of no value.
  b. Pyruvate dehydrogenase complex deficiency
    (1) Variable metabolic acidosis
    (2) Elevated blood and CSF lactate
    (3) Treatment is symptomatic
  c. Citric acid cycle defects. Congenital lactic acidemias, including phosphate dehydrogenase deficiency, pyruvate carboxylase deficiency, citric acid cycle defects, and respiratory chain defects, are all very difficult to distinguish clinically and biochemically. Organic acid analysis may be helpful, but not always. Diagnosis is made by a combination of biochemical features, MRI findings, muscle histopathology, and enzyme or DNA analysis depending on the specific defect.
    (1) Encephalopathy, hypotonia
    (2) Metabolic acidosis
    (3) Lactic acidosis
    (4) Elevated fumarase if there is a defect in fumarase
  d. Respiratory chain defects
    (1) Cytochrome *c* oxidase deficiency may present in infancy
  e. Other mitochondrial disorders
    (1) Leigh disease
    (2) Alpers disease
    (3) Leber's optic neuropathy
K. Ketosis. Ketosis and ketonuria are uncommon in sick neonates because of increased ketone conservation in the newborn. Thus, absence of ketosis or ketonuria does not rule out any metabolic defects. Ketonuria can be measured with Ketostick or Acetest tablets for acetone and the 2,4-dinitrophenylhydrazone (DNPH) reaction for alpha keto acids. If these are present, consider:
  1. The organic acidemias (e.g., maple syrup urine disease)
  2. Defects of glycogenolysis (glycogen storage disease, type I)
  3. Citric acid cycle defects
L. Hyperammonemia
  1. The **organic acidemias** (with metabolic acidosis) (See **III.D.**)
  2. Urea cycle defects (See **III.E.1.**)
  3. Transient hyperammonemia of the newborn
M. Abnormal odor of sweat or urine
  1. Ketosis: sweet odor due to acetone
  2. Maple syrup urine disease: maple syrup odor due to branched-chain ketoacids
  3. Isovaleric acidemia: sweaty feet odor due to isovaleric acid
  4. Tyrosinemia, type I: rancid butter odor due to alpha-keto-gamma-methiol butyrate
  5. Beta-methylcrotonyl-coenzyme A carboxylase deficiency: cat's urine odor due to beta-hydroxyisovalerate
  6. Trimethylaminuria: rotten fish odor due to trimethylamine
N. Reducing substances in urine (with the involved compound). Clinitest tablets detect all reducing substances including glucose; urine dipsticks detect glucose only
  1. Diabetes mellitus (glucose)
  2. Essential fructosuria (fructose)
  3. Fanconi syndrome with or without associated metabolic liver disease (glucose)

4. **Galactokinase deficiency** (galactose)
5. **Galactosemia** (galactose)
6. **Hereditary fructose intolerance** (glucose, fructose)
7. **Pentosuria** (xylulose)
8. **Renal glycosuria** (glucose)
9. **Severe liver disease** with secondary galactose intolerance (galactose)

O. **Positive ferric chloride reaction in urine** (with the color of the reaction)
   1. **Phenylketonuria** (green)
   2. **Tyrosinemia** (green, fading rapidly)
   3. **Maple syrup urine disease** (gray-green)
   4. **Histidinemia** (blue-green)
   5. **Alkaptonuria** (dark brown)
   6. **Ketosis** (light green)
   7. **Melanoma** (black)
   8. **Pheochromocytoma** (blue-green)
   9. **Formiminotransferase deficiency** (gray-green)
   10. **Drug intoxication** (purple, red-brown, or green)
   11. **Conjugated hyperbilirubinemia** (green)

P. **Primary lactic acidemia** [9]
   1. Considered primary when it is due to a defect in pyruvic acid metabolism or the respiratory chain as opposed to when it is secondary to poor muscle perfusion in shock.
      a. Metabolic acidosis.
      b. Encephalopathy.
      c. Seizures.
      d. Hypoglycemia if the defect affects gluconeogenesis (although this is rare in pyruvate carboxylase deficiency).
      e. Some patients with pyruvate dehydrogenase deficiency have malformations of the central nervous system and face.
      f. Patients with respiratory chain defects may have any combination of hypotonia and cardiomyopathy, liver disease, renal Fanconi syndrome, pigmentary retinopathy, or sensorineural hearing loss.
      g. Determination of lactic and pyruvate acid in blood and CSF, MRI of head, screens of organ function, ±muscle biopsy for light microscopy, electron microscopy, respiratory chain analysis, ±mitochondrial DNA analysis.
      h. Rarely respond to dietary or vitamin treatment.

III. **Inborn errors of metabolism that are potentially lethal in the newborn**
   A. **Galactosemia** [13]
      1. **Symptoms**
         a. Jaundice (mostly unconjugated in the first week, thereafter increasingly conjugated)
         b. Hepatomegaly, bleeding, coagulopathy
         c. Lethargy
         d. Weight loss, feeding intolerance
         e. Gram-negative sepsis
         f. Cataracts
         g. Hypoglycemia
         h. Renal Fanconi syndrome
      2. **Diagnosis** may be missed in mild cases or when feeding intolerance has been treated with a nonlactose milk.
         a. In galactosemia, after the ingestion of milk (lactose), the urine tests positive for reducing substances (Clinitest) but negative for glucose (glucose-oxidase dipstick test).
         b. Semiquantitative assay of blood for galactose-1-phosphate uridyltransferase (G_1PUT) (Beutler test). Metabolic assay of blood for galactose and G_1PUT can be performed on a newborn screening (PKU) blood filter screening program. Newborns deficient in G_1PUT who have been fed lactose-free formulas from birth may be missed

on screening programs that test only for galactose but do not measure the enzyme.

c. Abnormal liver function test results (SGOT, SGPT, PT, PTT)

3. **Treatment.** Elimination of lactose from the diet is the primary treatment.

B. **Hereditary fructose intolerance** (autosomal recessive)
   1. **Symptoms.** Problems after eating sucrose (such as in soy formulas) or fructose include the following:
      a. Fructose-1-phosphate aldolase deficiency in the liver, kidney, and small intestine
      b. Vomiting, abdominal pain
      c. Hypoglycemia
      d. Seizures
      e. Coma
      f. Hepatomegaly and hepatic failure
      g. Jaundice
      h. Coagulopathy
      i. Renal Fanconi syndrome
      j. Death
   2. **Diagnosis**
      a. Acute hypoglycemia after ingestion of sucrose or fructose
      b. Measurement of hepatic fructose-1-phosphate aldolase activity
      c. Molecular analysis of fructose-1-phosphate aldolase gene
   3. **Treatment.** Elimination of fructose and sucrose from the diet
   4. **Hereditary fructose 1,6 bisphosphate deficiency,** characterized by hyperventilation, apnea, hypoglycemia, ketosis, and lactic acidosis is very rare. It may be lethal in the newborn.

C. **Branched-chain ketoaciduria (maple syrup urine disease)**
   1. **Signs and symptoms** usually appear during the first week of life and are variable
      a. Lethargy
      b. Poor feeding, vomiting
      c. Episodes of decreased muscle tone alternating with increased tone
      d. Seizures
      e. Coma
   2. **Diagnosis**
      a. Maple syrup odor of urine and body
      b. Metabolic acidosis
      c. Ketoacidosis, ketonuria
      d. Green-gray urine color with the ferric chloride test
      e. Urine test with 2,4-dinitrophenylhydrazine for abnormal ketoacids
      f. Blood filter paper specimen obtained for newborn screening (PKU) cards for leucine by bacterial inhibition assay, used in newborn screening programs by states and regions that screen for MSUD
      g. Plasma quantitative amino acid analysis
      h. Assay of branched-chain ketoacid dehydrogenase in leukocytes or skin fibroblasts
   3. **Treatment.** Protein restriction, thiamine supplementation

D. **Organic acidemias: methylmalonic acidemia, propionic acidemia, isovaleric acidemia, and other organic acidemias**
   1. **Signs and symptoms**
      a. Poor feeding
      b. Vomiting
      c. Lethargy
      d. Coma
      e. Hypotonicity
      f. Spasticity
      g. Seizures
      h. Tachypnea

i. Hepatomegaly with liver dysfunction
2. **Diagnosis**
   a. Metabolic acidosis with anion gap
   b. Ketoacidosis, ketonuria
   c. Hyperammonemia (only with propionic, methylmalonic, sometimes present in isovaleric acidemia)
   d. Hypoglycemia
   e. Gas-liquid chromatography mass spectrometry of urine for organic acids
   f. Quantitative plasma amino acid analysis for increased glycine in propionic, methylmalonic, sometimes abnormal in isovaleric acidemia
3. **Treatment.** Immediate: hydration, sodium bicarbonate, IV dextrose, carnitine, vitamins may help. Long-term low protein, high calorie diet, carnitine, vitamins may help.
E. **Hyperammonemia syndromes** [20,24,27]
   1. **Urea cycle disorders, including**
      a. Carbamyl phosphate synthetase deficiency (CPS)
      b. Ornithine transcarbamylase deficiency (OTC) (X-linked)
      c. Argininosuccinate synthetase deficiency (citrullinemia) (AS)
      d. Argininosuccinate lyase deficiency (AL)
      e. N-acetylglutamate synthetase deficiency
   2. **Organic acidemias including** (see **III.D**)
      a. Organic acidemias: propionic, methylmalonic, sometimes present in isovaleric acidemia (see **III.D**)
   3. **Severe perinatal asphyxia**
   4. **Total parenteral nutrition** (excessive protein administration)
   5. **Liver failure** (end-stage)
   6. **Rare miscellaneous disorders** such as
      a. Lysinuric protein intolerance
      b. Hyperornithinemia-hyperammonemia-homocitrullinuria (HHH) syndrome
   7. **Transient hyperammonemia** of a severe degree has been described in **premature infants,** manifested by respiratory distress in the first day of life, coma by the second day of life, and an elevated ammonia level with a normal anion gap. Citrulline is often mildly elevated [5,10,26,27,30].
      a. Signs and symptoms
         (1) Feeding difficulties
         (2) Tachypnea
         (3) Irritability
         (4) Lethargy
         (5) Hypotonicity
         (6) Coma
         (7) Convulsions
      b. Diagnosis [5,10,24,27]
         (1) Hyperammonemia
         (2) Blood gases, electrolytes, bicarbonate, quantitative amino acids, carnitine, lactate, pyruvate
         (3) Urine ketones, quantitative amino acids, organic acids, orotic acid
         (4) Primary respiratory alkalosis is often seen unless perfusion becomes a problem, then a metabolic acidosis occurs.
   8. **Treatment** [2,4,6,18,22,24] of hyperammonemia involves four elements (see **IV**):
      a. Control production of ammonia by stopping protein intake and providing enough calories to prevent tissue catabolism. Intravenous solutions should contain at least 10% dextrose and should be infused at greater than maintenance rates.
      b. Provide adequate hydration as the necessary first step for excretion of ammonia. Removal of excess ammonia can be done by **peritoneal**

dialysis, preferably by **hemodialysis.** Hemodialysis is the treatment of choice. Exchange transfusion should be used only in an emergency on a temporary basis when dialysis is not immediately available, but it should not be implemented if transfusion will delay transfer of a patient to a center where dialysis can be performed.

- **c.** **Provide alternate pathways for nitrogen excretion:** sodium benzoate, sodium phenylacetate, and/or L-arginine may be indicated in urea cycle disorders when ammonia levels are over 600 µg/dl.
- **d.** **Treat any cause of catabolism,** such as infection or asphyxia, vigorously.
- **e.** Infants with transient hyperammonemia of the premature may respond to hemodialysis as well as intravenous glucose and lipids to decrease catabolism of protein.

F. Nonketotic hyperglycinemia
  1. **Signs and symptoms**
     a. Lethargy
     b. Poor feeding
     c. Seizures
     d. Profound hypotonicity
     e. Hiccoughs
     f. Death
  2. **Diagnosis** is made by documenting an elevated ratio of CSF and plasma glycine in plasma and spinal fluid amino acid analysis. In some infants the glycine is elevated only in the CSF. A burst-suppression pattern may be seen on EEG. Enzyme analysis may be done on liver tissue.
  3. **Treatment.** Anticonvulsants, benzoate

G. Pyridoxine-dependent convulsions
  1. **Symptom:** seizures
  2. Test for therapeutic response (see Chap. 27, Neonatal Seizures)
  3. **Treatment** involves pyridoxine (see Chap. 27, Neonatal Seizures)

H. Adrenogenital syndrome (see Chap. 30)
  1. **Diagnosis**
     a. Vomiting, dehydration, hyponatremia, hyperkalemia
     b. Ambiguous genitalia
  2. **Treatment** involves fluid and electrolyte therapy as well as corticosteroids

I. Other potentially lethal defects are hereditary tyrosinemia, molybdenum cofactor deficiency, mitochondrial defects (respiratory chain defects), peroxisomal defects, systemic carnitine deficiency, and glutaric acidemia, type II.

IV. Inborn errors of metabolism that are not usually lethal in the newborn.
  A. Infant of mother with PKU [14,17,19]
  1. **Signs and symptoms**
     a. Microcephaly
     b. Low birth weight
     c. Congenital heart disease (12 to 15%)
  2. **Diagnosis** is by plasma amino acid determination for phenylalanine or filter paper PKU test of the mother.
  3. **Treatment.** Supportive for baby; counseling to mother about dietary treatment during future pregnancies.

  B. Cystic fibrosis
  1. **Symptom:** intestinal obstruction by meconium ileus
  2. **Diagnosis:** sweat test (buccal cell DNA analysis) [21]
  3. **Treatment:** respiratory therapy, antibiotics, diet, sodium replacement, pancreatic enzymes
  4. Carrier testing and prenatal diagnosis are now available.

V. Management of infant with a suspected metabolic disorder (adapted from the protocol developed by Mark Korson, M.D., Metabolism Service, Children's Hospital, Boston, MA)

A. When a sibling has had symptoms consistent with a metabolic disorder, or has died of a metabolic disorder, the following steps should be taken:
1. **Preliminary considerations**
   a. Old hospital charts and postmortem material should be reviewed.
   b. There should be a prenatal discussion of possible diagnoses, and the parents and relatives should be screened for possible clues.
   c. When a diagnosis is known, intrauterine diagnosis by measurement of abnormal metabolites in the amniotic fluid or by enzyme assay of amniocytes obtained by amniocentesis should be considered (see Chaps. 1, 8).
   d. The baby should be delivered in a facility equipped to handle potential metabolic or other complications, preferably closely associated with a laboratory capable of performing or arranging the necessary diagnostic tests.
2. **Initial evaluation** includes a careful physical examination, seeking any of the signs described in **I.B.** All nonmetabolic causes of symptoms such as infection or asphyxia should be excluded. Careful examination of the eyes, skin, and liver should also be performed. Tests should be targeted toward the hereditary anomaly if it is known. **Blood tests** for CBC, platelet count, glucose, pH, carbon dioxide, electrolytes, liver function, PT, PTT, ammonia, lactate, pyruvate, amino acids, carnitine, and very-long-chain fatty acids should be done as appropriate. **Urine** should be examined for color, odor, sediment, pH, glucose, reducing substances, and reaction to ferric chloride and dinitrophenylhydrazine (DNPH). Urinary amino acids and organic acids should be analyzed. If appropriate, spinal fluid should be analyzed for amino acids (e.g., hyperglycinemia has increased spinal fluid: blood ratio of glycine), lactate, and pyruvate. It is important to obtain these specimens at the time of presentation before starting treatment for metabolic disease. The specimens can be frozen (plasma, urine) and analysis performed later.
3. **Sophisticated tests.** All abnormal substances found in the blood or urine should be identified. Quantitative amino acid, organic acid, or blood and urine analysis by column chromatography, thin-layer or paper chromatography, or gas chromatography and mass spectrometry should be performed by personnel who are aware of their uses and limitations. Avoid amino acid or organic acid "screens," which rarely provide a complete analysis. Enzyme assay or DNA analysis of red blood cells, white blood cells, fibroblasts, or liver tissue may be done for confirmation of diagnosis [8,11,22,24].
4. **Initial feedings** for the asymptomatic infant at risk for metabolic disease will vary with the diagnosis; e.g., in disorders of protein metabolism the infant may be given IV glucose or fed 10% glucose or dextrose polymer (Polycose Ross Laboratories, Columbus, OH) as tolerated. This may be followed by fat in the form of medium chain triglycerides (e.g., Nil Prote product 80056, Mead Johnson Laboratories, Evansville, IN). If the results of tests performed at 48 hours are all negative, protein may be introduced in the form of breast milk or any low-protein milk.

   The tests are repeated after 48 hours of protein intake. If no abnormalities are found (as would be expected in 75% of offspring from those who carry genes for autosomal-recessive disorders), the child may be cautiously fed. If metabolic abnormalities are found, the specific problem should be identified and the appropriate diet or treatment started.

   The initial feeding will vary with the type of suspected disorder. Many special products are available for various metabolic diseases, e.g., products in the Ross Metabolic Formula System can be ordered by calling 1-800-For-Ross. The Ross Metabolic Nutrition Support Protocol Manual (A6224) and the Ross Metabolics Ready Reference (G680) can be ordered from the Ross Laboratories, Columbus, OH 83216. Mead Johnson of Evansville, IN, and Scientific Hospital Supply, Gaithersburg, MD, have similar formulas and information.

B. When an infant has signs or symptoms of an acute metabolic disease (see **I.B**), the condition should be managed as follows:

1. **Other causes** of the symptoms should be ruled out, e.g., asphyxia, infection, or intracranial hemorrhage. Even when one of these is the likely cause, if an inborn error cannot be ruled out, obtain acute specimens and keep frozen.

2. **Tests** as in **V.A.2** and **V.A.3** should be performed. *Note:* Organic acids and ammonia are toxic to the brain, and accumulation of these substances may result in cerebral edema. Caution should be exercised when the need for lumbar puncture is considered in a situation where sepsis should be ruled out.

3. The **therapy** for acute metabolic decompensation in these disorders includes
   a. Hydration
   b. Correction of the biochemical abnormalities (metabolic acidosis, hyperammonemia, hypoglycemia)
   c. Reversal of catabolism/promotion of anabolism
   d. Elimination of toxic metabolites, e.g., by hemodialysis
   e. Treatment of the precipitating factor when possible (e.g., infection, excess protein ingestion)
   f. Cofactor supplementation

4. The baby should be adequately **hydrated** at 1¼ to 1½ times maintenance volume with glucose (and in some cases lipids) to prevent catabolism and with alkali to treat acidosis
   a. The baby should be kept NPO for 1 to 2 days with intravenous glucose in high doses. Added insulin should be considered if metabolic stability cannot be achieved (see Hypoglycemia and Hyperglycemia, above). If a diagnosis is not available, a protein source at 0.5 gm/kg/day by parenteral nutrition (PN) or enteral formula is given with other nonnitrogenous caloric supplements (carbohydrates and fats) (see **V.A.4.**).
   In galactosemia the infant can be fed a lactose-free formula immediately. Ringer's lactate should *not* be used for fluid or electrolyte therapy in a child with a known or suspected metabolic disorder.
   b. In undiagnosed cases of acidosis, when the lactate and pyruvate are markedly elevated, the possibility of a disorder of pyruvate metabolism must be considered. In **pyruvate dehydrogenase deficiency,** specifically, excess glucose will make the acidosis worse. Glucose and lactate levels should be monitored. In this disorder, lipids are given to prevent catabolism. Small amounts of glucose are given only to keep the blood glucose normal (see Hypoglycemia, above).

5. If the infant is acidotic (pH <7.22) or the bicarbonate level is <14 mEq/L, give $NaHCO_3$ (1 mEq/kg) as a bolus followed by a continuous infusion of bicarbonate. If hypernatremia is a problem, use potassium acetate as part of the solution (see Chap. 9).

6. Correct hypoglycemia (see Hypoglycemia, above).

7. **Lipid.** Intralipid may be given to supply extra calories. Intralipid is composed of even-chain fatty acids, so it is not contraindicated in propionic and methylmalonic acidemia.

8. **Calories.** Caloric consumption during a period of decompensation, in order to support anabolism, should be about 20% greater than that needed for ordinary maintenance. One must remember that withholding natural protein from the diet also eliminates this source of calories, which should be replaced using other dietary or nutritional (nonnitrogenous) sources.

Table 29-3. Organic acidemias with their respective offending amino acids

Disorder	Offending amino acid
Propionic acidemia	Methionine, isoleucine, valine
Methylmalonic acidemia	Threonine
Isovaleric acidemia	Leucine
β-Methylcrotonyl-CoA carboxylase deficiency	Leucine
Maple syrup urine disease	Leucine, isoleucine, valine
Glutaric acidemia, type I	Lysine, tryptophan

9. **Insulin.** Insulin is a potent anabolic hormone, promoting protein and lipid synthesis. It is probably a useful adjunct in reducing flux through defective catabolic catharays and facilitating the uptake of offending amino acid precursors. It will allow extra glucose to be metabolized and prevent hyperglycemia (see Hyperglycemia, above).

10. **Protein.** All natural protein (containing amino acids) should be withheld for 48 to 72 hours while the patient is acutely ill. Afterward, amino acid therapy may be very beneficial in facilitating clinical improvement, but it should be implemented only under the supervision of a physician/nutritionist with expertise in metabolic management. Table 29-3 contains a list of organic acidemias with their respective offending amino acids. Special parenteral amino acid solutions and specialized formulas are available for many disorders.

11. **Elimination of toxic metabolites.** Correction of acute metabolic perturbations (acidosis, hypoglycemia, dehydration) may help clear some of the factors contributing to the encephalopathy associated with acute metabolic crisis. However, large quantities of toxic intermediate metabolites, believed to be toxic to the brain as well, are not cleared with glucose or bicarbonate. Hydration promotes renal excretion of toxins. Consideration should be given to providing the means to facilitate the excretion of these compounds.

   a. **L-Carnitine.** Free carnitine levels are low in the organic acidemias because of increased esterification with organic acid metabolites. While the benefit of carnitine supplementation is controversial, there is evidence that carnitine facilitates excretion of these metabolites. If administered, it should be mixed in 10% glucose and given as an infusion to provide 25–100 mg/kg per 24-hour period. When oral fluids are tolerated, carnitine may be administered PO at a dose of 100–400 mg/kg/day. Diarrhea is the primary adverse effect of oral carnitine.

   b. **Antibiotics.** For certain organic acidemias (e.g., propionic acidemia, methylmalonic acidemia), gut bacteria are a significant source of organic acid synthesis (e.g., propionic acid). Eradicating the gut flora with a short course of a broad-spectrum antibiotic (e.g., neomycin, metronidazole) orally or intravenously may speed the recovery of a patient in acute crisis. In a newborn with galactosemia there is a significant risk of sepsis. Acute propionicacidemia and methylmalonic acidemia are often associated with neutropenia as well as thrombocytopenia.

   c. In hyperammonemia due to a urea cycle disorder, a mixture of sodium benzoate and sodium phenylactate may be used in addition to glucose, lipids, and electrolytes to facilitate the removal of ammonia. (This treatment is under FDA experimental approval through Saul Brusilow, M.D., at The Johns Hopkins Medical Institute: 410-

Table 29-4. Cofactor supplementation: pharmacologic doses of appropriate cofactors in cases of vitamin-responsive enzyme deficiencies

Disorder	Cofactor daily dose
Propionic acidemia	Biotin 5 mg (probably not effective)
β-Methylcrotonyl deficiency	Biotin 5 mg
Holocarboxylase synthetase deficiency	Biotin 5 mg
Biotinidase deficiency	Biotin 5 mg
Methylmalonic acidemia	Hydroxo-cobalamin (vitamin B_{12}) 1 mg intramuscularly
Maple syrup urine disease	Thiamine 10–50 mg

955-0885.) Arginine is given in all the urea cycle defects except arginase deficiency to prevent arginine deficiency and to stimulate further excretion of waste nitrogen by stimulating the activity of ornithine transcarboxylase. When ammonia levels exceed 500 to 600 mg/dl, dialysis is far more effective in reducing them.

   d. **Hemodialysis** is indicated in cases of intractable metabolic acidosis, unresponsive hyperammonemia (>600 to 700 μg/dl), coma, or severe (usually iatrogenic) electrolyte disturbances.

12. **Treatment of precipitating factors.** Infection should be treated vigorously when possible. Neutropenia (and thrombocytopenia) frequently accompany metabolic decomposition. Bone marrow recovery can be expected once the levels of toxic metabolites have diminished significantly.

13. **Cofactor supplementation.** Pharmacologic doses of appropriate cofactors may be useful in cases of vitamin-responsive enzyme deficiencies (see Table 29-4).

14. **Monitoring the patient**
   a. Clinical parameters
      (1) Mental status
      (2) Fluid balance
      (3) Evidence of bleeding (if thrombocytopenic)
      (4) Symptoms of infection (if neutropenic)
   b. Biochemical parameters
      (1) Electrolytes, measured CO_2, glucose, ammonia, blood gases, CBC with differential, platelets, urine for ketones at every voiding, urine specific gravity

15. **Recovery.** The patient should be kept NPO until his or her mental status is more stable. Anorexia, nausea, and vomiting during the acute crisis period make significant oral intake unlikely. If the patient is not significantly neurologically compromised, consideration should be given to providing the patient (PO or by NG tube) with a modified formula preparation containing all but the offending amino acids. When the infant is able to take oral feedings, a specific diet must be used. The diet will be individualized for each child and his/her metabolic defect.

VI. **Postmortem diagnosis.** If an infant is dying or has died of what may be a metabolic disease, it is very important to make a specific diagnosis in order to help the parents with genetic counseling for future reproductive planning. Sometimes families that will not permit a full autopsy will allow the collection of some premortem or immediately postmortem specimens that may help in diagnosis. Specimens that should be collected include the following:
   A. **Blood,** both clotted and heparinized. The specimen should be centrifuged and the plasma frozen. Lymphocytes may be saved for culture.
   B. **Urine,** refrigerated.

C. Spinal fluid, refrigerated.
D. Skin biopsy for fibroblast culture to be used for chromosomal analysis or enzyme assay. Two samples should be taken from a well-perfused area in the torso. The skin should be well cleaned, but any residual cleaning solution should be washed off with sterile water. The skin can be placed briefly in sterile saline until special media are available.
E. Liver biopsy samples, both premortem samples and generous-size postmortem samples, should be flash frozen to preserve enzyme integrity as well as tissue histology.
F. Other. Depending on the nature of the disease, other tissues such as skeletal muscle, cardiac muscle, brain, and kidney should be preserved.
Photographs should be taken and a full skeletal radiologic screening done of any infant with dysmorphic features. A full autopsy should be done. Information on the proper handling of the tissue should be obtained from one of the regional information centers (see **VIII**).
VII. Prenatal diagnosis (see Chaps. 1, 8)
  A. Fetal testing during first and second trimesters
   1. Analysis of amniotic fluid
   2. Enzyme analysis of cells obtained from amniotic fluid or chorionic villus biopsy
   3. Fetal liver biopsy
  B. Detectable disorders include galactosemia, maple syrup urine disease, organic acidemias, urea cycle disorders, homocystinuria, hyperglycinemia, and tyrosinemia. This is a rapidly changing field, and disorders are regularly added to the prenatally detectable list. Consult with your regional center as to what disorders are detectable (see Chap. 8) and the prenatal test of choice.
VIII. Regional information centers. Metabolic problems in the newborn are complicated and require sophisticated diagnosis and treatment. There are regional centers for assistance with these problems.
  A. New England
  Metabolism Service
  Children's Hospital
  300 Longwood Avenue
  Boston, MA 02115
  (617) 355-6394
  B. Mid-Atlantic states
  Pediatric Genetics Clinic
  1004 CMSC
  The Johns Hopkins Hospital
  Baltimore, MD 21205
  (410) 955-4260
  C. Southeast
  Emory Genetic Clinic
  Emory University School of Medicine
  2040 Ridgewood Drive, NE
  Atlanta, GA 30322
  (404) 727-5731
  D. Southwest
  Department of Pediatrics
  University of Texas Medical School
  P.O. Box 20708
  Houston, TX 77025
  (713) 792-4784
  E. Pacific states
  Medical Genetics Clinic
  Children's Hospital of Los Angeles
  P.O. Box 54700
  Los Angeles, CA 90054

(213) 669-2152
F. Northwest
PKU and Metabolic Birth Defects Center
University of Oregon Health Sciences Center
P.O. Box 574
Portland, OR 97297
(503) 494-7859
G. Rocky Mountain area
Inherited Metabolic Disease Clinic
University of Colorado Health Sciences Center
4200 East Ninth Avenue
Denver, CO 80262
(303) 861-6847
H. Midwest
Metabolic Clinic
Waisman Center on Mental Retardation and Human Development
1500 Highland Avenue
Madison, WI 53706
(608) 263-5993

IX. Routine screening. Each state, province, and country mandates the diseases that are tested for in its newborn screening program. Massachusetts routinely screens filter-paper blood specimens on all newborns for phenylketonuria, maple syrup urine disease, homocystinuria, galactosemia, hypothyroidism, sickle cell disease, congenital adrenal hyperplasia, biotinidase deficiency, hemoglobinopathies, and congenital toxoplasmosis. The state or regional department of health can provide information regarding a specific screening program. See Chap. 5 and references 1, 9, 15, and 29 for articles on newborn screening.

References
1. American Academy of Pediatrics Committee on Genetics. Issues in newborn screening. *Pediatrics* 89:345, 1992.
2. Bachmann, C. Treatment of congenital hyperammonemias. *Enzyme* 32:56, 1984.
3. Batshaw, M. L. Inborn errors of urea synthesis. *Ann. Neurol.* 35:133, 1994.
4. Batshaw, M. L., et al. Use of citrulline as a diagnostic marker in the prospective treatment of urea cycle disorders [see comments]. *J. Pediatr.* 118:914, 1991.
5. Batshaw, M. L., et al. Neurologic outcome in premature infants with transient asymptomatic hyperammonemia. *J. Pediatr.* 108:271, 1986.
6. Brusilow, S. W., et al. Treatment of episodic hyperammonemia in children with inborn errors of urea synthesis. *N. Engl. J. Med.* 310:1630, 1984.
7. Burton, B. K. Inborn errors of metabolism: The clinical diagnosis in early infancy. *Pediatrics* 79:359, 1987.
8. Cederbaum, S. D. Role of recombinant DNA in inborn errors of the urea cycle. Short review. *Enzyme* 45:75, 1991.
9. Goodman, S. I., et al. Metabolic disorders of the newborn. *Pediatr. Rev.* 14:359, 1994.
10. Hudak, M. L., et al. Differentiation of transient hyperammonemia of the newborn and urea cycle enzyme defects by clinical presentation. *J. Pediatr.* 107:712, 1985.
11. Kmiselly, D. S. Hemochromatosis. *Clin. Pediatr.* 39:383, 1992.
12. Ledley, F. D. Perspectives on methylmalonic acidemia resulting from molecular cloning of methylmalonyl CoA mutase. *Bioessays* 12:335, 1990.
13. Levy, H. L. Inborn errors of metabolism. In: H. W. Taeusch, et al. (eds.). *Diseases of the Newborn,* 6th ed. Philadelphia: W. B. Saunders, 1991, 120–146.
14. Levy, H. L. Maternal phenylketonuria. *Prog. Clin. Biol. Res.* 281:227, 1988.
15. Levy, H. L. Screening of the newborn. In: H. W. Taeusch, et al. (eds.). *Diseases of the Newborn,* 6th ed. Philadelphia: W. B. Saunders, 1991, 111–119.

16. Levy, P., et al. State of the art of biochemical genetics. *Am. J. Dis. Child.* 147:1153, 1993.
17. Luke, B., et al. The challenge of maternal phenylketonuria screening and treatment. *J. Reprod. Med.* 35:667, 1990.
18. Maestri, N. E., et al. Prospective treatment of urea cycle disorders. *J. Pediatr.* 119:923, 1991.
19. Matalon, R., et al. Phenylketonuria: Screening, treatment and maternal PKU. *Clin. Biochem.* 24:337, 1991.
20. Ozand, P. T., et al. Organic acidurias: A review. Part 2. *J. Child. Neurol.* 6:288, 1991.
21. Parad, R. B. Use of buccal cell DNA obtained by cheekbrush for rapid molecular genetics diagnosis of cystic fibrosis in preterm and term infants. *Pediatr. Res.* 35:246A, 1994.
22. Rosenberg, L. E. Treating genetic diseases: Lessons from three children. *Pediatr. Res.* S10, 1990.
23. Seashore, M. R., et al. Metabolic disease of the neonate and young infant. *Semin. Perinatol.* 17:318, 1993.
24. Sperl, W. Diagnosis and therapy of organic acidurias. *Padiatr. Padol.* 28:3, 1993.
25. Tada, K., et al. Non-ketotic hyperglycinaemia: Molecular lesion, diagnosis and pathophysiology. *J. Inherit. Metab. Dis.* 16:691, 1993.
26. Tuchman, M., et al. Transient hyperammonemia of the newborn: A vascular complication of prematurity? *J. Perinatol.* 12:234, 1992.
27. Watford, M. The urea cycle: A two-compartment system. *Essays Biochem.* 26:49, 1991.
28. Ward, J. C. Inborn errors of metabolism of acute onset in infancy. *Pediatr. Rev.* 2:205, 1990.
29. Wu, J. T. Screening for inborn errors of amino acid metabolism. *Ann. Clin. Lab. Sci.* 21:123, 1991.
30. Yoshino, M., et al. A nationwide survey on transient hyperammonemia in newborn infants in Japan: Prognosis of life and neurological outcome. *Neuropediatrics* 22:198, 1991.
31. Scriver, C. R., et al. (eds.). The molecular and metabolic bases of inherited disease, Vols. I–III. New York: McGraw-Hill, 1995.

16. Levy JH, et al: Role of the nitric oxide in the maintenance and ... (ref illegible). 1992.

17. Lake CR, et al: Electrochange in arterial pressure related to ... (ref illegible). Pharmacol Neural. New Series, 2000.

18. Mosley ... et al: Anaphylactoid reactions to ... (ref illegible). 1991.

19. Shulman R, et al: Perspectives in Anesthesiology. (ref illegible). 901.

20. Quaal V T, et al: Increased potentiation ... (ref illegible). 1981.

21. Gibson B: Deoxygenation of DNA ... and hydrolysis of low-mol-wt ... (ref illegible). J Anesth, 1990.

22. Lindberg GK: Investigating the dynamical factors from the children. 2 Am ... Rev Res, 1989.

23. Robertson, et al: Metabolic changes of the metabolism during ... anesthesia (ref illegible). 1992.

24. Sewell W: Diagnosis and therapy of operative ... (ref illegible). 1992.

25. Tom ... et al: ... the hypotension ... (ref illegible). Lancet 10.801, 1989.

26. Prosman M, et al: ... hypersensitivity of the near ... (ref illegible). 2 Anesthesiol 2 Zen, 1992.

27. Nolan M: The mechanism of work on anesthetic ... (ref illegible). 1990.

28. Ward J D: Inhibition of ... anesthetic. (ref illegible). Mosby, Boston, 1992. (partly illegible).

29. Bertocchi, et al: ... of anesthetic ... (ref illegible). 1991.

30. Cushing, et al: A worldwide survey on intraoperative ... (ref illegible). Proceedings of ... and International Anesthesia (ref illegible). 1991.

31. Gero JT, et al (eds): The principles and the basis of the ... anesthesia. Vols 1–II. New York, McGraw Hill, 1993.

30. AMBIGUOUS GENITALIA

Mary Deming Scott

I. **Definition.** The term *ambiguous genitalia* applies to any confusing appearance of the external genitalia. This includes any infant with
  1. A phallus but bilaterally unpalpable testes
  2. Unilateral cryptorchidism and hypospadias
  3. Penoscrotal or perineoscrotal hypospadias, even if the testes are descended

    In these cases, the correct sex for rearing cannot be determined from external appearance, and a thorough evaluation is required. The normal full-term male infant should have a phallus at least 2.5 cm long (Fig. 30-1). The normal full-term female infant should have a clitoris under 1 cm and no posterior labial fusion. Testes usually migrate into the scrotum during the last 6 weeks of gestation.
II. **Assignment of a sex for rearing.** Speed in the determination of sex assignment is essential for the parents' peace of mind. Sex assignment depends on anatomy and functional endocrinology rather than on chromosomes. Comments such as "It looks like a boy" or "We'll know when we get the chromosomes" should be avoided. Initial hasty statements by unthinking professionals can haunt families and can have profound psychosocial

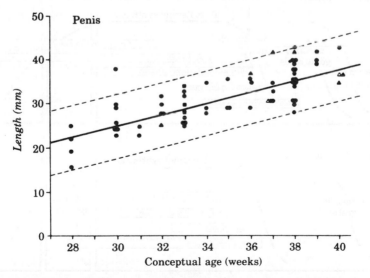

Fig. 30-1. Stretched phallic length of normal premature and full-term babies (closed circles), showing lines of mean 2 standard deviations. Correlation coefficient is 0.80. Superimposed are data for two small-for-gestational-age infants (open triangles), seven large-for-gestational-age infants (closed triangles), and four twins (closed boxes), all of whom are in the normal range. (From K. W. Feldman and D. W. Smith. Fetal phallic growth and penile standards for newborn male infants. *J. Pediatr.* 1975;86:395.)

consequences. Parents should be told that the child's genitalia are incompletely formed but that reconstructive surgery and hormonal support should enable the child to live a normal life. No promises should be made about fertility. A team approach between the pediatric endocrinologist and the pediatric surgeon is generally necessary. If endocrine evaluation shows partial testosterone resistance and the infant has microphallus, a female sex should be assigned, and appropriate external reconstructive surgery should be performed as soon as possible.

III. **Normal sexual development.** A timetable of sexual development is given in Fig. 30-2 and Table 30-1. Sex determination progresses in stages. At fertilization, a **genetic sex** is determined, and this in turn determines **gonadal sex.** The testis-determining factor is located on the short arm of the Y chromosome [4]. 46XX males and 46XY females are created by aberrant X-Y interchange during paternal meiosis [7]. A region necessary for spermatogenesis has been localized to the proximal long arm of the Y chromosome. Gonadal differentiation and sex hormone secretion effect internal genital tract development and external genital development, and a **phenotypic sex** is established at the end of the first trimester. **Psychologic sex** identity is formed by sociologic imprinting within a few years after birth. Prenatal hormonal secretion may have psychologic implications. At puberty, the appearance of secondary sex characteristics reinforces gender identity.

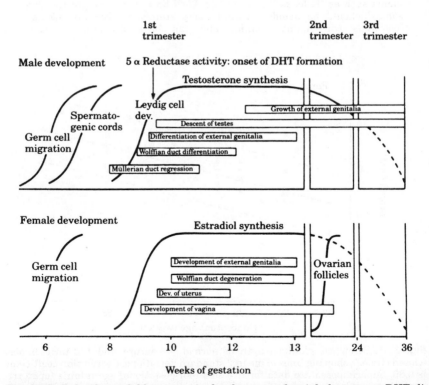

Fig. 30-2. Role of gonadal hormones in development of secial phenotypes. DHT, dihydroxytestosterone; Dev, development. (From J. D. Wilson et al. Relation between differentiation of gonads and anatomic differentiation of human male and female embryos. *Hum. Genet.* 1981;58:78.)

Table 30-1. Timetable of sexual development

Days after conception	Events of sexual development
19	Primordial germ cells migrate to the genital ridge
40	Genital ridge forms an undifferentiated gonad
44	Müllerian ducts appear; testes develop
62	Müllerian inhibitor (from testes) becomes active
71	Testosterone synthesis begins (induced by placental chorionic gonadotropin)
72	Fusion of the labioscrotal swellings
73	Closure of the median raphe
74	Closure of the urethral groove
77	Müllerian regression is complete

IV. **Nursery evaluation of a newborn with ambiguous genitalia**
  A. **History**
    1. **Family history** of hypospadias, cryptorchidism, infertile aunts, consanguinity.
    2. **Maternal drug exposure** in pregnancy (progestogens, danazol, testosterone, phenytoin, aminoglutethimide).
    3. **Maternal virilization in pregnancy.**
    4. **Repeated neonatal deaths** (adrenogenital syndrome).
    5. **Placental insufficiency** (human chorionic gonadotropin (HCG) initiates the synthesis of testosterone in the fetal testis.
  B. **Physical examination**
    1. The examiner should note phallic size, position of the urethral orifice, any fusion of the labia or scrotum, and the descent and size of the gonads.
    2. Bimanual rectal examination may reveal a palpable uterus in the midline.
    3. Associated anomalies. The syndrome of Wilms' tumor, hemihypertrophy, aniridia, genital ambiguity, and gonadoblastoma may be autosomal dominant or due to sporadic deletion of 11p13 [6].
    4. If a uterus and a vagina are present and the external genitalia would necessitate a several-stage hypospadias repair, the child should be raised as a girl.
  C. **Diagnostic tests**
    1. **Pelvic ultrasound** will determine whether a uterus and ovaries are present. An MRI may be needed to locate intraabdominal testes.
    2. The voiding orifice should be injected with radiopaque dye **(cystourethrography)**. This procedure may reveal fallopian tubes, a uterus, or a vagina emerging from the urogenital sinus.
    3. Quinacrine stains of white cells for Y body fluorescence give quick results but are not completely accurate. R-C- and Q-banding and G11 staining may reveal anomalies of the Y chromosome [2]. **Chromosome determinations** take 2 to 5 days.
V. **XX females with genital ambiguity.** With XX chromosomes, the diagnosis may be true hermaphroditism, adrenogenital syndrome due to 21-hydroxylase deficiency, 11-hydroxylase deficiency, or 3-beta hydroxysteroid dehydrogenase deficiency; maternal drug ingestion; or masculinizing tumors of the mother or fetus. If excessive androgens are present before 12 weeks of gestation, labial fu-

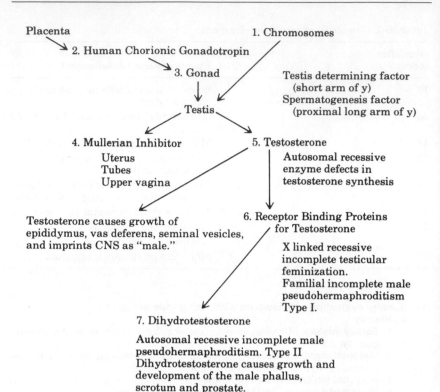

Placenta   1. Chromosomes
   ↘ 2. Human Chorionic Gonadotropin
                    ↘ 3. Gonad   Testis determining factor
                             ↓ ↙   (short arm of y)
                          Testis   Spermatogenesis factor
                        ↙   ↘   (proximal long arm of y)

4. Mullerian Inhibitor   5. Testosterone
   Uterus   Autosomal recessive
   Tubes   enzyme defects in
   Upper vagina   testosterone synthesis
        ↙
Testosterone causes growth of   6. Receptor Binding Proteins
epididymus, vas deferens, seminal vesicles,   for Testosterone
and imprints CNS as "male."
                                       X linked recessive
                                       incomplete testicular
                                       feminization.
                                       Familial incomplete male
                                       pseudohermaphroditism
                                       Type I.
        ↙
7. Dihydrotestosterone

Autosomal recessive incomplete male
pseudohermaphroditism. Type II
Dihydrotestosterone causes growth and
development of the male phallus,
scrotum and prostate.

Note that fetal gonadotropins do not have a significant role in male genital
formation. LH (FSH) and growth hormone seem to cause lengthening of the
phallus in later gestation.

Fig. 30-3. Possible defects in male genital development. Note that fetal gonadotropins do not have a significant role in male genital formation. Luteinizing
hormone (follicle-stimulating hormone) and growth hormone seen to cause a
lengthening of the phallus in later gestation. (CNS = central nervous system.)

sion may occur. After the first trimester, however, clitoral hypertrophy will be
the only sign of excessive androgen exposure.
   A. Determination of **17-hydroxyprogesterone (17-OHP) level,** 17-pregnenolone level, dehydroepiandrosterone level, and testosterone level should be
   made. Electrolytes must be monitored every 3 days in potential salt-losers
   who are discharged before the results of laboratory tests are known. In 90%
   of girls with adrenogenital syndrome, the 17-OHP will be elevated [8].
   Worldwide newborn filter-paper screening programs for 17-OHP show an
   incidence of 1:14,554 births, varying by country. Salt-losers outnumber non–
   salt-losers by 3:1. The male:female sex ratio is 1:1. False positive results occur in sick, premature, and low-birth-weight infants, with a false positive
   rate of up to 0.19% and a recall rate of up to 0.2%. Normal values must be
   determined for each individual program, since they depend on the filter paper thickness and the radioimmunoassay used [8].
   B. If the results of laboratory investigations are normal, ultrasound examination of the ovaries or computed tomography of the adrenals may reveal a

masculinizing tumor. Laparotomy or gonadal biopsy or both may be required to diagnose the rare true hermaphrodite.

VI. XY chromosomes. Even if the chromosomes are XY, the parents should not be hastily told that the child is a boy. Rearing the child as a girl may be appropriate in many cases.

A. Diagnostic possibilities

1. Chromosomal disorders

a. True hermaphroditism (10% are XY, 10% are mosaic, and 80% are XX). Sex assignment should be based on the external and internal genitalia. Generally, if a patent uterus and a vagina are present, these infants should be raised as girls. Two-thirds of them will menstruate.

B. Mixed gonadal dysgenesis. This disorder has 45X-46XY chromosomal complement. The genitalia may range from predominantly male to completely female, and a uterus and a fallopian tube are generally present. The external genitalia are usually asymmetric, with a gonad palpable in one labioscrotal fold and a streak gonad present intra-abdominally. Human chorionic gonadotropin (HCG) stimulation tests should be done to evaluate gonadal function. Gonadal neoplasia (gonadoblastoma) may arise in the first 20 years of life in up to 20% of these children; therefore, streak gonads should always be removed in infancy. Other features of the disorder are webbed neck, lymphedema, short stature, and occasional cardiac defects, specifically coarctation of the aorta. Mixed gonadal dysgenesis is thought to be due to meiotic nondisjunction, with no increased risk of recurrence in subsequent pregnancies.

C. XY "Pure" gonadal dysgenesis. Infants with XY gonadal dysgenesis fail to masculinize, owing to incomplete failure of testicular differentiation. The genitalia usually appear female, but clitoromegaly may occur, and streak gonads are present. Up to 30% of patients with XY gonadal dysgenesis will develop gonadoblastoma or dysgerminoma, so streak gonads should be removed in infancy. The uterus and vagina function well. Abnormalities of the SRY gene (testis-determining factor) are the cause of pure gonadal dysgenesis [5].

1. Male pseudohermaphroditism [9 11, 14]

Possible defects in male genital development are given in Fig. 30-3 and in Tables 30-2 and 30-3. They include the following:

a. Hereditary disorders [11]

(1) Enzyme defects in testosterone synthesis (autosomal recessive)

Table 30-2. Causes of male pseudohermaphroditism

Abnormal gonadal differentiation
  Mixed gonadal dysgenesis
  True hermaphroditism
Abnormal gonadal function
  Placental or fetal pituitary gonadotropin deficiency
  Leydig-cell agenesis
  Congenital anorchia (vanishing testes syndrome)
  Abnormalities of antimüllerian hormone synthesis or action (persistent oviduct syndrome)
Defective testosterone synthesis
Abnormal testosterone metabolism
  5-Alpha-reductase deficiency
Abnormal testosterone action
  Testicular feminization (complete or incomplete)

Source: Modified from P. Saenger, Pseudohermaphroditism. *Pediatr. Ann.* 10:15, 1981.

Table 30-3. Undermasculinization of the genetic male

| | Defects in adrenal and testis | | | Defects in testis | | Defects in end-organ response | | | |
| | | | | | | | | Testicular feminization | |
	20,22-Desmolase	3-Beta-HSD	17-Alpha-reductase	17,20-Desmolase	17-KS reductase	Transient defects	5-Alpha-reductase	Partial	Complete
External genitalia	Ambiguous F > M	Ambiguous M > F	Ambiguous F > M	Ambiguous F > M	Ambiguous F > M	Ambiguous F > M	Ambiguous M > F	Ambiguous M > F	Female
Müllerian ducts	No uterus or fallopian tubes, since Müllerian-inhibiting factor production is normal								
Wolffian ducts	Variably present, depending on severity of enzymatic defect						Epididymis and vas	Abnormal	None
Gonads	Testes in scrotal, inguinal, or abdominal locations								
Fertility	Impaired because of low intratesticular testosterone level					Possible	Possible	Possible	No
Tumors	Possibly increased incidence, but difficult to evaluate because of small numbers of patients with precise diagnoses					Possible	Rare	Rare	Various types: 4% at 20 years, 33% at 50 years
Puberty Virilization	Possible	Common	Possible	Possible	Possible	Common	Common	Sparse	No
Breasts	No	Common	Possible	Possible	Common	Rare	No	Common	Yes
Karyotype	46,XY by definition in undermasculinized genetic males								
Inheritance	AR	AR	AR	AR or XL	AR	?AR	AR	XL	XL

Table 30-3 (*Continued*)

| | Defects in adrenal and testis | | | Defects in testis | | Defects in end-organ response | | | |
| | 20, 22-Desmolase | 3-Beta-HSD | 17-Alpha-reductase | 17, 20-Desmolase | 17-KS reductase | Transient defects | 5-Alpha-reductase | Testicular feminization | |
								Partial	Complete
Elevated plasma steroids	None	17-Hydroxypregnenolone, androstenediol	Corticosterone	17-Hydroxyprogesterone	Androstenedione, estrone	None	High testosterone-to-dihydrotestosterone ratio	Testosterone-estradiol	Testosterone
Additional features	Salt loss	Salt loss	Hypertension	None	None	None	Sparse sexual hair		

Key: 3-beta-HSD = 3-beta-hydroxysteroid dehydrogenase; KS = ketosteroids; F = female; M = male; AR = autosomal recessive; XL = X-linked.
Source: Modified from J. S. Parks, Intersex. In S. A. Kaplan (ed.). *Clinical Pediatric and Adolescent Endocrinology.* Philadelphia: W. B. Saunders, 1982, 327.

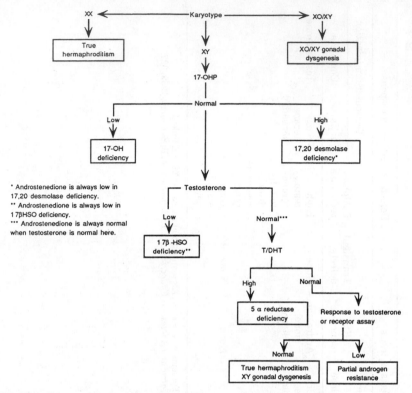

Fig. 30-4. Diagnostic algorithms for patients with ambiguous genitalia in whom gonads are palpable **(A)** or are not palpable **(B)** on physical examination. It is essential to realize that variations of the classical appearance of these defects occur and that details found in the text or other sources should be consulted in addition to this simplified plan. (From D.M. Styne: The testes: Disorders of sexual differentiation and puberty. In S.A. Kaplan (ed.): *Clinical pediatrics and adolescent endocrinology.* Philadelphia, W. B. Saunders, 1990.)

      (2) Partial end-organ resistance to testosterone (X-linked recessive, incomplete testicular feminization)
      (3) Adrenogenital syndrome (autosomal recessive)
      (4) Defects in testosterone metabolism (autosomal recessive)
   b. Nonhereditary disorders
      (1) Maternal drug ingestion (progesterone, phenytoin)
      (2) Placental insufficiency (HCG deficiency)
D. Laboratory evaluation in infants with XY chromosomes will determine the ability to synthesize testosterone and convert it to dihydrotestosterone. Blood is obtained for follicle-stimulating hormone (FSH), leutinizing hormone (LH), testosterone, dihydrotestosterone, dehydroepiandrosterone, androstenedione, cortisol, and 17-OHP. After blood sampling, HCG, 500 IU, is given intramuscularly each day for 3 days, and then the preceding laboratory tests are repeated. Serum sodium and potassium levels should be monitored periodically for the first several weeks of life before a diagnosis of salt-losing adrenogenital syndrome is ruled out.

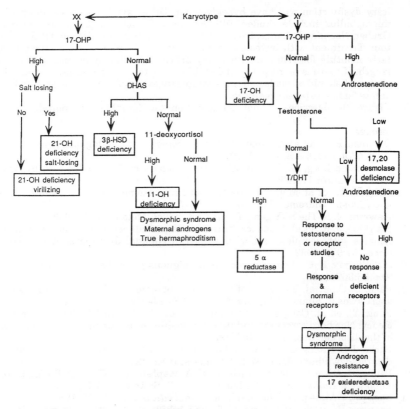

Fig. 30-4. *Continued.*

E. **Testosterone resistance.** If the laboratory tests mentioned above show initial high levels of testosterone that do not increase when HCG is given, the infant probably has incomplete testicular feminization (androgen resistance). Such children should never be raised as boys because they do not masculinize adequately, despite hormone therapy, and will feminize at adolescence.

VII. **Bilateral cryptorchidism** [12]. Bilateral cryptorchidism occurs in 3:1000 infants at birth, most of whom are premature. By 1 month of life, the testes remain undescended in 1:1000. Fewer than 1:1000 term infants have bilaterally nonpalpable undescended testes. Ultrasound or MRI may reveal an intra-abdominal location. If testicular tissue cannot be found, 500 to 1500 IU of HCG should be given intramuscularly daily for 3 days, and levels of FSH, LH, and testosterone should be determined before and after dosing to determine the presence and activity of gonadal tissue. Elevated gonadotropins and no rise in testosterone suggest absent or nonfunctioning testes. A surgeon should be consulted, and early orchidopexy (by 1 year) attempted. If abdominal testes cannot be brought into the scrotum, they should be removed because of the three- to tenfold risk of germ cell cancer in cryptorchidism. Cryptorchidism is seen in congenital ichthyosis, anencephaly, neural tube defects, Prader-Willi, Laurence-Moon-Biedl, Aarskog, Cockayne, Fanconi, Noonan, trisomy 21, and Klinefelter.

VIII. **Microphallus** [10]. Infants with microphallus (<2.5 cm in a full-term boy) and/or cryptorchidism may have hypothalamic-hypopituitary disorders, such as septo-optic dysplasia or Kallman syndrome. Over half of patients with pituitary dysfunction will have hypoglycemia. Other syndromes associated with microphallus include Prader-Willi, Robinow, Klinefelter, Carpenter, Meckel-Gruber, Noonan, de Lange, trisomy 21, Fanconi pancytopenia, and fetal hydantoin. Treatment with testosterone enanthate, 25 to 50 mg given intramuscularly monthly for 1 to 3 months, may provide significant increases in penile length. If there is no response, the child has testosterone resistance. Sex reassignment should be made and the appropriate external surgery be performed to create female external genitalia.

IX. Figure 30-4 describes an approach to patients with ambiguous genitalia.

References

1. Donahoe, P. K., et al. Evaluation of the newborn with ambiguous genitalia. *Pediatr. Clin. North Am.* 23:361, 1976.
2. Drummond-Borg, M., et al. Nonfluorescent dicentric Y in males with hypospadias. *J. Pediatr.* 113:469, 1988.
3. Jadresic, L., et al. Molecular analysis of chromosome region 11p13 in patients with Drash syndrome. *Hum. Genet.* 86:487, 1991.
4. Hawkins, J. R. The SRY gene. *Trend Endocrinol. Metab.* 4:328, 1993.
5. Hawkins, J. R., et al. Evidence for increased prevalence of SRY mutation in XY females with complete rather than partial gonadal dysgenesis. *Am. J. Hum. Genet.* 51:979, 1992.
6. McGillivray, B. C. Genetic aspects of ambiguous genitalia. *Pediatr. Clin. North Am.* 38:307, 1992.
7. Page, D. C., et al. Exchange of terminal proportions of X and Y chromosomal short arms in human XX males. *Nature* 328:427, 1987.
8. Pang, S., et al. Congenital adrenal hyperplasia due to 21 hydroxylase deficiency: Newborn screening and its relationship to the diagnosis and treatment of the disorder. *Screening* 2:105, 1993.
9. Parks, J. S. Intersex. In S. A. Kaplan (ed). *Clinical Pediatric and Adolescent Endocrinology.* Philadelphia, W. B. Saunders, 1982, 327.
10. Penny, R. Disorders of the testis. In S. A. Kaplan, (ed). *Clinical Pediatric and Adolescent Endocrinology.* Philadelphia, W. B. Saunders, 1982, 314.
11. Saenger, P. Male pseudohermaphroditism. *Pediatr. Ann.* 10:15, 1981.
12. Saenger, P., et al. Management of cryptorchidism. *Trends Endocrinol. Metab.* 3:249, 1992.
13. Saenger, P. Turner's syndrome. *N. Engl. J. Med.* 335:1789, 1996.
14. Styne, D. M. The testes: Disorders of sexual differentiation and puberty. In S. A. Kaplan, (ed). *Clinical Pediatric and Adolescent Endocrinology.* Philadelphia, W. B. Saunders, 1990, 376.

31. RENAL CONDITIONS

Melanie S. Kim and Francesco Emma

I. Renal embryogenesis and functional development

A. Embryology

1. Three paired renal systems develop from the nephrogenic ridge of the mesoderm.

2. The first two systems, the **pronephros** and the **mesonephros,** have limited function in the human being and are transient. The mesonephric tubules and duct form the efferent ductules of the epididymis, the vas deferens, the ejaculatory ducts, and the seminal vesicles in the male. In the female they result in the vestigial epoophoron and the paroophoron.

3. The **metanephros** is the third and final excretory system and appears in the 5th week of gestation. The metanephros is made up of two different cell types. These differentiate into the **pelvicalyceal system,** which is well delineated by the 13th or 14th week, and the **nephrons,** which continue to form up to the 35th week of gestation to a final complement of one million nephrons per kidney. Urine is produced by the 12th week.

4. Disruption of normal renal development may lead to renal malformations such as renal agenesis, renal hypoplasia, renal ectopy, and renal dysplasia.

B. Functional development

At birth, the kidney replaces the placenta as the major homeostatic organ, maintaining fluid and electrolyte balance and removing harmful waste products. This transition occurs with changes in renal blood flow, glomerular filtration rate and tubular functions

1. **Renal blood flow (RBF)** remains low in the fetus, accounting for only 2 to 3% of cardiac output. At birth, RBF rapidly increases because of (1) a decrease in renal vascular resistance, which is proportionally greater in the kidney compared to other organs and (2) an increase in systemic blood pressure.

2. **Glomerular filtration** begins soon after the first nephrons are formed and glomerular filtration rate (GFR) increases in parallel with body and kidney growth (approximately 1 ml/min/kg of body weight). Once all the glomeruli are formed by 34 weeks' gestation, the GFR continues to increase until birth because of decreases in renal vascular resistance. After birth, the GFR rises quickly, doubling by 2 weeks of age and reaching adult levels by 1 year of age. GFR is not altered by premature birth and increases at the same rate as if the infant were still in utero.

3. **Tubular function**

   a. **Sodium (Na) handling:** The capacity to reabsorb Na is developed by 24 weeks' gestation. However, tubular resorption of Na is low until 34 weeks' gestation, with fractional excretion of sodium (FeNa, Table 31-1) ranging from 5 to 10%. In severely ill infants, urinary Na losses can be very high, with FeNa reaching 15%. Very premature infants cannot conserve Na even when Na balance is negative. Hence, infants below 34 weeks' gestation receiving formula or breast milk without Na supplementation can develop hyponatremia. After 34 weeks' gestation, Na reabsorption becomes more efficient, so that 99% of filtered Na can be reabsorbed, resulting in a FeNa of less than 1%. Neonates are also limited in their ability to excrete a Na load because of their low GFR.

Table 31-1. Commonly used equations and formulas

$$\text{CrCl (ml/min/1.73 m}^2) = K \times \frac{\text{Length (cm)}}{P_{Cr}}$$

$K = 0.34$ in premature infants <34 wks and 0.44 in infants from 35 wks to term

$$\text{CrCl (ml/min/1.73 m}^2) = \frac{U_{Cr} \times U_{vol} \times 1.73}{P_{Cr} \times \text{BSA}}$$

$$\text{FeNa} = 100 \times \left(\frac{U_{Na} \times P_{Cr}}{P_{Na} \times U_{Cr}} \right)$$

$$\text{TRP} = 100 \times \left(1 - \frac{U_{P} \times P_{Cr}}{P_{P} \times U_{Cr}} \right)$$

$$\text{Calculated } P_{osm} \geq 2 \times \text{plasma [Na}^+] + \frac{\text{[glucose]}}{18} + \frac{\text{BUN}}{2.8}$$

Plasma anion gap = $[\text{Na}^+] - [\text{Cl}^-] - [\text{HCO}^-_3]$

Abbreviations: CrCl = creatinine clearance, U_{Cr} = urinary creatinine, U_{vol} = urinary volume per minute, P_{Cr} = plasma creatinine, P_{Na} = plasma sodium, BSA = body surface area, FeNa = fractional excretion of sodium, TRP = tubular reabsorption of phosphorus, P_{osm} = plasma osmolarity.

---

    b. Water handling: The newborn infant has a limited ability to concentrate urine. The maximal urine osmolality is 500 mOsm/L in premature infants and 800 mOsm/L in term infants. Although this is of little consequence in infants receiving appropriate amounts of water, it can become clinically relevant in infants receiving high osmotic loads. In contrast, both premature and full-term infants can dilute their urine with a minimal urine osmolality of 25 to 35 mOsm/L. Their low GFR, however, limits their ability to handle water loads.

    c. Potassium (K) handling: The limited ability of premature infants to excrete large K loads is primarily related to their low GFR.

    d. Acid and bicarbonate handling are limited by a low serum bicarbonate threshold in the proximal tubule (14 to 16 mEq/L in premature infants, 18 to 21 mEq/L in full-term infants). In addition, the production of ammonia in the distal tubule and the excretion of titratable acids is not fully developed in preterm infants, further limiting their ability to eliminate an acid load. Very-low-birth-weight infants can develop mild metabolic acidosis during the second to fourth week that is treated by administration of sodium bicarbonate.

II. Clinical assessment of renal function

Assessment of renal function is based on the patient's history, physical examination, and appropriate laboratory and radiologic tests.

  A. History

    1. Prenatal history includes any maternal illness, drug use, or exposure to known and potential teratogens.

      a. Maternal use of captopril and indomethacin has been associated with neonatal renal failure.

      b. Oligohydramnios may indicate a decrease in fetal urine production. It is often associated with renal agenesis, renal dysplasia, polycystic kidney disease, or severe obstruction of the urinary tract system. Polyhydramnios may be a result of renal tubular dysfunction with inability to fully concentrate urine. Elevated serum and amniotic fluid alpha-feto-protein have been associated with congenital nephrotic syndrome.

2. **Family history:** The risk of renal disease is increased if there is a family history of urinary tract anomalies, polycystic kidney disease, consanguinity, or inherited renal tubular disorders.

3. **Delivery history:** Fetal distress, perinatal asphyxia, or shock due to volume loss may lead to ischemic or anoxic damage, resulting in acute tubular necrosis.

4. **Micturition:** 17% of newborns void in the delivery room, 93% void by 24 hours, and 98% void by 48 hours. The rate of urine formation ranges from 0.5 to 5.0 ml/kg/hr at all gestational ages. The most common cause of delayed or decreased urine production is inadequate perfusion of the kidneys; however, delay in micturition may be due to intrinsic renal abnormalities or obstruction of the urinary tract.

B. **Physical examination**

Careful examination will detect abdominal masses in 0.8% of neonates. The majority of these masses are either renal in origin or related to the genitourinary system.

Other congenital anomalies detected by physical examination and associated with renal abnormalities include low-set ears, ambiguous genitalia, anal atresia, abdominal wall defect, vertebral anomalies, aniridia, meningomyelocele, pneumothorax, hemihypertrophy, persistent urachus, hypospadias, and cryptorchidism (Table 31-2). Edema may be present in infants with congenital nephrotic syndrome or renal failure and fluid overload. Spontaneous pneumothorax is associated with an increased risk of renal abnormalities.

C. **Laboratory evaluation**

Renal function tests must be interpreted in relationship to gestational and postnatal age (Tables 31-3 and 31-4).

1. **Urinalysis** reflects the developmental stages of renal physiology.
   a. **Specific gravity:** Full-term infants have a limited concentrating ability with a maximum specific gravity of 1.021 to 1.025.
   b. **Protein excretion** varies with gestational age. Urinary protein excretion is higher in premature infants and decreases progressively with postnatal age. In normal full-term infants, protein excretion is minimal after the 2nd week of life.
   c. **Glycosuria** is commonly present in premature infants of less than 34 weeks' gestation. The tubular resorption of glucose is less than 93% in infants born before 34 weeks' gestation compared with 99% in infants born after 34 weeks' gestation. Glucose excretion rates are highest in infants born before 28 weeks' gestation.
   d. **Hematuria** is abnormal and may indicate intrinsic renal damage (see III.F).

2. **Method of collection**
   a. **Suprapubic aspiration** is the most reliable method of detecting urinary tract infection.
   b. **Bladder catheterization** is used if an infant has failed to pass urine by 36 to 48 hours and is not hypovolemic (see III.B).
   c. **Bag collections** are adequate for most studies such as determinations of specific gravity, pH, electrolytes, protein, glucose, and sediment. It is the preferred method for detecting red blood cells in the urine.
   d. **Diaper urine specimens** are reliable for estimation of pH and qualitative determination of the presence of glucose, protein, and blood.

3. **Evaluation of renal function**
   a. **Serum creatinine** at birth reflects maternal renal function. In infants, serum creatinine levels fall quickly from 0.8 mg/dl at birth to 0.5 mg/dl at 5 to 7 days and reach a stable level of 0.3 to 0.4 mg/dl by nine days. The rate of decrease in serum creatinine in the first few weeks is slower in decreasing gestational age, as GFR is lower in the premature

able 31-2. Congenital abnormalities with renal components

Dysmorphic disorders, sequences, and associations	General features	Renal abnormalities
Oligohydramnios sequence (Potter syndrome)	Altered facies, pulmonary hypoplasia, abnormal limb and head position	Renal agenesis, severe bilateral obstruction, severe bilateral dysplasia, autosomal recessive polycystic kidney disease
VATER and VACTERL syndrome	Vertebral anomalies, anal atresia, tracheo-esophageal fistula, radial dysplasia, cardiac and limb defects	Renal agenesis, renal dysplasia, renal ectopia
MURCS association and Rokitansky sequence	Failure of paramesonephric ducts, vaginal and uterus hypoplasia/atresia, cervicothoracic somite dysplasia	Renal hypoplasia/agenesis, renal ectopia, double uterers
Prune belly	Hypoplasia of abdominal muscle, cryptorchidism	Megaureters, hydronephrosis, dysplastic kidneys, atonic bladder
Spina bifida	Meningomyelocele	Neurogenic bladder, vesicoureteral reflux, hydronephrosis, double ureter, horseshoe kidney
Caudal dysplasia sequence (caudal regression syndrome)	Sacral (and lumbar) hypoplasia, disruption of the distal spinal cord	Neurogenic bladder, vesicoureteral reflux, hydronephrosis, renal agenesis
Anal atresia (high imperforate anus)	Rectovaginal, rectovesical, or rectourethral fistula tethered to the spinal cord	Renal agenesis, renal dysplasia
Hemihypertrophy	Hemihypertrophy	Wilms' tumor, hypospadias
Aniridia	Aniridia, cryptorchidism	Wilms' tumor
Drash syndrome	Ambiguous genitalia	Mesangial sclerosis, Wilms' tumor
Small deformed or low-set ears		Renal agenesis/dysplasia
Hereditary disorders	**General features**	**Renal abnormalities**
Autosomal recessive		
Cerebrohepatorenal syndrome (Zellweger syndrome)	Hepatomegaly, glaucoma, brain anomalies, chondrodystrophy	Cortical renal cysts

Table 31-2 (*continued*).

Hereditary disorders	General features	Renal abnormalities
Jeune syndrome (thoracic asphyxiating dystrophy)	Small thoracic cage, short ribs, abnormal costochondral junctions, pulmonary hypoplasia	Cystic tubular dysplasia, glomerulosclerosis, hydronephrosis, horseshoe kidneys
Meckel-Gruber syndrome (dysencephalia splanchnocystica)	Encephalocele, microcephaly, polydactyly, cryptorchidism, cardiac anomalies, liver disease	Polycystic/dysplastic kidneys
Johanson-Blizzard syndrome	Hypoplastic alae nasi, hypothyroidism, deafness, imperforate anus, cryptorchidism	Hydronephrosis, caliectasis
Schinzel-Giedon syndrome	Short limbs, abnormal facies, bone abnormalities, hypospadias	Hydronephrosis, megaureter
Short rib–polydactyly syndrome	Short horizontal ribs, pulmonary hypoplasia, polysyndactyly, bone and cardiac defects, ambiguous genitalia	Glomerular and tubular cysts
Bardet-Biedl syndrome	Obesity, retinal pigmentation, polydactyly	Interstitial nephritis
Autosomal dominant		
Tuberous sclerosis	Fibrous-angiomatous lesions, hypopigmented macules, intracranial calcifications, seizures, bone lesions	Polycystic kidneys, renal angiomyolipomata
Melnick-Fraser syndrome (branchio-otorenal [BOR] syndrome)	Preauricular pits, branchial clefts, deafness	Renal dysplasia, duplicated ureters
Nail-patella syndrome (hereditary osteoonychodysplasia)	Hypoplastic nails, hypoplastic or absent patella, other bone anomalies	Proteinuria, nephrotic syndrome
Townes syndrome	Thumb, auricular and anal anomalies	Various renal abnormalities
X-Linked		
Oculocerebrorenal syndrome (Lowe's syndrome)	Cataracts, rickets, mental retardation	Fanconi syndrome
Oral-facial-digital (OFD) syndrome, type I	Oral clefts, hypoplastic alae nasi, digital asymmetry (X-linked, lethal in male)	Renal microcysts

Chromosomal abnormalities	General features	Renal abnormalities
Trisomy 21 (Down syndrome)	Abnormal facies, brachycephaly, congenital heart disease	Cystic dysplastic kidney and other renal abnormalities

Table 31-2 (*continued*).

Chromosomal abnormalities	General features	Renal abnormalities
X0 syndrome (Turner syndrome)	Small stature, congenital heart disease, amenorrhea	Horseshoe kidney, duplications and malrotations of the urinary collecting system
Trisomy 13 (Patau syndrome)	Abnormal facies, cleft lip and palate, congenital heart disease	Cystic dysplastic kidneys and other renal anomalies
Trisomy 18 (Edwards syndrome)	Abnormal facies, abnormal ears, overlapping digits, congenital heart disease	Cystic dysplastic kidneys, horseshoe kidney, or duplication
XXY, XXX syndrome (Triploidy syndrome)	Abnormal facies, cardiac defects, hypospadias and cryptorchidism in male, syndactyly	Various renal abnormalities
Partial trisomy 10q	Abnormal facies, microcephaly, limb and cardiac abnormalities	Various renal abnormalities

infant and creatinine is not cleared as rapidly as in the full-term infant (see Table 31-4).

 b. Serum urea nitrogen (BUN) is a useful indicator of renal function. However, BUN can be elevated as a result of increased production of urea nitrogen in hypercatabolic states, sequestered blood, tissue breakdown, hemoconcentration, or increased protein intake. Renal insufficiency is suspected if BUN is greater than 20 mg/dl or rises at a rate of 5 mg/dl/day or higher.

 c. Glomerular filtration rate can be measured by clearance studies of either exogenous substances (inulin, Cr-EDTA, sodium iothalamate) or endogenous substances such as creatinine. Practical considerations such as frequent blood sampling, urine collection or infusion of an exogenous substance limit their use. GFR can be estimated from serum creatinine and body length (see Table 31-1).

 d. Measurement of serum and urine electrolytes is used to guide fluid and electrolyte management and in assessing renal tubular function.

D. Radiological studies

 1. Ultrasound is the initial imaging study to delineate renal parenchymal architecture. Color flow Doppler techniques can estimate renal blood flow. The length of the kidneys in millimeters is approximately the gestational age in weeks. The renal cortex has echogenicity similar to that of the liver or spleen in the neonate, in contrast to the hypoechoic renal cortex seen in adults and older children. In addition, the medullary pyramids in the neonate are much more hypoechoic than the cortex and hence are more prominent in appearance.

 2. Intravenous pyelography (IVP) is rarely used in the newborn period, since the neonate has a limited concentrating ability and difficulty in excreting a highly osmolar load.

 3. Voiding cystourethography (VCUG), with fluoroscopy, is indicated in infants with urinary tract infections to rule out vesicoureteral reflux (VUR)

Table 31-3. Normal urinary and renal values in term and preterm infants

	Preterm infants <34 wks	Term infants at birth	Term infants 2 wks	Term infants 8 wks
GFR (ml/min/1.73 m²)	13–58	15–60		63–80
FeNa (%) (oliguric patient)	>1%	<1%	<1%	<1%
Bicarbonate threshold (mEq/L)	14–16	21	21.5	
TRP (%)	>85%	>95%		
Protein excretion (mg/m²/24h) (mean ± 1 SD)	60 ± 96	31 ± 44		
Maximal concentration ability (mOsmol/L)	500	800	900	1200
Maximal diluting ability (mOsmol/L)	25–30	25–30	25–30	25–30
Specific gravity	1.002–1.015	1.002–1.020	1.002–1.025	
Dipstick				
pH	5.0–8.0	4.5–8.0	4.5–8.0	4.5–8.0
Proteins	Neg to ++	Neg to +	Neg	Neg
Glucose	Neg to ++	Neg	Neg	Neg
Blood	Neg	Neg	Neg	Neg
Leukocytes	Neg	Neg	Neg	Neg

Table 31-4. Normal serum creatinine values in term and preterm infants (mean ±95th percentile)

Age (days)	<28 wk	29–32 wk	33–36 wk	>37 wk
7	0.95 (1.31)	0.94 (1.40)	0.77 (1.25)	0.56 (0.96)
14	0.81 (1.17)	0.78 (1.14)	0.62 (1.02)	0.43 (0.65)
28	0.66 (0.94)	0.59 (0.97)	0.40 (0.68)	0.34 (0.54)

From: Rudd, P. T., Hughes, E. A., Platczek, M. M., and Hodes, D. T. Reference ranges for plasma creatinine during the first month of life. *Arch. Dis. Child.* 58:212, 1983.

and in neonates with obstructive uropathy to define the underlying anatomical defect more specifically. Radionuclide cystography is often used to evaluate VUR because of its lower radiation dose. However, VCUG produces better static imaging for anatomical defects and is preferred for the initial evaluation of obstructive uropathy.

4. **Radionuclide scintigraphy** is useful in demonstrating the position and relative function of the kidneys. Isotopes such as technetium-99m-diethylene triamine pentacetic acid (DTPA) or mercaptoacetyltriglycine (MAG 3) are handled by glomerular filtration and can be used to assess renal blood flow and renal function. In conjunction with intravenously administered furosemide, it can help differentiate obstructive from nonobstructive hydronephrosis. Isotopes that bind to the renal tubules, such as technetium-99m-dimercaptosuccinic acid (DMSA), produce static images of the renal cortex. This may be helpful for assessing acute pyelonephritis and renal scarring from renal artery emboli, and to quantify the amount of renal cortex in patients with renal dysplasia and hypoplasia.

III. **Common clinical renal problems**
A. **Prenatal ultrasound**
1. Routine maternal ultrasound screening detects an incidence of fetal genitourinary abnormalities of 0.3 to 0.5%.
2. The most common finding is **hydronephrosis,** reported in over 80% of the cases. Approximately 75% of the cases are confirmed postnatally.
   a. Initial management of a newborn with prenatally identified hydronephrosis depends on the clinical condition of the patient and the suspected nature of the lesion.
   b. Unilateral hydronephrosis is more common and is not associated with systemic or pulmonary complications if the contralateral kidney is normal. Postnatal ultrasound confirmation may be carried out electively at about one month, depending on severity. It is important to avoid the first few days after birth, when hydronephrosis may not be detected because of physiologic dehydration.
   c. Bilateral hydronephrosis is more worrisome, especially if oligohydramnios or pulmonary disease is present. In the male infant, postnatal evaluation (VCUG and ultrasound) should be performed within the first day to rule out the possibility of posterior urethral valves (PUV). With post-bladder obstruction such as PUV, ultrasound will often demonstrate a trabeculated and thickened bladder wall.
   d. Prophylactic antibiotics (amoxicillin 20 mg/kg orally every day) is recommended before VCUG is performed, as hydronephrosis may be due to vesicoureteral reflux.
3. Routine prenatal ultrasound has increased the diagnosis of multicystic dysplastic kidney (MCDK), especially with unilateral involvement. Infants with unilateral MCDK are usually asymptomatic, and the affected kidney has no renal function as demonstrated by DMSA renal scan. There is general agreement that surgical removal is indicated in cases with associated hypertension or infection, or with respiratory compromise sec-

ondary to abdominal compression by the abnormal kidney. In asymptomatic patients, the relative merits of conservative observation versus surgical removal remain controversial.

B. Acute renal failure may be secondary to prenatal, intrinsic, or postrenal disorders (Table 31-5). **Prerenal failure** is due to hypoperfusion to the kidneys. This is the most common cause of renal failure in the neonate, and if not corrected it may lead to intrinsic renal damage. **Intrinsic renal failure** implies direct damage to the kidneys from an insult or congenital anomaly. **Postrenal failure** results from obstruction to urinary flow in both kidneys. In boys, the most common lesion occurs in the posterior urethral valves. Renal function may be abnormal even after correction of the obstruction.

  1. Diagnosis and management should proceed simultaneously to correct the defect as quickly as possible, so that compromise of the kidney will be limited.

    a. Suspect renal failure if oliguria is present (urine flow less than 0.5 ml/kg/hr) and/or if serum creatinine is elevated 2 standard deviations above the mean value for gestational age (see Table 31-3) or rising (0.3 mg/dl/day).

    b. Evaluate history for oligohydramnios, perinatal asphyxia, or maternal drug use, and identify abdominal mass or congenital anomaly.

Table 31-5. Causes of renal failure in the neonatal period

I. Prerenal
  A. Reduced effective circulatory volume
    Hemorrhage
    Dehydration
    Sepsis
    Necrotizing enterocolitis
    Congenital heart disease
    Hypoalbuminemia
  B. Increased renal vascular resistance
    Polycythemia
    Indomethacin
    Adrenergic drugs (e.g., tolazoline)
  C. Hypoxia/asphyxia
II. Intrinsic or renal parenchymal
  A. Sustained hypoperfusion leading to acute tubular necrosis
  B. Congenital anomalies
    Agenesis
    Hypoplasia/dysplasia
    Polycystic kidney disease
  C. Thromboembolic disease
    Bilateral renal vein thrombosis
    Bilateral renal arterial thrombosis
  D. Nephrotoxins
    Aminoglycosides
    Radiographic contrast media
III. Obstructive
  A. Urethral obstruction
    Posterior urethral valves
    Stricture
  B. Ureterocele
  C. Ureteropelvic/ureterovesical obstruction
  D. Extrinsic tumors
  E. Neurogenic bladder
  F. Megacystis or megaureter syndrome

    c. Perform ultrasound exam of genitourinary system.

    d. Catheterize the bladder to rule out lower urinary tract obstruction, measure residual urine volume, collect urine for analysis, and monitor subsequent urinary flow rate.

    e. To rule out prerenal failure, we give a fluid challenge of normal saline 10 to 20 ml/kg over 1 hour if there is no evidence of heart failure or volume overload, and administer a diuretic (furosemide, 1 mg/kg). No response suggests intrinsic or postrenal failure. We often infuse low-dose dopamine to improve renal blood flow and urine output.

    f. Table 31-6 lists laboratory tests that are helpful in differentiating prerenal from intrinsic renal failure in the oliguric patient.

2. Management

    a. Discontinue or minimize potassium (K). A low K formula such as Similac PM 60/40 or K-free solution is used. Treatment of hyperkalemia (K >6 mEq/L) is as follows:

        (1) Sodium polystyrene sulfonate (Kayexalate) is administered rectally in a dose of 1.0 to 1.5 gm/kg (dissolved in normal saline at 0.5 gm/ml saline) or orally in a dose of 1.0 gm/kg (dissolved in dextrose 10% in water) every 4 to 6 hours. The enema tube, a thin Silastic feeding tube, is inserted 1 to 3 cm. If possible, we avoid using Kayexalate in low-birth-weight infants. One gram/kg of resin removes 1 mEq/e of potassium.

        (2) Calcium is given as 1 to 2 ml/kg of calcium gluconate 10% over 2 to 4 minutes while the electrocardiogram (ECG) is monitored.

        (3) Sodium bicarbonate, 1 mEq/kg given intravenously over 5 to 10 minutes, will decrease serum potassium by 1 mEq/L.

        (4) Glucose and insulin: Begin with a bolus of regular human insulin (0.05 units/kilogram) and dextrose 10% in water (2 ml/kilogram) followed by a continuous infusion of dextrose 10% in water at 2 to 4 ml/kilogram per hour and human regular insulin (10 units/100 ml) at 1 ml/kg per hour. Monitor blood glucose level frequently. Maintain a ratio of 1 or 2 units of insulin to 4 gm glucose.

        (5) Furosemide 1 mg/kg is given when renal function is adequate because kaliuresis as well as natriuresis occurs with this diuretic.

        (6) Dialysis is considered when hyperkalemia cannot be controlled or if anuria is present.

    b. Fluid management is based on the patient's fluid status and should be limited to replacement of insensible losses and urine output (see Chap. 9).

    c. Sodium (Na) is restricted and Na concentration is monitored, accounting for fluid balance. Hyponatremia is usually secondary to excess free water.

    d. Phosphorus is restricted by using a low-phosphorus formula (e.g., Similac PM 60/40). Calcium carbonate can be used as a phosphate-binding agent.

    e. Calcium supplementation is given if ionized calcium is decreased or the patient is symptomatic. In infants with chronic renal failure, pro-

Table 31-6. Renal failure indices in the oliguric neonate

Indices	Prerenal failure	Intrinsic renal failure
Urine sodium (mEq/L)	10–50	30–90
Urine/plasma creatinine	29.2 ± 1.6	9.7 ± 3.6
FeNa[1]	0.9 ± 0.6	4.3 ± 2.2

[1]Fractional excretion of sodium defined in Chap. 9 (pp. 39).
Modified from Mathew, O. P., et al. Neonatal renal failure: Usefulness of diagnostic indices. *Pediatrics* 65:57, 1980.

vide 1,25-dihydroxyvitamin D or its analog to prevent renal osteodystrophy (see Chap. 29).

f. Metabolic acidosis is usually mild unless significant tubular dysfunction exists (see **III.I**). Use sodium bicarbonate or sodium citrate to correct severe metabolic acidosis.

g. Nutrition is limited by severe fluid restriction. Infants who can take oral feedings are given a low-phosphate formula with a low renal solute load (e.g., Similac PM 60/40). Caloric density is increased to a maximum of 50 kcal/ounce with glucose polymers (Polycose) and corn oil. Parenteral nutrition is given when oral feeding is not tolerated. Protein is limited to 0.5 gm/kg/day and is increased as tolerated.

h. Hypertension (see **III.C**)

i. Drugs that are renally excreted must have their dosing schedule adjusted in accordance with the patient's renal function. Potential nephrotoxic drugs such as indomethacin and aminoglycosides should be avoided.

j. Dialysis is indicated when conservative management has been unsuccessful in correcting severe fluid overload, hyperkalemia, acidosis, and uremia. Inadequate nutrition because of severe fluid restriction in the anuric infant is a relative indication. This procedure must be performed in centers where the staff have experience in infants.

C. **Blood pressure** in the newborn is related to weight and gestational age. Blood pressure rises with postnatal age, 1 to 2 mm Hg per day during the first week and 1 mm Hg per week during the next 6 weeks in both the preterm and full-term infant.

1. Normative values of blood pressure are shown for full-term infants and premature infants in Tables 31-7, 31-8, and 31-9.

2. **Hypertension** is defined as persistent blood pressure greater than 2 standard deviations above the mean. Premature infants with bronchopulmonary dysplasia or who have undergone umbilical artery catheterization are at increased risk for hypertension. The clinical signs and symptoms, which may be absent or nonspecific, include cardiorespiratory abnormalities such as tachypnea, cardiomegaly, or congestive heart failure; neurologic findings such as irritability, lethargy, or seizure; failure to thrive; or gastrointestinal difficulties.

3. Neonatal hypertension has many causes (Table 31-10), which may be determined by history and physical examination and a review of fluid status, medications, use and location of umbilical arterial catheter, maternal history, and other clinical findings such as intracranial hemorrhage and chronic lung disease. If a particular cause is suspected, proceed with appropriate laboratory evaluation. Otherwise, focus initial evaluation on renovascular and renal causes, which are most commonly responsible for

Table 31-7. Normal longitudinal blood pressure in full-term infants (mm Hg)

Age	Boys		Girls	
	Systolic	Diastolic	Systolic	Diastolic
1st day	67 ± 7	37 ± 7	68 ± 8	38 ± 7
4th day	76 ± 8	44 ± 9	75 ± 8	45 ± 8
1 month	84 ± 10	46 ± 9	82 ± 9	46 ± 10
3 months	92 ± 11	55 ± 10	89 ± 11	54 ± 10
6 months	96 ± 9	58 ± 10	92 ± 10	56 ± 10

From Gemeilli, M., Managanaro, R., Mami, C., et al. Longitudinal study of blood pressure during the 1st year of life. *Eur. J. Pediatr.* 149:318, 1990.

Table 31-8. Systolic and diastolic blood pressure ranges in infants of 500–2000 grams birth weight at 3–6 hours of life

Birth weight (gm)	Systolic (mm Hg)	Diastolic (mm Hg)
501–750	50–62	26–36
751–1000	48–59	23–36
1001–1250	49–61	26–35
1251–1500	46–56	23–33
1501–1750	46–58	23–33
1751–2000	48–61	24–35

From Hegyi, T., et al. Blood pressure ranges in premature infants. 1. The first hours of life. *J. Pediatr.* 124:627–633, 1994.

neonatal hypertension. Obtain urinalysis, renal function studies, serum electrolyte levels, and renal ultrasound examination. Color Doppler flow studies may detect aortic or renal vascular thrombosis. A DMSA renal scan may detect segmental renal arterial infarctions. Plasma renin levels are difficult to interpret in newborns.

4. Management is directed at correcting the underlying cause whenever possible. Antihypertensive therapy (Table 31-11) is administered for sustained hypertension not related to volume overload or medications.

D. **Renal vascular thrombosis** (see Chap. 26)

1. **Renal artery thrombosis (RAT)** is often related to the use of indwelling umbilical artery catheters. Management is controversial. The options include surgical thrombectomy, thrombolytic agents, and conservative medical care including antihypertensive therapy. The surgical renal salvage rate is no better than medical management, as it has a considerable mortality rate of 33%. Patients with unilateral RAT who received conservative medical treatment were normotensive by 2 years of age, were no longer receiving antihypertensive medications, and had normal creatinine clearance, although some have unilateral renal atrophy with compensatory contralateral hypertrophy.

2. **Renal vein thrombosis (RVT)** has the predisposing conditions of hyperosmolarity, polycythemia, hypovolemia, and hypercoagulable states. The clinical findings include gross hematuria, enlarged kidneys, hypertension, and thrombocytopenia. The diagnosis of RVT is confirmed by ultrasound, which typically shows an enlarged kidney with diffuse homogenous hyperechogenicity; Doppler flow studies may detect thrombi in the inferior vena

Table 31-9. Mean arterial blood pressure (MAP) in infants of 500–1500 grams birth weight

Birth weight (gm)	MAP ± SD (mm Hg)		
	Day 3	Day 17	Day 31
501–750	38 ± 8	44 ± 8	46 ± 11
751–1000	43 ± 9	45 ± 7	47 ± 9
1001–1250	43 ± 8	46 ± 9	48 ± 8
1251–1500	45 ± 8	47 ± 8	47 ± 9

From Klaus, M. H., and Fanaroff, A. A. (eds.). *Care of the High-risk Neonate.* Philadelphia: W.B. Saunders, 1993, p. 497.

Table 31-10. Causes of hypertension in the neonate

Vascular
  Renal artery thrombosis
  Renal vein thrombosis
  Coarctation of the aorta
  Renal artery stenosis
  Idiopathic arterial calcification
Renal
  Obstructive uropathy
  Polycystic kidney disease
  Renal insufficiency
  Renal tumor
    Wilms' tumor
  Glomerulonephritis
  Pyelonephritis
Endocrine
  Congenital adrenal hypoplasia
  Primary hyperaldosteronism
  Hyperthyroidism
Neurologic
  Increased intracranial pressure
  Cushing's disease
  Neural crest tumor
  Cerebral angioma
  Drug withdrawal
Pulmonary
  Bronchopulmonary dysplasia
Drugs
  Corticosteroids
  Theophylline
  Adrenergic agents
  Phenylephrine
Other
  Fluid/electrolyte overload
  Abdominal surgery
  Associated with extracorporeal membrane oxygenation (ECMO)

cava or renal vein. The management of RVT is also controversial. Initial therapy should focus on the underlying predisposing clinical condition. Assessment of the coagulation status includes platelet count, prothrombin time, partial thromboplastin time, fibrinogen, and fibrin split products. No consensus exists on the use of heparin. Our approach depends on the patient's clinical status. If there is unilateral involvement without evidence of disseminated intravascular coagulation (DIC), we use conservative management. If there is bilateral involvement and evidence of DIC, we initiate heparin therapy with an initial bolus of 50 to 100 units/kg followed by continuous infusion at 25 to 50 units/kg to maintain PTT of 1.5 times normal.

Thrombolytic therapy with streptokinase and urokinase have been used in both RAT and RVT, with variable success (see Chap. 26).

E. **Proteinuria** in newborns is frequently normal. After the first week, persistent proteinuria greater than 250 mg/m^2/24 hours should be investigated (see Table 31-3).

  1. In general, **mild proteinuria** reflects a vascular or tubular injury to the kidney. Administration of large amounts of colloid can exceed the reabsorptive capacity of the neonatal renal tubules and may result in mild proteinuria. **Massive proteinuria** (>1.5 g/m^2/24 hours), hypoalbuminemia with serum albumin levels less than 2.5 g/dl, and edema are all compo-

Table 31-11. Antihypertensive agents for the newborn (see Appendix)

	Dose	Comment
Diuretics		
Furosemide	0.5–1.0 mg/kg/dose IV, IM, PO	May cause hyponatremia, hypokalemia, hypercalciuria
Chlorothiazide	20–50 mg/kg/day; divided qd or bid	May cause hyponatremia, hypokalemia, hypochloremia
Vasodilators		
Hydralazine	1–8 mg/kg/day; divided q 6–8 hr	May cause tachycardia
Nitroprusside	0.2–6 μg/kg/min	Monitor isothiocyanate levels
Calcium channel blockers		
Nifedipine	0.2 mg/kg/dose SL[1], PO	Limited use in neonates; may cause tachycardia
Beta receptor antagonist		
Propranolol	0.5–5.0 mg/kg/day PO; divided q 6–8 hr	May cause bronchospasm
Alpha/beta receptor antagonist		
Labetalol	0.5–1.0 mg/kg/dose IV, q 4–6 hr	Limited use in neonates
ACE[2] inhibitor		
Captopril	0.15–2.0 mg/kg/day PO, divided q 8–12 hr	May cause oliguria, hyperkalemia, renal failure
Enalapril	5–10 μg/kg/dose IV, q 8–24 hr	May cause oliguria, hyperkalemia, renal failure

[1]Sublingual.
[2]Angiotensin-converting enzyme.

nents of congenital nephrotic syndrome. A renal biopsy is often required for final diagnosis. Prenatal diagnosis of Finnish-type nephrotic syndrome is possible before the 20th week of gestation by detection of elevated maternal and amniotic alpha-fetoprotein levels.

2. No specific treatment is required for mild proteinuria. Treat the underlying disease and monitor the proteinuria until resolved.

F. **Hematuria** is defined as greater than 5 red blood cells per high-power field. It is uncommon in newborns and should always be investigated.

1. Hematuria has many causes (Table 31-12). The differential diagnosis for hematuria includes urate staining of the diaper, myoglobinuria, or hemoglobinuria. A negative dipstick with benign sediment suggests urates, while a positive dipstick with negative sediment for RBCs indicates the present of globin pigments. Vaginal bleeding in girls or a severe diaper rash is also a possible cause of blood in the diaper or positive dipstick for heme.

2. Evaluation of neonatal hematuria depends on the clinical situation. In most cases, the initial investigation includes the following tests: urinalysis with examination of the sediment, urine culture, ultrasound of the upper and lower urinary tract, evaluation of renal function (serum creatinine and BUN), and coagulation studies.

G. **Urinary tract infection (UTI)** (see Chap. 23)

1. Infections of the urinary tract in newborns can result in asymptomatic bacteriuria or can lead to pyelonephritis and/or sepsis. A urine culture should be obtained from every infant with fever, poor weight gain, poor feeding, unexplained prolonged jaundice, or any clinical signs of sepsis.

2. The diagnosis is confirmed by positive urine culture obtained by suprapubic bladder aspiration or catheterized specimen with a colony count exceeding 1000 colonies per millimeter. A blood culture should also be obtained, even from asymptomatic infants. Although most newborns with UTIs have leukocytes in the urine, an infection can be present in the absence of leukocyturia.

3. *Escherichia coli* accounts for approximately 75% of the infections. The remainder are caused by other gram-negative bacilli (*Klebsiella, Enterobacter, Proteus*) and by gram-positive cocci (enterococci, *Staphylococcus epidermidis, Staphylococcus aureus*).

Table 31-12. Etiology of hematuria in the newborn

Acute tubular necrosis
Cortical necrosis
Vascular diseases
  Renal vein thrombosis
  Renal artery thrombosis
Bleeding and clotting disorders
  Disseminated intravascular coagulation
  Severe thrombocytopenia
  Clotting factors deficiency
Urological anomalies
Urinary tract infection
Glomerular diseases (see proteinuria)
Tumors
  Wilms' tumor
  Neuroblastoma
  Angiomas
Nephrocalcinosis
Trauma
  Suprapubic bladder aspiration
  Urethral catheterization

4. Evaluation of the urinary tract by ultrasound and VCUG is needed to detect urological abnormalities. Vesicoureteral reflex occurs in 40% of neonates with UTIs and predominates slightly in boys. If renal abnormality is detected, a renal scan is done to assess renal cortex and function. Inadequate therapy, particularly in the presence of urological abnormalities, could lead to renal scarring with potential development of hypertension and loss of renal function.

5. The initial treatment is antibiotics, usually a combination of ampicillin and gentamicin, given parenterally. The final choice of antibiotic is based on the sensitivity of the cultured organism. Treatment is continued for 10 to 14 days, and amoxicillin prophylaxis (20 mg/kg/day) is administered until a VCUG is performed. If VUR is present, prophylactic treatment should continue until the reflux has resolved.

H. Fanconi syndrome is a group of disorders with generalized dysfunction of the proximal tubule resulting in excessive urinary losses of amino acids, glucose, phosphate, and bicarbonate. The glomerular function is usually normal.

1. Clinical and laboratory findings
   a. Hypophosphatemia is due to the excessive urinary loss of phosphate. In these patients the tubular reabsorption of phosphate (TRP) is abnormally low. Rickets and osteoporosis are secondary to hypophosphatemia and can appear in the neonatal period.
   b. Metabolic acidosis is secondary to bicarbonate wasting (type II renal tubular acidosis).
   c. Aminoaciduria and glycosuria do not result in significant clinical signs or symptoms.
   d. These infants are often polyuric and therefore at risk for dehydration. Hypokalemia, due to increased excretion by the distal tubule to compensate for the increased sodium reabsorption, is also frequent and sometimes profound.

2. Etiology: The primary form of Fanconi syndrome is rare in the neonatal period and is a diagnosis of exclusion. Although familial cases (mainly autosomal dominant) have been reported, it is generally sporadic. Most secondary forms of the syndrome in the neonatal period are related to inborn errors of metabolism, including cystinosis, hereditary tyrosinemia, hereditary fructose intolerance, galactosemia, glycogenosis, and Lowe syndrome (oculocerebro-renal syndrome). Cases associated with heavy metal toxicity have also been described.

I. Renal tubular acidosis (RTA) is defined as metabolic acidosis resulting from the inability of the kidney to excrete hydrogen ions or to reabsorb bicarbonate. Poor growth may result from RTA.

1. **Distal RTA (type I)** is caused by a defect in the secretion of hydrogen ions by the distal tubule. The urine cannot be acidified below a pH of 6. It is frequently associated with hypokalemia and hypercalciuria. Nephrocalcinosis is common later in life. In the neonatal period, distal RTA may be primary, due to a genetic defect, or secondary to several disorders including nephrocalcinosis, obstructive uropathies, drugs such as amphotericin B, heavy metals, and hereditary elliptocytosis.

2. **Proximal RTA (type II)** is a defect in the proximal tubule with reduced bicarbonate reabsorption leading to bicarbonate wasting. Serum bicarbonate concentration falls until the abnormally low threshold for bicarbonate reabsorption is reached in the proximal tubule (generally below 16 mEq/L). Once this threshold has been reached, no significant amount of bicarbonate reaches the distal tubule, and the urine can be acidified at that level. Proximal RTA can occur as an isolated defect or in association with Fanconi syndrome (see **III.H**).

3. **Hyperkalemic RTA (type IV)** is a result of a combined impaired ability of the distal tubule to excrete hydrogen ions and potassium. In the neonatal period, this disorder is seen in infants with aldosterone deficiency, adrenogenital syndrome, reduced tubular responsiveness to aldosterone,

or associated obstructive uropathies. It can also be induced by treatment with angiotensin-converting enzyme (ACE) inhibitors or spironolactone.

4. The treatment of RTA is based on correction of the acidosis with alkaline therapy. Sodium bicarbonate, 2 to 3 mEq/kg/day in divided doses, is usually sufficient to treat type I and type IV RTA. The treatment of proximal RTA often requires more than 10 mEq/kg/day bicarbonate. In secondary forms, the treatment of the primary cause often results in the resolution of the RTA.

J. **Nephrocalcinosis (NC)** is detected by renal ultrasound examinations (see Chap. 29).

1. NC is generally associated with a hypercalciuric state. Drugs that are associated with NC and increased urinary calcium excretion include loop diuretics such as furosemide, methylxanthines, glucocorticoids, and vitamin D in pharmacological doses. In addition, hyperoxaluria, often associated with parenteral nutrition, and hyperphosphaturia facilitate the deposition of calcium crystals in the kidney.

2. Renal stones and NC secondary to primary oxalosis, renal tubular acidosis, or urinary tract infections are rare in newborns.

3. Few follow-up studies of NC in premature infants are available. In general, renal function is not significantly impaired, and most cases resolve spontaneously within the first year of life as demonstrated by ultrasound. However, significant tubular dysfunction at 1 to 2 years of age has been reported.

4. It is unclear whether NC requires a specific treatment. If possible, drugs that cause hypercalciuria should be discontinued.

K. The principal differential diagnosis of **polycystic kidney disease** in the newborn includes autosomal recessive polycystic kidney disease (ARPKD), the infantile form of autosomal dominant polycystic kidney disease (ADPKD), and glomerulocystic kidney disease (which in some affected families represents a variant of ADPKD).

1. In ARPKD, the kidneys appear markedly enlarged and hyperechogenic by ultrasound, with a typical "snowstorm" appearance. In contrast, macroscopic cysts are usually detected in cases of ADPKD and glomerulocystic disease. The clinical findings are variable and include renal insufficiency, which usually progresses to renal failure and severe renin-mediated hypertension. Infants with more severe cases may have oligohydramnios with pulmonary hypoplasia and Potter's syndrome. ARPKD is always associated with liver involvement. The diagnosis is confirmed by renal biopsy, unless the family history is certain.

2. In ADPKD, abnormal gene PKD1 has been identified and located on the short arm of chromosome 16.

3. Other hereditary syndromes that can manifest as renal cystic disease include tuberous sclerosis; von Hippel-Lindau disease; Jeune's asphyxiating thoracic dysplasia; oral-facial-digital syndrome, type 1; and brachymesomelia-renal syndrome.

L. The decision for **circumcision** is based primarily on cultural or ethnic background. Circumcision is medically indicated when urinary retention is due to adhesions of the foreskin or to tight phimosis. Circumcision is avoided in cases of hypospadias, ambiguous genitalia, and bleeding disorders (see Chap. 5).

Reference

1. Bailie, M.D. (ed.). Renal function and disease. *Clin. Perinatol.* 19(1), 1992 (entire issue).

32. NECROTIZING ENTEROCOLITIS

Karen R. McAlmon

I. **Background. Necrotizing enterocolitis (NEC)** is an acute intestinal necrosis syndrome of unknown etiology. Our understanding of the pathophysiology is largely speculative. Its pathogenesis, however, is probably complex and multifactorial. Inflammatory mediators may play a crucial role. Current clinical practice is directed toward prompt, early diagnosis and rapid institution of proper intensive care management.

A. **Epidemiology.** NEC is the most common serious surgical disorder among infants in a neonatal intensive care unit (NICU) and is a significant cause of neonatal morbidity and mortality.

1. The **incidence** of NEC varies from center to center and from year to year within centers. There are endemic and epidemic occurrences. An estimated 0.3 to 2.4 cases occur in every 1000 live births. In most centers, NEC occurs in 2–5% of all NICU admissions and 5–10% of VLBW infants. If infants who die early are excluded and only infants who have been fed included, the incidence is approximately 15%.

2. Sex, race, geography, climate, and season do not appear to play any determining role in the incidence or course of NEC.

3. **Prematurity** is the single greatest risk factor. Decreasing gestational age is associated with an increased risk for NEC. The mean gestational age of infants with NEC is 30–32 weeks, and the infants are generally appropriate for gestational age. Approximately 10% of infants are full-term. The postnatal age at onset is inversely related to birth weight and gestational age. The mean age at onset is 12 days, and the mode is 3 days. More than 90% of infants have been fed prior to the onset of this disease.

4. Infants exposed to **cocaine** have a 2.5 times increased risk of developing NEC. The vasoconstrictive and hemodynamic properties of cocaine may promote intestinal ischemia (see Chap. 19).

5. The overall **mortality** is 9–28% regardless of surgical or medical intervention. The mortality for infants weighing less than 1500 grams is up to 45%; for those weighing less than 750 grams, it ranges from 40 to 100%. The introduction of standardized therapeutic protocols with criteria for medical management and surgical intervention, as well as a high index of suspicion for the disease and general improvements in neonatal intensive care, have decreased the mortality rate. Infants exposed to cocaine who develop NEC have a significantly higher incidence of massive gangrene, perforation, and mortality than do infants not exposed.

6. Case-controlled epidemiologic studies have revealed that almost all previously described risk factors for NEC, including maternal disorders (e.g., toxemia), the infant's course [e.g., asphyxia, patent ductus arteriosus (PDA)], and the type of management (e.g., umbilical artery catheterization), simply describe a population of high-risk neonates. Excluding cocaine exposure, no maternal or neonatal factors other than prematurity are known to increase the risk of NEC. This suggests that immaturity of the gastrointestinal tract is the greatest risk factor.

B. **Pathogenesis**

1. The **causes** of NEC are not well defined. NEC is likely a heterogeneous disease resulting from complex interactions between mucosal injury secondary to a variety of factors, including ischemia, luminal substrate, and infection, and poor host protective mechanism(s) in response to injury.

2. The concept of a **hypoxic or hemodynamic insult,** resulting in splanchnic vasoconstriction and reduced mesenteric flow, inducing bowel mucosal hypoxia and rendering the intestine susceptible to injury, has long been considered a probable cause of NEC. The pathologic findings resemble those seen in older individuals with vascular compromise. However, in a significant number of cases no hypoxic or ischemic problems could be identified, and the temporal sequence of events does not support an ischemic event alone. Indocin use has been associated with NEC (see Chap. 25).

3. **Enteral feedings** have been implicated in the pathogenesis of NEC, potentially serving as a substrate for microbiologic flora and producing intestinal inflammation and injury. Factors that have been considered include osmolality of the formula, the lack of immunoprotective factors in the formula, and the timing, volume, and rate of feeding. In animal studies, breast milk has been shown to have protective factors; however, breast milk alone does not protect against NEC. Some studies have shown that very slow introduction of feedings and avoidance of large day-to-day volume increases may lower the incidence of NEC. However, the exact rate of feeding increment that predisposes infants to NEC has not been identified, and the mechanism by which excessive volumes predispose to the development of NEC is not known.

4. The **microbiologic flora** involved in NEC are not unique but represent the predominant bowel organisms present in the infant at the time of onset. Various bacterial and viral agents have been included in the microbial picture that is sometimes associated with NEC, especially with epidemic NEC, but none has yet been proved to be causal. Release of endotoxin and cytokines by proliferation of colonizing bacteria, and bacterial fermentation with gaseous distention, may play a role.

5. Increasing evidence supports a critical role for **platelet activating factor (PAF)** and other inflammatory mediators in the pathophysiology of NEC. Animal studies show that exogenous administration or endogenous increased production of PAF causes ischemic bowel necrosis pathologically similar to NEC. Several factors may promote (e.g., leukotrienes, oxygen radicals, tumor necrosis factor) or inhibit (e.g., acetylhydrolase, steroids, nitric oxide, prostacyclin) PAF-induced intestinal injury. PAF antagonists, including dexamethasone and PAF acetylhydrolase, prevent this histologic necrosis. All the NEC risk factors—prematurity, hypoxia, feeding, and bacteria—tend to increase the concentration of circulating or local PAF.

6. **Histopathologic examination** of tissue after surgery or autopsy indicates that the terminal ileum and ascending colon are the most frequently involved areas, but in the most severe cases the entire bowel may be involved. This localization has implications for long-term sequelae (see **IV**). The pathologic lesions consist of coagulation necrosis, bacterial overgrowth, inflammation, and reparative changes. These suggest that the disease is initiated by subtotal ischemia and gradual tissue compromise that results in bacterial invasion and inflammation.

II. Diagnosis. Early diagnosis of NEC is the most important factor in determining outcome. This is accomplished by careful clinical observation for nonspecific signs in infants at risk.

A. **Clinical characteristics.** There is a broad spectrum of disease manifestations. The clinical features of NEC can be divided into systemic and abdominal signs. Most infants have a combination of both.

1. **Systemic signs:** Respiratory distress, apnea or bradycardia (or both), lethargy, temperature instability, irritability, poor feeding, hypotension (shock), decreased peripheral perfusion, acidosis, oliguria, bleeding diathesis.

2. **Abdominal (enteric) signs:** Abdominal distention, abdominal tenderness, gastric aspirates (feeding residuals), vomiting (of bile, blood, or both), ileus (decreased or absent bowel sounds), abdominal wall ery-

thema or induration, persistent localized abdominal mass, ascites, bloody stools.

3. The **course of the disease** varies among infants. Most frequently, it will appear (a) as a fulminant, rapidly progressive presentation of signs consistent with intestinal necrosis and sepsis or (b) as a slow, paroxysmal presentation of abdominal distention, ileus, and possible infection. The latter course will vary with the rapidity of therapeutic intervention and require consistent monitoring and anticipatory evaluation [4] (see **III**).

B. **Laboratory features.** The diagnosis is suspected from clinical presentation but must be confirmed by diagnostic radiographs, surgery, or autopsy. No laboratory tests are specific for NEC; nevertheless, some tests are valuable in confirming diagnostic impressions.

1. **Roentgenograms.** The abdominal roentgenogram will often reveal an abnormal gas pattern consistent with ileus. Both anteroposterior (AP) and cross-table lateral or left lateral decubitus views should be included. These films may reveal bowel wall edema, a fixed-position loop on serial studies, the appearance of a mass, pneumatosis cystoides intestinalis (the radiologic hallmark used to confirm the diagnosis), portal or hepatic venous air, pneumobilia, or pneumoperitoneum.

2. **Blood studies.** Thrombocytopenia, persistent metabolic acidosis, and severe refractory hyponatremia constitute the most common triad of signs and help to confirm the diagnosis.

3. **Analysis of stool** for blood and carbohydrate has been used to detect infants with NEC based on changes in intestinal integrity. Although grossly bloody stools may be an indication of NEC, occult hematochezia does not correlate well with NEC. Carbohydrate malabsorption, as reflected in a positive stool Clinitest result, can be a frequent and early indicator of NEC within the setting of signs noted in **A.**

C. **Bell staging criteria** with the Walsh and Kleigman modification allow uniformity of diagnosis and treatment based on severity of illness.

1. **Stage I** (suspect) clinical signs and symptoms, nondiagnostic radiographs

2. **Stage II** (definite) clinical signs and symptoms, pneumatosis intestinalis on radiograph
   a. Mildly ill
   b. Moderately ill with systemic toxicity

3. **Stage III** (advanced) clinical signs and symptoms, pneumatosis intestinalis on radiograph, and critically ill
   a. Impending intestinal perforation
   b. Proven intestinal perforation

D. **Differential diagnosis**

1. **Pneumonia and sepsis** are common and frequently are associated with an abdominal ileus. The abdominal distention and tenderness characteristic of NEC will be absent, however.

2. **Surgical abdominal catastrophes** include malrotation with obstruction (complete or intermittent), malrotation with midgut volvulus, intussusception, ulcer, gastric perforation, and mesenteric vessel thrombosis (see Chap. 26, Hematologic Problems). The clinical presentation of these disorders may overlap with that of NEC. Occasionally, the diagnosis is made only at the time of exploratory laparotomy.

3. **Infectious enterocolitis** is rare in this population but must be considered if diarrhea is present. *Campylobacter* species have been associated with bloody diarrhea in the newborn. These infants lack any other systemic or enteric signs of NEC.

4. Severe forms of **inherited metabolic disease** (e.g., galactosemia with *Escherichia coli* sepsis) may lead to profound acidosis, shock, and vomiting and may initially overlap with some signs of NEC.

5. **Feeding intolerance** is a common but ill-defined problem in premature infants. Despite adequate gastrointestinal function in utero, some premature infants will have periods of gastric residuals and abdominal dis-

tention associated with advancing feedings. The differentiation of this problem from NEC can be difficult. Cautious evaluation by withholding enteral feedings and administering intravenous fluids and antibiotics for 72 hours may be indicated until this benign disorder can be distinguished from NEC.

E. Additional diagnostic considerations

1. Since the early features are often nonspecific, a high index of suspicion is the most reliable approach to early diagnosis. The entire picture of history, physical examination, and laboratory features must be considered in the context of the particular infant's course. Isolated signs or laboratory values often indicate the need for a careful differential diagnosis, despite the obvious concern over NEC.

2. **Diarrhea** is an uncommon presentation of NEC in the absence of bloody stools. This sign should point away from NEC.

3. **Roentgenographic findings** can often be subtle and confusing. For example, perforation of an abdominal viscus will not always cause pneumoperitoneum, and conversely, pneumoperitoneum does not necessarily indicate abdominal perforation from NEC. Careful serial review of the roentgenograms with a pediatric radiologist is indicated to assist in interpretation and to plan for further appropriate studies.

III. Management

A. Immediate medical management. Treatment should begin promptly when signs suggestive of NEC are present. Therapy is based on intensive care measures and the anticipation of potential problems.

1. **Respiratory function.** Rapid assessment of ventilatory status (physical examination, arterial blood gases) should be made, and supplemental oxygen and mechanical ventilatory support should be provided as needed.

2. **Cardiovascular function.** Rapid assessment of circulatory status (physical examination, blood pressure) should be made, and circulatory support should be provided as needed. In critically ill infants, we use fresh-frozen plasma (dose 10 ml/kg), since this is also a good source of clotting factors (see **6**). Pharmacologic support may be necessary; in this case, we use low doses of dopamine (3 to 5 gm/kg/min) to optimize the effect on splanchnic and renal blood flow. Impending circulatory collapse will often be reflected by poor perfusion and oxygenation, even though arterial blood pressure may be maintained. Intraarterial blood pressure monitoring is often necessary, but the proximity of the umbilical arteries to the mesenteric circulation precludes the use of these vessels. In fact, any umbilical artery catheter should be promptly removed and peripheral artery catheters used. Further monitoring of central venous pressure (CVP) may become necessary if additional pharmacologic support of the circulation or failing myocardium is needed (see Chap. 17).

3. **Metabolic function.** Severe metabolic acidosis will generally respond to volume expansion but may require treatment with sodium bicarbonate (dose 2 mEq/kg q6–8h). The blood pH should be carefully monitored; in addition, serum electrolyte levels and liver function should be measured. Blood glucose levels should be watched closely (see Chap. 9).

4. **Nutrition.** All gastrointestinal feedings are discontinued, and the bowel is decompressed by suctioning through a nasogastric tube. Parenteral nutrition (PN) is given through a peripheral vein as soon as possible, with the aim of providing 90 to 110 cal/kg per day once amino acid solutions and Intralipid are both tolerated. A central venous catheter may be necessary to provide adequate calories in the very-low-birth-weight infant. We wait to place a central catheter for this purpose until the blood cultures are negative for 3 days, during which time adaptation to peripheral PN can take place.

5. **Infectious disease.** Blood, urine, stool, and cerebrospinal fluid (CSF) specimens are obtained, examined carefully for indications of infection,

and sent for culture and sensitivity. We routinely begin broad-spectrum antibiotics as soon as possible, utilizing ampicillin, gentamicin, and clindamycin to cover most enteric flora. With changing antibiotic sensitivities, one must be aware of the predominant NICU flora, the organisms associated with NEC, and their resistance patterns and adjust antibiotic coverage accordingly. Stool should be tested for aminoglycoside-resistant organisms. Antibiotic therapy is adjusted on the basis of culture results, but only 10 to 40% of blood cultures will be positive, necessitating continued broad coverage in most cases. Treatment is generally maintained for 14 days. There is no evidence to support the use of enteral antibiotics.

6. **Hematologic aspects.** Analysis of the complete blood count and differential, with examination of the blood smear, is always indicated. We use platelet transfusions to correct severe thrombocytopenia and packed red blood cells to maintain the hematocrit above 35%. Neutropenia may be severe, and in extreme cases we treat it with whole blood exchange transfusion (see Chap. 26, Hematologic Problems). The prothrombin time, partial thromboplastin time, fibrinogen, and platelet count should be evaluated for evidence of disseminated intravascular coagulation. Fresh-frozen plasma is used to treat coagulation problems. In addition, we administer vitamin K to these infants (see Chap. 10, Nutrition), since they are not fed enterally for a long time.

7. **Renal function.** Oliguria often accompanies the initial hypotension and hypoperfusion of NEC; careful evaluation of urine output is essential. In addition, serum blood urea nitrogen (BUN), creatinine, and serum electrolyte levels should be monitored. Impending renal failure from acute tubular necrosis, coagulative necrosis, or vascular accident must be anticipated, and fluid therapy must be adjusted accordingly (see Chap. 31).

8. **Neurologic function.** Evaluation of the infant's condition is difficult given the degree of illness, but one must be alert to the problems of associated meningitis and intraventricular hemorrhage. Seizures may occur secondary to either of these problems or from the metabolic perturbations associated with NEC. These complications must be anticipated and promptly recognized and treated.

9. **Gastrointestinal function.** Physical examination and serial (every 6 to 8 hours during the first 2 to 3 days) roentgenograms are used to assess ongoing gastrointestinal damage. Unless perforation occurs or full-thickness necrosis precipitates severe peritonitis, the management of this system will be medical. The evaluation for surgical intervention, however, is an important and complex management issue (see **B**).

10. **Family support.** Any family of an infant in the NICU may be overwhelmed by the crisis. Infants with NEC present a particular challenge because the disease often causes sudden deterioration for "no apparent reason." Furthermore, the impending possibility of surgical intervention and the high mortality and uncertain prognosis make this situation most difficult for parents. Careful anticipatory sharing of information must be utilized by the staff to establish a trusting alliance with the family.

B. **Surgical intervention**
1. **Prompt consultation** should be obtained with a pediatric surgeon. This will allow the surgeon to become familiar with the case and will provide an additional evaluation by another skilled individual.
2. **Gastrointestinal perforation** is generally agreed on as an indication for intervention. Unfortunately, there is no reliable or absolute indicator of imminent perforation; therefore, careful monitoring is necessary. Perforation occurs in 20 to 30% of patients, usually 12 to 48 hours after the onset of NEC, although it can occur later. In some cases, the absence of pneumoperitoneum on the abdominal radiograph can delay the diagnosis, and paracentesis may aid in establishing the diagnosis. In general, an infant with increasing abdominal distention, an abdominal mass, a worsening clinical picture despite medical management, or a persistent

fixed loop on serial roentgenographic studies may have a perforation and may require operative intervention.

3. **Full-thickness necrosis of the gastrointestinal tract** may require surgical intervention, although this diagnosis is difficult to establish in the absence of perforation. In most cases, the infant with bowel necrosis will have signs of peritonitis, such as ascites, abdominal mass, abdominal wall erythema, induration, persistent thrombocytopenia, progressive shock from third-space losses, or refractory metabolic acidosis. Improvement may not occur until the necrotic bowel has been surgically removed. Paracentesis may help to identify these patients before perforation occurs.

4. At **surgery,** the goal is to excise necrotic bowel while preserving as much bowel length as possible. Peritoneal fluid is examined for signs of infection and sent for culture, necrotic bowel is resected and sent for pathologic confirmation, and viable bowel ends are exteriorized as stomas. All sites of diseased bowel are noted, whether or not removal is indicated. If there is extensive involvement, a "second look" operation is done within 24 to 48 hours to determine whether any areas that appeared necrotic are actually viable. The length and areas of removed bowel are recorded. If large areas are resected, the length and position of the remaining bowel are noted, since this will affect the long-term outcome. In approximately 14% of infants with this condition, NEC totalis (bowel necrosis from duodenum to rectum) is found. In these cases mortality is certain.

C. **Long-term management.** Once the infant has been stabilized and effectively treated, feedings can be reintroduced. We generally begin this process after 2 weeks of treatment by stopping nasogastric decompression. If infants can tolerate their own secretions, feedings are begun very slowly while parenteral alimentation is gradually tapered. No conclusive data are available on the best method or type of feeding. We sometimes use an elemental lactose-free formula. The occurrence of strictures may complicate feeding plans. The incidence of recurrent NEC is 4% and does not appear to be related to any type of management. Recurrent disease should be treated as before and will generally respond similarly. If surgical intervention was required and an ileostomy or colostomy was created, intestinal reanastomosis can be electively undertaken after an adequate period of healing. Before reanastomosis, a contrast study of the distal bowel is obtained to establish the presence of a stricture that can be resected at the time of ostomy closure.

IV. **Prognosis.** Few detailed and accurate studies are available on prognosis. In uncomplicated cases of NEC, the long-term prognosis may be comparable with that of other low-birth-weight infants; however, those with Stage IIB and Stage III NEC have a higher incidence of growth delay (delay in growth of head circumference is of most concern). NEC requiring surgical intervention may have more serious sequelae, including increased morbidity and mortality secondary to infection, respiratory failure, parenteral nutrition–associated hepatic disease, rickets, and significant developmental delay.

A. **Sequelae** of NEC can be directly related to the disease process or to the long-term NICU management often necessary to treat it. Gastrointestinal sequelae include strictures, enteric fistulas, short bowel syndrome, malabsorption and chronic diarrhea, dumping syndromes related to loss of terminal ileum and ileocecal valve, fluid and electrolyte losses with rapid dehydration, and hepatitis or cholestasis related to long-term PN. Strictures occur in 25 to 35% of patients with or without surgery and are most common in the large bowel. Short bowel syndrome occurs in approximately 10 to 20% following surgical treatment. Metabolic sequelae include failure to thrive, metabolic bone disease, and problems related to CNS function in the very-low-birth-weight infant.

B. **Prevention of NEC is the ultimate goal.** Unfortunately, this can best be accomplished only by preventing premature birth. If prematurity cannot be avoided, several preventive strategies may be of benefit:

1. **Induction of gastrointestinal maturation.** The incidence of NEC is significantly reduced after prenatal steroid therapy.
2. **Alteration of the immunologic status of the intestine.** Oral immunoglobulins may have potential benefit, and in one study IgA and IgG supplementation of feedings reduced the incidence of NEC. Breast milk contains many immunoprotective factors; however, no study has convincingly demonstrated that breast milk alone can prevent NEC.
3. **Optimization of enteral feedings** (Chap. 10). Very slow introduction of feedings may be useful, but more data are required, including the possible harmful effects of this nutritional approach.
4. **Reduction or antagonism of inflammatory mediators.** Since many of the factors associated with NEC promote increased PAF concentrations and the subsequent inflammatory cascade resulting in bowel injury, trials of oral PAF antagonists may reduce the incidence and severity of NEC.

References

Czyrko, C., Del Pin, C. A., O'Neill, J. A., et al. Maternal cocaine abuse and necrotizing enterocolitis: Outcome and survival. *J. Pediatr. Surg.* 26:414–421, 1991.

Kliegman, R. M., Walker, W. A., Yolken, R. H. Necrotizing enterocolitis: Research agenda for a disease of unknown etiology and pathogenesis. *Pediatr. Res.* 34:701–708, 1993.

Stoll, B. J., Kliegman, R. M., eds. Necrotizing enterocolitis. *Clin. Perinatol.* Philadelphia: W. B. Saunders, 21(2): 1994.

33. SURGICAL EMERGENCIES IN THE NEWBORN [1,3,5]

Steven A. Ringer

I. **Fetal manifestations**
   A. **Polyhydramnios** (amniotic fluid volume >2 liters) occurs in 1 in 1000 births.
      1. **Gastrointestinal (GI) obstruction** (including esophageal atresia) is the most frequent surgical cause of polyhydramnios.
      2. **Other causes** of polyhydramnios include abdominal wall defects (omphalocele and gastroschisis), anencephaly, diaphragmatic hernia, tight nuchal cord, fetal death, inability of the fetus to concentrate urine, maternal diabetes, and anything causing an inability of the fetus to swallow.
      3. All women in whom polyhydramnios is suspected should have an ultrasonographic examination. In experienced hands, these studies are the method of choice for the diagnosis of intestinal obstruction, abdominal wall defects, and diaphragmatic hernia, as well as abnormalities leading to an inability of the fetus to swallow.
      4. If an obstructing intestinal lesion is diagnosed antenatally and there is no evidence of dystocia, vaginal delivery is acceptable. Pediatric surgical consultation should be obtained prior to delivery.
   B. **Dystocia** may result from fetal intestinal obstruction, abdominal wall defect, genitourinary anomalies, or fetal ascites (see **I.D**).
   C. **Meconium peritonitis**
      1. A **plain film of the abdomen** will show scattered calcific shadows. Most congenital lesions causing intestinal obstruction (see **IV.A**) have, on occasion, produced meconium peritonitis.
      2. **Meconium peritonitis** is often associated with an antenatal perforation of the intestinal tract.
   D. **Fetal ascites** (see **VI**) is usually associated with urinary tract anomalies (lower urinary tract obstruction due to posterior urethral valves). Other causes are hemolytic disease of the newborn, any severe anemia (e.g., alpha-thalassemia), peritonitis, thoracic duct obstruction, cardiac disease, hepatic or portal vein obstruction, hepatitis, and congenital infection (e.g., syphilis or TORCH infections; see Chap. 23) as well as other causes of hydrops fetalis (see Chap. 18). After birth, ascites may be seen in the congenital nephrotic syndrome. **Prenatal ultrasound** is important in light of recent advances of fetal surgery, which might allow decompression of either the bladder or a hydronephrotic kidney and can save renal parenchyma (see Chaps. 1, 31).
   E. **Oligohydramnios** is usually associated with intrauterine growth retardation, postmaturity, or fetal distress, but it may indicate absent kidneys (Potter's syndrome; see Chap. 31) or amniotic fluid leak.
II. **Postnatal manifestations** [25]
   A. **Respiratory distress** (see **III.B** and **C** and Chaps. 4, 24)
      1. **Choanal atresia.** If bilateral, the baby is unable to breathe nasally (see **III.C.6**).
      2. Laryngotracheal clefts (see **III.C.4**)
      3. Tracheal agenesis
      4. Esophageal atresia with or without tracheoesophageal fistula (TEF) (see **III.A**)
      5. Diaphragmatic hernia (see **III.B**)
      6. Congenital lobar emphysema

7. Cystic adenomatoid malformation of the lung.
8. Biliary tracheobronchial communication (extremely rare)
B. Scaphoid abdomen
1. Diaphragmatic hernia (see **III.B**)
2. Esophageal atresia without TEF (see **III.A**)
C. Excessive mucus and salivations—esophageal atresia (see **III.A**)
Some clinicians advocate passing an orogastric tube in all newborns shortly after delivery to rule out esophageal atresia. We wait for clinical symptoms rather than screen routinely.
D. Pneumoperitoneum
1. **Perforated stomach** is associated with large amounts of free intraabdominal air. At times it is necessary to aspirate air from the abdominal cavity to relieve respiratory distress prior to definitive surgical repair. The lesion is associated with localized ischemia of the stomach and requires simple closure.
2. **Perforated Meckel's diverticulum** in the newborn is associated with free intraabdominal air.
3. **Perforated appendix** is associated with free intraabdominal air in the newborn.
4. Air from a pulmonary air leak may dissect into the peritoneal cavity in infants on ventilators.
5. Any perforation of the bowel may cause pneumoperitoneum (see Chap. 32).
E. Gaseous distention has a rapid onset in the left upper quadrant when there is complete duodenal obstruction. Lower obstruction causes more generalized distention, which varies with location. Gaseous distention can occur where there is esophageal atresia with TEF (see **III.A**). In the normal infant, the progression of the air column seen on an x-ray film of the abdomen is as follows: **1 hour** after birth the air is past the stomach into the upper jejunum; **3 hours** after birth it is at the cecum; by **8 to 12 hours** after birth it is at the rectosigmoid. The movement of air through the bowel is slower in the premature infant.
F. Vomiting. The causes of vomiting can be differentiated by the presence or absence of bile. The presence of bile-stained vomit in the newborn should be treated as a life-threatening emergency, with at least 20% of such infants requiring surgical intervention immediately after evaluation. Surgical consultation should be obtained immediately.
1. **Bile-stained vomitus.** Intestinal obstruction may result from malrotation with or without volvulus; duodenal, jejunal, ileal, or colonic atresias; annular pancreas; Hirschsprung's disease; aberrant superior mesenteric artery; preduodenal portal vein; peritoneal bands—persistent omphalomesenteric duct; or duodenal duplication. Bile-stained vomitus is occasionally seen in infants without intestinal obstruction. In these cases the bile-stained vomiting will only occur one or two times and will present without abdominal distention.
2. **Non-bile-stained vomitus**
a. Overfeeding (feeding excessive volume)
b. Milk or formula intolerance
c. Sepsis
d. Central nervous system (CNS) lesion
e. Lesion above ampulla of Vater
(1) Pyloric stenosis
(2) Upper duodenal stenosis
(3) Annular pancreas (rare)
G. Failure to pass meconium can occur in sick babies with decreased tone and in premature infants. It also may be the result of the following disorders:
1. Imperforate anus
2. Functional intestinal obstruction (see **IV.C**)
H. Failute to develop transitional fecal stools after the passage of meconium

   1. Volvulus
   2. Malrotation
 I. **Hematemesis and bloody stools**
   1. Necrotizing enterocolitis (most frequent cause of hematemesis and bloody stool in premature infants; see Chap. 32)
   2. Gastric and duodenal ulcers (due to stress) and Cushing-Rokitansky–type ulcer (e.g., CNS disease, meningitis, kernicterus, and CNS tumors)
   3. Coagulation disorder (see Chap. 26, Bleeding)
   4. Disseminated intravascular coagulation (DIC) (see Chap. 26, Bleeding)
   5. Duodenal stenosis
   6. Meckel's diverticulum
   7. Duplications of the small intestine
   8. Volvulus
   9. Intussusception
   10. Polyps, hemangiomas
   11. Cirsoid aneurysm
   12. Formula intolerance (usually protein intolerance)
   13. Maternal blood
       a. **Maternal blood** is sometimes swallowed by the newborn during labor and delivery. This can be diagnosed by an Apt test performed on blood aspirated from the infant's stomach (see **X.C** and Chap. 26, Anemia).
       b. In breast-fed infants, if blood obtained from the infant's stomach is adult blood, inspection of the mother's breasts or having the mother express milk from her breasts may reveal the source of blood. If the stomach is aspirated before a feeding and no blood is found, the baby should then nurse and the stomach should be aspirated after the feeding to document the breast as the source of the blood.
 J. **Abdominal masses** (see **VIII**)
   1. Genitourinary anomalies (see **VI** and Chap. 31)
   2. Tumors (see **VII**)
   3. Distended bladder
 K. **Birth trauma** (see Chap. 20)
   1. Lacerated solid organs—liver, spleen
   2. Spinal cord transection with quadriplegia
III. **Lesions causing respiratory difficulty**
 A. **Esophageal atresia** can occur with or without TEF.
   1. Esophageal atresia occurs with TEF in at least 85% of infants [5]. These infants may present with respiratory distress due to airway obstruction secondary to excess secretions, abdominal distention and diaphragmatic elevation, or both. Respiratory distress also can occur from the reflux of gastric contents up the distal esophagus into the lung by way of the fistula. Excessive salivation and vomiting soon after feedings are often the first clue in the nursery.
   2. **Esophageal atresia** itself is diagnosed by the inability to pass a catheter into the stomach. To confirm that the esophagus is patent, a catheter is passed and air is injected into the catheter while one listens over the stomach. The diagnosis is confirmed by x-ray studies showing the catheter coiled in the upper esophageal pouch. Plain x-ray films may demonstrate a distended blind upper esophageal pouch filled with air that is unable to progress into the stomach. Some infants may have associated vertebral anomalies of the cervical or upper thoracic region of the spine. Pushing 50 ml of air into the catheter under fluoroscopic examination may show dilatation and relaxation of the upper pouch, thus avoiding contrast studies.
   3. Rarely, esophageal atresia may occur without a TEF or with the fistula connecting with the upper esophagus. No GI gas will be seen on x-ray examination, and the abdomen is scaphoid. Respiratory difficulties are less acute. Diagnostic maneuvers are the same as in **2**.

4. TEF without esophageal atresia (H-type fistula) is extremely rare and usually presents after the neonatal period. Diagnosis is suggested by a history of frequent pneumonias or respiratory distress temporally related to meals. This disorder can often be demonstrated with administration of nonionic water-soluble contrast medium (iohexol [Omnipaque]) and cinefluoroscopy. The definitive examination is combined fiberoptic bronchoscopy and esophagoscopy with passage of a fine balloon catheter from the trachea into the esophagus. The H-type fistula is usually high in the trachea (cervical area).

5. Babies with esophageal atresia with or without TEF are often of low birth weight. Approximately 21% of these babies are premature (five times the normal incidence), and 19% are small for gestational age (eight times the normal incidence). Other anomalies may be present, including the syndrome of vertebral and vascular defects, imperforate anus, TEF with esophageal atresia, renal dysplasia, renal defects (VATER syndrome), and chromosomal anomalies.

6. **Management.** A **multiple end-hole suction catheter (Replogle)** should be placed in the proximal pouch and put under intermittent suction at the time the diagnosis is made. Prior to transportation of an infant with esophageal atresia with TEF, a suction cannula must be placed in the proximal pouch. Guidelines for intubation are the same as for other types of respiratory distress (see Chap. 36). If intubation is required, ventilation should be at an increased rate with low pressure to prevent gastric and intestinal distention. In the usual TEF, the fistula to the trachea is near the carina. Care must be taken to avoid accidental intubation of the fistula. If possible, it is best to avoid mechanical ventilation of these babies until the fistula is closed bcause the abdomen may become very distended, presenting a risk of compromising ventilation. The baby should be transported in the upright position (at about 45 degrees) to diminish reflux of gastric contents into the fistula. Surgical therapy usually involves immediate placement of a gastrostomy tube. As soon as the infant can tolerate further surgery, the fistula is divided, and primary repair of the esophagus is performed. Many infants with esophageal atresia are premature or have other defects that make it advisable to delay primary repair. They will need careful nursing care to prevent aspiration and total parenteral nutrition to allow growth until repair. We usually do the primary repair when the infant's weight is 2000 gm. **Mechanical ventilation** and nutritional management may be difficult in these infants because of the TEF. This problem has occasionally forced us to do the repair before the infant weighs 2000 gm. If the infant has cardiac disease requiring surgery, it is usually best to repair the fistula before cardiac surgery; if not, the postoperative ventilatory management will be very difficult.

B. **Diaphragmatic hernia**

1. Respiratory distress associated with a scaphoid abdomen and development of bowel sounds in a hemithorax are pathognomonic of diaphragmatic hernia. The most common site is the left hemithorax, with the defect in the diaphragm being posterior (foramen of Bochdalek in 70% of infants). It also can occur on the right, with either an anterior or a posterior defect.

2. The **incidence** is between 1 in 2000 to 5000. Fifty percent of these hernias are associated with other malformations, especially neural tube defects, cardiac defects, and intestinal malrotation. In some families diaphragmatic hernia recurs. Diaphragmatic hernia has been associated with trisomies 13 and 18, and 45,XO, and has been reported as part of Goldenhar's, Beckwith-Wiedemann, Pierre Robin, Goltz-Gorlin, and the rubella syndromes.

3. **Symptoms.** Infants with large diaphragmatic hernias may present at birth with cyanosis, respiratory distress, a scaphoid abdomen, de-

creased or absent breath sounds on the side of the hernia, and heart sounds displaced to the side opposite the hernia. Small hernias, right-sided hernias, and substernal hernias of Morgagni may have a more subtle onset, manifested by feeding problems and mild respiratory distress.

4. **Diagnosis.** The diagnosis is confirmed by x-ray study. A radiopaque marker should be placed on one side of the chest to aid interpretation of the x-ray film. The diagnosis is often made prenatally by ultrasonic studies, which may be precipitated by the occurrence of polyhydramnios. Diagnosis earlier in gestation because of some fetal symptom (e.g., polyhydramnios) may be correlated with a poorer prognosis. However, a prenatal diagnosis should lead to delivery in a center equipped to optimize chances for survival. If delivery before term is likely, fetal lung maturity should be assessed. If these indices are immature, maternal therapy with betamethasone should be given (see Chap. 24).

5. **Treatment**
   a. **Intubation.** A large sump nasogastric tube should be inserted immediately at the time of delivery if the diagnosis has been made antenatally, or at the time of postnatal diagnosis. It is safest to immediately intubate all diagnosed infants antenatally at delivery. If assisted ventilation is required in infants diagnosed after birth, it should be given by means of endotracheal tube. Bag and mask ventilation is contraindicated. All infants requiring transport should be intubated. Care must be taken with assisted ventilation to keep inspiratory pressures low to avoid damage or rupture of the contralateral lung. Umbilical venous and arterial lines should be placed as rapidly as possible. Pancuronium and fentanyl were used by us in the past, but recently we have had better results when letting the infants breathe spontaneously.
   b. **Preoperative management** is focused on minimizing pulmonary hypertension and avoiding barotrauma. High-frequency oscillatory ventilation and assist-control modes of ventilation have shown promise.

6. **Surgical repair** is through either the abdomen or the chest, with reduction of intestine into the abdominal cavity. Diaphragmatic hernia is frequently associated with intestinal malrotation. Small babies may require abdominal mesh if the abdominal cavity is too small for the intestines.

7. **Mortality and prognosis**
   a. **Mortality** from diaphragmatic hernia, while improved with modern therapy, is as high as 40% [12]. Although repair of the defect itself is relatively straightforward, the underlying pulmonary hypoplasia and pulmonary hypertension are largely responsible for overall mortality (see Chap. 24, Persistent Pulmonary Hypertension of the Newborn).
   b. **Prognosis.** Avoidance of hypoxia and acidosis will aid in minimizing pulmonary hypertension, and initial oxygen tension (PO_2) and carbon dioxide tension (PCO_2) after institution of therapy are predictive of prognosis. In addition, the later the onset of postnatal symptoms, the higher the survival rate. Newer therapies, including extracorporeal membrane oxygenation and nitric oxide inhalation therapy, offer the promise of improved survival (see Chap. 24, Extracorporeal Membrane Oxygenation).

C. **Other mechanical causes for respiratory difficulty**
   1. **Congenital lobar emphysema** may be due to a malformation, a cyst in the bronchus, or a mucous or meconium plug in the bronchus. These lesions cause air trapping, compression of surrounding structures, and respiratory distress. There may be a primary malformation of the lobe **(polyalveolar lobe).** Overdistention from mechanical ventilation may

cause lobar emphysema. Extrinsic pressure on a bronchus also can cause obstruction. Congenital lobar emphysema usually affects the upper and middle lobes on the right and the upper lobe on the left. Diagnosis is by chest x-ray studies.

   a. High-frequency ventilation may resolve the lobar emphysema (see Chap. 24).

   b. Elective intubation of the opposite bronchus may decompress the lobe if overinflation is thought to be the cause and if the infant can tolerate it. When the tube is withdrawn to the trachea after 8 to 12 hours, the lobar emphysema may not recur. Occasionally, selective suctioning of the bronchus on the side of the lesion may remove obstructing mucus or meconium and resolve the pulmonary problem. Treatment of acquired lobar emphysema (from inflammation of a bronchus) has included dexamethasone, 0.5 mg/kg per day for 3 days. If the child is symptomatic and conservative measures fail, the child should undergo an operation. Bronchoscopy should be performed to remove any obstructing material or rupture a bronchogenic cyst; if this procedure fails, the involved lobe should be resected.

  2. Cystic adenomatoid malformation of the lung may be confused with a diaphragmatic hernia. Respiratory distress is related to the effect of the mass on the uninvolved lung. This malformation can cause shifting of the mediastinal structures.

  3. Vascular rings. The symptomatology of vascular rings is related to the architecture of the ring. Both respiratory (stridor) and GI symptoms (vomiting, difficulty swallowing) may occur, depending on the anatomy of the ring. Barium swallow radiography is diagnostic.

  4. Laryngotracheal clefts. The length of the cleft determines the symptoms. The diagnosis is made by instillation of contrast material into the esophagus and is confirmed by bronchoscopy. Very ill newborns should undergo immediate bronchoscopy without contrast studies.

  5. Tracheal agenesis. This rare lesion is suspected when a tube cannot be passed down the trachea and the infant is ventilated by way of bronchi coming off the esophagus. Diagnosis is by use of contrast material in the esophagus and by endoscopy.

  6. Choanal atresia. Respiratory distress in the delivery room is associated with bilateral lesions. Infants are obligate nose breathers until the approximate age of 4 months. An oral airway is satisfactory initial treatment. Definitive therapy includes burrowing a hole through the bony plate, which can be accomplished with a laser, if available.

  7. Robin anomaly (Pierre Robin syndrome) consists of a hypoplastic mandible associated with a midline cleft palate. Airway obstruction often occurs secondary to the tongue occluding the airway. Forcibly pulling the tongue forward will relieve the obstruction. The neonate is best cared for in the prone position. These infants often improve after placement of a nasopharyngeal or endotracheal tube. If the infant can be helped for a few days, he or she will sometimes adapt, and aggressive procedures can be avoided. Button procedures have been utilized to avoid a tracheostomy (this button procedure is rarely indicated). A gastrostomy may be necessary for feeding, but a specialized feeder (Breck) can be used to feed the child. Some children will require tracheostomy and gastrostomy.

  8. Laryngeal web occludes the larynx. Perforation of the web by a stiff endotracheal tube or bronchoscopy instrument may be lifesaving.

IV. Lesions causing mechanical intestinal obstruction [10]. The most critical lesion to rule out is **malrotation with volvulus.** All patients with suspected intestinal obstruction should have a nasogastric sump catheter placed without delay.

  A. Congenital mechanical obstruction [10]

    1. Intrinsic types include atresia, stenosis, hypertrophic pyloric stenosis, meconium ileus (associated with cystic fibrosis or a rare form [familial

or nonfamilial] that is not associated with cystic fibrosis [10]), cysts within the lumen of the bowel, and imperforate anus.
   2. **Extrinsic** forms include malrotation with or without midgut volvulus, volvulus without malrotation, congenital peritoneal bands with or without malrotation, incarcerated hernia (premature infants), annular pancreas, duplications of the intestine, aberrant vessels (usually the mesenteric artery or preduodenal portal vein), hydrometrocolpos, and obstructing bands (persistent omphalomesenteric duct).
B. **Acquired mechanical obstruction**
   1. Malrotation with volvulus
   2. Intussusception
   3. Peritoneal adhesions
      a. After meconium peritonitis
      b. Idiopathic
      c. After an operation
   4. Mesenteric thrombosis
   5. Meconium and mucous plugs
   6. Necrotizing enterocolitis (acute and secondary to scarring and healing)
   7. Formation of abnormal intestinal concretions not associated with cystic fibrosis
C. **Functional intestinal obstruction** constitutes the major cause of intestinal obstruction seen in any neonatal unit.
   1. **Immaturity of large bowel**
   2. **Defective innervation (Hirschsprung's disease)**
   3. **Paralytic ileus**
      a. Induced by maternal drug ingestion
         (1) Narcotics
         (2) Hexamethonium bromide
         (3) Hypermagnesemia due to prenatal use of magnesium sulfate
      b. Sepsis
      c. *Pseudomonas* enteritis
   4. **Meconium plug syndrome**
   5. **Endocrine disorders**
      a. Hypothyroidism
      b. Adrenal insufficiency
   6. **Intrinsic defects in the bowel wall**
   7. **Other disorders** (e.g., sepsis, CNS disease, necrotizing enterocolitis)
D. **Other disorders associated with intestinal obstruction**
   1. **Duodenal atresia** in 70% of infants is associated with other malformations, including Down syndrome, cardiovascular anomalies, and such other GI anomalies as annular pancreas, esophageal atresia, malrotation of the small intestine, small-bowel atresias, and imperforate anus.
      a. There may be a history of polyhydramnios.
      b. Prenatal diagnosis is commonly made by ultrasound.
      c. Vomiting of bile-stained material usually begins a few hours after birth.
      d. Abdominal distention is limited to the upper abdomen.
      e. The infant may pass meconium in the first 24 hours of life; then bowel movements cease.
      f. Aspiration of the stomach returns more than 30 ml of gastric contents prior to feeding.
      g. A plain x-ray film of the abdomen will show air in the stomach and upper part of the abdomen ("double bubble") with no air in the small or large bowel.
      h. The neonate may be jaundiced in the presence of intestinal obstruction.
      i. Preoperative management includes nasogastric suction. Contrast radiographs of the upper intestine are not mandatory preoperatively.

2. **Pyloric stenosis** typically presents with nonbilious vomiting after the age of 2 to 3 weeks, but it has been seen in the first week of life. X-ray examination will show a large stomach; little or no gas is found below the duodenum. Often the pyloric mass cannot be felt in the newborn. The infant may have associated jaundice and hematemesis. An upper GI series is diagnostic. Real-time ultrasonography is used increasingly in diagnosis.

3. **Meconium ileus** is a frequent cause of meconium peritonitis. In most other obstructions, flat and upright x-ray films will demonstrate fluid levels. This is not the case for meconium ileus if fetal perforation has not occurred. Instead, the distended bowel may be granular in appearance or may show tiny bubbles mixed with meconium.

   a. No meconium will pass through the rectum, even after digital stimulation.

   b. Rare cases (both familial and nonfamilial) of meconium ileus are not associated with cystic fibrosis but display the clinical picture and x-ray findings described in **IV.C**.

   c. Cheek brushing for DNA analysis is becoming the standard initial screening for cystic fibrosis [24]. If the results are negative or equivocal, a sweat test should be performed.

   d. Results of tests of stool trypsin activity are negative with cystic fibrosis, but they are also negative with all types of complete obstruction (see **X.E**).

   e. Contrast enemas can be both diagnostic and therapeutic. Meglumine diatrizoate (Gastrografin) can be used in an adequately hydrated neonate. Diatrizoate sodium (Hypaque) also can be used. Both of these contrast agents are hypertonic. The baby should be well hydrated, and fluids should be run at two to three times the maintenance level. Meglumine diatrizoate is often diluted 1 : 4 before use.

   f. If the diagnosis is certain and the neonate stable, repeat enemas with a hyperosmolar, ionic contrast material meglumine diatrizoate or diatrizoate sodium may be used to relieve the impaction.

   g. Nasogastric suction should be used to prevent further distention.

   h. Distal atresias can accompany meconium ileus and require surgical therapy.

   i. Surgical therapy is required if the contrast enema fails to relieve the obstruction.

4. **Imperforate anus** is often associated with other anomalies such as esophageal atresia with or without TEF and is a component of the VATER syndrome. Infants with imperforate anus may pass meconium if a rectovaginal or rectourinary fistula exists; in these infants, the diagnosis may be missed.

   There are two types of imperforate anus: low and high. Eighty percent of females with imperforate anus have the low type; 50% of males have the low type.

   a. Low imperforate anus. The rectum has descended through the puborectalis sling and exists on the perineum as a fistula.

   (1) Meconium may be passed into the vagina.

   (2) Meconium may be visualized on the perineum. In males it may be found in the rugal folds of the scrotum.

   (3) Perineal fistulas may be dilated to temporarily relieve intestinal obstruction and allow passage of meconium.

   b. High imperforate anus. The rectum ends above the puborectalis sling. No perineal fistula is present. The fistula may enter the urinary tract or vagina.

   (1) The presence of meconium particles in the urine is diagnostic of a rectovesical fistula. Vaginal examination with a nasal speculum or cystoscope may reveal a fistula.

(2) A cystogram may show a fistula and the level of rectal descent. Injection of dye into the most distal portion of the pouch may show the level of rectal descent. Use of the Wangensteen-Rice technique of taking anteroposterior and lateral films in the upside-down position at the age of 48 hours may be misleading if the distal rectum is filled with meconium [5].

(3) Ultrasound is often helpful in defining the distal level of the rectum.

(4) Temporary colostomy is necessary in all neonates with a high imperforate anus with or without fistula.

5. **Volvulus with or without malrotation of the bowel**
   a. Malrotation may be associated with other GI abnormalities such as diaphragmatic hernia, annular pancreas, and bowel atresias.
   b. If this condition develops during fetal life, it may cause the appearance of a large midabdominal calcific shadow on x-ray examination; this results from calcification of meconium in the segment of necrotic bowel.
   c. After birth there is a sudden onset of bilious vomiting in an infant who has had some normal stools. If the level of obstruction is high, there may not be much abdominal distention.
   d. Signs of shock and sepsis are often present.
   e. Plain x-rays will show a dilated small bowel.
   f. If a malrotation is present, barium enema may show failure of barium to pass beyond the transverse colon or may show the cecum in an abnormal position.
   g. Demonstration of an absent or abnormal position of the ligament of Treitz confirms the diagnosis of malrotation. An upper GI series for localization of the ligament of Treitz is the most reliable diagnostic study for malrotation.
   h. Malrotation as the cause of intestinal obstruction is a surgical emergency because intestinal viability is at stake.

6. **Annular pancreas** may be nonobstructing but associated with duodenal atresia or stenosis. It presents as a high intestinal obstruction.

7. **Hydrometrocolpos**
   a. The hymen bulges.
   b. Accumulated secretions in the uterus may cause intestinal obstruction by bowel compression.
   c. Meconium peritonitis or hydronephrosis may occur.
   d. Edema and cyanosis of the legs may be observed.
   e. If hydrometrocolpos is not diagnosed at birth, the secretions will decrease, the bulging will disappear, and the diagnosis will be missed until puberty.

8. **Meconium and mucous plug syndrome** is seen in premature babies, infants of diabetic mothers, and sick babies (see also **IV.D.3**); it also can be caused by functional immaturity of the bowel with a small left colon, as seen in infants of diabetic mothers; meconium or mucous plug; or Hirschsprung's disease (see **IV.D.9**), which should always be considered when a newborn has difficulty passing stools. **Treatment** consists of glycerin suppository and one-half normal warm saline enemas (5 to 10 ml/kg) and stimulation with soft rubber catheter. A normal stooling pattern should follow evacuation of a plug. Contrast enema with a hyperosmolar contrast material may be both diagnostic and therapeutic.

9. **Hirschsprung's disease** should be suspected in any newborn who fails to pass meconium spontaneously by 24 to 48 hours after birth and who develops distention relieved by rectal stimulation. This is especially so if the infant is not premature or is not the infant of a diabetic mother or has the problems seen in **IV.C**. The diagnosis should be considered until future development shows sustained normal bowel function.

    a. Parents taking home a newborn suspected of having Hirschsprung's disease must understand the importance of immediately reporting obstipation, diarrhea, poor feeding, distention, lethargy, or fever. A toxic megacolon may be fatal.

    b. Barium enema frequently does not show the characteristic transition zone in the neonate. Suction rectal biopsy can be helpful if ganglion cells are found in a submucosal zone, thereby ruling out Hirschsprung's disease.

    c. Histochemical tests of biopsy specimens show an increase in acetylcholine. Formal full-thickness rectal biopsy is the definitive method for diagnosis.

    d. Obstipation can be relieved by gentle rectal irrigations with warm saline solution.

    e. Neonates require colostomy when diagnosis is made. Definitive repair is postponed until the infant is between the age of 8 and 12 months or weighs between 7.5 and 9.0 kg.

V. Other surgical problems

  A. Appendicitis is extremely rare in newborns. Its presentation may be that of pneumoperitoneum. The appendix usually perforates prior to the diagnosis; therefore, the baby may present with intestinal obstruction, sepsis, or even DIC related to the intraabdominal infection. Rule out Hirschsprung's disease.

  B. Omphalocele [11]. **The sac may be intact or ruptured.** The diagnosis is often made by prenatal ultrasound. Cesarean section may prevent rupture of the sac, but is not specifically indicated unless the defect is large (>5 cm) or contains liver.

    1. Intact sac. Emergency treatment includes the following:

      a. Nasogastric sump sunction

      b. Cover sac with warm, saline-soaked gauze.

      c. Wrap sac on abdomen with Kling gauze and cover with plastic wrap so as to support the intestinal viscera on the abdominal wall.

      d. Thoroughly wrap the neonate to prevent heat loss.

      e. Keep the infant warm.

      f. There should be no attempt to reduce the sac because this can cause rupture of the sac, interfere with venous return from the sac, and cause respiratory distress.

      g. Place a reliable intravenous line **in an upper extremity.**

      h. Start broad-spectrum antibiotics (ampicillin and gentamicin).

      i. Arrange a surgical consultation; definitive surgical therapy should be delayed until the baby is thoroughly resuscitated. Monitor temperature and pH. In the presence of other more serious abnormalities (respiratory or cardiac), definitive care can be postponed as long as the sac remains intact.

    2. Ruptured sac

      a. Nasogastric sump suction

      b. Place a saline-soaked gauze over the exposed intestine, and then wrap the baby in a dry, sterile towel to prevent heat loss.

      c. Monitor temperature and pH.

      d. Start a reliable intravenous line in an upper extremity.

      e. Start broad-spectrum antibiotics (ampicillin and gentamicin).

      f. Arrange emergency surgical treatment to cover the intestine.

      g. Bowel viability may be compromised with a small defect and an obstructed segment of eviscerated intestine. Prior to transfer, the defect must be enlarged in these circumstances by incising the abdomen cephalad or caudad to relieve the strangulated viscera.

    3. Omphalocele may be associated with other anomalies such as chromosomal defects, malrotation of the colon, congenital heart disease, or extrophy of the cloaca. A careful search must be made for associated problems. The Beckwith-Wiedemann syndrome includes omphalocele, macroglossia, hypoglycemia, and hemihypertrophy.

C. Gastroschisis [15], by definition, contains no sac and the intestine is eviscerated.
  1. Nasogastric sump suction
  2. Monitor temperature and pH.
  3. Cover exposed intestine with saline-soaked gauze, and wrap the baby in a dry, sterile towel to prevent heat loss.
  4. Start a reliable intravenous line in an upper extremity.
  5. Get immediate surgical evaluation.
  6. Ten percent of infants with gastroschisis have intestial atresia. Other anomalies should be searched for.
VI. Renal disorders (see Chap. 31)
  A. Genitourinary abnormalities should be suspected in babies with abdominal distention, ascites, flank masses, persistently distended bladder, poor nutrition, bacteriuria, or pyuria. All male infants, and especially those displaying symptoms, should be observed for voiding patterns. Normal voiding is forceful; voiding occurs by 24 hours in 92% of term babies and in 90% of premature babies (it occurs by 48 hours in 99% of normal babies).
    1. Posterior urethral valves may cause obstruction.
    2. Spontaneous pneumomediastinum or pneumothorax in infants not being given ventilatory assistance has been associated with obstructive urinary tract disease.
  B. Renal vein thrombosis. Hematuria with a flank mass suggests the diagnosis of renal vein thrombosis.
    1. Renal ultrasound will initially show a large kidney on the side of the thrombosis. In time the kidney will become small.
    2. Doppler ultrasound will show no blood flow.
    3. **Treatment** in the past was usually nephrectomy. Treatment in most centers now consists of supporting the patient medically and avoiding surgery. Heparin is not usually used by us in this disorder but has been advocated by some (see Chaps. 31, 26, Major Arterial and Venous Thrombosis Management).
  C. Extrophy of the bladder ranges from an epispadias to complete extrusion of the bladder on the abdominal wall. Currently, most centers are attempting bladder turn-in within the first 48 hours of life.
    1. **Preoperative Management**
      a. Use moist, fine-mesh gauze or petroleum jelly–impregnated gauze to cover the exposed bladder.
      b. Intravenous pyelography (IVP) is not required preoperatively, although renal ultrasound is useful.
      c. Transport the infant to a facility for definitive care within 48 hours.
    2. **Intraoperative management.** Surgical management of an extrophied bladder includes turn-in of the bladder to preserve bladder function. The symphysis pubis is approximated. The penis is lengthened. Iliac osteotomies are not necessary if repair is accomplished within 48 hours. No attempt is made to make the bladder continent at this procedure.
  D. Cloacal exstrophy is a complex GI and genitourinary anomaly that includes vesicointestinal fissure, omphalocele, extrophied bladder, hypoplastic colon, imperforate anus, absence of vagina in females, and microphallus in males.
    1. **Preoperative management**
      a. **Genetic counseling.** It is surgically easier to rear the child as a female, regardless of genotype.
      b. Nasogastric suction relieves partial intestinal obstruction. The baby excretes stool through a vesicointestinal fissure that is often partially obstructed.
      c. A series of complex operations is required in stages to achieve the most satisfactory results.
    2. **Surgical management**
      a. The initial procedure includes division of the vesicointestinal fissure and establishment of fecal and urinary stomas.

      b. The bladder can be closed during the initial procedure if the baby is stable.

      c. Subsequent procedures are designed to reduce the number of stomas.

VII. Tumors [7,13,16]

  A. Neuroblastoma is the most common malignant neonatal tumor, making up about 50% of neonatal malignant tumors [4]. It may be massive or minute, irregular, and stony hard. There are many sites of origin; the adrenal-retroperitoneal area is the most common. This tumor can, on rare occasions, cause diarrhea or hypertension by the release of tumor by-products, especially catecholamines or vasointestinal peptides. Tests should be performed to determine levels of catecholamines and their metabolites. Calcifications can often be seen on plain radiographs. Ultrasound is the most useful test. Prenatal diagnosis by ultrasound improves prognosis [6].

  B. Wilms' tumor is the second most common malignant tumor in the newborn. It presents as a smooth, flat mass and may be bilateral. One should palpate gently to avoid rupture. Ultrasound is the most useful diagnostic test.

  C. Teratomas are the most common tumor in the neonatal period. They are most commonly found in the sacrococcygeal area. Some occur in the retroperitoneal area, and some arise in the ovaries. They can arise anywhere. Approximately 10% contain malignant elements. Prenatal diagnosis is often made by ultrasound. After delivery, rectal examination, ultrasound, computed tomography (CT), magnetic resonance imaging (MRI), as well as serum alpha-fetoprotein and beta-human chorionic gonadotropin measurements are used in evaluation. Calcifications are often seen on x-ray films. Excessive heat loss, platelet trapping, and dystocia are often seen.

  D. Sarcoma botryoides. This grapelike tumor arises from the edge of the vulva or vagina. It may be small and thus be confused with a normal posterior vaginal tag. IVP is an important test preoperatively, especially to avoid confusing the lesion with an obstructing ureterocele.

  E. Other tumors

    1. Hemangiomas

    2. Lymphangiomas

    3. Hepatoblastomas

    4. Hepatomas

    5. Hamartomas

    6. Nephromas

VIII. Abdominal masses [2]

  A. Renal masses (see **VI** and Chap. 31), polycystic kidneys, multicystic dysplastic kidney, hydronephrosis, renal vein thrombosis

  B. Tumors (see **VII**)

  C. Adrenal hemorrhage

  D. Ovarian tumor or cysts

  E. Pancreatic cyst

  F. Choledochal cyst

  G. Hydrometrocolpos

  H. Mesenteric or omental cyst

  I. Intestinal duplications

IX. Inguinal hernia [7,11] is found in 5% of premature infants weighing under 1500 gm, and as many as 30% of infants weighing less than 1000 gm at birth. It is more common in small-for-gestational-age infants and male infants. In females the ovary is often in the sac.

  A. Surgical repair. Inguinal hernia repair is the most common operation performed on premature infants. In general, in premature infants, hernias that are easily reducible and are causing no problems are repaired shortly before discharge home.

    1. Immediate repair. It may be a difficult operation and should be performed by an experienced pediatric surgeon. We have the infant's primary nurse and neonatologist go to the operating room with the infant to assist in the details of intraoperative management (see **XII**). The postoperative care is usually done by this same team. These infants should not be sent home on the day of surgery. They should be monitored overnight for apnea.

2. **Scheduled repair.** We have occasionally had well-instructed parents bring their babies home, and then have them admitted later for repair. This method of management has had poor results on occasion but has not been fully evaluated. Infants with pulmonary disease, such as bronchopulmonary dysplasia, are often best repaired at a later time when their respiratory status has improved. The use of spinal anesthesia has simplified the care of the infants with respiratory problems. It should be done by experienced anesthesiologists. In a term infant, repair should be scheduled when the diagnosis is made. An incarcerated hernia can usually be reduced with sedation, steady firm pressure, and elevation of the feet. If a hernia has been incarcerated, it should be repaired as soon as the edema is gone.

X. **Tests used in diagnosis**
   A. **X-ray examinations.** A flat plate radiograph of the abdomen usually will suffice. A left lateral decubitus radiograph is done to ascertain the presence of free air in the abdomen.
      1. **Barium enema** may sometimes (but not always) be diagnostic in suspected cases of Hirschsprung's disease. It may reveal microcolon in the infant with complete obstruction of the small intestine and may show a narrow segment in the sigmoid in the infant with meconium plug syndrome due to functional immaturity.
      2. **Barium swallow** with meglumine diatrizoate may be used to demonstrate H-type TEF without esophageal atresia.
      3. Some infants with Hirschsprung's disease will have problems passing barium after a barium enema. Gentle rectal saline washes are helpful in removing trapped air and barium.
      4. In patients with suspected malrotation, a combination of contrast studies may be necessary. A barium enema may show malposition of the cecum but will not always rule out malrotation. In combination with air or contrast media, an upper GI series will determine the presence or absence of the normally placed ligament of Treitz. Neonates with intestinal obstruction presumed secondary to malrotation require urgent surgery to relieve possible volvulus of the midgut.
   B. **Ultrasonography** is the preferred method of evaluating abdominal masses in the newborn. It is useful for defining the presence of masses, together with their size, shape, and consistency.
   C. The **Apt test** differentiates maternal from fetal blood. A small amount of bloody material is mixed with 5 ml of water and centrifuged. One part 0.25N sodium hydroxide is added to five parts of pink supernatant. The fluid remains pink in the presence of fetal blood but rapidly becomes brown if maternal blood is present. The test is useful only if the sample is not contaminated by pigmented material (e.g., meconium).
   D. **Cheek brush sampling for DNA analysis** is the initial test for cystic fibrosis, and will detect the majority of cases [8]. When the test result is negative but clinical suspicion remains high, a **sweat test** should be done. This test will not be accurate if less than 100 mg of sweat is collected. It may be necessary to repeat the test when the infant is 3 to 4 weeks old if inadequate sweat is collected.
   E. **Test for stool trypsin activity.** A negative result is not diagnostic of cystic fibrosis, since in any type of complete bowel obstruction the stool will be without enzyme activity. The method involves making 1 : 5 and 1 : 10 dilutions of meconium or stool and placing them on the gelatin side of undeveloped x-ray films. They should be incubated at 37°C for 1 hour. If trypsin activity is present, the gelatin will be dissolved.

F. CT is an excellent modality to evaluate abdominal masses as well as their relationship to other organs. Contrast enhancement can outline the intestine, blood vessels, kidneys, ureter, and bladder.

G. IVP use should be restricted to evaluating genitourinary anatomy if other modalities (ultrasound and contrast CT) are not available. The IVP dye is poorly concentrated in the newborn.

H. Radionuclide scan of the kidneys can aid in determining function. This is especially useful in assessing complex genitourinary anomalies and in evaluating the contribution of each kidney to renal function.

I. MRI is useful to better define the anatomy and location of masses.

XI. Management

A. Bilious vomiting and abdominal distention

1. Gastric suction with a sump catheter is mandatory if intestinal obstruction is suspected. All babies with presumed intestinal obstruction should be transported with a nasogastric suction catheter in place. A catheter-tip syringe (Becton-Dickinson catheter-tip 60-ml syringe no. 5664) should be available for continuous aspiration of gastric contents. Failure to decompress the stomach could lead to gastric rupture, aspiration, or respiratory compromise secondary to diaphragmatic compression. This is especially important in infants who are to be transported by air ambulance, since loss of cabin pressure may be associated with rupture of an inadequately drained viscus.

2. **Shock, dehydration, and electrolyte imbalance** should be treated if present, or measures should be taken to prevent these problems. The baby should be resuscitated with the appropriate fluids and electrolytes (see Chap. 9).

3. **Antibiotics** are used if there is suspicion of volvulus or any question about bowel integrity; broad coverage is indicated (ampicillin and gentamicin); clindamycin is used if there is perforation.

4. **Studies** that should be performed include the following:
   a. Hematocrit
   b. Electrolytes
   c. Blood gases and pH
   d. Clotting studies (e.g., prothrombin time, partial thromboplastin time, and platelet count)
   e. Continuous monitoring of oxygen saturation, blood pressure, and urine output is often indicated.

B. Nonbilious vomiting with distention. Many babies with nonbilious vomiting and distention respond to glycerin suppositories, half-strength saline enemas (5 ml/kg body weight), rectal stimulation with a soft rubber catheter, or a combination of these measures. It is important to rule out other nonfunctional causes of distention. Limited feedings, stimulation to the rectum, and care for the general condition of the baby will solve most of these problems. Plain x-ray studies are helpful. Barium enema should be used with caution because it may be difficult to evacuate the barium.

C. Vomiting without distention

1. If the baby's general condition is good, feedings of dextrose and water should be attempted. If these are tolerated, milk should be given again. If vomiting recurs, the baby should be given a trial of nonmilk formula. If this is successful, a trial of a milk formula should be undertaken in 2 weeks.

2. The mechanics of feeding the baby should be observed. Rapid feeding, difficult burping, and excessive volumes are all causes of nonbilious vomiting without distention.

3. The functional and mechanical causes must be ruled out.

D. Masses. The following steps may be taken for the diagnosis of the cause of abdominal masses:

1. X-ray examination of the chest and abdomen with the infant supine and upright

2. Abdominal ultrasonography
3. Contrast-enhanced CT
4. MRI
5. Determination of the level of catecholamines and their metabolites
6. Complete blood cell count and urinalysis
7. Angiography—venous and arterial
8. Surgical consultation

XII. **Intraoperative management**
A. **Monitoring devices**
1. Temperature probe
2. Electrocardiogram (ECG)
3. Arterial cannula to monitor blood gases and pressure. Transcutaneous PO_2 (see Chap. 24, Blood Gas Monitoring and Pulmonary Function Tests) is helpful but can be inaccurate when anesthetic agents that dilate skin vessels are used.
4. Pulse oximetry
B. **Well-functioning intravenous line.** In babies with omphalocele or gastroschisis, the intravenous line needs to be in the upper extremity or neck.
C. **Maintenance of body temperature**
1. Warmed operating room
2. Humidified, warmed anesthetic agents
3. Cover exposed parts of the baby, especially the head.
4. Warmed preparation solution, blood, and fluids used intraperitoneally
D. **Fluid replacement**
1. Replace lost blood with warmed packed cells if the loss is more than 15% of total blood volume.
2. Replace ascites loss milliliter per milliliter to maintain pressure.
3. The neonate loses approximately 5 ml of fluid per kilogram for each hour that the intestine is exposed. This should be replaced by Ringer's lactate or fresh-frozen plasma.
E. **Anesthetic management** of the neonate is reviewed in ref. 30 and Chap. 37.
F. **Postoperative pain management** is discussed in ref. 31 and Chap. 37.
G. Postoperatively, the newborn fluid requirement is two-thirds the standard maintenance level for the first 24 to 48 hours, plus continuing losses which must be replaced.

References

1. Altman, R. P., et al. Pediatric surgery. *Pediatr. Clin. North Am.* 40:1121, 1993.
2. Brodeur, A. E., et al. Abnormal masses in children: Neuroblastoma, Wilms tumor, and other considerations. *Pediatr. Rev.* 12:196, 1991.
3. Dillon, P. W., and Cilley, R. E. Newborn surgical emergencies. *Pediatr. Clin. North Am.* 40:1289, 1993.
4. Grosfeld, J. Neuroblastoma: A 1990 review. *Pediatr. Surg. Int.* 6:9, 1991.
5. Guzzetta, P. C., et al. General surgery. In G. B. Avery (Ed.), *Neonatology.* Philadelphia: Lippincott, 1994.
6. Ho, P. T., et al. Prenatal detection of neuroblastoma: A ten year experience from the Dana-Farber Cancer Institute and Children's Hospital. *Pediatrics* 92:358, 1993.
7. Nakayama, D. K., et al. Inguinal hernia and the acute scrotum in infants and children. *Pediatr. Rev.* 11:87, 1989.
8. Parad, R. B. Buccal cell DNA mutation analysis for diagnosis of cystic fibrosis in newborns and infants inaccessible to sweat chloride measurement. *Pediatrics* (in press).
9. Ringer, S. A., and Stark, A. S. Management of neonatal emergencies in the delivery room. *Clin. Perinatol.* 16:23, 1989.
10. Ross, A. J. Intestinal obstruction in the newborn. *Pediatr. Rev.* 15:338, 1994.
11. Sherer, L. R., III, et al. Inguinal hernias and umbilical anomalies. *J. Pediatr. Surg.* 40:1121, 1993.

12. West, K. N., et al. Delayed surgical repair and ECMO improves survival in congenital diaphragmatic hernia. *Ann. Surg.* 216:454, 1992.

34. SKIN CARE

Susan D. Izatt

I. **Skin care** in the newborn period must be given careful consideration [2,7]. Because the skin is a protective organ and because any break in integrity may create an opportunity for infection, care should involve cleaning that will offer protection and prevent infection. The term newborn infant is covered with **vernix caseosa,** a combination of secretions of the sebaceous glands and decomposing epidermis that is believed to be protective of the newborn skin. Preservation of the **acid mantle** of the skin is also important, as the skin surface pH of 4.95 has bacteriostatic effects.

   A. There should be **minimum manipulation of the skin to** prevent the following:
   1. Heat loss
   2. Trauma
   3. Exposure of the infant to agents that may have potentially harmful side effects (e.g., hexachlorophene)

   B. **Bathing** of the newborn
   1. Cleansing should be performed only after the infant has a stable body temperature.
   2. Blood and meconium should be removed from the face, neck, and perianal area by careful rinsing with water and a sterile cotton sponge. The remainder of the skin can be left alone unless it is grossly stained.
   3. Vernix caseosa should be removed from the face; it can remain on the rest of the body, to be removed by clothing and bedding.
   4. The diaper area should be cleaned with a water-soaked cotton sponge when soiled.
   5. Term infants may be bathed with warm water and a low-alkaline soap (BASIS, Lowella, Aveeno). Premature infants weighing less than 2000 gm should be bathed with warm sterile water only for the first week of life. Premature infants weighing less than 1000 gm should be washed with water only for the first 2 weeks of life. After these times, a low-alkaline soap can be used occasionally.
      We occasionally use Eucerin in small amounts if the skin develops cracks or fissures.

   C. Umbilical cord care in term infants involves exposure of the cord to the air and application of alcohol to the cord two times per day to aid drying and possibly to prevent infection. Care should be taken to limit the spillage of alcohol on the skin as it may be absorbed. After the cord has fallen off, the alcohol applications can be stopped. For infants who will be in the hospital more than a few days, topical antibiotic ointments are not used because use may encourage the emergence of bacteria that are resistant to multiple antibiotics.

   D. **Endotracheal tubes and catheters** placed in umbilical or peripheral vessels should be secured in place by adhesive tape on the skin that has been prepared with benzoin tincture. When this tape is removed, the edge of the tape is lifted and the skin-adhesive interface is wiped with an adhesive tape remover (Clinipad adhesive tape remover contains 1,1,1-trichloroethane, petroleum naphtha, and hexadecyl alcohol. Available from the Clinipad Corporation, Guilford, CT 06437). For small premature infants, we do not use the benzoin tincture or adhesives. We use Hollihesive (see **II.A.1**).

   E. Less important equipment can be attached to the skin by paper tape or by a hypoallergenic cloth tape that is less adherent (Dermicel. Available from Johnson & Johnson Products, Patient Care Division, 501 George Street, New Brunswick, NJ 08903).

F. Electrodes attached to the skin of premature infants should be secured by a gel adhesive that has been trimmed down to the minimum needed to hold the electrode.

G. Topical agents applied to the skin of infants may be absorbed and have systemic effects. Agents should not be used on newborn skin without attention to possible toxic effects from absorption.

II. Alterations in barrier function occur due to physical injury of the skin, immaturity, or skin disease [4].

A. Physical injury can result from a variety of insults. The decreased epidermal thickness due to the thin stratum corneum and the decreased cohesion between the epidermis and dermis place the premature infant at increased risk for injury. Damage to the protective barrier of the skin contributes to an increased risk of infection and possible scar formation [6].

1. **Epithelial damage and epidermal stripping** may occur with the use of adhesive agents. A pectin-based barrier (Hollihesive, Hollister, 2000 Hollister Drive, Libertyville, IL 60048) between the adhesive agent and the skin minimizes damage caused by removal and reapplication of tape, probes, and monitors [5].

2. **Chemical burns** may result from the use of disinfectants such as iodine and alcohol applied topically (see Chap. 2, Thyroid Diseases, on absorption of iodine solutions). Minimal exposure of the skin surface to these agents and careful removal with sterile water after use minimize the risk.

3. **Infiltration of intravenous solutions** containing caustic substances including dopamine, bicarbonate, calcium, and parenteral nutrition may cause tissue necrosis and sloughing. Treatment of dopamine infiltrations with **phentolamine** (Regitine, CIBA-GEIGY, Summit, NJ 07901) may decrease the localized vasoconstriction. Inject subcutaneously a 1 mg/ml solution of phentolamine in normal saline solution into the affected area. The amount needed (usually 1 to 5 ml) depends on the size of the infiltrate (see ref. 9 and Appendix). **Hyaluronidase** (Wydase, Wyeth-Ayerst Laboratories, Philadelphia, PA 19101) injected subcutaneously around the periphery of the site of infiltration of parenteral nutrition nafcillin, calcium, or bicarbonate may decrease tissue necrosis by temporarily destroying the interstitial barrier and increasing the absorptive area. Inject 1 ml (15 units) as five separate 0.2-ml injections around the periphery of the extravasation site with a 25 to 26 gauge needle (see ref. 9 and Appendix). Infiltration may require the use of bacitracin ointment and xeroform dressing for wound care. Benefit may be derived from consultation with a plastic surgeon for both acute wound care and the need for future skin grafting.

4. **Thermal injury** may occur from warming devices such as heel warmers and warming packs. Heated electrodes used with transcutaneous oxygen monitoring may cause erythema and crater formation in the premature skin.

5. **Pressure necrosis** can result from identification bands, endotracheal tubes, or pressure from intravenous boards or casts.

6. **Wound care** for areas that have broken down can be provided using primary wound dressing. **Vigilon** (Bard Products, Murray Hill, NJ 07974) applied to a dermal wound may support improved healing while minimizing infection and scarring.

7. Fragile intact skin at risk of breaking down can be protected with Opsite (Smith and Nephew LTD, Hull-HU3-2BN England). We often use this prophylactically in infants weighing less than 800 gm. All skin barriers pose some risk of bacterial or fungal growth between the bandage and the skin.

B. Immaturity of the skin in the premature infant contributes to increased insensible water loss and increased permeability of topical substances. Water loss and permeability are very high in the very-low-birth-weight infant during the first 3 days, owing to the underdeveloped stratum corneum of the epidermis. After birth of the premature infant, epidermal maturation accelerates so that by 2 weeks of life barrier function is similar to that of a term infant (see Chap. 9).

C. **Skin diseases** including ichthyosis and epidermolysis bullosa may be associated with increased insensible water loss and increased infection due to an ineffective skin barrier.

D. **Insensible water loss** in the premature infant or the infant with skin damage can be minimized (see Chap. 9).

1. Radiant warmers cause a 50 to 80% increase in insensible water loss as compared to incubators.

2. Plastic sheeting over an infant on a radiant warmer can reduce insensible water loss. Caution should be used to prevent suffocation, avoiding placement of the sheeting over the head unless the infant is intubated.

3. Humidification in the range of 40 to 60% can reduce insensible water loss as well as decrease evaporative heat loss.

E. **Increased skin permeability** to topical substances has been demonstrated in the premature infant. The term infant demonstrates permeability characteristics similar to an adult, except in the scrotal area. However, the increased skin surface–body volume ratio in term infants increases the risk of a higher blood level of toxic substances. Caution should be used with the application of any topical agent. When applied topically, steroids, alcohol, iodine, hexachlorophene, estrogen, and boric acid have systemic side effects [8].

III. **Transient cutaneous lesions** are common in the neonatal period. Some of the more frequent are listed.

A. **Milia.** Many infants, especially those born at term, have multiple pearly white or pale yellow papules or cysts. These cysts are known as milia and are scattered about on the face, especially the nose, chin, and forehead. Histologically, milia are epidermal cysts (up to 1 mm in diameter) developing in connection with the pilosebaceous follicle. They will exfoliate and disappear within the first few weeks of life. No treatment is necessary.

B. **Sebaceous gland hyperplasia** is similar to milia, but the lesions are smaller, more numerous, and usually confined to the nose, upper lip, and chin. These lesions are present mainly in full-term babies and, like milia, they disappear within a few weeks after birth. They are related to maternal androgen stimulation.

C. **Erythema toxicum.** The rash of erythema toxicum, which usually appears on the first or second day of life, is a scattering of macules, papules, and even some vesicles, usually occurring on the trunk but frequently on the extremities and face as well. The condition is not serious and is self-limited, but it may cause alarm when papules and vesicles are numerous, especially when the lesions are considered to be pustular.

1. If the vesicles are opened and the contents smeared and stained with Wright stain, and examined microscopically, they are found to contain almost exclusively eosinophils. Cultures are sterile except for an occasional contaminant such as *Staphylococcus epidermidis*.

2. The **cause** of erythema toxicum is not really known, although some allergic or immediate hypersensitivity reaction is suspected.

3. Although erythema toxicum may occur in 50 to 70% of full-term babies in a nursery, this figure decreases as the gestational age decreases. Infants less than 1500 gm or less than 30 weeks' gestational age rarely exhibit erythema toxicum. No treatment is needed.

D. **Transient neonatal pustular melanosis** is a benign, self-limited disorder seen at birth in 2 to 5% of term black infants and under 1% of term white infants. The lesions consisting of small papules, vesicles, pustular lesions, and hyperpigmented spots occur most commonly on the forehead, neck, lower back, and shins. The lesions rupture easily, revealing white scales surrounding a hyperpigmented macule. Staining the contents of an open lesion with Wright stain will reveal neutrophils, few to no eosinophils, and cellular debris with no organisms. Transient neonatal pustular melanosis should be differentiated from pustules caused by staphylococci, candida, or herpes. The lesions resolve in 1 to 2 days, leaving a hyperpigmented macule that slowly disappears.

IV. **Abnormalities of pigmentation** frequently are noted in the newborn. Sometimes they are cutaneous clues to underlying disease.

A. **Flat lesions**

1. **Mongolian spots** are pigmented lesions often found at birth. They are seen in over 90% of the black and Native American population, 81% of the Asian population, 70% of the Hispanic population, and 10% of the white population. The area most commonly involved is the lumbosacral region, but the upper part of the back, shoulders, arms, buttocks, legs, and face are occasionally included. The lesions may be small or large, grayish blue or bluish black, and irregularly round; they are never elevated or palpable. Mongolian spots occur as the result of an infiltration of melanocytes deep in the dermis. Although they frequently fade as the child gets older, this is probably the result of decreasing transparency of the overlying skin rather than a true disappearance of the lesions. They present no danger.

2. **Café au lait** spots are flat, brown, round or oval lesions with smooth edges. They are found anywhere on the body. They occur in 10% of normal individuals. These lesions are somewhat darker in color in black than in white infants. Many appear after birth. As the infant grows older, they do not resolve. A few small spots are of little or no significance, but larger ones (or increasing numbers) may indicate the presence of neurofibromatosis. A biopsy may reveal differences in the appearance of melanosomes within the melanocytes. The presence of giant pigment granules is characteristic of neurofibromatosis (see **IV.A.3**). Many other diseases including **tuberous sclerosis** may be associated with café au lait spots.

3. **Neurofibromatosis (von Recklinghausen's disease)** is a hereditary disease resulting from an autosomal gene, characterized by the development of multiple mixed neural and fibrous tumors in late childhood and adolescence. The café au lait spots that eventually develop in over 90% of patients are occasionally present at birth, but they usually develop during the first years of life. Neurofibromatosis should be strongly suspected in any newborn with more than three café au lait spots (especially if any of the spots is larger than 3 cm). Groups of spots in the axillary area are characteristic of neurofibromatosis.

4. **Albright's syndrome** is characterized in the newborn by the presence of a large, very irregular, ragged pigmented area, as much as 9 to 12 cm in extent. Other features, appearing later, are bony lesions and endocrine disorders.

5. **Junctional nevi** are brown or black and are flat to slightly raised. They are present at birth. Junctional nevi are composed of nests of cuboidal cells with melanocytes and occur at the border of the dermis and epidermis. They are benign lesions, needing no treatment unless excision is desired for cosmetic reasons.

6. **Peutz-Jeghers syndrome.** At birth, individuals with this condition show multiple, scattered hyperpigmented macules, especially around the nose and mouth, but also on the hands and fingers, and frequently on the mucous membrane of the mouth. The more serious part of the syndrome appears later, with the development of polyposis of the small bowel and subsequent episodes of intussusception.

B. **Raised lesions**

1. **Giant hairy nevi (bathing trunk nevi)** are present at birth and may be huge (involving 20 to 30% of the body surface); they are leathery and hard and brown to black, with a large amount of hair. Other pigmentary abnormalities are frequently present on the remaining skin. Occasionally, deeper structures, including the central nervous system (CNS), may

be involved as well. Surgical removal, although sometimes an extremely difficult procedure, is indicated, not only for cosmetic reasons but also because a significant number of these lesions (more than 10%) progress to malignant melanoma.

2. **Compound nevi** are very similar to junctional nevi in that they are composed of melanocytes. Compound nevi tend to be larger, however, and are often hairy; they involve the dermis as well as the epidermis. Treatment involves surgical removal, if technically feasible, at age 5 or 6 because of the possibility of a later change to a malignant lesion.

3. **Other raised lesions.** Epidermal nevi, blue nevi, and juvenile melanoma are other forms of raised lesions rarely seen in the newborn; they require no treatment except occasional diagnostic excision.

C. **Diffuse hyperpigmentation**
  1. Melanism
  2. Progressive familial hyperpigmentation
  3. Congenital Addison's disease
  4. Fanconi's syndrome
  5. Generalized hereditary lentiginosis
  6. Androgen excess

D. **Hypopigmentation**
  1. **Albinism** is a hereditary disease caused by an autosomal recessive gene that leads to a defect in tyrosinase activity. This defect, in turn, produces a pronounced defect in pigment production throughout the body. The defect is most noticeable in the skin, the hair, and the eyes (iris). No treatment is effective; the infant must be protected from ultraviolet light.
  2. **Piebaldism,** also known as **partial albinism,** is probably caused by an autosomal dominant gene with decreased penetrance. In this condition the skin and hair are involved in a patchy way, with some areas being hypomelanotic and some normal. A white "forelock" of hair, as in Waardenburg's syndrome, is a feature of this disorder.
  3. **Vitiligo** is characterized by patchy areas of decreased or absent pigmentation. The lesions are occasionally present at birth, but may develop in later infancy or childhood. The characteristic appearance under the microscope shows few or no melanocytes in the junctional layer.
  4. **Hypopigmented macules (white spots)** are of concern because of the association of these spots with tuberous sclerosis. The typical white spot seen in tuberous sclerosis is small (2 to 3 cm) with an irregular border and is usually seen on the trunk and buttocks. The number of spots is variable. The lesion differs from the lesion of vitiligo in that there are many melanocytes present, but the melanosomes are poorly pigmented. In fair-skinned infants, it may be difficult to demonstrate the white macule without the use of a Wood's lamp. Many infants with tuberous sclerosis also have at least one café au lait spot. Magnetic resonance imaging (MRI) of the brain and examination of the eye by slit lamp may confirm the diagnosis of tuberous sclerosis.
  5. **Waardenburg's syndrome and Chediak-Higashi syndrome** are other examples of inherited conditions in which pigmentary deficits form part of the clinical picture but are not primarily responsible for the problems associated with the disease. The main problems in these disorders are immune deficiencies in Chediak-Higashi syndrome and congenital deafness in Waardenburg's syndrome.

V. **Vascular abnormalities** occur in up to 40% of newborns.
  A. A **salmon patch, nevus simplex,** or **macular hemangioma** is a flat pink macular lesion found on the forehead, upper eyelid, nasolabial area, glabella, or nape of the neck (stork bite). It is the most common vascular lesion of the newborn, occurring in 30 to 40% of infants. Examination of the nevus reveals distended dermal capillaries representing persistence of the fetal pattern. Except for those on the neck, most resolve by 1 year of life.

Crying will often make a fading lesion transiently more prominent. They are more or less bilateral.

B. A **port-wine stain,** or **nevus flammeus,** is a flat or mildly elevated reddish purple lesion most commonly found on the face. It is often unilateral. The lesion is a vascular malformation of dilated capillary-like vessels. Port-wine stains do not involute. They are often associated with hemangiomas of the underlying structures. The association of nevus flammeus (port-wine stain) in the region of the first branch of the trigeminal nerve with cortical lesions in the brain is known as the **Sturge-Weber syndrome.** Of the three trigeminal sensory areas, only involvement of area V1, the ophthalmic area, is accompanied by neuroocular involvement (Sturge-Weber syndrome). When the skin lesions occur only in the maxillary (V2) or mandibular (V3) areas, no ocular or intracranial lesion is found. When coverage of the ocular (V1) area is complete (high-risk group), 60% have CNS lesions. If **Sturge-Weber syndrome** is suspected, the brain should be imaged and the eyes evaluated. Ocular involvement may result in glaucoma. The skin lesions can be obliterated with pulse-dye laser therapy. Treatment, which may necessitate several stages, should be started in early infancy so that it can be completed before the child starts school.

C. **Strawberry hemangiomas** may not be present at birth or may present as a pale macule with irregular margins. There are often a few blood vessels in the center of the macule. They are more common in the head, neck, and trunk but can occur anywhere. They are more common in premature infants and are not usually noticed until the infant is 1 to 2 weeks old. Strawberry hemangiomas grow rapidly during the first 6 months and continue to grow until 1 year. The majority subsequently involute completely with no scar by age 4 to 5. A strawberry hemangioma involving the eyelid may need treatment to prevent amblyopia.

D. A **cavernous hemangioma** is a deep strawberry hemangioma composed of large, mature vascular elements. It is often present at birth. A cavernous hemangioma also grows during the first year of life, but regression is often less complete. Most regress but some do not. A small number of cavernous hemangiomas are associated with significant complications that may be life-threatening. These infants may have hemangiomas anywhere in the body. The dangers are hemorrhage due to platelet trapping (Kasabach-Merritt syndrome), hypertrophy of involved structures (Klippel-Trénaunay syndrome), heart failure due to arteriovenous anastomoses, and infection in infants with large venous lakes. Treatment may involve surgery, occlusion, laser therapy, steroids, and more recently alpha interferon.

E. Other syndromes with cavernous hemangiomas are diffuse neonatal hemangiomatosis, blue rubber bleb nevus syndrome, and Riley-Smith syndrome.

F. Cutis marmorata telangiectica congenita (congenital generalized phlebectasia)

G. Familial annular erythema

H. Periarteritis nodosa

I. **Disorders of lymphatic vessels**
   1. Lymphangiomas (simple, lymphangioma circumscriptum, and cavernous lymphangioma)
   2. Cystic hygroma
   3. Lymphedema
   4. Milroy's disease (congenital hereditary lymphedema)

J. **Purpura** can result from one of the following conditions:
   1. Infectious disorders such as TORCH infections or bacterial infections (see Chap. 23)
   2. Giant hemangioma with thrombocytopenia
   3. Congenital leukemia
   4. Congenital Letterer-Siwe disease

5. Immune disorders (isoimmune thrombocytopenia) (see Chap. 26, Thrombocytopenia)
6. Maternal drug ingestion
7. Congenital megakaryocytic hypoplasia (see Chap. 26, Thrombocytopenia)
8. Inherited thrombocytopenias (see Chap. 26, Thrombocytopenia)
9. Coagulation defects (see Chap. 26, Bleeding)

VI. Trauma (see Chap. 20). Various forms of contusions, abrasions, and ecchymoses occur as the result of forces associated with delivery.

A. **Caput succedaneum** is a collection of edema and frequently small or large hemorrhages in the skin of the scalp over the presenting part. Similar areas may appear over the buttocks, scrotum, or vulva in breech presentations. The edema usually disappears in a day or two, but the ecchymosis may take longer; if the ecchymosis is large, it may contribute to hyperbilirubinemia.

B. **Forceps application and extraction,** especially if forceps rotation is required, may lead to varying degrees of trauma to the skin and subcutaneous tissues of the face, neck, and scalp. **Abrasions and ecchymoses** from forceps are quite common and of no serious consequence, except as a possible path of entry for infection. Occasionally deeper lacerations may need surgical repair, however. Injury to the facial nerve may result but the injury usually resolves.

C. **Subcutaneous fat necrosis.** Small, firm, movable masses can occur over bony prominences of the mandible or zygoma as the result of pressure, usually from forceps. These lumps are often not discovered for several days, and then may persist for weeks. They eventually disappear without treatment.

D. Areas of **pressure necrosis** of the scalp (similar to subcutaneous fat necrosis) can occur over the parietal bosses. These masses occasionally break down and drain, and they may become secondarily infected, thereby necessitating antibiotic treatment.

E. **Sucking blisters** may be present at birth, usually on a hand or wrist (sometimes both). They may be filled with clear fluid, or they may be open and in the process of healing. Some may even be so old as to be more like calluses than blisters. Observations of fetuses in utero by ultrasonography show that they do suck frequently, and may suck on any part that comes easily to the mouth. Treatment is not necessary.

F. **Bruising and abrasions** of the legs and feet caused by difficult breech extraction are now largely lesions of the past. Although these usually clear with remarkable rapidity, the resorption of blood breakdown products from the tissues may lead to an elevation of serum bilirubin.

G. **Ecchymosis** of the back, buttocks, and feet has resulted from overvigorous physical stimulation as part of resuscitation; fortunately, this is seldom seen in the modern nursery.

H. **Small puncture wounds** (sometimes multiple) of the scalp are new lesions that result from advances in medical care. The puncture wounds are caused by the placement of an internal monitoring electrode or by the sampling of fetal blood to detect fetal distress. These lesions are usually insignificant, but occasionally they lead to superficial infection. Similar wounds, or scars of wounds, can also result from amniocentesis needles.

VII. Development abnormalities of skin

A. **Skin dimples and sinuses** can occur on any part of the body, but they are most common over bony prominences such as the scapula, knee joint, and hip. They may be simple depressions in the skin (of no pathologic significance) or actual sinus tracts connecting to deeper structures. In the sacral area there may be a pilonidal dimple or sinus. Usually if one can see to the bottom of the dimple, it is of no significance. A sinus that is deep but does not communicate to underlying structures usually does not cause problems. At puberty, if hair grows in the depths of the sinus, a cyst may form. The cyst occasionally gets infected and needs excision. This does not happen until adolescence.

If the sinus connects to the CNS, serious infection can occur but is rare. Occasionally, a dimple, sometimes accompanied by a nevus or hemangioma, may signify an underlying spinal disorder such as diastematomyelia. Diagnosis of these connections usually requires ultrasound computed tomography (CT), or MRI.

Dermal sinuses or cysts along the cheek or jawline, or extending into the neck, may represent remnants of the branchial cleft structures of the early embryo.

The most common dermal sinus is the **preauricular sinus,** which is a leftover from the first branchial cleft. It appears in the most anterior upper portion of the tragus of the external ear. Preauricular sinuses may be unilateral or bilateral; they usually require no treatment unless secondary infection develops, in which case surgical excision is recommended. In my experience, preauricular sinuses rarely cause problems in the newborn period.

Sinuses or cysts in the sides of the neck usually arise from the second branchial cleft. They may or may not open into the mouth or pharynx.

B. Small skin tags can occur on the chest wall near the breast. They usually have a narrow base and can be "twirled" off.

C. Redundant skin also can be considered an anomaly. This usually occurs as loose folds of excess skin in the posterior part of the neck. It is a common finding in some chromosomal disorders, such as trisomy 18, Down syndrome, trisomy 13, and especially Turner's syndrome.

D. Hemihypertrophy is a condition in which one side of the body is larger than the other. The asymmetry is often apparent at birth, but it becomes more and more obvious as growth takes place.

   1. The **skin** is only one of many systems involved, and anomalous development of the extremity on the larger side is frequent. The skin on the hypertrophied side usually feels thicker and may sweat more. The hypertrophied side is also more prone to the development of anomalies such as nail defects, hypertrichosis, pigmentation abnormalities, nevi, and vascular anomalies.

   2. Asymmetry of the face may be more striking than that of the rest of the body, especially with involvement of one eye and the tongue. Treatment is for both cosmetic and symptomatic reasons.

   3. Mental retardation, occasionally with seizures, occurs in some of these patients. Children with hemihypertrophy are also more prone to the development of embryonal tumors of the kidney, adrenal, and liver.

E. Aplasia cutis (congenital absence of skin) is seen most frequently in the midline of the posterior part of the scalp. It is usually a round, punched-out lesion 1 or 2 cm in diameter that is present at birth. The area is devoid of hair; it is sometimes covered with a thin membrane and is sometimes crusted and weeping. Rarely, other parts of the body may be involved, but the scalp is the most common site. Treatment is simply protection from trauma and infection; healing is usually slow. Plastic surgical repair might be considered for the rare occasion when the scar cannot be adequately covered by growing hair. Multiple areas of scalp aplasia are associated with trisomy 13 and trisomy 18.

VIII. Scaling disorders

   A. Harlequin fetus (ichthyosis)

   B. Ichthyosis vulgaris

   C. Sex-linked ichthyosis

   D. Nonbullous congenital ichthyosiform erythroderma

   E. Bullous congenital ichthyosiform erythroderma

   F. Ichthyosis linearis circumflexa

   G. Erythrokeratodermia variabilis

   H. Other syndromes with scaling

1. Netherton's syndrome
2. Sjögren-Larsson syndrome
3. Rud's syndrome
4. Conradi's syndrome
5. Refsum's syndrome
6. Tay's syndrome
I. **Keratoderma of palms and soles**
   1. Tylosis
   2. Mutilating keratoderma
   3. Progressive keratoderma
   4. Mal de Meleda
   5. Papillon-Lefèvre syndrome
J. Psoriasis
K. **Zinc deficiency** recently was determined to be a leading cause, or perhaps *the* cause, of **acrodermatitis enteropathica;** therefore, a more complete discussion is presented here.
   1. **Etiology.** The condition previously was considered to be a hereditary autosomal recessive disorder; however, recent reports document remarkable responses to intravenous or oral doses of zinc sulfate only slightly in excess of the recommended daily requirement. In the newborn period, zinc deficiency has been found almost exclusively in infants receiving total parenteral nutrition with solutions containing either no zinc or inadequate amounts of zinc. Most infants have had increased zinc losses in gastric or ileostomy fluids and increased requirements due to sepsis. There have been a few reports of zinc deficiency occurring in otherwise healthy breast-fed infants whose mother's milk, for unknown reasons, was exceptionally low in zinc content.
   2. **Clinical features.** The skin lesions of acrodermatitis enteropathica may be dry or moist; they are scaling and impetiginous and appear primarily around the nose, mouth, and perineum, as well as around ostomy wounds They frequently spread to adjacent areas and especially to the fingers and toes. The condition is often accompanied by severe diarrhea, irritability, and failure to thrive despite theoretically adequate nutritional intake. Sepsis is frequently associated with acrodermatitis enteropathica. Response to zinc therapy is prompt and dramatic.
   3. **Therapy.** Guidelines established by the American Medical Association Department of Foods and Nutrition suggest that term babies receive zinc at 0.1 mg/kg per day, and that premature infants (low birth weight) of less than 3 kg receive 0.3 mg/kg per day. Current formulas, as well as human milk, contain approximately 0.35 mg of zinc per deciliter, which should be adequate under most circumstances. Human milk is also believed to contain a factor that enhances the absorption of zinc from the gastrointestinal tract (see Chap. 10).
L. **Neonatal lupus erythematosus** can occur in infants born to mothers with systemic lupus erythematosus. Skin lesions typical of discoid lupus, dry, scaly and reddened areas, may appear on the face, trunk, or extremities or may be present at birth. Congenital heart block occurs in about half the affected infants and is the only complication resulting in significant morbidity and mortality. If persistent, the heart block may require implementation of a permanent pacemaker (see Chap. 25).
IX. **Vesicobullous eruptions**
   A. **Hereditary causes (nonscarring)**
      1. Epidermolysis bullosa simplex
      2. Epidermolysis bullosa letalis
      3. Bullous eruption of hands and feet (Cockayne-Weber syndrome)
   B. **Hereditary causes (scarring)**
      1. Epidermolysis bullosa dystrophica (dominant)
      2. Epidermolysis bullosa dystrophica (recessive)
   C. **Congenital porphyria**

D. **Incontinentia pigmenti**
E. **Juvenile dermatitis herpetiformis**
F. **Infiltrative diseases**
   1. **Mast cell diseases**
      a. Mastocytosis
      b. Urticaria pigmentosa
   2. Histiocytosis X
G. **Infections**
   1. **Bacterial infections**
      a. Staphylococcal infections
         (1) Bullous impetigo
         (2) Ritter's disease
      b. *Pseudomonas* infections
      c. Listeriosis
      d. Syphilis (congenital)
   2. **Viral infections**
      a. Varicella-zoster
      b. Herpes infections
      c. Rubella
   3. Candidal infections
   4. Toxoplasmosis

References

1. Esterly, N. B., et al. Dermatologic Conditions. In H. W. Taeusch, R. A. Ballard, and M. E. Avery (Eds.), *Schaffer and Avery's Diseases of the Newborn.* Philadelphia: Saunders, 1991. P. 973.
2. *Guidelines for Perinatal Care,* 3rd ed. AAP Committee on the Fetus and Newborn. Elk Grove, IL: ACOG Committee on Obstetrics: Maternal and Fetal Medicine, 1992.
3. Hurwitz, S. *Clinical Pediatric Dermatology.* Philadelphia: Saunders, 1993.
4. Lefrak-Okikawa, L., et al. Nursing Practice in the Neonatal Intensive Care Unit. In M. H. Klaus and A. A. Fanaroff (Eds.), *Care of the High-Risk Neonate.* Philadelphia: Saunders, 1993. P. 212.
5. Lund, C., et al. Evaluation of a pectin-based barrier under tape to protect neonatal skin. *J. Obstet. Gynecol. Neonatal Nurs.* 15:39, 1986.
6. Malloy, M. B., et al. Neonatal skin care: Prevention of skin breakdown. *Pediatr. Nurs.* 17:41, 1991.
7. Nurses Association of American College of Obstetrics and Gynecology. Neonatal skin care. *J. Obstet. Gynecol.* 20:1, 1992 [entire issue].
8. Rutter, N. Percutaneous drug absorption in the newborn: Hazards and uses. *Clin. Perinatol.* 14:911, 1987.
9. Young, T. E., et al. *Neofax® '97: A Manual of Drugs Used in Neonatal Care* (10th Ed.). Acorn Publishing USA, 1997.
10. Zenk, K. E., et al. Nafcillin extravasation injury: Use of hyaluronidase as an antidote. *Am. J. Dis. Child.* 135:1113, 1981.

35. AUDITORY AND OPHTHALMOLOGIC PROBLEMS

Retinopathy of Prematurity
Charles L. Anderson, Jr. and Jane E. Stewart

I. **Background.** **Retinopathy of prematurity (ROP)** is a multifactorial vasoprolifer-
ative retinal disorder that increases in incidence with decreasing gestational
age. Approximately 65% of infants with a birth weight less than 1250 gm and
80% of those with a birth weight less than 1000 gm will develop some degree of
ROP. In Massachusetts, ROP is the second most common cause of blindness for
children under 6 years old.

II. **Pathogenesis**
A. **Normal development.** After the sclera and choroid have developed, retinal
elements, including nerve fibers, ganglion cells, and photoreceptors, migrate from the optic disk at the posterior pole of the eye and move toward
the periphery. The photoreceptors have progressed 80% of the distance to
their resting place at the ora serrata by 28 weeks' gestation. Before the
retinal vessels develop, the avascular retina receives its oxygen supply by
diffusion across the retina from the choroid vessels. The retinal vessels,
which arise from the spindle cells of the adventitia of the hyaloid vessels at
the optic disk, begin to migrate outward at 16 weeks' gestation. Migration
is complete by 36 weeks on the nasal side and by 40 weeks on the temporal
side.

B. **Possible mechanisms of injury.** Clinical observations suggest that the onset
of ROP consists of two stages.
1. The **primary stage** involves an initial insult, such as hyperoxia, hypoxia,
or hypotension, at a critical point in retinal vascularization that results in
vasoconstriction and decreased blood flow to the developing retina with a
subsequent arrest in vascular development.
2. During the **second stage,** neovascularization occurs. This aberrant retinal vessel growth is thought to be driven by angiogenic factors released by
the ischemic avascular retina. New vessels grow through the retina into
the vitreous. These vessels are permeable and hemorrhage and edema can
occur. Extensive and severe extraretinal fibrovascular proliferation can
lead to retinal detachment and abnormal retinal function. In the majority
of affected infants, however, the disease process regresses and the retinopathy gradually resolves.

C. **Risk factors.** Many factors have been associated with ROP. The most consistent association has been with low gestational age, low birth weight, and
duration of mechanical ventilation. Other factors implicated in the pathogenesis include vitamin E deficiency, bright-light exposure, hypocapnia and
alkalosis, acidosis, intraventricular hemorrhage, bronchopulmonary dysplasia and oxygen exposure, fluctuation in blood gas tensions, sepsis, respiratory distress syndrome, dexamethasone exposure, and patent ductus arteriosus.

III. **Screening and diagnosis.** Because no early clinical signs or symptoms indicate
developing ROP, early and regular retinal examination is necessary. The timing
of the occurrence of ROP is related to the maturity of retinal vessels and thus
postmenstrual age. The median postmenstrual ages at the onset of stage 1 ROP,
prethreshold disease, and threshold disease (see **IV.B**) are 34, 36, and 37 weeks,
respectively. Preterm infants who are discharged from level III facilities before
they reach the postmenstrual age of highest incidence for severe ROP must continue to have ophthalmologic examinations until their retinal vessels have
reached maturity.

ROP is diagnosed by retinal examination with indirect ophthalmoscopy; this should be performed by a pediatric ophthalmologist when the infant is 4 to 6 weeks old. We screen all infants with a birth weight less than 1500 gm or gestational age less than 32 weeks. Infants who are born between 32 and 34 weeks' gestational age are examined if they have been ill (e.g., those who have had severe respiratory distress syndrome, hypotension requiring pressor support, or surgery in the first several weeks of life). Because the timing of ROP is related to postmenstrual age, infants who are born at 24 to 26 weeks' gestation are examined at the postnatal age of 6 weeks and those of more advanced gestational age are examined at the postnatal age of 4 weeks. Patients are examined every 2 weeks until their vessels have grown out to the ora serrata and the retina is considered mature. If ROP is diagnosed, the frequency of examination depends on the severity and rapidity of progression of the disease. Infants are examined more frequently until their retinopathy regresses and full maturity of vessels is noted or until they reach a threshold for treatment. (See **IV.B**)

IV. **Classification and definitions**

A. **Classification.** The International Classification of Retinopathy of Prematurity (ICROP) is used to classify ROP. This classification system consists of four components (Fig. 35-1).

1. **Location** refers to how far the developing retinal blood vessels have progressed. The retina is divided into three concentric circles or zones:

   a. **Zone 1** consists of an imaginary circle with the optic nerve at the center and a radius of twice the distance from the optic nerve to the macula.

   b. **Zone 2** extends from the edge of zone 1 to the equator on the nasal side of the eye and about half the distance to the ora serrata on the temporal side.

   c. **Zone 3** consists of the outer crescent-shaped area extending from zone 2 out to the ora serrata temporally.

2. **Severity** refers to the stage of disease.

   a. **Stage 1.** A demarcation line appears as a thin white line that separates the normal retina from the undeveloped avascular retina.

   b. **Stage 2.** A ridge of scar tissue with height and width replaces the line of stage 1. It extends inward from the plane of the retina.

   c. **Stage 3.** The ridge has extraretinal fibrovascular proliferation. Abnormal blood vessels and fibrous tissue develop on the edge of the ridge and extend into the vitreous.

   d. **Stage 4.** Partial retinal detachment may result when scar tissue pulls on the retina. Stage 4A is partial detachment outside the macula, so that the chance for vision is good if the retina reattaches. Stage 4B is partial detachment that involves the macula, thus limiting the likelihood of usable vision in that eye.

   e. **Stage 5.** Complete retinal detachment occurs. The retina assumes a funnel-shaped appearance and is described as open or narrow in the anterior and posterior regions.

3. **Plus disease** is an additional designation that refers to the presence of vascular dilatation and tortuosity of the posterior retinal vessels. This indicates a more severe degree of ROP and may be associated with iris vascular engorgement, pupillary rigidity, and vitreous haze. Plus disease that is associated with zone 1 ROP is termed **rush disease;** this type of ROP tends to progress extremely rapidly.

4. **Extent** refers to the circumferential location of disease and is reported as clock hours in the appropriate zone.

B. **Definition of threshold and prethreshold ROP**

1. **Threshold ROP** is five or more contiguous or eight cumulative clock hours (30-degree sectors) of stage 3 with plus disease in either zone 1 or 2. This is the level of severity at which the risk of blindness is predicted to approach 50% and thus treatment is recommended.

Children's Hospital
300 Longwood Ave., Boston, Massachusetts

OPHTHALMOLOGIC CONSULTATION FOR
RETINOPATHY OF PREMATURITY (ROP)

USE PLATE OR PRINT

MR. NO. _____ DATE _____

Gestational Age (wks) _____ Birth Weight _____ gm

PT. NAME

Date of Exam _____, Age (wks) _____

DATE OF BIRTH_____

Ophthalmologist _____ MD

EXAMINATION:

Right Eye
(O.D.)

Left Eye
(O.S.)

ORA SERRATA

COMMENTS

KEY

Stage 1 - line of demarcation
Stage 2 - ridge, elevated
Stage 3- ridge with ERVP
Stage 4 - partial detachment
Stage 5 - total detachment

SUMMARY DIAGNOSIS

O.D.   O.S.

_____ Mature Retina _____

_____ Immature, No ROP _____
Zone   Zone

ROP

Stage _____   Stage _____

Zone _____   Zone _____

clock hrs _____   # clock hrs _____

O.D.	Other Findings	O.S.
	(mark with an "X")	
_____	Dilatation/Tortuosity	_____
_____	Iris Vessel Dilatation	_____
_____	Pupil Rigidity	_____
_____	Vitreous Haze	_____
_____	Hemorrhages	_____

Other: _____

_____

_____

_____

Plan: Repeat Exam in : _____

Discussed with: _____ MD/NNP

Examined by: _____ MD

Routing: White - Medical Record   Yellow - Physician Copy

03241 10/96 25/PKG

Fig. 35-1. Sample of form for ophthalmologic consultation.

2. **Prethreshold ROP** is any of the following: zone 1 ROP of any stage less than threshold; zone 2 ROP with stage 2 and plus disease; zone 2 ROP with stage 3 without plus disease; or zone 2 ROP at stage 3 with plus disease with fewer than the threshold number of sectors of stage 3. Infants with prethreshold ROP have a 1 in 3 chance of needing surgical treatment and a 1 in 6 chance of extreme loss of vision if treatment is not done promptly when threshold is reached. With therapy, they have a 1 in 12 chance of extreme visual loss.

V. Prognosis

A. Short-term prognosis. Factors that increase the risk of reaching threshold ROP include posterior location of the ROP in zone 1 or posterior zone 2, increased severity of stage, circumferential involvement, the presence of plus disease, and rapid progression of disease. Most infants with stage 1 or 2 ROP will have regression. In a large study [2] of infants weighing less than 1250 gm at birth, the overall incidence of ROP was 65.8%; stage 1 was the highest stage reached in 25.2% and stage 2 was the highest stage in 21.7%. Prethreshold ROP was reached in 17.8% and threshold in 6.0%. Zone 3 disease has a good prognosis for complete recovery. Tables 35-1 and 35-2 show the risk of progression and poor visual outcome according to severity of ROP and postmenstrual age.

B. Long-term prognosis. Infants with ROP have an increased risk of myopia, high myopia and other refractive errors, strabismus, amblyopia, astigmatism, late retinal detachment, glaucoma, and vitreal hemorrhage. **Cicatricial disease** refers to residual scarring in the retina and may be associated with much later retinal detachment. The prognosis for stage 4 ROP depends on the involvement of the macula; the chance for functional vision is greater when the macula is not involved. Careful follow-up by a pediatric ophthalmologist is essential.

VI. Management

A. Prevention. Currently no proven methods are available to prevent ROP. When ROP is diagnosed early and followed closely, however, intervention can be made before detachment occurs. Once the retina has detached, the prognosis is poor even with surgical reattachment attempts.

B. Treatment

1. Cryotherapy. A multicenter trial designed to evaluate the benefit of cryotherapy for threshold ROP demonstrated a reduction in unfavorable outcome from 51.4% in control eyes to 31.1% in treated eyes [4]. That is, cryotherapy reduces the risk of extreme loss of vision by half, although these infants may not have normal vision. The procedure is usually done under general anesthesia. The cryoprobe is applied to the external surface of the sclera and areas are frozen until the entire anterior avascular retina has been treated. Approximately 20 to 70 applications are made in each eye. Vas-

Table 35-1. Probability of reaching cryotherapy criteria

	Postmenstrual age (wk)					
	≤32	33–34	35–36	37–38	39–40	41–42
Zone 1[a]						
Incomplete	33%	37%	7%	36%	b	b
Stage 1 −	18%	33%	b	b	b	b
All others	b	b	b	b	b	b
Zone 2[a]						
Incomplete	9%	6%	3%	1%	2%	0%
Stage 1 −	8%	6%	4%	2%	1%	1%
Stage 2 −	4%	6%	4%	2%	1%	1%
Stage 3 −	b	16%	13%	8%	2%	0%
Stage 1 +	b	83%	42%	b	b	b
Stage 2 +	b	44%	34%	25%	17%	0%
Stage 3 +	b	77%	61%	34%	31%	14%

[a]"+" means with plus disease; "−" means without plus disease.
[b]Too few to calculate risk.
Source: Modified from Schaffer, D. B., et al. Prognostic factors in the natural course of retinopathy of prematurity. The Cryotherapy for Retinopathy of Prematurity Group. *Ophthalmology* 100:230, 1993.

Table 35-2.   Probability of poor visual outcome (without cryotherapy)

Zone 2[a]	Postmenstrual age (wk)					
	≤32	33–34	35–36	37–38	39–40	41–42
Incomplete	7%	4%	1%	2%	2%	3%
Stage 1 −	6%	3%	2%	<1%	1%	0%
Stage 2 −	0%	3%	2%	1%	0%	2%
Stage 3 −	b	3%	2%	5%	4%	1%
Stage 1 +	b	b	b	b	b	b
Stage 2 +	b	27%	29%	20%	12%	33%
Stage 3 +	b	62%	48%	35%	30%	32%

[a]"+" means with plus disease; "−" means without plus disease.
[b]Not calculated due to small number.
Source: Modified from Schaffer, D. B., et al. Prognostic factors in the natural course of retinopathy of prematurity. The Cryotherapy for Retinopathy of Prematurity Group. *Ophthalmology* 100:230, 1993.

cularized regions are not treated. Close follow-up is required to detect continued progression and requirement of further cryotherapy.

2. **Laser therapy.** Laser photocoagulation therapy for ROP has become a preferred initial treatment in many centers. Laser therapy is technically difficult if there is vitreal hemorrhage obscuring the view of the retinal vessels or if there is a significant remnant of the tunica vasculosa lentis (the vascular layer enveloping the lens of the fetal eye) with remnants of hyaloid vessels obscuring the view through the lens. When these situations occur, cryotherapy is the preferred treatment. Laser treatment is delivered through an indirect ophthalmoscope and is applied to the avascular retina anterior to the ridge of extraretinal fibrovascular proliferation for 360 degrees. Approximately 400 to 2000 spots are placed in each eye. Both argon and diode laser photocoagulation have been successfully used in infants with severe ROP. The advantage of this technique is that the equipment is portable and the procedure can be performed in the newborn intensive care unit. Clinical observations suggest that it is as effective as cryotherapy in achieving favorable visual outcomes. Further long-term follow-up studies are still needed for both modalities.

3. **Retinal reattachment.** Buckling procedures have proved to be of limited value. The anatomic success rate is 53.3% in the early postoperative phase, but later decreases to 33.3%, with a functional success rate of 20% at follow-up (with perception of large forms). Lensectomy–vitrectomy has an anatomic success rate of 29.8% at 5.5 years of age. Only 15% had any functional vision at that time (light perception or low vision) and the rest were blind. Although these techniques are limited, the achievement of even minimal vision can result in a large difference in a child's overall quality of life.

4. **Supplemental oxygen.** Studies are in progress to test whether supplemental oxygen given to infants with prethreshold ROP limits the progression to threshold ROP.

References
1. Page, J. M., et al. Ocular sequelae in premature infants. *Pediatrics* 92:787,1993.
2. Palmer, E., et al. Incidence and early course of retinopathy of prematurity. *Ophthalmology* 98:1628, 1991.
3. Phelps. D. L. Retinopathy of prematurity. *Pediatr. Clin. North Am.* 40:705, 1993.

4. Cryotherapy for Retinopathy of Prematurity Cooperative Group. Multicenter trial of cryotherapy for retinopathy at prematurity. *Arch. Ophthalmol.* 108:195–209, 1990.
5. Quinn, G. E., et al. Visual acuity of eyes after vitrectomy for retinopathy of prematurity. *Ophthalmology* 103:595–600, 1996.

Hearing Loss in Neonatal Intensive Care Unit Graduates
Jeffrey W. Stolz

I. **Definition.** Neonatal intensive care unit (NICU) graduates are at high risk of developing sensorineural hearing loss associated with significant functional handicaps that may result in special educational requirements, articulation abnormalities, or need for hearing aids.

II. **Incidence.** Although the overall incidence of infant deafness is 1 in 1000 live births, 1.5 to 15.3% of low-birth-weight infants requiring neonatal intensive care will develop some degree of sensorineural hearing loss. The risk factor combination of low birth weight and neonatal seizures is associated with a 28.6% incidence of sensorineural impairment.

III. **Risk factors**
   A. Family history of childhood hearing loss
   B. Birth weight less than 1500 gm
   C. Central nervous system insult
      1. Hypoxic-ischemic injury
         a. Apgar score of 6 or less at 5 minutes
      2. Intracranial hemorrhage
      3. Neonatal seizures
      4. Infection (meningitis, encephalitis)
      5. No spontaneous respirations by 10 minutes after birth
   D. Otologic damage
      1. Inner-ear hemorrhage
      2. Hyperbilirubinemia (high enough to meet criteria for exchange transfusion)
      3. Ototoxic drugs (significant exposure to aminoglycosides, loop diuretics)
      4. Fetal alcohol syndrome
      5. Congenital viral infection, syphilis, or toxoplasmosis
      6. Persistent pulmonary hypertension
      7. Hyperventilation, respiratory alkalosis
   E. Malformations of the ear (including low-set ears, ear pits and tags, abnormalities of the pinna and ear canal).
   F. Craniofacial anomalies including abnormalities of the palate, lip, face, or neck.

IV. **Screening tests**
   A. **Auditory brainstem responses (ABRs).** At present, assessing ABRs is the preferred screening method for the evaluation of hearing loss in the NICU graduate. The technique is reliable after 34 weeks' postmenstrual age. Electrodes are placed on the mastoid process behind the ear and on the forehead in the midline, just below the hairline. Earphones are either held or allowed to rest on the ear to be tested, and short bursts of clicks are emitted. The characteristic waveform recorded from the electrodes becomes more well defined with increasing postconceptional age. The auditory threshold, the minimum intensity for a recognizable V wave, decreases with increasing gestational age; thus, the results must be compared to postconceptional age-adjusted norms. Thresholds 40 to 100 dB higher than expected at a given postconceptional age correspond to a moderate to profound hearing loss.
   B. **Evoked otoacoustic emissions (EOAEs).** This test records acoustic "feedback" from the cochlea through the ossicles to the tympanic membrane and ear canal following a click stimulus. Although the test is easy to administer, norms are not well established for premature or term infants. In addition,

there are more false-positive results than with ABR tests, making EOAE a less desirable initial screening test.

V. Screening recommendations
   A. Infants at risk should have ABRs tested prior to discharge. We currently screen infants with the risk factors listed in **III.** Because ABRs depend on the maturation of the auditory system, abnormal test results obtained while the infant is at a postmenstrual age of less than 34 weeks may reflect immaturity. We usually screen sick or premature infants just prior to discharge. If the test results are abnormal, we rescreen the infants at 40 weeks' postmenstrual age or 1 month later. At Brigham and Women's Hospital, 10% of NICU infants screened have abnormal ABRs. On follow-up, 25% of this group has significant neurosensory hearing impairment.
   1. Although few controlled studies evaluate the ototoxic effect of **aminoglycoside therapy** in infants, prolonged therapy in the very-low-birth-weight infant appears to be associated with increased risk of sensorineural hearing loss. Kanamycin and amikacin appear more toxic than gentamicin or tobramycin. In term infants, no proven association of hearing loss exists with short courses of gentamicin during which peak serum levels remain in the therapeutic range. We test hearing in full-term infants treated for more than 7 days even if serum medication levels were acceptable.
   2. Universal screening. As many as 50% of infants with permanent hearing loss may have no identifiable risk factors and thus be missed by risk-based screening. Unfortunately, universal screening of newborns will miss the late-onset hearing losses due to some viral infections or genetic syndromes. A panel of the National Institutes of Health has recommended universal screening of infants, and this will likely become standard practice.
   B. All infants with abnormal screening ABRs should have follow-up testing (repeat ABR testing, behavioral testing, Crib-O-Gram) by the age of 3 months.
   C. Infants with neonatal seizures, perinatal viral infection, or evidence of neurodevelopmental delay also should be retested by the age of 6 months, regardless of predischarge ABR results.
   D. Infants with persistently abnormal test results require close supervision by an audiologist and otolaryngologist. Early intervention programs geared to optimize hearing and communication skill acquisition should be instituted.
VI. Prognosis. The prognosis depends largely on the degree of impairment, as well as the time of diagnosis and treatment. Abnormalities in auditory threshold may be predictive of language delays. Fitting of hearing aids by the age of 6 months has been associated with improved speech outcome. Initiation of early intervention services before 3 months of age has been associated with improved cognitive developmental outcome at 3 years.

Reference
1. NIH Joint Committee on Infant Hearing. 1994 Position Statement. *Pediatrics* 95:152–156, 1994.

36. COMMON NEONATAL PROCEDURES

James E. Gray and Steven A. Ringer

Invasive procedures are a necessary but potentially risk-laden part of newborn intensive care. To provide maximum benefit, these techniques must be performed in a manner that both accomplishes the task at hand and maintains the patient's general well-being.

I. **General principles**
   A. **Consideration of alternatives.** For each procedure, all alternatives should be considered and risk-benefit ratios evaluated.
   B. **Monitoring and homeostasis.** Care providers should always maintain their primary focus on the patient, rather than on the procedure being performed. They must assess cardiorespiratory and thermoregulatory stability throughout the procedure, and apply interventions when needed. Continuous monitoring can be accomplished through a combination of invasive (e.g., arterial blood pressure monitoring) or noninvasive (e.g., oximeter) techniques. In addition, the operator should consider delegating the responsibility for monitoring and managing the patient to another care provider during the procedure.
   C. **Pain control.** Treatment of procedure-associated discomfort can be accomplished with pharmacologic or nonpharmacologic approaches (see Chap. 37). The potential negative impact of any medication on the patient's cardiorespiratory status should be considered.
   D. **Informing the family.** Whenever possible, we notify parents of the need for invasive procedures in their child's care before we perform them. We discuss the indications for and possible complications of each procedure. In addition, alternative procedures, where available, are also discussed.
   E. **Precautions.** The operator should use universal precautions, including use of gloves, impermeable gowns, and barriers to protect from exposure to blood and bodily fluids that may be contaminated with infectious agents.
   F. **Education and supervision.** Individuals should be trained in the conduct of procedures prior to performing the procedure on patients. This training should include a discussion of indications, possible complications and their treatment, alternatives, and the techniques to be used. Experienced operators should be available at all times to provide further guidance and needed assistance.
   G. **Documentation.** Careful documentation of procedures enhances patient care. For example, noting difficulties encountered at intubation or the size and positioning of an endotracheal tube used provides important information if the procedure must be repeated. We routinely write notes after all procedures, including unsuccessful attempts. We document the date and time, indications, techniques used, difficulties encountered, complications (if any), and results of any laboratory tests performed.
II. **Blood drawing.** The preparations for withdrawing blood depend somewhat on the blood studies that are required.
   A. **Capillary blood** is drawn when there is no need for many serial studies in close succession.
      1. **Applicable blood studies** include hematocrit, blood glucose (using glucose reagent strips or other methods), and electrolyte determinations, and occasionally blood gas studies.
      2. **Techniques**
         a. Better results will be obtained if the extremity to be used is warmed to increase peripheral blood flow.

    b. A lancet is probably adequate if only a small quantity of blood, 3 or 4 drops, is required. If more blood is necessary, a No. 11 scalpel blade should be used, resulting in increased blood flow and a more accurate determination of laboratory values.

    c. When a **capillary puncture of the foot** is performed, the operator should use the lateral side of the sole of the heel, avoiding previous sites if possible.

    d. The skin should be cleaned carefully with povidone-iodine and alcohol before puncture to avoid infection of soft tissue or underlying bone.

B. Catheter blood samples

  1. Umbilical artery or radial artery catheters are often used for repetitive blood samples, especially for blood gas studies.

  2. Techniques

    a. Needleless systems for blood sampling from arterial catheters are now available for neonatal intensive care unit (NICU) use and are recommended. Specific techniques for use vary with the product and the manufacturer's guidelines should be followed.

    b. For **blood gas studies,** a 1-ml preheparinized syringe is used to withdraw the sample. Alternatively, a standard 1-ml syringe rinsed with 0.5 ml of heparin can be used.

    c. The catheter must be adequately cleared of infusate prior to withdrawing samples, to avoid false readings. After the sample is drawn, the line is cleared with a small volume of heparinized saline flushing solution.

C. Venous blood for blood chemistry studies, blood cultures, and other laboratory studies is usually obtained from either the antecubital vein, the external jugular vein, or the saphenous vein. For blood cultures, the area should be cleaned with an iodine-containing solution; if the position of the needle is directed by using a sterile gloved finger, the finger should be cleaned in the same way. A new sterile needle should be used to insert the blood into the culture bottles.

III. Bladder tap

A. Since bladder taps are most often used to obtain urine for culture, a sterile technique is crucial. Careful cleaning with iodine and alcohol solution over the prepubic region is essential.

B. Technique. Bladder taps are done with a 5- to 10-ml syringe attached to a 22 or 23 gauge needle or to a 23 gauge butterfly needle. Before the tap, one should try to determine that the baby has not recently urinated. Ultrasound guidance is useful. One technique is as follows:

  1. The pubic bone is located by touch.

  2. The needle is placed in the midline, just superior to the pubic bone.

  3. The needle is slid in, aimed at the infant's coccyx.

  4. If the needle goes in more than 3 cm and no urine is obtained, one should assume that the bladder is empty and wait before attempting again.

IV. Intravenous therapy. The insertion and management of intravenous catheters require great care. As in older infants, hand veins are used most often, but veins in the scalp, foot, and ankle can be used. Transillumination can help identify a vein.

V. Arterial punctures are usually carried out by using the radial artery; occasionally, the brachial or posterior tibial artery is used. **Radial artery punctures** are most easily done using transillumination to assist in location of the vessel. The radial artery is visualized and entered with the bevel of the needle up and at a 15-degree angle against the direction of flow. The artery is transfixed, and then the needle is slowly withdrawn and the syringe filled. A 23 to 25 gauge scalp vein needle is most often used.

VI. Lumbar puncture

A. Technique

  1. The infant should be placed in the lateral decubitus position or in the sitting position with legs straightened. The assistant should hold the infant

firmly at the shoulders and buttocks so that the lower part of the spine is curved. Neck flexion should be avoided so as not to compromise the airway.
2. A sterile field is prepared and draped with towels.
3. A 22 to 24 gauge spinal needle with a stylet should be used. Use of a No. 25 butterfly needle may introduce skin into the subarachnoid space and is to be avoided.
4. The needle is inserted in the midline into the space between the fourth and fifth lumbar spinous processes. The needle is advanced gradually in the direction of the umbilicus, and the stylet is withdrawn frequently to detect the presence of spinal fluid. Usually a slight "pop" is felt as the needle enters the subarachnoid space.
5. The **cerebrospinal fluid (CSF)** is collected into three or four tubes, each with a volume of 0.5 to 1.0 ml.

B. Examination of the spinal fluid. CSF should be inspected immediately for turbidity and color. In many newborns the CSF may be mildly xanthochromic, but it should always be clear.
1. **Tube 1.** Cell count and differential should be determined from the unspun fluid in a counting chamber. The unspun fluid should be stained with methylene blue; it should be treated with concentrated acetic acid if there are numerous red blood cells (RBCs). The centrifuged sediment should be stained with Gram stain and Wright stain.
2. **Tube 2** should be sent for culture and sensitivity studies.
3. **Tube 3.** Glucose and protein determinations should be obtained.
4. **Tube 4.** The cells in this tube also should be counted if the fluid is bloody. The fluid can be sent for latex fixation tests for infectious agents.

C. Information obtainable
1. When the CSF is collected in three or four separate containers, an **RBC count** can be done on the first and last tubes to see if there is a difference in the number of RBCs/mm^3 between these specimens. With traumatic taps, the final tube will have fewer RBCs than the first. CSF in the newborn may normally contain up to 600 to 800 RBCs/mm^3.
2. **White blood cell (WBC) count.** The normal number of WBCs/mm^3 in newborns is a matter of controversy. We accept up to 5 to 8 lymphocytes or monocytes as normal if there are no polymorphonuclear WBCs. Others accept as normal up to 25 WBCs/mm^3, including several polymorphonuclear cells. Data obtained from high-risk newborns without meningitis (Table 36-1) show 0 to 32 WBCs/mm^3 in term infants and 0 to 29 WBCs/mm^3 in preterm infants with about 60% polymorphonuclear cells to be within the normal range. Higher WBC counts are generally seen with gram-negative meningitis than with group B streptococcal disease; as high as 50% of the latter group will have 100 WBCs/mm^3 or less. Because of the overlap between normal infants and those with meningitis, the presence of polymorphonuclear leukocytes in CSF deserves careful attention. Ultimately, the diagnosis depends on culture results and clinical course.
3. Data on glucose and protein levels in CSF from high-risk newborns are shown in Table 36-1. The CSF glucose level is about 80% of the blood glucose level for term infants and 75% for preterm infants. If the blood glucose level is high or low, there is a 4- to 6-hour equilibration period with the CSF glucose.

The normal level of CSF protein in newborns falls in a wide range. In full-term infants, levels below 100 mg/dl are acceptable. In premature infants, the acceptable level can be as high as 180 mg/dl. Values for high-risk infants are shown in Table 36-1. The level of CSF protein in the premature infant appears to be related to the degree of prematurity.

VII. Intubation
A. Endotracheal intubation. In most cases an infant can be adequately ventilated by bag and mask so that endotracheal intubation can be done as a controlled procedure.

Table 36-1. Cerebrospinal fluid examination in high-risk neonates without meningitis

Determination	Term	Preterm
White blood cell count (cells/μl)		
No. of infants	87	30
Mean	8.2	9.0
Median	5	6
Standard deviation	7.1	8.2
Range	0–32	0–29
± 2 Standard deviations	0–22.4	0–25.4
Percentage of polymorphonuclear cells	61.3%	57.2%
Protein (mg/dl)		
No. of infants	35	17
Mean	90	115
Range	20–170	65–150
Glucose (mg/dl)		
No. of infants	51	23
Mean	52	50
Range	34–119	24–63
Glucose in cerebrospinal fluid divided by blood glucose (%)		
No. of infants	51	23
Mean	81	74
Range	44–248	55–105

Source: From L. D. Sarff, L. H. Platt, and G. H. McCracken, Cerebrospinal fluid evaluation in neonates: Comparison of high-risk neonates with and without meningitis. *J. Pediatr.* 88:473, 1976.

1. **Tube size and length.** The correct tube size (see Chap. 4) and length (Fig. 36-1) can be estimated from the infant's weight.
2. **Route.** Contradictory data exist over the preferred route for endotracheal intubation (i.e., oral versus nasal). In most circumstances local practice should guide this selection with two exceptions. First, oral intubation should be performed in all emergent situations, as it is generally easier and quicker than nasal intubation. Second, a functioning endotracheal tube should never be electively changed simply to provide an alternate route.
3. **Technique**
   a. The patient should be preoxygenated with 100% oxygen. When possible, oxygen saturations higher than 98% should be achieved prior to laryngoscopy.
   b. Throughout the intubation procedure, observation of the patient and monitoring of the heart rate are mandatory. Pulse oximetry should also be used when available. Electronic monitoring with an audible pulse rate frees personnel to attend to other tasks. If bradycardia is observed, especially if accompanied by hypoxia, the procedure should be stopped and the baby ventilated with bag and mask. An anesthesia bag attached to the tube adapter can deliver oxygen to the pharynx during the procedure or free-flow oxygen at 5 liters per minute can be given from a tube placed ½ inch from the infant's mouth.
   c. The baby's head should be slightly lifted anteriorly with the baby's body aligned straight. The operator should stand looking down the midline of the body.
   d. The **laryngoscope** is held between the thumb and first finger of the left hand, with the second and third fingers holding the baby's chin and stabilizing the head. Pushing down on the larynx with the fifth

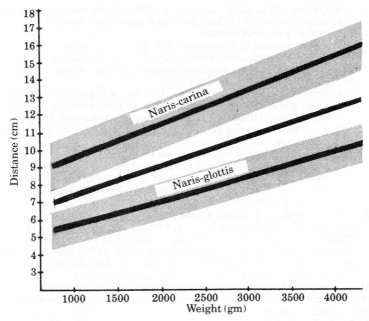

Fig. 36-1. The relationship of naris–carina and naris–glottis distance with body weight. The middle line represents the distance from naris to midtrachea. (Modified from J. Coldiron, Estimation of nasotracheal tube length in neonate. *Pediatrics* 41: 823, 1968. © 1968, American Academy of Pediatrics.)

finger of the left hand (or having an assistant do it) may help to displace the cords anteriorly and aid in visualization.

   e. The laryngoscope blade is passed into the right side of the mouth and then to the midline, swinging the tongue out of the way. It should be advanced into the vallecula. Keeping the infant's head straight will aid in visualization of the vocal cords. Care should be taken not to lever the laryngoscope blade against the upper gingiva.

   f. The **endotracheal tube** is held with the right hand and inserted between the vocal cords to about 2 cm below the glottis (less in extremely small infants). During nasotracheal intubation, Magill forceps can be useful in guiding the tube appropriately. If a finger is pressing on the trachea, the tube can be felt passing underneath.

   g. The anatomic structures of the larynx and pharynx have different appearances. The esophagus is a horizontal muscular slit; it should never be accidentally or mistakenly intubated if this is kept clearly in mind. The glottis, in contrast, consists of a triangular opening formed by the vocal cords meeting anteriorly at the apex. This orifice lies directly beneath the epiglottis, which is lifted away by gentle upward traction with the laryngoscope.

   h. The **tube position** is checked by auscultation of the chest to ensure equal aeration of both lungs and observation of chest movement with positive-pressure inflation. If air entry is poor over the left side of the chest, the tube should be pulled back until it improves.

4. Intubation in the delivery room is usually temporary, and the tube can be held in place by hand. For prolonged ventilation, the tube should be taped securely in place; the position of the tube is checked by x-ray studies or methods such as that mentioned above (see Chap. 34).

5. **Commonly observed errors**
   a. Focus is placed on the procedure and not the patient.
   b. The baby's neck is excessively extended. This displaces the cords anteriorly and obscures visualization or makes the passing of the endotracheal tube difficult.
   c. Excessive pressure is placed on the infant's upper gum by the laryngoscope blade. This results from the tip of the laryngoscope blade being tilted upward instead of traction being exerted parallel to the handle.
   d. The tube is inserted too far, resulting in intubation of the right mainstem bronchus.
   e. Laryngoscopy and intubation are made more difficult because of the level of patient activity. If not contraindicated by the patient's condition, consideration should be given to use of sedatives or muscle relaxants to facilitate intubation, but they should be used only by those skilled in airway management.

B. **Nasal continuous positive airway pressure.** Continuous distending pressure can be applied using nasal prongs as part of the ventilator circuit. These are simple to insert and are usually held on by a Velcro-fastened headset. Alternatively, an appropriately sized endotracheal tube can be passed nasally and advanced to a position just inferior to the uvula. This tube is then connected to the ventilator circuit as above.

VIII. **Thoracentesis and chest tube placement** (see Chap. 24, Air Leak)

IX. **Vascular catheterization** (see Fig. 36-2 for diagrams of the newborn venous and arterial systems)

A. **Types of catheters**
   1. **Umbilical artery catheters** are used (1) for frequent monitoring of arterial blood gases, (2) as a stable route for infusion of parenteral fluids, and (3) for continuous monitoring of arterial blood pressure.
   2. **Peripheral artery catheters** are used when frequent blood gas monitoring is still required and an umbilical artery catheter is contraindicated, cannot be placed, or is removed because of complications. Peripheral artery catheters must not be used to infuse alimentation solution or medications. They require that motion of the infant's arm be kept restricted.
   3. **Umbilical vein catheters** are used for exchange transfusions, monitoring of central venous pressure, infusion of fluids (when passed through the ductus venous and near the right atrium), and emergency vascular access for infusion of fluid, blood, or medications.
   4. **Central venous catheters,** used largely for prolonged parenteral nutrition and occasionally to monitor central venous pressure, also can be placed percutaneously through the external jugular, subclavian, basilic, or saphenous vein.

B. **Umbilical artery catheterization**
   1. **Guidelines.** In general, only seriously ill infants should have an umbilical artery catheter placed. If only a few blood gas measurements are anticipated, peripheral arterial punctures should be performed together with noninvasive oxygen monitoring, and a peripheral intravenous route should be used for fluids and medications.
   2. **Technique**
      a. **Sterile technique is used.** Before preparing cord and skin, make external measurements to determine how far the catheter will be inserted (Figs. 36-3–36-5). In a high setting, the catheter tip is placed between the eighth and tenth thoracic vertebrae; in a low setting, the tip is between the third and fourth lumbar vertebrae.
      b. The cord and surrounding area are washed carefully with an antiseptic solution, and the abdomen is draped with sterile towels. Avoid burns caused by allowing excess solution to remain on the skin by

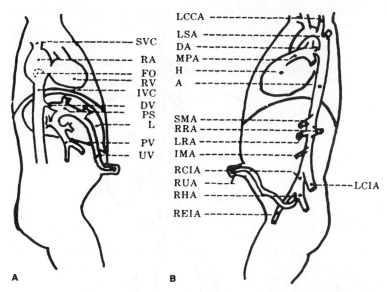

SVC
RA
FO
RV
IVC
DV
PS
L
PV
UV

LCCA
LSA
DA
MPA
H
A

SMA
RRA
LRA
IMA

RCIA
RUA
RHA

REIA

LCIA

A

B

Fig. 36-2. A. Diagram of the newborn umbilical venous system (SVC = superior vena cava; RA = right atrium; FO = foramen ovale; RV = right ventricle; IVC = inferior vena cava; DV = ductus venosus; PS = portal sinus; L = liver; PV = portal vein; UV = umbilical vein). **B.** Diagram of the newborn arterial system, including the umbilical artery (LCCA = left common carotid artery; LSA = left subclavian artery; DA = ductus arteriosus; MPA = main pulmonary artery; H = heart; A = aorta; SMA = superior mesenteric artery; RRA = right renal artery; LRA = left renal artery; IMA = inferior mesenteric artery; LCIA = left common iliac artery). (From J.A. Kitterman, R.H. Phibbs, and W.H. Tooley, Catheterization of umbilical vessels in newborn infants. *Pediatr. Clin. North Am.* 17:898, 1970.)

carefully cleaning the skin (including the back and trunk) with sterile water.
  c. Umbilical tape should be placed around the base of the cord. If it is placed on the skin, it must be loosened after the procedure. The tape is used to gently constrict the cord to prevent bleeding. The cord is cut cleanly with a scalpel to a length of 1.0 to 1.5 cm.
  d. The cord is stabilized with a forceps or hemostat, and the two arteries are identified.
  e. The open tip of an iris forceps is inserted into the artery lumen and gently used to dilate the vessel; and then the closed tip is inserted into the lumen of an artery to a depth of 0.5 cm. Tension on the forceps is released, and the forceps is left in place to dilate the vessel for about 1 minute. This pause may be the most useful step in insertion of the catheter.
  f. The forceps is withdrawn, and a sterile saline-filled 3.5F or 5F umbilical vessel catheter with an end hole is threaded into the artery. The smaller catheter is generally used for infants weighing less than 1500 gm. Increased resistance will be felt as the catheter passes through the base of the cord and as it navigates the umbilical artery–femoral artery junction. In about 5 to 10% of attempted umbilical artery catheterizations, one of the following problems may occur.

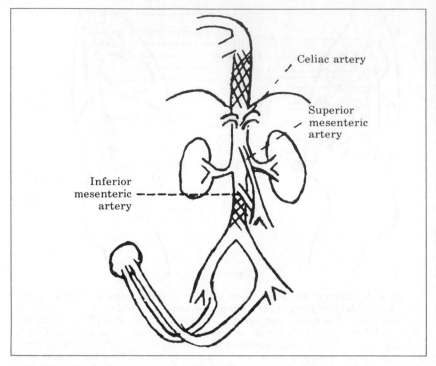

Fig. 36-3. Localization of umbilical artery catheters. The crosshatched areas represent sites in which complications are least likely. Either site may be used for placement of the catheter tip.

(1) The catheter will not pass into the abdominal aorta. Sometimes a double-catheter technique will allow successful cannulation in this situation.

(2) The catheter may pass into the aorta but head caudad to one of the iliac arteries and then down the other leg or out one of the arteries to the buttocks. There may be difficulty advancing the catheter and cyanosis or blanching of the leg or buttocks may occur. This happens more frequently when a small catheter (3.5F) is placed in a large baby. Sometimes using a larger, stiffer catheter (5.0F) will allow the catheter to advance up the aorta. Alternatively, removing the catheter from the aorta (while leaving it in the umbilical artery), twirling it, and reinserting it into the aorta will allow it to proceed cephalad. If this fails, the other umbilical artery can be tried. Sometimes the catheter goes up the aorta and then reverses itself and goes back down. This also happens more frequently in a large baby when a small catheter is used. The catheter may also enter any of the vessels coming off the aorta. If the catheter cannot be advanced to the desired position, the tip should be pulled to a low position or the catheter removed.

(3) There is persistent cyanosis, blanching, or poor distal extremity perfusion. If this occurs, the catheter should be removed.

g. When the catheter is advanced the appropriate distance, placement should be confirmed by x-ray examination.

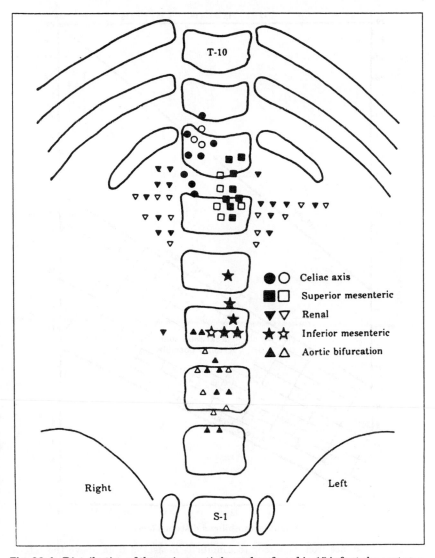

Fig. 36-4. Distribution of the major aortic branches found in 15 infants by aortography as correlated with the vertebral bodies. Filled symbols represent infants with cardiac or renal anomalies (or both); open symbols represent those without either disorder. Major landmarks appear at the following vertebral levels: diaphragm, T12 interspace; celiac artery, T12; superior mesenteric artery, L1 interspace; renal artery, L1; inferior mesenteric artery, L3; aortic bifurcation, L4. (From D.L. Phelps et al. The radiologic localization of the major aorta tributaries in the newborn. *J. Pediatr.* 81:336, 1972.)

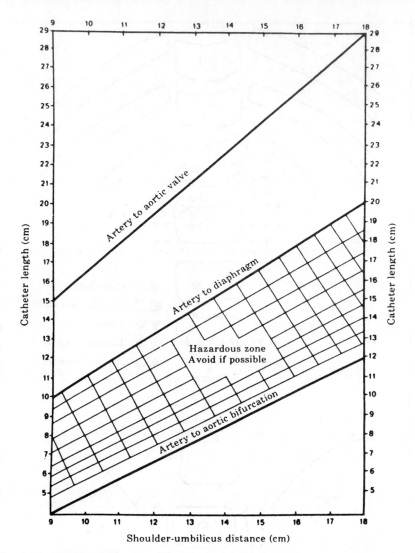

Fig. 36-5. Distance from shoulder to umbilicus measured from above the lateral end of the clavicle to the umbilicus, as compared with the length of umbilical artery catheter needed to reach the designated level. (From P.M. Dunn, Localization of the umbilical catheter by postmortem measurement. *Arch. Dis. Child.* 41:69, 1969.)

    h. The catheter can be fixed in place with a purse-string suture using silk thread, and it should be taped for further stability (see Chap. 34).

    i. Antibiotic ointment may be applied to the junction of the cord and catheter.

3. Catheter removal

    a. The umbilical artery catheter should be removed when either of the following criteria are met:

(1) The infant improves so that continuous monitoring and frequent blood drawing are not necessary.

(2) Complications are noted.

b. **Method of catheter removal.** The catheter is removed slowly over a period of 30 to 60 seconds, allowing the umbilical artery to constrict at its proximal end while the catheter is still occluding the distal end. This usually prevents profuse bleeding. Old sutures should be removed.

4. **Complications associated with umbilical artery catheterization.** Significant morbidity can be associated with complications of umbilical artery catheterization. These complications are mainly due to vascular accidents, including thromboembolic phenomena to the kidney, bowel, legs, or rarely the spinal cord. These may manifest as hematuria, hypertension, signs of necrotizing enterocolitis or bowel infarction, and cyanosis or blanching of the skin of the back, buttocks, or legs. Other complications seen are infection, disseminated intravascular coagulation, and vessel perforation. All these complications are indications for catheter removal. Close observation of the skin, monitoring of the urine for hematuria, measuring blood pressure, and following the platelet count may give clues to complications.

a. We perform ultrasound examination of the aorta and renal vessels to check for thrombi in infants in whom we are concerned about complications. If thrombi are observed, the catheter is removed.

b. If there are small thrombi without symptoms or with increased blood pressure alone, we usually remove the catheter, follow resolution of the thrombi by ultrasound examination, and treat hypertension if necessary (see Chap. 31). If there are signs of emboli or loss of pulses, or coagulopathy, and no intracranial hemorrhage is present, we consider heparinization, maintaining the partial thromboplastin time (PTT) at double the control value. If there is a large clot with impairment of perfusion, we consider the use of fibrinolytic agents (see Chap. 26, Major Arterial and Venous Thrombosis Management). Surgical treatment of thrombosis is not generally effective.

c. **Blanching of a leg** following catheter placement is the most common complication noted clinically. Although this often occurs transiently, it deserves careful attention. One technique that may reverse this finding is to warm the opposite leg. If the vasospasm resolves, the catheter may be left in place. If there is no improvement, the catheter should be removed.

5. **Other considerations**

a. **Use of heparin for anticoagulation to prevent clotting.** Whether the use of heparin in the infusate decreases the incidence of thrombotic complications is not known. We use dilute heparin 0.5 to 1.0 unit/ml of infusate.

b. **Positioning of the catheter tip.** Little helpful information convincingly supports the choice between high and low placement of umbilical artery catheters. A higher complication rate has been reported in infants with the catheter tip at L3 to L4, compared with T7 to T8, owing to more episodes of blanching and cyanosis of one or both legs. No difference between the high- and low-position groups was seen in the rate of complications requiring catheter removal. Renal complications and emboli to the bowel may be more common with catheter tips placed at T7 to T8 while catheters placed low (L3 to L4) are associated with complications such as cyanosis and blanching of the leg, which are easier to observe.

c. **Indwelling time.** The incidence of complications associated with umbilical artery catheterization appears to be directly related to the length of time the catheter is left in place.

6. **Infection and use of antibiotics.** We do not use prophylactic antibiotics for placement of umbilical artery catheters. In infants with umbilical

artery catheters, we use antibiotics whenever infection is suspected and after appropriate cultures have been obtained.

C. Umbilical vein catheterization (see Figs. 36-2 and 36-6)

1. **Indications.** We use umbilical vein catheterization for emergency vascular access and exchange transfusions; in these cases, the venous catheter is replaced by a peripheral intravenous catheter or other access as soon as possible. In critically ill infants, we also use an umbilical vein catheter to monitor central venous pressure and to infuse vasopressors or hypertonic solutions.

2. **Technique**

   a. The site is prepared as for umbilical artery catheterization after determining the appropriate length of catheter to be inserted (see Fig. 36-6).

   b. Any clots seen are removed with a forceps, and the umbilical vein is gently dilated as with the umbilical artery above.

   c. The catheter (3.5F or 5F) is prepared by filling it and an attached syringe with heparinized saline solution, 1 unit/ml of saline solution. The catheter should never be left open to the atmosphere because negative intrathoracic pressure could cause an air embolism.

   d. The catheter is inserted while gentle traction is exerted on the cord. Once the catheter is in the vein, one should try to slide the catheter cephalad just under the skin, where the vein runs very superficially. If the catheter is being placed for an exchange transfusion, it should be advanced only as far as is necessary to establish good blood flow (usually 2 to 5 cm). If the catheter is being used to monitor central venous pressure, it should be advanced through the ductus venosus into the inferior vena cava and its position verified by x-ray.

   e. Only isotonic solutions should be infused until the position of the catheter is verified by x-ray studies. If the catheter tip is in the inferior vena cava, hypertonic solutions may be infused.

D. Multiple-lumen catheters for umbilical venous catheterization

1. **Indications.** Placement of a double- or triple-lumen catheter into the umbilical vein can provide additional venous access for administration of incompatible solutions (e.g., those containing vasopressor agents, sodium bicarbonate, or calcium).

2. **Technique**

   a. **Modified Seldinger technique.** In patients with an indwelling single-lumen catheter, a wire exchange technique may be used to place a multiple-lumen catheter. While this method decreases the probability of catheter loss during exchange, it entails the risks of wire passage including cardiac dysrhythmias and perforation, and should be attempted only by those familiar with the Seldinger technique.

   b. **Direct placement.** Multiple-lumen catheters can be placed directly following the outline provided above for single-lumen catheters. The increased pliability of many of the multiple-lumen catheters makes passage into the hepatic veins more likely.

3. **Usage.** Where possible, infusions that should not be interrupted (e.g., vasopressors) are placed in the proximal lumen to allow measurement of central venous pressure from the distal port.

E. Percutaneous radial artery catheterization. Placement of an indwelling radial artery catheter is a useful alternative to umbilical artery catheterization for monitoring blood gas levels and blood pressure.

1. **Advantages**

   a. Accessibility (when the umbilical artery is inaccessible or has been used for a long period)

   b. Reflection of preductal flow (if the right radial artery is used)

   c. Avoidance of thrombosis of major vessels, which is sometimes associated with umbilical vessel catheterization

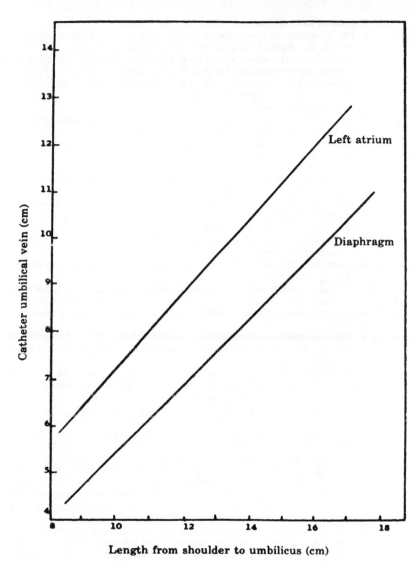

Fig. 36-6. Catheter length for umbilical vein catheterization. The catheter tip should be placed between the diaphragm and the left atrium. (From P.M. Dunn, Localization of the umbilical catheter by postmortem measurements. *Arch. Dis. Child.* 41:69, 1966.)

2. **Risks** are usually small if the procedure is performed carefully, but infection, air embolus, inadvertent injection of incorrect solution, and arterial occlusion may occur.
3. **Equipment** required includes a 22 or 24 gauge intravenous cannula with stylet, a T-connector, heparinized saline flushing solution (0.5 to 1.0 unit of heparin per milliliter of solution), and an infusion pump.

4. Method of catheterization

a. The adequacy of the ulnar collateral flow to the hand must be assessed. The radial and ulnar arteries should be simultaneously compressed, and the ulnar artery should then be released. The degree of flushing of the blanched hand should be noted. If the entire hand becomes flushed while the radial artery is occluded, the ulnar circulation is adequate. A high-intensity light may be used to view the radial and ulnar arteries.

b. The hand may be secured on an arm board with the wrist extended, leaving all fingertips exposed, to observe color changes.

c. The wrist is prepared with an iodine-containing solution, and the site of maximum arterial pulsation is palpated.

d. The intravenous cannula is inserted through the skin at an angle less than 30 degrees to horizontal and is slowly advanced into the artery. Transillumination may help delineate the vessel and its course. If the artery is entered as the catheter is advanced, the stylet is removed and the catheter is advanced in the artery. If there is no blood return, the artery may be transfixed. The stylet is then removed, and the catheter is slowly withdrawn until blood flow occurs; then it is advanced into the vessel.

5. Caution. Only heparinized saline solution, at a rate not exceeding 2 ml per hour, is infused into the catheter.

F. Percutaneous central venous catheterization is useful for long-term venous access for intravenous fluids, particularly parenteral nutrition.

1. Subclavian vein catheterization is useful in infants weighing more than 1200 gm.

a. **The equipment** required includes a 3.0F catheter with introducer needle and guidewire. Double-lumen 4.0F catheters may be used in larger infants (>2.5 kg).

b. **Technique.** The infant is sedated and placed supine with a roll between the scapulae. Generally, the patient should be ventilated and muscle relaxed to afford maximum chance of success. The head is turned away from the side of insertion. The shoulders should drop posteriorly. The skin is prepared with an iodine-containing solution and infiltrated with local anesthetic. The introducer needle is inserted through the skin and immediately beneath the clavicle, a third of the way from the shoulder to the midline. The needle should be almost parallel to the chest wall and aimed at the sternal notch. When blood flow is established, the guidewire is passed and the catheter is placed over the wire. Catheter position is determined radiographically. The catheter tip should lie at the junction of the superior vena cava and right atrium.

c. **Complications** include pneumothorax, hemothorax, and inadvertent subclavian artery puncture. The potential severity of these complications dictates that only those thoroughly familiar with this technique should attempt this form of venous cannulation.

2. Peripheral or external jugular vein catheterization is useful in infants weighing less than 1500 gm.

a. **The equipment** required includes a 1.9F to 2.1F silicone catheter cut to the appropriate length, an introducer needle, and iris forceps.

b. **Technique.** An appropriate vein of entry is selected. This may be an external jugular, basilic, or greater saphenous vein. The site is prepared with an iodine-containing solution, and the introducer needle is inserted into the vein until blood flows freely. The silicone catheter is inserted through the needle with forceps and is slowly advanced the predetermined distance for central venous positioning. The introducer needle is removed, the extra catheter length is coiled on the skin near the insertion site, and the site is covered with transparent surgical covering. The catheter tip is positioned at the junction of the vena cava and right atrium, as confirmed by radiography. Some physicians inject a small amount of isotonic contrast material to make visualization easier.

   c. Complications are rare but include infection, thrombosis, and thrombophlebitis.

X. **Abdominal paracentesis for removal of ascitic fluid**
   A. **Indications**
      1. Therapeutic indications include respiratory distress resulting from abdominal distention (e.g., hydropic infants, infants with urinary ascites) for which removal of ascitic fluid will ameliorate respiratory symptoms. In addition, interference with urine production or lower extremity perfusion resulting from increased intraabdominal pressure may be improved by paracentesis.
      2. Diagnostic indications include the evaluation of suspected peritonitis.
   B. **Technique**
      1. The equipment needed includes an 18 to 22 gauge intravenous catheter, three-way stopcock, and a 10- to 50-ml syringe.
      2. The lower abdomen is prepared with povidone-iodine solution and the area is draped. If the bladder is distended, it is drained with manual pressure or a urinary catheter. A local anesthetic such as 1% lidocaine (Xylocaine) is infiltrated into the subcutaneous tissues when possible. The catheter is inserted just lateral to the rectus sheath one-third of the distance between the umbilicus and the symphysis pubis. Alternatively the catheter can be inserted in the midline, during aspiration with the syringe. The catheter is advanced approximately 1 cm until the resistance of passing through the abdominal wall diminishes or fluid is obtained. Five to 10 ml of fluid is removed for diagnostic paracentesis while 10 to 20 ml/kg should be removed for therapeutic effects. The catheter is removed and the site bandaged.
   C. **Potential complications**
      1. Cardiovascular effects, including tachycardia, hypotension, and decreased cardiac output, may result from rapid redistribution of intravascular fluid to the peritoneal space following removal of large amounts of ascites.
      2. Bladder or intestinal aspiration may occur more frequently in the presence of a dilated bladder or bowel. These puncture sites usually heal spontaneously and without significant clinical findings.

Reference
Fletcher, M.A., McDonald M.G., and Avery, G.B. (Eds.), *Atlas of Procedures in Neonatology*. Philadelphia: Lippincott, 1994.

37. ANESTHESIA AND ANALGESIA

Charles Berde

Newborns can and should receive anesthesia and analgesia for surgery and invasive procedures. Safe methods of anesthesia are available for even the sickest and most premature of neonates, so that it is no longer valid to claim that anesthesia should be withheld from these newborns because of excessive risk. Newborns have sufficient neurologic development to process noxious sensation as distressing, and to respond to injury with behavioral signs of distress and physiologic signs of stress. (For a review, see refs. 1 through 5 and 15. For a detailed discussion, see ref. 6.)

I. **Preoperative laboratory testing.** Routine preoperative testing for comparatively healthy newborns should be extremely limited, unless tests are guided by abnormalities in the history and physical examination. A number of tests including chest x-ray, electrolyte, urinalysis, and coagulation studies have low predictive value for otherwise healthy infants undergoing relatively straightforward surgery.

The most prevalent recommendation at present is for routine hematocrit determinations. Hematocrit determinations may indicate a need for preoperative treatment of anemia in some circumstances, or may predict a greater likelihood of a requirement for transfusion in the circumstance of moderate blood loss in surgery. In addition, anemia may increase the risk of postoperative apnea in former premature infants [7].

In specific contexts, further testing or consultation is indicated. For example, for a neonate presenting for repair of esophageal atresia–tracheoesophageal fistula, there is a high likelihood of associated cardiac anomalies, and cardiac evaluation should be routine. As another example, for a 1-month-old with pyloric stenosis and protracted vomiting, hypochloremia, hypokalemia, and metabolic alkalosis are common, and electrolyte concentrations should be measured and corrected prior to surgery.

II. **Monitoring infants undergoing surgery** (Table 37-1). Newborns experience physiologic change more rapidly than do most adults undergoing anesthesia. Hypoxemia and hypotension may occur precipitously with changes in oxygen delivery and anesthetic depth, respectively. Basic monitoring of newborns undergoing both routine and major surgery includes a precordial or esophageal stethoscope, electrocardiography (ECG), noninvasive blood pressure measurement, pulse oximetry, capnometry, and monitoring of temperature. Specific modifications are required for many of these monitors. Small lightweight stethoscope attachments are useful, as are small ECG contact electrodes. Oscillometric measurement of blood pressure is effective in neonates with modifications of cuff sizes and analytic algorithms.

Pulse oximetry can be applied in most infants, although there may be difficulty with recording in states of low peripheral perfusion. Oximetry has a rapid response time that makes it useful for intraoperative monitoring. Oximetry is insensitive to hyperoxia, which may predispose premature infants to retinopathy. Capnometry is a useful measure of both ventilation and pulmonary perfusion. In newborns, many factors predispose to erroneous capnometry measurements, including circuit dead space, dilution of exhaled gases by fresh gas flow, and limitations of sampling rate at high respiratory rates. In selected cases, transcutaneous measurement of oxygen and carbon dioxide may be a useful adjunct to oximetry and capnometry.

Transcutaneous measurements have several limitations in intraoperative use, including a slow response time, a requirement for skin heating (for oxy-

667

Table 37-1.   Basic monitoring equipment for pediatric anesthesia

Precordial stethoscope
Pulse oximeter
Electrocardiograph
Noninvasive blood pressure device (oscillometric, aneroid, or other)
Temperature probe
Capnometer
Oxygen analyzer

gen, not carbon dioxide), and a potential for interference from inhalation anesthetics.

Neonates have a high potential for hypothermia or hyperthermia intraoperatively. Hypothermia can cause several problems, including (1) apnea, (2) increased bleeding, (3) inability to reverse neuromuscular blocking drugs, and (4) shivering and increased oxygen consumption upon emergence. Temperature monitoring is essential during anesthesia. Several methods are available for active warming, including (1) warming blankets, (2) fluid warmers, (3) convective warming blankets, (4) control of room temperature, or (5) active or passive warming of the breathing circuit. Convective warming is the most effective noninvasive method if aggressive warming is needed.

Arterial cannulation is helpful for procedures with the potential for major respiratory or hemodynamic derangement or major blood loss, or in the critically ill newborn. Percutaneous catheterization of radial, dorsalis pedis, or posterior tibial arteries can be accomplished with a very low risk of morbidity, though it may be technically difficult in infants with low blood pressure or previous vessel punctures. Where percutaneous peripheral arterial access is not feasible, alternatives include (1) umbilical artery cannulation, (2) percutaneous femoral artery cannulation, and (3) peripheral arterial cutdown. Arterial catheterization is useful for beat-to-beat measurement of blood pressure, for analysis of the waveform as an approximate measure of hemodynamic condition and volume status, and for repeated blood sampling.

Central venous catheterization is useful for (1) secure venous access in the child undergoing major surgery with a paucity of peripheral sites, (2) monitoring of central venous pressure in infants with major fluid shifts, (3) vasopressor infusion in critically ill neonates, and (4) situations where prolonged hyperalimentation is needed for nutritional support. Softer-tip catheters are preferred, to diminish the risk of vascular perforation. For short-term use, percutaneous catheters may be placed; for longer-term use, tunneled silicone elastomer catheters are widely preferred, to diminish the risk of infection, vascular perforation, and vessel thrombosis.

III. **Airway management.** Much of the morbidity and mortality in newborn anesthesia is related to difficulties with airway management. Anatomic and physiologic factors make newborns more susceptible to airway obstruction and respiratory insufficiency (Table 37-2).

Airway equipment must be tailored to the size of the newborn. Availability of appropriately sized masks, oral airways, laryngoscopes, and endotracheal tubes is crucial.

For most major operations requiring general anesthesia in newborns, endotracheal intubation is preferred. In most elective situations, our preference is to perform laryngoscopy and intubation following anesthetic induction because they are more easily accomplished and less traumatic for the newborn. Awake intubation may be associated with transient rises in blood pressure and intracranial pressure that may be a particular stress for the sick newborn at risk for intracranial hemorrhage. Nevertheless, intubation following anesthetic induction is predicated on a confidence that intubation can be readily accomplished, or at least that mask ventilation will be successful. Desaturation

Table 37-2. Developmental factors and their anesthetic implications

Physiologic variable	Implications
Immaturity of hepatic enzyme systems	Delayed clearance of intravenous anesthetics and opioids
Immaturity of renal clearance	Delayed clearance of pancuronium
High ratio of oxygen consumption and minute ventilation to functional residual capacity	Accelerated uptake and removal of inhalation anesthetics
Immature thermoregulatory reflexes	Increased potential for hypothermia or hyperthermia during surgery
Immature ventilatory reflexes	Increased potential for postanesthetic apnea
Immature baroreceptors, incomplete sympathetic nervous development	Increased risk of hypotension with inhalation anesthesia Lack of hypotension or bradycardia with spinal anesthesia

occurs much more rapidly in neonates following rapid induction of anesthesia, due to a lower ratio of functional residual capacity to oxygen consumption, in comparison with older children and adults. If anesthesia is induced or paralyzing agents are given and the newborn cannot be intubated or ventilated by mask, the results may be catastrophic. We prefer awake intubation when airway control may be extremely problematic, such as in newborns with Pierre Robin syndrome or other causes of macroglossia, micrognathia, narrow mouth opening, or related difficulties. A variety of techniques have been described for aiding intubation of the difficult airway in newborns, including fiberoptic laryngoscopy [8], use of the anterior commissure laryngoscope, or use of a specially modified "light wand" for blind intubation [9]. A recent development is the laryngeal mask airway, a device that is placed blindly into the pharynx and inflated and that facilitates ventilation or delivery of anesthetic gases [10]. The laryngeal mask has been used successfully in newborns with a variety of difficult airway conditions.

IV. Hemodynamics in the newborn. Newborns are at particular risk of hypotension and low cardiac output during anesthesia, due to a variety of factors, including (1) rate dependence of cardiac output, (2) poor ventricular compliance, (3) diminished baroreceptor function [11,12], (4) inadequate maturation of sympathetic responses, and (5) increased susceptibility to the myocardial depressant effects of volatile anesthetic agents. With the transitional circulation, they are prone to right-to-left shunting at either ductal or foraminal levels in the setting of hypoxemia or acidosis.

V. Anesthetic equipment for neonates
Breathing circuits [13]. Many of the "smart" alarms on contemporary anesthetic machines are tailored primarily to adults, and their response times and sensitivities are awkward for neonates. As with adults, anesthetic delivery systems should include oxygen analyzers to confirm delivered inspired oxygen concentrations.

Spontaneous ventilation during anesthesia is more likely to fail in the newborn than in the older child because of several factors, including (1) increased tendency to diaphragmatic fatigue, (2) increased airway resistance and work of breathing, and (3) diminished ventilatory reflexes to hypoxemia or hypercarbia.

Circle systems with one-way valves can be used for young infants and newborns receiving controlled ventilation. They are readily available in most operating rooms and permit heating, humidification, carbon dioxide absorption and scavenging of exhaled gases. In very small infants or in those with substantial lung disease, use of circle systems is more problematic, because of largely wasted ventilation due to high circuit compliance and circuit dead space. Pediatric circle systems may diminish dead space, but do not eliminate the problem of high circuit compliance. In very small infants or in infants with substantial lung disease, most pediatric anesthesiologists prefer circuits functionally similar to a Mapleson D, including the Bain circuit or the Jackson-Rees modification of the Ayres T-piece.

Although standard operating room ventilators can be used for comparatively healthy newborns, for the sicker and smaller newborns, we prefer use of dedicated ventilators such as those used in newborn intensive care. They can be used to deliver air and oxygen for a newborn receiving intravenous anesthesia, or they can be equipped to deliver anesthetic vapors as well.

VI. **Fluid management.** The purpose of preoperative fasting is to increase the likelihood of an empty stomach at the time of induction, to diminish the risk of aspiration of acidic fluid or particulates. Several studies suggested that newborns and infants can safely receive clear liquids (apple juice, flat ginger ale, glucose-electrolyte solutions) up to 2 hours before surgery [6,15]. Continued feeding of clear liquids has several benefits: (1) prevention of dehydration and hypoglycemia, and (2) reduced hunger, with less fussiness or crying at induction.

Intravenous infusions are recommended for all but the most brief of operative procedures. They are needed both for fluid replacement and as a route to administer emergency medications.

Isotonic or nearly isotonic solutions are preferred to hypotonic solutions in most cases. Hyperglycemia and hypoglycemia are to be avoided. Hyperglycemia during anesthesia has two primary causes: (1) inadequate depth of anesthesia leading to secretion of counterregulatory hormones and (2) rapid infusion of glucose-containing solutions. Although most newborns will not become hypoglycemic if glucose is omitted from infusions during anesthesia, a subgroup of newborns may have hypoglycemia, with catastrophic consequences. Thus it is recommended that rapid rehydration to replace deficits or to treat hypotension or mild blood loss employ isotonic electrolyte solutions such as lactated Ringer's, and that maintenance infusions that are infused slowly should include glucose. If glucose-containing solutions are not administered routinely, blood glucose concentrations should be measured.

VII. **Analgesic and anesthetic pharmacology.** Infants undergoing painful surgery deserve analgesics postoperatively. Analgesic pharmacology has received increasing attention in recent years. Newborns have a number of factors that influence drug disposition: (1) a higher percentage of body mass is water, and less is fat; (2) a higher percentage of body mass in the "highly perfused" tissue group (heart, brain, and viscera), and a lower percentage in the muscle tissue compartment; (3) delayed maturation of hepatic drug-metabolizing enzyme systems; and (4) delayed maturation of glomerular filtration.

A. **Acetaminophen.** Acetaminophen is the most commonly used analgesic for mild pain and fever control in pediatrics. Recommended dosing is based largely on doses effective for fever control, since analgesic studies to date have not confirmed the effective dose-response curve. Dosing of 15 mg/kg every 4 hours by mouth is quite safe for short-term (i.e., postoperative) use, even in neonates.

Rectal dosing appears much less efficient than previously believed. Recent studies by Rusy et al. in our group using 35 mg/kg [14] revealed peak concentrations in the therapeutic range for fever control. Peak concentrations were not achieved until typically 45 to 60 minutes after administration.

Although acetaminophen is quite useful and has a wide safety margin, it is a mistake to regard it as effective as the sole analgesic for extensive operations in newborns.

B. Nonsteroidal agents. Nonsteroidal antiinflammatory drugs have become widely used for adults and older children. In newborns, they are used primarily for closure of the ductus arteriosus rather than for analgesia. Although they may provide analgesia in newborns, their use is currently limited by concerns regarding gastritis, nephropathy, and postoperative or intracranial bleeding. Further studies of their use in young infants are in progress.

C. Opioids. Opioids have a wide range of uses for newborns. For newborns undergoing major operations, particularly where postoperative mechanical ventilation is anticipated, opioids can form the major component of a general anesthetic technique. Robinson and Gregory [16] initially showed that prematures undergoing ligation of the ductus arteriosus under fentanyl anesthesia tolerated the procedure with excellent hemodynamic stability. Subsequent studies by Anand et al. [2] and Hickey et al. [17] in Oxford and Boston showed that anesthesia with synthetic opioids (fentanyl, sufentanil, alfentanil) can be performed with excellent outcomes. Since opioids provide analgesia but not immobility, they generally are administered either with neuromuscular blocking drugs (e.g., pancuronium) or with lower concentrations of inhalation anesthetics. Yaster et al. [18] found that to achieve complete anesthesia for noncardiac operations in premature infants, incremental doses of 10 μg of fentanyl per kilogram provided adequate suppression of autonomic responses to surgery. Anand et al. showed in a series of studies that high-dose fentanyl or sufentanil anesthesia attenuates hormonal and metabolic responses to surgical stress in high-risk newborns [2].

The primary concern with opioids lies in their potential for postoperative hypoventilation, particularly in less extensive procedures that permit extubation postoperatively. The susceptibility of newborns to respiratory depression probably involves both pharmacokinetic and pharmacodynamic factors. Newborns metabolize and excrete opioids somewhat more slowly than do older children and adults. In abdominal surgery, where there is a reduction of hepatic blood flow intraoperatively and postoperatively, the clearance of opioids such as fentanyl can be severely delayed.

Continuous infusions of opioids can provide excellent postoperative analgesia for major operations in newborns. Based on the pharmacokinetic data and clinical experience of Koren et al. [19] and Lynn et al. [20], starting morphine infusion rates are recommended to be 0.015 mg/kg per hour.

D. Inhalation anesthetics [21]. Vapor inhalation anesthetics commonly used for children include the potent vapors halothane and isoflurane and the weaker gas anesthetic nitrous oxide. Uptake and induction are more rapid for infants than for older subjects, and following discontinuation of the anesthetics, clearance and awakening are also more rapid for infants than for older children. Inhalation anesthesia is widely chosen for infants because of the ease of inhalation induction, particularly in infants with difficult venous access, and because of rapid awakening. Inhalation anesthesia is also preferred when spontaneous breathing is required, as with some critical airway conditions. Halothane hepatitis and malignant hyperthermia, which are rare conditions in older subjects, are virtually never seen in the newborn.

Nitrous oxide is a useful adjunctive anesthetic, particularly for short procedures because of its rapid onset and offset. It is inadequate as a sole anesthetic. Nitrous oxide can diffuse into gas-filled spaces such as the lumen of the bowel, and may be contraindicated for prolonged abdominal surgery. Its use is also limited when there is a need to use high concentrations of oxygen, such as thoracic operations.

A limitation of the potent inhalation anesthetics is their tendency in newborns to produce myocardial depression and hypotension at alveolar concentrations close to those required to produce immobility. Anesthetic depth must be judged carefully.

E. Intravenous anesthetics. All of the commonly used intravenous anesthetics have their actions terminated by redistribution and subsequently by hepatic metabolism. Hepatic metabolism is delayed in newborns, leading to prolonged residual sedation following induction doses for most agents.

Ketamine is a useful induction agent in sick newborns. It is quite analgesic and is associated with good hemodynamic stability in the great majority of patients [22]. Pulmonary arteriolar constriction appears unimportant, particularly if hypercarbia is avoided.

Thiopental can be used in newborns for rapid sequence induction. Hypotension may occur with large doses in the setting of hypovolemia or cardiac disease. Delayed clearance may produce comparatively prolonged sedation following thiopental use in newborns.

Propofol is the newest of the commonly used intravenous agents. It permits extremely rapid emergence. Studies by Schrum et al. [23], Hannallah et al. [24], and others [25] suggested that younger infants recieving propofol emerge more quickly and with fewer airway difficulties than do infants receiving thiopental induction. Propofol has some potential for hypotension, particularly in infants with congenital heart disease or hypovolemia.

F. Neuromuscular blocking drugs. Neuromuscular blocking drugs (muscle relaxants) provide immobility but no analgesia or amnesia. Their use in the absence of adequate anesthesia or analgesia is deplorable and should be condemned.

A common technique is to use opioids or vapor anesthetics in combination with muscle relaxants. Since the alveolar concentrations of vapor anesthetics required to produce unconsciousness are generally less than those required for immobility (roughly 50%), this technique is useful for providing good operating conditions without hypotension or movement. There remains a concern for ensuring unconsciousness and analgesia based solely on autonomic signs in the absence of signs of movement.

Because of a larger volume of distribution, the initial dose of muscle relaxants required per kilogram to produce a given degree of blockade may be larger in newborns than in older infants [26]. The duration of action of nondepolarizing relaxants in newborns is prolonged, especially with repeated dosing, because of either immaturity of renal excretion (e.g., pancuronium) or immaturity of hepatic metabolism (e.g., vecuronium). Train-of-four monitoring of adductor pollicis twitches following stimulation of the ulnar nerve is a useful noninvasive measure of degrees of neuromuscular blockade. For all the reasons described earlier, newborns are at increased risk of ventilatory depression due to residual concentrations of muscle relaxants following surgery. Antagonism of residual blockade using acetylcholinesterase inhibitors (e.g., neostigmine and edrophonium) and anticholinergics (atropine and glycopyrrolate) is recommended unless prolonged ventilation is anticipated.

G. Local anesthetics [27,28]. Local anesthetics are extremely useful for providing analgesia for procedures (cut-down, chest tube insertion) and operations. They can provide analgesia with excellent preservation of alertness, respiratory drive, and hemodynamic stability.

When infiltration blockade is used in newborns, concentrations should be diluted greatly. For example, lidocaine is quite effective for infiltration in concentrations ranging from 0.3 to 0.5%; 1 to 2% solutions are unnecessary and may predispose to systemic toxicity (Table 37-3).

For infiltration blockade, aspiration through a small needle may not always exclude intravascular injection, since veins may collapse on aspiration. It is more reliable to infiltrate with a constantly moving needle tip, so that the tip is highly unlikely to remain in a vessel for any appreciable portion of the dose.

Peripheral nerve blockade and wound infiltration have become widely used for infants undergoing a variety of surgical procedures, including inguinal hernia repair. In the case of circumcision [29], penile blockade can be an effective anesthetic in awake newborns. Do not use epinephrine with local anesthesia for circumcision.

Table 37-3. Maximum local anesthetic dosing in newborns

Drug	Single dose		Infusion rate
	Without epinephrine	With epinephrine	
Lidocaine	4 mg/kg	6 mg/kg	1 mg/kg/hr
Bupivacaine	1.5–2 mg/kg	2 mg/kg	0.2 mg/kg/hr

For major thoracoabdominal and pelvic surgery in infants, epidural analgesia using local anesthetics and opioids can provide outstanding analgesia
and can facilitate a rapid recovery [30]. Combined epidural–light general
anesthetic techniques are particularly useful to facilitate early extubation
[31]. Regional anesthesia for newborns requires particular expertise on the
part of pediatric anesthesiologists, and requires an ongoing system of management such as an acute pain service [32] with close communication between neonatologists, surgeons, and anesthesiologists.

Excessive dosing of local anesthetics can lead to seizures, arrhythmias,
and myocardial depression. Dosing guidelines need to be adhered to strictly,
and with an awareness that the warning signs of impending toxicity in
newborns may be absent [33].

For operations below the umbilicus, such as inguinal hernia repair, spinal
[34] or continuous caudal epidural anesthesia [35] may be used as the sole
form of anesthesia in unsedated neonates, particularly in former premature
infants who are at risk of apnea [36]. The ester local anesthetic 2-chloropro-
caine is uniquely useful for epidural anesthesia in this setting [35], since its
clearance is extremely rapid even in the newborn, permitting large enough
doses to achieve good surgical conditions without high plasma concentrations as is seen with either lidocaine or bupivacaine.

Skin analgesia may be delivered via a transdermal preparation known as
EMLA (eutectic mixture of local anesthetics). Although not currently rec-
ommended for neonates, preliminary studies suggest safety and efficacy of
EMLA for needle procedures [4] and even circumcision [37,41].

VIII. Anesthetic risk. Although in expert hands anesthesia can be performed safely
in critically ill or healthy newborns, several studies found that morbidity and
mortality are higher among newborns undergoing surgery than among older
children or healthy adults [38–40]. One retrospective study found that morbidity is reduced when anesthesia is administered by experienced pediatric anesthesiologists.

It is commonly recommended that elective procedures be delayed until infants are several months old. More problematic decisions arise when surgical
outcomes are likely to be improved by earlier intervention. Cleft lip and palate
repairs, inguinal hernias, and craniosynostosis repairs are examples of situations where relative risks related to anesthesia must be weighed against benefits in terms of surgical results.

General pediatricians, neonatologists, and pediatric surgeons need to advocate for availability of expert neonatal anesthetic services.

References

1. Anand, K. J. S., et al. Pain and its effects in the human neonate and fetus. *N.
   Engl. J. Med.* 317:1321, 1987.
2. Anand, K. J. S., et al. Hormonal-metabolic stress responses in neonates undergoing cardiac surgery. *Anesthesiology* 73:661, 1990.
3. Anand, K. J., et al. The neuroanatomy, neurophysiology, and neurochemistry of
   pain, stress, and analgesia in newborns and children [Review]. *Pediatr. Clin.
   North Am.* 36:795, 1989.

4. Fitzgerald, M., et al. Cutaneous hypersensitivity following peripheral tissue damage in newborn infants and its reversal with topical anaesthesia. *Pain* 39:31, 1989.
5. Fitzgerald, M. Development of pain mechanisms [Review]. *Br. Med. Bull.* 47:667, 1991.
6. Schecter, N. L., Berde, C. B., and Yaster, M., eds. *Pain in Infants, Children, and Adolescents.* Baltimore: Williams & Wilkins, 1993.
7. Welborn, L. G., et al. Anemia and postoperative apnea in former preterm infants. *Anesthesiology* 74:1003, 1991.
8. Roth, A. G., et al. Comparison of a rigid laryngoscope with the ultrathin fibreoptic laryngoscope for tracheal intubation in infants. *Can. J. Anaesth.* 41:1069, 1994.
9. Holzman, R. S., et al. Lightwand intubation in children with abnormal upper airways. *Anesthesiology* 69:784, 1988.
10. Mason, D. G., et al. The laryngeal mask airway in children [see comments]. *Anaesthesia* 45:760, 1990.
11. Murat, I., et al. Effects of fentanyl on baroreceptor reflex control of heart rate in newborn infants. *Anesthesiology* 68:717, 1988.
12. Murat, I., et al. Isoflurane attenuates baroreflex control of heart rate in human neonates. *Anesthesiology* 70:395, 1989.
13. Coté, C. J. Pediatric breathing circuits and anesthesia machines [Review]. *Int. Anesthesiol. Clin.* 30:51, 1992.
14. Rusy, L. M., et al. A double-blind evaluation of ketorolac tromethamine versus acetaminophen in pediatric tonsillectomy: Analgesia and bleeding. *Anesth. Analg.* 80:226, 1995.
15. Wetzel, R. C. Pediatric anesthesia. *Pediatr. Clin. North Am.* 41:1, 1994.
16. Robinson, S., and Gregory, G. A. Fentanyl-air–oxygen anesthesia for ligation of patent ductus arteriosis in preterm infants. *Anesthesiology* 60:331, 1981.
17. Hickey, P. R., et al. Fentanyl- and sufentanil-oxygen-pancuronium anesthesia for cardiac surgery in infants. *Anesth. Analg.* 63:117, 1984.
18. Yaster, M. The dose response of fentanyl in neonatal anesthesia. *Anesthesiology* 66:433, 1987.
19. Koren, G., et al. Postoperative morphine infusion in newborn infants: Assessment of disposition characteristics and safety. *J. Pediatr.* 107:963, 1985.
20. Lynn, A. M., et al. Morphine pharmacokinetics in early infancy. *Anesthesiology* 66:136, 1987.
21. LeDez, K. M., et al. The minimum alveolar concentration (MAC) of isoflurane in preterm neonates. *Anesthesiology* 67:301, 1987.
22. Hickey, P. R., et al. Pulmonary and systemic hemodynamic responses to ketamine in infants with normal and elevated pulmonary vascular resistance. *Anesthesiology* 62:287, 1985.
23. Schrum, S. F., et al. Comparison of propofol and thiopental for rapid anesthesia induction in infants. *Anesth. Analg.* 78:482, 1994.
24. Hannallah, R. S., et al. Propofol: Effective dose and induction characteristics in unpremedicated children. *Anesthesiology* 74:217, 1991.
25. Westrin, P. The induction dose of propofol in infants 1–6 months of age and in children 10–16 years of age [see comments]. *Anesthesiology* 74:455, 1991.
26. Fisher, D. M., et al. Pharmacokinetics and pharmacodynamics of d-tubocurarine in infants, children and adults. *Anesthesiology* 57:203, 1982.
27. Strichartz, G. R., et al. Local Anesthetics. In R. D. Miller (Ed.), *Anesthesia* (4th Ed.). New York: Churchill-Livingstone, 1994. P. 489–521.
28. Sethna, N., et al. Pediatric Regional Anesthesia. In G Gregory (Ed.), *Pediatric Anesthesia* (3rd Ed.). New York: Churchill-Livingstone, 1994. Pp. 281–317.
29. Maxwell, L. G., et al. Penile nerve block reduces the physiologic stress to newborn circumcision. *Anesthesiology* 65:A432, 1986.
30. Meignier, M., et al. Postoperative dorsal epidural analgesia in the child with respiratory disabilities. *Anesthesiology* 59:473, 1983.
31. Murrell, D., et al. Continuous epidural analgesia in newborn infants undergoing major surgery. *J. Pediatr. Surg.* 28:548, 1993.

32. Berde, C. B., et al. Regional analgesia on pediatric medical and surgical wards. *Intensive Care Med.* 28(Suppl.):S40, 1989.
33. Berde, C. B. Toxicity of local anesthetics in infants and children. *J. Pediatr.* 122:S14, 1993.
34. Abajian, J., et al. Spinal anesthesia for surgery in the high-risk infant. *Anesth. Analg.* 63:359, 1984.
35. Henderson, K. H., et al. Continuous caudal anesthesia with 2-chloroprocaine for premature infants undergoing inguinal hernia repair. *Anesthesiology* 75(Suppl.): A916, 1991.
36. Welborn, L. G., et al. Postoperative apnea in former preterm infants: Prospective comparison of spinal and general anesthesia. *Anesthesiology* 72:838, 1990.
37. Benini, F., et al. Topical anesthesia during circumcision in newborn infants. *JAMA* 270:850, 1993.
38. Morray, J. P., et al. A comparison of pediatric and adult anesthesia closed malpractice claims. *Anesthesiology* 78:461, 1993.
39. Cohen, M. M., et al. Pediatric anesthesia morbidity and mortality in the perioperative period. *Anesth. Analg.* 70:160, 1990.
40. Holzman, R. S. Morbidity and mortality in pediatric anesthesia [Review]. *Pediatr. Clin. North Am.* 41:239, 1994.
41. Taddio, A., et al. Efficacy and safety of lidocaine-prilocaine for pain during circumcision. *N. Engl. J. Med.* 336:1197, 1997.

APPENDIX: DRUGS IN COMMON USAGE IN NEONATAL INTENSIVE CARE UNITS

Acetaminophen (Tylenol, Tempra, Liquiprin)

Indications: Antipyretic-analgesic. Useful in newborns with hemostatic disturbance and upper GI disease. **Dosage (mg/kg/dose)/Dosage Interval: PO:** 10–15, q6–8h. **PR:** 20–25, q6–8h. **Precautions:** Rectal suppositories associated with erratic release characteristics. **Contraindications:** G6PD deficiency. **Adverse Reactions:** Blood dyscrasias (thrombocytopenia, leukopenia, pancytopenia, and neutropenia). Adverse reactions are associated with excessive dosages. Acute effects include hepatic necrosis, transient azotemia, and renal tubular necrosis. Chronic effects include anemia, renal damage, and GI disturbances. **Truog:** *Clin Perinatol* 1989;16:74. **Johnson:** *The Harriet Lane Handbook,* 1993, p. 376.

Acetazolamide (Diamox)
Dosage/Dosage Interval

Indication	Dosage (mg/kg/dose)/route/frequency
Diuresis	5, PO, IV (administer over 2 min), qday–qod
Decrease CSF production	10, Increase as tolerated to 25, PO, IV, q6–8h
Anticonvulsant	2–7.5, PO, q6–8h
Alkalinize urine (RTA)	5, IV, IM, PO, q8–12h

Precautions: Adjust dose for renal impairment. IM administration painful due to alkaline pH. Tolerance to diuretic effect occurs with long-term administration. **Monitoring:** Acid–base status, daily intake/output, weight, and weekly head circumference. **Adverse Reactions:** Hyperchloremic metabolic acidosis, hypokalemia, and bone marrow suppression. **Gomella:** *Neonatology,* 1994, p. 467. **Johnson:** *The Harriet Lane Handbook,* 1993, p. 377.

Acetylcysteine (Mucomyst, Mucosil)

Indications: Treatment of atelectasis associated with mucous plugging. Treatment of bowel obstruction due to meconium ileus or its equivalent.
Dosage/Dosage Interval

Indications	Dosage/frequency/precautions
Nebulization: treatment of atelectasis	3–5 ml of 20% solution + 3–5 ml of 0.9% normal saline, q4–6h, or 6–10 ml of 10% solution. *To prevent bronchospasm, administer with, or precede acetylcysteine therapy with a bronchodilator*
Meconium ileus therapy	5–30 ml of 10% solution, PO, PR, q4–8h; usual dose is 10 ml q6h

Adverse Reactions: Bronchospasm, hemoptysis, stomatitis, and rhinorrhea.

Johnson: *The Harriet Lane Handbook,* 1993, p. 378. **Bibi:** *Acta Paediatr* 1992;81:335–339.

Acyclovir (Zovirax)
Dosage/Dosage Interval

Indications	Dosage (mg/kg/day)/route/frequency
Neonatal HSV infection	30–40, IV, divided q8h (dilute to final conc. of 5 mg/ml, and infuse over 1–3 h). 10–21 day duration of treatment
Neonatal HSV infection—premature infant	20, IV, divided q12h. Duration of treatment = 10–21 days
HSV encephalitis	40, IV, divided q8h. Duration of treatment = 10 days
Topical therapy	Apply to lesion q4–6h, for 7 days. *Not for ophthalmic application. Use gloves for topical applications*

Drug Interactions

Drug	Drug interaction
Dopamine/dobutamine	Do not infuse with acyclovir-containing fluids
Concurrent probenecid usage	Decreased acyclovir excretion
Paraben-containing bacteriostatic water	Precipitate formation

Precautions: Reduce dosage for impaired renal function. **Monitoring:** Renal and hepatic function. **Adverse Reactions:** Nephrotoxicity, bone marrow suppression, fever, thrombocytosis, and transitory increase of serum creatinine and liver enzymes. Rare encephalopathy associated with rapid IV administration (lethargy, obtundation, agitation, tremor, seizure, and coma). **American Academy of Pediatrics (AAP):** *Report of the Committee on Infectious Diseases,* 1997, pp. 266–277. **Nelson:** *Pocketbook of Pediatric Antimicrobial Therapy,* 1995, p. 66.

Adenosine (Adenocard)
Indications: Treatment of supraventricular tachycardia (SVT). **Dosage/Dosage Interval:** 0.05–0.2 mg/kg/dose rapid IV bolus followed by flush. If no response in 1–2 min, double the dose and continue to double the dose every 1–2 min until response occurs. **Maximum single dose:** 0.25 mg/kg. **Contraindications:** Second or third AV block, sick sinus syndrome. **Precautions:** Administer during continuous ECG monitoring. **Clinical Considerations:** Because adenosine effect may be temporary, follow initial adenosine therapy with a longer-acting agent such as digoxin. **Drug Interactions:** More severe degrees of heart block reported with concurrent carbamazepine therapy. Methylxanthines are competitive antagonists and may necessitate larger doses of adenosine. **Adverse Reactions:** Short-duration first-, second-, or third-degree heart block; bronchospasm, dyspnea, and hypotension. **American Heart Association (AHA):** *JAMA* 1992;268:2262–2275. **Johnson:** *The Harriet Lane Handbook,* 1993, p. 379.

Albumin, Human (Albuminar, Albutein, Buminate, Plasbumin-5, Human Albumin)
Dosage/Dosage Interval

Indications	Dosage (g/kg/dose)	Route/frequency
Hypoproteinemia	0.5–1.0, repeat q1–2days or as calculated to replace ongoing losses. *For sodium restriction, use dextrose solutions*	IV; infuse × 2–4 h, or at 0.05–0.1 g/min. **Max. dose: 6 g/kg/day**
Hypovolemia	0.5–1.0 (10–20 ml/kg). **Max. dose: 6 g/kg/day**	IV bolus, repeat PRN. Administer as fast as necessary for shock, and over 2–4 h for mild hypotension

Contraindications: Severe anemia or congestive heart failure (CHF); 25% solutions contraindicated due to increased risk of IVH. **Precautions:** Use with caution in hypervolemia states (maximum dose 6 g/24 h). If >6 g/24 h is required, consider blood products for treatment of hypovolemia. **Adverse Reactions:** Chills, fever, and urticaria. Rapid infusion (>1.0 g/min) may precipitate CHF due to hypervolemia, pulmonary edema due to CHF or extravasation of albumin from pulmonary circulation. **Johnson:** *The Harriet Lane Handbook,* 1993, p. 380. **Gomella:** *Neonatology,* 1994, p. 468.

Albuterol (Proventil, Ventolin, Salbutamol)
Indications: Acute bronchodilator for bronchopulmonary dysplasia (BPD)
Dosage/Dosage Interval

Route	Dosage/frequency/comments
Nebulization	Initial: 0.1–0.5 mg/kg/dose of 5 mg/ml solution + 1.5 ml normal saline, q2–6h. Increase to 0.5 mg/kg/dose PRN. Hold or decrease dose for heart rate >180 bpm. Can be given as continuous aerosol
Continuous IV infusion	0.5–5 mcg/kg/min
Oral administration	0.1–0.3 mg/kg/dose, q6–8h

Monitoring: Monitor response to albuterol, serum potassium, electrocardiogram, and heart rate (withhold albuterol for heart rate >180 bpm). **Drug Interactions:** Antagonized by beta-adrenergic blocking agents and potentiated by MAO inhibitors. **Adverse Reactions:** Tachycardia, arrhythmias, CNS stimulation, hyperactivity, hypokalemia, and irritability **Fanaroff:** *Neonatal Perinatal Medicine,* 1992, p. 1426. **Johnson:** *The Harriet Lane Handbook,* 1993, p. 380.

Alprostadil—See Prostaglandin E₁

Amikacin Sulfate (Amikin)
Classification: Aminoglycoside. **Indications:** Reserved for infections with gram-negative organisms resistant to other aminoglycosides.

Dosage (mg/kg/dose)/Dosage Interval: IM, IV (final concentration of 5 mg/ml, infused over 30 min); IM absorption is erratic, especially in VLBW infants)

Weight <1200 g		Weight 1200–2000 g		Weight >2000 g	
Postnatal age (PNA) ≤4 wk	PNA ≤7 days	PNA >7 days	PNA ≤7 days	PNA >7 days	
7.5–24 h	7.5 q12–18h	7.5 q8–12h	10, q12h	10, q8h	

Precautions: Adjust dose for renal impairment.

Drug Interactions

Drug or clinical condition	Interaction
Neuromuscular blocking agent	Increased neuromuscular blockade
Hypermagnesemia	Increased neuromuscular blockade
Loop diuretics (ethacrynic acid, furosemide, bumetanide), vancomycin	Potentiate aminoglycoside-induced ototoxicity/nephrotoxicity
Penicillins, cephalosporins	Blunting of amikacin serum peak concentration if administered simultaneously with these agents; administer as a separate infusion from pencillin-containing solutions

Monitoring: Monitor renal function before and during therapy and auditory function after completion of therapy. Adjust dosage according to serum peak and trough levels. Draw serum levels around the fourth maintenance dose. Draw serum peak levels 30 min after the end of infusion, or 1 h after IM injection. Draw serum trough levels 30 min before the next dose. **Therapeutic levels** (μg/ml): **Peak:** 25–35, **Trough:** <10. **Adverse Reactions:** Bone marrow suppression, eosinophilia. Vestibular and auditory ototoxicity associated with serum peak concentration >35–40 μg/ml. Nephrotoxicity associated with serum trough concentrations >10 μg/ml. **Nelson:** *Pocketbook of Pediatric Antimicrobial Therapy,* 1995, p. 16. **Prober:** *Pediatr Infect Dis J* 1990;9:111.

Aminophylline
Dosage/Dosage Interval

Indications	Dosage (mg/kg/dose)/route/frequency*
Apnea of prematurity	Load: 4–6, IV (infuse over 30 min), or PO Maintenance: 1–3, IV, PO, q8–12h. Start maintenance dose 8–12 h after loading dose.
Bronchodilator	IV Load: 6, IV (infuse over 30 min). Each 1 mg/kg raises the serum theophylline concentration 2 mg/L Maintenance: continuous IV (mg/kg/h): Neonate: 0.2, 6 wk–6 mo: 0.2–0.9. Intermittent dosing: divide total daily dose from continuous IV drip, and administer q4–6h, IV PO: see theophylline

*When switching from IV to PO aminophylline, consider increasing the dose by 20%.

Precautions: IM administration causes intense local pain and sloughing. **Monitoring:** Monitor heart rate and check blood glucose periodically during loading-dose therapy. Assess for agitation and feeding intolerance. Withhold next dose if heart rate exceeds 180 bpm. After maintenance therapy is established, monitor serum trough levels on day 4 of therapy and then 1–2 times weekly. Check serum trough level when suspecting toxicity or when apnea spells increase in frequency. If apnea is severe prior to the fourth day of therapy, obtain a serum trough level; if low, give a partial bolus: Give 1.0 mg/kg for each desired 2 mg/ml in serum theophylline concentration. **Therapeutic ranges:** Apnea of prematurity: 5–15 mcg/ml; bronchospasm: 10–20 mcg/ml. **Adverse Reactions:** GI upset, arrhythmias, seizures, tachycardia (HR >180 bpm warrants determination of serum levels to detect excessive aminophylline levels). **Johnson:** *The Harriet Lane Handbook*, 1993, p. 384. **Fanaroff:** *Neonatal-Perinatal Medicine*, 1992, p. 1426.

Amphotericin-B
Indications: Antifungal agent of choice for systemic antifungal therapy.
Dosage/Dosage Interval

Dosage/indications	Dosage/route/frequency	Comments
Initial dose	0.25–0.5 mg/kg IV, diluted in D10W to conc. of 0.1 mg/10 ml; infuse over 2–6 h, q24h	Associated fever/chills prevented with antipyretic or antihistamine pretreatment
Maintenance dose	Daily dose increased by 0.125 to 0.25 mg/kg/day q24–48h until max daily dose of 0.5–1 mg/kg q24–48h. Infuse over 2–6 h	Total dose of 30–35 mg/kg administered over 4–6 wk
Intrathecal (usually not needed)	0.01 mg Initial dose; diluted in nonbacteriostatic sterile water to final conc. <0.25 mg/ml	Gradually increase over 5–7 days to 0.1 mg q72 h *Further dilution in CSF is recommended*

Precautions: Incompatible with sodium chloride. **Monitoring:** Serum concentrations not routinely monitored due to poorly defined therapeutic range. Daily monitoring of renal, liver, and hematologic functions until dosage stabilized, then weekly. Discontinue if BUN >40 mg/dl, serum creatinine >0.4 mg/dl, or if liver function tests are abnormal. Resume at lower dosage or administer less frequently after values normalize. **Adverse Reactions:** Pancytopenia, electrolyte imbalance, cardiovascular instability, hepatic and renal failure, and bone marrow suppression with reversible decline in hematocrit. CSF pleocytosis (arachnoiditis) associated with intrathecal administration.
Remington: *Infectious Diseases of the Fetus and Newborn Infant*, 1990, pp. 501–502. **Nelson:** *Pocketbook of Pediatric Antimicrobial Therapy*, 1995, p. 95.

Ampicillin (Omnipen, Polycillin, Principen, Totacillin, Ancil, Amplin)
Classification: Semisynthetic penicillinase-sensitive penicillin.
Indications: Combined with either an aminoglycoside or cephalosporin for the prevention and treatment of infections with group B streptococci,

group D streptococci, and *Listeria monocytogenes*. **Dosage (mg/kg/dose)/ Dosage Interval:** IM, IV (final concentration of 50 mg/ml, infused over 10 min, maximum infusion rate: 100 mg/min). **Meningitis:** We usually start with 150 mg/kg/dose q12h, regardless of birth weight or postnatal age (max. dose: 400 mg/kg/day), for the treatment of presumed group B streptococcal meningitis. When meningitis is ruled out the dose is changed to 50–100 mg/kg/dose. The higher dose is used for group B streptococcal infections.

Postconceptual age (wk)	Postnatal age (days)	Dosage interval (h)
≤29	0–28	q12
	>28	q8
30–36	0 to 14	q12
	>14	q8
37–44	0 to 7	q12
	>7	q8
≥45	All postnatal ages	q6

Precautions: Dosage adjustment for renal impairment. **Drug Interactions:** Blunting of peak aminoglycoside concentration if administered simultaneously with ampicillin. **Test Interactions:** False-positive urinary glucose levels (Benedict's solution, Clinitest). **Adverse Reactions:** Diarrhea, hypersensitivity reaction (rubella-like rash and fever), nephritis (typically preceded by eosinophilia), elevated transaminases, and penicillin encephalopathy (CNS excitation and seizure activity associated with large or rapidly administered doses). **Young TE:** *Neofax '97*, pp. 8–9. **Johnson:** *The Harriet Lane Handbook*, 1993, p. 388.

Ampicillin/Sulbactam (Unasyn)
Classification: Bactericidal spectrum of ampicillin extended to include beta-lactamase-producing strains of *Staphylococcal aureus* organisms. **Dosage/Dosage Interval: IM or IV (final concentration of 50 mg/ml, infused over 15–30 min)**

Indications	Postnatal age/dosage (mg/kg/day)/frequency
Meningitis	0–7 Days: 100–200, divided q12h >7 Days: 200–300, divided q6–8h. Max. dose: 400 mg/kg/day
Nonmeningitic infections	0–7 Days: 50, div. q12h. >7 Days: 75, divided q12h

Precautions and side effects—See Ampicillin.
Gomella: *Neonatology*, 1994, p. 470.

Atracurium Besylate (Tracurium)
Indications: Nondepolarizing neuromuscular blocking agent. **Dosage/Dosage Interval:** IM administration causes tissue irritation. **Initial:** 0.3–0.4 mg/kg/dose, IV. **Maintenance:** 0.05–0.06 mg/kg/dose, IV, q15–30 min. **Continuous infusion:** 2–10 mcg/kg/min (ideal for continuous infusion due to short duration of action and constant rate of elimination). **Clinical Considerations:** No dosage adjustment necessary in renal and hepatic disease due to elimination by Hofmann degradation. Because sensation remains intact, administer concurrent sedation. **Precautions:** Re-

duce dose in neonates in whom substantial histamine release would be potentially hazardous (cardiovascular disease or reactive airway disease). **Adverse Reactions:** Histamine release-associated bradycardia and bronchospasm. **Overdose: Symptoms:** Respiratory depression, cardiovascular collapse. **Treatment:** Neostigmine, pyridostigmine, or edrophonium administered immediately after atropine.
Rudolph: *Rudolph's Pediatrics,* 1991, p. 1964. **Fanaroff:** *Neonatal-Perinatal Medicine,* 1992, p. 1428.

Atropine Sulfate
Dosage/Dosage Interval

Indications	Dosage (mg/kg/dose)/frequency
Prolonged CPR/bradycardia	IV: 0.01–0.03, q10–15 min, × 2–3 doses, PRN; minimal dose: 0.1 mg; Max. dose: 0.5 mg; administer undiluted form for IV, and ETT administration PO: 0.02–0.09, q4–6h (use IV formulation diluted to final concentration of 0.08 mg/ml) ETT: 2–3 times IV dose; add normal saline to total volume of 1–2 ml
Preanesthetic	0.04, administer 30 min to 1 h preoperatively
Nebulization (BPD)	0.05–0.08 mg, + 2.5 ml normal saline q4–6h; Min. dose: 0.25 mg; Max. dose: 1 mg
Nondepolarizing muscle relaxant reversal	Atropine 10–20 mcg/kg. Administered before edrophonium

Clinical Considerations: Adequate oxygenation and ventilation must precede atropine treatment of bradycardia. Low doses may cause paradoxical bradycardia secondary to central action. **Contraindications:** Tachycardia, narrow-angle glaucoma, thyrotoxicosis, GI or GU obstruction. **Precautions:** Spastic paralysis or CNS damage. **Adverse Reactions:** Tachycardia, mydriasis, abdominal distention/ileus, urinary retention, arrhythmias, and esophageal reflux. **Antidote:** Physostigmine.
Gomella: *Neonatology,* 1994, p. 471. **Johnson:** *The Harriet Lane Handbook,* 1993, pp. 390–391.

Aztreonam (Azactam)
Classification: Monobactam antibiotic.
Indications: Bactericidal against *Pseudomonas aeruginosa* and most *Enterobacteriaceae;* minimal activity against gram-positive aerobic bacteria or anaerobic bacteria.
Dosage (mg/kg/dose)/Dosage Interval: IM, IV (final IV concentration of 20 mg/ml infused over 30 min)

Weight <1200 g	Weight 1200–2000 g		Weight >2000 g	
Postnatal age (PNA) ≤4 wk	PNA ≤7 days	PNA >7 days	PNA ≤7 days	PNA >7 days
30 q12h	30 q12h	30 q8h	30 q8h	30 q6h

Precautions: Reduce dosage in renal impairment. **Drug Interactions:** Avoid antibiotics that induce beta-lactamase production. **Test Interactions:** Increases AST, SGPT, alkaline phosphatase, creatinine, and LDH. **Ad-**

verse Reactions: Diarrhea, rash, pancytopenia, eosinophilia, hypotension, increased prothrombin time, and seizures.
Nelson: *Pocketbook of Pediatric Antimicrobial Therapy,* 1995, p. 16. **Johnson:** *The Harriet Lane Handbook,* 1993, pp. 391–392.

Bicarbonate—See Sodium Bicarbonate

Bumetanide (Bumex)
Indications: Management of edema associated with congenital heart disease, congestive heart failure, hepatic or renal disease. **Dosage/Dosage Interval:** 0.015–0.1 mg/kg/day qday-QOD, IV, IM, PO, q24h. Give IV over 1–2 min, and IM as undiluted injection. Well-absorbed PO. Administer maintenance doses on an intermittent schedule (qod or every 2–3 days, alternating with 1–2 day bumetanide-free periods). Doses for oral and intravenous therapy are the same. **Contraindications:** Anuria or increasing azotemia. **Clinical Considerations:** Potency 40 times greater than furosemide, but equipotent in causing ototoxicity and liver damage. **Monitoring:** Because Bumex is 40 times more potent than furosemide, excessive dosages can lead to profound diuresis with fluid and electrolyte loss. Closely monitor serum electrolytes, urine output, and daily weight. Closely monitor neonates receiving digoxin for possible potassium depletion. **Test Interactions:** Increased BUN, creatinine, ammonia, amylase, glucose, and uric acid. Decreased Na, Ca, Cl, and K. **Drug Interactions:** Lithium, indomethacin, probenicid, and potassium-wasting agents. **Adverse Reactions:** Electrolyte imbalance, hyperuricemia, cardiovascular instability, glucose intolerance, metabolic alkalosis, excessive volume depletion (dehydration and hemoconcentration), ototoxicity, encephalopathy, possible association with blood dyscrasias, and hepatotoxicity. Displaces bilirubin from albumin binding sites when given in high doses or for prolonged periods.
Gomella: *Neonatology,* 1994, p. 472. **Johnson:** *The Harriet Lane Handbook,* 1993, p. 395.

Caffeine Citrate
Indications: Apnea of prematurity.
Dosage/Dosage Interval: Loading dose: 10 mg/kg caffeine base (20 mg/kg caffeine citrate) PO, IV, ×1 dose. **Maintenance dose:** 2.5–5 mg/kg/dose of caffeine base PO, IV, q24h (started 24 h after the loading dose). 2 mg caffeine citrate = 1 mg caffeine base. **Clinical Considerations:** Initial half-life is 90–100 h, decreasing to 6 h after 60 weeks postconceptual age. **Monitoring:** Therapeutic trough levels (obtain before 5th dose): = 5 to 25 mcg/ml. Cardiovascular, neurologic, or GI toxicity reported with levels >40 to 50 mcg/ml. Monitor heart rate and hold and then reduce dose if HR >180 bpm. Assess for agitation and response to therapy. **Precautions:** An increased risk of kernicterus exists with caffeine sodium benzoate due to uncoupling of albumin-bilirubin binding. **Adverse Reactions:** Restlessness, agitation, vomiting, and tachycardia. Overdose symptoms include arrhythmias and tonic-clonic seizures.
Bhutani: *Clin Perinatol* 1992;19:649–671. **Johnson:** *The Harriet Lane Handbook,* 1993, pp. 395–396.

Calcium Chloride, 10%
Dosage/Dosage Interval

Indications	Dosage/route/frequency
Symptomatic hypocalcemia: Acute treatment*	35–70 mg/kg/dose (0.35–0.70 ml/kg/dose). Dilute and infuse over 30 min (IV push not to exceed 100 mg/min). Stop if bradycardia occurs.
Maintenance therapy*	75–300 mg/kg/day (0.75–3 ml/kg/day). Closely monitor serum levels. Dilute in feedings: administer PO in 4 divided doses. Treatment duration = 3–5 days
Exchange transfusion*	33 mg or 0.33 ml per 100 ml of exchanged citrated blood
Cardiac arrest (with documented hypocalcemia)	20–30 mg/kg/dose (0.15–0.30 ml/kg/dose) of 10% IV solution, q10 min PRN

*Calcium gluconate is usually used for these indications.

Clinical Considerations: Hypocalcemia is defined as serum ionized calcium concentrations <3.5 mg/dl (or total serum calcium <7.0 mg/dl). Treatment is usually reserved for symptomatic hypocalcemia. Correct concurrent hypomagnesemia. Calcium chloride 10% injection contains 27 mg/ml or 1.36 mEq/ml of elemental calcium. Calcium chloride is preferred to gluconate during cardiac arrest. See Calcium Glubionate for information regarding PO administration of calcium products. **Contraindications:** Hypercalcemia, renal calculi, ventricular fibrillation. **Precautions:** Not to be given SC or IM. Intestinal bleeding and/or lower-extremity tissue necrosis reported with bolus infusions via umbilical artery catheter. Gastric irritation and diarrhea may occur with oral therapy. Necrotizing enterocolitis has been reported with oral administration of hyperosmolar solutions. Use with caution in premature neonates, digitalized infants, respiratory failure, or acidosis. **Drug Interactions:** May potentiate digoxin-related arrhythmias. Precipitates when mixed with sodium bicarbonate. **Monitoring:** Continuously monitor ECG and stop infusion for heart rate <100 bpm. **Adverse Reactions:** Vasodilatation, cardiovascular instability, ventricular fibrillation (associated with rapid administration), lethargy, coma, elevated serum amylase and serum/urine calcium, and decreased serum magnesium. Extravasation may lead to cutaneous necrosis or calcium deposition (consider hyaluronidase treatment). **Fanaroff:** *Neonatal-Perinatal Medicine,* 1992, p. 1427. **Johnson:** *The Harriet Lane Handbook,* 1993, p. 397. **Broner CW:** *J Pediatr* 1990;117:986.

Calcium Glubionate (Neocalglucon)
Indications: Treatment and prevention of hypocalcemia. (6.5% calcium glubionate.) **Dosage (mg/kg/day)/Dosage Interval:** Neonatal hypocalcemia: 500, divided q3–4h, PO (administer before feedings). **Maintenance:** 150, divided q3–4h, PO × 9 days (maximum 9 g/day). **Contraindications:** Hypercalcemia, renal calculi, ventricular fibrillation. **Clinical Considerations:** 6.5% Calcium glubionate syrup contains 23 mg/ml of elemental calcium and has an osmolarity of 2500 mosm/L. Supplement premature infants to a total intake of 150 mg/kg/day of calcium (including the calcium content of feedings). To minimize osmotic diarrhea, gradually reduce the dose and administer in divided doses. **Drug Interactions:** Tetracycline,

digoxin, and sodium bicarbonate. **Monitoring:** Monitor for GI intolerance, and correct concurrent hypomagnesemia. Avoid hypercalcemia (ionized calcium is the preferred measurement) and hypercalciuria. **Adverse Reactions:** GI irritation, hypercalcemia, hypercalciuria, and constipation. High osmotic load of syrup (20% sucrose) may cause diarrhea. **Taeusch:** *Schaffer and Avery's Diseases of the Newborn*, 1991, p. 1049. **Johnson:** *The Harriet Lane Handbook*, 1993, p. 397.

Calcium Gluconate, 10% (see Chap. 29)
Dosage/Dosage Interval: (100 mg/ml final concentration, infused at 100 mg/min, or 0.465 mEq/min)

Indications	Dosage/route/frequency	Clinical considerations
Symptomatic hypocalcemia	100–200 mg/kg/dose, IV (1–2 ml/kg/dose)	Administer IV over 10 min
Acute therapy	10–12 mg/kg elemental calcium	Monitor heart rate and stop infusion if <100 bpm
Maintenance therapy	200–800 mg/kg/day or 2–8 ml/kg/day	IV as continuous infusion or diluted with feedings in divided doses
Exchange transfusion	100 mg or 1 ml/100 ml of citrated exchanged blood	IV
CPR	100 mg/kg/dose, IV, q10 min	IV
Hyperkalemia	50 mg/kg/dose, IV, over 5–10 min	IV

Contraindications: Hypercalcemia, renal calculi, ventricular fibrillation. **Drug Interactions:** May potentiate digitalis-induced arrhythmias. Precipitates when mixed with sodium bicarbonate. **Precautions:** Use with caution in digitalized patients, respiratory failure, or acidosis. IM or SC administration may result in severe tissue necrosis or sloughing. Use of scalp veins not recommended. **Clinical Considerations:** Preferred in neonates (nonarrest situations) because calcium gluconate produces less acidosis than calcium chloride; 10% calcium gluconate = 9.3 mg/ml or 0.46 mEq/ml elemental calcium, and osmolarity = 700 mosm/L. Must be metabolized to release calcium ion. **Adverse Reactions:** Refer to adverse reactions for both calcium chloride and calcium glubionate. **Rudolph:** *Rudolph's Pediatrics*, 1991, p. 1966. **Johnson:** *The Harriet Lane Handbook*, 1993, p. 398.

Carbamazepine (Tegretol)
Indications: Anticonvulsant.
Dosage/Dosage Interval: Initial: 10 mg/kg/day, PO, divided q12–24h.
Dosage Increment: 10 mg/kg/day. Gradually increase dose to compensate for "autoinduction" phenomenon, and titrate dose to achieve a serum concentration of 4–12 mcg/ml (20–40 nmol/L).
Drug Interactions

Drug(s) combinations	Drug interaction
Erythromycin, verapamil, INH, cimetidine	Associated with increased carbamazepine levels

| Phenobarbital, phenytoin, primidone, (singly or in combination) | Associated with decreased carbamazepine levels |
| Theophylline, warfarin, phenytoin, benzodiazepines, ethosuximide, and valproic acid | Carbamazepine may decrease serum levels of these drugs |

Test Interactions: Asymptomatic increase in serum transaminases. **Monitoring:** Obtain pretreatment CBC. Monitor for renal, hematologic, and hepatic toxicity. **Adverse Reactions:** Aplastic anemia, neutropenia, urinary retention, SIADH, anaphylaxis, platelet dysfunction, electrolyte imbalance, and Stevens-Johnson syndrome. **Fanaroff:** *Neonatal-Perinatal Medicine,* 1992, p. 1424. **Johnson:** *The Harriet Lane Handbook,* 1993, pp. 399–400.

Cardioversion
Indications: Symptomatic supraventricular tachycardia or ventricular tachycardia accompanied by cardiovascular instability. **Dosage/Dosage Interval:** Initial dose is 0.5 J/kg; double dose each time for a total of three attempts (range, 0.25–2 wt-s/kg). If IV access is available, administer adenosine before cardioversion, but do not delay cardioversion while attempting to obtain IV access. Correct acidosis, hypoxemia, and hypothermia before, during, and after cardioversion attempts. **Adverse Reactions:** Energy doses of 5–6 J/kg can result in severe myocardial burns, congestive cardiomyopathy secondary to reduced contractility, and death. **AHA:** *JAMA* 1992;268:2262-2275.

Carnitine (Carnitor, Vitacam)
Dosage/Dosage Interval (oral DL carnitine doses)

Indications	Dosage/route/frequency
Carnitine deficiency	50–100 mg/kg/day, PO. Initial dose: 50 mg/kg/day, slowly increase to 100 mg/kg/day. Max. dose 3 g/day.
Cardiomyopathy: load	100 mg/kg/dose, PO
Cardiomyopathy: maintenance	200 mg/kg/day, PO

Monitoring: Blood chemistries and serum carnitine level. Normal serum carnitine levels are 22.6–33.9 μmol/L. Normal cord blood levels are 30–50 nmol/ml. **Clinical Considerations:** The recommended dose of L-carnitine enteral liquid is 50–100 mg/kg/day. Administer higher doses with caution and only if clinical and biochemical considerations make it likely that they will be of benefit. **Adverse Reactions:** Transient diarrhea. **Steenhout:** *J Inherit Metabol Dis* 1990;13:69–75. **Winter:** *Am J Dis Child* 1987;141:660–665.

Cefazolin (Ancef, Kefzol, Zolicef)
Classification: First-generation cephalosporin.
Indications: Good activity against gram-positive cocci (except enterococci).
See **Cephalosporin-associated Drug Resistance** comments.

Dosage (mg/kg/dose)/Dosage Interval: IM or IV (100 mg/ml final concentration, infused over 30 min)

Weight <1200 g	Weight 1200–2000 g		Weight >2000 g	
Postnatal age (PNA) ≤4 wk or >4 wk	PNA ≤7 days	PNA >7 days	PNA ≤7 days	PNA >7 days
20 q12h	20 q12h	20 q12h	20 q12h	20 q8h

Precautions: Dosage reduction in renal impairment. **Clinical Considerations:** Contains 2 mEq Na/g cefazolin. **Monitoring:** CBC, liver function tests. **Adverse Reactions:** Fever, allergic reactions, positive Coombs' test, pancytopenia, eosinophilia, and transient elevation of liver enzymes. Excessive dosages (especially in association with renal impairment) may cause CNS irritation (delirium, seizures).
Nelson: *Pocketbook of Pediatric Antimicrobial Therapy,* 1995, p. 16. **Prober:** *Pediatr Infect Dis* 1990;9:111.

Cefotaxime Sodium (Claforan)
Classification: Third-generation cephalosporin.
Indications: Reserved for suspected or documented gram-negative meningitis or sepsis. When used as empiric therapy, combined with ampicillin or aqueous penicillin G for gram-positive coverage.
See **Cephalosporin-associated Drug Resistance** comments.
Dosage (mg/kg/dose)/Dosage Interval: IM or IV (50 mg/ml final concentration, infused over 30 min)

Weight <1200 g		Weight 1200–2000 g		Weight >2000 g	
PNA ≤4 wk	PNA ≥4 wk	PNA ≤7 days	PNA >7 days	PNA ≤7 days	PNA >7 days
50 q12h	50 q8h	50 q12h	50 q8h	50 q12h	50 q8h
Specific infections					
Gonococcal conjunctivitis			Meningitis		
25 mg/kg/dose, IV, IM, q12h × 7 days			50 mg/kg/dose IV q6h × 14–21 days		

PNA = postnatal age

Precautions: Dosage modification for impaired renal function. **Monitoring:** CBC, BUN, creatinine, and liver enzymes. **Drug Interactions:** Blunting of peak aminoglycoside concentration if administered <2 h before/after cefotaxime. **Adverse Reactions:** Leukopenia, granulocytopenia, pseudomembranous colitis, positive direct Coombs' test, serum-sickness-like reaction, and transient elevation of BUN, creatinine, eosinophils, and liver enzymes.
Nelson: *Pocketbook of Pediatric Antimicrobial Therapy,* 1995, p. 16. **Prober:** *Pediatr Infect Dis J* 1990;9:111.

Ceftazidime (Fortaz, Tazidime, Tazicef, Ceptaz)
Classification: Third-generation cephalosporin.
Indications: Broad-spectrum cephalosporin and the only antipseudomonal cephalosporin. Indicated for treatment of gram-negative meningitis.
See **Cephalosporin-associated Drug Resistance** comments.

Dosage (mg/kg/dose)/Dosage Interval: IM or IV (50 mg/ml final concentration, infused over 30 min)

Weight <1200 g		Weight 1200–2000 g		Weight >2000 g	
PNA ≤4 wk	PNA ≥4 wk	PNA ≤7 days	PNA >7 days	PNA ≤7 days	PNA >7 days
50 q12h	50 q8h	50 q12h	50 q8h	50 q8h	50 q8h

PNA = postnatal age

Clinical Considerations: Treat serious pseudomonal infections with ceftazidime in combination with an aminoglycoside. **Precautions:** Modify dosage for renal impairment. **Drug Interaction:** Blunting of peak aminoglycoside concentration if administered simultaneously with ceftazidime. **Monitoring:** CBC, renal and liver function tests. **Adverse Reactions:** Transient leukopenia and bone marrow suppression, positive direct Coombs' test, candidiasis, hemolytic anemia, pseudomembranous colitis, and transient elevation of eosinophils, platelets, and renal/liver function tests. **Nelson:** *Pocketbook of Pediatric Antimicrobial Therapy,* 1991, p. 16. **Prober:** *Pediatr Inf Dis* 1990;9:111.

Ceftriaxone Sodium (Rocephin)
Classification: Third-generation cephalosporin.
Indications: Good activity against both gram-negative and gram-positive organisms except for *Pseudomonas* spp., enterococci, methicillin-resistant staphylococci, and *Listeria monocytogenes.* Indicated for treatment of gonococcal meningitis and conjunctivitis.
See **Cephalosporin-associated Drug Resistance** comments.
Dosage (mg/kg/dose)/Dosage Interval: IV (25 mg/ml final concentration, infused over 30 min), or IM (reconstitute with 1% lidocaine without epinephrine to reduce pain at injection site)

Weight <1200 g	Weight 1200–2000 g		Weight >2000 g	
Postnatal age (PNA) ≤4 wk or >4 wk	PNA ≤7 days	PNA >7 days	PNA ≤7 days	PNA >7 days
50 q24h	50 q24h	50 q24h	50 q24h	75 q24h

Specific Infections

Indications	Dosage/route/frequency
Prevention of gonococcal ophthalmia See Chap. 23	Premature infant: 25–50 mg/kg single dose IM, IV Term infant: 125 mg single dose, IM, IV
Disseminated gonococcal infection gonococcal and ophthalmia	50 mg/kg/day, IM, IV, divided q12h × 7 days

Precautions: Gallbladder, biliary tract, liver, or pancreatic disease. Not recommended for use in neonates with hyperbilirubinemia. **Clinical Considerations:** Do not use as sole therapy for staphylococcal or pseudomonal infections. Combine with ampicillin for initial empiric therapy of meningitis. **Monitoring:** CBC, electrolytes, and renal/liver function tests. **Adverse Reactions:** Leukopenia, anemia, GI intolerance, and rash. Transient increase in eosinophils, platelets, bleeding time, free serum bilirubin concen-

tration, and renal/liver function tests. Transient formation of gallbladder precipitates characterized by vomiting and cholelithiasis. GI tract bacterial or fungal overgrowth.
Nelson: *Pocketbook of Pediatric Antimicrobial Therapy*, 1995, p. 16. **Prober:** *Pediatr Infect Dis* 1990;9:111.

Cephalosporin-associated Drug Resistance:
Routine or frequent use of cephalosporins in the neonatal intensive care unit will quickly result in the emergence of resistant enteric organisms. Clinicians are advised to use aminoglycosides combined with ampicillin or penicillin for initial empiric therapy of suspected or proven neonatal sepsis.
Nelson: *Pediatr Infect Dis J* 1988;14:1, *Am J Dis Child* 1985;139:1079, *Am J Dis Child* 1987;62:148.

Cephalothin (Keflin)
Classification: First-generation cephalosporin.
Indications: Better activity against gram-positive organisms than second-generation cephalosporins.
See **Cephalosporin-associated Drug Resistance** comments.
Dosage (mg/kg/dose)/Dosage Interval: IV: (final concentration of 20 mg/ml infused over 30 min); IM administration painful, IV route preferred

Weight <1200 g	Weight 1200–2000 g		Weight >2000 g	
Postnatal age (PNA) ≤4 wk or ≥4 wk	PNA ≤7 days	PNA >7 days	PNA ≤7 days	PNA >7 days
20 q12h	20 q12h	20 q8h	20 q8h	20 q6h

Precautions: Dosage reduction for renal failure. Contains 2.8 mEq sodium/g.
Test Interactions: False elevation of creatinine. **Adverse Reactions:** Hypersensitivity reactions, serum sickness-like reaction with prolonged use, neutropenia, leukopenia, and transient elevation of AST.
Nelson: *Pocketbook of Pediatric Antimicrobial Therapy*, 1995, p. 16. **Prober:** *Pediatr Infect Dis J* 1990;9:111.

Chloral Hydrate (Noctec, Somnos, Aquachloral)
Dosage/Dosage Interval

Indications	Dosage (mg/kg/dose)/route/frequency
Sedative/hypnotic	25–50, PO, PR, q6–8h PRN, Max. dose: 50; to reduce gastric irritation, dilute in feedings or administer after feedings.

Precautions: Rectal suppositories are not recommended due to unreliable release characteristics. Use caution with concurrent administration of furosemide and anticoagulants. **Clinical Considerations:** Because chloral hydrate has no analgesic properties, excitation may occur instead of sedation in infants with pain. Carefully assess level of sedation. Accumulation of the toxic metabolite (trichloroethanol) and direct hyperbilirubinemia occur with routine-schedule use and/or long-term administration. **Contraindications:** Hepatic or renal impairment. **Adverse Reactions:** Paradoxical excitation, GI intolerance, allergic manifestations, leukopenia, eosinophilia, vasodilation, cardiopulmonary depression (especially when coadministered with barbiturates and opiates), and cardiac arrhythmias. **Rudolph:** *Rudolph's Pediatrics,* 1991, p. 1968. **Johnson:** *The Harriet Lane Handbook,* 1993, p. 407.

Chloramphenicol (Chloromycetin)

Indications: Broad-spectrum antimicrobial agent. Bactericidal against *Haemophilus influenzae* and *Neisseria meningitis.*
Dosage (mg/kg/dose)/Dosage Interval: IV: (100 mg/ml final concentration, infused over 30 min), PO

Weight <1200 g		Weight 1200–2000 g		Weight >2000 g	
Postnatal age (PNA) ≤4 wk or >4 wk	PNA ≤7 days	PNA >7 days	PNA ≤7 days	PNA >7 days
25 q24h	25 q24h	25 q24h	25 q24h	25 q12h

If necessary, bioavailability is reportedly adequate by the PO route, but do not administer IM. **Ophthalmic:** One drop in each eye q6–12h. **Warnings:** Avoid chloramphenicol use if other options are available (the third-generation cephalosporins have decreased the need for chloramphenicol). Serious and fatal blood dyscrasias reported with both short- and long-term therapies. **Monitoring:** Close monitoring of serum concentration is mandatory. Draw peak levels 3 h after a dose and maintain at 10–20 μg/ml for most infections and 15–25 μg/ml for meningitis. Monitor CBC, platelets, and reticulocyte counts every other day, and closely monitor renal and hepatic function and serum iron levels at least twice weekly. **Drug Interactions:** Chlorpropamide, phenytoin, oral anticoagulants, and phenobarbital. **Adverse Reactions:** "Gray baby" syndrome occurs with peak serum concentrations greater than 50 mcg/ml. Typical symptoms include hyperammonemia, unexplained metabolic acidosis, hypotonia, gray skin color, vomiting, hypothermia, shallow and irregular respirations, abdominal distention, cyanosis, vasomotor collapse, and death. Reversible bone marrow suppression also occurs, and typical manifestations include increased serum iron concentration, increased saturation of iron-binding capacity, decreased hematocrit, thrombocytopenia, leukopenia, and vacuolization of bone marrow elements. Chloramphenicol-induced aplastic anemia is irreversible, rare, and not dose-related and may occur anytime either during or after cessation of therapy. Fungal overgrowth is also reported.
Nelson: *Pocketbook of Pediatric Antimicrobial Therapy,* 1995, p. 16. **Prober:** *Pediatr Infect Dis J* 1990;90:111.

Chlorothiazide (Diuril, Diurigen)

Indications: Fluid overload, pulmonary edema, BPD, CHF, and hypertension. **Dosage/Dosage Interval:** 20–40 mg/kg/day PO, IV, divided q12h. IM and SC administration not recommended due to local pain and irritation. **Contraindications:** Anuria or hepatic dysfunction. **Drug Interactions:** Reduced antihypertensive effect with concurrent NSAID use. **Monitoring:** Serum electrolytes, calcium, blood glucose, urine output, blood pressure, and daily weight. **Adverse Reactions:** Hypochloremic alkalosis, prerenal azotemia, volume depletion, blood dyscrasias, decreased serum potassium and magnesium levels, and increased levels of glucose, uric acid, lipids, bilirubin, and calcium.

Gomella: *Neonatology,* 1994, p. 477. Johnson: *The Harriet Lane Handbook,* 1993, p. 409.

Cholestyramine Resin (Questran, Cholybar)

Indications: Treatment of diarrhea associated with excess fecal bile acids, ileal resection, or pseudomembranous colitis. **Dosage/Dosage Interval:** 240 mg/kg/day PO, divided q8h. Administer with formula, water, or juice. **Clinical Considerations:** Useful only in infants with limited ileal resections; use in neonates with extensive resections can cause further depletion of bile acid pool and exacerbate steatorrhea. **Contraindications:** Complete biliary obstruction. **Precautions:** Use with caution in neonates with constipation. Do not give other oral medications within 1 h before and 6 h after cholestyramine. **Drug Interactions:** Binds with digoxin and warfarin resulting in decreased absorption of both drugs. **Adverse Reactions:** Steatorrhea, GI dysfunction, malabsorption of fat-soluble vitamins, constipation, and vomiting. Hyperchloremic acidosis may result from excessive doses/prolonged use. **Johnson:** *The Harriet Lane Handbook,* 1993, p. 410. **Hay:** *Neonatal Nutrition and Metabolism,* 1991, p. 444.

Cimetidine (Tagamet)

Indications: Duodenal and gastric ulcers, hypersecretory conditions, and gastroesophageal reflux. **Dosage/Dosage Interval:** 10–20 mg/kg/day divided q6h. PO, IV (IV final concentration of 6 mg/ml infused over 20 min). IV/PO dosing titrated to maintain gastric pH >5. **Precautions:** Reserve use for specific indications due to limited experience with the use of cimetidine in newborns and because of concern over possible endocrinologic toxicities. Cimetidine effectively increases gastric pH. Increased gastric pH may result in gastric colonization with pathogenic bacteria and yeast. Modify dosage for renal impairment. **Drug Interactions:** May increase effects or toxicity of chlordiazepoxide, diazepam, lidocaine, phenytoin, procainamide, carbamazepine, propranolol, morphine, quinidine, theophylline (reduce theophylline dose 50%), and warfarin. Antacids may reduce absorption of cimetidine. **Adverse Reactions:** CNS toxicity, cholestatic jaundice, diarrhea, neutropenia and elevated creatinine, SGOT, and SGPT levels. **Johnson:** *The Harriet Lane Handbook,* 1995, p. 411. **Gomella:** *Neonatology,* 1994, p. 478.

Cisapride (Domperidone)

Indications: Increases gastric emptying and GI motility. Treatment of gastroesophageal reflux. **Dosage/Dosage Interval: Gastroesophageal reflux:** 0.1–0.3 mg/kg/dose, PO/PG, q6–12h (preferably 30 ac and hs). **Clinical Considerations:** Cisapride has several advantages over metoclopramide, including no associated CNS toxicity and improved prokinetic activity at all levels of the GI tract. **Monitoring:** Measure gastric residuals. **Drug Interactions:** Enhances absorption of diazepam, cimetidine, and ranitidine, and both cimetidine and ranitidine increase cisapride bioavailability. **Adverse Reactions:** Transient abdominal cramping, borborygmi, and diarrhea. **Malfroot A:** *Pediatr Pulmonol* 1987;3:208–213. **Janssens G:** *J Pediatr Gastroenterol Nutr* 1990;11:420. **Wiseman LR:** *Drugs* 1994;47:116.

Citrate Mixtures, Oral
Indications: Metabolic acidosis.
Content (mEq) in each ml of citrate mixture

	Na	K	Citrate
Polycitra	1	1	2
Polycitra-K	0	2	2
Bicitra	1	0	1
Oracit	1	0	1

Dosage/Dosage Interval: 5–15 ml/kg/dose q6–8h, PO or 2–3 mEq/kg/day divided q6–8h. Adjust dose to maintain desired urine pH; 1 mEq citrate equivalent to 1 mEq HCO_3. **Precautions:** Use with caution in infants receiving potassium supplements. **Adverse Reactions:** Laxative effect.
Johnson: *The Harriet Lane Handbook,* 1993, p. 412.

Clindamycin (Cleocin)
Indications: Treatment of *B. fragilis* septicemia or peritonitis. Not indicated for meningitis.
Dosage (mg/kg/dose)/Dosage Interval: PO: Reconstitute with sterile water to a concentration of 75 mg/5 ml, IV (final concentration of 10 mg/ml infused over 30 min); IM administration associated with sterile abscess formation

Weight <1200 g		Weight 1200–2000 g		Weight >2000 g	
PNA ≤4 wk	PNA ≥4 wk	PNA ≤7 days	PNA >7 days	PNA ≤7 days	PNA >7 days
5 q12h	5 q8h	5 q12h	5 q8h	5 q8h	5 q6h

PNA = postnatal age

Contraindications: Hepatic impairment. **Warnings:** Can cause severe and possibly fatal pseudomembranous colitis characterized by severe persistent diarrhea and possibly the passage of blood and mucus. If bloody diarrhea occurs, discontinue clindamycin, begin bowel rest and total parenteral nutrition, and consider oral vancomycin therapy. **Drug Interactions:** Tubocurarine, pancuronium. **Adverse Reactions:** Pseudomembranous colitis, Stevens-Johnson syndrome, glossitis, pruritus, granulocytopenia, thrombocytopenia, hypotension, and elevation of liver enzymes.
Nelson: *Pocketbook of Pediatric Antimicrobial Therapy,* 1995, p. 16. **Prober:** *Pediatr Infect Dis J* 1990;9:111. **Faix:** *J Pediatr* 1988;112:271–277.

Codeine
Indications: Narcotic analgesic for mild to moderate pain. **Dosage/Dosage Interval:** 0.5–1.5 mg/kg/dose, q4–6h, IM, SC, PO. IV use not recommended due to histamine release. **Drug Interactions:** CNS depressants may potentiate, and phenothiazines may antagonize the analgesic effect of codeine. **Contraindications:** Do not use as an antitussive in children <2 years old. **Clinical Considerations:** Causes less sedation and constipation than morphine sulfate. Poor analgesic alone; thus, it should be used with Tylenol or aspirin for oral analgesia therapy. **Adverse Reactions:** CNS and respiratory depression, GI intolerance, cardiovascular instability, his-

tamine release, increased intracranial pressure, biliary or urinary tract spasm, and antidiuretic hormone release. **Johnson:** *The Harriet Lane Handbook,* 1993, p. 415. **Rudolph:** *Rudolph's Pediatrics,* 1991, p. 1970.

Colfosceril Palmitate (Exosurf) (see Chap. 24)

Indications: Prophylactic therapy: Infants weighing <1350 g at risk for developing respiratory distress syndrome (RDS) and >1350 g with evidence of pulmonary immaturity. **Rescue therapy:** Treatment of infants with RDS based on respiratory distress not attributable to any other causes based on clinical and laboratory assessments or chest radiographic findings consistent with the diagnosis of RDS. **Dosage/Dosage Interval: Prophylactic treatment:** 5 ml/kg as soon as possible. Administer the second and third doses 12 and 24 h after the first dose. **Rescue treatment:** After diagnosing RDS, administer 5 ml/kg, follow with the second dose 12 h later. After ET suctioning, administer using the sideport of supplied ET tube adapter without interrupting mechanical ventilation. With the neonate's head in the midline position, administer each 2.5 ml/kg dose over 1–2 min in small bursts timed with inspiration. After the first half-dose, turn the head and torso 45 degrees to the right for 30 s. Return the neonate to the midline position, administer the second 2.5 ml/kg in the same fashion, and then turn 45 degrees to the left for 30 s. Withhold suctioning for 2 h following administration, except when clinically indicated. **Precautions:** Exosurf may rapidly affect oxygenation and lung compliance. **Monitoring:** Continuously monitor oxygen saturation, ECG, and blood pressure. Obtain frequent blood gas analyses to detect and correct abnormalities of oxygenation and/or ventilation. **Adverse Reactions:** Mucous plugging and hypoxemia. Pulmonary hemorrhage reported in 2% to 4% of treated infants. **Product Information, Burroughs Wellcome Co., 1990.**

Cromolyn Sodium (Intal, Nasalcrom, Opticrom, Gastrocrom)

Indications: Prevention of bronchospasm in neonates with bronchopulmonary dysplasia. **Dosage/Dosage Interval: Metered dose inhaler (MDI):** 2 puffs q6h. (Although intrapulmonary deposition is greater with MDI administration, consider the fact that the long-term hazards of chlorofluorocarbon exposure are unknown, and that a hypoxic condition may be created by the mixture of propellant and ventilator gases.) **Nebulization:** 10–20 mg q6–8h. **Contraindications:** Do not use for treatment of acute bronchospasm episodes. **Precautions:** Renal or hepatic dysfunction. **Clinical Considerations:** Allow 2–4 weeks for adequate determination of treatment effect. **Adverse Reactions:** Rash, cough, bronchospasm, nasal congestion, urticaria, and vomiting. **Johnson:** *The Harriet Lane Handbook,* 1993, p. 417. **Bhutani:** *Clin Perinatol* 1992;19:649–671.

Defibrillation

Indications: Treatment of ventricular fibrillation or pulseless ventricular tachycardia. **Dosage/Dosage Interval:** 1–2 Watt-seconds/kg initial dose; double with each successive attempt to a maximum of 10 Watt-seconds/kg. Perform the first three defibrillation attempts in rapid succession. Correct acidosis, hypoxemia, and hypothermia before, during, and after defibrillation attempts. Administer lidocaine and epinephrine to increase coarseness of the fibrillation, and repeat defibrillation at 4 J/kg. **Clinical Considerations:** Suggested paddle diameter is 4.5 cm for infants. **Adverse Reactions:** Fatal arrhythmias, hypotension, myocardial injury, emboli, pulmonary edema, and increased levels of SGOT, LDH, and CPK. **AHA:** *JAMA* 1992;268:2262–2275.

Dexamethasone (Decadron) (see Chapter 23)

Dosage/Dosage Interval: IM: Preferred route of administration unless in shock or acutely ill; PO, IV (IV solution diluted in equal volume of diluent and infused over 10 min (see Chap. 24)

Indications	Dosage/frequency
Extubation	0.25–0.1 mg/kg/dose, q6h PRN for airway edema. Max. dose: 1 mg/kg/day. Begin 24 h prior to extubation, and continue for 3–4 doses afterwards
Refractory neonatal hypoglycemia	0.25 mg/kg/dose IV, PO, q12h, PRN
Cerebral edema	Load: 0.5–1.5 mg/kg, IV, IM Maintenance: 0.2–0.5 mg/kg/day q6h, IV, IM; administer for 5 days, then taper
Bronchopulmonary dysplasia	0.5 mg/kg/day divided q12h × 3 days, then 0.3 mg/kg/day divided q12h × 3 days. Decrease dose by 0.1 mg/kg/day q72h until reaching 0.1 mg/kg/day, then administer qod for 1 wk and discontinue; all doses given IV and administered q12h

Bronchopulmonary dysplasia (BPD) Therapy: Because benefit is usually evident after 5 days, failed response necessitates a search for infection or other pathology and cessation of further steroid therapy. **Clinical Considerations:** Suppression of the hypothalamic-pituitary-adrenal axis (HPAA) occurs in 50–100% of premature infants given treatment regimens lasting a week or longer. This suppression may last from several weeks to months and necessitates careful consideration of the need for stress-dose steroid therapy for surgery or intercurrent infections. **Monitoring:** Prior to starting therapy, confirm the absence of infection (systemic and pulmonary) and patent ductus arteriosus. Obtain baseline blood pressure, blood glucose, growth parameters, and stool occult blood tests. During therapy, monitor blood pressure, guaiac gastric aspirates, and assess for hyperglycemia, hypertension, and glycosuria. **Precautions:** Hypothyroidism, hypertension, congestive heart failure, or thromboembolic disorder. Infants with a gastric pH <2 may benefit from an H2-receptor antagonist. **Contraindications:** Active untreated infections. **Drug Interactions:** Barbiturates, phenytoin, rifampin, vaccines, and toxoids. **Adverse Reactions:** Hyperglycemia, glycosuria, and hypertension occur frequently during the first few days of therapy. **Short-term adverse effects:** Seizures, hypokalemia, leukocytosis, hypocalcemia, alkalosis, sodium and water retention, gastric and duodenal ulceration/perforation, and GI hemorrhage. **Long-term adverse effects:** Nephrolithiasis, osteopenia/osteoporosis, fractures, Cushing's syndrome, pituitary-adrenal axis suppression, growth suppression, cataracts, transient hypertrophic cardiomyopathy, and pseudotumor cerebri. **Johnson:** *The Harriet Lane Handbook,* 1993, p. 422. **Gomella:** *Neonatology,* 1994, p. 479.

Dextrose (see Chap. 29)
Indications: Treatment of hypoglycemia. **Dosage/Dosage Interval:** 2–5 ml/kg (0.2–0.5 g/kg) D10W initially, followed by constant infusion of D10W at 100 ml/kg/day (8 mg/kg/min). **Monitoring:** Monitor blood glucose levels 30 min after bolus, q30min until stable, then according to unit policy. **Rudolph:** *Rudolph's Pediatrics,* 1991, p. 1973. **Yeh:** *Neonatal Therapeutics,* 1991, p. 245.

Diazepam (Valium)
Dosage/Dosage Interval

Indications	Dosage/route/frequency
Status epilepticus	IV: 0.1–0.3 mg/kg/dose, q15–30 min. to max. dose: 2–5 mg. PR: 0.3–0.5 mg/kg/dose × 1 dose
Continuous refractory seizures	0.1–0.3 mg/kg/dose as IV bolus; follow with continuous infusion of 0.3 mg/kg/h (dilute in saline to 0.1 mg/ml). Do not exceed 1–2 mg/kg/min IV infusion rate
Sedation/muscle relaxation	PO: 0.12–0.8 mg/kg/day q6–8h. IM/IV: 0.04–0.3 mg/kg/dose q2–4h; Max: 0.6 mg/kg within 8h period
Drug withdrawal	0.1–0.8 mg/kg/dose, PO, IV, q6–8h
Hyperglycinemia	1.5–3 mg/kg/day, PO divided q6–8h. Administer in combination with sodium benzoate 125–200 mg/kg/day, PO, divided q6–8h

Contraindications: Coma or preexisting CNS depression. **Precautions:** Be prepared for possible respiratory depression. Do not mix with other IV medications. Because the vehicle for IV diazepam contains sodium benzoate, and sodium benzoate displaces bilirubin from albumin binding sites, use caution during diazepam therapy in the icteric-premature neonate. Neonates tend to be resistant to the sedative effect of diazepam and require higher doses than older infants. **Adverse Reactions:** Laryngospasm and phlebitis. Rapid IV administration is associated with bradycardia, apnea, cardiac arrest, respiratory arrest, hypotension, bradycardia, and cardiovascular collapse.
Gomella: *Neonatology,* 1994, p. 479. **Johnson:** *The Harriet Lane Handbook,* 1993, p. 423.

Diazoxide (Hyperstat, Proglycem)
Dosage/Dosage Interval (see Chap. 29)

Indications	Dosage/route/frequency
Hypertensive crisis	IV: 1–3 mg/kg/dose × 1. Repeat q15–20 min PRN, then q4–24h. Rapid injection not required. PO: 8–15 mg/kg/day divided q8–12h
Hyperinsulinemic hypoglycemia	PO, IV: 8–15 mg/kg/day, divided q8–12h

Clinical Considerations: Initial treatment of hypoglycemia consists of IV glucose. Diazoxide used only for glucose-refractory hypoglycemia. **Contraindications:** Compensatory hypertension associated with aortic coarc-

tation or arteriovenous shunts. **Precautions:** Diabetes mellitus, renal or liver disease. May displace bilirubin from albumin. **Monitoring:** Blood pressure, CBC, and serum uric acid levels. **Drug Interactions:** Phenytoin. **Adverse Reactions:** Hyperglycemia (insulin reverses diazoxide-induced hyperglycemia), ketoacidosis, sodium and water retention, hypotension, hyponatremia, extrapyramidal symptoms, seizures, arrhythmias, leukopenia, thrombocytopenia, and hyperosmolar coma.
Johnson: *The Harriet Lane Handbook,* 1993, p. 424. **Fanaroff:** *Neonatal-Perinatal Medicine,* 1991, p. 1173.

Digoxin (Lanoxin)

Indications: Heart failure, paroxysmal A-V nodal tachycardia, atrial and atrial fibrillation/flutter. **Dosage/Dosage Interval:** Reserve total digitalizing dose (TDD) for treatment of arrhythmias and acute congestive heart failure. Administer TDD over 24 h as three divided doses: 1st dose = 1/2 TDD, 2nd dose = 1/4 TDD administered 8 h after 1st dose, and 3rd dose = 1/4 TDD administered 8 h after 2nd dose. Administer IV doses over 10 minutes. Utilize maintenance dose schedule for nonacute arrhythmia and CHF conditions. Do not administer IM. **Pediatric formulation:** 100 μg/ml IV, 50 μg/ml PO.

Postconceptional age (wk)	Total digitalizing dose		Maintenance dose		
	IV (μg/kg)	PO (μg/kg)	IV (μg/kg)	PO (μg/kg)	Interval (h)
≤29	15	20	4	5	24
30–36	20	25	5	6	24
37–48	30	40	4	5	12
≥49	40	50	5	6	12

15 μg = 0.015 mg

Precautions: Reduce dose for renal and hepatic impairment. Cardioversion or calcium infusion may precipitate ventricular fibrillation in the digoxin-treated neonate (may be prevented by lidocaine pretreatment). **Monitoring:** Monitor heart rate and rhythm closely to assess for both desired effects and signs of toxicity. Monitor closely for increased/decreased serum calcium and magnesium (especially in neonates receiving diuretics and amphotericin B, both of which predispose to digoxin toxicity). **Therapeutic levels:** 0.8–2 μg/ml. Neonates may have falsely elevated digoxin levels due to maternal digoxin-like substances. **Contraindications:** A-V block, idiopathic hypertrophic subaortic stenosis, ventricular dysrhythmias, atrial fibrillation or flutter with slow ventricular rates, or constrictive pericarditis. **Drug Interactions:** Amiodarone, erythromycin, cholestyramine, indomethacin, spironolactone, quinidine, verapamil, and metoclopramide. **Adverse Reactions:** Feeding intolerance, vomiting (persistent vomiting is the most common sign of digoxin toxicity in infants), diarrhea, and lethargy. **Nontoxic cardiac effects:** Shortening of QTc interval, sagging ST segment, diminished T-wave amplitude and bradycardia. **Toxic cardiac effects:** Prolongation of PR interval, sinus bradycardia or S-A block, atrial or nodal ectopic beats, and ventricular arrhythmias. Toxicity enhanced by hypokalemia. Treat life-threatening digoxin toxicity with Digoxin Immune Fab.
Young TE: *Neofax '97,* p. 100. **Johnson:** *The Harriet Lane Handbook,* 1993, p. 427.

Digoxin Immune Fab (Digibind)

Indications: Antidote for digoxin intoxication. **Dosage/Dosage Interval:** Fab (mg) = Total body digoxin load × 66.7. Diluted to a final concentration of 1 mg/ml and infused over 20 min through a 0.22-μm filter. Given as rapid bolus injection if cardiac arrest is imminent. **Total body digoxin load** = serum digoxin level (ng/ml) × 5.6 × wt (kg) divided by 1000. Treat hypokalemia with potassium chloride. **Contraindications:** Renal or cardiac failure. **Clinical Considerations:** May rapidly cause severe hypokalemia. Reinstitute digoxin therapy 3 to 7 days after correction of toxicity. **Johnson:** *The Harriet Lane Handbook,* 1993, p. 428. **Woolf:** *N Engl J Med* 1992;326:1739–1744.

Dobutamine (Dobutrex) (see Chap. 17)

Supplied as 12.5 mg/ml.
Indications: Short-term support of neonates with shock and hypotension. **Dosage/Dosage Interval:** 2.5–25 mcg/kg/min. **Maximum recommended dose:** 40 mcg/kg/min. Suggested drip administration = [6 × infant's weight (kg) × (desired dose (mcg/kg/min)/desired fluid rate (ml/hr))] = mg dobutamine per 100 ml solution. For example, 1 kg to get 5 mcg/kg/min if IV rate is 3 ml/hr; [6 × 1 kg × (5 mcg/kg/min)/(3 ml/hr)] = 10 mg dobutamine added to 100 ml solution. **Clinical Considerations:** Unlike dopamine, dobutamine does not cause release of endogenous norepinephrine, nor does it have any effect on dopaminergic receptors, which are two features that render dobutamine a useful alternative if dopamine-associated tachycardia is undesirable. **Contraindications:** Idiopathic hypertrophic subaortic stenosis. **Precautions:** Correct hypovolemia before use. Do not administer dobutamine or other vasopressors via UAC. **Warnings:** Increases A-V conduction and may precipitate ventricular ectopy. Increases myocardial oxygen consumption. **Monitoring:** Continuously monitor heart rate and blood pressure. **Adverse Reactions:** Hypotension (in setting of hypovolemia), arrhythmias, tachycardia (with high doses), cutaneous vasodilation, hypertension, and dyspnea. Extravasation may cause tissue necrosis (treat with phentolamine). **Johnson:** *The Harriet Lane Handbook,* 1993, p. 431. **AHA:** *JAMA* 1992;268:2262–2275.

Dopamine (Intropin, Dopastat) (see Chap. 17)

Supplied as 40 mg/ml.
Indications: Adjunctive therapy for shock refractory to adequate volume replacement. Dose related stimulation of dopaminergic, beta, and alpha receptors with resultant dose related inotropic and vasopressor effects. **Dosage/Dosage Interval: Low dose** (2–5 mcg/kg/min IV): Dopaminergic stimulation. "Renal dose" promotes splanchnic blood flow and renal cortical redistribution of blood flow. Increases urine output, fractional excretion of sodium, and creatinine clearance. **Intermediate dose** (5–15 mcg/kg/ min IV): Cardiotonic dose. Prominent beta-agonist effect. Increased cardiac contractility and blood pressure at lower dose; increased heart rate with higher dose. Inotropic response varies with gestational age and baseline stroke volume. **High dose** (>20 mcg/kg/min IV): Pressor dose. Prominent alpha agonist effect causes increased systemic and pulmonary vascular resistance. Decreases renal perfusion. Doses >20 mcg/kg/min may result in excessive vasoconstriction and loss of renal vasodilating effects. Either epinephrine or dobutamine is preferable to a dopamine infusion of 20 mcg/kg/min. Suggested drip administration = [6 × infant's weight (kg) × (desired dose

(mcg/kg/min)/desired fluid rate (ml/hr))] = mg dopamine per 100 ml solution. (See example for dobutamine.) **Precautions:** Max dose recommended: 20–25 mcg/kg/min IV. Correct hypovolemia to augment pressor effectiveness of dopamine. **Contraindications:** Pheochromocytoma, tachyarrhythmias, or hypovolemia. Because dopamine may increase pulmonary artery pressure, use caution when treating newborns with PPHN. **Warnings:** Do not administer via UAC. **Drug Interactions:** Concurrent administration of phenytoin may exacerbate bradycardia and hypotension. **Monitoring:** Continuously monitor heart rate and blood pressure. Assess urine output, peripheral perfusion, and IV site for blanching/infiltration hourly. **Adverse Reactions:** Arrhythmias, tachycardia, vasoconstriction, hypotension, widened QRS complex, bradycardia, hypertension, excessive diuresis, and azotemia. Reversible suppression of prolactin and thyrotropin secretion; IV infiltration may result in tissue sloughing/necrosis (treat with phentolamine). **American Heart Association:** *JAMA* 1992;268:2262–2275. **Young TE:** *Neofax '97,* p. 104.

Doxapram (Dopram)

Indications: Idiopathic apnea of prematurity refractory to therapeutic levels of methylxanthines. **Dosage/Dosage Interval:** Dilute to a concentration of 1–2 mg/ml. **Loading dose:** 2–3 mg/kg followed by 0.5–1.5 mg/kg/h in D5W; 0.5 mg/kg/h-stepwise increase in dosage at 24–48 h intervals until response or neonate has received 2.5 mg/kg/h for 48 h. After achieving apnea control, decrease infusion rate. **Max. dose:** 2.5 mg/kg/h. **Precautions:** Contains benzyl alcohol 0.9% as preservative. **Contraindications:** Contraindicated in first few days of life when possible occurrence of hypertensive episodes could increase risk of intraventricular hemorrhage. **Monitoring:** Narrow therapeutic range necessitates close monitoring of serum drug levels. Follow aminophylline recommendations for timing of serum samples. Minimum effective serum concentration is 1.5 mcg/ml. Therapeutic range is 5 mcg/ml. Dosage ranges >2–2.5 mg/kg/h are associated with increased risk of adverse reactions. **Adverse Reactions:** Hypertension, tachycardia, skeletal muscle hyperactivity, abdominal distention, increased gastric residuals, vomiting, glucose intolerance, and seizures. **Pellowski:** *J Pediatr* 1990;116:648–653. **Gomella:** *Neonatology,* 1994, p. 481.

DT Vaccine (Pediatric) (see Chap. 23)

Indications: Immunoprophylaxis against diphtheria and tetanus in infants who have a contraindication to pertussis vaccine. **Dosage/Dosage Interval:** 0.5 ml, IM in anterolateral thigh. First dose at 2 months of age (≥6 wk of age). Give second and third doses at 2-month intervals (≥4 wk apart). Immunize premature infants based on postnatal age. **Clinical Considerations:** Vaccinations are appropriate in infants with stable neurological conditions (including well-controlled seizures). When giving multiple vaccines, use a separate syringe for each and give at different sites. **Precautions:** Infants who have had prior seizures are at increased risk for seizures following DT vaccination. Administer acetaminophen to prevent postvaccination fever. **Monitoring:** Observe injection site for erythema, induration (common), palpable nodule (uncommon), and sterile abscess (rare). **Adverse Reactions:** Fever, drowsiness, agitation, anaphylaxis, and anorexia have been reported. **Advisory Committee on Immunization Practices: Diphtheria, tetanus, and pertussis.** *MMWR* 1991;40(RR-10):1.

aDTP Vaccine (acellular)

Indications: Immunoprophylaxis against diphtheria, tetanus, and pertussis. **Dosage/Dosage Interval:** 0.5 ml IM in the anterolateral thigh. First dose given at 2 months of age. Give second and third doses at 2-month intervals. Immunize premature infants based on postnatal age. When giving multiple vaccines, use a separate syringe for each and give at different sites. **Precautions:** Delay the initial aDTP dose until the neurologic status and effects of treatment are clear in infants with evolving neurologic disorders. aDTP doses are appropriate in infants with stable neurologic conditions (including well-controlled seizures), although infants with a history of seizures are at increased risk for seizures following aDTP vaccination. Administer acetaminophen to prevent postvaccination fever. **Precautions to further aDTP vaccination:** (1) Temperature $\geq$40.5°C within 48 h of administration and not due to another cause; (2) hypotonic-hyporesponsive collapse or shock-like state within 48 h; (3) inconsolable crying ($\geq$3 h) occurring within 48 h; and (4) convulsions with or without fever occurring within 3 days. **Contraindications to further aDTP vaccination:** An immediate anaphylactic reaction or encephalopathy occurring within 7 days following aDTP vaccination. **Adverse Reactions:** Injection site erythema, induration, palpable nodule, or sterile abscess. Other adverse reactions include drowsiness, agitation, and anorexia. Moderate to severe systemic reactions include high fever, collapse, short-duration seizures, and inconsolable crying (>3 h).
Advisory Committee on Immunization Practices: *MMWR* 1991;40(RR-10):1.
AAP: *Redbook,* 1997;395.

aDTP/Hib Conjugate Combination Vaccine

Indications: Immunoprophylaxis against infections caused by diphtheria, tetanus, pertussis, and *Haemophilus influenzae* type B. **Dosage/Dosage Interval:** First dose given at 2 months of age ($\geq$6 wk of age). Give second and third doses at 2-month intervals ($\geq$4 wk intervals). Immunize premature infants based on postnatal age. When giving multiple vaccines, use a separate syringe for each and give at different sites. Follow specific preparation and administration recommendations for tetraimmune and Acti-HiB products. **Monitoring/Adverse Reactions/Precautions/Contraindications:** Refer to DTP data.
Committee on Infectious Diseases, American Academy of Pediatrics. *Pediatrics,* 1993;92:480. **Advisory Committee on Immunization Practices.** *MMWR* 1993;42 (RR-13):1.

Enalapril Maleate (Vasotec), Enalaprilat (Vasotec IV)

Indications: Treatment of moderate to severe hypertension. Afterload reduction in newborns with congestive heart failure (CHF). **Dosage/Dosage Interval: Severe CHF:** Enalapril maleate: Initial dose: 0.1 mg/kg/day, PO; increase according to response to 0.12–0.43 mg/kg/day, PO. PO suspension prepared by dissolving a crushed 2.5-mg tablet in 12.5 ml of sterile water, yielding final concentration of 0.2 mg/ml (200 mcg/ml).
Neonatal hypertension: Enalaprilat: 5–10 mcg/kg/dose (0.005–0.010 mg/kg/dose), IV, q8–24h. **Precautions:** Impaired renal function. **Monitoring:** Blood pressure. Frequent assessment of renal function and serum electrolytes. **Adverse Reactions:** Transient or prolonged episodes of hypotension, oliguria, mild nonoliguric renal failure, hypotension in volume-

depleted neonates, and hyperkalemia in neonates receiving potassium supplements and/or potassium-sparing diuretics. **Young TE:** *Neofax '97,* p. 102. **Frennaux M:** *Arch Dis Child* 1989;64:219–223. **Wells TG:** *J Pediatr* 1990;117:664–667.

Epinephrine HCL (Adrenalin) 1:10,000 (0.1 mg/ml) for individual doses. **Indications:** Cardiac arrest, refractory hypotension, bronchospasm. **Dosage/Dosage Interval**

Severe bradycardia and hypotension	IV, push 0.1 to 0.3 ml/kg of **1:10,000** concentration; may repeat 2–3 times q3–5 min. **Second and subsequent doses for unresponsive asystolic and pulseless arrest should be 0.1–0.2 mg/kg (0.1–0.2 ml/kg of 1:1000 solution), administered q3–5 min.** *Endotracheal tube (ETT):* 0.1 mg/kg (0.1–0.3 ml/kg of 1:1000 solution), use a 1:1 dilution with normal saline.
Continuous IV [(Final conc. of 4 mcg/ml in D5W or NS (1 mg/250 ml), use 1:1000 solution]: Start with 0.1 mcg/kg/min titrated up to 1.5 mcg/kg/min. *If asystolic or pulseless arrest* continues, administer up to 20 mcg/kg/min, until cardiac activity returns. After restoration of effective perfusion, decrease infusion rate by 0.1 mcg/kg/min and titrate to desired response.	To make IV infusion: $6 \times \text{wt (kg)} \times \dfrac{\text{desired dose (mcg/kg/min)}}{\text{desired fluid rate (ml/hr)}}$ = mg epinephrine to be added to 100 ml IV solution For example, 1 kg to get 0.5 mcg/kg/min at 3 ml fluid/hr. $6 \times 1 \text{ kg} \times \dfrac{0.5 \text{ mcg/kg/min}}{3 \text{ ml/hr}}$ = 1 mg epinephrine added to 100 ml of IV solution
Nebulization (racemic epinephrine alternative)	0.5 m/kg of 1:1000 (1 mg/ml) concentration diluted in 3 ml normal saline.

Monitoring: Continuous heart rate and blood pressure monitoring. **Drug Interactions:** Incompatible with alkaline solutions (sodium bicarbonate). **Precautions:** Note the differences in concentration for usual and high dose/continuous IV epinephrine doses. High doses of preservative-containing epinephrine will necessitate caution in selection of epinephrine preparations. Always use as a 1:10,000 concentration (0.1 mg/ml) for individual doses. Use the 1:1000 concentration for preparation of continuous infusions. ETT doses, and for the high-dose regimen. Correction of acidosis prior to administration of catecholamines enhances their effectiveness. **Contraindications:** Hyperthyroidism, hypertension, and diabetes. **Adverse Reactions:** Ventricular arrhythmias, tachycardia, pallor and tremor, severe hypertension with possible intraventricular hemorrhage, myocardial ischemia, hypokalemia, and decreased renal and splanchnic blood flow. IV infiltration may cause tissue ischemia and necrosis (consider treatment with phentolamine). **AHA:** *JAMA* 1992;268:2262–2275. **Gomella:** *Neonatology,* 1994, p. 482.

Epinephrine Racemic (Vaponefrin, Micronefrin, AsthmaNefrin) Indications: Treatment of postextubation stridor. **Dosage/Dosage Interval:** Stridor/croup: 0.05 ml/kg/dose diluted with 3 ml normal saline. Given by nebulizer q2h PRN (maximum dose: 0.5 ml). **Clinical Considerations:**

Observe neonate closely for rebound airway edema. Closely monitor heart rate (discontinue for heart rate >180 bpm) and blood pressure during administration. **Adverse Reactions:** Tachyarrhythmias, hypokalemia. **Johnson:** *The Harriet Lane Handbook,* 1993, p. 436. **Rudolph:** *Rudolph's Pediatrics,* 1991, p. 1976.

Ergocalciferol (Vitamin D₂, Drisdol, Calciferol) (see Chap. 29)

Indications: Refractory rickets; hypophosphatemia; hypoparathyroidism.

Dosage/Dosage Interval

Indications	Dosage/route/frequency
Dietary supplement	Preterm: 12–20 µg/day (400–800 IU/day) Term infant: 10 µg/day (400 IU/day), PO. IM administration for fat malabsorption.

Ergocalciferol 1.25 mg provides 50,000 IU of vitamin D activity. **Contraindications:** Hypercalcemia and evidence of vitamin D toxicity. **Monitoring:** Serum calcium, phosphorus, and alkaline phosphatase levels. Excessive doses may lead to hypervitaminosis D manifested by hypercalcemia, azotemia, elevated serum creatinine, mild hypokalemia, diarrhea, polyuria, metastatic calcification, and nephrocalcinosis. **Adverse Reactions:** Acidosis, polyuria, nephrocalcinosis, hypertension, and arrhythmias. **Johnson:** *The Harriet Lane Handbook,* 1993, p. 437. **Gomella:** *Neonatology* 1994, p. 514.

Erythromycin (EES, Pediamycin, Ilosone) (see Chap. 23)

Indications: Antibiotic treatment of infections caused by *Chlamydia, Mycoplasma,* and *Ureaplasma.* Treatment and prophylaxis of *Bordetella pertussis* and ophthalmia neonatorum.

Dosage (mg/kg/dose)/Dosage Interval for Systemic Infections: PO: 10 mg/kg/dose: E. Estolate (Ilosone): q8h; E. ethylsuccinate (E.E.S., EryPed): q6h. **IV:** Severe systemic infections or PO route unavailable: 5–10 mg/kg/dose, q6h. (Dilute to 1–5 mg/ml and infuse over 1 h.) IV lactobionate formulations may contain benzyl alcohol.

Specific Infections

Indications	Dosage/route/frequency
Ophthalmia neonatorum	Prophylaxis: 0.5–1 cm ribbon of 0.5% ointment into each conjunctival sac × 1 application
Chlamydia conjunctivitis	0.5–1 cm ribbon of 0.5% ointment into each conjunctival sac q6h. PO therapy is preferable to topical therapy for eradication of nasopharyngeal carrier state. Treat mother and her sexual partner
Ureaplasma urealyticum	Use PO or IV dose schedules and treat for 10–14 days

Administer with infant formula to enhance absorption of *E. ethylsuccinate* and to reduce possible GI upset. **Precautions:** Do not administer IM. IM administration causes pain and necrosis. Cholestatic jaundice occurs with estolate, although hepatotoxicity is uncommon. **Contraindications:** Preexisting hepatic dysfunction. **Drug Interactions:** Increased blood levels of carbamazepine, digoxin, cyclosporine, warfarin, methylprednisolone, and theophylline. **Test Interactions:** False positive urine catecholamines. **Mon-

itoring: Liver function tests, and CBC (eosinophilia). **Adverse Reactions:** Anaphylaxis, rash, stomatitis, candidiasis, hepatotoxicity, ototoxicity (high-dose erythromycin), intrahepatic cholestasis, and vomiting. **Young TE:** *Neofax '97*, p. 24. **Waites KB:** *Pediatr Infect Dis J* 1994;13:287.

Exosurf—See Colfosceril Palmitate

Fentanyl Citrate (Sublimaze, Duragesic)
Dosage (mcg/kg/dose)/Dosage Interval

Indications	Dosage (mcg/kg/dose)/route/frequency
Sedation	1–4, IM, slow IV push, q2–4h, PRN, or continuous IV at 0.5–1 mcg/kg/h, titrated to effect
Analgesia	Initial: 2, q2–4h, PRN, or continuous IV 1–5 mcg/kg/h. Tachyphylaxis occurs rapidly with continuous infusions
Anesthesia	5–50

Monitoring: Respiratory and cardiovascular status. Observe for fentanyl-induced ileus (abdominal distention, loss of bowel sounds) and muscle rigidity. **Clinical Considerations:** Tolerance rapidly develops to sedating effects, necessitating escalation of doses; 0.1 mg fentanyl equivalent to 10 mg morphine or 75 mg meperidine. Adherence to ECMO membranes may necessitate dosage increase. **Precautions:** Give IV dose over 3–5 min to avoid apnea and fentanyl-induced decreased total lung and chest wall compliance. Muscle relaxants are used to prevent fentanyl-induced decreased lung and chest wall compliance. Respiratory depression occurs with doses >5 mcg/kg and also may occur unexpectedly due to redistribution (naloxone should be at the bedside to reverse adverse effects). **Adverse Reactions:** CNS and respiratory depression, skeletal/thoracic muscle rigidity, vomiting, constipation, peripheral vasodilation, miosis, biliary or urinary tract spasm, and ADH release. Tolerance rapidly develops in association with continuous IV infusions. Significant withdrawal symptoms occur with use of continuous infusions >5 days. **Arnold JH:** *Anesthesiology* 1990;73:1136. **Gomella:** *Neonatology*, 1994, p. 483.

Ferrous Sulfate (Ferinsol, Fer iron)
Dosage (mg/kg/day of elemental iron)/Dosage Interval

Indications	Dosage/route/frequency
Iron deficiency anemia	PO: 3–6, divided q6h. PO dose diluted in formula
Treatment prophylaxis	Premie: 2, PO. Term: 1–2, PO. Maximum dose: 15 mg; iron supplementation may increase hemolysis without adequate vitamin E therapy

Start iron therapy no later than 2 months of age for both premature and term infants. **Clinical Considerations:** Absorption is variable. Ferrous sulfate elemental iron content: drops: 15 mg/0.6 ml; syrup: 18 mg/5 ml; elixir: 44 mg/5 ml. Vitamin C, 200 mg per 30 mg elemental iron, enhances iron absorption. **Contraindications:** Peptic ulcer disease, ulcerative colitis, enteritis, hemochromatosis, and hemolytic anemia. **Drug Interactions:** Decreased absorption of both iron and tetracycline when given together. Antacids and chloramphenicol decrease iron absorption. **Monitoring:** Hemoglobin and reticulocyte counts during therapy. Observe stools (may color the stool black and cause false-positive guaiac test for blood), and monitor for constipation. **Adverse Reactions:** Constipation, diarrhea, and GI irritation. **Overdose:** Serum iron level >300 μg/ml usually requires treatment due to severe toxicity; acute GI irritation, erosion of GI mucosa, hematemesis, lethargy, acidosis, hepatic and renal dysfunction, circulatory collapse, coma, and death. Antidote is deferoxamine chelation therapy. Gastric lavage with 1–5% sodium bicarbonate or sodium phosphate solution prevents additional absorption of iron. **Gomella:** *Neonatology,* 1994, p. 484. **Fanaroff:** *Neonatal-Perinatal Medicine,* 1992, p. 1428.

Fluconazole (Diflucan)

Indications: Treatment of amphotericin-resistant systemic fungal infections and severe superficial mycoses.

Dosage/Dosage Interval: 6 mg/kg/dose PO or IV (infused over 1–2 h)

GA (wk) ≤29		GA 30–36		GA 37–44		GA ≥45
PNA ≤14 days	PNA >14	PNA ≤14	PNA >14	PNA ≤7	PNA >7	ALL PNA
q72h	q48h	q48h	q24h	q48h	q24h	q24h

GA = gestational age; PNA = postnatal age.

Clinical Considerations: Well-absorbed PO. Good CSF penetration by both IV and PO routes. **Precautions:** Adjust dosage for impaired renal function. **Drug Interactions:** Warfarin, phenytoin, oral antidiabetic agents, rifampin. Possible interference with metabolism of caffeine and theophylline. **Monitoring:** Renal and liver function tests. **Adverse Reactions:** Vomiting, diarrhea, exfoliative skin disorders, and reversible elevation of AST, ALT, and alkaline phosphatase. **Young TE:** *Neofax '97,* p. 26. **Saxen H:** *Clin Pharmacol Ther* 1993;54:269.

Flucytosine (Ancoban, 5-FC, 5-Fluorocytosine)

Indications: Antifungal agent used with amphotericin B for treatment of *Candida* and *Cryptococcus* strains. Routine use of flucytosine with amphotericin B not recommended. **Dosage/Dosage Interval:** 50–150 mg/kg/day divided q6h, PO. **Precautions:** Dosage reduction for renal impairment. Should not be used as single agent in treatment of fungal sepsis because of rapid development of resistance. **Monitoring:** Assess renal function and GI status closely. Obtain weekly CBC, electrolytes, platelets, and liver function tests. Follow amikacin recommendations for timing of serum samples. Desired peak serum concentration ranges from 50–80 mcg/ml. Toxicity occurs with levels above 100 mcg/ml and is reversible after discontinuing flucytosine or with dosage reduction. **Drug Interactions:** Concurrent amphotericin B may increase toxicity by decreasing renal excretion. **Adverse Reactions:** Fatal bone marrow depression (related to fluorouracil production), CNS disturbance (confusion and sedation), anemia, increased BUN and creatinine, leukopenia, thrombocytopenia, and hepatotoxicity. **Nelson:** *Pocketbook of Pediatric Antimicrobial Therapy,* 1995, p. 96. **Fanaroff:** *Neonatal-Perinatal Medicine,* 1992, p. 1425.

Furosemide (Lasix, Furomide)

Indications: Management of edema associated with congestive heart failure, and hepatic or renal disease; management of infants with bronchopulmonary dysplasia.

Dosage/Dosage Interval (direct IV injection administered over 1–2 min)

Route/dosage (mg/kg/dose)	Frequency/clinical considerations
PO: initial: 2, range: 1–6, mg/kg/dose, q12–24h	Increase dose in 1–2 mg/kg/day increments. Poor bioavailability by PO
Maintenance: Same as initial dose	route. Max. dose: 6 mg/kg/day
IV/IM: initial: 1, range: 1–2 mg/kg/dose, q12–24h	Increase dose in 1 mg/kg increments. Max. dose: 6 mg/kg/dose. Dosage
Rapid diuresis for CHF: 1–3, repeated PRN	frequency: premie: q24h. Term: q12–24h, term >1 mo of age: q6–8h.
Fluid overload and PDA: 1, q12–24h	Consider qod therapy for long-term use.

Monitoring: Follow daily weight changes, urine output, serum phosphate, and serum electrolytes. Closely monitor potassium levels in neonates receiving digoxin. **Precautions:** Hepatic and renal disease. **Adverse Reactions:** Fluid and electrolyte imbalance, hypocalcemia/hypercalciuria, hypochloremic alkalosis, nephrocalcinosis (associated with long-term therapy), potential ototoxicity (especially in infants also receiving aminoglycosides), prerenal azotemia, hyperuricemia, agranulocytosis, anemia, thrombocytopenia, interstitial nephritis, pancreatitis, and cholelithiasis (in infants with bronchopulmonary dysplasia or CHF who receive long-term total parenteral nutrition and furosemide therapy).
Rush MG: *J Pediatr* 1990;117:112. **Gomella:** *Neonatology,* 1994, p. 484.

Gamma Globulin Intravenous (see Chap. 23)

Indications	Dosage/route/frequency
Hepatitis A exposure	0.15 ml/kg, IM one dose
Treatment of severe neonatal sepsis See Chap. 23	500–750 mg/kg/dose over 2–6 hours
Prevention of late onset sepsis See Chap. 23	500–750 mg/kg/dose; start day 3–7; repeat every 7–14 days
Neonatal autoimmune thrombocytopenia See Chap. 26	400 mg/kg/day for 2–5 days
Neonatal alloimmune thrombocytopenia See Chap. 26	400 mg/kg/day for 2–5 days

All donor units are nonreactive to HBsAg and HIV. **Precautions:** Product preparation and administration rates vary with each product; refer to manufacturer-supplied product insert prior to use. **Monitoring:** Continuous heart rate and blood pressure monitoring during administration. **Adverse Reactions:** Transient hypoglycemia, tachycardia, and hypotension (resolved with cessation of infusion). Tenderness, erythema, and induration at injection site and allergic manifestations. Rare hypersensitivity reactions reported with rapid IV administration.
Gomella: *Neonatology,* 1994, p. 485. **Kinney:** *Am J Dis Child* 1991;145:1233–1238.

Gentamicin Sulfate (Garamycin)
Classification: Aminoglycoside. **Indications:** Active against gram-negative aerobic bacteria; some activity against coagulase-positive staphylococci; ineffective against anaerobes and streptococci. **Dosage/Dosage Interval:** 2.5 mg/kg/dose IM, IV. Verify that a pediatric dosage vial (concentration of 10 mg/ml) is used. Administer a final concentration of 2 mg/ml infused over 30 min. IM absorption is variable, especially in the VLBW infant.

Postconceptual age (wk)	Postnatal age (days)	Dosage interval (h)
≤30 (or significant asphyxia,	<7	q24
or impaired renal function)	>7	q18
30–36	<7	q18
	>7	q12
≥37	0–7	q12
	>7	q8

Specific Indications

Route	Dosage/frequency
Ophthalmic therapy	1 drop OU q4–12h; ointment: q6–8h

Precautions: Dosage modification for renal impairment. Do not use aminoglycosides as solo therapy for gram-positive organisms. **Monitoring:** Some have suggested monitoring creatinine levels in children who need therapy more than 72 h. If gentamicin levels are measured, the level of gentamicin will be a good index of renal function. If levels exceed the therapeutic trough and peak, this suggests some problem with clearance of the medicine and should warn of problems with renal function; the dose given or the interval between doses should be changed. Measure serum gentamicin levels around the second dose for infants under 30 weeks' gestation and in infants who may have problems with renal function, including infants on a q18 or q24h dosage schedule. Other premature or sick infants should have levels measured around the third dose. In term infants >37 weeks who are asymptomatic and who are receiving antibiotics to rule out sepsis, for whom there is no concern about renal function, gentamicin levels should be obtained around the third to the fifth dose. The practical effect is if the gentamicin level is to be obtained around the fifth dose, most of these infants will be off antibiotics and the levels will not be required. Levels should be measured twice weekly. **Therapeutic serum concentrations: Peak:** 30 min. after IV infusion, 60 min. after IM injection, 5–10 mcg/ml. **Trough:** 1–2 mcg/ml.
Drug Interactions

Drug(s)	Drug interactions
Penicillins, cephalosporins, amphotericin B	Blunting of gentamicin serum peak concentration if administered <2 h before or after these agents
Loop diuretics (furosemide, bumetanide), vancomycin	Potentiates gentamicin-induced ototoxicity and/or nephrotoxicity
Hypermagnesemia, concurrent neuromuscular blocking agent use	Increased neuromuscular blockade

Adverse Reactions: Vestibular and auditory ototoxicity (associated with high peak and trough levels) and renal toxicity (occurs in the proximal tubule, associated with high trough levels, usually reversible). **Young TE:** *Neofax '97,* pp. 27–30. **Johnson:** *The Harriet Lane Handbook,* 1993, p. 450.

Glucagon
Indications: Treatment of hypoglycemia when parenteral dextrose is unavailable or in cases of documented glucagon deficiency. **Dosage/Dosage Interval:** 25–300 mcg/kg/dose (0.025–0.3 mg/kg/dose) IV push IM, SC, q20 min PRN. Maximum dose: 1 mg. **Continuous IV:** Administer in D10W solution, starting at 0.5 mg/day. Add hydrocortisone if no response within 4 h. Further dosage increases >2 mg/day unlikely to be effective. After effect seen, slowly taper over at least 24 h. **Infant of diabetic mother: Initial dose:** 0.3 mg/kg/dose up to 1 mg total as standard dose. Compatible with dextrose solutions. **Contraindications:** Should not be used in small-for-gestational-age infants. **Precautions:** Do not delay starting glucose infusion while awaiting effect of glucagon. Use caution in infants with history of insulinoma or pheochromocytoma. Incompatible with electrolyte-containing solutions. **Monitoring:** Serum glucose concentration. **Adverse Reactions:** Vomiting, tachycardia, and GI upset. **Fanaroff:** *Neonatal-Perinatal Medicine,* 1992, p. 1422. **Johnson:** *The Harriet Lane Handbook,* 1993, p. 451.

Haemophilus b (Hib) Conjugate Vaccine
Indications: Immunoprophylaxis against disease caused by *Haemophilus influenzae* type b. **Dosage/Dosage Interval:** 0.5 ml IM in the anterolateral thigh. Give the first dose of either HbOC or PRP-OMP at 2 months of age. Immunize premature infants according to postnatal age. **HbOC:** Give the second and third doses at 2-month intervals and the fourth dose at age 15 months. **PRP-OMP:** Give the second dose after a 2-month interval and the third dose at age 15 months. **Clinical Considerations:** When giving multiple vaccines, use a separate syringe for each and administer at separate sites. **Monitoring:** Observe the injection site for local reactions. **Adverse Reactions:** Pain at the injection site with local erythema, swelling, tenderness; fever. **Committee on Infectious Diseases, AAP:** Haemophilus influenzae type b conjugate vaccines. *Pediatrics* 1993;92:480.

Heparin Sodium (see Chap. 26)
Indications: Prophylaxis and treatment of thromboembolic disorders.
Dosage/Dosage Interval: 1 mg heparin = 100 U

Indications	Dosage/route/frequency
Catheter patency (intravenous, intraarterial)	0.5–1.0 U/ml of IV fluid

Systemic heparinization	Initial dose: 50 U/kg/, IV bolus
	Maintenance: Continuous IV: 5–35 U/kg/h.
	  Intermittent dose: 50–100 U/kg/dose, q4h, IV.
	  PTT of 1.5–2.5 times pretherapy control
	  values or clotting time of 20–30 min

Disseminated intravascular coagulation (DIC) associated	Bolus: 50 U/kg/h. Continuous infusion: <1.5 kg: 20–25 U/kg/h, >1.5 kg: 25–30 mg/kg/h.

with large vessel thrombosis: high-dose therapy	Monitor whole blood clotting time or APTT and keep at 1 1/2 times pretreatment level. Administer replacement therapy (FFP, cryoprecipitate, platelets) if pretreatment screening levels are abnormal
DIC-associated ischemia and necrosis: low-dose therapy	10–15 U/kg/h + appropriate replacement therapy

Administer replacement therapy with fresh frozen plasma, cryoprecipitate, and platelets if pretreatment screening levels are abnormal. **Contraindications:** Platelet count <50,000/mm^3, suspected intracranial hemorrhage, GI bleeding, shock, severe hypotension, and uncontrolled bleeding. **Precautions:** Risk factors for hemorrhage include IM injections, venous and arterial blood sampling, and peptic ulcer disease. Use preservative-free heparin in neonates. To avoid systemic heparinization in small neonates, use more dilute heparin flush concentrations. **Monitoring:** Follow platelet counts every 2 to 3 days. Closely follow PTT, or clotting time during titration of dose, and then daily. Assess for signs of bleeding and thrombosis. **Drug Interactions:** Thrombolytic agents and IV nitroglycerin. **Adverse Reactions:** Heparin-induced thrombocytopenia (HIT) reported in some heparin-exposed newborns. Other adverse reactions include hemorrhage, fever, urticaria, vomiting, elevated liver enzymes, osteoporosis, and alopecia. **Antidote:** Protamine sulfate (1 mg/100 U of heparin given in the previous 4 h). **Behrman:** *Nelson Textbook of Pediatrics,* 1992, p. 225. **Johnson:** *The Harriet Lane Handbook,* 1993, p. 453. **Spadone D:** *J Vasc Surg* 1992;15:306.

Hepatitis B Immune Globulin (H-BIG, Hep-B Gammagee, HyperHep)

Indications: Immunoprophylaxis of newborns whose mothers have acute hepatitis B infections at the time of delivery, or who are HBsAg positive. **Dosage/Dosage Interval:** Do not administer IV; 0.5 ml in the anterolateral thigh as soon as possible after birth, preferably within the first 12 h of life. If a mother is positive, HBIG may still be of value after this time. Use a separate syringe and injection site when administered with hepatitis B vaccine. **Contraindications:** IgA deficiency, thrombocytopenia, or coagulopathy. **Precautions:** Follow universal precautions with all neonates before and after removal of maternal blood and secretions. **Adverse Reactions:** Local pain and tenderness may occur at injection site. IV administration may result in serious systemic reactions. **AAP:** *Report of the Committee on Infectious Diseases,* 1997, p. 247. **Gomella:** *Neonatology,* 1994, p. 486.

Hepatitis B Vaccine (Recombivax-HB, Heptavax B, Engerix-B) (see Chap. 23)

Indications: Immunoprophylaxis against hepatitis B. Administer in anterolateral thigh.
Dosage/Dosage Interval (Both products are interchangeable. A product different from that given for the initial immunization may be used for subsequent immunizations)

Indications	Dosage/route/frequency
Maternal HBsAg negative	Engerix-B: 0.5 ml (10 mcg) or Recombivax HB: 0.25 ml (2.5 mcg)
Maternal HBsAg positive	Engerix-B: 0.5 ml (10 mcg) or Recombivax HB: 0.5 ml (5 mcg); at birth or before 12 h of age (Administered with HBIG)

Unknown maternal HBsAg status at delivery	Follow schedule for maternal HBsAg positive. Additional HBIG administration will depend on results of maternal serologic screening done within 12 h after delivery
Preterm infants	The optimal time to initiate hepatitis B immunization in premature infants with birth weight <2 kg has not been determined. Seroconversion rates in very-low-birth-weight infants in whom vaccination was initiated shortly after birth have been reported in some studies to be lower than those in preterm infants vaccinated at an older age or in term infants vaccinated shortly after birth. Therefore, for preterm infants weighing <2 kg at birth and born to HBsAg-negative women, initiation of vaccination should be delayed until just before hospital discharge if the infant weighs >2 kg or until about 2 mo of age when other routine immunizations are given. These infants do not need to have serologic testing for anti-HBs performed routinely after the third dose All premature infants born to HBsAg-positive mothers should receive immunoprophylaxis (HBIG and vaccine) beginning as soon as possible after birth, followed by appropriate postvaccination testing

Recommended Routine Hepatitis B Immunization Schedules

Maternal HBsAg	Dose no.	Age
Negative*	1	0–2 days
*Alternative schedule:	2	1–2 Mo
dose 1: 1–2 mo of age; dose 2: 4 mo;	3	6–18 Mo
dose 3: 6–18 mo		
Positive	1 (administered with HBIG)	0 Days
	2	1 Mo
	3	6 Mo

Precautions: If administered with HBIG at birth, give in opposite anterolateral thigh with a different syringe to ensure vaccine absorption and avoidance of neutralization. *Do not administer intravenously or intradermally.* **Clinical Considerations:** Safe for use in an infant born to an HIV-positive mother. **Monitoring:** Test for immunity 3 months after completion of the vaccination series for infants born to HBsAg-positive mothers, HIV-positive mothers, and premature infants who receive a first dose before they are term-postconceptional age. **Adverse Reactions:** Local reaction at injection site (pain, erythema, swelling, warmth), allergic reactions (urticaria, angioedema, pruritus), and neuropathic effects (optic neuritis, transverse myelitis, Guillain-Barré syndrome, paresthesias). **AAP:** *Redbook* 1977, p. 247. **Gomella:** *Neonatology,* 1994, p. 487.

Hyaluronidase (Wyadase) (see Chap. 34)
Indications: Prevention of tissue injury caused by IV extravasation of hyperosmolar or extremely alkaline solutions. **Dosage/Dosage Interval: Subcutaneous or intradermal:** Dilute to 150 U/ml in normal saline. Inject

four or five 0.25-ml injections into the leading edge of the infiltrate. Use a 25- or 26-gauge needle and change after each injection. Elevate the extremity. *Do not apply heat and do not administer IV.* Best results are obtained when used within 1 h of extravasation. May repeat if necessary. **Clinical Considerations:** Some agents for which hyaluronidase is effective include aminophylline, amphotericin, calcium, diazepam, erythromycin, gentamicin, methicillin, nafcillin, oxacillin, phenytoin, KCl, sodium bicarbonate, tromethamine, vancomycin, TPN, and concentrated IV solutions. **Warnings:** Hyaluronidase is neither effective nor indicated for treatment of extravasations of vasoconstrictive agents (phentolamine is the preferred agent for treatment of extravasation with vasoconstrictive agents). **Rudolph:** *Rudolph's Pediatrics,* 1991, p. 1979. **Gomella:** *Neonatology,* 1994, p. 487. **Raszka WW:** *J Perinatol* 1990;10:146.

Hydralazine (Apresoline)
Dosage/Dosage Interval

Indications	Dosage/route/frequency
Hypertensive crisis, Afterload reduction in congestive heart failure, antihypertensive therapy in acute renal failure	0.1–0.5 mg/kg/dose IM, or IV push over 5 min, q3–6h PRN for blood pressure control; increase dose by 0.1 mg/kg until blood pressure control achieved, or maximum dose of 2 mg/kg achieved. Maintenance: 0.75–3 mg/kg/day divided q6–12h, IM, IV, PO. Max. dose: 7.5 mg/kg/day. Oral suspension prepared by crushing a 50 mg tablet and dissolving in 4 ml of 5% mannitol. Add 46 ml of sterile water to yield a final concentration of 1 mg/ml

Precautions: Severe renal and cardiac disease. **Clinical Considerations:** May cause reflex tachycardia. Concurrent β-blocker therapy recommended to reduce the magnitude of reflex tachycardia and to enhance antihypertensive effect. Maximum effect occurs in 3–4 days. Tachyphylaxis reported with chronic therapy. **Drug Interactions:** Concurrent use with other antihypertensives allows reduced dosage requirements of hydralazine to <0.15 mg/kg/dose. **Monitoring:** Daily monitoring of heart rate, blood pressure, urine output, and daily weight. Guaiac all stools, and obtain CBC at least twice weekly. **Adverse Reactions:** Tachycardia, vomiting, diarrhea, orthostatic hypotension, edema, GI irritation and bleeding, anemia, and agranulocytosis. May cause a lupus-like syndrome that is usually reversible with discontinuation of hydralazine (keep daily dose <200 mg to avoid lupus-like syndrome). **Rudolph:** *Rudolph's Pediatrics,* 1991, p. 1979. **Johnson:** *The Harriet Lane Handbook,* 1993, p. 454. **Young TE:** *Neofax '97,* p. 110.

Hydrochlorothiazide (Esidrix, Hydro-T, Thiuretic, Hydrodiuril)
Dosage/Dosage Interval

Indications	Dosage/route/frequency
Mild to moderate edema and hypertension	2–5 mg/kg/day, PO, div.q12h; administer with formula to enhance absorption; avoid IM administration

Diuretic therapy for BPD	Hydrochlorothiazide: 2 mg/kg/dose, PO, q12h

Contraindications: Anuria, hyperkalemia, and renal or hepatic failure. **Monitoring:** Serum electrolytes, blood glucose, urine output, and blood pressure. **Drug Interactions:** Hydrochlorothiazide effects increase when used in combination with furosemide or spironolactone. **Adverse Reactions:** Increased blood levels of calcium, bilirubin, glucose, and uric acid; decreased blood levels of potassium and magnesium; blood dyscrasias; and pancreatitis. **Rush:** *Clin Perinatol* 1992;19:563–590. **Fanaroff:** *Neonatal-Perinatal Medicine,* 1992, p. 900.

Hydrocortisone (Solu-Cortef)

Dosage/Dosage Interval: Na Succinate used for IV dosing, NA phosphate used for IM, SC, or IV dosing. **Acute Adrenal Insufficiency: IM, IV** (final concentration of 1 mg/ml, infused over 30 min); *1–2 mg/kg/dose* or 50 mg/m^2 bolus over 3–5 min, followed by 50–100 mg/m^2/day (25–50 mg/kg/day) continuous IV, or divided q4–6h. **Congenital Adrenal Hyperplasia: PO:** Individualize dose according to the degree of adrenal androgen suppression. **Initial:** 30–36 mg/m^2/day divided q8h; alternative schedule: 0.5–0.7 mg/kg/day divided 1/4 a.m., 1/4 noon, 1/2 night. **Maintenance:** 15–20 mg/m^2/day divided q8h. Alternative schedule: 0.3–0.4 mg/kg/day divided 1/4 a.m., 1/4 noon, 1/2 night. **Anti-inflammatory/ Imunosuppressive: IV:** 0.8–4 mg/kg/day divided q6h. **PO:** 2.5–10 mg/kg/day divided q6–8h. **Gram-negative Shock:** 35–50 mg/kg/dose IV bolus, then 50–150 mg/kg/day IV divided q6h × 48–72 h. **Hypoglycemia:** 10 mg/kg/day divided q12h, IV, IM, PO. **Indications:** (1) if plasma glucose values are not above 40 mg/dl despite adequate IV dextrose therapy, (2) if hypoglycemia recurs, or (3) if IV dextrose concentrations >12 mg/kg/min are required. As the net effect of hydrocortisone may require several hours, increasing glucose infusion rates may be necessary. After normoglycemia is maintained for 48–72 h, taper IV fluids first and continue hydrocortisone until the infant is stable for 48 h off IV fluids. Hydrocortisone therapy usually continues for 5 to 7 days. Infants who do not respond to hydrocortisone may need additional or alternate therapy, depending on the cause of hypoglycemia. **Precautions:** Acute adrenal insufficiency may occur with abrupt withdrawal following long-term therapy or during periods of stress. Use a corticoid with less mineralocorticoid activity for prolonged therapy. See **Dexamethasone,** comments concerning monitoring of serum cortisol levels. **Adverse Reactions:** Hypertension, edema, cataracts, peptic ulcer, immunosuppression, hypokalemia, hyperglycemia, dermatitis, Cushing's syndrome, and skin atrophy.

Fanaroff: *Neonatal-Perinatal Medicine,* 1992, pp. 1172–1173. **Johnson:** *The Harriet Lane Handbook,* 1993, p. 455.

Imipenem/Cilastin (Primaxin)

Indications: Active against a broad spectrum of aerobic and anaerobic gram-positive and gram-negative bacteria.

Dosage (mg/kg/dose)/Dosage Interval: IM (use lidocaine 1% as diluent-IM formulation not for IV use), **IV** (final concentration of 5 mg/ml infused over 30–60 min)

Weight ≤1200 g		Weight 1200–2000 g		Weight ≥2000 g	
PNA ≤4 wk	PNA ≥4 wk	PNA ≤7 days	PNA >7 days	PNA ≤7 days	PNA >7 days
20 q24h	20 q18h	20 q12h	20 q12h	20 q12h	20 q8h

PNA = Postnatal age

Precautions: The IM formulation is not for IV use. **Monitoring:** Complete blood count, liver function tests. **Adverse Reactions:** Pruritus, vomiting, diarrhea, seizures, hypotension, elevated LFTs, blood dyscrasias, and penicillin allergy.
Nelson: *Pocketbook of Pediatric Antimicrobial Therapy,* 1995, p. 16. **Prober:** *Pediatr Infect Dis J* 1990;9:111. **Johnson:** *The Harriet Lane Handbook,* 1993, p. 457.

Indomethacin (Indocin)
Indications: Pharmacologic alternative to surgical closure of ductus arteriosus.
Dosage (mg/kg/dose)/Dosage Interval (IV dosing only—PO dosing not recommended)

Age at first dose	1st dose	2nd dose	3rd dose
≤48 Hours	0.2	0.1	0.1
2–7 Days	0.2	0.2	0.2
3–8 Days	0.2	0.25	0.25

Given by IV infusion pump over 30 min; three doses per course with a usual maximum of two courses; given at 12- to 24-h intervals. Slow, continuous infusions (11 mcg/kg/h for 36 h) reportedly reduce indomethacin-caused reductions in cerebral blood flow velocity. Some infants require a longer treatment course (0.2 mg/kg q24h for 5 to 7 days). **Contraindications:** Impaired renal function (BUN ≥30 mg/dl, urine output <0.6 ml/kg/h for preceding 8 h and creatinine ≥1.8 mg/dl), active bleeding, IVH within preceding 7 days (controversial), ulcer disease, necrotizing enterocolitis or stool hematest >3+, platelet count <60,000/mm^3, and coagulation defects. **Precautions:** IV is the preferred route of administration for PDA closure. Use with caution in neonates with cardiac dysfunction and hypertension. Because indomethacin causes decreases in renal and GI blood flow, withhold enteral feedings during therapy. Reduction in cerebral flow reported with IV infusions of <5-min duration. **Monitoring:** Monitor urine output (keep >0.6 ml/kg/h), serum electrolytes, serum BUN and creatinine, and platelet counts. Closely assess pulse pressure, cardiopulmonary status, and PDA murmur for evidence of success/failure of therapy. Guaiac all stools and gastric aspirates to detect GI bleeding. Observe for prolonged bleeding from puncture sites. **Drug Interactions:** Concurrent administration with digoxin and/or with aminoglycosides results in increased plasma concentrations of these respective agents. **Adverse Reactions:** Decreased platelet aggregation, ulcer, GI intolerance, hemolytic anemia, bone marrow suppression, agranulocytosis, thrombocytopenia, ileal perforation, transient oliguria, electrolyte imbalance, hypertension, hypoglycemia, indirect hyperbilirubinemia, and hepatitis.
Hammerman: *Pediatrics* 1995;95:244–248. **Johnson:** *The Harriet Lane Handbook,* 1993, p. 459. (see Chap. 25)

Insulin, Regular
Dosage/Dosage Interval

Indications	Dosage/route/frequency	Clinical considerations
Hyperglycemia See Chap. 29	Load: 0.1 U/kg/dose regular insulin, IV × 15–20 min; Maintenance: 0.02–0.1 U/kg/h, regular insulin; Intermittent dose: 0.1–0.2 U/kg, q6–12h, SC	Dilute initial concentration to 0.1–1 U/ml in 0.9% normal saline
VLBW with hyperglycemia See Chap. 29	0.02–0.4 U/kg/h, IV; adjust conc. to keep infusion rates ≤0.1 ml/h	Titrate to keep blood glucose: 100–150
Hyperkalemia See Chap. 9	First administer calcium gluconate 50 mg/kg/dose IV, + sodium bicarbonate: 1 mEq/kg/dose IV; follow with dextrose 300–600 mg/kg/dose + regular insulin 0.2 U/kg/dose IV (3–4:1 glucose to insulin ratio)	Use a 3–4:1 glucose: insulin ratio

Monitoring: Follow blood glucose concentration, q30 min after starting infusion and after changes in infusion rate. Follow these parameters of q2–4h after achieving a stable euglycemic state. **Clinical Considerations:** Reduce loss of insulin due to adsorption to the plastic tubing by flushing tubing with the insulin solution prior to beginning the infusion or by adding albumin 0.3 g/100 ml of solution. **Adverse Reactions:** Hyperglycemic rebound (Somogyi effect), urticaria, anaphylaxis; may rapidly induce hypoglycemia. Insulin resistance may develop with prolonged use and necessitate an increased dose.
Gomella: *Neonatology,* 1994, p. 489. **Collins:** *J Pediatr* 1991;118:921–927. (See Chap. 29)

Ipratropium Bromide (Atrovent)
Indications: Bronchodilator treatment of reactive airways disease in ventilator-dependent neonates with chronic lung disease. **Dosage/Dosage Interval: Metered dose inhaler (MDI) with spacer:** 36–72 mcg q6–8h; **Aerosol:** 75–175 mcg, q6–8h. Although intrapulmonary deposition is greater with MDI administration, consider that the long-term hazards of chlorofluorocarbon exposure is unknown and that a hypoxic condition may be created by the mixture of propellant and ventilator gases. **Clinical Considerations:** Not indicated for the initial treatment of acute bronchospasm. The combination of ipratropium with a beta-agonist bronchodilator (e.g., albuterol) produces greater bronchodilatation than either agent alone. Peak effect occurs 1–2 h after administration and lasts for 4–6 h. **Contraindications:** Narrow-angle glaucoma, obstructive uropathy, tachycardia, and thyrotoxicosis. **Adverse Reactions:** Tachycardia, constipation, urinary retention, restlessness, and fever. Ipratropium is poorly absorbed into the systemic circulation from both the lungs and the GI tract.
Young TE: *Neofax '97,* p. 152. **Lee H:** *Arch Dis Child* 1994;70:F218.

Isoniazid (INH, Nydrazid, Laniazid)

Indications: Treatment of susceptible tuberculosis infections and prophylaxis for neonates exposed to tuberculosis. **Dosage (mg/kg/day)/Dosage Interval:** PO, IM: **Prophylaxis:** 10–15, q24h; or 20, twice weekly (after 1 month of daily therapy) for a total of 9 months of therapy. **Treatment:** 10–20, PO, IM, divided q8–12h; or 20–40, twice weekly with rifampin for 9 months. Given IM when PO therapy is not feasible. **Precautions:** Combine with rifampin for treatment of tuberculosis. Risk of hepatic damage increases with combined rifampin and isoniazid therapy in dosages 15 mg/kg of each daily. Administer supplemental pyridoxine (1–2 mg/kg/day). Use with caution in neonates with renal impairment. **Contraindications:** Acute liver disease. **Drug Interactions:** Dosage reductions of carbamazepine, diazepam, phenytoin, and prednisone may be necessary. **Test Interactions:** False-positive urine glucose test with Clinitest. Mild elevations of ALT commonly occur in the first weeks of therapy but resolve with continued administration. **Adverse Reactions:** Seizure, hepatitis (although hepatotoxicity in neonates is rare, check LFTs monthly), blood dyscrasias, vomiting, and hyperglycemia. INH toxicity antidote is Vitamin B_6.

Johnson: *The Harriet Lane Handbook,* 1993, p. 463. **Nelson:** *Pocketbook of Pediatric Antimicrobial Therapy,* 1995, p. 95.

Isoproterenol (Isuprel)

Indications: Reversible airway obstruction; A-V nodal block; hemodynamically compromised or atropine-resistant bradyarrhythmias; low cardiac output; vasoconstrictive shock states.

Dosage/Dosage Interval

Route	Dosage/frequency/comments
Continuous IV (final concentration of 2–10 mcg/ml)	(mcg/kg/min): 0.05–0.5 mcg/kg/min. Begin with 0.05 and increase by 0.05 mcg/kg/min q5–10 min until either desired effect, arrhythmia, or heart rate >180 bpm occurs. Max. dose: 2 mcg/kg/min. Refer to dobutamine calculations to determine number of mgs isoproterenol to add to 100 ml of IV solution
Nebulized solution	0.1–0.25 ml/dose of 1:200 solution + 2 ml of normal saline q4–6h, PRN
Metered-dose inhaler (MDI)	1–2 Puffs up to 5 times a day. Although intrapulmonary deposition is greater with MDI administration, consider the fact that the long-term hazards of chlorofluorocarbon exposure are unknown and that a hypoxic condition may be created by the mixture of propellant and ventilator gases

Contraindications: Preexisting ventricular arrythmias, A-V block due to digoxin intoxication, hypertension, degenerative heart disease, and hyperthyroidism. **Precautions:** Correct acidosis before beginning infusion. Use caution in newborns with diabetes, renal, or cardiovascular disease (CHF, ischemia, or aortic stenosis). Isoproterenol is not an inotropic agent of choice because it increases cardiac oxygen consumption out of proportion to increases in cardiac output (possibly resulting in myocardial ischemia). May precipitate arrhythmias when used in combination with epinephrine or theophylline. **Monitoring:** Continuous cardiac and oxygen saturation monitoring is required. **Adverse Reactions:** Cardiac arrhythmias, tachycardia, hypotension, systemic vasodilation, tremor, vomiting, hypoxemia, and hypoglycemia. **Johnson:** *The Harriet Lane Handbook,* 1993, pp. 463–464. **Gomella:** *Neonatology,* 1994, p. 490. **Young TE:** *Neofax '97,* p. 114.

Kanamycin (Kantrex) (Rarely used)
Classification: Aminoglycoside. **Indications:** Activity identical to gentamicin. Active against gram-negative aerobic bacteria including some *Pseudomonas* sp. Some activity against staphylococci and mycobacteria. Not active against other gram-positive organisms or anaerobes.
Dosage (mg/kg/dose)/Dosage Interval (IM, IV (final IV concentration of 6 mg/ml infused over 30 min); direct IV push not recommended; maximum dose 500 mg/kg)

Weight <1200 g		Weight 1200–2000 g		Weight >2000 g	
PNA ≤4 wk	PNA ≥4 wk	PNA ≤7 days	PNA >7 days	PNA ≤7 days	PNA >7 days
7.5 q24h	7.5 q18h	7.5 q12–18h	7.5 q8–12h	10 q12h	10 q8h

PNA = postnatal age

Optimal dose based on determination of serum concentrations, especially in low-birth-weight (<1.5 kg) neonates. Poor GI absorption renders it useful for treatment of GI bacterial overgrowth. **Monitoring:** Monitor BUN and creatinine at least weekly. Obtain serum drug levels around the third dose. Monitor serum peak levels 30 min after a 30-min infusion and serum trough levels 30 min prior to the next dose. Therapeutic serum peak levels are 15–30 mg/L, and trough levels are 5–10 mg/L. Measure serum creatinine level at least twice weekly. **Precautions:** Dosage reduction for renal impairment. **Adverse Reactions:** Excessive serum peak concentrations associated with ototoxicity and excessive serum trough concentrations associated with nephrotoxicity (usually reversible with cessation of therapy). **AAP:** *Pediatrics* 1988;81:904–907. **Nelson:** *Pocketbook of Pediatric Antimicrobial Therapy,* 1995, p. 16.

Kayexalate—See Sodium Polystyrene Sulfonate

Levothyroxine Sodium (Levothroid, Synthroid, T4)
Indications: Replacement or supplementary therapy for hypothyroidism.

Use L-thyroxine	Dose/route/frequency	Clinical considerations
	Initial PO dose: 10–15 mcg/kg/day q24h; adjust in 12.5 mcg increments every 2 weeks until T4 is 10–15 µg/dl and TSH is	PO route preferred: Use IV when PO route unavailable or with myxedema stupor/coma.

<15 μU/ml; usual final dose for term infant is 37.5 to 50 mcg/day	
Initial IV dose: 5–10 mcg/μg/day, q24h increased every 2 weeks by 5–10 mcg as in PO treatment.	PO tablets 25–300 mcg/tablets
Usually have switched to PO after the first week	Don't use IM
IV dose: 75% of PO dose/day	Read package insert with IV preparations

Contraindications: Thyrotoxicosis and uncorrected adrenal insufficiency. **Precautions:** Use with caution in infants receiving anticoagulants. In infants with cardiac disease, begin with 1/4 of usual maintenance dose and increase weekly (100 μg levothyroxine = 65 mg thyroid USP). To avoid differences in bioavailability, use the same brand of thyroid hormone. **Monitoring:** Adjust dosage based on clinical status and serum T_4 and TSH. Obtain serum T_4, free T_4 index, and TSH, 12–24 h after last dose of T_4. Adjust T_4 dose during the first few months to keep free T_4 index in 10–14 mcg/dl range. Adequate therapy should suppress TSH values to <15 μU/ml within 3–4 months of starting therapy. Closely assess for signs of hypothyroidism: lethargy, poor feeding, constipation, intermittent cyanosis, and prolonged neonatal jaundice. Also closely assess for signs of thyrotoxicosis: hyperreactivity, tachycardia, tachypnea, fever, exophthalmos, and goiter. Periodically assess growth and bone-age development. **Adverse Reactions:** Hyperthyroidism, rash, weight loss, diarrhea, tachycardia, cardiac arrhythmias, tremors, fever, and hair loss. Prolonged overtreatment can produce premature craniosynostosis and acceleration of bone age.
Johnson: *The Harriet Lane Handbook,* 1993, p. 468. **Fisher:** *Pediatrics* 1989;83:785–789. **Germak JA:** *J Pediatr* 1990;83:785. **Young TE:** *Neofax '97,* p. 196. (See Chap. 2)

Lidocaine Hydrochloride (Xylocaine)
Dosage/Dosage Interval (administer IV push slowly, undiluted, as a bolus dose over 5 min; continuous infusions diluted to 2 mg/ml in D5W)

Indications	Dosage/route/frequency
Ventricular arrhythmias See Chap. 25	IV bolus: 0.5–2 mg/kg/dose IV (over 5 min), repeat q10 min for 3 doses to a maximum of 5 mg/kg; maintenance infusion: 10–50 μg/kg/min. Refer to dobutamine calculations to determine number of milligrams of lidocaine to add to 100 ml of IV solution
Local injection See Chap. 37	Injection: Max. dose: 4 mg/kg/dose without epinephrine q2h.

Contraindications: Severe degrees of S-A, A-V, or intraventricular heart block (without a pacemaker). **Precautions:** Keep infusion rate below 1 mg/kg/h (20 mcg/kg/min) due to reduced drug clearance in neonates with hepatic disease, renal disease, heart failure, and hypovolemia or shock. Also use caution in neonates with hypoxemia, severe respiratory failure, incomplete heart block or bradycardia, and atrial fibrillation. **Monitoring:** Prolonged infusion (≥24 h) may result in toxic accumulation of lidocaine. **Therapeutic levels:** 1.5–5.0 μg/L. Bradycardia or QRS widening >0.2 s suggests toxicity and occurs with levels >7 μg/L. **Drug Interactions:** Concomitant cimetidine or propranolol administration may result in increased serum lidocaine concentrations with resultant toxicity. **Adverse Reactions:** Early signs of CNS toxicity include drowsiness, agitation, vomiting, and muscle twitching. Late signs include respiratory depression, apnea, loss of consciousness, and seizures. Cardiac toxicity is manifested by hypotension, asystole, bradycardia, heart block, arrhythmias, and cardiovascular collapse. **Johnson:** *The Harriet Lane Handbook,* 1993, p. 469. **AHA:** *JAMA* 1992;268:2262. (See Chap. 25)

Lorazepam (Ativan)
Dosage (mg/kg/dose)/Dosage Interval: PO, IM, IV

Indications	Dosage (mg/kg/dose)/route/frequency
Status epilepticus refractory to conventional therapy	Initial dose: 0.05–0.1, IV over 2–3 min, repeat in 10–15 min. if necessary. Max. dose: 4 mg/dose. Maintenance dose: 0.05, q6–24h depending on response. Use the injectable form for PR doses. Max. dose: 4 mg, q6h
Anxiety and sedation	0.05–0.1 (over 2 min), IM, IV, PO, administer 2 h before procedure, q4–8h PRN

Contraindications: Preexisting CNS depression or severe hypotension. **Precautions:** Stereotypic movements observed in several premature infants treated with IV lorazepam. Some preparations contain 2% benzyl alcohol and may be hazardous to neonates in high doses. Dilute prior to IV use with equal volume of compatible diluent normal saline or sterile water (to minimize benzyl alcohol content). Use with caution in infants with renal or hepatic impairment or myasthenia gravis. **Monitoring:** Monitor respiratory status closely during and after administration of lorazepam. Therapeutic range is 50–240 ng/ml. **Adverse Reactions:** CNS depression, bradycardia, circulatory collapse, constipation, urinary retention, respiratory depression, blood pressure instability, and GI symptoms. Discontinue therapy if syncope and paradoxic CNS stimulation occur. Overdose treated with flumazenil (Romazicon) 5–10 mg/kg/dose IV. **Johnson:** *The Harriet Lane Handbook,* 1993, pp. 471–472. **Cronin MG:** *Pediatrics* 1992;89:1129–1130. **Gomella:** *Neonatology,* 1994, p. 492. (See Chap. 27)

Magnesium Sulfate
Indications: Treatment and prevention of hypomagnesemia; treatment of refractory hypocalcemia. Supplied as injectable 100 mg (0.8 mEq/ml), 125 mg (1.0 mEq/ml), 250 mg (2.0 mEq/ml), 500 mg (4.0 mEq/ml).
Dosage/Dosage Interval

Indications	Dosage/route/frequency
Hypomagnesemia or hypocalcemia acute treatment	IM, IV (final concentration of 10 mg/ml (1%) infused over 10 min): (mEq/kg/dose) 0.2 mEq q6h until serum Mg level normal-

| | ized or symptoms resolved or 0.8–1.6, PO, q6h |
| maintenance therapy | 0.25–0.5 mEq/kg/24h IV (add to 24 h maintenance IV infusion), or 30–60 mg/kg/24 h. Repeat PRN until Mg level normalized |

Contraindications: Parenteral administration contraindicated in heart block or myocardial damage and serious renal impairment. **Precautions:** Renal insufficiency or digoxin therapy. **Drug Interactions:** CNS depressants, neuromuscular blocking agents, and digoxin. **Monitoring:** Blood pressure, serum Ca, Mg, and PO_4 levels, and knee-jerk reflex (decrease or stop administration and check serum Mg level if decreased knee-jerk reflex becomes evident). **Adverse Reactions:** Hypotension, respiratory depression, and hypermagnesemia. Magnesium intoxication associated with circulatory collapse, CNS depression, and respiratory paralysis. Antidote is IV calcium gluconate.
Johnson: *The Harriet Lane Handbook,* 1993, p. 473. **Gomella:** *Neonatology,* 1994, p. 492.

Methadone
Indications: Treatment of neonatal opiate withdrawal. **Dosage/Dosage Interval:** Initial dose: 0.05–0.2 mg/kg/dose, PO or slow IV push, q12–24h. Titrate dose based on neonatal abstinence score. Wean dose by 10–20% per week over 4–6 week period. PO solution prepared by diluting 1 ml of 10 mg/ml concentration solution with 19 ml of sterile water to yield a final concentration of 0.5 mg/ml. **Monitoring:** Closely monitor respiratory and cardiac status. **Drug Interactions:** Methadone metabolism accelerated by rifampin and phenytoin and this may precipitate withdrawal symptoms. **Adverse Reactions:** Respiratory depression, ileus, and delayed gastric emptying.
Young TE: *Neofax '97,* p. 164. **Tobias JD:** *Crit Care Med* 1990;18:1292. (See Chap. 19)

Methicillin (Staphcillin)
Classification: Penicillinase-resistant penicillin. **Indications:** Mechanism of action the same as other beta-lactam antibiotics. Active against both penicillinase-positive and penicillinase-negative staphylococci, with no activity against enterococci. Less effective than penicillin G against other gram-positive cocci. **Dosage (mg/kg/dose)/Dosage Interval: IM, IV:** final concentration of 20 mg/ml infused at 200 mg/min.
Meningitis

Weight <1200 g		Weight 1200–2000 g		Weight >2000 g	
PNA ≤4 wk	PNA ≥4 wk	PNA ≤7 days	PNA >7 days	PNA ≤7 days	PNA >7 days
50 q12h	50 q12h	50 q12h	50 q8h	50 q8h	50 q6h

Nonmeningitic infections

Weight <1200 g		Weight 1200–2000 g		Weight >2000 g	
PNA ≤4 wk	PNA ≥4 wk	PNA ≤7 days	PNA >7 days	PNA ≤7 days	PNA >7 days
25 q12h	25 q12h	25 q12h	25 q8h	25 q8h	25 q6h

PNA = postnatal age

Clinical Considerations: Low protein binding suggests potential advantage in neonates with hyperbilirubinemia. In cases of methicillin resistance, vancomycin is the antistaphylococcal drug of choice. **Monitoring:** CBC, renal function tests, and urinalysis. **Precautions:** Dosage adjustment for renal impairment. **Drug Interactions:** Blunting of peak aminoglycoside concentration when administered simultaneously with methicillin. **Adverse Reactions:** Interstitial nephritis occurs more often with methicillin than with other penicillins and is associated with hematuria, albuminuria, and casts in the urine. Bone marrow depression, eosinophilia, hypersensitivity reactions, anemia, leukopenia, thrombocytopenia, and hemorrhagic cystitis in poorly hydrated neonates. Extravasation treated with hyaluronidase.
Nelson: *Pocketbook of Pediatric Antimicrobial Therapy,* 1995, p. 17. **Prober:** *Pediatr Inf Dis J* 1990;9:111.

Methylene Blue
Indications: Treatment of methemoglobinemia.
Dosage/Dosage Interval: Methemoglobinemia: 0.1–0.2 mg/kg/dose of 1% solution IV over 5 min (inject slowly to prevent high local concentrations of methylene blue and additional production of methemoglobin). Repeat in 1 h if needed. **Contraindications:** Renal insufficiency and G6PD deficiency. **Warnings:** Do not administer either intramuscularly or intrathecally. Methylene blue is a reducing agent and may decrease hemoglobin oxygen-carrying capacity. **Adverse Reactions:** Vomiting, hypertension, and diaphoresis. Blue-green discoloration of urine and feces frequently occurs.
Tauesch: *Schaffer and Avery's Diseases of the Newborn* 1991, p. 1052. **Johnson:** *The Harriet Lane Handbook,* 1993, p. 479.

Metoclopramide (Reglan, Clopra, Maloxon)
Indications: Improve gastric emptying and GI motility. **GI dysmotility:** 0.03–0.5 mg/kg/day divided q6h PO, IM, IV (IV administered over 10–15 min); administered 30 min before meals and at bedtime. **Maximum dose:** 0.5 mg/kg/day. **Contraindications:** GI obstruction, pheochromocytoma, history of seizure disorder. **Drug Interactions:** Anticholinergic agents and opiate analgesics. **Monitoring:** Measure gastric residuals. **Adverse Reactions:** Drowsiness, restlessness, agitation, diarrhea, methemoglobinemia, and extrapyramidal symptoms (usually occur following IV administration of large doses and within 24–48 h of starting therapy; respond rapidly to Benadryl and subside within 24 h after stopping metoclopramide). **Overdose:** Associated with doses >1 mg/kg/day, characterized by drowsiness, ataxia, extrapyramidal reactions, seizures, and methemoglobinemia (treat with methylene blue). IV given as 0.1 mg/ml, PO available as 1 mg/ml and 10 mg/ml.
Johnson: *The Harriet Lane Handbook,* 1993, p. 480. **Reed:** *Semin Perinatol* 1992;16:21–31.

Metronidazole (Flagyl, Protostat, Metric)
Indications: Treatment of intraabdominal infections, ventriculitis, meningitis, and endocarditis caused by penicillin-resistant anaerobes.

Dosage (mg/kg/dose)/Dosage Interval (final concentration of 5 mg/ml infused over 1 h): IV, PO

Weight <1200 g		Weight 1200–2000 g		Weight >2000 g	
PNA ≤4 wk	PNA ≥4 wk	PNA ≤7 days	PNA >7 days	PNA ≤7 days	PNA >7 days
7.5 q48h	7.5 q36h	7.5 q24h	7.5 q12h	7.5 q12h	15 q12h

PNA = postnatal age

Precautions: Blood dyscrasias, liver disease, or renal disease (GFR <10 ml/min). **Drug Interactions:** Potentiates anticoagulant effect of warfarin anticoagulants. **Test Interactions:** Falsely decreased AST and SGPT levels. **Clinical Considerations:** Reddish brown urine discoloration frequently occurs following initiation of metronidazole therapy. **Monitoring:** During therapy for CNS infections. Obtain CSF trough levels and maintain at a level greater than the minimum inhibitory concentration. **Adverse Reactions:** Diarrhea, thrombocytopenia, leukopenia, seizures, vomiting, and urticaria.
Nelson: *Pocketbook of Pediatric Antimicrobial Therapy,* 1995, p. 17. **Johnson:** *The Harriet Lane Handbook,* 1993, p. 481. **Young TE:** *Neofax '97,* p. 36.

Mezlocillin (Mezlin)
Classification: Semisynthetic extended-spectrum penicillin. **Indications:** Principally active against gram-negative organisms, and also active against many anaerobes.
Dosage (mg/kg/dose)/Dosage Interval: IM, IV (final concentration of 20–40 mg/ml administered over 30 min)

Weight <1200 g		Weight 1200–2000 g		Weight >2000 g	
PNA ≤4 wk	PNA ≥4 wk	PNA ≤7 days	PNA >7 days	PNA ≤7 days	PNA >7 days
75 q12h	75 q8h	75 q12h	75 q8h	75 q12h	75 q8h

PNA = postnatal age

Precautions: Dosage modification for impaired renal function. **Monitoring:** CBC, renal and liver function tests. Desired serum concentrations with IV administration are peak 150 mcg/ml and trough 15–50 mcg/ml. **Drug Interactions:** Aminoglycosides (blunting of peak aminoglycoside concentration when administered simultaneously with mezlocillin), probenecid, and vecuronium. **Adverse Reactions:** Eosinophilia, serum-sickness-like reaction, positive direct Coombs' test, hemolytic anemia, neutropenia, prolonged bleeding time, interstitial nephritis, hypokalemia, seizures, thrombocytopenia, and elevated BUN, creatinine, and liver enzymes. **Overdosage:** Characterized by neuromuscular hypersensitivity and seizures.
Nelson: *Pocketbook of Pediatric Antimicrobial Therapy,* 1995, p. 17. **Prober:** *Pediatr Infect Dis J* 1990;9:111.

Midazolam (Versed)
Indications: Preoperative sedation; conscious sedation during mechanical ventilation. **Dosage/Dosage Interval: Preoperative sedation:** 0.07–0.2 mg/kg/dose IM, IV, or 0.3 mg/kg/dose PR. Final concentration of ≤0.5 mg/ml infused over 2–5 min q2–4h PRN. **Continuous IV infusion:** 0.2 mg/kg bolus, continuous IV, 0.4–0.6 mcg/kg/min. The presence of 1% ben-

zyl alcohol preservative necessitates caution with prolonged continuous IV infusions. **Contraindications:** Preexisting CNS depression or shock. **Precautions:** Congestive heart failure and renal impairment. Contains 1% benzyl alcohol (minimize neonate exposure by diluting the 5 mg/ml concentration to 0.5 mg/ml). **Monitoring:** Respiratory status, heart rate, and blood pressure. **Drug Interactions:** CNS depressants, anesthetic agents, cimetidine, and theophylline. Decrease dose by 25% during concurrent narcotic administration. **Adverse Reactions:** Sedation, respiratory depression, apnea, cardiac arrest, hypotension, bradycardia, and seizures (following rapid bolus administration and in neonates with underlying CNS disorders). Encephalopathy reported in several infants sedated for 4 to 11 days with midazolam and fentanyl. Encephalopathy symptoms include poor social interaction, decreased visual attentiveness, dystonic postures, and choreoathetosis. **Silvasi:** *Anesth Analg* 1988;67:286–288. **Bergman:** *J Pediatr* 1991;119:644–649. **Johnson:** *The Harriet Lane Handbook,* 1993, p. 484.

Morphine Sulfate
Indications: Analgesia, sedation, supplement to anesthesia, treatment of tetralogy of Fallot hypercyanotic spells, and opiate withdrawal.
Dosage/Dosage Interval

Indications	Dosage (mg/kg/dose)/route/frequency
Analgesia/tetralogy of Fallot (cyanotic) spells	0.05–0.2, IM, slow IV, SC, q2–4h, PRN Continuous IV: 0.025–0.05 mg/kg/h, start with lower dose and titrate to effect. Max. dose: 20 μg/kg/h; PO: 0.5, q6h; IM/IV dose is equivalent to 6 times the PO dose
Opiate withdrawal See Chap. 19	0.08–0.2 mg/dose q3–4h, using 0.4 mg/ml solution using either a concentrated oral morphine solution or deodorized tincture of opium

Contraindications: Severe respiratory depression and severe liver or renal insufficiency. **Clinical Considerations:** Neonates may require higher doses due to decreased amounts of active metabolites. Naloxone should be readily available to reverse CNS and respiratory depression. **Monitoring:** Urine output; respiratory and cardiovascular status. Examine neonate frequently for loss of bowel sounds, and abdominal or bladder distention. **Drug Interactions:** Morphine potentiation with CNS depressants and antagonism with phenothiazines. **Adverse Reactions:** CNS and respiratory depression, hypotension, seizures, bradycardia, histamine release, increased intracranial pressure, miosis, biliary or urinary tract spasm, antidiuretic hormone release, and physical dependence. **Rudolph:** *Rudolph's Pediatrics,* 1991, p. 1989. **Johnson:** *The Harriet Lane Handbook,* 1993, p. 485.

Mupirocin (Bactroban, Pseudomonic Acid A)
Indications: Topical antibiotic. **Dosage/Dosage Interval:** Apply to affected area q8h for 3–5 days. **Warnings:** Absorption of potentially toxic amounts of polyethylene glycol in very-low-birth-weight neonates with immature epidermal-dermal layers or in neonates with disrupted skin barriers. **Pre-**

cautions: Impaired renal function. **Adverse Reactions:** Minor local burning, stinging, pruritis, rash, erythema, tenderness, and swelling. **Johnson:** *The Harriet Lane Handbook,* 1993, p. 486. **Behrman:** *Nelson's Textbook of Pediatrics,* 1992, p. 1838.

Nafcillin (Unipen, Nafcil, Nalipen)
Classification: Semisynthetic penicillinase-resistant penicillin.
Indications: Primarily active against staphylococci, spectrum identical to that of methicillin. Reserve for penicillin-resistant *S. aureus* infections.
Dosage (mg/kg/dose)/Dosage Interval: IV (final concentration of 25 mg/ml infused over 30 min)

Weight <1200 g		Weight 1200–2000 g		Weight >2000 g	
PNA ≤4 wk	PNA >4 wk	PNA ≤7 days	PNA >7 days	PNA ≤7 days	PNA >7 days
25 q12h	25 q8h	25 q12h	25 q8h	25 q8h	25 q6h

PNA = postnatal age

Precautions: Dosing interval increased with hepatic dysfunction. Oral route not recommended due to poor absorption. Avoid IM administration if possible. **Monitoring:** CBC, BUN, creatinine, and liver function tests. Observe for hematuria and proteinuria. **Clinical Considerations:** Better CSF penetration than methicillin. Methicillin is the preferred anti-staphylococcal agent in the newborn because lower protein binding offers a potential advantage in neonates with hyperbilirubinemia. **Drug Interactions:** Blunting of peak aminoglycoside concentration when administered simultaneously with nafcillin. **Adverse Reactions:** Agranulocytosis hypersensitivity, granulocytopenia, and nephrotoxicity (eosinophilia may precede renal damage). Treat extravasation with hyaluronidase.
Nelson: *Pocketbook of Pediatric Antimicrobial Therapy,* 1995, p. 17. **Prober:** *Pediatr Infect Dis J* 1990;9:111. **Johnson:** *The Harriet Lane Handbook,* 1993, p. 486.

Naloxone (Narcan)
Indications: Treatment of narcotic induced respiratory depression. **Dosage and Administration:** 0.1–0.2 mg/kg/dose IV push (over 30 s), ETT, or IM. IV and ET preferred. Repeat as necessary q3–5 min. **Continuous IV infusion:** Dilute to final concentration of 0.4 mg/ml. Do not mix in alkaline solution. After titrating initial doses for effectiveness, add 75–100% of last effective dose to 1 h of maintenance IV fluids to run over 1 h. Wean in 50% increments over the next 6–12 h. Weaning period >48 h frequently required for methadone. If symptoms recur, rebolus and resume 100% of last effective dose. **Precautions:** The 0.04 mg/ml concentration is the recommended dosage strength. May precipitate withdrawal symptoms (vomiting, diaphoresis, seizures, tachycardia, hypertension, and tremulousness) in neonates addicted to opiates. Because duration of action of some narcotics may exceed that of naloxone, keep neonates under continued surveillance and administer repeated doses of naloxone as needed. **Adverse Reactions:** Vomiting, sweating, hypotension, tachycardia, ventricular arrhythmias, cardiac arrest, and seizures. Does not cause respiratory depression.
Johnson: *The Harriet Lane Handbook,* 1993, p. 487. **Bloom:** *Textbook of Neonatal Resuscitation,* 1994, pp. 6–25. (See Chap. 19)

Neostigmine Methylsulfate (Prostigmin)

Indications: Diagnosis and treatment of neonatal transient and persistent (congenital) myasthenia gravis; reversal of effects of nondepolarizing neuromuscular blocking agents after surgery.

Dosage (mg/kg/dose)/Dosage Interval

Indications	Dosage/route/frequency
Myasthenia gravis [transient and persistent (congenital)] diagnosis	IM, SC: 0.05–1.0, 30 min AC; or 0.02, IV × 1. PO: 1 mg, administered 2 h AC. Edrophonium is the preferred agent for myasthenia gravis diagnosis.
Myasthenia gravis: treatment	IM, IV, SC: 0.01–0.04, q2–3h PRN; PO: 2 mg/kg/day, divided q3–4h
Reversal of nondepolarizing neuromuscular blockade	0.02–0.08, IV, in conjunction with atropine (0.01–0.04 mg/kg); do not attempt reversal for at least 30 min after last dose of neuromuscular blocking agent

Contraindications: GU or GI obstruction, bradycardia, or hypotension. **Precautions:** Adjust dose for renal impairment. Epilepsy, reactive airways disease, bradycardia, hyperthyroidism, cardiac arrhythmias, or peptic ulcer disease. **Monitoring:** Respiratory and cardiovascular status. **Adverse Reactions:** Cholinergic crisis, seizures, tremor, fasciculations, bronchoconstriction, bradycardia, hypotension, bradyarrhythmias, asystole, hyperperistalsis, and vomiting. **Antidote:** Atropine 0.01–0.04 mg/kg/ dose. **Rudolph:** *Rudolph's Pediatrics,* 1991, p. 1990. **Johnson:** *The Harriet Lane Handbook,* 1993, p. 489. **Gomella:** *Neonatology,* 1994, pp. 496–497.

Nitroprusside Sodium (Nipride, Nitropress)

Indications: Severe hypertension and hypertensive crisis, pulmonary hypertension, and congenital heart disease. **Dosage and Administration:** 0.25–6 μg/kg/min (usual dose is ≤2 μg/kg/min). Double rate q15–20 min until desired effect, adverse effects (hypotension, tachycardia), or achieve maximum infusion rate of 6 μg/kg/min. Discontinue nitroprusside infusion if no beneficial effect occurs after 2–4 h of maximum recommended dose. If beneficial response occurs, reduce dose 15–25% every 6–12 h and continue until reaching 0.5 μg/kg/min; then discontinue infusion. **Contraindications:** Decreased cerebral perfusion, hypertension associated with arteriovenous shunt, or coarctation of the aorta. **Precautions:** Severe renal impairment, hepatic failure, or hypothyroidism. Administer by IV infusion pump and continuously monitor blood pressure. Although it is necessary to protect solution from light, it is not necessary to wrap administration set. **Monitoring:** Nitroprusside metabolism involves nonenzymatic conversion to cyanide, with further metabolism to thiocyanate. Monitor thiocyanate levels for prolonged infusions (>48 h), high-dose therapy (≥4 μg/kg/min), or impaired renal function. Therapeutic levels are <5 mg/dl, toxicity reported with plasma levels of approximately 5–10 mg/dl, and mortality reported with levels ≥20. Closely monitor acid-base status to detect acidosis associated with cyanide toxicity. **Adverse Reactions:** Thiocyanate toxicity causes hyperreflexia, seizures, and coma. Cyanide toxicity causes acidosis, increased mixed venous oxygen tension, tachycardia, altered mental status, coma, convulsions, and almond smell on breath. Other reported adverse reactions are profound hypotensive response, vomiting, restlessness, diaphoresis, thrombocytopenia, and thyroid suppression. **Antidote:** Treat thiocyanate toxicity with 20% sodium thiosulfate (10 mg/kg/min over 15 min). **Rasoulpour:** *Clin Perinatol* 1992;19:121–137. **Gomella:** *Neonatology,* 1994, p. 497. **Johnson:** *The Harriet Lane Handbook,* 1993, p. 492. **Young TE:** *Neofax '77,* p. 122.

Nystatin (Mycostatin, Nilstat)
Indications: Treatment of susceptible cutaneous, mucocutaneous, and oropharyngeal fungal infections caused by *Candida* species.
Dosage/Dosage Interval

Route	Age/administration/frequency
PO therapy (use 100,000 U/ml suspension)	Apply suspension with swab to each side of mouth q6h (after feedings). Preterm Infant: 0.5 ml (50,000 U). Term Infant: 1 ml (100,000 U)
Topical therapy	Apply ointment or cream q6h.

Continue PO therapy and topical application for 3 days beyond resolution of fungal infection. **Clinical Considerations:** Combination therapy for candidal perineal infections with oral and topical nystatin is possible because of nystatin's poor absorption in the GI tract and because the GI tract serves as the reservoir for fungi causing perineal infection. Eliminate factors contributing to fungal growth (wet, occlusive diapers, and the use of contaminated nipples). **Adverse Reactions:** Irritation, contact dermatitis, diarrhea, and vomiting.
Johnson: *The Harriet Lane Handbook,* 1993, p. 492. **Baley:** *Clin Perinatol* 1991;18:263.

Oxacillin Sodium (Bactocil, Prostaphin)
Indications: Treatment of infections caused by penicillinase-producing staphylococci.
Dosage (mg/kg/dose)/Dosage Interval (final concentration of 50 mg/ml administered over 30 min): Double doses for meningitis and severe systemic infections

Infants <1 wk of age		Infants ≥1 wk of age	
Birth weight		Birth weight	
≤2000 g	>2000 g	≤2000 g	>2000 g
25 q12h	25 q8h	25 q8h	25 q6h

Precautions: Methicillin is the preferred penicillinase-resistant agent in neonates because of less displacement of bilirubin from albumin. Avoid IM administration due to associated sterile abscess formation. **Monitoring:** CBC, BUN, creatinine, and urinalysis (observe for hematuria and/or proteinuria). **Drug Interactions:** Probenecid and aminoglycosides (blunting of peak aminoglycoside concentration when administered simultaneously with oxacillin). **Adverse Reactions:** Diarrhea, vomiting, interstitial nephritis (associated with eosinophilia, albuminuria, and hematuria), leukopenia, elevated AST, agranulocytosis, hepatotoxicity, and extravasation (consider hyaluronidase therapy). **AAP:** *Report of the Committee on Infectious Diseases,* 1997, p. 607. **Johnson:** *The Harriet Lane Handbook,* 1993, p. 494.

Pancuronium Bromide (Pavulon)
Indications: Skeletal muscle relaxation; increased pulmonary compliance during mechanical ventilation; facilitate endotracheal intubation. **Dosage/Dosage Interval: Initial:** 0.05–1.0 mg/kg/dose IV (administer undiluted over 5 min). May repeat twice q5–10 min PRN. **Maintenance:** 0.04–0.10 mg/kg/dose q1–4h PRN. **Continuous infusion:** 0.05–0.2 mg/kg/h. **Precautions:** Preexisting pulmonary, hepatic, or renal impairment. In neonates with myasthenia gravis, small doses of pancuronium may have profound effects. **Monitoring:** Continuous cardiac and blood pressure monitoring. Because sensation remains intact, administer concurrent sedation and analgesia as needed.
Factors Influencing Duration of Neuromuscular Blockade

Potentiation	Antagonism
Acidosis, hypothermia, neuromuscular disease, hepatic disease, renal failure, cardiovascular disease, aminoglycosides, succinylcholine, hypermagnesemia, and hypokalemia	Pyridostigmine, neostigmine, or edrophonium in conjunction with atropine, alkalosis, epinephrine, and hyperkalemia

Adverse Reactions: Tachycardia, hypertension, hypotension, excessive salivation, rashes, and bronchospasm. **Antidote:** Neostigmine 0.025 mg/kg IV (with atropine 0.02 mg/kg).
Fanaroff: *Neonatal-Perinatal Medicine,* 1992, p. 1428. **Johnson:** *The Harriet Lane Handbook,* 1993, p. 496.

Penicillin G Preparations, Aqueous: Potassium and Sodium
Indications: Treatment of neonatal meningitis and bacteremia, group B streptococcal infections, and congenital syphilis. **Dosage (U/kg/day)/ Dosage Interval: IM, IV:** Final concentration of 50,000 U/ml infused over 20–60 min.
Aqueous Penicillin G for IV treatment
Bacteremia: 25,000 to 50,000 u/μg/dose infused over 30 minutes
Meningitis: 75,000 to 100,000 u/μg/dose

Postconceptual age	Postnatal age	Dose interval in hours
<29 weeks	0–4 weeks	12
	>4 weeks	8
30–36 weeks	0–2 weeks	12
	>2 weeks	8
37–44 weeks	0–1 week	12
	>1 week	8
>45 weeks	all	6

Group B streptococcal infections: 200,000 μ/μg/d for Bacteremia
400,000 μ/μg/d for Meningitis
When treating bacteremia use the meningitis dose until meningitis is ruled out.

Monitoring: Serum potassium and sodium for renal failure and high-dose therapy. Weekly CBC, BUN, and creatinine. **Precautions:** Dosage adjustment for renal failure. **Drug Interactions:** Blunting of peak aminoglycoside serum concentration if administered simultaneously with penicillin G preparations. T1/2 = 30 minutes and may be prolonged with probenecid. **Test Interactions:** Positive direct Coombs' test. **Adverse Reactions:** Bone marrow suppression, granulocytopenia, anaphylaxis, hemolytic anemia, interstitial nephritis, Jarisch-Herxheimer reaction, change in bowel flora (candida superinfection and diarrhea) and CNS toxicity.
Nelson: *Pocketbook of Pediatric Antimicrobial Therapy,* 1995, p. 17. **Zenker:** *Pediatr Infect Dis J* 1991;10:516–522. **AAP/ACOG:** *Guidelines for Perinatal Care,* 1992, pp. 165–166. (See Chap. 23)

Penicillin G Benzathine (Permapen, Bicillin L-A)
Indications: Treatment of asymptomatic congenital syphilis.
Dosage/Dosage Interval (Rarely used)

Indications	Dosage/route/frequency
Congenital syphilis, asymptomatic See Chap. 23	50,000 U/kg/dose IM × 1 dose Max. dose: 2.4 million units
Prophylaxis for neonates exposed during group A streptococcal epidemic	50,000 U/kg/dose IM × 1 dose

Precautions: Do not administer IV. Dosage adjustment for renal failure. Contains 1.7 mEq sodium per million units, necessitating caution in neonates with congestive heart failure or hypernatremia. **Monitoring:** Weekly CBC, BUN, and creatinine. **Test Interactions:** Positive Coombs' reaction. **Adverse Reactions:** Jarisch-Herxheimer reaction, CNS toxicity (convulsion, drowsiness, myoclonus), hemolytic anemia, interstitial nephritis, and hypersensitivity reaction.
Nelson: *Pocketbook of Pediatric Antimicrobial Therapy,* 1995, p. 17. **AAP/ACOG:** *Guidelines for Perinatal Care,* 1992, pp. 165–166.

Penicillin G Procaine (Crystacillin, Wycillin)
Dosage/Dosage Interval

Indications	Dosage/route/frequency
Moderate to severe infections due to penicillin G-sensitive organisms; usually use IV penicillin G	50,000 U/kg/day IM q24h (IM route generally avoided in neonates due to sterile abscess formation, and possibility of procaine toxicity)
Symptomatic/asymptomatic congenital syphilis See Chap. 23	50,000 U/kg/day IM q24h × 10–14 days *or* penicillin G 50,000 U/kg/dose, IV; ≤7 days of age: q12h, >7 days of age: q8h

Precautions: Contains 120 mg procaine/300,000 U, which may cause allergic reaction, myocardial depression, and systemic vasodilation. **Drug Interactions:** Probenecid, tetracycline, and aminoglycosides (blunting of peak aminoglycoside concentration when administered simultaneously with procaine penicillin G). **Test Interactions:** Positive direct Coombs' test. **Adverse Reactions:** Sterile abscess at injection site, CNS stimulation, seizures, myocardial depression, vasodilation, conduction disturbances, pseudoanaphylactoid reactions, Jarisch-Herxheimer reaction, interstitial nephritis, myoclonus, and hemolytic anemia. **Nelson:** *Pocketbook of Pediatric Antimicrobial Therapy,* 1995, pp. 8, 17. **Prober:** *Pediatr Infect Dis J* 1990;90:111.

Pentobarbital Sodium
Indications: Sedative/hypnotic. **Dosage and Administration: Sedative:** IV push: 2–6 mg/kg slow IV push until asleep. **PO, PR, IM:** 2–6 mg/kg/day, divided q8h. **Hypnotic:** 3–5 mg/kg/dose. **Clinical Considerations:** Inject IV dose slowly in fractional doses. No advantage over phenobarbital for seizure control. May cause drug-related isoelectric EEG. **Contraindications:** Liver failure or latent porphyria. **Precautions:** Hypovolemic shock, congestive heart failure, hepatic and renal impairment. Pentobarbital has no analgesic effects, necessitating concurrent analgesia. Because tolerance and dependence occur with continued use, consider limiting pentobarbital therapy to less than 2 weeks. **Drug Interactions:** Chloramphenicol, cimetidine. Enhances metabolism of phenytoin, sodium valproate, and corticosteroids by microsomal enzyme induction. **Monitoring:** Blood pressure and respiratory status. **Therapeutic serum levels:** Sedation = 1–3 mg/L, hypnosis = 5–15 mg/L, coma = 20–40 mg/L. **Adverse Reactions:** Hypotension (associated with rapid administration), hypothermia, oliguria, cardiac arrhythmias, respiratory depression, CNS excitation or depression, and vomiting.
Taeusch: *Schaffer and Avery's Diseases of the Newborn,* 1991, p. 1052. **Johnson:** *The Harriet Lane Handbook,* 1993, p. 505.

Phenobarbital (Luminal)
Dosage/Dosage Interval

Indications	Dosage/route/frequency
Seizures: loading therapy (mg/kg/dose) See Chap. 27	20, IV over 10 min (<1 mg/kg/min). Administer additional doses of 5 mg/kg q5 min until cessation of seizures or a total dose of 40 mg/kg is administered. To achieve the blood level obtained with IV therapy, the IM dose must be 10–15% greater than the IV dose. Use the IV route if possible
Seizures: maintenance therapy (mg/kg/day) See Chap. 27	3–5, IV, IM, PO divided q12h. Begin maintenance therapy 12 h after loading dose. Parenteral dose preferred for seriously ill neonate. See above comments about necessary adjustments to IM dose
Cholestasis (See Chap. 18)	4–5 mg/kg/day, IV, IM, PO for 4–5 days.

Neonatal withdrawal syndrome (See Chap. 19) Administer loading dose then titrate based on abstinence score. Loading dose = 15–20 mg/kg/dose; closely follow blood levels, and after stabilization of abstinence symptoms for 24–48 h, decrease the daily dose to allow drug level reduction by 10–20% per day	Dosage (mg/kg/day) titrated based on abstinence score (AS): IM, IV, PO

AS	Dosage/frequency
8–10	6, divided q8h
11–13	8, divided q8h
14–16	10, divided q8h
>17	12, divided q8h

Clinical Considerations: Hyperbilirubinemia: More effective in reducing bilirubin levels in full-term infants than premature infants. **Neonatal withdrawal syndrome:** Phenobarbital will not resolve vomiting and diarrhea, and may aggravate poor sucking and feeding. If gastrointestinal symptoms are prominent, phenobarbital is not the appropriate drug. **Warnings:** Abrupt discontinuation in infants with epilepsy may precipitate status epilepticus. **Precautions:** Hepatic or renal impairment. **Monitoring:** Therapeutic serum concentration: 15–30 mcg/ml. Monitor respiratory status during administration and observe IV site for phlebitis and extravasation. **Drug Interactions:** Benzodiazepines, primidone, warfarin, corticosteroids, and doxycycline. Increased serum concentrations with concurrent phenytoin or valproate. **Adverse Reactions:** Respiratory depression (with serum concentrations >60 mcg/ml), hypotension, circulatory collapse, paradoxical excitement, megaloblastic anemia, hepatitis, and exfoliative dermatitis. Sedation reported at serum concentrations >40 mcg/ml. **Volpe:** *Neurology of the Newborn,* 1987, pp. 150–151. **Gomella:** *Neonatology,* 1994, p. 500. **Finnegan:** Neonatal Abstinence Syndrome. *Current Therapy in Neonatal-Perinatal Medicine,* 1990;2:318.

Phentolamine Mesylate (Regitine)
Dosage/Dosage Interval

Indications	Dosage/route/frequency
Vasoconstrictor extravasation Prevention	Add 10 mg phentolamine/liter of vasoconstrictor-containing solution; phentolamine will not alter the pressor effect(s) of these agents
Treatment	Phentolamine, 5 mg, diluted in 4 ml of 0.9% normal saline to concentration of 1 mg/ml. Using a 25- or 26-gauge needle, inject 0.2 ml at 5 sites around edge of infiltration. Best results if used within 30 min after extravasation occurrence; repeat if necessary
Pheochromocytoma diagnosis	0.01–0.02 mg/kg/dose, IV

Clinical Considerations: Topical 2% nitroglycerin ointment used for significantly swollen extremity. **Contraindications:** Renal impairment. **Precautions:** Gastritis or peptic ulcer. **Monitoring:** Assess affected area for reversal of ischemia. Closely monitor blood pressure, and heart rate/rhythm. **Adverse Reactions:** Hypotension, tachycardia, arrhythmias, nasal congestion, vomiting, diarrhea, and exacerbation of peptic ulcer. **Rudolph:** *Rudolph's Pediatrics,* 1991, p. 1193. **Fanaroff:** *Neonatal-Perinatal Medicine,* 1992, p. 1421.

Phenytoin (Dilantin)
Dosage and Administration: Precipitate formation can be reduced by employing the following precautions: (1) Use 0.9% NaCl infusion solution, (2) dilute to <6.7 mg/ml, (3) start infusion immediately after preparation, (4) infuse over 30 min, (5) use a 0.22 μm in-line filter, and (6) observe for precipitates. Even with these precautions, do not administer in central lines.

Indications	Dosage/route/frequency
Status epilepticus (mg/kg/dose) See Chap. 27	Load: 15–20, IV at rate ≤1 mg/kg/min. If possible divide the loading dose into 10 mg/kg increments, separated by approximately 20 min, to avoid excessive blood levels and disturbance of cardiac function. Maintenance: 4–8 mg/kg/day, PO, IV divided q12h. IM administration associated with erratic absorption and muscle necrosis
Antiarrhythmic digitalis-induced arrhythmias See Chap. 25 selected supraventricular and ventricular arrhythmias	Load: 10 mg/kg IV × 30–60 min Maintenance: 5–10 mg/kg/day IV divided q12h PO therapy: load: 10–15 mg/kg/day divided q6h. Maintenance: 5 mg/kg/day divided q12h

Contraindications: Heart block, sinus bradycardia. **Monitoring:** Therapeutic serum concentration: 10–20 mg/L (free + bound phenytoin), or 1–2 mg/L (free phenytoin only). Obtain trough level 48 h after loading dose. Closely monitor for bradycardia arrhythmias, and hypotension during infusion. Slow rate of infusion if heart rate decreases by >10 bpm. **Clinical Considerations:** Bilirubin displaces phenytoin from albumin-binding sites, increasing the percentage of unbound drug, and may result in elevated free-drug levels. **Drug Interactions: Increased phenytoin levels:** Cimetidine, chloramphenicol, INH, sulfonamides, and trimethoprim. **Decreased phenytoin levels:** Antineoplastic agents, and theophylline. Phenytoin induces hepatic microsomal enzymes leading to decreased effectiveness of drugs metabolized by this system. **Adverse Reactions:** Hypersensitivity reaction, arrhythmias, hypotension, lymphoid hyperplasia, hyperglycemia, cardiovascular collapse, liver damage, blood dyscrasias, dermatitis, Stevens-Johnson and a systemic lupus erythematosus-like syndrome. Extravasation may cause dermal necrosis and tissue sloughing (consider hyaluronidase therapy). Seizures reported with high serum concentrations.
Volpe: *Neurology of the Newborn,* 1995, pp. 150–151. **Fyler:** *Nadas' Pediatric Cardiology,* 1992, p. 762.

Piperacillin Sodium (Pipracil)
Classification: Semisynthetic extended-spectrum penicillin.
Indications: Good activity against *Pseudomonas aeruginosa.* Spectrum same as mezlocillin. Useful for neonates in whom sodium restriction is necessary and in neonates with bleeding problems in whom it would be desirable to minimize antibiotic-associated hemostatic impairment.

Dosage (mg/kg/day) and Dosage Interval: IM, IV (final concentration of 40 mg/ml infused over 30 min)

Postnatal age: ≤1 wk of age		Postnatal age: >1 wk of age	
Birth weight		Birth weight	
≤2000 g	>2000 g	≤2000 g	>2000 g
150 divided q12h	225 divided q8h	225 divided q8h	300 divided q6h

Avoid IM use where possible. Piperacillin reserved for ticarcillin-resistant organisms. **Precautions:** Dosage modification for impaired renal function. **Warnings:** Has the potential to cause neuromuscular hyperirritability or seizures. Limited experience in newborns. **Drug Interactions:** Aminoglycosides (blunting of peak aminoglycoside concentration when administered simultaneously with piperacillin), neuromuscular blocking agents, and probenecid). **Test Interactions:** False-positive urinary and serum proteins, positive direct Coombs' test. **Adverse Reactions:** Eosinophilia (usually precedes onset of piperacillin-induced renal injury), serum-sickness-like reaction, hemolytic anemia, neutropenia, prolonged bleeding time, interstitial nephritis, hypokalemia, seizures, hyperbilirubinemia, and extravasation (consider hyaluronidase therapy). Causes elevations in ALT, AST, BUN, and creatinine. **Overdose:** Neuromuscular hypersensitivity and seizures. Hemodialysis may be effective in drug removal from the circulation; treatment is otherwise supportive and symptom directed. **Gomella:** *Neonatology,* 1994, p. 502. **AAP:** *Report of the Committee on Infectious Diseases,* 1997, p. 151.

Poliovirus Vaccine, Inactivated (IPV)

Indications: Immunoprophylaxis against poliomyelitis for hospitalized infants and for infants with contraindications for OPV (immunodeficiency, HIV positive, or infants with immunodeficient contacts). We use only IPV in the neonatal period. **Dosage/Dosage Interval:** 0.5 ml injected subcutaneously in the midlateral thigh. Administer the first dose at 2 months of age (minimum 6 weeks), the second dose 4–8 weeks later; the third dose 6–12 months after second dose; and a fourth dose at age 4–6 years. Immunize premature infants according to postnatal age. When administering multiple vaccines, use a separate syringe for each and give at different sites. **Adverse Reactions:** Trace components may cause allergic reactions. Occasionally causes erythema and tenderness at injection site. **Committee on Infectious Diseases:** *Report of the Committee on Infectious Diseases (Red Book),* 24th ed., Elk Grove Village, Ill: American Academy of Pediatrics, 1997, p. 426. (See Chaps. 5, 6)

Potassium Chloride (KCl)

Indications: Maintenance potassium therapy, correct hypokalemia and hypochloremia. **Dosage/Dosage Interval: Acute symptomatic hypokalemia:** 0.5–1 mEq/kg, IV diluted in a 6–8 h volume of IV solution, and administered over 1 h. Reassess after initial replacement. **Maximum KCl concentrations:** peripheral vein = 40 mEq/L and central vein = 80 mEq/L. **Maintenance:** PO, IV: 2–4 mEq/kg/day diluted in 24-h maintenance IV solution or divided into feedings. **Contraindications:** Severe renal impairment, hyperkalemia, or severe tissue trauma. Do not administer liquid preparations to infants with esophageal compression or delayed gastric

emptying time. **Precautions:** Potassium-sparing diuretics. **Warnings:** Limit potassium supplements in infants with inadequate urine output. Use caution during concurrent use of potassium-sparing diuretics. **Monitoring:** Continuous ECG monitoring is mandatory during acute treatment of symptomatic hypokalemia with IV potassium (infants receiving >0.5 mEq/kg/h). Observe closely for signs of extravasation during IV therapy and for signs of GI intolerance during PO replacement therapy. Closely monitor serum potassium and urine output. **Adverse Reactions:** Excessive dose and/or rate may cause arrhythmias (peaked T waves, widened QRS flattened P waves, bradycardia, and heart block), respiratory paralysis, and hypotension. Thrombophlebitis reported with peripheral IV administration of concentrated potassium solutions. Consider hyaluronidase for treatment of extravasations. Manifestations of GI irritation include diarrhea, vomiting, and bleeding. Division of oral doses and administration with feedings will minimize GI irritation.
Rudolph: *Rudolph's Pediatrics,* 1991, p. 1994. **Johnson:** *The Harriet Lane Handbook,* 1993, p. 515. (See Chap. 9)

Procainamide Hydrochloride (Pronestyl)
Dosage/Dosage Interval

Indications	Dosage/route/frequency
Atrial and ventricular arrhythmias IV loading therapy	1.5–2 mg/kg/dose. Diluted to 10 mg/ml in dextrose solution, and infused over 10–30 min. Repeat as needed to max. Dose of 10–15 mg/kg
Maintenance therapy	Continuous IV: 20–60 µg/kg/min. IM: 20–30 mg/kg/day divided q4–6h; PO: 5–15 mg/kg/day, divided q3–6 h.

Precautions: Continuous ECG and blood pressure monitoring. **Contraindications:** Complete heart block; second- or third-degree heart block without pacemaker; "les torsades de pointes" ventricular tachycardia. **Warnings:** Prolonged administration may lead to the development of a positive antinuclear antibody test and may progress to a systemic lupus erythematosus (SLE)-like syndrome. To avoid a possible paradoxical increase in ventricular rate, do not use in atrial fibrillation or flutter until ventricular rate is adequately controlled. **Precautions:** Marked A-V conduction disturbances, bundle-branch block or severe digitalis toxicity, ventricular arrhythmias in infants with organic heart disease, renal or hepatic failure, myasthenia gravis, and supraventricular tachyarrhythmias (unless concurrent digitalis levels are sufficient to prevent a marked increase in ventricular rate). Be prepared for bradycardia and hypotension, and have phenylephrine available to treat hypotension. Quinidine is generally used for long-term therapy because it has less associated toxicity. **Monitoring:** Monitor blood pressure and ECG when using IV therapy. **Therapeutic levels:** 4–10 mg/L for procainamide (toxicity associated with levels >12 mg/L) or 10–30 mg/L for procainamide and NAPA levels combined (toxicity associated with levels >30 mg/L). **Adverse Reactions:** GI irritation, drug fever, agranulocytosis, tachycardia, arrhythmias, increased or decreased A-V block, SLE-like syndrome, hepatomegaly, positive Coombs' test, and thrombocytopenia. Serious toxic effects if given rapidly IV (asystole, myocardial depression, ventricular fibrillation, and hypotension). **Overdose** (widening of QRS interval by more than 0.02; or significant ventricular slowing): Hypotension, widening of QRS complex, junctional tachycardia, intraventricular conduction delay, oliguria, and lethargy. **Gomella:** *Neonatology,* 1994, p. 504. **AAP:** *Pediatrics* 1988;81:464. **Johnson:** *The Harriet Lane Handbook,* 1993, p. 520. (See Chap. 25)

Propranolol (Inderal)
Dosage/Dosage Interval

Indications	Dosage/route/frequency
Arrhythmias	IV: 0.01–0.1 mg/kg/dose IV push × 10 min (<1 mg/min). Max. dose: 1 mg/dose. PO: 0.5–4 mg/kg/day divided q6–8h (may increase to ≥1 mg/kg q6h as tolerated.
Hypertension	PO: Initial dose: 0.25–3.5 mg/kg/dose, PO q6–8h. May repeat q15 min. PRN. IV: Initial dose: 0.01–0.15 mg/kg/dose, q6–8h. Max. dose: 0.15 mg/kg/dose, q6–8h
Tetralogy of Fallot hypercyanotic ("Tet") spells	IV: 0.15–0.25 mg/kg/dose, slow IV, repeat q15 min PRN. PRN therapy: 1–2 mg/kg/dose, PO, q6h
Thyrotoxicosis See Chap. 2	2 mg/kg/day, PO, divided q6h

Contraindications: Uncompensated congestive heart failure, cardiogenic shock, bradycardia, heart block, hypoglycemia, and reactive airway disease. **Monitoring:** Continuous ECG monitoring during initial IV therapy. Closely monitor blood pressure, blood glucose, and changes in airway resistance during initiation of therapy and after dosage changes. **Therapeutic levels:** 30–100 ng/ml. **Precautions:** Dosage reduction for renal or hepatic failure. **Drug Interactions: Decreased propranolol activity:** Barbiturates, indomethacin, or rifampin. **Increased propranolol activity:** Cimetidine, hydralazine, chlorpromazine, or verapamil. Aluminum-containing compounds may reduce GI absorption of propranolol. **Adverse Reactions:** Hypoglycemia, hypotension, bronchospasm, heart block, impaired myocardial contractility, and lethargy. Abrupt cessation associated with withdrawal syndrome (tachycardia, agitation, diaphoresis). **Antidote:** Atropine. **Johnson:** *The Harriet Lane Handbook,* 1993, p. 522. **Fyler:** *Nadas' Pediatric Cardiology,* 1992, p. 763. **Rasoulpour:** *Clin Perinatol* 1992;19:121–137. **Karlowicz:** *Clin Perinatol* 1992;19:139–158. (See Chaps. 2, 25)

Prostaglandin E₁ (Alprostadil, PGE₁, Prostin VR)
Indications: Promote patency of the ductus arteriosus in infants with congenital heart lesions that are dependent on ductal patency for oxygenation or perfusion. **Dosage/Dosage Interval:** Continuous IV infusion into either a vein or umbilical artery catheter positioned near the ductus arteriosus opening. **Initial:** 0.05–0.4 μg/kg/min. Titrate dose based on infant's response (improved oxygenation versus adverse effects). **With therapeutic response:** Reduce rate to lowest effective dose (can be reduced to as little as 0.01 mg/kg/min). **With unsatisfactory response:** Gradually increase dose. Higher initial doses are usually no more effective and are associated

with a higher incidence of averse effects. **Usual maintenance dose:** 0.01–0.4 µg/kg/min. **Monitoring:** Closely monitor cardiovascular, respiratory, and oxygenation status. **Precautions:** Persons skilled in neonatal intubation/resuscitation should be immediately available during alprostadil administration. **Contraindications:** Coagulation abnormalities. **Adverse Reactions:** Apnea, bradycardia, hypotension, hypocalcemia, cardiac arrest, seizure-like activity, cutaneous flushing, decreased platelet function (DIC, hemorrhage). Gastric outlet obstruction and reversible long bone cortical proliferation (reported following administration of ≥120 h). **Fyler:** *Nadas' Pediatric Cardiology,* 1992, p. 767. **Peled:** *N Engl J Med* 1992;327:505–510. **Johnson:** *The Harriet Lane Handbook,* 1993, p. 525. (See Chap. 25) **Young TE:** *Neofax '97,* p. 120.

Protamine Sulfate

Indications: Treatment of heparin overdose. Neutralize heparin effect during surgery or dialysis procedures. **Dosage and Administration: Heparin antidote:** 1 mg will neutralize approximately 90 U (bovine origin) or 100 U (porcine origin) of heparin. For IV heparin therapy, protamine dose is based on amount of heparin received in the previous 2 h. <30 min since last dose: 1 mg/100 U IV; 30–60 min: 0.5–0.75 mg/100 U IV; >120 min: 0.25–0.375 mg/100 U IV. **Maximum rate:** <5 mg/min. **Monitoring:** Monitor vital signs, clotting functions, and blood pressure continuously during therapy. Observe closely for bleeding. **Adverse Reactions:** Hypotension, bradycardia, dyspnea, transitory flushing, pulmonary hypertension, hypersensitivity reactions. Heparin rebound has been occasionally reported. Protamine exerts an anticoagulant effect when given alone and when given in excessive doses beyond that needed to reverse heparin effect. **Johnson:** *The Harriet Lane Handbook,* 1993, p. 525. **Gomella:** *Neonatology,* 1994, p. 505.

Pyridoxine (Vitamin B6)

Indications: Prevention and treatment of pyridoxine deficiency, pyridoxine-dependent seizures, drug-induced neuritis, and sideroblastic anemia. **Dosage/Dosage Interval**

Indications	Dosage/route/frequency
Pyridoxine deficiency	Prevention: 100 µg/L of ingested formula. Treatment: 2–5 mg/day divided q6h for several weeks
Daily pyridoxine requirements (RDA)	Premature: 400 µg, PO. Full-term: 35 µg, PO. Human milk supplies 77 µg/day, which is adequate intake if maternal diet is pyridoxine supplemented. 1 ml PolyViSol & ViDaylin supplies 400 µg
Pyridoxine-dependent seizures See Chap. 27	50–100 mg IV over 1 min, or IM (with EEG monitoring), as a single test dose; followed by 30 min observation period. If response seen, begin maintenance dose of 50–100 mg, PO, qday
Sideroblastic anemia	200–600 mg/24 h for 1–2 mo

Monitoring: EEG monitoring recommended during initial therapy for pyridoxine-dependent seizures. **Precautions:** Risk of profound sedation and respiratory depression. Ventilatory support may be required. **Adverse Reactions:** Sedation, increased AST, decreased serum folic acid level, and allergic reaction. Seizures reported following IV administration of very large doses. **Gomella:** *Neonatology,* 1994, p. 505. **Johnson:** *The Harriet Lane Handbook,* 1993, p. 527. **Tsang:** *Nutrition During Infancy,* 1988, p. 239.

Quinidine (Atabrine, Mepacrine HCl)

Indications: Prevention and treatment of supraventricular and ventricular arrhythmias. **Dosage/Dosage Interval: IM, PO:** Test dose for idiosyncrasy: 2 mg/kg PO. **Therapeutic dose:** Total daily dose: 10–30 mg/kg. **PO:** 5–15 mg/kg/dose q6h. **IM:** 2–4 mg/kg/dose q2–4 h PRN. *IV administration not recommended.* **Clinical Considerations:** Quinidine gluconate (62% quinidine), quinidine sulfate (83% quinidine). Procainamide is the preferred parenteral, and quinidine is the preferred oral antiarrhythmic agent in neonates. **Contraindications:** Complete A-V nodal block, intraventricular conduction defects, and digitalis-induced A-V conduction disorders. **Precautions:** Myocardial depression, sick-sinus syndrome, incomplete A-V block, digitalis-induced intoxication, hepatic or renal insufficiency, myasthenia gravis, G6PD deficiency, and SLE syndrome.
Drug Interactions

Drug(s)	Drug interaction
Amiodarone, cimetidine	Increased quinidine effect
Barbiturates, phenytoin, rifampin	Decrease quinidine effect
Nondepolarizing and depolarizing muscle relaxants	Potentiated by quinidine
Digoxin	Concurrent quinidine therapy produces increased plasma digoxin concentrations; may require reduction in digoxin dosage by as much as 50% with initiation of quinidine therapy; closely monitor digoxin levels (5–7 days required for new steady-state digoxin plasma concentration)

Monitoring: Weekly CBC, liver and renal function tests. **Therapeutic quinidine level:** 2–5 μg/ml, toxic >7. **Adverse Reactions:** Quinidine-induced syncope has been reported, and its occurrence necessitates discontinuation of therapy. GI disturbances, hypotension, tachycardia, arrhythmias, blood dyscrasias, thrombotic thrombocytopenic purpura, and cardiac arrest. Idiosyncratic response (respiratory depression, ventricular tachycardia, vascular collapse, and angioedema) reported with low serum quinidine levels, especially when initiating therapy. Quinidine-induced hepatotoxicity (granulomatous hepatitis, increased AST and alkaline phosphatase, jaundice) is also reported. **Overdosage: Symptoms:** Lethargy, respiratory distress, apnea, severe hypotension, anuria, absence of P waves, ventricular arrhythmias, seizures, and widening of QRS complex (≥ 0.02 s), PR and QT intervals. **Management:** Initial therapy: Skip dose or stop quinidine. Other options include supportive therapy, cardiac pacing, urine acidification. Sodium lactate therapy is used to reduce cardiotoxic effects of quinidine.

Fyler: *Nadas' Pediatric Cardiology,* 1992, p. 761. **Johnson:** *The Harriet Lane Handbook,* 1993, p. 529. **Rudolph:** *Rudolph's Pediatrics,* 1991, p. 1997.

Ranitidine (Zantac)
Indications: Duodenal and gastric ulcers, gastroesophageal reflux, and hypersecretory conditions. **Dosage (mg/kg/dose)/Dosage Interval: PO:** 2–4, q8–12h. **IV: Dilution/administration rate: direct IV injection:** ≤2.5 mg/ml over 5 min. **Intermittent IV infusion:** ≤0.5 mg/ml over 20 min. IV = 0.1–0.8, q6h. **Continuous infusion (for gastric bleeding):** 0.6 mg/kg followed by 0.1 mg/kg/h. Titrate dose to a gastric pH >4. **Clinical Considerations:** Due to the absence of possible endocrine toxicity and drug interactions, ranitidine is the preferred H_2 receptor antagonist. Ranitidine effectively increases gastric pH. Increased gastric pH may promote the development of gastric colonization with pathogenic bacteria or yeast. **Precautions:** IV formulation contains 0.5% phenol; no short-term toxicity has been reported. Caution for liver impairment and dosage modification for renal impairment. **Drug Interactions:** May increase serum levels of theophylline, warfarin, and procainamide. **Monitoring:** Monitor gastric pH to assess ranitidine efficacy. **Test Interactions:** False-positive urine protein using Multistix. **Adverse Reactions:** GI disturbance, sedation, thrombocytopenia, hepatotoxicity, vomiting, and bradycardia or tachycardia.
Reed: *Semin Perinatol* 1992;16:21–31. **Fontana M:** *Arch Dis Child* 1993;68:602. **Johnson:** *The Harriet Lane Handbook,* 1993, p. 531. **Young TE:** *Neofax '97,* p. 204.

Rifampin (Rifadin, Rimactane)
Action: Effective against mycobacteria, Neisseria, and gram-positive cocci. Because resistance rapidly develops, rifampin should always be used as part of combined therapy for tuberculosis.
Dosage/Dosage Interval

Indications	Dosage/route/frequency
Management of active tuberculosis See Chap. 23	10–20 mg/kg/dose, PO, qday or twice weekly.
Meningitis prophylaxis: *H. influenzae* (mg/kg/day)	≤1 mo of age: 10 mg/kg/day, PO, qday × 4 days >1 mo of age: 20 mg/kg/day, PO, qday × 4 days Max. dose: 600 mg/day qday × 4 days
Meningitis prophylaxis: *N. meningitidis* (mg/kg/day)	≤1 mo of age: 10 mg/kg/day, divided q12h × 48 h >1 mo of age: 20 mg/kg/day divided q12h, PO × 48 h. Administer 1 h before or 2 h after meals. IV dose same as PO dose

Clinical Considerations: Because resistance develops rapidly, rifampin should always be used in combination with other agents for synergistic effect. Causes red discoloration of urine, saliva, and tears. **Precautions:** Liver impairment. **Drug Interactions:** Rifampin use associated with decreased serum concentrations of verapamil, methadone, corticosteroids, oral anticoagulants, ketoconazole, phenytoin, phenobarbital, theophylline, and digoxin. Close monitoring of serum concentrations is necessary. **Adverse Reactions:** Vomiting, diarrhea, pruritus, stomatitis, eosinophilia, hepatitis, blood dyscrasias, elevated BUN and uric acid, and renal failure.

Johnson: *The Harriet Lane Handbook,* 1993, p. 532. **Gomella:** *Neonatology,* 1994, p. 506.

Silver Nitrate, 1% Ophthalmic Solution

Indications: Prophylaxis against gonococcal ophthalmia. **Dosage/Dosage Interval:** Immediately after birth (for both vaginal and cesarean section-delivered infants) cleanse the child's eyes with a sterile-water soaked cotton pledget. Use a separate pledget for each eye and cleanse the unopened lids from the nose outwards. Separate the lids and instill two drops of 1% solution into each eye. Irrigation of the eyes following instillation of silver nitrate does not reduce chemical conjunctivitis and may reduce antibacterial effectiveness.

AAP: *Report 'of the Committee on Infectious Diseases,* 1997, p. 601. (See Chap. 23)

Sodium Bicarbonate

Indications: Treatment of metabolic acidosis, documented metabolic acidosis during prolonged CPR after establishment of effective ventilation and renal tubular acidosis. Adjunctive treatment of hyperkalemia.

Dosage and Administration (final concentration of 0.18 mEq/ml, infused at 1–2 mEq/kg/min)

Indications	Dosage/route/frequency
Cardiac arrest See Chap. 4	Initial dose: 1–2 mEq/ml; using 1:1 dilution of 1 mEq/ml $NaHCO_3$ or undiluted 0.5 mEq/ml $NaHCO_3$. Administer <1 mEq/min. May repeat with 0.5 mEq/kg q10 min or as indicated by acid-base status
Metabolic acidosis See Chaps. 9, 31	$NaHCO_3$ dose (mEq) = body weight (kg) × base deficit (mEq/L) × 0.35. Administer half of calculated dose IV (at <1 mEq/min) or PO, then reassess
Renal tubular acidosis See Chap. 31	Distal: 2–3 mEq/kg/day, PO, IV. Proximal: 5–10 mEq/kg/day, PO, IV

Contraindications: Alkalosis, hypocalcemia, inadequate ventilation during CPR. **Warnings:** Effective ventilation must precede and accompany the administration of sodium bicarbonate. Do not mix with calcium salts, catecholamines, or atropine. **Precautions:** Most studies failed to demonstrate that sodium bicarbonate administration improves the outcome of cardiac arrest. Treatment priorities for the infant in cardiac arrest include intubation, ventilation, and restoration of effective systemic perfusion. Sodium bicarbonate is used in the infant with prolonged cardiac arrest after effective ventilation is achieved and epinephrine and cardiac compressions have been instituted. Monitor acid/base status, oxygenation, ventilation, and electrolytes closely. **Monitoring:** Acid/base and ventilation status. **Adverse Reactions:** Metabolic alkalosis resulting from excessive sodium bicarbonate administration produces a leftward shift of the oxyhemoglobin dissociation curve with impaired tissue oxygen delivery, acute intracellular shifts of potassium, decreased plasma ionized calcium concentration, decreased fibrillation threshold, and impaired cardiac function. Other reported adverse reactions include hypernatremia, hypokalemia, hypocalcemia, edema, cerebral hemorrhage, intracranial acidosis, and tissue necrosis following extravasation (consider hyaluronidase treatment).

AHA: *JAMA* 1992;268:2262–2275. **Bloom:** *Textbook of Neonatal Resuscitation,* 1994, pp. 6–19.

Sodium Polystyrene Sulfonate (Kayexalate)
Indications: Treatment of hyperkalemia.
Dosage (g/kg/dose)/Dosage Interval: PO: 1, q6h. **PR** (in 20–25% sorbitol solution): 1, q2–6h. Cation exchange resin. Each gram of resin exchanges 1 mEq sodium for each mEq potassium removed. Calcium, magnesium, and other cations are also bound. **Clinical Considerations:** PR therapy reduces the serum potassium faster than PO therapy, but the PO route results in a greater overall reduction. PR dose is administered with 20–25% sorbitol to prevent intestinal obstruction; however, this concentration of sorbitol may be injurious to the intestinal mucosa of very-low-birth-weight infants. **Precautions:** Severe congestive heart failure, hypertension, renal failure, or edema. **Drug Interactions:** Concurrent administration with antacids or laxatives containing Mg or Al may result in systemic alkalosis. **Adverse Reactions:** Vomiting, constipation, intestinal necrosis, hypokalemia, hypocalcemia, hypernatremia, and hypomagnesemia. Large doses may cause fecal impaction.
Johnson: *The Harriet Lane Handbook,* 1993, p. 535. **Taeusch:** *Schaffer and Avery's Diseases of the Newborn,* 1991, p. 1053. (See Chap. 9)

Spironolactone (Aldactone)
Indications: Mild diuretic with potassium-sparing effects. Used in conjunction with thiazide diuretics in the treatment of congestive heart failure, hypertension, edema, and BPD when prolonged diuresis is desirable. More expensive/effective than potassium supplements. **Dosage and Administration:** 1–3 mg/kg/day PO divided q12h. Adjust dose for desired effect. **BPD therapy:** Hydrochlorothiazide: 2 mg/kg/dose q12h, PO, × 8 wk + spironolactone: 1.5 mg/kg/dose q12h PO, × 8 wk. **Contraindications:** Renal failure, anuria, hyperkalemia. **Monitoring:** Serum and urine potassium levels. **Drug Interactions:** May potentiate ganglionic blocking agents and other antihypertensive agents. **Adverse Reactions:** Hyperkalemia, vomiting, diarrhea, hyperchloremic metabolic acidosis, dehydration, and hyponatremia.
Taeusch: *Schaffer and Avery's Diseases of the Newborn,* 1991, p. 1053. **Johnson:** *The Harriet Lane Handbook,* 1993, p. 535. (See Chaps. 24, 25)

Streptokinase (Streptase, Kabikinase)
Indications: Treatment of thrombosis in major artery, vein, or shunt.
Dosage/Dosage Interval: Loading dose: 1500–2000 IU/kg/h (final concentration of 1000 IU/ml in D5W or D10W, infused over 30–60 min). **Maintenance:** 1000 IU/kg/h as continuous infusion × 24–72 h. Titrate to maintain thrombin time at 2–5 times normal and PT/PTT at 1.5–2 times normal. Usual duration of therapy is 4–5 days. At the end of streptokinase therapy, begin IV heparin therapy. **Contraindications:** Internal bleeding, recent spinal or intracranial surgery. **Warnings:** Avoid IM injections. **Drug Interactions:** Anticoagulants, antiplatelet agents. **Monitoring:** Before starting therapy, obtain baseline thrombin time, PT, PTT, hematocrit, and platelet count and continue to monitor these parameters q12h. **Adverse Reactions: Hemorrhage:** external, internal, and intracranial, flushing, hypersensitivity and anaphylactoid reactions, fever (common), hypotension, arrhythmias, and chills. **Antidote:** Aminocaproic acid (loading dose:

200 mg/kg IV, PO. **Maintenance dose:** 100 mg/kg/dose IV, PO q6h until hemorrhagic adverse reactions terminated. **Gomella:** *Neonatology,* 1994, p. 507. **Johnson:** *The Harriet Lane Handbook,* 1993, p. 536. (See Chap. 26)

Survanta (Beractant)

Indications: Prophylaxis: Infants with high risk for RDS, defined in clinical trials as a birth weight <1250 g, and larger infants with evidence of pulmonary immaturity. **Rescue Therapy:** Infants with moderate to severe RDS, defined in clinical trials as requirement for mechanical ventilation and FiO_2 above 40%. **Dosage/Dosage Interval:** Administered intratracheally by instillation into a 5 French end-hole catheter inserted into the infant's endotracheal tube with the tip of the catheter protruding just beyond the end of the endotracheal tube and above the infant's carina. **Prophylactic Therapy:** 4 ml/kg/dose intratracheally as soon as possible; up to four doses may be administered at intervals no shorter than q6 hours during the first 48 h of life. **Rescue Therapy:** 4 ml/kg/dose intratracheally immediately following the diagnosis of RDS. Each dose is divided in four 1 ml/kg aliquots; administer 1 ml/kg into each of four different positions (slight Trendelenburg with head turned to the right, then to the left; slight reverse Trendelenburg with head turned to the right, then to the left). **Monitoring:** Assess ET tube patency and correct anatomic location prior to administration of survanta. Monitor oxygen saturation and heart rate continuously during administration of doses. After administration of each dose monitor abg's frequently to detect and correct postdose abnormalities of ventilation and oxygenation. **Precautions:** A videotape demonstrating survanta administration procedure is available from Ross Laboratories and should be viewed prior to use of this product. **Adverse Reactions:** Transient bradycardia, hypoxemia, pallor, vasoconstriction, hypotension, endotracheal tube blockage, hypercapnia, apnea, and hypertension may occur during the administration process. **Ross Laboratories, Columbus, Ohio 43216, 1991.** (See Chap. 24)

Terbutaline Sulfate (Brethine, Bricanyl)

Indications: Acute bronchodilator therapy for BPD.
Dosage and Administration

Route	Dosage/frequency/comments
Nebulized aerosol	0.1 mg/kg in 2.5 ml normal saline q4–6h Injectable form used for inhalation.
Metered-dose inhaler (MDI)	2 Puffs with spacer device, q4–6h. Although intrapulmonary deposition is greater with MDI administration, consider the fact that the long-term hazards of chlorofluorocarbon exposure is unknown, and that a hypoxic condition may be created by the mixture of propellant and ventilator gases
Continuous IV infusion	Load: 2–5 mcg/kg Maintenance: 2–12 mcg/kg/h

Warnings: Paradoxical bronchoconstriction may occur with excessive use; if it occurs discontinue terbutaline immediately. Administration limited by tachycardia; decrease dose or discontinue administration if heart rate exceeds 180 bpm. **Drug Interactions:** Beta-receptor blocking agents block the action of terbutaline and other beta-agonist bronchodilators. **Adverse Reactions:** Tremor, tachycardia, arrhythmias, hypertension, and drowsiness. **Fanaroff:** *Neonatal-Perinatal Medicine,* 1992, p. 1426. **Johnson:** *The Harriet Lane Handbook,* 1993, p. 543.

Tetanus Immune Globulin, Human (Hyper-TET, TIG)

Indications: Prevention and/or treatment of tetanus neonatorum. **Dosage/Dosage Interval: IM:** 3000–6000 U × 1; optimal dosage not established for newborns. **Clinical Considerations:** Tetanus immune globulin is preferred over tetanus antitoxin for the prevention and/or treatment of tetanus neonatorum. The formulation in use in the United States is not licensed for intrathecal or intravenous use. **Taeusch:** *Schaffer and Avery's Diseases of the Newborn,* 1991, p. 1054. **AAP:** *Report of the Committee on Infectious Diseases,* 1991, p. 466.

Theophylline
Dosage/Dosage Interval: IV, PO

Indications	Dosage (mg/kg/dose)/route/frequency
Neonatal apnea: loading dose	4–6 mg/kg/dose, PO, for preterm and term infants or IV over 30 min
Neonatal apnea: maintenance dose (mg/kg/day)	Start 8–12h after loading dose 4–8 mg/kg/day PO-IV divided q8–12h; older infants may require 10–12 mg/kg/day; when switching from IV to PO, consider increasing the dose 20%
Ventilator weaning: (mg/kg/dose)	Load: 4–6 mg, IV. Maintenance: 2–4 mg, q12h, IV

Administer doses around the clock rather than on a qid, tid, or bid basis. **Contraindications:** Uncontrolled arrhythmias, hyperthyroidism. **Clinical Considerations:** Consider caffeine therapy for theophylline-resistant apnea of prematurity. Consider albuterol or terbutaline in preference to theophylline for initial therapy of infants with reactive airway disease. **Precautions:** Peptic ulcer, hypertension, and compromised cardiac function. Some elixir preparations may contain alcohol. **Drug Interactions: Increased theophylline elimination:** Carbamazepine, isoproterenol, phenytoin, phenobarbital, and rifampin. **Decreased theophylline elimination:** Erythromycin, quinolones, calcium channel blockers, nonselective beta-blockers, and cimetidine. **Monitoring:** Monitor heart rate and check blood glucose periodically during loading dose therapy. Assess for agitation and feeding intolerance. Withhold next dose if heart rate exceeds 180 bpm or gastric upset occurs. Monitor serum levels on day 4 of therapy, then 1–2 times weekly after maintenance therapy is established. Levels should be checked anytime toxicity is suspected or when apnea spells increase in frequency. If apnea is severe prior to the fourth day of therapy, a serum level should be drawn; if low, a partial bolus should be given: 0.8 mg/kg is given for each desired 2 mg/L increase in serum theophylline level. **Therapeutic ranges:** Apnea of prematurity: 5–15 mcg/ml; bronchospasm: 10–20 mcg/ml. **Adverse Reactions:** Vomiting, sinus tachycardia, hyperglycemia, diuresis, dehydration, feeding intolerance, CNS irritability, and gastroesophageal reflux. **Overdosage:** Tachycardia, vomiting, seizures, circulatory failure, failure to gain weight, hyperreflexia, and encephalopathy. **Theophylline toxicity treatment:** Activated charcoal, 1 g/kg slurry via gavage tube q2–4h. Sorbitol-containing preparations used for toxicity treatment may cause osmotic diarrhea and should be avoided. **Johnson:** *The Harriet Lane Handbook,* 1993, p. 545. **Gomella:** *Neonatology,* 1994, p. 509. (See Chap. 24)

Thiamine Hydrochloride (Vitamin B$_1$)
Indications: Treatment of thiamine deficiency.
Dosage/Dosage Interval

Indications	Dosage/route/frequency
Thiamine RDA	300 mcg/day for preterm and term infants
Thiamine deficiency: preventive dose	0.5–1.0 mg/day, PO
Thiamine deficiency: therapeutic dose	5–10 mg/day, divided q6–8h
	Therapeutic range: 1.6–4.0 mg/dl
Thiamine sources	1 ml of PolyViSol or ViDaylin supplies 500 mcg. Human milk supplies 56 μg/day

Drug Interactions: Thiamine requirements increased with high carbohydrate diets or high-concentration IV dextrose solutions. **Test Interactions:** False-positive uric acid and urobilinogen; large doses may interfere with spectrophotometric determination or serum theophylline. **Adverse Reactions:** Allergic reaction, angioedema, and cardiovascular collapse. Severity and frequency of adverse reactions increase with parenteral route of administration. **Tsang:** *Nutrition During Infancy,* 1988, pp. 241–242. **Johnson:** *The Harriet Lane Handbook,* 1993, p. 547.

Ticarcillin (Ticar)
Classification: Extended-spectrum, semisynthetic penicillin.
Indications: Good antipseudomonal activity. Action and spectrum similar to that of mezlocillin. Drug of choice when considering an extended spectrum penicillin.
Dosage (mg/kg/dose)/Dosage Interval: IM, IV (final concentration of 10–50 mg/ml infused over 30 min; avoid IM use if possible)

Weight <1200 g	Weight 1200–2000 g		Weight >2000 g	
Postnatal age (PNA) ≤4 wk or ≥4 wk	PNA ≤7 days	PNA >7 days	PNA ≤7 days	PNA >7 days
75 q12h	75 q12h	75 q8h	75 q8h	75 q6h

Meningitis: 0–7 days: 150–225 mg/kg/day divided q8–12h. 8–28 days: 225–300 mg/kg/day divided q6–8h. **Precautions:** Each gram of ticarcillin contains 5.2–6.5 mEq sodium, necessitating caution in neonates with congestive heart failure, edema, or renal failure. Ceftazidine is a suitable alternative. **Warnings:** Avoid concurrent aminoglycoside administration in the same administration setup. **Monitoring:** Serum sodium and potassium levels 2 or 3 times a week. **Adverse Reactions:** Decreased platelet aggregation, bleeding diathesis, hypernatremia, hypocalcemia, rash, and increased AST.

Prober: *Pediatr Infect Dis J* 1990;9:111. **Nelson:** *Pocketbook of Pediatric Antimicrobial Therapy,* 1995, p. 17.

Ticarcillin/Clavulanate (Timentin)
Indications: Antipseudomonal activity similar to ticarcillin with additional coverage of lactamase-producing species, particularly gram-positive cocci. **Dosage/Dosage Interval, Precautions, Warnings, Monitoring, and Adverse Reactions:** As per Ticarcillin. **Test Interactions:** May interfere with urine protein measurement.
Nelson: *Pocketbook of Pediatric Antimicrobial Therapy,* 1995, p. 17. **Prober:** *Pediatr Infect Dis J* 1990;9:111.

Tobramycin (Nebcin, Tobrex)
Indications: Treatment of documented or suspected *Pseudomonas aeruginosa* infection. Action and spectrum identical to that of gentamicin.
Dosage (mg/kg/dose)/Dosage Interval: IM, IV (final concentration of 2 mg/ml infused over 30 min). IM absorption variable in VLBW infant.

Weight ≤1200 g		Weight 1200–2000 g		Weight ≥2000 g	
PNA ≤4 wk	PNA ≥4 wk	PNA ≤7 days	PNA >7 days	PNA ≤7 days	PNA >7 days
2.5 q24h	2.5 q18h	2.5 q12–18h	2.5 q8–12h	2.5 q12h	2.5 q8h

PNA = postnatal age

Meningitis: 0–7 days: 4 mg/kg/day divided q12h; 8–28 days: 6 mg/kg/day divided q8h. **Ophthalmic: Drops:** 1–2 drops OU 2 to 6 times a day. **Ointment:** OU q3–4h until improvement occurs. Reduce treatment prior to discontinuance. **Precautions:** Dosage modification for impaired renal function. Optimal dosage based on serum concentrations, especially in low-birth-weight (<1.5 kg) infants. In very-low-birth-weight infants (<1 kg) once = daily dosing may be appropriate in the first week of life. Administer as a separate infusion from penicillin-containing solutions. **Drug Interactions:** Increased nephrotoxicity and ototoxicity when administered concurrently with other nephrotoxic and ototoxic drugs. Increased neuromuscular blockade when administered concurrently with neuromuscular blocking agents and in neonates with hypermagnesemia. **Monitoring:** Obtain drug levels around the third dose. Peak level is obtained 30 min after 30-min infusion or 1 h after IM injection and is kept at 4–8 µg/ml. The trough level is drawn 30 min before the next dose and is kept at 0.5–2 µg/ml. **Adverse Reactions:** Ototoxicity (related to drug dose and duration of treatment), nephrotoxicity (usually reversible), neuromuscular blockade, rash, myelotoxicity, and allergy.
Nelson: *Pocketbook of Pediatric Antimicrobial Therapy,* 1995, p. 17. **AAP:** *Report of the Committee on Infectious Diseases,* 1991, p. 551.

Tolazoline Hydrochloride (Priscoline) (Barely used)
Indications: Vasodilator used to decrease pulmonary vascular resistance in persistent pulmonary hypertension of the newborn. **Dosage and Administration:** Dissolve 50 mg/kg × wt (kg) in 50 ml D5W (ml/hr = mg/kg/h). **Pulmonary hypertension:** Administered via right arm vein or scalp vein. **Test dose:** 1–2 mg/kg IV over 10 min. Significant increase in postductal PaO$_2$ or saturation is considered a positive response and should

occur within 30 min after the test dose. **Constant infusion:** 0.2–2 mg/kg/hr IV. **Contraindications:** Renal failure, hypotension, shock, and intraventricular hemorrhage. **Warnings:** Stimulates gastric secretion and may activate stress ulcers. H_2-receptor blockers should not be used for tolazoline-induced gastric hemorrhage, due to possible concurrent antagonism of tolazoline-induced pulmonary vasodilation. **Drug Interactions:** See H_2-receptor blocker comments. Large doses of tolazoline administered concurrently with epinephrine or norepinephrine may cause paradoxical hypotension, followed by an exaggerated rebound hypertension. Should be treated with volume replacement, ephedrine, or dopamine, not epinephrine or norepinephrine (large doses of tolazoline may cause "epinephrine reversal," a further reduction in blood pressure, followed by an exaggerated rebound). **Monitoring:** Monitor blood pressure, renal status, and bone marrow status. Heme-test gastric aspirates to detect GI bleeding. **Adverse Reactions:** Agranulocytosis, pancytopenia, vomiting, diarrhea, hypertension or hypotension, tachycardia, arrhythmias, pulmonary hemorrhage, and GI bleeding. **Overdosage:** See drug interactions.
Johnson: *The Harriet Lane Handbook,* 1993, p. 550. **Gomella:** *Neonatology,* 1994, p. 511. (See Chap. 23)

Tromethamine (THAM)

Indications: Sodium-free organic buffer used to correct metabolic acidosis, primarily in neonates who have received maximum sodium bicarbonate therapy or who have hypercarbia or hypernatremia. **Dosage/Dosage Interval: Loading dose:** 3–16 ml/kg of undiluted solution (0.3M) infused over 5 min, or dose (ml) = wt (kg) × 1.1 × base deficit (mEq/L). Use 0.3 M solution for dosage calculations. **Maintenance:** 3 ml/kg/h undiluted solution (0.3M) or prepared as 10–50% solution in D5W as continuous infusion. Do not administer for longer than 24 h. **Contraindications:** Chronic respiratory acidosis, metabolic acidosis due to bicarbonate deficiency, anuria, or uremia. **Warnings:** Infusion into UAC should be avoided. **Precautions:** Reduce dosage and monitor pH carefully in renal impairment. **Monitoring:** Follow abg's closely to assess therapeutic efficacy and follow urine output. Closely monitor for respiratory depression, hypoglycemia, and hyperkalemia during large dose or rapid infusion therapy. **Adverse Reactions:** Hyperosmolality, hepatotoxicity, hyperkalemia, hypoglycemia, hypocalcemia, respiratory depression, apnea, thrombophlebitis, venospasm, and tissue irritation/necrosis with extravasation (inject 1% procaine [to which 75 U of hyaluronidase has been added]) into the affected area, and infuse 0.1 mg/kg of phentolamine mesylate into the vasospastic area). Hepatic necrosis reported with UVC administration of tromethamine.
Gomella: *Neonatology,* 1994, p. 512. **Fanaroff:** *Neonatal-Perinatal Medicine,* 1992, p. 318.

Urokinase (Abbokinase, Breokinase)

Indications: Management of vascular thromboses either spontaneous or catheter-associated. **Dosage/Dosage Interval: Aortic Thrombosis:** Visualization of thrombotic vessel a prerequisite. **Loading dose:** 4000 IU/kg IV over 20 min by constant infusion. Avoid shaking during reconstitution to minimize filament formation, and terminally filter through a 0.45-μm filter to remove filaments or precipitates. **Maintenance dose:** 4000–6000 IU/kg/h IV as a continuous infusion. **Occluded IV Catheter:** Aspiration method: Use 5000 IU/ml concentration. Instill 5000 IU into each lumen

over 1–2 min using a 1-ml tuberculin syringe, and gently aspirate with a 5-ml syringe every 5 min × 6. If the catheter remains occluded, leave in place for 1–4 h, then repeat aspiration procedure. May repeat with 10,000 IU into each lumen if 5000 IU fails to clear catheter. When patency is restored, aspirate 5 ml of blood-residual clot and discard. Gently irrigate with NS before resuming infusion of fluids. **Warnings:** If heparin has been given, it should be discontinued and urokinase therapy deferred until the thrombin time and PTT are less than twice normal values. **Contraindications:** Major abdominal, thoracic, or CNS surgery up to 10 days prior to the thromboembolic event, preexisting severe bleeding (intracranial, pulmonary, gastrointestinal), intracranial neoplasm, arteriovenous malformation, or aneurysm. **Monitoring:** Baseline thrombin time, PT, PTT, hematocrit, and platelet count before starting therapy, then every 12 h. Prolongation of thrombin time or PT or decreased plasminogen or fibrinogen levels are indicative of a fibrinolytic state but otherwise correlate poorly with therapeutic effects. **Adverse Reactions:** Allergic reactions, rash, fever, and bronchospasm. Discontinue administration if signs of bleeding occur.
Johnson: *The Harriet Lane Handbook,* 1993, p. 552. **Fanaroff:** *Neonatal-Perinatal Medicine,* 1992, p. 1424. (See Chap. 26)

Vancomycin Hydrochloride

Indications: Antibiotic of choice for serious infections caused by methicillin-resistant staphylococci and penicillin-resistant pneumococci. Oral therapy for colitis caused by *Clostridium difficile.*
Dosage (mg/kg/dose)/Dosage Interval: IV (final concentration of 5 mg/ml infused >1 h)

Weight <1200 g		Weight 1200–2000 g		Weight >2000 g	
PNA ≤4 wk	PNA ≥4 wk	PNA ≤7 days	PNA >7 days	PNA ≤7 days	PNA >7 days
15 q24h	15 q18–24h	15 q12–18h	15 q8–12h	15 q12h	15 q8h

PNA = postnatal age

Clostridium difficile colitis: **PO:** Dilute parenteral product with 10 ml of sterile water for injection to a concentration of 5 mg/ml and administer via a feeding tube. Dose is 40–50 mg/kg/day, divided q6h, × 5–7 days. Intraventricular therapy for shunt-related infections: 4–5 mg/kg/dose q48–72h, irrespective of concurrent systemic therapy. Obtain pre- and postdose CSF vancomycin levels: Trough CSF levels maintained <20 mcg/ml. **Clinical Considerations:** If staphylococci exhibit vancomycin tolerance, combine vancomycin and an aminoglycoside with or without rifampin. Remove catheters in infants with septicemia secondary to an infected indwelling catheter; shunt hardware in infants with shunt-related meningitis. **Duration of therapy:** Uncomplicated septicemia: 10–14 days; uncomplicated meningitis and NEC: 14 days. **Precautions:** Dosage reduction for renal failure. **Drug Interactions:** Anesthetic agents and aminoglycosides (enhances nephrotoxicity and ototoxicity). **Monitoring:** Obtain drug levels around the fourth dose; peak levels drawn 1 h after completion of a 1-h infusion; troughs are obtained just before the third dose. **Therapeutic levels: Peak:** 20–40 µg/ml, trough: 5–10 µg/ml. Assess renal function and observe IV site for extravasation and phlebitis. **Adverse Reactions:** Ototoxicity (associated with prolonged serum concentrations >60 μg/ml), nephrotoxicity, allergic reactions, neutropenia (associated with administration >3 weeks), phlebitis (minimized by slowing infusion rate and/or further dilution of drug), extravasation (consider hyaluronidase therapy), and eosinophilia. "Red man syndrome" (intense pruritus, tachycardia, sudden and profound hypotension, rash involving the face, neck, upper trunk, back, and upper arms) is associated with rapid IV infusions and is not an allergic reaction (reversible with diphenhydramine). **Nelson:** *Pocketbook of Pediatric Antimicrobial Therapy*, 1995, p. 17. **Johnson:** *The Harriet Lane Handbook*, 1993, p. 554.

Varicella-Zoster Immune Globulin (V-ZIG)

Indications: (1) Infants born to mothers who have had the onset of chickenpox within 5 days before or 2 days after delivery. (2) Postnatally exposed preterm infants <1 kg or <28 weeks regardless of maternal history. (3) Postnatally exposed premature infants with maternal history negative for varicella. **Dosage/Dosage Interval:** <10 kg: 125 U (minimum dose) as a single dose injected at one site. IM administration only. **Clinical Considerations:** Best results achieved if administered within 96 h after exposure. Passive immunity through infusion of IgG antibody. Protection lasts 1 month or longer. V-ZIG does not reduce the incidence but does decrease the complications associated with varicella. **Adverse Reactions:** Pain, erythema, swelling, and rash at injection site. Anaphylaxis rare. **Gomella:** *Neonatology*, 1994, p. 513. **AAP:** *Report of the Committee on Infectious Disease*, 1997, p. 578. **Johnson:** *The Harriet Lane Handbook*, 1993, p. 555.

Vecuronium Bromide (Norcuron)

Indications: Skeletal muscle relaxation in neonates requiring mechanical ventilation. **Dosage/Dosage Interval: Initial dose:** 0.08–0.1 mg/kg/dose IV. **Incremental dose:** 0.05–1 mg/kg q1–2h to maintain paralysis. **Continuous infusion:** 0.5–1 mg/kg/min. **Clinical Considerations:** Less tachycardia and hypotension in comparison to pancuronium bromide. Associated with minimal cardiovascular effects and histamine release. **Precautions:** Duration of action increased in newborns with hepatic or renal impairment. Use with caution in neonates with neuromuscular disease. Eye lubrication/protection provided to pavulon-treated neonates. Because sensation remains intact, concurrent sedation is required and analgesia should be administered for painful procedures. Due to vecuronium's lack of vagal blocking effects, bradycardia and hypotension may occur with concurrent narcotic administration. **Drug Interactions: Increased potency and duration of neuromuscular blockade:** Aminoglycosides, metronidazole, tetracyclines, bacitracin, acidosis, hypothermia, neuromuscular disease, hepatic disease, hypokalemia, hypermagnesemia, renal failure, calcium channel blockers, and clindamycin. **Decreased potency and duration of neuromuscular blockade:** Alkalosis, epinephrine, and hyperkalemia. **Monitoring:** Continuous monitoring of blood pressure, and heart rate/rhythm. **Adverse Reactions:** Skeletal muscle weakness, respiratory insufficiency, urticaria, and bronchospasm. **Antidotes:** Neostigmine, pyridostigmine, or edrophonium. **Fanaroff:** *Neonatal-Perinatal Medicine*, 1992, p. 1428. **Johnson:** *The Harriet Lane Handbook*, 1993, pp. 556–557.

Vidarabine (Vira-A) (Adenine Arabinoside, Ara-A)
Indications: Treatment of acute keratoconjunctivitis and epithelial keratitis due to herpes simplex virus; treatment of herpes simplex systemic virus infection or encephalitis.
Dosage/Dosage Interval

Indications	Dosage/route/frequency
Keratoconjunctivitis	Topical therapy: 3% 1/2-in ointment ribbon to lower conjunctival sac q3h, 5 times a day. Discontinue if no improvement in 7 days
HSV encephalitis: IV therapy (mg/kg/day)	15–30, qday × 10 days. (Final concentration of 0.50 mg/ml, filtered through ≤0.45 micron in-line filter, and infused over 12–24 h)
Neonatal HSV infection: IV therapy (mg/kg/day)	<1 mo of age: 15–30, 18–24h infusion; >1 mo of age: 15, 12–18h infusion; 10–21 day duration of treatment
Varicella or zoster in immunocompromised host: IV therapy (mg/kg/day)	10, 12–24 h infusion; duration of treatment: 5–10 days

Clinical Considerations: Document HSV infection prior to therapy. Rarely used due to large volume of diluent required for administration. Acyclovir is agent of choice for treatment of HSV and varicella infections. **Precautions:** Do not dilute in biologic or colloid solutions. **Monitoring:** Monitor hematologic and hepatic status. **Adverse Reactions:** Decreased reticulocyte count, white blood cell count, and platelet count. Elevation of total bilirubin and AST. Topical therapy associated with burning, lacrimation, and keratitis.
AAP: *Report of the Committee on Infectious Disease,* 1997, p. 266. **Gomella:** *Neonatology,* 1994, p. 514.

Vitamin B₁—See Thiamine

Vitamin B2 (Riboflavin)
Dosage/Dosage Interval

Indications	Dosage/route/frequency
Riboflavin daily requirements (RDA)	Premature: 400 µg PO Full-term: 60 µg PO
Riboflavin deficiency: therapy	IV therapy (VLBW): 0.15 mg/kg/day
Riboflavin sources	Human milk supplies 88 µg/day 1 ml PolyViSol or ViDaylin supplies 600 µg

Clinical Considerations: Riboflavin deficiency affects glucose, fatty acid, and amino acid metabolism. **Drug Interactions:** GI absorption of riboflavin is increased with food intake and decreased with liver dysfunction and concurrent probenecid usage. **Test Interactions:** Large doses may interfere with urinalysis based on spectrometry and may cause false elevations in fluorimetric determinations of catecholamines and urobilinogen.

Tsang: *Nutrition During Infancy,* 1988, p. 239. **Greene:** *J Am Col Nutr* 1991;10:281–287.

Vitamin B₆—See Pyridoxine Hydrochloride

Vitamin C (Ascorbic Acid)
Dosage/Dosage Interval

Indications	Dosage/route/frequency
Daily requirements (RDA)	Premature: 50–100 mg/day, PO, IM Full-term: 25–50 mg/day, PO, IM
Vitamin C deficiency	Therapeutic dose: 100 mg PO, IM, q4h for ≥2 wk
Vitamin C sources	Human milk supplies 14 mg/day; 1 ml PolyViSol or ViDaylin supplies 35 mg

Adverse Reactions: Vomiting, flushing, diarrhea, and hyperoxaluria. **Taeusch:** *Schaffer and Avery's Diseases of the Newborn,* 1991, p. 1054. **Tsang:** *Nutrition During Infancy,* 1988, p. 242. (See Chap. 10)

Vitamin D₂—See Ergocalciferol

Vitamin E (Aquasol E)
Indications: Prevention and treatment of vitamin E deficiency. Investigational use for treatment or prevention of anemia of prematurity.
Dosage/Dosage Interval (PO, IV with IV multivitamin preparations)

Indications	Dosage/route/frequency
Daily requirements	Premature: 1 U/g linoleic acid Full-term: 0.3 IU/100 Kcal or 0.7 IU/g linoleic acid; 1 mg of Aquasol E provides 1.00 IU of vitamin E
Anemia of prematurity: Prevention generally requires only adequate intake of vitamin E	Prophylaxis: 25–50 U/day, PO, until 2–3 mo of age Treatment: 50–200 U/day, PO for 2 wk VLBW (<1.5 kg): 2.9–3.5 mg α-tocopherol/kg/day, IV

Precautions: Because Aquasol E is very hyperosmolar (3000 mosm), a 1:4 dilution with sterile water is required. Poorly absorbed in malabsorption disorders. **Monitoring:** Physiologic serum levels for premature infants are 1–2 mg/dl and should be monitored during administration of pharmacologic doses of vitamin E. **Clinical Considerations:** Requirements for vitamin E increase as the intake of polyunsaturated fatty acids increases. **Adverse Reactions:** Liver failure reported in several premature infants receiving 25–100 mg/day.
Gomella: *Neonatology,* 1994, p. 514. **Greene:** *J Am Col Nutr* 1991;10:281–287.

Vitamin K₁ (Phytonadione, Aquamephyton, Mephyton)
Indications: Prevention and treatment of hemorrhagic disease of the newborn and hypoprothrombinemia caused by drug-induced or anticoagulant-induced vitamin K deficiency.

Dosage/Dosage Interval: (for IV use dilute in D5W and infuse no faster than 1 mg/min)

Indications	Dosage/route/frequency
Prophylaxis (administered at birth)	<1 kg: 0.5 mg, IM, SC >1 kg: 1 mg IM, SC
Severe hemorrhagic disease	Initial treatment: 1–10 mg/dose IM, SC, PO, slow IV (<1 mg/min) Vitamin K deficiency treatment: 1 mg dose, PO, IM, slow IV (<1 mg/min)
Oral anticoagulant overdose	1–2 mg/dose IV (<1 mg/min), q4–8h, PRN: assess response with serial PT and PTT

Warnings: Ineffective in hereditary hypoprothrombinemia or hypoprothrombinemia caused by severe liver disease. Severe hemolytic anemia or hyperbilirubinemia reported in neonates following administration of doses >20 mg. IM administration not associated with an increased risk of childhood cancer. **Precautions:** Despite proper dilution and rate of administration, severe anaphylactoid or hypersensitivity-like reactions (including shock and cardiac/respiratory arrest) have been reported to occur during or immediately after IV administration. IV administration restricted to emergency use and should not exceed 1 mg/min and should occur with a physician in attendance. Use with caution in neonates with severe hepatic disease. **Drug Interactions:** Antagonizes action of warfarin. **Monitoring:** Monitor PT and PTT if giving maintenance therapy. Allow a minimum of 2–4 h to detect measurable improvement in these parameters.
Gomella: *Neonatology,* 1992, p. 487. **Rudolph:** *Rudolph's Pediatrics,* 1991, p. 2005. **American Academy of Pediatrics:** *Pediatrics* 1993;91:1001. (See Chap. 26)

Warfarin Sodium (Coumadin Sodium, Panwarfin)
Indications: Prophylaxis and treatment of thromboembolic disorders. **Dosage (mg/kg/day)/Dosage Interval: PO:** 0.1, qday. **Maintenance dose:** 0.05–0.34, PO, qday. Adjust dose to achieve desired prothrombin time (1.25–1.5 times normal). **Contraindications:** Severe liver or kidney disease, uncontrolled bleeding, GI ulcers, and neurosurgical procedures. **Drug Interactions:** Amiodarone, metronidazole, chloramphenicol, cimetidine, urokinase, sulfonamides, and barbiturates. Decreased warfarin effect is associated with concomitant use of vitamin K. Increased warfarin effect associated with ethacrynic acid, indomethacin, phenylbutazone, and salicylates. **Adverse Reactions:** Hemorrhage, vomiting, fever, diarrhea, skin lesions, and hemolysis. **Antidote:** Vitamin K, fresh-frozen plasma.
Gomella: *Neonatology,* 1994, p. 515. **Rudolph:** *Rudolph's Pediatrics,* 1991, p. 2005.

Zidovudine (Azidothymidine, AZT, Retrovir)
Indications: Approved for use in asymptomatic HIV-infected infants, who have laboratory evidence of HIV-related immunosuppression and infants born to HIV-infected mothers. **Dosage (mg/kg/dose)/Dosage Interval:** Final concentration <4 mg/ml, infused over 1 h. IM administration not recommended. **PO:** ≤2 wk of age: 2, q6h, and >2 wk of age: 3, q6h. IV formulation of ZDV given undiluted or diluted in 5–10 ml of sucrose/water or apple juice. Avoid administration from 30 min before to 60 min after a feeding. **IV:** 1.5 mg/kg/dose, q6h infused over 60 min. PO and IV therapy is administered for 6 weeks, with subsequent treatment contingent on clini-

cal status and results of HIV studies. **Precautions:** Impaired renal or hepatic function. **Drug Interactions:** Acetaminophen, acyclovir (increased toxicity), ganciclovir (increased hematological toxicity), cimetidine, indomethacin, and lorazepam. Coadministration with other drugs metabolized by glucuronidation increases toxicity of either drug, and increases granulocytopenia. **Monitoring:** Weekly CBC and differential to detect anemia, pancytopenia, neutropenia, and thrombocytopenia. **Adverse Reactions:** Pancytopenia, anemia, neutropenia, thrombocytopenia, seizures, cholestatic hepatitis, and rash. **Conner:** *N Engl J Med* 1994;331:1173. **Boucher:** *J Pediatr* 1993;122:137. (See Chap. 23)

Subject Index

A

Abdomen
  birth trauma, 231
  masses, 628, 631
  physical examination in neonate, 33–34
ABO hemolytic disease, 207–208
ABR. See Auditory brain stem response
Acetaminophen, 670, 677
Acetazolamide, 677
Acetylcysteine, 677
Acquired immunodeficiency syndrome (AIDS), 246
Acrodermatitis enteropathica, 641
Acyclovir, 259–260, 678
Adenosine
  arrhythmia treatment, 448–449, 678
aDTP/Hib conjugate combination vaccine, 700
aDTP vaccine, 700
AIDS. See Acquired immunodeficiency syndrome, 246
Air leak, 347, 358–359
  pneumomediastinum, 362
  pneumopericardium, 362–363
  pneumoperitoneum, 363–364, 618
  pneumothorax, 359–361
  pulmonary interstitial emphysema, 362
  subcutaneous emphysema, 364
  systemic air embolism, 364
  ventilator strategy, 347
Albumin, 679
Albuterol, 679
Alpha-fetoprotein, 1, 533
Alprostadil. See Prostaglandins
Ambiguous genitalia. See Genitalia
Amikacin sulfate, 679–680
Aminocaproic acid
  extracorporeal membrane oxygenation application, 352
Aminophylline
  apnea treatment, 376
  recommendations for use, 680–681
Amniocentesis
  amniotic fluid analysis, 2
  fetal cell analysis, 2–3
Amphotercin-B, 298, 681
Ampicillin, 289, 681–682
Amrinone, 440–441
Anaerobic infection

  pathogens and treatment, 299
Analgesia. See specific drugs
Anemia
  anemia of prematurity, 453–454
  blood loss etiologies, 454–455
  diagnosis, 456–457
  hemolysis etiologies, 455–456
  prophylaxis, 459
  transfusion
    blood products, 458–459
    indications, 456, 458
Anesthesia, neonates
  airway management, 668–669
  breathing circuits, 669–670
  fluid management, 670
  monitoring of infants, 667–668
  pharmacology
    inhalation anesthetics, 671
    intravenous anesthetics, 672
    local anesthetics, 672–673
    muscle relaxants, 672
  preoperative laboratory testing, 667
  risks, 673
Antiobiotics. See specific antibiotics
Anus
  inperforate anus, 624–625
Aorta
  coarctation, 412–414
  interrupted aortic arch, 414–417
  stenosis, 412
  thrombosis, 487
Apgar score
  assigning, 55–64
Apnea
  definition, 374
  incidence, 374
  monitoring and evaluation, 375
  pathophysiology, 347, 374–375
  persistent apnea and sudden infant death syndrome prevention, 377–378
  treatment
    aminophylline, 376, 680
    caffeine, 377
    continuous positive airway pressure, 376
    doxapram, 377
    theophylline, 376–377, 741

Weight (mass) (pounds [lb] and ounces [oz] to grams [gm])

Example: To obtain gm equivalent to 6 lb, 8 oz, read 6 on top scale, 8 on side scale; equivalent is 2948 gm.

Ounces (oz)	Pounds (lb) 0	1	2	3	4	5	6	7	8	9	10
0	0	454	907	1361	1814	2268	2722	3175	3629	4082	4536
1	28	482	936	1389	1843	2296	2750	3203	3657	4111	4564
2	57	510	964	1417	1871	2325	2778	3232	3685	4139	4593
3	85	539	992	1446	1899	2353	2807	3260	3714	4167	4621
4	113	567	1021	1474	1928	2381	2835	3289	3742	4196	4649
5	142	595	1049	1503	1956	2410	2863	3317	3770	4224	4678
6	170	624	1077	1531	1984	2438	2892	3345	3799	4252	4706
7	198	652	1106	1559	2013	2466	2920	3374	3827	4281	4734
8	227	680	1134	1588	2041	2495	2948	3402	3856	4309	4763
9	255	709	1162	1616	2070	2523	2977	3430	3884	4337	4791
10	283	737	1191	1644	2098	2551	3005	3459	3912	4366	4819
11	312	765	1219	1673	2126	2580	3033	3487	3941	4394	4848
12	340	794	1247	1701	2155	2608	3062	3515	3969	4423	4876
13	369	822	1276	1729	2183	2637	3090	3544	3997	4451	4904
14	397	850	1304	1758	2211	2665	3113	3572	4026	4479	4933
15	425	879	1332	1786	2240	2693	3147	3600	4054	4508	4961

Note: 1 lb = 453.59237 gm; 1 oz = 28.349523 gm; 1000 gm = 1 kg. Gram equivalents have been rounded to whole numbers by adding 1 when the first decimal place is 5 or greater.

Temperature (Fahrenheit [F] to centigrade [C])

°F	°C	°F	°C	°F	°C	°F	°C
95.0	35.0	98.0	36.7	101.0	38.3	104.0	40.0
95.2	35.1	98.2	36.8	101.2	38.4	104.2	40.1
95.4	35.2	98.4	36.9	101.4	38.6	104.4	40.2
95.6	35.3	98.6	37.0	101.6	38.7	104.6	40.3
95.8	35.4	98.8	37.1	101.8	38.8	104.8	40.4
96.0	35.6	99.0	37.2	102.0	38.9		
96.2	35.7	99.2	37.3	102.2	39.0		
96.4	35.8	99.4	37.4	102.4	39.1		
96.6	35.9	99.6	37.6	102.6	39.2		
96.8	36.0	99.8	37.7	102.8	39.3		
97.0	36.1	100.0	37.8	103.0	39.4		
97.2	36.2	100.2	37.9	103.2	39.6		
97.4	36.3	100.4	38.0	103.4	39.7		
97.6	36.4	100.6	38.1	103.6	39.8		
97.8	36.6	100.8	38.2	103.8	39.9		

Note: $°C = (F - 32) \times \frac{5}{9}$. Centigrade temperature equivalents rounded to one decimal place by adding 0.1 when second decimal place is 5 or greater.
The metric system replaces the term *centigrade* with *Celsius* (the inventor of the scale).

Length (inches [in.] to centimeters [cm])

1-in. increments
Example: To obtain cm equivalent to 22 in., read *20* on top scale, *2* on side scale; equivalent is 55.9 cm.

In.	0	10	20	30	40
0	0	25.4	50.8	76.2	101.6
1	2.5	27.9	53.3	78.7	104.1
2	5.1	30.5	55.9	81.3	106.7
3	7.6	33.0	58.4	83.8	109.2
4	10.2	35.6	61.0	86.4	111.8
5	12.7	38.1	63.5	88.9	114.3
6	15.2	40.6	66.0	91.4	116.8
7	17.8	43.2	68.6	94.0	119.4
8	20.3	45.7	71.1	96.5	121.9
9	22.9	48.3	73.7	99.1	124.5

One-quarter (¼)-in. increments
Example: To obtain cm equivalent to 14¾ in., read *14* on top scale, ¾ on side scale; equivalent is 37.5 cm.

10-15 in.	10	11	12	13	14	15
0	25.4	27.9	30.5	33.0	35.6	38.1
¼	26.0	28.6	31.1	33.7	36.2	38.7
½	26.7	29.2	31.8	34.3	36.8	39.4
¾	27.3	29.8	32.4	34.9	37.5	40.0

16-21 in.	16	17	18	19	20	21
0	40.6	43.2	45.7	48.3	50.8	53.3
¼	41.3	43.8	46.4	48.9	51.4	54.0
½	41.9	44.5	47.0	49.5	52.1	54.6
¾	42.5	45.1	47.6	50.2	52.7	55.2

Note: 1 in. = 2.540 cm. Centimeter equivalents rounded one decimal place by adding 0.1 when second decimal place is 5 or greater; for example, 33.48 becomes 33.5.